Textbook of
GLAUCOMA

THIRD EDITION

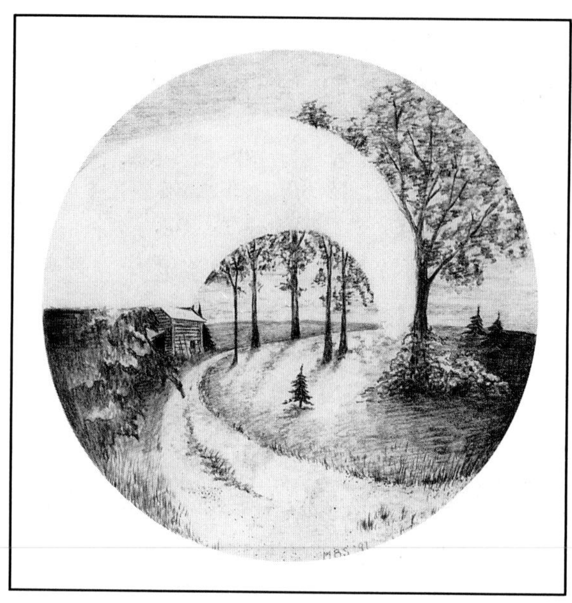

APPROACHING DARKNESS III

Dusk in the Carolina piedmont is superimposed on visual field loss of glaucoma. Dawn will come again to this country road, but not to the person blinded by glaucoma.

Textbook of GLAUCOMA

THIRD EDITION

M. Bruce Shields, M.D.

Professor of Ophthalmology
Duke University Medical Center
Durham, North Carolina

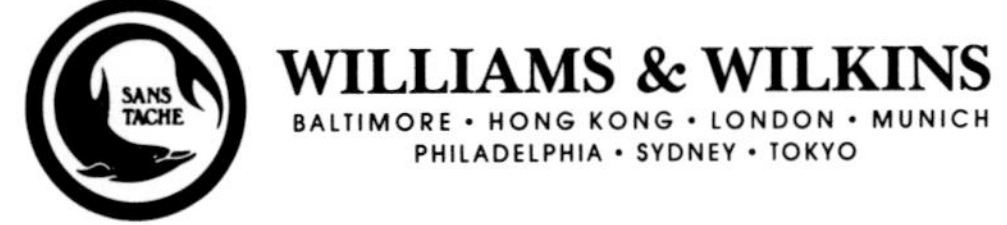

Editor: Carol-Lynn Brown
Managing Editor: Victoria M. Vaughn
Copy Editor: Dana L. Knighten
Designer: Norman W. Och
Illustration Planner: Wayne Hubbel
Production Coordinator: Kathleen C. Millet

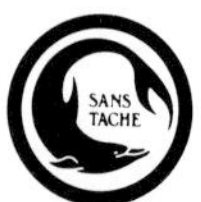

428 East Preston Street
Baltimore, Maryland 21202, USA

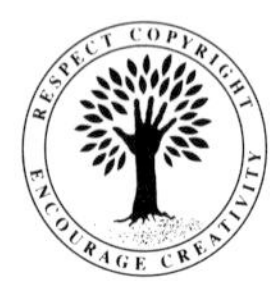

Accurate indications, adverse reactions, and dosage schedules for drugs are provided in this book, but it is possible that they may change. The reader is urged to review the package information data of the manufacturers of the medications mentioned.

Printed in the United States of America

First Edition 1982
Second Edition 1987

Library of Congress Cataloging in Publication Data

Shields, M. Bruce.
Textbook of glaucoma / M. Bruce Shields.—3rd ed.
p. cm.
Includes bibliographical references and index.
ISBN (invalid) 0-683-07965-8
1. Glaucoma. I. Title.
[DNLM: 1. Glaucoma. WW 290 S555s]
RE871.S447 1992
617.7'41—dc20
DNLM/DLC
for Library of Congress 91-12138
CIP

91 92 93 94
1 2 3 4 5 6 7 8 9 10

To

ROBERT MACHEMER, M.D.

My Chairman, 1978–1991

My Friend, Forever

PREFACE TO THE THIRD EDITION

One of the drawbacks to writing a medical textbook is that it is never current. The author must choose, therefore, to either let his or her work fade into oblivion or continually update it with new editions. However, while the need for new editions may be a disadvantage of textbook writing on one hand, it is also a major advantage in that it always offers one more chance to do it better.

Working on this third edition over the last couple of years was a humbling experience. In rereading the second edition for the first time in awhile, I was disappointed with confusing wording and poor organization of some topics, not to mention outright errors (some of which were pointed out by thoughtful readers, for which I am very grateful). For me, therefore, the advantages of writing a new edition clearly outweigh the disadvantages, and I only hope that this third edition will be better than those that came before it.

The main change in this edition, as always, is the updating of the literature. A little more than 1000 new journal articles have been added to the new edition, which represents only a fraction of the glaucoma papers published since the second edition. Topics receiving the most attention during this time period, as evidenced by substantial expansion of the corresponding chapters, include the optic nerve head and visual fields. There has been continued interest in the mechanism of glaucomatous optic atrophy, as well as the clinical recognition of disc and nerve fiber layer change, including computerized image analysis. Automated perimetry continues to be an area of considerable study, although other aspects of visual function in glaucoma are also receiving increasing attention. The expanded scope of study in both of these major areas has necessitated changing the titles of the two chapters.

The medical and surgical management of glaucoma have also continued to be areas of primary interest in recent years, especially with regard to laser surgery and modulation of wound healing for filtering surgery. The ever expanding role of laser surgery in the treatment of glaucoma is such that it is no longer reasonable to discuss laser and incisional surgery in separate chapters. As a result, the surgical chapters in this edition have been reorganized to combine the various laser and incisional techniques under common chapter titles.

A few general changes have also been made in the format of the new edition. A brief outline is provided at the beginning of most chapters to give the reader a quick overview of the content and organization of that chapter. A summary is also provided at the end of the chapter. Illustrations have been updated, with new schematic drawings and photographs, and a set of color plates has been provided, for the first time, in the back of the book.

As always, I am indebted and sincerely grateful to a number of thoughtful and talented people who helped in the preparation of this edition. Mr. Stanley M. Coffman and Ms. Susan Tanner, of the Duke University Medical Center Division of Audiovisual Education, provided the new schematic drawings and the excellent full-color illustrations. The new photographs were made by our highly professional Duke Eye Center photographers, Ms. Ruth Schirmer and Ms. Beth Ann Benetz. The many drafts of each chapter were typed in the Word Center of our department under the expert supervision of Ms. India Cain, with her superb team of Ms. Wanda Ellis, Ms. Diane Evans, and Mr. Joseph McCullum. Ms. Cain was also a great help in proofreading each draft. Once again I was fortunate to have access to the many talents of my secretary, Ms. Robin Goodwin, which included modeling for many of the pictures in this edition.

Finally, my sincere thanks to those without whom these editions would never have been possible. First, to my chairman and friend, Dr. Robert Machemer, who encouraged me to embark on this work more than a decade ago and has provided strong support ever since. Second, to my editor, Ms. Carol-Lynn Brown, and all the people at Williams & Wilkins who have contributed their many talents to the preparation of this book. But most of all, I thank the readers for their kind and encouraging comments over the years, which have been my primary motivation to continue this work. I only hope that these efforts will help all of us, in some small way, as we attempt to prevent the blindness of glaucoma.

M. Bruce Shields, M.D.
Durham, North Carolina

PREFACE TO THE FIRST EDITION

The primary intent of this book is to provide an introduction to the subject of glaucoma, as well as a framework on which to expand the study of that discipline. The content of the text has been organized in modified outline form to facilitate its use as a study guide. Presentation of the material begins with the most fundamental aspects of glaucoma and builds on successive levels of knowledge. In keeping with the simplicity of the format, illustrations have been limited to schematic line drawings and are used only where they are felt to clarify material in the text.

A moderately extensive bibliography has also been included in the study guide, and it is hoped that this may serve at least two purposes. First, it provides the student with a reading list from which he can select material for more detailed study of specific subjects on glaucoma. In addition, it may be of value to the practitioner as a reference source to help him stay abreast of the current concepts regarding the diagnosis and management of the glaucomas. Along with the classic literature on glaucoma, an effort has been made to provide an up-to-date bibliography, insofar as this is possible for a field of medicine in which knowledge is expanding so rapidly.

A valid criticism of this study guide will be the confusion created by attempting to present more than one viewpoint on many issues. However, the complex nature of glaucoma is such that many questions remain unanswered, and the best one can do in these areas is to become familiar with the leading theories. With a few exceptions, an effort has been made to avoid imposing the author's bias into this text, but rather to present, as objectively as possible, the various schools of thought in areas where controversy exists.

It is in no way intended that this study guide should compete with the many excellent textbooks that are currently available on the various aspects of glaucoma. Rather, it is hoped that this book may supplement the others by filling what is felt to be a need for a study guide and limited reference source on glaucoma. During the course of initial study or in refreshing oneself on this subject, both student and practitioner are urged to take full advantage of the wealth of outstanding textbooks on glaucoma, most of which are referenced throughout this study guide.

I am deeply indebted to a large number of talented and thoughtful people who helped me in many ways during the preparation of this text. To each of these individuals I wish to express my most sincere gratitude.

The collection and organization of reference materials used in this study guide was started during my time with W. Morton Grant at the Massachusetts Eye and Ear Infirmary. I am grateful to Dr. Grant for allowing access to his files and for the excellent teaching he and his staff provided.

The first several drafts of this book were prepared as outlines to accompany a series of lectures given to the residents at the Duke University Eye Center. The concept of developing this material into a study guide for publication was prompted by the kind words and encouragement of the Duke residents and senior staff. I am very indebted to all of these individuals, and especially to

Robert Machemer, who urged me to embark on the project and was a strong source of support throughout its preparation.

The following experts kindly agreed to critically review preliminary drafts of certain chapters in this study guide: A. Robert Bellows, Richard F. Brubaker, David G. Campbell, David L. Epstein, Keith Green, B. Thomas Hutchinson, Michael Kahn, Gordon K. Klintworth, Marvin L. Kwitko, William E. Layden, Alan I. Mandell, Samuel D. McPherson, Jr., Arthur H. Neufeld, Charles D. Phelps, Irvin P. Pollack, Harry A. Quigley, Robert Ritch, Richard J. Simmons, George L Spaeth, E. Michael Van Buskirk, David S. Walton, Martin Wand, Myron Yanoff, and Thom J. Zimmerman. Their helpful comments and suggestions were invaluable in preparing the final draft of each chapter.

I was extremely fortunate to receive the highly professional and conscientious assistance of the following individuals: Robert L. Blake, medical illustration; Margaret L. Hayes, manuscript typing; David L. Smith, library research; and Lori S. Fields and Pamela S. Weinert, secretarial assistance. I also wish to thank the publishers, Williams & Wilkins, and especially Barbara C. Tansill for her invaluable help.

M. Bruce Shields, M.D.
Durham, North Carolina

CONTENTS

SECTION ONE: THE BASIC ASPECTS OF GLAUCOMA

SECTION TWO: THE CLINICAL FORMS OF GLAUCOMA

SECTION THREE: THE MANAGEMENT OF GLAUCOMA

Chapter 1

AN OVERVIEW OF GLAUCOMA

THE SIGNIFICANCE OF GLAUCOMA

Glaucoma is a leading cause of irreversible blindness throughout the world. Based on an evaluation of government and commercial statistics, this group of disorders is estimated to affect approximately 1.4 million individuals in the United States.[1] Although it more commonly afflicts the elderly, glaucoma occurs in all segments of our society, with significant health and economic consequences.[2,3] Figures from a 1977 survey suggest that more than $400 million was spent that year in direct treatment costs for glaucoma, and that another $1.9 billion was lost in productive work time.[4] These figures provide some appreciation for the significance of glaucoma as a major public health problem.

A DEFINITION OF GLAUCOMA

A Group of Diseases. The most fundamental fact concerning glaucoma is that it is not a single disease process. Rather, it is a large group of disorders that are characterized by widely diverse clinical and histopathologic manifestations. This point is not commonly appreciated by the general public, or even by a portion of the medical community, which frequently leads to confusion. For example, a patient may have difficulty understanding why she has no symptoms with her glaucoma, when a friend experienced sudden pain and redness with a disease of the same name. Another individual may avoid the use of cold medications because the package insert cautions against it in patients with glaucoma, and he was not informed that this relates only to certain types of glaucoma.

Terminology. The term *glaucoma* should be used only in reference to the entire group of disorders, just as the term cancer is used to refer to another discipline of medicine that encompasses many diverse clinical entities with certain common denominators. Whenever referring to the diagnosis of a patient, one of the more precise terms, such as *primary open-angle glaucoma,* should be used, which relates to the specific type of glaucoma that that individual is believed to have.

The Common Denominators. If we were to attempt a definition that would encompass all the glaucomas, it might be "those situations in which the intraocular pressure (IOP) is too high for the normal functioning of the optic nerve head." This definition, however, is a gross oversimplification of a highly complex and only partly understood discipline of medicine. For example, we do not know what level of IOP will lead to glaucomatous damage from one patient to the next, nor do we fully understand the mechanism by which the optic atrophy occurs. We do know, however, that the damage to the optic nerve head is associated with a progressive loss of the visual field, which can lead to total, irreversible blindness if the condition is not diagnosed and treated properly. These three common denominators (*IOP, optic nerve head damage,* and *visual field loss*) represent the common pathway to blindness with all forms of glaucoma and also provide the basis for our understanding of this large group of disorders. In *Section One,* these parameters will be discussed as they relate in general to the study of glaucoma.

THE PREVENTION OF BLINDNESS FROM GLAUCOMA

Once the blindness of glaucoma has occurred, no known treatment will restore the lost vision. However, in nearly all cases, blindness from glaucoma is preventable.

This prevention requires early detection and proper treatment. Detection depends on the ability to recognize the early clinical manifestations of the various glaucomas. In *Section Two,* we will consider the many forms of glaucoma and the clinical and histopathologic features by which they are characterized. Appropriate treatment requires an understanding of the pathogenic mechanisms involved, as well as a detailed knowledge of the drugs and operations that are used to control the IOP. In *Section Three,* we will consider these medical and surgical modalities that are used in the treatment of glaucoma.

References

1. National Center for Health Statistics: Prevalence of selected chronic conditions, United States, 1979–1981. Vital and Health Statistics, series 10, no. 155. Washington, D.C.: Government Printing Office, 1986. (Publication no. DHHS (FHS) 86-1583)
2. Leske, MC: The epidemiology of open-angle glaucoma. A review. Am J Epidemiol 118:166, 1983.
3. Ghafour, IM, Allan, D, Foulds, WS: Common causes of blindness and visual handicap in the west of Scotland. Br J Ophthal 67:209, 1983.
4. Roden, DR: The prevalence and cost of glaucoma. In: Glaucoma Detection and Treatment. Proceedings of the First National Glaucoma Conference, Sponsored by the National Society to Prevent Blindness, Tarpon Springs, Florida, 1980, p. 20.

Section One

The Basic Aspects of Glaucoma

Chapter 2

AQUEOUS HUMOR DYNAMICS I. ANATOMY AND PHYSIOLOGY

The study of glaucoma deals primarily with the consequences of elevated intraocular pressure (IOP). A logical place to begin this study, therefore, is with the physiologic factors that control the IOP, which are the dynamics of aqueous humor flow.

HOW AQUEOUS HUMOR DYNAMICS INFLUENCE INTRAOCULAR PRESSURE

To reduce a highly complex and only partly understood situation to its simplest form, IOP is a function of the rate at which aqueous humor enters the eye (inflow) and the rate at which it leaves the eye (outflow). When inflow equals outflow, a steady state exists, and the pressure remains constant.

Inflow is related to the rate of aqueous humor production, while outflow depends on the resistance to the flow of aqueous from the eye and the pressure in the episcleral veins. The control of IOP, therefore, is a function of: (1) production of aqueous humor; (2) resistance to aqueous humor outflow; and (3) episcleral venous pressure.

The remainder of this chapter deals with these three parameters and their complex interrelationship with the IOP.

AN OVERVIEW OF THE ANATOMY

Aqueous humor is involved with virtually all portions of the eye, although the two main structures related to aqueous humor dynamics are the *ciliary body,* the site of aqueous production, and the *limbus,* the principal site of aqueous outflow. The stepwise construction of a schematic model, as shown in Figure 2.1 (A–D), illustrates the close relationship between these two structures and the surrounding anatomy:

A. The *limbus* is the transition zone between the cornea and the sclera. On the inner surface of the limbus is an indentation, the scleral sulcus, which has a sharp posterior margin, the *scleral spur,* and a sloping anterior wall that extends to the peripheral cornea.

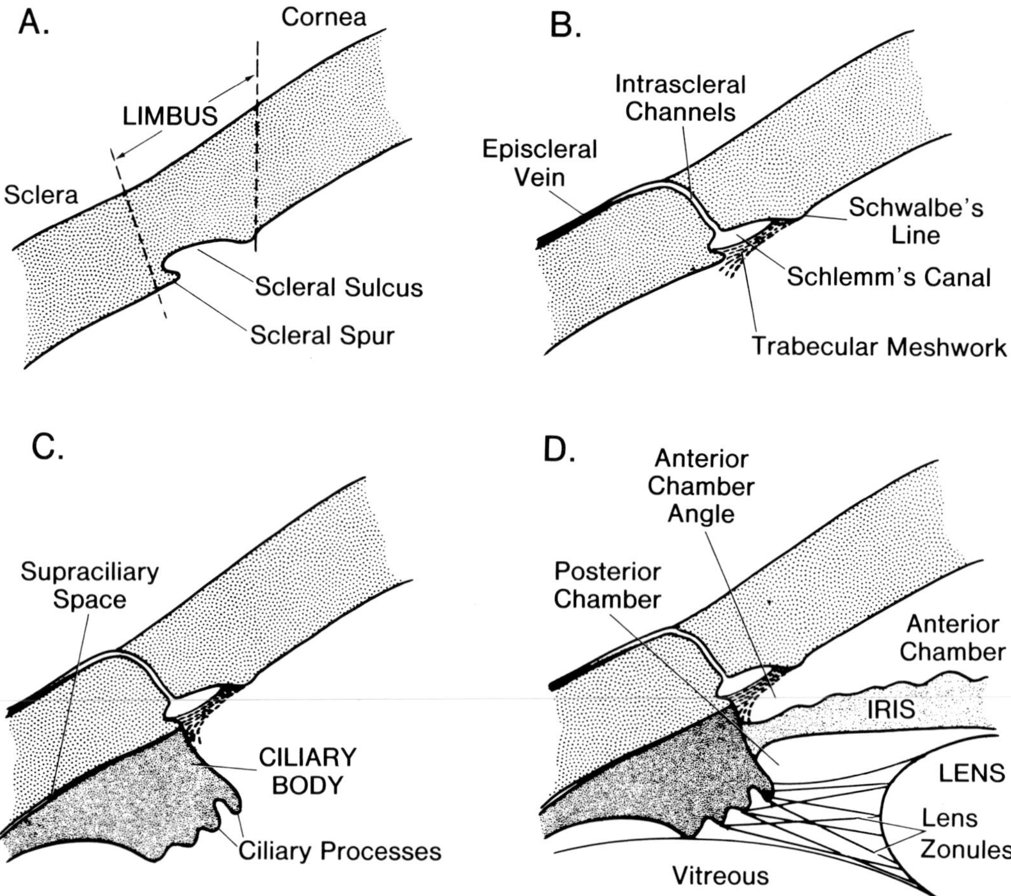

Figure 2.1. Stepwise construction of a schematic model, depicting the relationship of structures involved in aqueous humor dynamics: **A,** limbus; **B,** main route of aqueous outflow; **C,** ciliary body (site of aqueous production); **D,** iris and lens.

B. A sieve-like structure, the *trabecular meshwork,* bridges the scleral sulcus and converts it into a tube, called *Schlemm's canal*. Where the meshwork inserts into the peripheral cornea, a ridge is created, known as *Schwalbe's line*. Schlemm's canal is connected by intrascleral channels to the episcleral veins. The trabecular meshwork, Schlemm's canal, and the intrascleral channels comprise the main route of aqueous humor outflow.

C. The *ciliary body* attaches to the scleral spur and creates a potential space, the supraciliary space, between itself and the sclera. On cross-section, the ciliary body has the shape of a right triangle, and the *ciliary processes* (the actual site of aqueous production) occupy the innermost and anteriormost portion of this structure, extending back for approximately 2 mm in the region called the pars plicata (or corona ciliaris). The ciliary processes consist of approximately 70 radial ridges (major ciliary processes) between which are interdigitated an equal number of smaller ridges (minor or intermediate ciliary processes)[1] (Fig. 2.2). The posterior 4 mm of the ciliary body, the pars plana (or orbicularis ciliaris), has a flatter inner surface and joins the choroid at the ora serrata.

D. The *iris* inserts into the anterior side of the ciliary body, leaving a variable width of the latter structure visible between the root of the iris and scleral spur, referred to as the *ciliary body band*. The *lens* is suspended from the ciliary body by zonules and sepa-

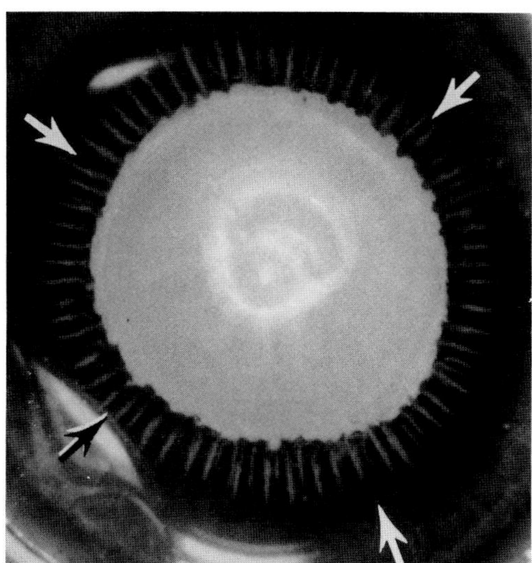

Figure 2.2. Gross anatomical view of the ciliary body showing the radial ridges of the ciliary processes (*arrows*).

rates the vitreous, posteriorly, from the aqueous, anteriorly. The iris separates the aqueous compartment into a posterior and an anterior chamber, and the angle formed by the iris and the cornea is called the *anterior chamber angle*. Further details regarding the gonioscopic appearance of the anterior chamber angle are considered in Chapter 3.

PRODUCTION OF AQUEOUS HUMOR

Histology of the Ciliary Body

The ciliary body is one of three portions of the uveal tract, or vascular layer of the eye, the other two structures in this system being the iris and choroid. The ciliary body measures 6 mm from the scleral spur to the ora serrata and is composed of (1) muscle, (2) vessels, and (3) epithelia (Fig. 2.3).

Ciliary Muscle

The ciliary muscle consists of two main portions: the *longitudinal* and the *circular* fibers. It is the longitudinal fibers that attach the ciliary body to the limbus at the scleral spur. This portion of muscle then runs posteriorly to insert into the suprachoroidal lamina (fibers connecting choroid and sclera) as far back as the equator or beyond. The circular fibers occupy the anterior and inner portion of the ciliary body and run parallel to the limbus. A third portion of the ciliary muscle has been described as radial fibers, which connect the longitudinal and circular fibers.

Ciliary Vessels

Traditional teaching holds that the vasculature of the ciliary body is supplied by the *anterior ciliary arteries* and the *long posterior ciliary arteries* that anastomose near the root of the iris to form the *major arterial circle,* from whence branches supply the iris, ciliary body, and anterior choroid. More recent studies with vascular casting techniques and sequential microdissection in primates have shown this to be a complex vascular arrangement with collateral circulation on at least three levels.[2] (1) The anterior ciliary arteries on the surface of the sclera send out lateral branches that supply the episcleral plexus and anastomose with branches from adjacent anterior ciliary arteries to form an *episcleral circle.* (2) The anterior ciliary arteries then perforate the limbal sclera. In the ciliary muscle, branches of these arteries anastomose with each other as well as with branches from the long posterior ciliary arteries to form the *intramuscular circle.* Divisions of the anterior ciliary arteries also provide capillaries to the ciliary muscle and iris, and send recurrent ciliary arteries to the anterior choriocapillaris. (3) The "*major arterial circle*" is actually the least consistent of the three collateral systems. Although the primate studies reveal a contribution from perforating anterior ciliary arteries, microvascular casting studies of human eyes,[3] as well as those of several non-primate animals,[4,5] indicate that this circle is formed exclusively by paralimbal branches of the long posterior ciliary arteries. In any case, this arterial circle is the immediate vascular supply of the iris and ciliary processes.

Contrary to traditional teaching, there is evidence from human studies that blood flows in the anterior ciliary arteries from the inside of the eye to the outside. This is based on studies with rapid sequence fluorescein angiography[6] and the observations that an

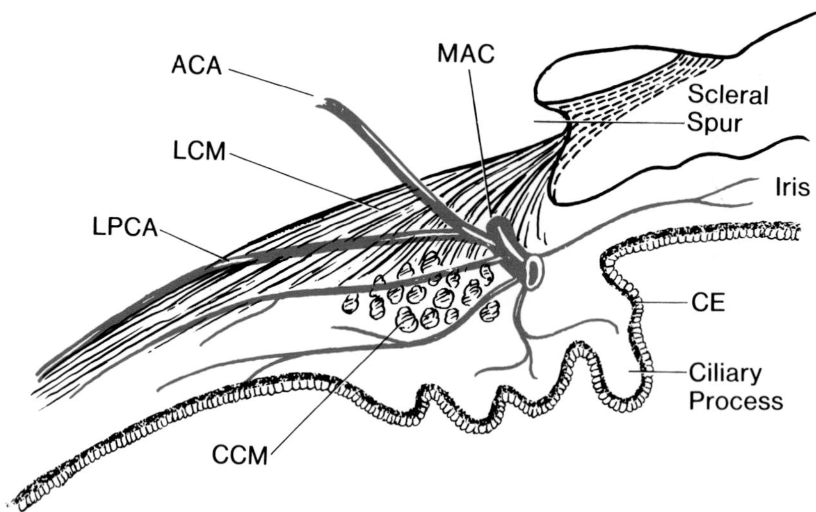

Figure 2.3. Three major components of the ciliary body. (1) The ciliary muscle, composed of longitudinal (*LCM*) and circular (*CCM*) fibers. (2) The vascular system, formed by branches of the anterior ciliary arteries (*ACA*) and long posterior ciliary arteries (*LPCA*), which form the major arterial circle (*MAC*). (3) The ciliary epithelium (*CE*), composed of an outer pigmented and an inner nonpigmented layer.

increase in IOP is associated with a decrease in anterior ciliary arterial pressure[7,8] and an increase in the diameter of these vessels.[8]

The ciliary processes in primates are supplied by two types of branches from the major arterial circle: the anterior and posterior ciliary process arterioles.[9] *Anterior ciliary process arterioles* supply the anterior and marginal (innermost) aspects of the major ciliary processes. These arterioles have luminal constrictions before producing irregularly dilated capillaries within the processes, suggesting precapillary arteriolar sphincters. This may represent the anatomic site of adrenergic neural influence on aqueous humor production by regulation of blood flow through the ciliary processes in response to physiologic and pharmacologic mediators.[4,5] The *posterior ciliary process arterioles* supply the central, basal, and posterior aspects of the major ciliary processes, as well as all portions of the minor processes. These arterioles are of larger caliber than the anterior arterioles and lack the constrictions seen in the latter vessels. Both populations of arterioles have interprocess anastomoses. Venous drainage is into choroidal veins, either from the posterior aspects of the major and minor processes or by direct communication from the interprocess connections (Figs. 2.4 and 2.5).

A similar dual arteriolar supply to the ciliary processes has been observed in rabbits,[4] whereas other species studied (cows, pigs, sheep, goats, dogs, cats, rats, and guinea pigs) have only one type of arteriole, which extends posteriorly from the major arterial circle to the iris root, where it gives rise to the ciliary process arterioles.[5]

Ciliary Epithelia

Two layers of epithelium line the inner surface of the ciliary processes and the pars plana: (1) pigmented epithelium comprises the outer layer, adjacent to the stroma, and is composed of low cuboidal cells, while (2) nonpigmented epithelium makes up the inner layer, adjacent to the aqueous in the posterior chamber, and consists of columnar cells (see further details under "Ultrastructure").

Ultrastructure of the Ciliary Processes

Each ciliary process is composed of (1) capillaries, (2) stroma, and (3) epithelia (Fig. 2.6):

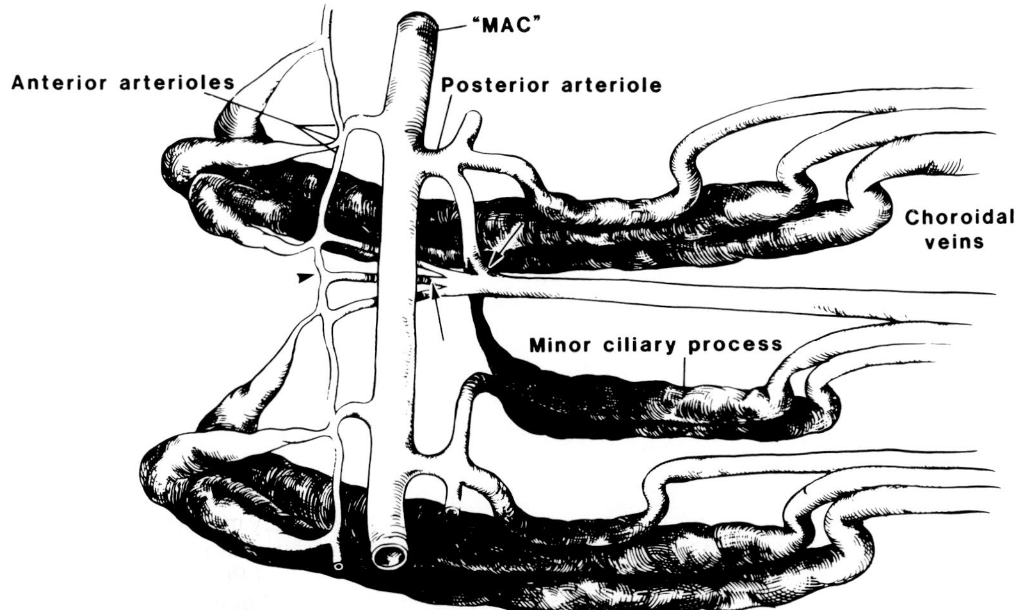

Figure 2.4. Vascular interconnections of two contiguous major ciliary processes. Lateral anterior arteriolar branches join to form interprocess capillary networks (*arrowhead*) that provide communication between major processes. Laterally directed posterior arterioles form posterior interprocess networks through which the minor ciliary processes receive blood. In addition, both anterior and posterior interprocess networks drain directly into the choroidal veins (*arrows*). "*MAC*," major arterial circle. (Reprinted by permission from Morrison JC, Van Buskirk EM: Am J Ophthal 97:372, 1984.)

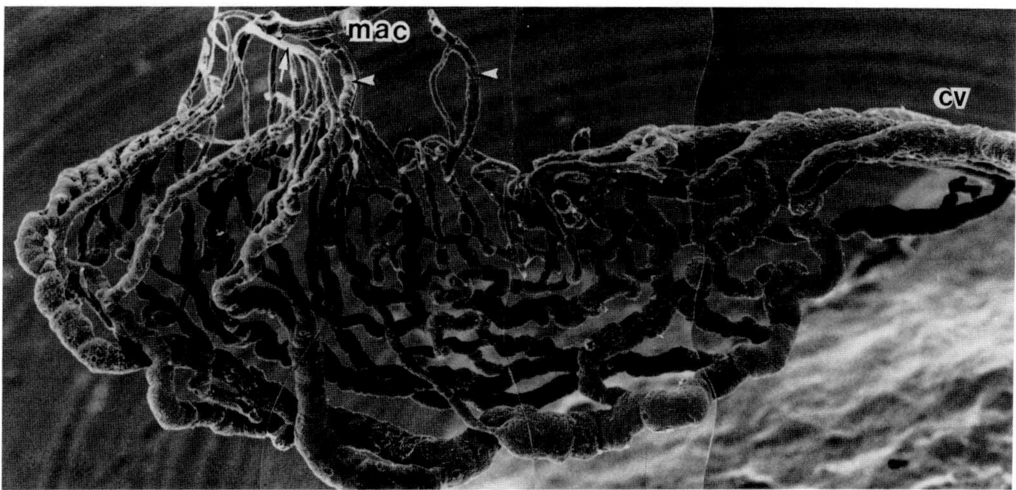

Figure 2.5. Microvascular casting of a single ciliary process. Constricted anterior arterioles (*arrows*) enter the anterior portion of the process to provide large irregular vein-like capillaries that occupy the margins of the process. Posteriorly, larger caliber arterioles (*arrowheads*) originate and enter the middle of the process to divide into smaller capillaries that in general are confined to the base of the process. All capillaries travel posteriorly to drain into the choroidal veins (*CV*). *MAC*, major arterial circle. (Original magnification, × 150.) (Reprinted by permission from Morrison JC, Van Buskirk EM: Am J Ophthal 97:372, 1984.)

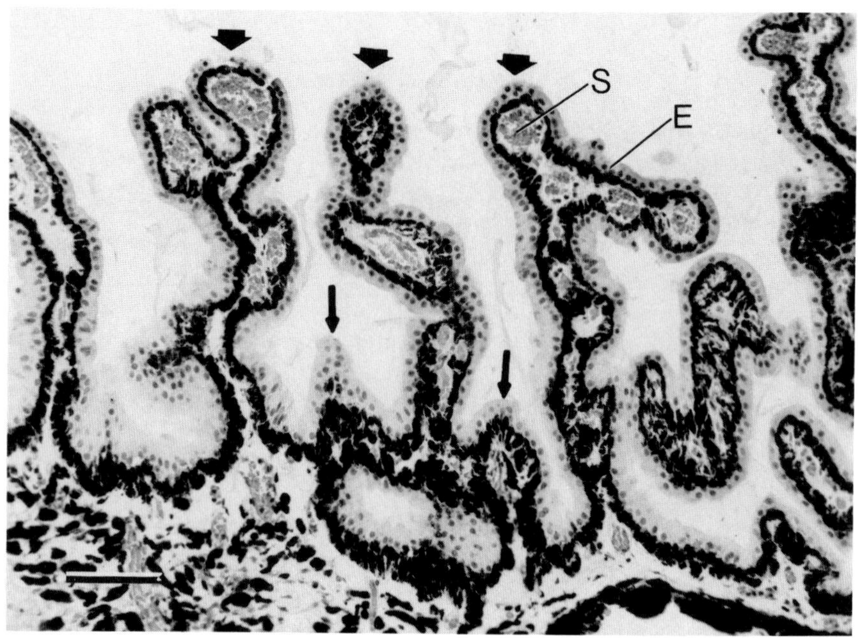

Figure 2.6. Light microscopic view of ciliary processes, sectioned perpendicular to radial ridges, showing major ciliary processes (*large arrows*) and minor ciliary processes (*small arrows*). Note vascular stroma (*S*) surrounded by outer pigmented and inner nonpigmented epithelium (*E*). (Hematoxylin, eosin; bar = 100 μm.)

Ciliary Process Capillaries

The network of capillaries occupies the center of each process. The endothelium is very thin, with fenestrae, or false "pores," that represent areas of absent cytoplasm with fusion of the plasma membranes and that may be the site of increased permeability. A basement membrane surrounds the endothelium, and mural cells, or pericytes, are located within the basement membrane.[10]

Ciliary Process Stroma

A very thin stroma surrounds the capillary network and separates it from the epithelial layers. The stroma is composed of ground substance, consisting of mucopolysaccharides, proteins and solute of plasma (except those of large molecular size), a very few collagen connective tissue fibrils, and wandering cells of connective tissue and blood origin.[10] Tubular microfibrils with and without elastin have been demonstrated in bovine ciliary body, especially in the stroma of the pars plana, in relationship to lens zonules.[11]

Ciliary Process Epithelia

Two layers of epithelium surround the stroma, with the apical surfaces of the two cell layers in apposition to each other (Fig. 2.7).[10,12–14]

Pigmented epithelium is characterized by numerous melanin granules in the cytoplasm and an atypical basement membrane on the stromal side.

Nonpigmented epithelium. The basement membrane is composed of fibrils in a glycoprotein. This membrane, which faces the aqueous, is also called the *internal limiting membrane* and fuses with the lens zonules. Numerous mitochondria are seen in the cytoplasm, along with poorly developed rough and smooth endoplasmic reticulum, and a scant number of ribosomes. Rows of vesicles near the free surface, called "pinocytic vesicles," are seen only with osmium tetroxide fixation and are believed to represent artifactual tubules cut on end.[12] The

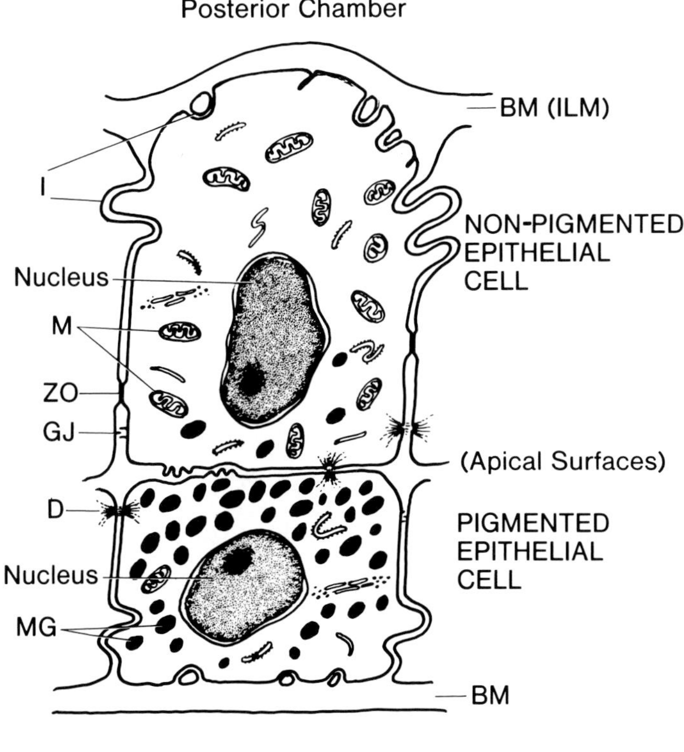

Figure 2.7. The two layers of the ciliary epithelium. Apical surfaces are in apposition to each other. Basement membrane (*BM*) lines the double layer and constitutes the internal limiting membrane (ILM) on the inner surface. The nonpigmented epithelium is characterized by mitochondria (*M*), zonula occludens (*ZO*), and lateral and surface interdigitations (*I*). The pigmented epithelium contains numerous melanin granules (*MG*). Additional intercellular junctions include desmosomes (*D*) and gap junctions (*GJ*).

nucleus has a nucleolus that appears to contain ribosomes. The cell membrane is 200 Å thick and is characterized by infoldings or interdigitations, especially surface infoldings on the free surface and lateral interdigitations, which are actually different cuts of the same structure.

A variety of *intercellular junctions* have been described that connect adjacent cells within each epithelial layer, as well as the apical surfaces of the two layers.[15,16] Electrophysiologic studies of rabbit ciliary epithelium suggest that all of the cells in the epithelium function as a syncytium.[17,18] Tight junctions create a permeability barrier between the nonpigmented epithelial cells, which forms part of the *blood-aqueous barrier*. These tight junctions are said to be the "leaky" type, in contrast to the "non-leaky" type in the blood-retinal barrier, and may be the main diffusional pathways for water and ion flow.[19,20] Microvilli separate the two layers of epithelial cells. In addition, *ciliary channels* have been described as spaces between the two epithelial layers.[21] They are believed to be related to the formation of aqueous humor, since they develop between the 4th and 6th months of gestation, corresponding to the start of aqueous production.

Theories of Aqueous Humor Production

Aqueous humor appears to be derived from plasma within the capillary network of the ciliary processes. To reach the posterior chamber, therefore, the various constituents of aqueous must traverse the three tissue layers of the ciliary processes; i.e., the capillary wall, stroma, and epithelia. The principal barrier to transport across these tissues is the cell membrane and related junctional complexes, and substances appear to pass through this structure by one of three mechanisms:[22] (1) *diffusion* (lipid-soluble substances are transported through the lipid portions of the membrane proportional to a concentration gradient across the membrane); (2) *ultrafiltration* (water and water-soluble substances, limited by size and charge, flow through theoretical "micropores" in the protein of the cell membrane in response to an osmotic gradient or hydrostatic pressure); and (3) *secretion* (water-soluble substances of larger size or greater charge are actively transported across the cell membrane). The latter mechanism is believed to be mediated by globular proteins in the membrane and requires the expenditure of energy. All three transport mechanisms are probably involved in aqueous production, possibly in accordance with the following simplified three-part scheme:

1. Accumulation of Plasma Reservoir. Tracer studies suggest that most plasma substances pass easily from the capillaries of the ciliary processes, across the stroma, and between the pigmented epithelial cells before accumulating behind the tight junctions of the nonpigmented epithelium.[23,24] Studies with normal rats suggest that pericapillary permeability of the ciliary processes is influenced by the presence of fixed anionic groups that favor the penetration and accumulation of cationic tracers.[25] This movement takes place primarily by ultrafiltration, and drugs that alter ciliary perfusion may exert their influence on IOP at this level.[3,4,5,9,26]

2. Transport Across Blood-Aqueous Barrier. The tight junctions between the nonpigmented epithelial cells create part of the blood-aqueous barrier, and certain substances appear to be actively transported across this barrier into the posterior chamber, thereby establishing an osmotic gradient. Studies with isolated rabbit ciliary processes suggest that aqueous humor could be secreted by the generation of a modest osmotic gradient across the nonpigmented cell basal membrane.[27] There is a specific secretory pump for *sodium* ions,[28,29] and approximately 70% of this electrolyte is actively transported into the posterior chamber,[30] while the remainder enters by passive ultrafiltration[22] or diffusion.[30] The active transport of Na^+ is Na^+K^+-activated ATPase-dependent,[31] but does not appear to be related to the concentration of Na^+ in the plasma.[32]

A much smaller percentage of the *chloride* ion is actively transported, and this appears to be dependent on the presence of sodium, as well as the pH.[33,34] *Potassium* ions are transported by secretion and diffusion.[35] One proposed model for the exit of Na^+ and Cl^- into the aqueous humor is that Na^+K^+-ATPase pumps Na^+ in exchange for K^+ in the aqueous. K^+ recycles through K^+ channels, and Cl^- passively diffuses through Cl^- channels into the aqueous.[36] Electrolyte movement across the ciliary epithelium is measured primarily by electrochemical gradients, but studies with rabbit ciliary epithelium have demonstrated electrically silent Na^+ and Cl^- fluxes, suggesting an additional pathway for electrolyte movement.[37]

Ascorbic acid is secreted against a large concentration gradient,[30] with a probable small contribution from passive diffusion.[38] *Amino acids* are secreted by at least three carriers.[39] The rapid interconversion between *bicarbonate* and CO_2, which is catalyzed by carbonic anhydrase, makes it difficult to determine the relative proportions of these two substances. However, bicarbonate formation has been shown to influence fluid transport through its effect on Na^+,[40] possibly by regulating the pH for optimum active transport of Na^+.[22]

3. Osmotic Flow. The osmotic gradient across the ciliary epithelium, which results from the active transport of the above substances, leads to the movement of other plasma constituents by ultrafiltration and diffusion. There is evidence that sodium is the ion primarily responsible for the movement of water into the posterior chamber.[26,28,41]

The precise location of aqueous humor production appears to be predominantly in the anterior portion of the pars plicata along the tips or crests of the ciliary processes, since this region has been shown to have (1) increased basal and lateral interdigitations, mitochondria, and rough endoplasmic reticulum in the nonpigmented ciliary epithelium, (2) more numerous fenestrations in the capillary endothelium, (3) a thinner layer of ciliary stroma, and (4) an increase in cell organelles and gap junctions between pigmented and nonpigmented epithelia.[42,43] Furthermore, when sodium fluorescein is administered systemically and the ciliary body is observed with a special gonioprism, fluorescein-stained aqueous is seen primarily at the tips of the ciliary processes.[44]

The site of active transport is considered to be the nonpigmented epithelial cells, especially in the cell membrane of the lateral interdigitations, since this area has (1) abundant $Na^{+}K^{+}$-activated ATPase and carbonic anhydrase,[45] (2) higher specific activity for glycolytic enzymes,[46] and (3) preferential incorporation of labeled sulfate into macromolecules (primarily glycolipids and glycoproteins).[47,48] The ciliary epithelium also contains alpha- and beta-adrenergic receptors, and drugs that act on these receptors or on enzymes, such as carbonic anhydrase, may influence aqueous production, and subsequently IOP, by altering the active transport mechanisms.[49]

Ultrastructural studies of primates suggest that the ciliary epithelium, in addition to actively transporting aqueous humor, produces a secretory material that diffuses into the ciliary body stroma and possibly enters the blood stream.[50]

Rate of Aqueous Humor Production

The rate at which aqueous humor is formed (inflow) is measured in microliters per minute (μL/min). The actual value in the human eye varies somewhat according to the measurement techniques, which are discussed in the next chapter. A figure of approximately 2.0 μL/min is generally quoted,[30] although fluorophotometric studies, which may provide the most reliable estimates, give a mean value of approximately 2.4 ± 0.6 μL/min in the undisturbed human eye.[51]

Many factors have been evaluated with regard to an influence on the rate of aqueous production. An elevation of IOP was once thought to be associated with a decline in aqueous production, which was referred to as *pseudofacility*.[52–57] More recent studies, however, indicate that aqueous formation is relatively pressure-insensitive and a possible explanation for conflicting findings is that earlier work involved a relatively short period of observation, whereas a longstanding rise in IOP has less effect on the rate of aqueous flow.[58–61]

Fluorophotometric studies support the traditional concept that aqueous production decreases with age,[62] although the degree of this change is less than previously thought, amounting to only 2% (0.06 μL/min) per decade of age.[51,63] The formation of aqueous humor is actually much more stable than the IOP or anterior chamber volume with respect to aging changes.[63] Aqueous flow has also been shown to be reduced in diabetic patients, which is independent of the type of diabetes.[64]

Aqueous humor flow is lower during sleep, with a mean suppression of 45 ± 20%.[65,66] The diurnal fluctuation in the rate of aqueous flow in humans appears to be driven by changes in the concentration of endogenous epinephrine available to the ciliary epithelia, primarily due to the influence on beta-adrenergic receptors.[67,68]

Inflammation (iridocyclitis) causes a decrease in inflow,[69] possibly related to a disruption in ciliary epithelium.[70] Aqueous production is reduced during the acute phase of hypotony following cyclodialysis but not with chronic cyclodialysis if unassociated with iridocyclitis.[69] Choroidal detachment in a hypotonous eye is often associated with, but does not appear to cause, reduced inflow.[69] Retinal detachment is commonly associated with a reduction in the IOP, although it is not clear how much of this results from a decrease in aqueous production[71] or an increase in aqueous outflow by an unconventional, posterior route.[69] Pharmacologic agents that reduce inflow are discussed in Section Three.

FUNCTION AND COMPOSITION OF AQUEOUS HUMOR

Function

In addition to its role in maintaining a proper IOP, aqueous humor is associated with important metabolic functions that provide substrates for and remove metabolites from the avascular cornea and lens. For example, the cornea takes glucose and oxygen from the aqueous and releases lactic acid and a small amount of CO_2 into the aqueous.[30,72] The lens also uses glucose and generates lactate and pyruvate.[30] In addition, it is reported that potassium and amino acids in the aqueous may be taken up by the lens, while sodium moves from the lens to the aqueous.[39] The metabolism of the vitreous and retina also appears to be associated with the aqueous humor in that substances such as amino acids and glucose pass into the vitreous from the aqueous.[30,39]

Table 2.1.
General Character of Human Aqueous Humor (Expressed relative to plasma)

Slightly hypertonic
Acidic
Marked excess of ascorbate
Marked deficit of protein
Slight excess of:
Chloride
Lactic acid[a]
Slight deficit of:
Sodium (rabbit study)
Bicarbonate[a]
Carbon dioxide
Glucose
Other reported constituents/features:
Amino acids (variable concentrations)
Sodium hyaluronate
Norepinephrine
Coagulation properties
Tissue plasminogen activator
Latent collagenase activity

[a] Varies with measurement technique.

Composition

From the discussion above, it may be seen that the composition of aqueous humor depends not only on the nature of its production, but also on the constant metabolic interchanges that occur throughout its intraocular course. However, close similarities in aqueous composition between the phakic and aphakic eye of the same individual suggest that lens metabolism has practically no influence on the composition of aqueous.[73] Diffusional exchange across the iris may be a more significant factor in the changing composition of the aqueous between the posterior and anterior chambers, although there appears to be considerable species variation. Studies in rabbit eyes indicate that the total concentration of dissolved substances, pH, and osmotic pressure are the same in the posterior and anterior chambers, while the actual composition of the aqueous in the two chambers is different.[74] This difference appears to be related to active transport in the posterior chamber and passive transfer in the anterior chamber, where the iris vessels are permeable to anions and nonelectrolytes.[74] Tracer studies in primates suggest that a unidirectional vesicular transport in iris vessels is responsible for the selective movement of anionic substances from the tissues of the eye to the bloodstream.[75] In the rhesus monkey, however, the complexity of the interendothelial junctions in the blood vessels of the iris strongly suggests that these vessels participate only minimally in aqueous humor dynamics.[76,77]

The following statements, summarized in Table 2.1, describe only the general character of aqueous humor, expressed relative to plasma.[72–74,78–81] Aqueous of both the anterior and posterior chamber is slightly *hypertonic* compared with plasma. It is *acidic,* with a pH in the anterior chamber of 7.2.[79] The two most striking characteristics of aqueous humor are (1) a marked *excess of ascorbate* (15 times greater than that of arterial plasma), and (2) a marked *deficit of protein* (0.02% in aqueous as compared with 7% in plasma). In a study of 22 species of mammals, a wide range of ascorbic acid levels was found, although it was generally higher in diurnal than nocturnal animals, suggesting that it may play a protective role against light-induced damage.[82]

Studies of intravenously injected fluoresceinated horseradish peroxidase in normal rabbits suggest that the proteins in the aqueous humor pass through the ciliary body and iris to the anterior iris surface.[83] Protein content of the aqueous humor has both quantitative and qualitative differences in comparison with that of serum, which may explain the observed characteristic of aqueous to obstruct flow through artificial membranes with pore sizes similar to those found in the aqueous outflow pathway.[84,85] The albumin/globulin ratio is the same as that of plasma, although there is less gamma globulin. Human aqueous has been found to contain IgG, but no IgD, IgA, or IgM.[86] Protein and antibodies in the aqueous equilibrate with those in plasma to form a *plasmoid aqueous* when the eye is inflamed. In addition, following aspiration of aqueous, the newly formed fluid has a high protein content, which is suggested by monkey studies to result from new gaps in the inner wall endothelial lining of Schlemm's canal and enlarged extracellular spaces in the ciliary epithelium of the anterior pars plicata.[87,88]

The relative concentrations of free amino acids in human aqueous varies, with aqueous/plasma concentrations ranging from 0.08 to 3.14, supporting the concept of active transport of amino acids.[89] The concentrations of most other ions and nonelectrolytes are very close to those in the plasma, and conflicting statements in the literature primarily represent differences with regard to species and measurement techniques. In general, human aqueous has a slight excess of chloride and a deficiency of bicarbonate.[79,80] However, several factors lead to rapid changes in aqueous bicarbonate levels, and the concentrations measured may not accurately reflect the relative concentration of bicarbonate transported by the ciliary epithelia. Lactic acid is reported to be in relative excess in human aqueous,[80] although this determination varies widely with the technique of measurement. Sodium in rabbits[78] and glucose in human eyes[80] show a relative deficiency in the aqueous. The total CO_2 content in aqueous has considerable species variation, with a deficiency in humans.[90]

Sodium hyaluronate in human aqueous humor, obtained before cataract extraction, is reported to have a mean value of 1.14 ± 0.46 mg/g, with no substantial difference in patients with diabetes or glaucoma.[91] Norepinephrine was found consistently in human aqueous and was higher in patients undergoing cataract surgery than those with glaucoma.[92] Human aqueous also appears to have coagulation properties as demonstrated by its ability to shorten ear lobe puncture bleeding time, prothrombin time, and partial thromboplastin time.[93] However, the ratio of tissue plasminogen activator to total protein in normal human aqueous is approximately 30 times greater than that in plasma, suggesting an important role in intraocular fibrinolysis.[94] A latent collagenase activity has also been demonstrated in normal human aqueous, which may participate in the extracellular matrix metabolism of the trabecular meshwork.[95]

AQUEOUS HUMOR OUTFLOW

As noted earlier in this chapter, most of the aqueous humor leaves the eye at the anterior chamber angle through the system consisting of trabecular meshwork, Schlemm's canal, intrascleral channels, and episcleral and conjunctival veins. It has been estimated that this pathway, often referred to as the *conventional system,* accounts for 83[96]–96%[97] of aqueous outflow in human eyes under normal circumstances. The other 5–15% of the aqueous leaves the eye by a number of systems that are only partly understood but include *uveoscleral*[97–99] and *uveo-vortex*[100] systems. Collectively, these alternate aqueous outflow pathways are referred to as the *unconventional system*[101] or secondary pathways.[102] Alternative terms might be *canalicular* for the conventional outflow system, involving Schlemm's canal, and *extracanalicular* for the other pathways of aqueous outflow.[a]

Histology of the Conventional Aqueous Outflow System

Scleral Spur-Roll

The posterior wall of the scleral sulcus is formed by a group of fibers, the scleral roll, that run parallel to the limbus and project inward to form the *scleral spur* (Fig. 2.1).[103] The scleral spur-roll is composed of 75–80% collagen and 5% elastic tissue.[104] It has been suggested that this circular structure prevents the ciliary muscle from causing Schlemm's canal to collapse.[103]

[a] Richard F. Brubaker, M.D., personal communication, 1981.

Schwalbe's Line

Just anterior to the apical portion of the trabecular meshwork is a smooth area, which varies in width from 50 μ to 150 μ and has been called *Zone S*.[105] The anterior border of this zone consists of the transition from trabecular to corneal endothelium and the thinning and termination of Descemet's membrane. The posterior border is demarcated by a discontinuous elevation, called *Schwalbe's line*, that appears to be formed by the oblique insertion of uveal trabeculae into limbal stroma.[105] Clusters of secretory cells, called *Schwalbe line's cells*, have been observed just beneath this ridge in monkey eyes and are believed to produce a phospholipid material that facilitates aqueous flow through the canalicular system.[106]

Trabecular Meshwork

As previously discussed, the scleral sulcus is converted into a circular channel, called *Schlemm's canal*, by the trabecular meshwork. This tissue consists of a connective tissue core surrounded by endothelium and may be divided into three portions: (1) uveal meshwork, (2) corneoscleral meshwork, and (3) juxtacanalicular tissue (Fig. 2.8–2.10).

Uveal Meshwork. The portion adjacent to the aqueous in the anterior chamber is arranged in bands or rope-like trabeculae that extend from the iris root and ciliary body to the peripheral cornea. The arrangement of the trabecular bands creates irregular openings that vary in size from 25–75 μ across.[107]

Corneoscleral Meshwork. This portion extends from the scleral spur to the anterior wall of the scleral sulcus and consists of sheets of trabeculae that are perforated by elliptical openings. These holes become progressively smaller as the trabecular sheets approach Schlemm's canal, with a range of 5–50 μ in diameter.[107]

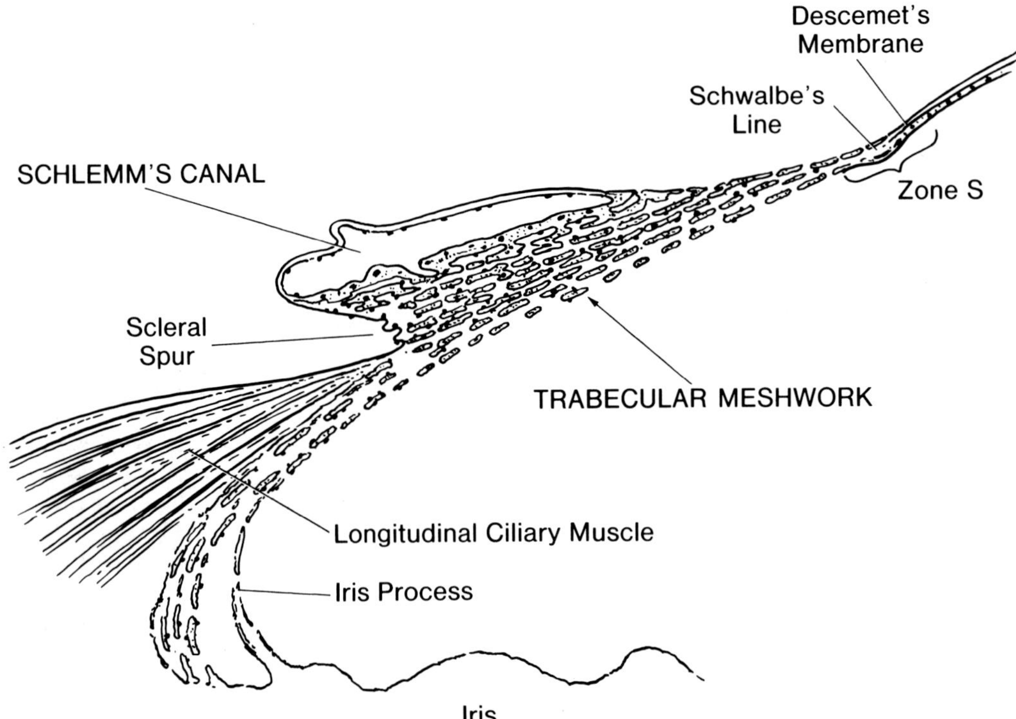

Figure 2.8. The trabecular meshwork extends from iris, ciliary body, and scleral spur to the sloping anterior wall of the scleral sulcus, converting the sulcus into Schlemm's canal.

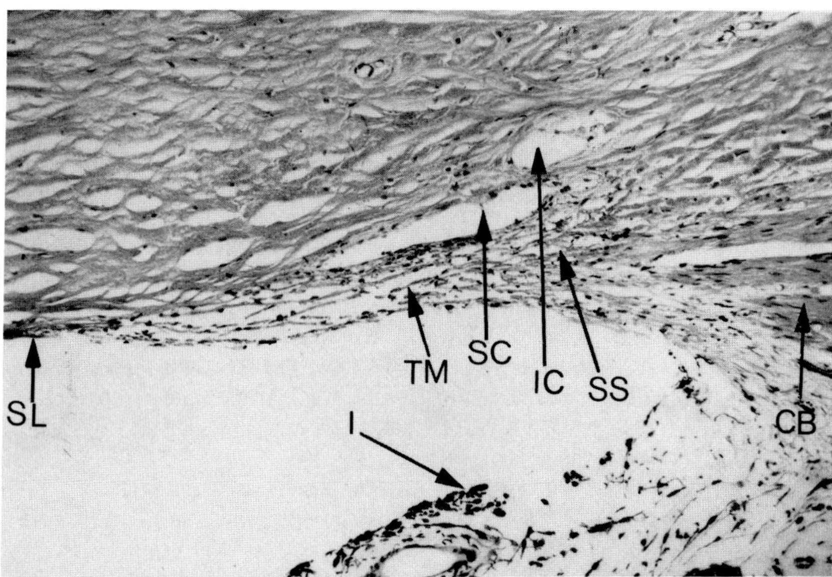

Figure 2.9. Light microscopic view of conventional aqueous outflow system: iris (*I*), ciliary body (*CB*), scleral spur (*SS*), trabecular meshwork (*TM*), Schlemm's canal (*SC*), intrascleral channels (*IC*), Schwalbe's line (*SL*). (Hematoxylin, eosin; original magnification, ×128.)

Juxtacanalicular Tissue. The outermost portion of the meshwork (adjacent to Schlemm's canal) consists of a layer of connective tissue lined on either side by endothelium.[108] The outer endothelial layer comprises the inner wall of Schlemm's canal, while the inner layer is continuous with the remainder of the trabecular endothelium.

Schlemm's Canal

This is an endothelial-lined channel averaging 190–370 μ in diameter.[109,110] It may be a single channel but occasionally branches into a plexus-like system.

Intrascleral Channels

Schlemm's canal is connected to episcleral and conjunctival veins by a complex system of vessels. Intrascleral aqueous vessels, the *aqueous veins of Ascher,*[111] have been defined as originating at the outer wall of Schlemm's canal and terminating in episcleral and conjunctival veins in a lamination of aqueous and blood, referred to as the *laminated vein of Goldmann.*[112] However, others refer to the proximal portion of these vessels as *outflow channels*[110,113] or *collector channels,*[109] since the structural pattern of the outer wall of Schlemm's canal extends into the first third of these channels.[113] Two systems of intrascleral vessels have been identified: (1) a direct system of large caliber vessels that run a short intrascleral course and drain directly into the episcleral venous system; and (2) an indirect system of more numerous, finer channels, which form an intrascleral plexus before eventually draining into the episcleral venous system.[109,110,113–115] The intrascleral aqueous channels do not connect with vessels of the uveal system, except for occasional fine communications with the ciliary muscle.[116] There are no arterial communications,[114–116] although arteriovenous anastomotic vessels may occur in the anterior episcleral system.[114–117]

Episcleral and Conjunctival Veins

The aqueous vessels join the episcleral venous system by several routes.[111] Most aqueous vessels are directed posteriorly with the majority of these draining into episcleral veins, while a few cross the subconjunctival tissue and drain into conjunctival veins. Some aqueous vessels proceed ante-

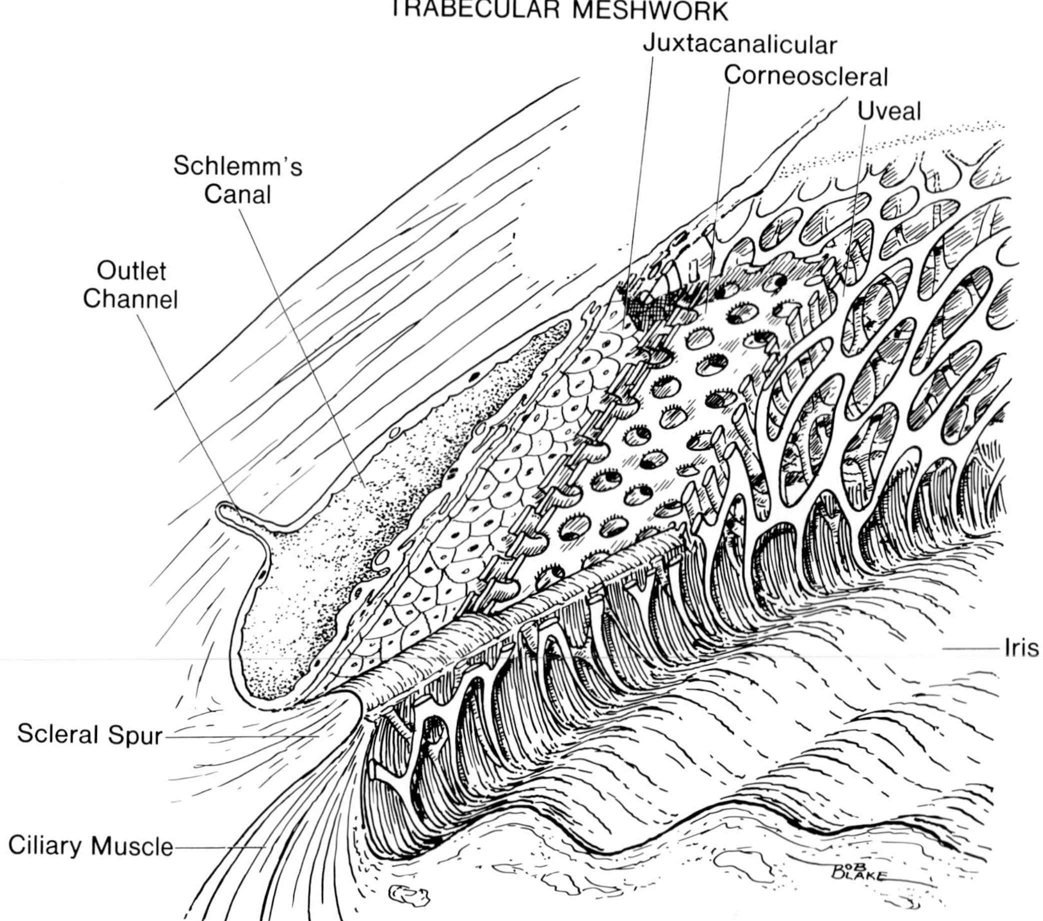

Figure 2.10. Three layers of trabecular meshwork (shown in cutaway views): (1) uveal; (2) corneoscleral; and (3) juxtacanalicular.

riorly to the limbus, with most of these running a short course parallel to the limbus before turning posteriorly to conjunctival veins. Other vessels make a sharp loop to join conjunctival veins or rarely extend a short distance into the cornea before turning posteriorly (Figs. 2.11, 2.12). In the rhesus monkey, the conjunctival vessels have a diameter consistent with that of capillaries, while most of the vessels in the episcleral plexus are the size of venules.[118] Both types of vessels have simple walls composed of endothelium and a discontinuous layer of pericytes, through which horseradish peroxidase (and presumably aqueous) freely diffuses into subconjunctival and episcleral loose connective tissue.[118] The episcleral veins drain into the cavernous sinus via the anterior ciliary and superior ophthalmic veins, while the conjunctival veins drain into superior ophthalmic or facial veins via the palpebral and angular veins.[112]

Ultrastructure of Trabecular Meshwork and Schlemm's Canal

Uveal and Corneoscleral Meshwork

Although the gross structure of these two trabecular subunits differs, as previously discussed, their ultrastructure is the same. Each trabecular band or sheet is composed of four concentric layers:[119]

1. An inner connective tissue core is composed of typical collagen fibers, with the usual 640 Å periodicity.[119] Indirect immunofluorescent studies of human trabecular

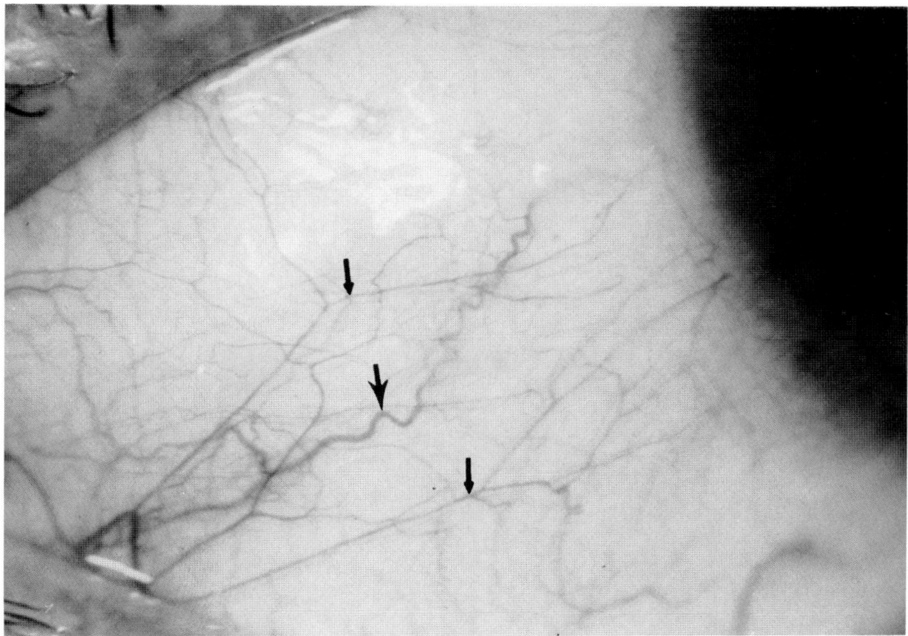

Figure 2.11. Slit-lamp view of normal episcleral and conjunctival vessels. Note typically large, serpiginous anterior ciliary artery (*large arrow*) and thinner, straighter episcleral and conjunctival veins (*small arrows*). (Courtesy of Douglas E. Gaasterland, M.D.)

meshwork indicate that the central core contains collagen types I and III and elastin.[120,121]

2. "Elastic" fibers are actually composed of otherwise typical collagen, arranged in a spiraling pattern with an apparent periodicity of 1000 Å.[122] These spiral fibrils may wind loosely or tightly, and may provide flexibility to the trabeculae.[123]

3. Glass membrane is a name given to the layer between the spiraling collagen and the basement membrane of the endothelium.[119] It is a broad zone composed of delicate filaments embedded in a ground substance.[121]

4. An endothelial layer provides a continuous covering over the trabeculae. The cells are larger, more irregular, and have less prominent borders than corneal endothelial cells.[105] They are joined by gap junctions and desmosomes, which provide stability but allow aqueous humor to freely traverse the patent endothelial clefts.[123,124] Two types of microfilaments have been found in the cytoplasm of human trabecular endothelium.[125,126] Six-nm filaments are located primarily in the cell periphery, around the nucleus, and in cytoplasmic processes. These appear to be actin filaments[126] that are involved in cell contraction and motility, phagocytosis and pinocytosis, and cell adhesion. Tissue culture studies suggest that actin filaments are important in regulating the shape and cytoskeletal organization of human,[127] monkey,[128] and bovine[129] trabecular cells. Intermediate filaments of 10 nm are more numerous in the cells and are composed of vimentin and desmin, according to immunocytochemical studies of cultured human trabecular cells, suggesting that these cells possess muscle cell-like functions.[130]

Animal studies of trabecular meshwork tissue indicate that the cells synthesize a heterogeneous mixture of glycosaminoglycans and glycoproteins,[131,132] which are distributed throughout the trabecular meshwork.[131–138] Human trabecular meshwork contains hyaluronic acid, chondroitin sulfate, dermatan sulfate, keratan sulfate,[137] and heparan sulfate.[120,139–142] Other components of the extracellular matrix of human trabecular meshwork include fibronectin and laminin (glycoprotein basement mem-

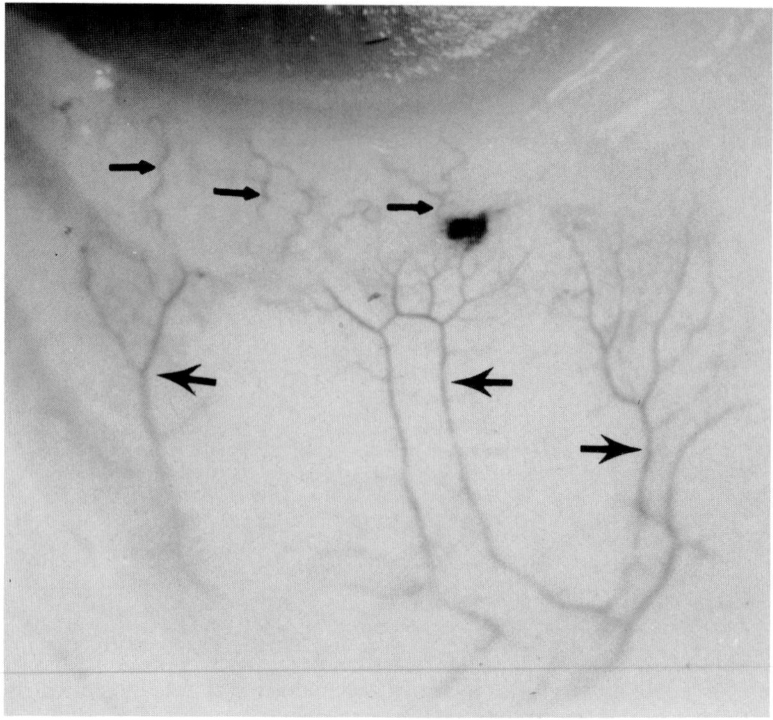

Figure 2.12. India ink perfusion of anterior chamber in human autopsy eye demonstrates filling of episcleral (*large arrows*) and conjunctival (*small arrows*) veins from aqueous veins.

brane components) and collagen types III, IV, and V in the basement membrane.[120,143–145] Human trabecular meshwork has also been shown to contain cells that express class II glycoproteins of the major histocompatibility complex, suggesting an important role in the initiation and regulation of ocular immunity.[146,147] Neuron-specific enolase has been found in the trabecular meshwork of monkey eyes, which may be evidence of neuroregulatory cells.[148]

The trabecular endothelial cells have been shown to phagocytose and degrade foreign material,[103,149–153] or to engulf debri, detach from the trabecular core, and leave through Schlemm's canal.[154] The amount of pigment in the trabecular meshwork, however, does not appear to correlate with the cellularity or morphology of the tissue.[155]

Juxtacanalicular Tissue

The portion of the trabecular meshwork adjacent to Schlemm's canal (and that actually makes up the inner wall of the canal) differs histologically from the other parts of the meshwork and has been given various names, depending on how one defines the anatomical limits of the tissue (e.g., *juxtacanalicular connective tissue, pore tissue,* and *endothelial meshwork*). In the broadest sense, this structure has three layers,[156] discussed here beginning with the innermost portion (Figs. 2.13, 2.14):

1. **A trabecular endothelial layer** is continuous with the endothelium of the corneoscleral meshwork and might be considered a part of this layer.

2. **A central connective tissue layer** of variable thickness is unfenestrated and has several layers of parallel, spindle-shaped cells loosely arranged in a connective tissue ground substance.[108,122,157] This tissue contains collagen type III, but no collagen type I or elastin.[120] Connective tissue cells in human and rabbit trabecular meshwork have been shown to contain coated pits and coated vesicles in the plasma membrane

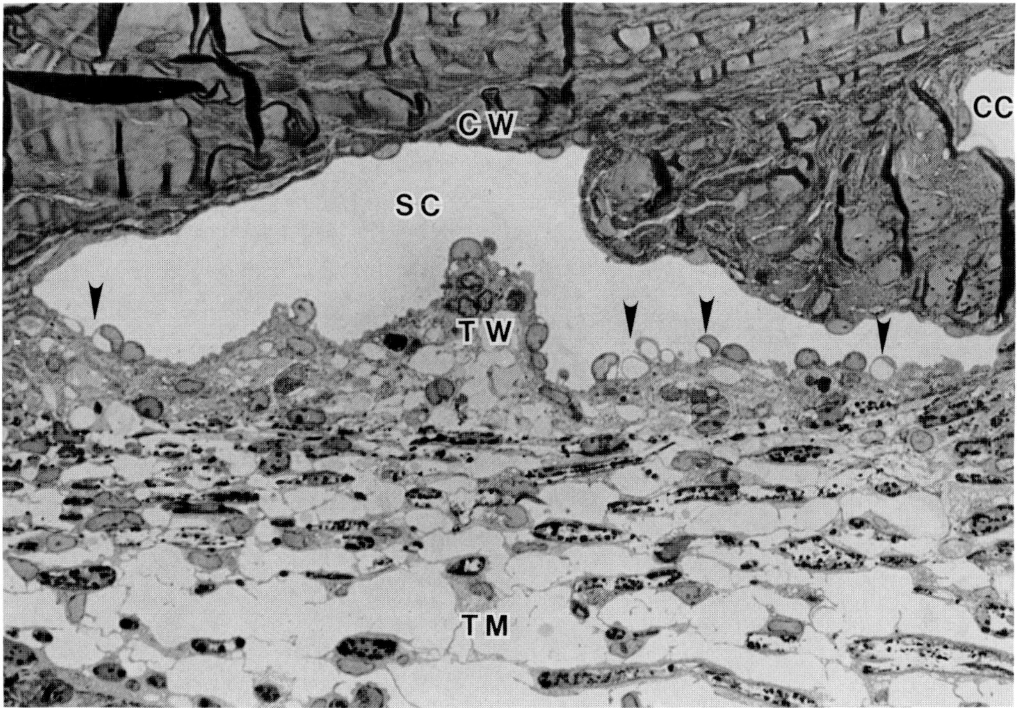

Figure 2.13. Light microscopic view of Schlemm's canal (*SC*) and adjacent trabecular meshwork (*TM*) of normotensive rhesus monkey eye. Trabecular wall of Schlemm's canal (*TW*) with prominent vacuolated cells (*arrows*); corneoscleral wall of Schlemm's canal (*CW*); and collector channel (*CC*). (Toluidine blue; original magnification, ×1030.) (Reprinted with permission from Tripathi RC: Exp Eye Res 7:335, 1968.)

that are involved in receptor-mediated endocytosis.[158,159]

3. The inner wall endothelium of Schlemm's canal is also the outermost portion of the trabecular meshwork (i.e., the last tissue that aqueous must traverse before entering the canal). This endothelial layer has significant morphologic characteristics, which distinguish it from the rest of the endothelium in both the trabecular meshwork and in Schlemm's canal. The surface is bumpy because of protruding nuclei,[157] cyst-like vacuoles,[160] and finger-like projections[161] bulging into the canal. The finger-like projections have been described as endothelial tubules with patent lumens, although there is lack of agreement as to whether they communicate between the anterior chamber and Schlemm's canal[161] or have no significant openings.[162] Actin filaments, as previously described in the uveal and corneoscleral trabecular endothelium, are also present in the inner wall endothelium of Schlemm's canal.[126]

The intercellular spaces are 150–200 Å wide and the adjacent cells are connected by a variety of intercellular junctions.[122,157] It is not clear as to how tightly these junctions maintain the intercellular connections, although it has been shown that they will open to permit the passage of red blood cells.[157] Zonulae occludentes have been demonstrated in primate studies, which are traversed by meandering channels of extracellular space or slit pores, although it is estimated that this accounts for only a small fraction of the aqueous humor that leaves the eye by the conventional route.[124] The endothelial cells are anchored by cytoplasmic processes to underlying subendothelial cells and trabecular meshwork.[163]

Openings in the endothelial cells have been described by many investigators. Considerable controversy has arisen as to the

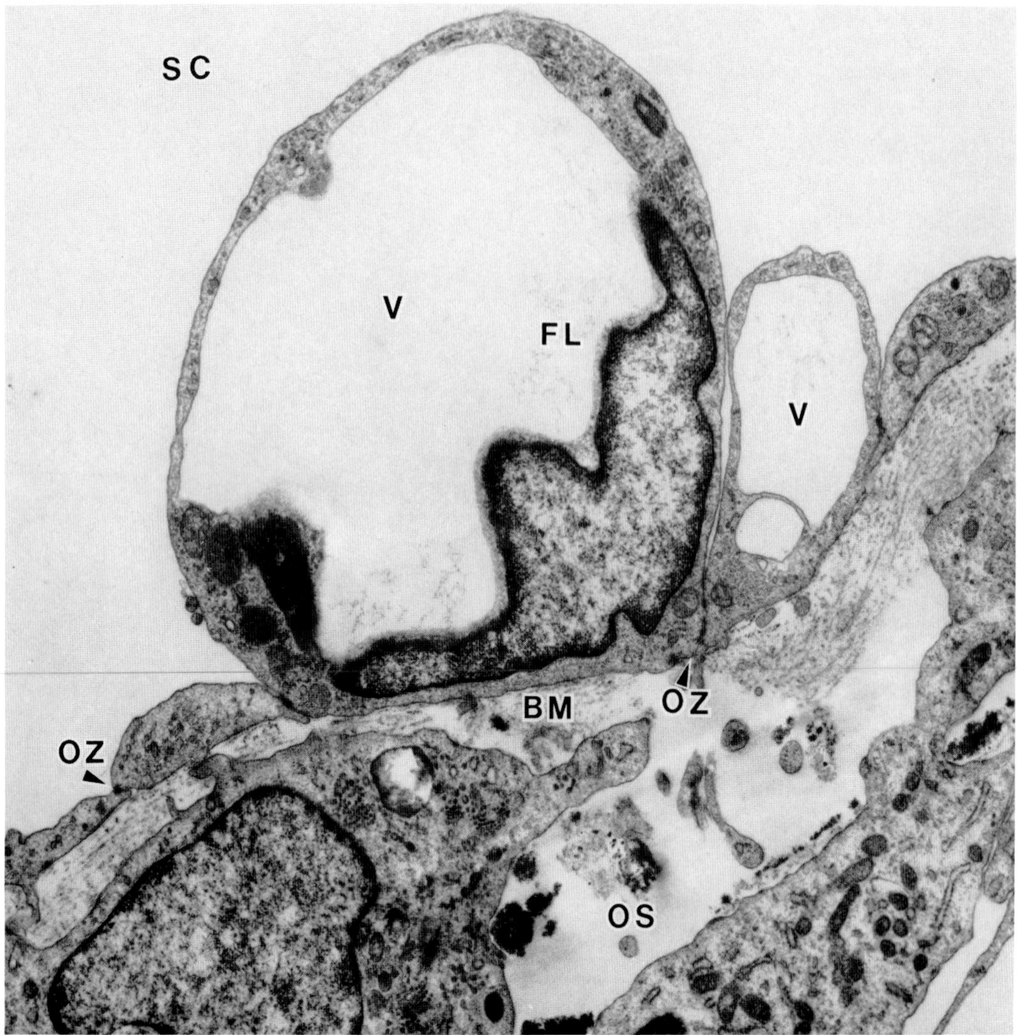

Figure 2.14. Electron microscopic view of trabecular wall of Schlemm's canal (*SC*) of normotensive human eye, showing vacuolated endothelial cells (*V*) containing flocculent material (*FL*). Occluding zonules (*OZ*), basement membrane (*BM*), open spaces in endothelial meshwork (*OS*). (Original magnification, ×15,000) (Reprinted with permission from Tripathi RC: Trans Ophthal Soc UK 89:449, 1969.)

morphology and function of these structures. In general, the openings consist of minute *pores* and large or *giant vacuoles*. The reported sizes of the pores vary considerably, although most are in the range of 0.5–2.0 μ.[107,109,164–170] Tracer studies have shown that these pores communicate between the intertrabecular spaces and Schlemm's canal.[168,169] The giant vacuoles in the endothelial cells were once thought to be postmortem artifacts,[171] but numerous studies have confirmed their existence and suggest that they are involved in aqueous outflow.[156,172–175] It may be that the pores and vacuoles represent different parts of the same transcellular channels.[168] The possible significance of these structures in resistance to aqueous outflow will be discussed later in this chapter.

Sondermann's "canals," although originally described as endothelial-lined channels communicating between Schlemm's canal and intertrabecular spaces,[176] have subsequently been interpreted as tortuous communications wandering irregularly and obliquely through the meshwork,[177] or as deep grooves on cross-section,[156] slit-like spaces between cells,[178] or artifacts.[107] It is unlikely that the structures, if they exist, play a significant role in aqueous outflow.

The Outer Wall of Schlemm's Canal

The endothelium of the outer wall is a single cell layer that is continuous with the inner wall endothelium.[122] The surface is smoother than that of the inner wall and has larger, less numerous cells[179] and no pores,[164,165] but numerous large *outlet channels,* as previously described. Smooth muscle myosin-containing cells have been localized in the human aqueous outflow pathway adjacent to the collector channels, slightly distal to the outer wall of Schlemm's canal.[180] Torus, or lip-like thickenings, have been observed around the openings of the outlet channels,[110,113] and septae have been noted to extend from these openings to the inner wall of Schlemm's canal, which presumably help to keep the canal open.[109,110,113] The endothelium is separated from the collagenous bundles of the limbus by a basement membrane[122] and layers of fibrocytes and fibroblasts.[113]

Age-Related Changes

The normal human trabecular meshwork undergoes several changes with age. The general configuration changes from a long, wedge shape to a shorter, more rhomboidal form.[181] The scleral spur becomes more prominent, the uveal meshwork becomes more compact, and localized closures in Schlemm's canal become more common.[181] The trabecular beams progressively thicken, and the endothelial cellularity declines[181,182] at the rate of approximately 0.58% of cells per year,[183] occasionally leading to trabecular denuding.[181] A decrease in the number of giant vacuoles was associated with a decreased cell count in Schlemm's canal, although both vacuole and cell decline were explained by an age-related reduction in the size of Schlemm's canal.[184] A narrowing of the intertrabecular spaces and an increase in extracellular material, especially of electron-dense plaques near the juxtacanalicular tissue, are also seen with increasing age.[181,182]

Additional observations regarding the trabecular meshwork and Schlemm's canal that may relate to aqueous outflow resistance are considered later in this chapter, while those associated with possible drug responses are discussed in the pharmacology chapters in Section Three.

Unconventional Aqueous Outflow Pathways

As discussed earlier in this chapter, aqueous humor diffuses throughout virtually every portion of the eye. It is likely, therefore, that many ocular tissues, such as retina and cornea, participate in unconventional outflow by absorbing small quantities of aqueous. However, the only structure in which this has been studied in detail is the uveal tract. Two pathways have been identified whereby aqueous leaves the eye following absorption by the anterior uvea.

Uveoscleral Outflow

Tracer studies in human[96] and animal[97–101] eyes suggest that aqueous may pass through the root of the iris and interstitial spaces of the ciliary muscle to reach the suprachoroidal space. From there it passes to episcleral tissue via scleral pores surrounding ciliary arteries and nerves, through vessels of optic nerve membranes, or through the actual collagen substance of the sclera. Studies with cynomolgus monkeys revealed a lower hydrostatic pressure in the suprachoroidal space as compared with that in the anterior chamber, and it was suggested that this pressure differential is the driving force for uveoscleral outflow.[185]

Uveovortex Outflow

It has also been demonstrated by tracer studies in primates that iris vessels allow unidirectional flow into the lumen of the vessel by vesicular transport, which is not energy dependent.[186] The tracer can penetrate vessels of the iris, ciliary muscle, and anterior choroid to eventually reach the vortex veins.[99]

A computed tomographic study of perfused radiopaque contrast media in rhesus monkeys suggested that the unconventional aqueous drainage pathways are cleared immediately by circulating blood in the uvea and possibly the extraocular muscles, since posterior movement of contrast media through the globe wall was not seen in the living animal, but appeared immediately after death when the IOP was maintained artificially.[187]

Normal Resistance to Aqueous Outflow

Assuming an average normal IOP of 15 mm Hg and an episcleral venous pressure of approximately 10 mm Hg, a resistance to aqueous outflow of 5 mm Hg must be accounted for to explain the equilibrium between inflow and outflow in the normal steady state. Grant[188,189] demonstrated that a 360° incision in the trabecular meshwork of nonglaucomatous, enucleated human eyes eliminated 75% of the resistance to aqueous outflow. The exact site and nature of this resistance within the conventional outflow system is uncertain. The following observations, however, provide some insight into this important question.

Resistance in the Trabecular Meshwork

Studies with tracer elements show relatively free flow through the trabecular spaces and juxtacanalicular connective tissue until reaching the inner surface of the inner wall endothelium of Schlemm's canal.[157,168,169,173] It would appear, therefore, that this endothelial layer accounts for the majority of any resistance to outflow that the meshwork may provide, although other portions of the system may also contribute to the regulation of aqueous outflow.

Pores and giant vacuoles in the inner wall endothelium of Schlemm's canal, as previously discussed, appear to be parts of a transcellular system for aqueous outflow, since tracer elements injected into the anterior chamber are seen in the vacuoles and pores.[157,168,169,173,190] The observation that the concentration of tracer material in the giant vacuoles is not always the same as in the juxtacanalicular connective tissue[157] suggests a dynamic system in which the vacuoles intermittently open and close to transport aqueous from the juxtacanalicular tissue to Schlemm's canal (Fig. 2.15).[173] Whether this transport is active or passive has been controversial.

Indirect evidence for a theory of active transport has included the demonstration of enzymes[191] and electron microscopic structures[192] compatible with an active transport system in or near the endothelial layer. However, the bulk of evidence supports the theory of passive (pressure-dependent) transport, since the number and size of the vacuoles have been shown to increase with progressive elevation of the IOP.[193–196] Furthermore, this phenomenon is reversible in the enucleated eye,[193] and hypothermia has no effect on the development of the vacuoles in the enucleated eye.[197]

It may be, therefore, that potential transcellular spaces exist in the inner wall endothelium of Schlemm's canal, which open as a system of vacuoles and pores, primarily in response to pressure, to transport aqueous from the juxtacanalicular connective tissue to Schlemm's canal. The actual resistance to aqueous outflow provided by this system is unclear, although it has been calculated, based on the estimated size and total number of pores in the inner wall endothelium of Schlemm's canal, that resistance to outflow through the endothelial cells is a small fraction of the total resistance to outflow.[198–201]

The following possibilities have been considered to explain the inability of the observed morphology of the inner wall endothelium of Schlemm's canal to account for the 5 mm Hg pressure drop across this tissue: (1) the major resistance might be located elsewhere in the trabecular meshwork (for which there is no strong evidence);[200] (2) shrinkage of tissue during preparation for electron microscopy might cause artificial enlargement of the natural lumina[200] (which is taken into account in most theoretical models); (3) tissue preparation might also alter or remove extracellular materials;[200,201] (4) proteins or glycoproteins in aqueous humor might cause a greater resistance to flow than would isotonic saline;[202] and (5) only a portion of the juxtacanalicular tissue might actually filter.[200] It is likely that a combination of these factors (especially the last three) explains the discrepancies be-

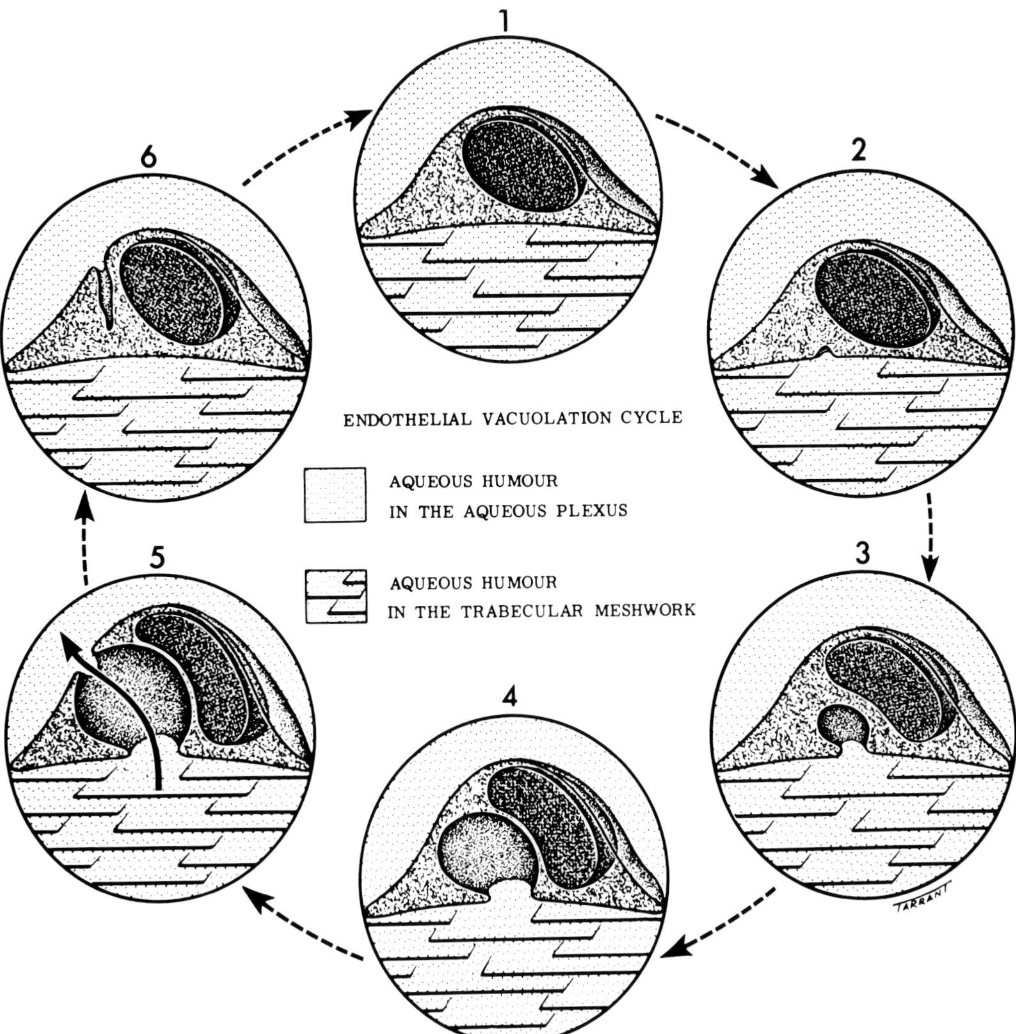

Figure 2.15. Theory of transcellular aqueous transport, in which series of pores and giant vacuoles open (probably in response to transendothelial hydrostatic pressure) on connective tissue side of juxtacanalicular meshwork (**2–4**). Fusion of basal and apical cell plasmalemma creates a temporary transcellular channel (**5**) that allows bulk flow of aqueous into Schlemm's canal. (Reprinted with permission from Tripathi RC: Exp Eye Res 11:116, 1971.)

tween calculated and measured aqueous outflow resistance. Some of these possibilities will now be considered in more detail.

Glycosaminoglycans (acid mucopolysaccharides) that are present in large concentrations within the trabecular beams, on the surface of the trabecular endothelial cells, and in the juxtacanalicular tissue[139–141] may contribute significantly to aqueous outflow resistance in the trabecular meshwork.[200,201] These polysaccharide chains in covalent association with protein form highly polymerized complexes, which exert osmotic forces that may help to maintain hydration of the trabecular meshwork. In addition, a strong negative charge influences electromagnetic properties of tissues, which may determine the directional transport of ions in the aqueous humor.

The precise mechanism by which glycosaminoglycans contribute to the resistance and regulation of aqueous humor flow through the trabecular meshwork is not clear. It has been suggested that enzymes that catabolize glycosaminoglycans are released by lysosomes in the meshwork, to depolymerize the glycosaminoglycans, thereby reducing this cause of resistance to outflow.[203,204] *Hyaluronidase* decreases aqueous outflow resistance in nonprimate species, suggesting a glycosaminoglycans barrier to aqueous outflow, although similar evidence in primate and human eyes is inconclusive.[189,205,206] Another species difference has been seen with prolonged perfusion of eyes, which causes a gradual increase in outflow facility in canine eyes, apparently caused by a "washout" of a hyaluronidase-sensitive component of the barrier to aqueous outflow.[207,208] In primates, however, a decrease in facility occurs with prolonged perfusion.[209] The difference may relate to the pectinate ligament in the canine eye, which appears to compartmentalize glycosaminoglycans in the spaces of Fontana.[210] Perfusion studies with enucleated monkey eyes, using a trabeculotomy and hyaluronidase, suggest that outflow resistance due to glycosaminoglycans is only slightly related to the trabecular meshwork.[211]

Glucocorticoid receptors have been demonstrated in the trabecular meshwork of trabeculectomy specimens from human glaucomatous eyes, nonglaucomatous autopsy eyes,[212] and cultured human trabecular cells,[213] suggesting that glucocorticoids may influence the outflow facility by means of a direct effect on the metabolism of these cells. This effect may be on the incorporation of precursors of extracellular matrix components, leading to an increase in collagen synthesis or a decreased synthesis of glycosaminoglycans, glycoproteins, or possibly glycolipids.[214] Glucocorticoids also inhibit the synthesis of prostaglandins,[215] the production of which has been seen in cultured human trabecular cells.[215,216] Prostaglandins have been shown to cause increased IOP in high doses, but reduced ocular tension in moderate to low concentrations.[217]

Contractile microfilaments, as previously described, occur in the inner wall endothelium of Schlemm's canal as well as the endothelium lining the trabeculae. Perfusing monkey eyes with substances that are known to disrupt the microfilaments, such as cytochalasin B,[218–221] cytochalasin D,[221] or EDTA,[222,223] significantly reduces the resistance to aqueous outflow, and histologic studies suggest that this is primarily due to an alteration in the trabecular meshwork or inner wall of Schlemm's canal.[219,220,222,223]

Sulfhydryl groups in trabecular cells also appear to modulate aqueous outflow by several mechanisms. Perfusion with certain sulfhydryl reagents, including iodoacetic acid,[224] iodoacetamide,[225] and N-ethylmaleimide,[226] increases facility of outflow. Apparently this is not due to a metabolic inhibitory action but to an alteration of cell membrane sulfhydryl groups at multiple sites in the endothelial lining of Schlemm's canal.[227] Conversely, mercurial sulfhydryl agents cause a decrease in aqueous outflow, presumably due to cellular swelling of the trabecular meshwork.[228] Another mechanism by which sulfhydryl groups modulate aqueous outflow may involve hydrogen peroxide, a normal constituent of aqueous humor that may reduce outflow through oxidative damage of the trabecular meshwork. Calf trabecular meshwork has been shown to contain the sulfhydryl compound glutathione[229] as well as the enzyme glutathione peroxidase,[230] which catalyzes the reaction between glutathione and hydrogen peroxide, thereby detoxifying the latter and presumably protecting the meshwork from its harmful effects.[231]

Fibrinolytic activity has been demonstrated in the endothelium of Schlemm's canal,[232] but no evidence of coagulation factors has been found.[233] Tissue plasminogen activator, which is responsible for the conversion of plasminogen to plasmin, thereby mediating the lysis of formed fibrin, has been demonstrated in many ocular tissues, including the trabecular meshwork of human and animal eyes.[234–236] This suggests that a hemostatic balance, displaced toward fibrinolysis, protects this portion of the outflow system from occlusion by fibrin and platelets.[232–236] In addition to facilitating the resolution of hyphema, tissue plasminogen activator may also influence resistance to aqueous outflow under normal circumstances by altering the glycoprotein content of the extracellular matrix.[200,201]

Resistance in Schlemm's Canal

Once aqueous has entered Schlemm's canal, resistance to continued flow into the intrascleral outlet channels may depend on the spatial configuration of the canal. There is controversy as to whether the canal is normally entirely open and whether it allows circumferential flow. Perfusion studies in enucleated human adult eyes suggest that aqueous cannot flow more than 10° within the canal,[237] although there is less resistance to circumferential flow in infant eyes.[238] However, studies of segmental blood reflux into Schlemm's canal imply that the canal is normally entirely open and that there is circumferential flow.[239]

Pressure-dependent changes in aqueous outflow facility appear to be related to a collapse of Schlemm's canal. Elevation of IOP is associated with increased resistance to outflow,[193,240–242] which is most likely due to collapse of the canal. Histologic studies of eyes perfused at different pressures suggest that compromise of the canal lumen with elevated IOP is due to distention of the trabecular meshwork,[193,243,244] an increase in endothelial vacuoles,[194–196] and a ballooning of the inner wall endothelial cells into the canal.[163] Perfusion studies also suggest that the resistance to aqueous outflow may normally depend in part on an intact, unyielding outer wall of Schlemm's canal, against which the intact inner wall is pressed by the IOP,[245] probably as a result of blockage of the intrascleral outlet (collector) channels by the canal's inner wall.[246] However, significant differences in the response to elevated perfusion pressure have been found among different mammalian eyes, and it has been suggested that factors other than, or in addition to, collapse of Schlemm's canal may be important regarding the influence of elevated IOP on resistance to outflow.[247]

As might be expected from the above observations, resistance to outflow is decreased by expanding Schlemm's canal. The trabecular meshwork has been described as a three-dimensional set of diagonally crossing collagen fibers, which respond to backward, inward displacement with a widening of Schlemm's canal.[248] The effect of tensing the meshwork has been demonstrated by deepening of the anterior chamber during perfusion studies when an iridectomy is not made,[188] by posterior depression of the lens,[237,246,249–252] or by tension on the choroid.[253] With each experimental model, the tension on the trabecular meshwork is associated with increased outflow facility, which appears to be due to widening of Schlemm's canal[250,252] and an increase in canal inner wall porosity.[250]

As previously noted, a 360° incision of the trabecular meshwork (trabeculotomy) eliminates approximately 75% of the normal outflow resistance.[188,189] However, when such an eye is perfused at 7 mm Hg, the trabeculotomy eliminates only half the resistance, with further decrease in resistance of 2% per mm Hg rise in the IOP.[254] This suggests that a significant fraction of aqueous outflow resistance is in the distal aspects of the outflow system, and that this resistance decreases with increasing IOP.

Resistance in the Intrascleral Outflow Channels

The remainder of the resistance to aqueous outflow appears to be within the intrascleral outflow channels. One monkey study has suggested that 60–65% of outflow resistance is in the trabecular meshwork, 25% is in the inner one-third to one-half of the sclera, and 15% is in the outer one-half to two-thirds of the sclera.[255]

Resistance to Unconventional Outflow

Unlike the conventional outflow system, unconventional outflow has been reported to improve with an elevation of the IOP, presumably as a result of ultrafiltration of aqueous into uveal vessels.[97] It has also been shown that outflow by this route is reduced by miotics.[96] It should be noted that our understanding of the unconventional outflow system is based more on physiology than on anatomy, and further study is needed to correlate function and anatomy in this system.

Episcleral Venous Pressure

As discussed earlier in this chapter, another factor that contributes to the IOP is the episcleral venous pressure. The precise interrelationship between episcleral venous pressure and aqueous humor dynamics is complex and only partly understood. It has been commonly held that the IOP rises mm Hg for mm Hg with an increase in episcleral venous pressure, although it may be that the magnitude of IOP rise is greater than the rise in venous pressure.[256] The normal episcleral venous pressure is reported to be within the range of 8–11 mm Hg,[257–261] and one study found that this does not vary with age.[261] However, these values are influenced considerably by the particular technique of measurement,[262] which will be discussed in the next chapter.

SUMMARY

Intraocular pressure is the result of a complex interplay of the components of aqueous humor dynamics, especially the rate of aqueous production, the resistance to aqueous outflow, and the episcleral venous pressure. Aqueous humor is produced by the ciliary processes through ultrafiltration of plasma from capillaries, active transport of certain constituents of the plasma across an epithelial barrier, and flow of other plasma components across the epithelium as a result of an osmotic gradient that is created by the active transport. The aqueous enters the posterior chamber, between the iris and lens, and undergoes metabolic interchanges with virtually all ocular structures, especially the cornea, iris, lens, vitreous, and retina. The bulk of aqueous, however, flows through the pupil into the anterior chamber and leaves the eye via structures in the anterior chamber angle, primarily through the trabecular meshwork and Schlemm's canal (conventional outflow), with a small contribution from anterior uveal absorption. From Schlemm's canal, aqueous passes through intrascleral channels to reunite with the blood system in the episcleral veins.

References

1. Hogan, MF, Alvarado, JA, Weddell, JE: Histology of the Human Eye. Philadelphia, WB Saunders, 1971, p. 269.
2. Morrison, JC, Van Buskirk, EM: Anterior collateral circulation in the primate eye. Ophthalmology 90:707, 1983.
3. Woodlief, NF: Initial observations on the ocular microcirculation in man. I. The anterior segment and extraocular muscles. Arch Ophthal 98:1268, 1980.
4. Morrison, JC, DeFrank, MP, Van Buskirk, EM: Regional microvascular anatomy of the rabbit ciliary body. Invest Ophthal Vis Sci 28:1314, 1987.
5. Morrison, JC, DeFrank, MP, Van Buskirk, EM: Comparative microvascular anatomy of mammalian ciliary processes. Invest Ophthal Vis Sci 28:1325, 1987.
6. Talusan, ED, Schwartz, B: Fluorescein angiography. Demonstration of flow patterns of anterior ciliary arteries. Arch Ophthal 99:1074, 1981.
7. Sakimoto, G, Schwartz, B: Decrease of anterior ciliary arterial pressure with increased ocular pressure. Invest Ophthal Vis Sci 25:992, 1984.
8. Nanba, K, Schwartz, B: Increased diameter of the anterior ciliary artery with increased intraocular pressure. Arch Ophthal 104:1652, 1986.
9. Morrison, JC, Van Buskirk, EM: Ciliary process microvasculature of the primate eye. Am J Ophthal 97:372, 1984.
10. Smelser, GK: Electron microscopy of a typical epithelial cell and of the normal human ciliary process. Trans Am Acad Ophthal Otol 70:738, 1966.
11. Streeten, BW, Licari, PA: The zonules and the elastic microfibrillar system in the ciliary body. Invest Ophthal Vis Sci 24:667, 1983.
12. Tormey, JMcD: The ciliary epithelium: an attempt to correlate structure and function. Trans Am Acad Ophthal Otol 70:755, 1966.
13. Holmberg, A: Ultrastructure of the ciliary epithelium. Arch Ophthal 62:935, 1959.
14. Holmberg, A: Differences in ultrastructure of normal human and rabbit ciliary epithelium. Arch Ophthal 62:952, 1959.
15. Raviola, G, Raviola, E: Intercellular junctions in the ciliary epithelium. Invest Ophthal Vis Sci 17:958, 1978.
16. Smith, RL, Raviola, G: The structural basis of the blood-aqueous barrier in the chicken eye. Invest Ophthal Vis Sci 24:326, 1983.
17. Green, K: Physiology and pharmacology of aqueous humor inflow. Surv Ophthal 29:208, 1984.
18. Green, K, Bountra, C, Georgiou, P, House, CR: An electrophysiologic study of rabbit ciliary epithelium. Invest Ophthal Vis Sci 26:371, 1985.
19. Cunha-Vas, JG: The blood-ocular barriers. Invest Ophthal Vis Sci 17:1037, 1978.
20. Pederson, JE: Fluid permeability of monkey ciliary epithelium in vivo. Invest Ophthal Vis Sci 23:176, 1982.
21. Wulle, KG: Zelldifferenzierungen im Ciliarepithel wahrend der menschlichen Fetalentwicklung und ihre Beziehungen zur Kammerwasserbildung. Graefe's Arch Ophthal 172:170, 1967.

22. Richardson, KT: Cellular response to drugs affecting aqueous dynamics. Arch Ophthal 89:65, 1973.
23. Uusitalo, R, Palkama, A, Stjernschantz, J: An electron microscopical study of the blood-aqueous barrier in the ciliary body and iris of the rabbit. Exp Eye Res 17:49, 1973.
24. Smith, RS, Rudt, LA: Ultrastructural studies of the blood-aqueous barrier. 2. The barrier to horseradish peroxidase in primates. Am J Ophthal 76:937, 1973.
25. Peress, NS, Tompkins, DC: Pericapillary permeability of the ciliary processes. Role of molecular charge. Invest Ophthal Vis Sci 23:168, 1982.
26. Macri, JF, Cevario, SJ: The formation and inhibition of aqueous humor production. Arch Ophthal 96:1664, 1978.
27. Farahbakhsh, NA, Fian, GL: Volume regulation of non-pigmented cells from ciliary epithelium. Invest Ophthal Vis Sci 28:934, 1987.
28. Becker, B: The effect of hypothermia on aqueous humor dynamics. III. Turnover of ascorbate and sodium. Am J Ophthal 51:1032, 1961.
29. Berggren, L: Effect of composition of medium and of metabolic inhibitors on secretion in vitro by the ciliary processes of the rabbit eye. Invest Ophthal 4:83, 1965.
30. Sears, ML: The aqueous. In: Adler's Physiology of the Eye, 6th ed., Moses, RA, ed. CV Mosby, St. Louis, 1975, p. 232.
31. Bonting, SL, Becker, B: Studies on sodium-potassium activated adenosinetriphosphatase. XIV. Inhibition of enzyme activity and aqueous humor flow in the rabbit eye after intravitreal injection of ouabain. Invest Ophthal 3:523, 1964.
32. Cole, DF: Some effects of decreased plasma sodium concentration on the composition and tension of the aqueous humor. Br J Ophthal 43:268, 1959.
33. Holland, MG, Gipson, CC: Chloride ion transport in the isolated ciliary body. Invest Ophthal 9:20, 1970.
34. Holland, MG: Chloride ion transport in the isolated ciliary body. II. Ion substitution experiments. Invest Ophthal 9:30, 1970.
35. Bito, L, Davson, H: Steady-state concentrations of potassium in the ocular fluids. Exp Eye Res 3:283, 1964.
36. Helbig, H, Korbmacher, C, Wohlfarth, J, et al: Electrical membrane properties of a cell clone derived from human nonpigmented ciliary epithelium. Invest Ophthal Vis Sci 30:882, 1989.
37. Chu, T-C, Candia, OA: Electrically silent Na^+ and Cl^- fluxes across the rabbit ciliary epithelium. Invest Ophthal Vis Sci 29:594, 1988.
38. Chu, T-C, Candia, OA: Active transport of ascorbate across the isolated rabbit ciliary epithelium. Invest Ophthal Vis Sci 29:594, 1988.
39. Reddy, VN: Dynamics of transport systems in the eye. Invest Ophthal Vis Sci 18:1000, 1979.
40. Maren, TH: The rates of movement of Na^+, Cl^-, and HCO_3^- from plasma to posterior chamber: effect of acetazolamide and relation to the treatment of glaucoma. Invest Ophthal 15:356, 1976.
41. Cole, DF: Effects of some metabolic inhibitors upon the formation of the aqueous humor in rabbits. Br J Ophthal 44:739, 1960.
42. Hara, K, Lutjen-Drecoll, E, Prestele, H, Rohen, JW: Structural differences between regions of the ciliary body in primates. Invest Ophthal Vis Sci 16:912, 1977.
43. Ober, M, Rohen, JW: Regional differences in the fine structure of the ciliary epithelium related to accommodation. Invest Ophthal Vis Sci 18:655, 1979.
44. Mizuno, K, Asaoka, M: Cycloscopy and fluorescein cycloscopy. Invest Ophthal 15:561, 1976.
45. Lutjen-Drecoll, E, Lonnerholm, G, Eichhorn, M: Carbonic anhydrase distribution in the human and monkey eye by light and electron microscopy. Graefe's Arch Ophthal 220:285, 1983.
46. Russman, W: Levels of glycolytic enzyme activity in the ciliary epithelium prepared from bovine eyes. Ophthal Res 2:205, 1971.
47. Feeney, L, Mixon, R: Localization of ^{35}sulfated macromolecules at the site of active transport in the ciliary processes. Invest Ophthal 13:882, 1974.
48. Feeney, L, Mixon, RN: Sulfate and galactose metabolism in differentiating ciliary body and iris epithelia: autoradiographic and ultrastructural studies. Invest Ophthal 14:364, 1975.
49. Krupin, T, Wax, M, Moolchandani, J: Aqueous production. Trans Ophthal Soc UK 105:156, 1986.
50. Raviola, G: Evidence for a secretory process, distinct from that of the aqueous humor, in the ciliary epithelium of *Macaca mulatta*. Trans Ophthal Soc UK 105:140, 1986.
51. Brubaker, RF: The flow of aqueous humor in the human eye. Trans Am Ophthal Soc 80:391, 1982.
52. Brubaker, RF, Kupfer, C: Determination of pseudofacility in the eye of the rhesus monkey. Arch Ophthal 75:693, 1966.
53. Kupfer, C, Sanderson, P: Determination of pseudofacility in the eye of man. Arch Ophthal 80:194, 1968.
54. Bill, A: Aspects of suppressability of aqueous humour formation. Doc Ophthal 26:73, 1969.
55. Brubaker, RF: The measurement of pseudofacility and true facility by constant pressure perfusion in the normal rhesus monkey eye. Invest Ophthal 9:42, 1970.
56. Leydhecker, W, Rehak, S, Mathyl, J: Investigations on homeostasis: the effect of experimental changes of pressure on the production of aqueous

humour in the living rabbit eye. Klin Monatsbl Augenheilkd 159:427, 1971.
57. Kupfer, C, Ross, K: Studies of aqueous humor dynamics in man. 1. Measurements in young normal subjects. Invest Ophthal 10:518, 1971.
58. Bill, A: Effects of longstanding stepwise increments in eye pressure on the rate of aqueous humor formation in a primate (*Cercopithecus ethiops*). Exp Eye Res 12:184, 1971.
59. Carlson, KH, McLaren, JW, Topper, JE, Brubaker, RF: Effect of body positions on intraocular pressure and aqueous flow. Invest Ophthal Vis Sci 28:1653, 1985.
60. Moses, RA, Grodzki, WJ Jr, Carras, PL: Pseudofacility. Arch Ophthal 103:1653, 1985.
61. Brown, JD, Brubaker, RF: A study of the relation between intraocular pressure and aqueous humor flow in the pigment dispersion syndrome. Ophthalmology 96:1468, 1989.
62. Becker, B: The decline in aqueous secretion and outflow facility with age. Am J Ophthal 46:731, 1958.
63. Brubaker, RF, Nagtaki, S, Townsend, DJ, et al: The effect of age on aqueous humor formation in man. Ophthalmology 88:283, 1981.
64. Hayashi, M, Yablonski, ME, Boxrud, C, et al: Decreased formation of aqueous humour in insulin-dependent diabetic patients. Br J Ophthal 73:621, 1989.
65. Reiss, GR, Lee, DA, Topper, JE, Brubaker, RF: Aqueous humor flow during sleep. Invest Ophthal Vis Sci 25:776, 1984.
66. McLaren, JW, Trocme, SD, Relf, S, Brubaker, RF: Rate of flow of aqueous humor determined from measurements of aqueous flare. Invest Ophthal Vis Sci 31:339, 1990.
67. Topper, JE, Brubaker, RF: Effects of timolol, epinephrine, and acetazolamide on aqueous flow during sleep. Invest Ophthal Vis Sci 26:1315, 1985.
68. Gharagozloo, NZ, Larson, RS, Kullerstrand, LJ, Brubaker, RF: Terbutaline stimulates aqueous humor flow in human during sleep. Arch Ophthal 106:1218, 1988.
69. Pederson, JE: Ocular hypotony. Trans Ophthal Soc UK 105:220, 1986.
70. Howes, EL, Cruse, VK: The structural basis of altered vascular permeability following intraocular inflammation. Arch Ophthal 96:1668, 1978.
71. Dobbie, JG: A study of the intraocular fluid dynamics in retinal detachment. Arch Ophthal 69:53, 1963.
72. Cole, DF: Aqueous and ciliary body. In: Biochemistry of the Eye, Graymore, CN, ed. Academic Press, London, 1970, p. 114.
73. De Berardinis, E, Tieri, O, Iuglio, N, Polzella, A: The composition of the aqueous humour of man in aphakia. Acta Ophthal 44:64, 1966.
74. Kinsey, VE: Comparative chemistry of aqueous humor in posterior and anterior chamber of rabbit eye. Its physiologic significance. Arch Ophthal 50:401, 1953.
75. Raviola, G, Butler, JM: Asymmetric distribution of charged domains on the two fronts of the endothelium of iris blood vessels. Invest Ophthal Vis Sci 26:597, 1985.
76. Freddo, TF, Raviola, G: The homogeneous structure of blood vessels in the vascular tree of *Macaca mulatta* iris. Invest Ophthal Vis Sci 22:279, 1982.
77. Freddo, TF, Raviola, G: Freeze-fracture analysis of the interendothelial junctions in the blood vessels of the iris in *Macaca mulatta*. Invest Ophthal Vis Sci 23:154, 1982.
78. Reddy, DVN: Chemical composition of normal aqueous humor. In: Biochemistry of the Eye, Dardenna, MU, Nordmann, J, eds. Karger, Basel, 1968, p. 167.
79. Becker, B: Chemical composition of human aqueous humor. Effects of acetazolamide. Arch Ophthal 57:793, 1957.
80. De Berardinis, E, Tieri, O, Polzella, A, Iuglio, N: The chemical composition of the human aqueous humour in normal and pathological conditions. Exp Eye Res 4:179, 1965.
81. Kinsey, VE, Reddy, DVN: Chemistry and dynamics of aqueous humor. In: The Rabbit in Eye Research, Prince, JH, ed. Charles C Thomas, Springfield, Ill., 1964, p. 218.
82. Reiss, GR, Werness, PG, Zollman, PE, Brubaker, RF: Ascorbic acid levels in the aqueous humor of nocturnal and diurnal mammals. Arch Ophthal 104:753, 1986.
83. Freddo, TF, Bartels, SP, Barsotti, MF, Kamm, RD: The source of proteins in the aqueous humor of the normal rabbit. Invest Ophthal Vis Sci 31:125, 1990.
84. Pavao, AF, Lee, DA, Ethier, CR, et al: Two-dimensional gel electrophoresis of calf aqueous humor, serum, and filter-bound proteins. Invest Ophthal Vis Sci 30:731, 1989.
85. Ethier, CR, Kamm, RD, Johnson, M, et al: Further studies on the flow of aqueous humor through microporous filters. Invest Ophthal Vis Sci 30:739, 1989.
86. Sen, DK, Sarin, GS, Saha, K: Immunoglobulins in human aqueous humour. Br J Ophthal 61:216, 1977.
87. Okisaka, S: Effects of paracentesis on the blood-aqueous barrier: a light and electron microscopic study on cynomolgus monkey. Invest Ophthal 15:824, 1976.
88. Bartels, SP, Pederson, JE, Gaasterland, DE, Armaly, MF: Sites of breakdown of the blood-aqueous barrier after paracentesis of the rhesus monkey eye. Invest Ophthal Vis Sci 18:1050, 1979.
89. Dickinson, JC, Durham, DG, Hamilton, PB: Ion

exchange chromatography of free amino acids in aqueous fluid and lens of the human eye. Invest Ophthal 7:551, 1968.

90. Davson, H, Luck CP: A comparative study of the total carbon dioxide in the ocular fluids, cerebrospinal fluid, and plasma of some mammalian species. J Physiol 132:454, 1956.

91. Laurent, UBG: Hyaluronate in human aqueous humor. Arch Ophthal 101:129, 1983.

92. Trope, GE, Rumley, AG: Catecholamines in human aqueous humor. Invest Ophthal Vis Sci 26:399, 1985.

93. Khodadoust, AA, Stark, WJ, Bell, WR: Coagulation properties of intraocular humors and cerebrospinal fluid. Invest Ophthal Vis Sci 24:1616, 1983.

94. Tripathi, RC, Park, JK, Tripathi, BJ, Millard, CB: Tissue plasminogen activator in human aqueous humor and its possible therapeutic significance. Am J Ophthal 106:719, 1988.

95. Vadillo-Ortega, F, Gonzalez-Avila, G, Chevez, P, et al: A latent collagenase in human aqueous humor. Invest Ophthal Vis Sci 30:332, 1989.

96. Jocson, VL, Sears, ML: Experimental aqueous perfusion in enucleated human eyes. Arch Ophthal 86:65, 1971.

97. Bill, A, Phillips, CI: Uveoscleral drainage of aqueous humour in human eyes. Exp Eye Res 12:275, 1971.

98. Pederson, JE, Gaasterland, DE, MacLellan, HM: Uveoscleral aqueous outflow in the rhesus monkey: importance of uveal reabsorption. Invest Ophthal Vis Sci 16:1008, 1977.

99. Inomata, H, Bill, A: Exit sites of uveoscleral flow of aqueous humor in cynomolgus monkey eyes. Exp Eye Res 25:113, 1977.

100. Sherman, SH, Green, K, Laties, AM: The fate of anterior chamber fluorescein in the monkey eye. I. The anterior chamber outflow pathways. Exp Eye Res 27:159, 1978.

101. Inomata, H, Bill, A, Smelser, GK: Unconventional routes of aqueous humor outflow in cynomolgus monkey (*Macaca irus*). Am J Ophthal 73:893, 1972.

102. McMaster, PRB, Macri, FJ: Secondary aqueous humor outflow pathways in the rabbit, cat, and monkey. Arch Ophthal 79:297, 1968.

103. Moses, RA, Grodzki, WF Jr: The scleral spur and scleral roll. Invest Ophthal Vis Sci 16:925, 1977.

104. Moses, RA, Grodzki, WJ Jr, Starcher, BC, Galione, MJ: Elastin content of the scleral spur, trabecular mesh, and sclera. Invest Ophthal Vis Sci 17:817, 1978.

105. Spencer, WH, Alvarado, J, Hayes, TL: Scanning electron microscopy of human ocular tissues: trabecular meshwork. Invest Ophthal 7:651, 1968.

106. Raviola, G: Schwalbe line's cells: a new cell type in the trabecular meshwork of *Macaca mulatta*. Invest Ophthal Vis Sci 22:45, 1982.

107. Flocks, M: The anatomy of the trabecular meshwork as seen in tangential section. Arch Ophthal 56:708, 1957.

108. Fine, BS: Observations on the drainage angle in man and rhesus monkey: a concept of the pathogenesis of chronic simple glaucoma. A light and electron microscopic study. Invest Ophthal 3:609, 1964.

109. Hoffmann, F, Dumitrescu, L: Schlemm's canal under the scanning electron microscope. Ophthal Res 2:37, 1971.

110. Rohen, JW, Rentsch, FJ: Morphology of Schlemm's canal and related vessels in the human eye. Graefe's Arch Ophthal 176:309, 1968.

111. Ascher, KW: The Aqueous Veins. Biomicroscopic Study of the Aqueous Humor Elimination. Charles C Thomas, Springfield, Ill., 1961.

112. Last, RJ: Wolff's Anatomy of the Eye and Orbit, 5th ed. WB Saunders, Philadelphia, 1961, p. 49.

113. Rohen, JW, Rentsch, FJ: Electronmicroscopic studies on the structure of the outer wall of Schlemm's canal, its outflow channels and age changes. Graefe's Arch Ophthal 177:1, 1969.

114. Jocson, VL, Sears, ML: Channels of aqueous outflow and related blood vessels. I. *Macaca mulatta* (rhesus). Arch Ophthal 80:104, 1968.

115. Jocson, VL, Sears, ML: Channels of aqueous outflow and related blood vessels. II. *Cercopithecus ethiops* (Ethiopian green or green vervet). Arch Ophthal 81:244, 1969.

116. Jocson, VL, Grant, WM: Interconnections of blood vessels and aqueous vessels in human eyes. Arch Ophthal 73:707, 1965.

117. Gaasterland, DE, Jocson, VL, Sears, ML: Channels of aqueous outflow and related blood vessels. III. Episcleral arteriovenous anatomoses in the rhesus monkey eye (*Macaca mulatta*). Arch Ophthal 84:770, 1970.

118. Raviola, G: Conjunctival and episcleral blood vessels are permeable to blood-borne horseradish peroxidase. Invest Ophthal Vis Sci 24:725, 1983.

119. Ashton, N: The exit pathway of the aqueous. Trans Ophthal Soc UK 80:397, 1960.

120. Murphy, CG, Yun, AJ, Newsome, DA, Alvarado, JA: Localization of extracellular proteins of the human trabecular meshwork by indirect immunofluorescence. Am J Ophthal 104:33, 1987.

121. Gong, H, Trinkaus-Randall, V, Freddo, TF: Ultrastructural immunocytochemical localization of elastin in normal human trabecular meshwork. Curr Eye Res 8:1071, 1989.

122. Fine, BS: Structure of the trabecular meshwork and the canal of Schlemm. Trans Am Acad Ophthal Otol 70:777, 1966.

123. Yi, Y, Li, Y: Histochemical and electron microscopic studies of the trabecular meshwork in normal human eyes. Eye Sci 1:9, 1985.

124. Raviola, G, Raviola, E: Paracellular route of aqueous outflow in the trabecular meshwork and

canal of Schlemm. A freeze-fracture study of the endothelial junctions in the sclerocorneal angle of the macaque monkey eye. Invest Ophthal Vis Sci 21:52, 1981.

125. Grierson, I, Rahi, AHS: Microfilaments in the cells of the human trabecular meshwork. Br J Ophthal 63:3, 1979.

126. Gipson, IK, Anderson, RA: Actin filaments in cells of human trabecular meshwork and Schlemm's canal. Invest Ophthal Vis Sci 18:547, 1979.

127. Ryder, MI, Weinreb, RN, Alvarado, J, Polansky, JR: The cytoskeleton of the cultured human trabecular cell. Characterization and drug response. Invest Ophthal Vis Sci 29:251, 1988.

128. Weinreb, RN, Ryder, MI, Polansky, JR: The cytoskeleton of the cynomolgus monkey trabecular cell. Invest Ophthal Vis Sci 27:1312, 1986.

129. Grierson, I, Miller, L, Yong, JD, et al: Investigations of cytoskeletal elements in cultured bovine meshwork cells. Invest Ophthal Vis Sci 27:1318, 1986.

130. Iwamoto, Y, Tamura, M: Immunocytochemical study of intermediate filaments in cultured human trabecular cells. Invest Ophthal Vis Sci 29:244, 1988.

131. Knepper, PA, Collins, JA, Weinstein, HG, Breen, M: Aqueous outflow pathway complex carbohydrate synthesis in vitro. Invest Ophthal Vis Sci 24:1546, 1983.

132. Ohnishi, Y, Taniguchi, Y: Distributions of ^{35}S-sulfate and ^{3}H-glucosamine in the angular region of the hamster: light and electron microscopic autoradiography. Invest Ophthal Vis Sci 24:697, 1983.

133. Richardson, TM: Distribution of glycosaminoglycans in the aqueous outflow system of the cat. Invest Ophthal Vis Sci 22:319, 1982.

134. Rohen, JW, Schachtschabel, DO, Berghoff, K: Histoautoradiographic and biochemical studies on human and monkey trabecular meshwork and ciliary body in short-term explant culture. Graefe's Arch Ophthal 221:199, 1984.

135. Schachtschabel, DO, Berghoff, K, Rohen, JW: Synthesis and composition of glycosaminoglycans by explant cultures of human ciliary body and ciliary processes in serum-containing and serum-free defined media. Graefe's Arch Ophthal 221:207, 1984.

136. Polansky, JR, Wood, IS, Maglio, MT, Alvarado, JA: Trabecular meshwork cell culture in glaucoma research: evaluation of biological activity and structural properties of human trabecular cells in vitro. Ophthalmology 91:580, 1984.

137. Acott, TS, Westcott, M, Passo, MS, Van Buskirk, EM: Trabecular meshwork glycosaminoglycans in human and cynomolgus monkey eye. Invest Ophthal Vis Sci 26:1320, 1985.

138. Yue, BYJT, Elvart, JL: Biosynthesis of glycosaminoglycans by trabecular meshwork cells in vitro. Curr Eye Res 6:959, 1987.

139. Berggren, L, Vrabec, F: Demonstration of a coating substance in the trabecular meshwork of the eye and its decrease after perfusion experiments with different kinds of hyaluronidase. Am J Ophthal 44:200, 1957.

140. Armaly, MF, Wang, Y: Demonstration of acid mucopolysaccharides in the trabecular meshwork of the rhesus monkey. Invest Ophthal 14:507, 1975.

141. Grierson, I, Lee, WR: Acid mucopolysaccharides in the outflow apparatus. Exp Eye Res 21:417, 1975.

142. Mizokami, K: Demonstration of masked acidic glycosaminoglycans in the normal human trabecular meshwork. Jap J Ophthal 21:57, 1977.

143. Worthen, DM, Cleveland, PH: Fibronectin production by cultured human trabecular meshwork cells. Invest Ophthal Vis Sci 23:797, 1985.

144. Floyd, BB, Cleveland, PH, Worthen, DM: Fibronectin in human trabecular drainage channels. Invest Ophthal Vis Sci 26:797, 1985.

145. Hernandez, MR, Weinstein, BI, Schwartz, J, et al: Human trabecular meshwork cells in culture: morphology and extracellular matrix components. Invest Ophthal Vis Sci 28:1655, 1987.

146. Lynch, MG, Peeler, JS, Brown, RH, Niederkorn, JY: Expression of HLA class I and II antigens on cells of the human trabecular meshwork. Ophthalmology 94:851, 1987.

147. Latina, M, Flotte, T, Crean, E, et al: Immunohistochemical staining of the human anterior segment. 106:95, 1988.

148. Stone, RA, Kuwayama, Y, Laties, AM, Marangos, PJ: Neuron-specific enolase-containing cells in the rhesus monkey trabecular meshwork. Invest Ophthal Vis Sci 25:1332, 1984.

149. Grierson, I, Chisholm, IA: Clearance of debris from the iris through the drainage angle of the rabbit's eye. Br J Ophthal 62:694, 1978.

150. Grierson, I, Day, J, Unger, WG, Ahmed, A: Phagocytosis of latex microspheres by bovine meshwork cells in culture. Graefe's Arch Ophthal 224:536, 1986.

151. Barak, MH, Weinreb, RN, Ryder, MI: Quantitative assessment of cynomolgus monkey trabecular cell phagocytosis and absorption. Curr Eye Res 7:445, 1988.

152. Shirato, S, Murphy, CG, Bloom, E, et al: Kinetics of phagocytosis in trabecular meshwork cells. Flow cytometry and morphometry. Invest Ophthal Vis Sci 30:2499, 1989.

153. Johnson, DH, Richardson, TM, Epstein, DL: Trabecular meshwork recovery after phagocytic challenge. Curr Eye Res 8:1121, 1989.

154. Grierson, I, Lee, WR: Erythrocyte phagocytosis in the human trabecular meshwork. Br J Ophthal 57:400, 1973.

155. Johnson, DH: Does pigmentation affect the trabecular meshwork? Arch Ophthal 107:250, 1989.
156. Speakman, JS: Drainage channels in the trabecular wall of Schlemm's canal. Br J Ophthal 44:513, 1960.
157. Feeney, L, Wissig, S: Outflow studies using an electron dense tracer. Trans Am Acad Ophthal Otol 70:791, 1966.
158. Diaz, G, Orzalesi, N, Fossarello, M, et al: Coated pits and coated vesicles in the endothelial cells of trabecular meshwork. Exp Eye Res 35:99, 1982.
159. Diaz, G, Carta, S, Orzalesi, N: Nonrandom distribution of coated pits and vesicles in the connective tissue cells of the trabecular meshwork of rabbit. Graefe's Arch Ophthal 224:147, 1986.
160. Anderson, DR: Scanning electron microscopy of primate trabecular meshwork. Am J Ophthal 71:90, 1971.
161. Johnstone, MA: Pressure-dependent changes in configuration of the endothelial tubules of Schlemm's canal. Am J Ophthal 78:630, 1974.
162. Svedbergh, B: Protrusions of the inner wall of Schlemm's canal. Am J Ophthal 82:875, 1976.
163. Johnstone, MA: Pressure-dependent changes in nuclei and the process origins of the endothelial cells lining Schlemm's canal. Invest Ophthal Vis Sci 18:44, 1979.
164. Segawa, K: Electron microscopic observations on the replicas of Schlemm's canal. Acta Soc Ophthal Jap 73:2013, 1969.
165. Segawa, K: Scanning electron microscopic studies on the iridocorneal angle tissue in normal human eyes. Acta Soc Ophthal Jap 76:659, 1972.
166. Holmberg, A: The fine structure of the inner wall of Schlemm's canal. Arch Ophthal 62:956, 1959.
167. Holmberg, A: Schlemm's canal and the trabecular meshwork. An electron microscopic study of the normal structure in man and monkey (*Cercopithecus ethiops*). Doc Ophthal 19:339, 1965.
168. Inomata, H, Bill, A, Smelse, GK: Aqueous humor pathways through the trabecular meshwork and into Schlemm's canal in the cynomolgus monkey (*Macaca irus*). Am J Ophthal 73:760, 1972.
169. Segawa, K: Pores of the trabecular wall of Schlemm's canal. Ferritin perfusion in enucleated human eyes. Acta Soc Ophthal Jap 74:1240, 1970.
170. Segawa, K: Pore structures of the endothelial cells of the aqueous outflow pathway: scanning electron microscopy. Jap J Ophthal 17:133, 1973.
171. Shabo, AL, Reese, TS, Gaasterland, D: Postmortem formation of giant endothelial vacuoles in Schlemm's canal of the monkey. Am J Ophthal 76:896, 1973.
172. Tripathi, RC: Ultrastructure of the trabecular wall of Schlemm's canal in relation to aqueous outflow. Exp Eye Res 7:335, 1968.
173. Tripathi, RC: Mechanism of the aqueous outflow across the trabecular wall of Schlemm's canal. Exp Eye Res 11:116, 1971.
174. Tripathi, RC: Ultrastructure of the exit pathway of the aqueous in lower mammals (a preliminary report on the "angular aqueous plexus"). Exp Eye Res 12:311, 1971.
175. Tripathi, RC: Aqueous outflow pathway in normal and glaucomatous eyes. Br J Ophthal 56:157, 1972.
176. Sondermann, R: Beitrag zur entwicklung und morphologie des Schlemmschen kanals. Graefe's Arch Ophthal 124:521, 1930.
177. Ashton, N, Brini, A, Smith, R: Anatomical studies of the trabecular meshwork of the normal human eye. Br J Ophthal 40:257, 1956.
178. Iwamoto, T: Further observation on Sondermann's channels of the human trabecular meshwork. Graefe's Arch Ophthal 172:213, 1967.
179. Lutjen-Drecoll, E, Rohen, JW: Uber die endotheliale auskleidung des Schlemmschen kanals im silberimpragnationsbild. Graefe's Arch Ophthal 180:249, 1970.
180. de Kater, AW, Spurr-Michaud, SJ, Gipson, IK: Localization of smooth muscle myosin-containing cells in the aqueous outflow pathway. Invest Ophthal Vis Sci 31:347, 1990.
181. McMenamin, PG, Lee, WR, Aitken, DAN: Age-related changes in the human outflow apparatus. Ophthalmology 93:194, 1986.
182. Miyazaki, M, Segawa, K, Urakawa, Y: Age-related changes in the trabecular meshwork of the normal human eye. Jap J Ophthal 31:558, 1987.
183. Alvarado, J, Murphy, C, Polansky, J, Juster, R: Age-related changes in trabecular meshwork cellularity. Invest Ophthal Vis Sci 21:714, 1987.
184. Ainsworth, JR, Lee, WR: Effects of age and rapid high-pressure fixation on the morphology of Schlemm's canal. Invest Ophthal Vis Sci 31:745, 1990.
185. Emi, K, Pederson, JE, Toris, CB: Hydrostatic pressure of the suprachoroidal space. Invest Ophthal Vis Sci 30:233, 1989.
186. Raviola, G, Butler, JM: Unidirectional transport mechanism of horseradish peroxidase in the vessels of the iris. Invest Ophthal Vis Sci 25:827, 1984.
187. Butler, JM, Raviola, G, Beers GJ, Carter AP: Computed tomography of aqueous humor outflow pathways. Exp Eye Res 39:709, 1984.
188. Grant, WM: Further studies on facility of flow through the trabecular meshwork. Arch Ophthal 60:523, 1958.
189. Grant, WM: Experimental aqueous perfusion in enucleated human eyes. Arch Ophthal 69:783, 1963.
190. Tripathi, RC, Tripathi, BJ: The mechanism of aqueous outflow in lower mammals. Exp Eye Res 14:73, 1972.
191. Tarkkanen, A, Niemi, M: Enzyme histochemis-

try of the angle of the anterior chamber of the human eye. Acta Ophthal 45:93, 1987.
192. Vegge, T: Ultrastructure of normal human trabecular endothelium. Acta Ophthal 41:193, 1963.
193. Johnstone, MA, Grant, WM: Pressure-dependent changes in structure of the aqueous outflow system of human and monkey eyes. Am J Ophthal 75:365, 1973.
194. Grierson, I, Lee, WR: Changes in the monkey outflow apparatus at graded levels of intraocular pressure: a qualitative analysis by light microscopy and scanning electron microscopy. Exp Eye Res 19:21, 1974.
195. Grierson, I, Lee, WR: Pressure-induced changes in the ultrastructure of the endothelium lining Schlemm's canal. Am J Ophthal 80:863, 1975.
196. Kayes, J: Pressure gradient changes on the trabecular meshwork of monkeys. Am J Ophthal 79:549, 1975.
197. Van Buskirk, EM, Grant, WM: Influence of temperature and the question of involvement of cellular metabolism in aqueous outflow. Am J Ophthal 77:565, 1974.
198. Bill, A, Svedbergh, B: Scanning electron microscopic studies of the trabecular meshwork and the canal of Schlemm—an attempt to localize the main resistance to outflow of aqueous humor in man. Acta Ophthal 50:295, 1972.
199. Moseley, H, Grierson, J, Lee, W: Mathematical modeling of aqueous humor outflow from the eye through the pores in the lining endothelium of Schlemm's canal. Clin Phys Physiol Meas 4:47, 1983.
200. Seiler, T, Wollensak, J: The resistance of the trabecular meshwork to aqueous humor outflow. Graefe's Arch Ophthal 223:88, 1985.
201. Ethier, CR, Kamm, RD, Palaszewski, BA, et al: Calculations of flow resistance in the juxtacanalicular meshwork. Invest Ophthalmol Vis Sci 27:1741, 1986.
202. Johnson, M, Ethier, CR, Kamm, RD, et al: The flow of aqueous humor through micro-porous filters. Invest Ophthal Vis Sci 27:92, 1986.
203. Francois, J: The importance of the mucopolysaccharides in intraocular pressure regulation. Invest Ophthal 14:173, 1975.
204. Hayasaka, S, Sears, ML: Distribution of acid phosphatase, beta-glucuronidase, and lysosomal hyaluronidase in the anterior segment of the rabbit eye. Invest Ophthal Vis Sci 17:982, 1978.
205. Grierson, I, Lee, WR, Abraham, S: A light microscopic study of the effects of testicular hyaluronidase on the outflow system of a baboon (*Papio cynocephalus*). Invest Ophthal Vis Sci 18:356, 1979.
206. Knepper, PA, Farbman, AI, Telser, AG: Exogenous hyaluronidase and degradation of hyaluronic acid in the rabbit eye. Invest Ophthal Vis Sci 25:286, 1984.
207. Van Buskirk, EM, Brett, J: The canine eye: in vitro dissolution of the barriers to aqueous outflow. Invest Ophthal Vis Sci 17:258, 1978.
208. Van Buskirk, EM, Brett, J: The canine eye: in vitro studies of the intraocular pressure and facility of aqueous outflow. Invest Ophthal Vis Sci 17:373, 1978.
209. Kaufman, PL, Erickson, KA, Bárány, EH: Effect of repeated anterior chamber perfusion on intraocular pressure and total outflow facility in the cynomolgus monkey. Invest Ophthal Vis Sci 24:159, 1983.
210. Morrison, JC, Van Buskirk, EM: The canine eye: pectinate ligaments and aqueous outflow resistance. Invest Ophthal Vis Sci 23:726, 1982.
211. Peterson, WS, Jocson, VL: Hyaluronidase effects of aqueous outflow resistance. Quantitative and localizing studies in the rhesus monkey eye. Am J Ophthal 77:573, 1974.
212. Hernandez, MR, Wenk, EJ, Weinstein, BI, et al: Glucocorticoid target cells in human outflow pathway: autopsy and surgical specimens. Invest Ophthal Vis Sci 24:1612, 1983.
213. Weinreb, RN, Bloom, E, Baxter, JD, et al: Detection of glucocorticoid receptors in cultured human trabecular cells. Invest Ophthal Vis Sci 21:403, 1981.
214. Hernandez, MR, Weinstein, BI, Wenk, EJ, et al: The effect of dexamethasone on the in vitro incorporation of precursors of extracellular matrix components in the outflow pathway region of the rabbit eye. Invest Ophthal Vis Sci 24:704, 1983.
215. Weinreb, RN, Mitchell, MD, Polansky, JR: Prostaglandin production by human trabecular cells: in vitro inhibition by dexamethasone. Invest Ophthal Vis Sci 24:1541, 1983.
216. Weinreb, RN, Polansky, JR, Alvarado, JA, Mitchell, MD: Arachidonic acid metabolism in human trabecular meshwork. Invest Ophthal Vis Sci 29:1708, 1988.
217. Bito, LZ, Draga, A, Blanco, J, Camras, CB: Long-term maintenance of reduced intraocular pressure by daily or twice daily topical application of prostaglandins to cat or rhesus monkey eyes. Invest Ophthal Vis Sci 24:312, 1983.
218. Kaufman, PL, Bárány, EH: Cytochalasin B reversibly increases outflow facility in the eye of the cynomolgus monkey. Invest Ophthal Vis Sci 16:47, 1977.
219. Svedbergh, B, Lutjen-Drecoll, E, Ober, M, Kaufman, PL: Cytochalasin B-induced structural changes in the anterior ocular segment of the cynomologus monkey. Invest Ophthal Vis Sci 17:718, 1978.
220. Johnstone, M, Tanner, D, Chau, B, Kopecky, K: Concentration-dependent morphologic effects of cytochalasin B in the aqueous outflow system. Invest Ophthal Vis Sci 19:835, 1980.
221. Kaufman, PL, Erickson, KA: Cytochalasin B and

D dose-outflow facility response relationships in the cynomolgus monkey. Invest Ophthal Vis Sci 23:646, 1982.

222. Kaufman, PL, Svedbergh, B, Lutjen-Drecoll, E: Medical trabeculocanalotomy in monkeys with cytochalasin B or EDTA. Ann Ophthal 11:795, 1979.
223. Bill, A, Lutjen-Drecoll, E, Svedbergh, B: Effects of intracameral Na_2EDTA and EGTA on aqueous outflow routes in the monkey eye. Invest Ophthal Vis Sci 19:492, 1980.
224. Barany, EH: In vitro studies of the resistance to flow through the angle of the anterior chamber. Acta Soc Med Uppsal 59:260, 1954.
225. Epstein, DL, Hashimoto, JM, Anderson, PJ, Grant, WM: Effect of iodoacetamide perfusion on outflow facility and metabolism of the trabecular meshwork. Invest Ophthal Vis Sci 20:625, 1981.
226. Epstein, DL, Patterson, MM, Rivers, SC, Anderson, PJ: N-ethylmaleimide increases the facility of aqueous outflow of excised monkey and calf eyes. Invest Ophthal Vis Sci 22:752, 1982.
227. Lindenmayer, JM, Kahn, MG, Hertzmark, E, Epstein, DL: Morphology and function of the aqueous outflow system in monkey eyes perfused with sulfhydryl reagents. Invest Ophthal Vis Sci 24:710, 1983.
228. Freddo, TF, Patterson, MM, Scott, DR, Epstein, DL: Influence of mercurial sulfhydryl agents on aqueous outflow pathways in enucleated eyes. Invest Ophthal Vis Sci 25:278, 1984.
229. Kahn, MG, Giblin, FJ, Epstein, DL: Glutathione in calf trabecular meshwork and its relation to aqueous humor outflow facility. Invest Ophthal Vis Sci 24:1283, 1983.
230. Scott, DR, Karageuzian, LN, Anderson, PJ, Epstein, DL: Glutathione peroxidase of calf trabecular meshwork. Invest Ophthal Vis Sci 25:599, 1984.
231. Nguyen, KPV, Chung, ML, Anderson, PJ, et al: Hydrogen peroxide removal by the calf aqueous outflow pathway. Invest Ophthal Vis Sci 29:976, 1988.
232. Pandolfi, M, Kwaan, HC: Fibrinolysis in the anterior segment of the eye. Arch Ophthal 77:99, 1967.
233. Pandolfi, M: Coagulation Factor VIII localization in the aqueous outflow pathways. Arch Ophthal 94:656, 1976.
234. Tripathi, BJ, Geanon, JD, Tripathi, RC: Distribution of tissue plasminogen activator in human and monkey eyes. Ophthalmology 94:1434, 1987.
235. Park, JK, Tripathi, RC, Tripathi, BJ, Barlow, GH: Tissue plasminogen activator in the trabecular endothelium. Invest Ophthal Vis Sci 28:1341, 1987.
236. Shuman, MA, Polansky, JR, Merkel, C, Alvarado, JA: Tissue plasminogen activator in cultured human trabecular meshwork cells. Predominance of enzyme over plasminogen activator inhibitor. Invest Ophthal Vis Sci 29:401, 1988.
237. Van Buskirk, EM, Grant, WM: Lens depression and aqueous outflow in enucleated primate eyes. Am J Ophthal 76:632, 1973.
238. Van Buskirk, EM: Trabeculotomy in the immature, enucleated human eye. Invest Ophthal Vis Sci 16:63, 1977.
239. Moses, RA, Hoover, GS, Oostwouder, PH: Blood reflux in Schlemm's canal. I. Normal findings. Arch Ophthal 97:1307, 1979.
240. Ellingsen, BA, Grant, WM: The relationship of pressure and aqueous outflow in enucleated human eyes. Invest Ophthal 10:430, 1971.
241. Ellingsen, BA, Grant, WM: Influence of intraocular pressure and trabeculotomy on aqueous outflow in enucleated monkey eyes. Invest Ophthal 10:705, 1971.
242. Brubaker, RF: The effect of intraocular pressure on conventional outflow resistance in the enucleated human eye. Invest Ophthal 14:286, 1975.
243. Grierson, I, Lee, WR: The fine structure of the trabecular meshwork at graded levels of intraocular pressure. (1) Pressure effects within the near-physiological range (8–30 mm Hg). Exp Eye Res 20:505, 1975.
244. Grierson, I, Lee, WR: The fine structure of the trabecular meshwork at graded levels of intraocular pressure. (2) Pressure outside the physiological range (0 and 50 mm Hg). Exp Eye Res 20:523, 1975.
245. Ellingsen, BA, Grant, WM: Trabeculotomy and sinusotomy in enucleated human eyes. Invest Ophthal 11:21, 1972.
246. Moses, RA: The conventional outflow resistances. Am J Ophthal 92:804, 1981.
247. Hashimoto, JM, Epstein, DL: Influence of intraocular pressure on aqueous outflow facility in enucleated eyes of different mammals. Invest Ophthal Vis Sci 19:1483, 1980.
248. Moses, RA, Arnzen, RJ: The trabecular mesh: a mathematical analysis. Invest Ophthal Vis Sci 19:1490, 1980.
249. Van Buskirk, EM: Changes in the facility of aqueous outflow induced by lens depression and intraocular pressure in excised human eyes. Am J Ophthal 82:736, 1976.
250. Moses, RA, Etheridge, EL, Grodzki, WJ Jr: The effect of lens depression on the components of outflow resistance. Invest Ophthal Vis Sci 22:37, 1982.
251. Van Buskirk, EM: Anatomic correlates of changing aqueous outflow facility in excised human eyes. Invest Ophthal Vis Sci 22:625, 1982.
252. Rosenquist, RC Jr, Melamed, S, Epstein, DL: Anterior and posterior axial lens displacement and human aqueous outflow facility. Invest Ophthal Vis Sci 29:1159, 1988.
253. Moses, RA, Grodzki, WJ Jr: Choroid tension and

facility of aqueous outflow. Invest Ophthal Vis Sci 16:1062, 1977.

254. Rosenquist, R, Epstein, D, Melamed, S, et al: Outflow resistance of enucleated human eyes at two different perfusion pressures and different extents of trabeculotomy. Curr Eye Res 8:1233, 1989.

255. Peterson, WS, Jocson, VL, Sears, ML: Resistance to aqueous outflow in the rhesus monkey eye. Am J Ophthal 72:445, 1971.

256. Kollarits, CR, Gaasterland, D, Di Chiro, G, et al: Management of a patient with orbital varices, visual loss, and ipsilateral glaucoma. Ophthal Surg 8:54, 1977.

257. Brubaker, RF: Determination of episcleral venous pressure in the eye. A comparison of three methods. Arch Ophthal 77:110, 1967.

258. Podos, SM, Minas, TF, Macri, FJ: A new instrument to measure episcleral venous pressure. Comparison of normal eyes and eyes with primary open-angle glaucoma. Arch Ophthal 80:209, 1968.

259. Krakau, CET, Widakowich, J, Wilke, K: Measurements of the episcleral venous pressure by means of an air jet. Acta Ophthal 51:185, 1973.

260. Phelps, CD, Armaly, MF: Measurement of episcleral venous pressure. Am J Ophthal 85:35, 1978.

261. Zeimer, RC, Gieser, DK, Wilensky, JT, et al: A practical venomanometer. Measurement of episcleral venous pressure and assessment of the normal range. Arch Ophthal 101:1447, 1983.

262. Gaasterland, DE, Pederson, JE: Episcleral venous pressure: a comparison of invasive and noninvasive measurements. Invest Ophthal Vis Sci 24:1417, 1983.

Chapter 3

AQUEOUS HUMOR DYNAMICS II. TECHNIQUES FOR EVALUATING

EVALUATION OF AQUEOUS PRODUCTION

Cycloscopy

This technique allows direct visualization of ciliary processes under special circumstances, such as the presence of an iridectomy, wide iris retraction, aniridia, and some cases of aphakia (Fig. 3.1). Although special contact prisms with scleral indentors have been developed for cycloscopy,[1,2] the procedure is still limited by the small percentage of eyes in which circumstances are favorable for good visualization of the ciliary processes. The main value of the technique thus far has been in research studies of the ciliary processes[1,2] and in conjunction with laser therapy to the ciliary processes (transpupillary cyclophotocoagulation), which is discussed in Section Three.

Measuring the Rate of Aqueous Production

Fluorophotometry

Fluorescein techniques involve instillation of fluorescein into the anterior chamber by iontophoresis, with subsequent measurement of either (1) the flow of unstained aqueous from the posterior to anterior chamber using photogrammetric methods[3] or (2) the change in concentration of fluorescein in the anterior chamber by fluorophotometry.[4–9] Of these two approaches, fluorophotometry has become the most commonly used and is currently the standard research technique by which the rate of aqueous humor flow is calculated in normal human subjects and glaucoma patients under various circumstances, including the response to glaucoma drugs.[9]

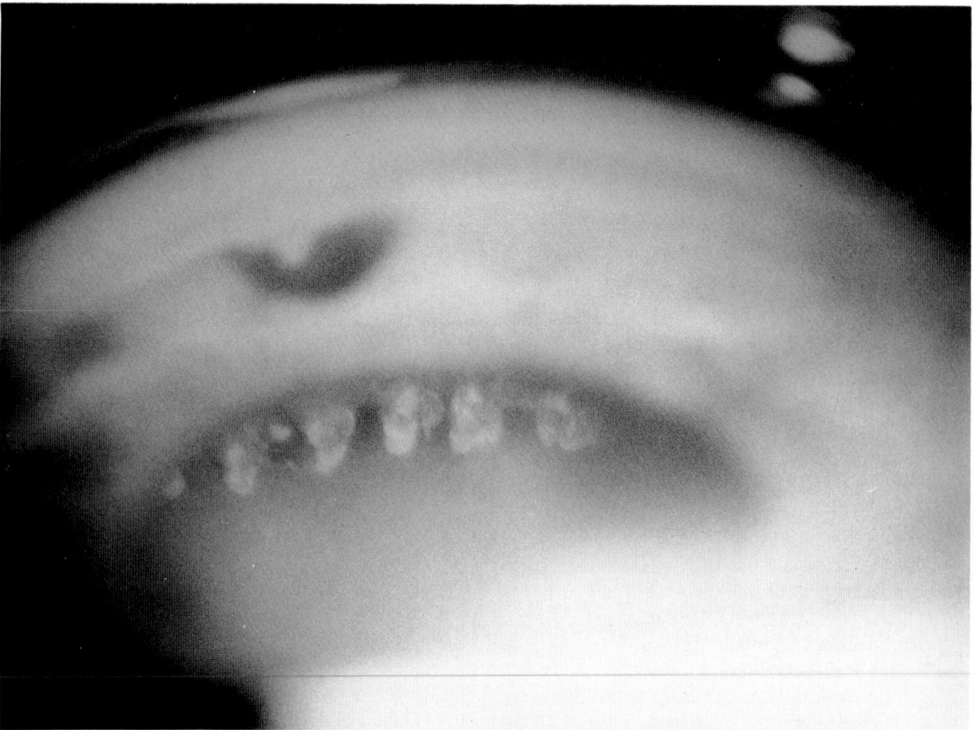

Figure 3.1. Transpupillary view of ciliary processes as seen by cycloscopy in eye with neovascular glaucoma in which fibrovascular membrane has caused dilation and anterior displacement of iris.

Other Techniques for Calculating Inflow

Radioactive-labeled isotopes have been used to measure inflow in animals by observing either (1) the accumulation of the isotope in the anterior chamber[10] or (2) the decay rate of the intracamerally injected isotope.[11] Perfusion of eyes at a constant pressure can also be used to determine the inflow in animals.[12]

GONIOSCOPY

Gonioscopy is a clinical technique that is used to examine structures in the anterior chamber angle. In the management of glaucoma, gonioscopic assessment is necessary to establish the type of glaucoma, which is essential in planning the appropriate therapy, since the treatment for one type of glaucoma may be ineffective or contraindicated in another form. The present discussion is limited to technique and normal anatomic findings, while the gonioscopic alterations associated with the various forms of glaucoma will be considered in Section Two.

Historical Background[13]

In 1907, Trantas visualized the angle in an eye with keratoglobus by indenting the limbus. He later coined the term *gonioscopy*. Salsmann introduced the goniolens in 1914, and Koeppe improved it 5 years later by designing a steeper lens. Troncoso also contributed to gonioscopy by developing the gonioscope for magnification and illumination of the angle. In 1938, Goldmann introduced the gonioprism, and Barkan established the use of gonioscopy in the management of glaucoma.

The Principle of Gonioscopy (Fig. 3.2)[14]

The problem is the *critical angle*. When light passes from a medium with a greater

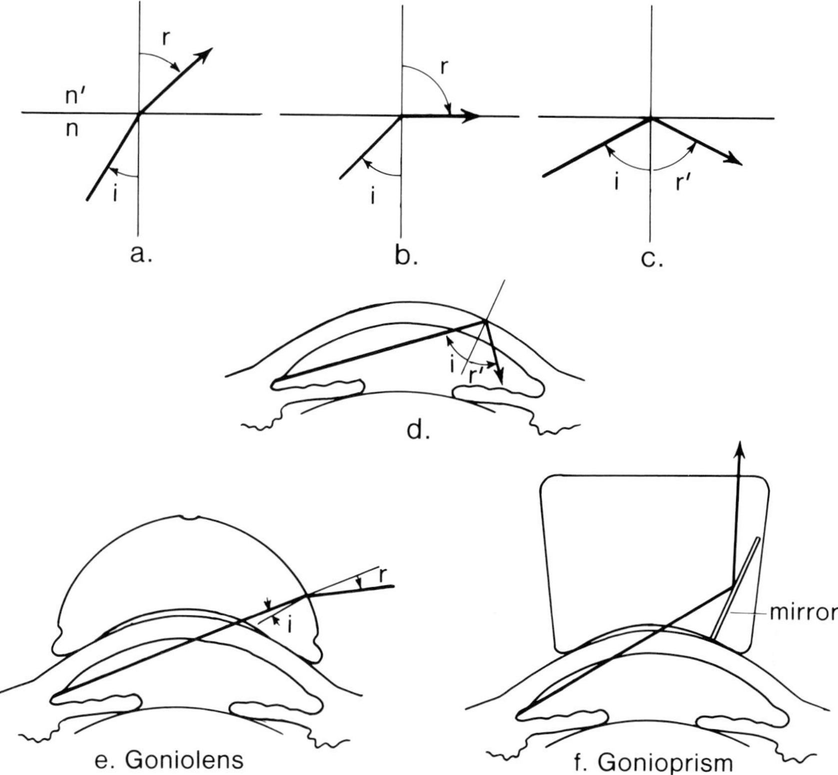

Figure 3.2. Principle of gonioscopy: **a.** Light ray is refracted when angle of incidence (*i*) at interface of two media with different indices of refraction (*n* and *n′*) is less than the critical angle. **b.** Angle of refraction (*r*) is 90° when i equals the critical angle. **c.** Light is reflected when i exceeds the critical angle. **d.** Light from anterior chamber angle exceeds the critical angle at the cornea-air interface and is reflected back into the eye. **e** and **f.** Contact lenses have an index of refraction (n) similar to that of the cornea, allowing light to enter the lens and then be refracted (*goniolens*) or reflected (*gonioprism*) beyond contact lens-air interface.

to one with a lesser index of refraction, the angle of refraction (*r*) will be larger than the angle of incidence (*i*). When *r* equals 90°, *i* is said to have attained the critical angle. When *i* exceeds the critical angle, the light is reflected back into the first medium. The critical angle for the cornea-air interface is approximately 46°. Light rays coming from the anterior chamber angle exceed this critical angle and are, therefore, reflected back into the anterior chamber, preventing visualization of the angle.

The solution to this problem is to eliminate the cornea (optically). Since the index of refraction of a contact lens approaches that of the cornea, there is minimal refraction at the interface of these two media, which eliminates the optical effect of the front corneal surface. Therefore, light rays from the anterior chamber angle enter the contact lens and are then made to pass through the new contact lens-air interface by one of two basic designs. In *direct gonioscopy,* the anterior curve of the contact lens (goniolens) is such that the critical angle is not reached, and the light rays are refracted at the contact lens-air interface. In *indirect gonioscopy,* the light rays are reflected by a mirror in the contact lens (gonioprism) and leave the lens at nearly a right angle to the contact lens-air interface. The more commonly used goniolenses and gonioprisms are listed in Table 3.1.

Table 3.1.
Contact Lenses for Gonioscopy

	Lens	Description/Use
I. Goniolenses (Direct Gonioscopy)	1. Koeppe	1. Prototype diagnostic goniolens
	2. Richardson-Shaffer	2. Small Koeppe lens for infants
	3. Layden	3. For premature infant gonioscopy
	4. Barkan	4. Prototype surgical and diagnostic lens
	5. Thorpe	5. Surgical and diagnostic lens for operating room
	6. Swan-Jacob	6. Surgical goniolens for children
II. Gonioprisms (Indirect Gonioscopy)	1. Goldmann single-mirror	1. Mirror inclined at 62° for gonioscopy
	2. Goldmann three-mirror	2. One mirror for gonioscopy; two for retina; coated front surface available for laser use
	3. Zeiss four-mirror	3. All four mirrors inclined at 64° for gonioscopy; requires holder (Unger); fluid bridge not required
	4. Posner four-mirror	4. Modified Zeiss four-mirror gonioprism with attached handle
	5. Sussman four-mirror	5. Hand-held Zeiss-type gonioprism
	6. Thorpe four-mirror	6. Four gonioscopy mirrors, included at 62°; requires fluid bridge
	7. Ritch trabeculoplasty lens	7. Four gonioscopy mirrors; two inclined at 59° and two at 62° with convex lens over two

Direct Gonioscopy

Instruments

The *Koeppe* lens is the prototype diagnostic goniolens and is available in different diameters and radii of posterior curvature (Fig. 3.3). A gonioscope, or hand biomicroscope, provides 15–20× magnification. It may be hand-held or suspended from the ceiling with a counterbalance or on an elastic belt.[15] The light source is usually a separate hand-held unit, such as the Barkan focal illuminator, although it may be attached to the gonioscope.

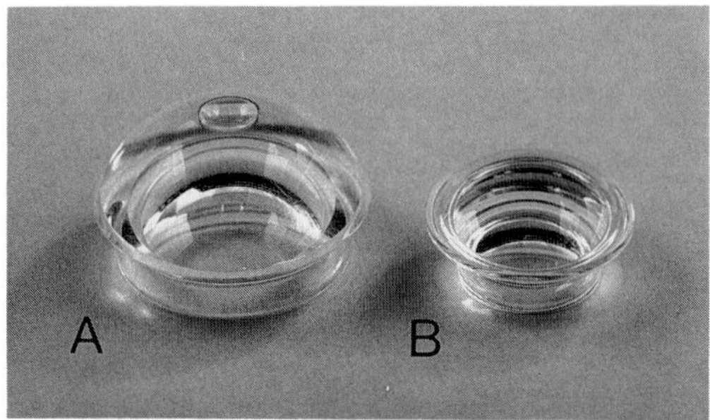

Figure 3.3. Koeppe goniolenses: **A,** Adult lens. **B,** Infant lens.

Technique

Direct gonioscopy is performed with the patient in a supine position, preferably on a movable diagnostic table. After application of a topical anesthetic, the goniolens is positioned on the cornea, using a bridge of balanced salt solution, a viscous preparation such as methylcellulose, or the patient's own tears. The examiner usually holds the gonioscope in one hand and a light source in the other (Fig. 3.4). Occasionally an assistant may be needed to move the goniolens to the desired position. Alternatively, a gonioscope with mounted light source may be used, which allows the examiner to control the goniolens with the other hand. In either case, the examiner scans the anterior chamber angle by shifting his or her position until all 360° have been studied.

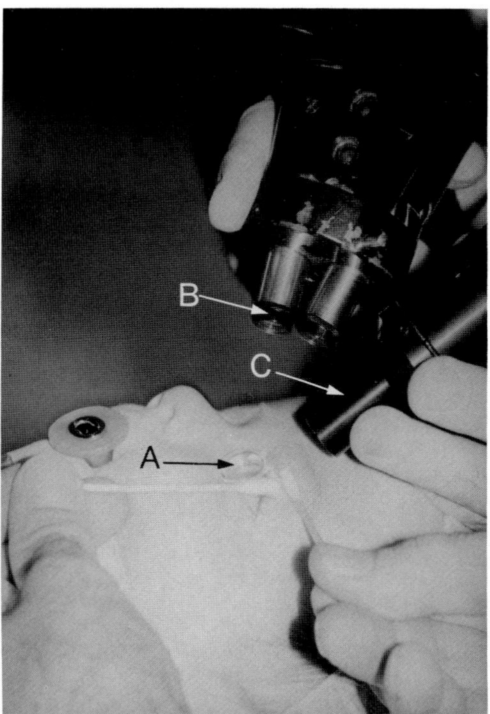

Figure 3.4. Technique of direct gonioscopy during examination of infant under anesthesia: **A,** Koeppe goniolens. **B,** Gonioscope. **C,** Focal illuminator.

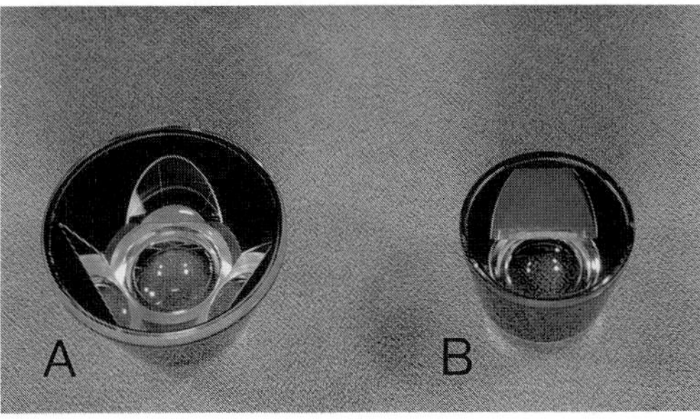

Figure 3.5. Goldmann gonioprisms: **A,** Three-mirror lens (domed mirror used for gonioscopy). **B,** Single-mirror lens.

Indirect Gonioscopy

Instruments

The gonioprism and a slit lamp are the only instruments needed for indirect gonioscopy. The *Goldmann* single-mirror lens is the prototype gonioprism (Fig. 3.5). The mirror in this lens has a height of 12 mm and a tilt of 62° from the plano front surface. The central well has a diameter of 12 mm and a posterior radius of curvature of 7.38 mm. A Goldmann three-mirror lens has two mirrors for examination of the fundus and one for the anterior chamber angle, which is tilted at 59°. The posterior radius of curvature of both standard Goldmann diagnostic gonioprisms is such that a viscous material must be used to fill the space between cornea and lens. However, a modified Goldmann-type lens has been developed with an 8.4 mm radius of curvature, which eliminates this problem.[16] Goldmann-type lenses have also been modified with antireflection coating for use with laser trabeculoplasty.

In the *Zeiss four-mirror* lens, all four mirrors are tilted at 64° for evaluation of the angle, thereby eliminating the need for rotating the lens. The original four-mirror lens is mounted on a holding fork (Unger holder), while newer models have a permanently attached holding rod (Posner lens) or are held directly (Sussman lens) (Fig. 3.6).[17] An adjustable slit lamp mount has also been developed for the Zeiss four-mirror gonioprism.[18] The posterior curvature of Zeiss lens is similar to that of the cornea, which allows the patient's own tears to be used as the fluid bridge.

The *Ritch trabeculoplasty lens* has four gonioscopy mirrors, two of which are tilted at 59° and two at 62° with a convex lens over one mirror of each set.[19] Another four-mirror lens, referred to as the *trabeculens,* has a 30-diopter convex contact lens in a hollow funnel, with four mirrors at 62° angles.[20] It can be used as a diagnostic gonioprism, as well as for laser trabeculoplasty and iridotomy. The use of gonioprisms in laser therapy is discussed further in Section Three.

With both Goldmann- and Zeiss-type instruments, the anterior chamber angle is viewed "indirectly" through a mirror 180° away. However, a gonioprism has been developed with double mirrors that allow direct viewing.[21]

Technique

The cornea is anesthetized and, with the patient positioned at the slit lamp, the gonioprism is placed against the cornea with or

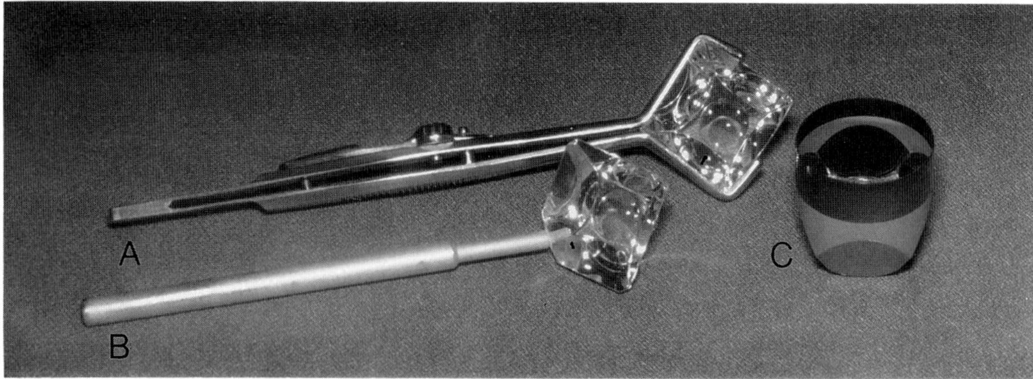

Figure 3.6. Four-mirror gonioprisms (all four mirrors for gonioscopy): **A,** Zeiss four-mirror lens with Unger holder. **B,** Posner lens. **C,** Sussman lens.

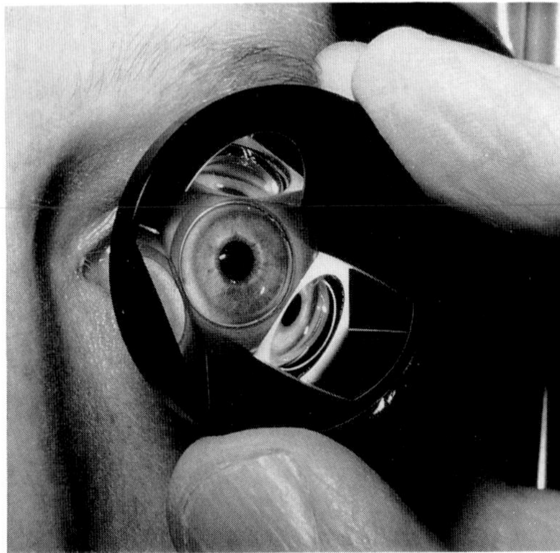

Figure 3.7. Technique of indirect gonioscopy with a Goldmann three-mirror lens.

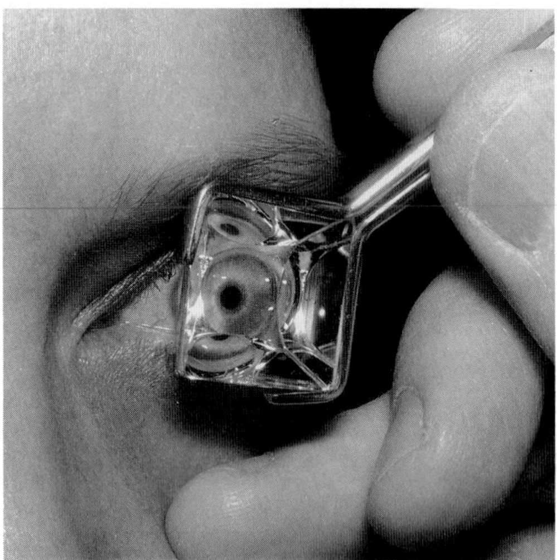

Figure 3.8. Technique of indirect gonioscopy with a Zeiss four-mirror lens.

without a fluid bridge, depending on the posterior radius of curvature of the instrument (Figs. 3.7, 3.8). The lens is then rotated to allow visualization of all 360° of the angle, or the quadrants are studied with the four mirrors. Visualization into a narrow angle can be enhanced by manipulating the gonioprism (e.g., asking the patient to look in the direction of the mirror being used), although such maneuvers must be used with caution, since they can distort the appearance of the angle depth.[22]

Comparison of Direct and Indirect Gonioscopy

There is no unanimity of opinion as to which basic method of gonioscopy is best. Advantages have been suggested for both approaches. With *direct gonioscopy,* the height of the observer may be changed to look more deeply into a narrow angle, while the gonioprism is limited in this regard by the height of the mirror. In addition, the goniolens may cause less distortion of the anterior chamber. Both features make it desirable when assessing the true depth of the anterior chamber angle.[23,24] A major advantage of direct gonioscopy, especially with the infant Koeppe lenses, is its use in sedated or anesthetized patients, as in the examination of children. These lenses are also useful in examining the fundus through a small pupil with a direct ophthalmoscope.

In *indirect gonioscopy,* the slit lamp may provide better optics and lighting, which could be an advantage when looking for subtle details in the angle.[25] Furthermore, the method requires less additional instrumentation and space (assuming the slit lamp is already a part of the routine office examination) and is probably faster than direct gonioscopy. The latter is particularly true of the Zeiss four-mirror lenses and modified Goldmann-type lenses in which a viscous bridge is not required. Gonioprisms with a posterior radius of curvature closer to that of the anterior corneal surface may also reduce corneal distortion.[22,26] In addition, gonioprisms with taller mirrors facilitate visualization of narrow angles.[22] The Zeiss four-mirror lens, because of the smaller diameter of corneal contact, also has the advantage of use in "compressive gonioscopy," which is explained in Section Two under *Angle Closure Glaucoma*.[27]

Cleaning of Diagnostic Contact Lenses

Any instrument that contacts the eye creates the potential hazard of transmitting bacterial and viral infection. This problem is considered in more detail in the next chapter with regard to tonometry, although the basic principles of instrument cleaning also apply to diagnostic contact lenses. In addition, a container has been developed that allows the diagnostic lens to stay in contact with a disinfectant solution.[28]

Gonioscopic Appearance of the Normal Anterior Chamber Angle

Starting at the root of the iris and progressing anteriorly toward the cornea, the following structures can be identified by gonioscopy in a normal open adult angle (Figs. 3.9, 3.10).

The Ciliary Body Band

This structure is the portion of ciliary body that is visible in the anterior chamber as a result of the iris insertion into the ciliary body. The width of the band depends on the level of iris insertion and tends to be wider in myopia and narrower in hyperopia. The color of the band is usually gray or dark brown.

Scleral Spur

This is the posterior lip of the scleral sulcus, which is attached to the ciliary body posteriorly and the corneoscleral meshwork anteriorly. It is usually seen as a prominent white line between the ciliary body band and functional trabecular meshwork, unless it is obscured by dense uveal meshwork or excessive pigment dispersion. Variable numbers of fine, pigmented strands may frequently be seen crossing the scleral spur from the iris root to the functional meshwork. These are referred to as *iris processes* and represent thickenings of the posterior uveal meshwork.

Functional Trabecular Meshwork

This is seen as a pigmented band just anterior to the scleral spur. Although the trabecular meshwork actually extends from the iris root to Schwalbe's line, it may be considered in two portions: (1) the anterior part, between Schwalbe's line and the anterior edge of Schlemm's canal, which is involved to a lesser degree in aqueous outflow; and (2) the posterior (or functional) part, which is the remainder of the meshwork and is the primary site of aqueous outflow (especially that portion immediately adjacent to Schlemm's canal).[29]

The appearance of the functional meshwork varies considerably depending upon the amount and distribution of pigment deposition. It has no pigment at birth, but develops color with age from faint tan to dark brown, depending on the degree of pigment dispersion in the anterior chamber. The distribution of pigment may be homogeneous for 360° in some eyes and irregular in others. In the functional portion of the meshwork, especially when lightly pigmented, blood reflux in Schlemm's canal may sometimes be seen as a red band.

Schwalbe's Line

This is the junction between the anterior chamber angle structures and the cornea. It is a fine ridge just anterior to the meshwork and is often identified by a small build-up of pigment, especially inferiorly.

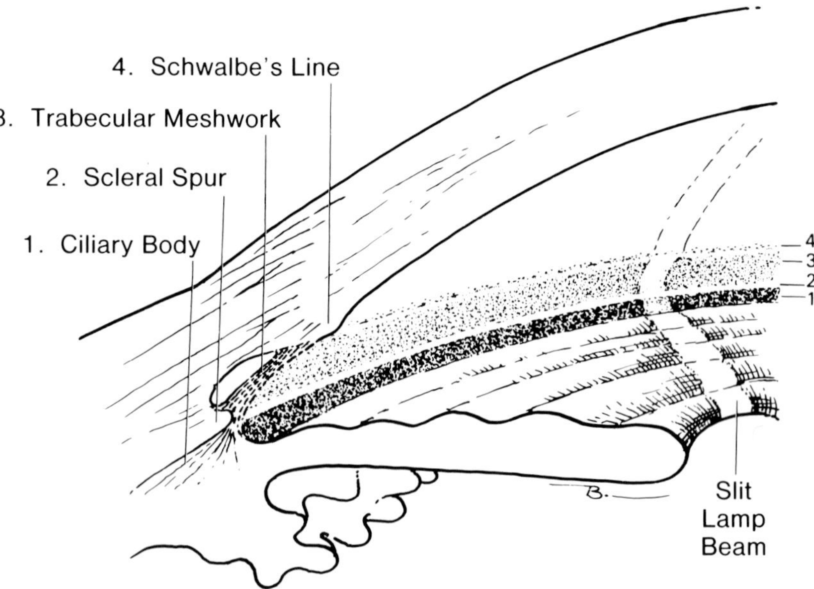

Figure 3.9. Normal adult anterior chamber angle showing gonioscopic appearance (*right*) and cross-section of corresponding structures (*left*): *1.* Ciliary body band; *2.* Scleral spur; *3.* Trabecular meshwork (degree of pigmentation varies); *4.* Schwalbe's line.

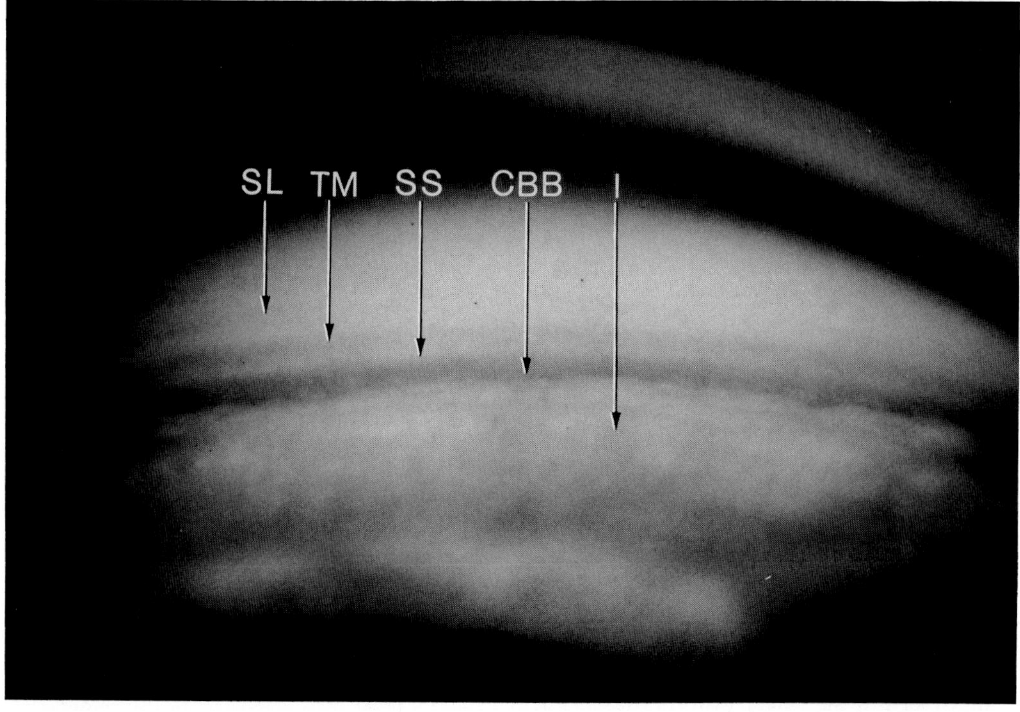

Figure 3.10. Gonioscopic view of normal anterior chamber angle, showing iris (*I*), ciliary body band (*CBB*), scleral spur (*SS*), trabecular meshwork (*TM*), and Schwalbe's line (*SL*).

Normal Blood Vessels

Blood vessels are normally not seen in the angle, although loops from the major arterial circle may appear in front of the ciliary body band and less commonly over the scleral spur and trabecular meshwork. These vessels typically take a circumferential route in the angle. In addition, an anterior ciliary artery may occasionally be seen as a more radially oriented vessel in the ciliary body band of lightly pigmented eyes. Circumferential and radial vessels may also occasionally be seen in the peripheral iris of lightly colored eyes. In a study of 100 patients with no known cause for abnormal anterior chamber angle vascularization, 16 had normal angle vessels in both eyes and 10 more had them in one eye.[30] Radial vessels were more common in the peripheral iris, while the circumferential type were more common on the ciliary body band.

Recording Gonioscopic Findings

A variety of classifications have been suggested for describing the width and appearance of the anterior chamber angle, and these will be discussed in Section Two under *Angle Closure Glaucoma*. However, descriptive words and drawings are probably the most useful technique for recording gonioscopic findings. The recorded data should include: (1) configuration of the angle; (2) depth of the angle on the basis of the most posterior structure that can be seen; (3) degree of pigmentation; and (4) presence of abnormal structures. For example, a normal angle might be recorded as "wide open, with visualization to a wide ciliary body band for 360° and moderate trabecular meshwork pigmentation." Drawings can also be placed on a chart with concentric circles to document more specific details.

TONOGRAPHY

Tonography is a clinical, noninvasive technique for estimating the facility of aqueous outflow. It has been extremely valuable in advancing our understanding of the mechanisms of glaucoma and the actions of antiglaucoma drugs, although its clinical usefulness in the detection and management of glaucoma remains a matter of controversy. Nevertheless, it is worth considering tonography in some detail, since an understanding of the involved physiology provides insight into the complex interplay of factors related to aqueous humor dynamics.

Historical Background

The 19th century French physician and physiologist Poiseuille (pronounced "pwah zoó e") pursued his interest in the circulation of blood by studying the flow of liquids in tubes of very small diameter.[31] This work led to the formulation of an equation, *Poiseuille's law,* that relates the velocity of flow (F) of fluid in a rigid tube to (1) the radius of the tube (r), (2) the pressure drop per length of tube (P1-P2/1), and (3) the coefficient of viscosity (n) of the fluid:[32]

$$F = \frac{\pi r^4}{8n} \cdot \frac{P1 - P2}{1}$$

In 1949, Goldmann sought to apply Poiseuille's law to aqueous outflow, suggesting that the rate of aqueous flow through the trabecular meshwork (F) is directly proportional to the IOP (Po) minus the episcleral venous pressure (Pv) and inversely proportional to the resistance to outflow (R):[33]

$$F = \frac{Po - Pv}{R}$$

The equation implied that aqueous flow in living ocular tissue could be expressed in the same linear terms as that of fluid in rigid tubes, a belief that would subsequently be proved inaccurate. Nevertheless, it was modifications of Poiseuille's law that led to the mathematical foundation for tonography.

At approximately the same time that Poiseuille was conducting his studies, Pagenstecher (1878) observed that massage of the eye lowered the IOP. In 1905, Schiøtz reported that repeated tonometry also lowered the pressure, although less so in eyes with glaucoma. Polak-van Gelder, applying these observations, described a technique in 1911 of repeated tonometer applications for 1–2 minutes to differentiate normal and glaucomatous eyes. Schoenberg modified this technique the following year by using a continuous application of the tonometer while reading the pressure fall on the scale of the instrument.[34]

In 1950, Grant[35] introduced the modern concept of tonography by combining a modification of Poiseuille's law with electronic techniques of continuous IOP measurement.

Mathematical Basis

Relationship of IOP to Outflow

As Goldmann[33] suggested, the rate of aqueous outflow (F), which is expressed in μl/min, is proportional to the IOP (Po), minus the episcleral venous pressure (Pv):

$$F \propto (Po - Pv)$$

Grant[35,36] proposed that the factors that convert this proportionality to equality be expressed collectively as the *coefficient of outflow facility* (C), which is given in μl/min/mm Hg:

$$F = C\,(Po - Pv)$$

The C-value is an expression of the degree to which a change in the IOP will cause a change in the rate of aqueous outflow, which is an indirect expression of the patency of the aqueous outflow system.

Estimation of the C-Value[35]

Tonography is a means of estimating the C-value by raising the IOP with the weight of an indentation tonometer and observing the subsequent decay curve in the IOP. (This discussion presupposes an understanding of indentation tonometry, and the reader may wish to see the next chapter for an explanation of that technique.) The weight of the tonometer plunger on the cornea raises the IOP from the baseline (Po) to a new, higher level (Pt). The elevated pressure causes an increased rate of aqueous outflow, leading to a change in the aqueous volume (V), which is inferred from Friedenwald's tables relating volume change to Schiøtz scale readings.[37] Direct measurements of intraocular fluid volume change in enucleated eyes have supported Friedenwald's calculations.[38] Assuming for the moment that the elevated pressure does not alter other ocular parameters, the rate of volume decrease (Δ V/T) equals the rate of outflow.

The standard tonographic technique is to measure the IOP for 4 minutes (i.e., T = 4). The change in IOP during this time is computed as an arithmetic average of pressure increments for successive half-minute intervals (Ave. Pt − Po). The C-value is then derived from Grant's equation:

$$C = \frac{V}{T(Ave.\ Pt - Po)}$$

Perfusion studies of enucleated human eyes have supported Grant's equation, although newer tables used in the formula have given C-values far higher than those generally accepted.[39]

Ocular Parameters That Influence Tonography

The tonographic calculation assumes that only the rate of aqueous outflow changes in response to a change in IOP. However, there are many other ocular parameters that respond to a pressure change, all of which can influence the tonographic result.

Aqueous production may decrease during the early phase of a rise in IOP, primarily as a result of an alteration in ultrafiltration.[40] Any subsequent IOP drop in response to reduced production of aqueous creates an impression of increased outflow and is called *pseudofacility*. This accounts for up to 20% of the total C-value.[40] Tonography measures the total C-value, without distinguishing between true facility and pseudofacility. More recent fluorophotometric studies suggest that aqueous production is relatively insensitive to long-term changes in IOP.[41]

Resistance to aqueous outflow increases with an increase in the IOP, the physiologic basis of which was discussed in Chapter 2. The tonographic result is that the C-value of an eye decreases with increasing IOP.[42] This phenomenon relates to the conventional route of aqueous outflow. The influence of unconventional outflow on the tonographic results is not fully understood.

Episcleral venous pressure rises an average of 1.25 mm Hg with the pressure elevation during tonography,[43] which is usually corrected for in the formula by adding 1.25 to Po. Episcleral venous pressure measurements throughout tonography indicate that the rise is greatest during the first half of tonography, with a return to a nearly pretonographic level by the end of the procedure and a mean change in episcleral venous pressure during this time of 0.44 mm Hg.[44]

Ocular rigidity is an expression of the "stretchability" of the eye in response to an increase in IOP and probably represents several characteristics of the eye. An average ocular rigidity of 0.0125 is used in calculating the tonographic C-value, although there is significant interpatient variation in this parameter, which leads to a potential source of error in tonography. For this reason it is useful to check the pressure by applanation tonometry before performing the tonography and to compare this with the Po obtained with the indentation tonometer, as a means of identifying any major discrepancy in ocular rigidity.

The expulsion of uveal blood in response to elevated IOP probably influences tonography, although the actual effect is uncertain.[45]

Technique of Tonography[34]

The standard tonography unit consists of an electronic indentation tonometer, which continuously records IOP on a paper strip (Fig. 3.11). With the recorder running, the tonometer is calibrated at scale readings of 0 and 7. The recording needle is then set at 0 for the subsequent readings. The patient is in a supine position, fixing on a target overhead. After instilling a topical anesthetic on the cornea, the IOP is measured with two brief applications of the electronic tonometer.

The 4-minute pressure tracing is then made by gently applying the tonometer to the cornea and maintaining this position until a smooth tracing has been obtained for a full 4 minutes. A good tracing will have fine oscillations and a gentle downward slope. If the slope is steeper or irregular during the first few seconds, which is not uncommon, the study should be continued until a good 4-minute tracing has been obtained. The slope of the tracing is then estimated by placing a free hand line through the middle of the oscillations (Fig. 3.12). The scale readings are noted at the beginning and end of the 4-minute tracing. Po and

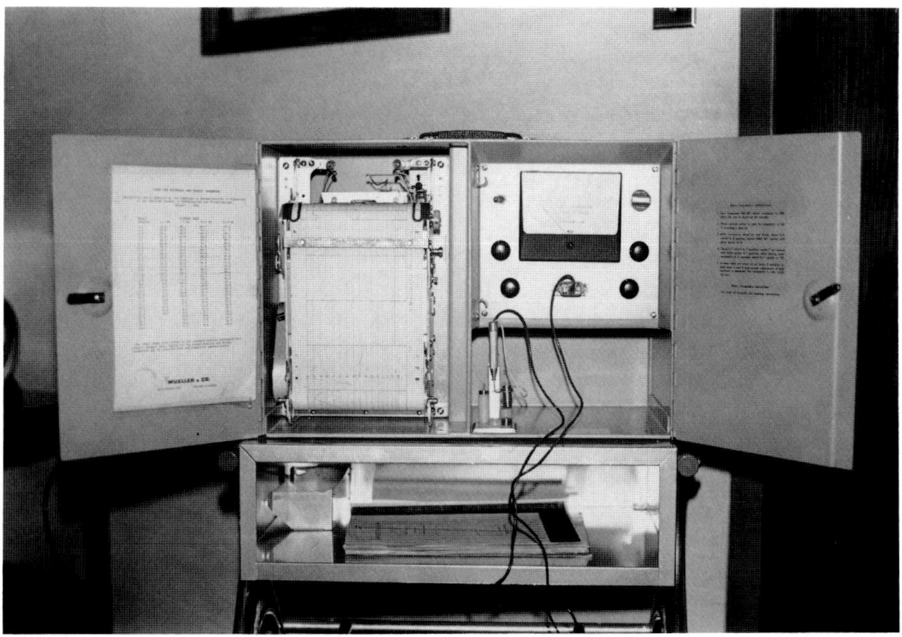

Figure 3.11. Tonography unit.

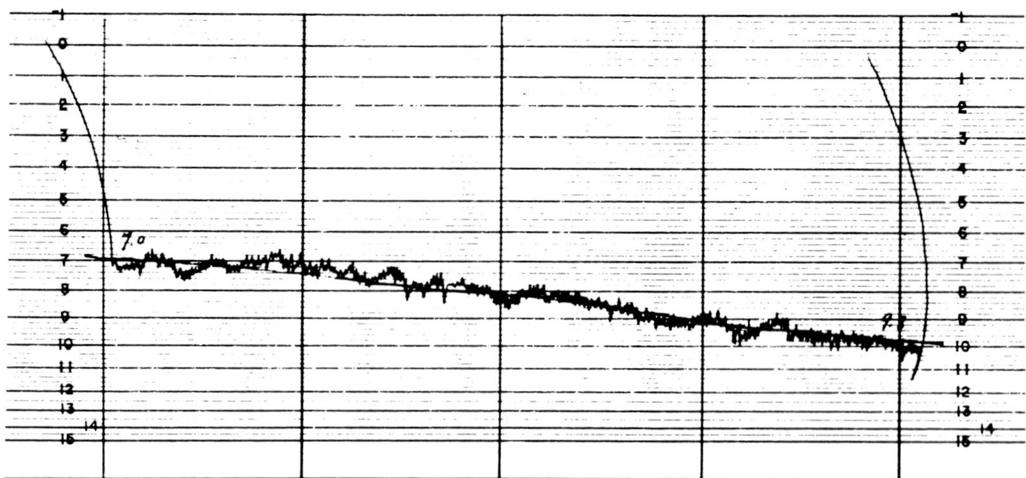

Figure 3.12. Tonographic tracing.

the change in scale readings over 4 minutes (R) are then used to obtain the C-value from special tonographic tables.

A basic assumption of tonography is that C-value calculations from each minute of the clinical tonogram do not differ significantly, although this has been shown to be invalid, with a trend toward highest values in the first minute and progressive reduction in the ensuing minutes.[46] A computer program has been developed to evaluate tonograms and assess the findings,[47] and a computerized tonography instrument has been devised, which gave mean outflow facilities that did not differ statistically significantly from those obtained with a standard tonography unit.[48]

Applanation tonometers cause less change in IOP, resulting in less effect on outflow resistance and on the other parameters influenced by pressure change. The use of applanation tonometers in tonography has been evaluated by using instruments that maintain a constant IOP level[49,50] or a constant diameter of tonometer contact with the cornea.[51] These techniques are still investigational. Tonography with a pneumatic tonometer (pneumotonography, described in Chapter 4) was compared with that with a Schiøtz tonometer in normal and glaucomatous subjects and was found to give virtually identical average C-values, but had significantly higher intrasubject and interobserver variability.[52]

Sources of Error in Tonographic Technique

Variations in corneal curvature from the assumed average of 7.8 mm may significantly influence the pressure measurements.[34]

Moses effect. The hole in the tonometer footplate must be slightly larger in electronic tonometers to prevent sticking. At low scale readings, the cornea may mold into the space between the plunger and hole, pushing the plunger up and leading to falsely high pressure readings.[53]

Variations in line voltage may produce an apparent drift in the IOP measurements, which can be minimized with line voltage stabilizers and by avoiding magnetic fields.[34]

Consensual pressure drop. The IOP has been shown to drop approximately 1 mm Hg in the fellow eye while tonography is being performed on the first eye. A neural etiology was once postulated for this phenomenon, but it was subsequently found to be secondary to the evaporation that results from keeping the eye open for fixation during the 4-minute test.[54] The problem can be eliminated by draping a plastic sheet over the fellow eye while the first eye is being tested.[54]

Eye movement under the tonometer can also influence the tonographic tracing.

Patient relaxation effect. During the first

15–20 seconds after the tonometer is placed on the cornea, the IOP will fall as the patient relaxes. Time should be allowed for this before starting the 4-minute tracing.

Operator error, including improper cleaning, calibration, or positioning of the instrument, as well as improper calculation of the tracing, can also lead to inaccurate results.

Interpreting Tonographic Results

Despite the many potentials for error in tonography and the possibility that currently accepted values may be grossly inaccurate, it is nevertheless necessary to be familiar with the values that might be anticipated with current techniques.

From a study of 1379 eyes, Becker[55] reported the following values:

C-Value. The mean in 909 normal eyes was 0.28 μl/min/mm Hg, and the prevalence of low C-values was:

C-Value	Normals (n = 909)	Glaucoma Patients (n = 250)	Family History of Glaucoma (n = 220)
<0.18	2.5%	65%	20%
<0.13	0.15%	43%	11%

Po/C Ratio. The mean of the normal population was 56, and the prevalence of high Po/C ratios was:

C-Value	Normals	Glaucoma Patients	Family History of Glaucoma
>100	2.5%	73%	21%
>138	0.15%	50%	14%

In a study of 7577 eyes, the C-value was found to decrease with age, with an average of 0.2932 for ages 41–45 years, compared with 0.2518 in the 81–85-year-old group. There was no sex difference at any age level.[56]

When the C-value and Po do not seem to correlate, the following possibilities should be considered.[34] A low C with a normal Po may be due to: (1) a sticky tonometer, (2) low ocular rigidity, or (3) hyposecretion. A high C with elevated Po may be due to: (1) an artificially elevated Po, (2) high ocular rigidity, (3) high pseudofacility, (4) elevated episcleral venous pressure, (5) angle-closure glaucoma (the force of the tonometer may open the angle), or (6) the Moses effect.

The wave components of a tonographic tracing include: (1) fine oscillations, which reflect the cardiac pulse; (2) large waves, which reflect the respiratory movement; and (3) still larger, irregular waves (Traube-Hering waves), which reflect periodic oscillations in the systemic blood pressure. Cardiac irregularities (e.g., extrasystoli, bigeminy, etc.) can also cause irregularities in the tonographic tracing.[57]

The Clinical Value of Tonography

As previously noted, there is controversy regarding the value of tonography in the detection and management of glaucoma. The following are the main situations in which tonography is believed by some physicians to have clinical value:

As an adjunct in diagnosing open-angle glaucoma, tonography is suggested to have predictive value regarding the development of nerve damage in patients with elevated IOP,[58,59] although this has not been confirmed in all studies.[60] The *Po/C* ratio is generally thought to be the more sensitive parameter in this situation,[58,59] and a prior water-drinking test (discussed in Chapter 9) has been suggested to further enhance the predictive value of tonography.[58] However, it has been stressed that abnormal tonometric and tonographic results do not make the diagnosis of glaucoma, but alert the ophthalmologist to follow the patient more closely.[61]

A wide diurnal fluctuation in IOP was believed to correlate with a low *C*-value, but a study of 388 eyes showed that a single tonometric reading correlated with the diurnal curve better than did the tonographic results.[62]

In angle-closure glaucoma, a 25–30% fall in the *C*-value may be used as adjunctive confirmation of a positive provocative test. In addition, once an acute attack is broken, a *C*-value of 0.10 or less suggests that a peripheral iridectomy alone may be insufficient.[34]

Ocular inflammation, as with surgery, trauma, disease, etc., may mask a compromised outflow system by temporarily reducing aqueous production, and tonography during this time can disclose the abnormal outflow.[34]

Myasthenia gravis may also be evaluated with tonography by observing a rise in IOP of 2–5 mm Hg in response to intravenous tensilon.[63]

Since both aqueous and blood are expelled from the eye in variable amounts during tonography, a future value of tonography may lie in its ability to assess the posterior half of the eye, the portion directly related to visual loss, by measuring the blood-ejection coefficient.[45,64]

MEASUREMENT OF EPISCLERAL VENOUS PRESSURE

A variety of techniques have been developed for measuring the pressure in the episcleral veins. All of these work on the principle of correlating partial collapse of the vein with the force required to achieve the alteration in blood flow. A *pressure chamber* technique utilizes a thin membrane stretched over the tip of a hollow applanating head, which is filled with air[65–67] or saline[68] (Fig. 3.13). The pressure in the chamber is raised until the bulging membrane produces the desired visible change in the adjacent vessel. Most of these instruments are mounted on a slit lamp, although a portable pressure transducer has been developed to measure episcleral venous pressure with a subject in various body positions.[69] A *torsion balance* instrument utilizes a clear plastic applanating head, attached to a torsion rod.[65,70] The applanating head is placed over a vein, and the pressure of the head against the vessel is raised until the desired endpoint in blood flow change is achieved. An *air jet* technique uses a stream of air to collapse the vessel.[71] When the first two methods were compared with direct cannulation of the episcleral vein, the pressure chamber method was found to be superior to the torsion technique.[65]

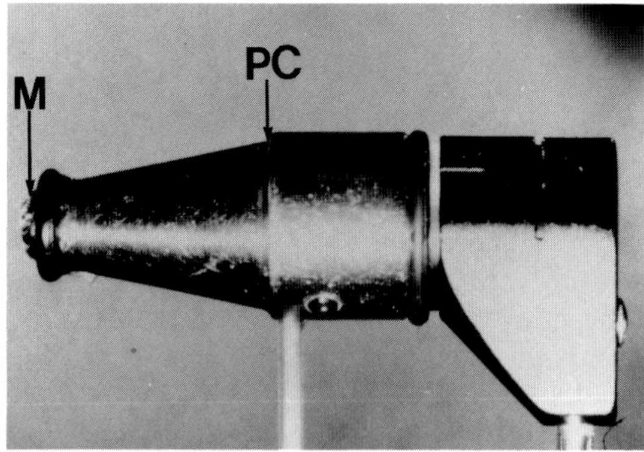

Figure 3.13. Head of instrument for measuring episcleral venous pressure, showing flexible membrane (*M*), which presses against episcleral vessel, and pressure chamber (*PC*), which transfers pressure to membrane. (Courtesy of Douglas E. Gaasterland, M.D.)

As noted in Chapter 2, the normal episcleral venous pressure is generally considered to be between 8 and 11 mm Hg. Two features that significantly influence the pressure measurement are the selected endpoint and the choice of vessel. When a pressure chamber technique was compared with direct cannulation, a slight indentation, rather than an intermittent or sustained collapse of the vein lumen, gave the most accurate reading.[68] It has been suggested that the best point of measurement is just distal to the junction of aqueous and episcleral veins, although this junction is often difficult to ascertain and it is more practical to take all measurements 3 mm from the limbus.[67]

SUMMARY

Instruments and techniques have been developed for evaluating aqueous humor inflow by directly visualizing the ciliary processes (cycloscopy) and by measuring the actual rate of aqueous production (fluorophotometry). Other instruments can be used to study aqueous humor outflow by direct visualization of the anterior chamber angle (gonioscopy), estimation of the resistance to aqueous outflow (tonography), and the measurement of episcleral venous pressure. Of these techniques, only gonioscopy is commonly used in the daily practice of ophthalmology, with the others currently having primary value as research tools.

References

1. Mizuno, K, Asaoka, M: Cycloscopy and fluorescein cycloscopy. Invest Ophthal 15:561, 1976.

2. Mizuno, K, Asaoka, M, Muroi, S: Cycloscopy and fluorescein cycloscopy of the ciliary process. Am J Ophthal 84:487, 1977.
3. Holm, O: A photogrammetric method for estimation of the pupillary aqueous flow in the living human eye. I. Acta Ophthal 46:254, 1968.
4. Brubaker, RF, Nagtaki, S, Townsend, DJ, et al: The effect of age on aqueous humor formation in man. Ophthalmology 88:283, 1981.
5. Jones, RF, Maurice, DM: New methods of measuring the rate of aqueous flow in man with fluorescein. Exp Eye Res 5:208, 1966.
6. Bloom, JN, Levene, RZ, Thomas, G, Kimura, R: Fluorophotometry and the rate of aqueous flow in man. Arch Ophthal 94:435, 1976.
7. Coakes, RL, Brubaker, RF: Method of measuring aqueous humor flow and corneal endothelial permeability using a fluorophotometry nomogram. Invest Ophthal Vis Sci 18:288, 1979.
8. Brubaker, RF, Coakes, RL: Use of xenon flash tube as the excitation source in new slit-lamp fluorophotometer. Am J Ophthal 86:474, 1978.
9. Brubaker, RF, McLaren, JW: Uses of fluorophotometry in glaucoma research. Ophthalmology 92:884, 1985.
10. Becker, B: The measurement of rate of aqueous flow with iodide. Invest Ophthal 1:52, 1962.
11. Macri, JF, Cevario, SJ: The formation and inhibition of aqueous humor production. Arch Ophthal 96:1664, 1978.
12. Wickham, MG, Worthen, DM, Downing, D: A randomized technique of constant-pressure infusion. Invest Ophthal 15:1010, 1976.
13. Becker, S: Clinical Gonioscopy—A Text and Stereoscopic Atlas. CV Mosby, St. Louis, 1972.
14. Rubin, ML: Optics for Clinicians, 2nd ed. Triad Scientific Publishing, Gainesville, Fla., 1974, p. 56.
15. O'Rourke, J, Lal, M, Kalwat, W: Weightless Koeppe gonioscopy. Arch Ophthal 99:1646, 1981.
16. Kapetansky, FM: A bubble-free goniolens. Ophthal Surg 19:414, 1988.
17. Sussman, W: A new instrument for gonioscopy. Ophthalmology 86:130, 1979.
18. Kaufman, PL, Neider, MW, Pankonin, WH: Slit-lamp mount for Zeiss gonioscopy lens. Arch Ophthal 99:1455, 1981.
19. Ritch, R: A new lens for argon laser trabeculoplasty. Ophthal Surg 16:331, 1985.
20. Mizuno, K: A new multipurpose goniolens. Arch Ophthal 106:1309, 1988.
21. Kapetansky, FM, Johnstone, MA: A direct-view goniolens. Am J Ophthal 93:242, 1982.
22. Becker, SC: Unrecognized errors induced by present-day gonioprisms and a proposal for their elimination. Arch Ophthal 82:160, 1969.
23. Hetherington, J Jr: Koeppe lens gonioscopy. In: Controversy in Ophthalmology, Brockhurst, FJ, Boruchoff, SA, Hutchinson, BT, Lessell, S, eds. WB Saunders, Philadelphia, 1977, p. 142.
24. Campbell, DG: A comparison of diagnostic techniques in angle-closure glaucoma. Am J Ophthal 88:197, 1979.
25. Schwartz, B: Slit lamp gonioscopy. In: Controversy in Ophthalmology, Brockhurst, RJ, Boruchoff, SA, Hutchinson, BT, Lessell, S, eds. WB Saunders, Philadelphia, 1977, p. 146.
26. Smith, RJH: An improved diagnostic contact lens. Br J Ophthal 63:482, 1979.
27. Forbes, M: Gonioscopy with corneal indentation. Arch Ophthal 76:488, 1966.
28. Vijfvinkel, G, de Jong, PTVM: Disinfectant container for diagnostic lenses. Am J Ophthal 99:600, 1985.
29. Inomata, H, Tawara, A: Anterior and posterior parts of human trabecular meshwork. Jpn J Ophthal 28:339, 1984.
30. Shihab, ZM, Lee, P-F: The significance of normal angle vessels. Ophthal Surg 16:382, 1985.
31. Bingham, EC: Biography of Dr. Jean Leonard Marie Poiseuille. Rheological Memoirs 1:vii, 1940.
32. Frank, NH: Introduction to Mechanics and Heat, 2nd ed. McGraw-Hill, New York, 1939, p. 246.
33. Goldmann, H: Augendruck and glaukom. Die Kammerwasservenen und das Poiseuille'sche Gesetz. Ophthalmologica 118:496, 1949.
34. Drews, RC: Manual of Tonography. CV Mosby, St. Louis, 1971.
35. Grant, WM: Tonographic method for measuring the facility and rate of aqueous flow in human eyes. Arch Ophthal 44:204, 1950.
36. Grant, WM: Clinical measurements of aqueous outflow. Arch Ophthal 46:113, 1951.
37. Friedenwald, JS: Some problems in the calibration of tonometers. Am J Ophthal 31:935, 1948.
38. Hetland-Eriksen, J, Odberg, T: Experimental tonography on enucleated human eyes. II. The loss of intraocular fluid caused by tonography. Invest Ophthal 14:944, 1975.
39. Hetland-Eriksen, J, Odberg, T: Experimental tonography on enucleated human eyes. I. The validity of Grant's tonography formula. Invest Ophthal 14:199, 1975.
40. Kupfer, C: Clinical significance of pseudofacility. Am J Ophthal 75:193, 1973.
41. Carlson, KH, McLaren, JW, Topper, JE, Brubaker, RF: Effect of body position on intraocular pressure and aqueous flow. Invest Ophthal Vis Sci 28:1346, 1987.
42. Moses, RA: Constant pressure applanation tonography. III. The relationship of tonometric pressure to rate of loss of ocular volume. Arch Ophthal 77:181, 1967.
43. Linnér, E: Episcleral venous pressure during tonograpy. Acta XVII Cong Ophthal 3:1532, 1955.
44. Leith, AB: Episcleral venous pressure in tonography. Br J Ophthal 47:271, 1963.

45. Fisher, RF: Value of tonometry and tonography in the diagnosis of glaucoma. Br J Ophthal 56:200, 1972.
46. Armaly, MF: On the consistency of tonography. II. One minute analysis of clinical tonogram. Klin Monatsbl Augenheilkd 184:299, 1984.
47. Strobel, J: A new method of evaluating tonograms. Klin Monatsbl Augenheilkd 183:301, 1983.
48. Teitelbaum, CS, Podos, SM, Lustgarten, JS: Comparison of standard and computerized tonography instruments on human eyes. Am J Ophthal 99:403, 1985.
49. Moses, RA: Constant pressure applanation tonography with the Mackay-Marg tonometer. I. A preliminary report. Arch Ophthal 76:20, 1966.
50. Moses, RA: Constant pressure applanation tonography with the Mackay-Marg tonometer. II. Limits of the instrument. Arch Ophthal 77:45, 1967.
51. Moses, RA, Grodzki, WJ Jr, Arnzen, RJ: Constant-area applanation tonography. Invest Ophthal Vis Sci 20:722, 1981.
52. Feghali, JG, Azar, DT, Kaufman, PL: Comparative aqueous outflow facility measurements by pneumatonography and Schiøtz tonography. Invest Ophthal Vis Sci 27:1776, 1986.
53. Moses, R: Tonometry—effect of tonometer footplate hole on scale reading. Further studies. Arch Ophthal 61:373, 1959.
54. Grant, WM, English, FP: An explanation for so-called consensual pressure drop during tonography. Arch Ophthal 69:314, 1963.
55. Becker, B: Tonography in the diagnosis of simple (open angle) glaucoma. Trans Am Acad Ophthal Otol 65:156, 1961.
56. Johnson, LV: Tonographic survey. Am J Ophthal 61:680, 1966.
57. Haik, GM, Perez, LF, Reitman, HS, Massey, JY: Tonographic tracings in patients with cardiac rhythm disturbances. Am J Ophthal 70:929, 1970.
58. Becker, B, Christensen, RE: Water-drinking and tonography in the diagnosis of glaucoma. Arch Ophthal 56:321, 1956.
59. Portney, GL, Krohn, M: Tonography and projection perimetry. Relationship according to receiver operating characteristic curves. Arch Ophthal 95:1353, 1977.
60. Pohjanpelto, PEJ: Tonography and glaucomatous optic nerve damage. Acta Ophthal 52:817, 1974.
61. Podos, SM, Becker, B: Tonography—current thoughts. Am J Ophthal 75:733, 1973.
62. Phelps, CD, Woolson, RF, Kolker, AE, Becker, B: Diurnal variation in intraocular pressure. Am J Ophthal 77:367, 1974.
63. Wray, SH, Pavan-Langston, D: A reevaluation of edrophonium chloride (Tensilon) tonography in the diagnosis of myasthenia gravis: with observations on some other defects of neuromuscular transmission. Neurology 21:586, 1971.
64. Spaeth, GL: Tonography and tonometry. In: Clinical Ophthalmology, Vol. 3, Ch. 47, Duane, TD, ed. Harper & Row, Hagerstown, Md., 1976.
65. Brubaker, RF: Determination of episcleral venous pressure in the eye. A comparison of three methods. Arch Ophthal 77:110, 1967.
66. Phelps, CD, Armaly, MF: Measurement of episcleral venous pressure. Am J Ophthal 85:35, 1978.
67. Zeimer, RC, Gieser, DK, Wilensky, JT, et al: A practical venomanometer. Measurement of episcleral venous pressure and assessment of the normal range. Arch Ophthal 101:1447, 1983.
68. Gaasterland, DE, Pederson, JE: Episcleral venous pressure: a comparison of invasive and noninvasive measurements. Invest Ophthal Vis Sci 24:1417, 1983.
69. Friberg, TR: Portable transducer for measurement of episcleral venous pressure. Am J Ophthal 102:396, 1986.
70. Podos, SM, Minas, TF, Macri, FJ: A new instrument to measure episcleral venous pressure. Comparison of normal eyes and eyes with primary open-angle glaucoma. Arch Ophthal 80:209, 1968.
71. Krakau, CET, Widakowich, J, Wilke, K: Measurements of the episcleral venous pressure by means of an air jet. Acta Ophthal 51:185, 1973.

Chapter 4

INTRAOCULAR PRESSURE AND TONOMETRY

INTRAOCULAR PRESSURE

What Is Normal?

Within the context of a discussion on glaucoma, "normal" intraocular pressure (IOP) might be defined as that pressure which does not lead to glaucomatous damage of the optic nerve head. Unfortunately, such a definition cannot be expressed in precise numerical terms, since all eyes do not respond the same to given pressure levels. The best we can do is to describe the distribution of IOP in general populations and in groups of individuals with glaucomatous damage to establish levels of risk for glaucoma within different pressure ranges. In this chapter, we will consider the distribution of IOP in the general population and the factors other than glaucoma that may influence IOP. In Section Two, the significance of various pressure levels within populations of patients with specific types of glaucoma is considered.

Distribution in General Populations

The most frequently cited population study is that by Leydhecker and associates[1] in which 10,000 persons with no known eye disease were tested with Schiøtz tonometers. These investigators obtained a distribution of pressures that resembled a Gaussian curve but was skewed toward the higher pressures, which they interpreted as two subpopulations: a large, "normal" group, and a smaller group that was believed to represent previously unrecognized glaucoma (this included individuals with and without established glaucomatous optic nerve damage). In the "normal" group, the mean IOP was 15.5 ± 2.57 mm Hg. Two standard deviations (2SD) above the mean was approximately 20.5 mm Hg, which the authors interpreted as the upper limit of "normal," since approximately 95% of the area under a Gaussian curve lies between the mean ± 2SD. However, the latter principle does not apply when a frequency distribution is skewed, and the concept of "normal" IOP limits must be viewed as only a rough approximation.[2]

Subsequent IOP screening studies, using either indentation or applanation tonometry (these techniques are explained later in the chapter), have generally agreed with Leydhecker's findings regarding pressure distribution in general populations, with small differences probably related to population selection and testing techniques (Table 4.1).[3–10] However, the division of IOP groups into normal and abnormal is not as simple as Leydhecker and associates[1] originally suspected, since there are many factors that influence the IOP. Furthermore, as previously noted, all eyes do not respond the same to given pressure levels. This leads to an overlapping of IOP distributions within nonglaucoma and glaucoma populations, which can be illustrated only theoretically (Fig. 4.1), since the precise boundaries of both groups are not known.

Factors Exerting Long-Term Influence on IOP

The following factors are believed to exert, to variable degrees, a sustained influence on IOP throughout the lifetime of the individual.

Genetics. The IOP within the general population appears to be under hereditary influence, possibly through a polygenic, multifactorial mode.[11–13] In addition, the IOP tends to be higher in individuals with an enlarged cup-disc ratio[10] and those who have relatives with open-angle glaucoma.[5,14]

Age. There are conflicting statements in the literature regarding the association of IOP and age. Young children may have lower pressures than the rest of the general population, although accurate measurements are difficult to obtain because of the influence of lid squeezing while they are awake and anesthetic agents when they are asleep. The mean IOP, using only topical anesthesia for the tonometry, has been reported to be 11.4 ± 2.4 mm Hg in newborns[15] and 8.4 ± 0.6 mm Hg in infants less than 4 months of age,[16] although another

Table 4.1.
Reported IOP Distributions in General Populations

Investigators	Number of Individuals	Ages (years)	IOP (mm Hg) Mean	S.D.
TESTED WITH SCHIØTZ TONOMETERS				
Leydhecker, et al. (1958)[1]	10,000	10–69	15.8	2.57
Johnson (1966)[3]	7,577	>41	15.4	2.65
Segal & Skwierczyńska (1967)[4]	15,695	>30	15.3–15.9 (women)	
			15.0–15.2 (men)	
TESTED WITH APPLANATION TONOMETERS				
Armaly (1965)[5]	2,316	20–79	15.91	3.14*
Perkins (1965)[6]	2,000	>40	15.2	2.5(OD)
			14.9	2.5(OS)
Loewen, et al. (1976)[7]	4,661	9–89	17.18	3.78
Ruprecht et al. (1978)[8]	8,899	5–94	16.25	3.45
Shiose and Kawase (1986)[9]	75,545 (men)	<70	14.60	2.52
	18,158 (women)		15.04	2.33
David, et al. (1987)[10]	2,504	40–70+	14.93	4.04

* Computed from data reported according to sex and age groups.

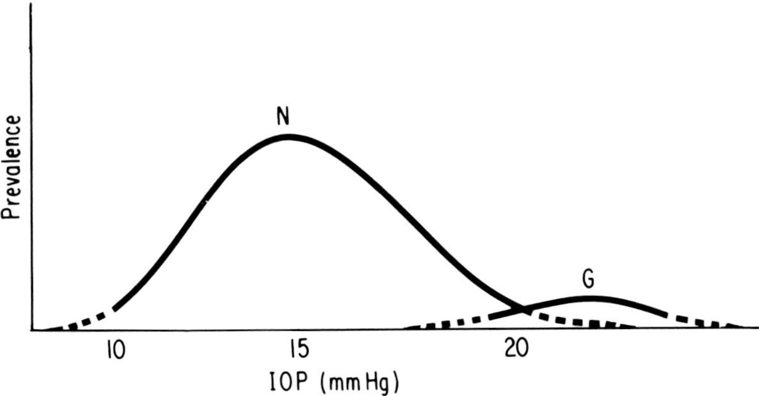

Figure 4.1. Theoretical distribution of intraocular pressures in nonglaucoma (*N*) and glaucoma (*G*) populations, showing overlap between the two groups (dotted lines represent uncertainty of extreme values in both populations).

study found a mean of 18 mm Hg in premature infants.[17] The use of general anesthesia or a hypnotic agent in older children may artificially lower the IOP (discussed later in this chapter). In one study, the mean IOP for children measured under halothane anesthesia was 7.8 ± 0.4 mm Hg at age 1 year, with a gradual increase of approximately 1 mm Hg per year of age to 11.7 ± 0.6 mm Hg at the age of 5 years.[16]

In the adult population, the IOP distribution is Gaussian between 20 and 40 years of age.[5] Thereafter, the curve begins to shift toward the higher pressures with advancing age.[5,7,8] Some investigators believe that this is due to a positive independent correlation between IOP and age.[5,10,18,19] Others, however, have found a weak[20,21] or negative[9,22] correlation and suggest that other factors such as pulse rate,[20] obesity,[9] or blood pressure[9,21,22] may be responsible for the apparent rise in IOP with increasing age. If a true positive correlation exists between IOP and age, it may be related to reduced facility of aqueous outflow, since aqueous production actually appears to decrease slightly with increasing age.[23–25]

Sex. IOP is equal between the sexes in ages 20–40 years. In older age groups, the apparent increase in the mean IOP with age is greater in females and coincides with the onset of menopause, while the increase in the standard deviation of the IOP distribution is equal between the sexes.[5]

Refractive Error. A positive correlation between IOP and both axial length of the globe[26] and increasing degrees of myopia[10,14,27,28] has been reported. However, another study of patients with anisometropic myopia found no difference in IOP between the two eyes.[29] Myopes also have a higher incidence of primary open-angle glaucoma, and it is hard to know whether the higher pressures in this group reflect the early glaucoma cases or a truly higher IOP distribution throughout the myopic population.

Race may occasionally influence IOP distribution. For example, full-blooded Indians in a New Mexico tribe were found to have a significantly lower mean IOP than did a control population.[30] Blacks have been reported to have slightly higher pressures than do whites,[18,19] and persons born in Africa or Asia were found to have higher mean IOPs than did those born in Europe or America.[10]

Factors Exerting Short-Term Influence on IOP

The following are factors that have been associated with a rise or fall in IOP, lasting from seconds to months.

Diurnal Variation. Like many biological parameters, the IOP is subject to cyclic fluctuations throughout the day. The reported mean amplitude of the daily fluctuation ranges from approximately 3[31]–6 mm Hg.[32]

An amplitude greater than 10 mm Hg is generally considered to be pathologic,[33] and glaucomatous eyes have been reported to exceed 30 mm Hg of diurnal variation.[33] The pattern of the daily cycle has classically been described as having the peak IOP in the morning hours.[31] However, subsequent studies have revealed many exceptions to this rule (if, indeed, it is the rule at all), with frequent peak pressures in the afternoon, as well as short-term fluctuations throughout the day.[32–35]

The obvious clinical significance of diurnal IOP variation is the risk of missing a pressure elevation with single readings. In one study using self-tonometry to obtain diurnal curves, half of the IOP peaks occurred at times outside of normal office hours, and more elevated readings were recorded in patients with suspected or documented progression of glaucomatous damage.[36] Using the same self-tonometry, the authors found that many patients have a significant drop in IOP between the time they awake and 30 minutes later,[37] suggesting that either the act of waking is associated with a transient pressure rise or significant IOP peaks may disappear before the patient is seen in the clinic.

The mechanism of diurnal IOP variation is uncertain. Results of tonographic studies have been conflicting, with one showing an inverse relationship between IOP and outflow facility,[38] and another showing no relationship.[33] A circadian rhythm of IOP in rabbits has been correlated with aqueous inflow.[39,40] A relationship between adrenocortical steroids and diurnal IOP variation has been suggested, since the diurnal variation of plasma cortisol has been observed to parallel that of the IOP, peaking 3–4 hours before the latter.[38,41] Furthermore, interruption of the normal daily corticosteroid cycle has been shown to alter the diurnal IOP curve,[38,42] and oral administration of metyrapone, an inhibitor of adrenal cortical biosynthesis, is associated with a decrease in IOP.[43]

Postural Variation. Most studies show that the IOP increases when changing from the sitting to the supine position, with reported average pressure differences of 0.3–6.0 mm Hg,[44–46] although some investigators have been unable to confirm these findings in normal eyes.[47,48] The postural influence on IOP is greater in eyes with glaucoma[44,46,49] and persists even after a successful trabeculectomy.[49] One study suggested that the postural variation is greatest in patients with low tension glaucoma,[50] although another study found that 15% of ocular hypertensives had an IOP rise of 5–9 mm Hg when going from the sitting to supine position, and that this rise was sustained throughout 4 hours of observation.[51] Postural variation is also higher in patients with central retinal vein occlusion,[48] and patients with systemic hypertension have a significantly higher IOP rise after 15 minutes in the supine position than do normotensive controls.[52] These observations may explain why retinal vascular occlusive events are most often discovered in the morning.

Whole-body, head-down tilt leads to a further increase in IOP, which correlates with the degree of inversion.[53] In one study, after 5 minutes of total inversion, the mean pressure rose from 16.8 ± 2.8 to 32.9 ± 7.9 mm Hg in normal eyes and from 21.3 ± 2.3 to 37.6 ± 5 mm Hg in glaucomatous eyes.[54] The mechanism of this phenomenon appears to be elevated episcleral venous pressure.[55]

Exertional Influences. Exertion may lead to either a lowering or an elevation of the IOP, depending on the nature of the activity. Prolonged exercise, such as running or bicycling, has been reported to lower the IOP.[56–61] This reduction was found to average 24% of the baseline IOP in normal individuals[57] and 30% in the open-angle glaucoma patients,[59] although reports vary. One study showed that short-term aerobic exercise in normotensive individuals was associated with a mean IOP decrease of 5.9 ± 0.6 mm Hg that lasted approximately 30 minutes, and that 4 months of exercise conditioning significantly reduced the baseline IOP but attenuated the hypotensive response to short-term exertion.[61] Theories of mechanism include increased serum osmolarity[58] and metabolic acidosis.[59] Salt loading in patients on a bicycle ergometer was associated with only a 1 mm Hg decrease in IOP.[62] Most investigators agree that many factors are probably involved in the influence of prolonged exertion on IOP.

Straining, as associated with Valsalva's maneuver[56,63] or electroshock therapy[64] has been reported to elevate the IOP. Mechanisms for this phenomenon likely include elevated episcleral venous pressure, especially with Valsalva's maneuver, and increased orbicularis tone.

Lid and Eye Movement. Blinking has been shown to raise the IOP 10 mm Hg, while hard lid squeezing may raise it as high as 90 mm Hg.[65] It has also been shown that repeated lid squeezing will lead to a slight reduction in IOP, although less so in glaucomatous eyes.[66] Voluntary lid fissure widening causes an increase in IOP of approximately 2 mm Hg, which may relate to an increased orbital volume from retraction of the upper lid into the orbit.[67] Reports differ as to whether decreased orbicularis tone, as with Bell's palsy or local facial nerve block, reduces IOP.[68,69] Patients with third neuron Horner's syndrome were found to have a slight reduction in IOP without alterations in aqueous humor dynamics.[70] Contraction of extraocular muscles also influences the IOP. Intraocular pressure has been shown to increase slightly in horizontal gaze position,[71] especially when full duction is restricted in patients with noncomitant strabismus.[72] During strabismus surgery, especially for eyes with thyroid ophthalmolopathy, the IOP has been recorded to rise as high as 84 mm Hg.[73]

Intraocular Conditions. In addition to the many ocular conditions that can lead to secondary glaucoma, which will be discussed in Section Two, some intraocular conditions may lead to a reduction in IOP. *Anterior uveitis,* as noted in Chapter Two, often leads to a slight reduction in IOP, as a result of a decrease in aqueous humor formation. *Rhegmatogenous retinal detachment* may also be associated with a reduced IOP, apparently as a result of reduced aqueous flow,[74] as well as a shunting of aqueous from the posterior chamber, through the vitreous and retinal hole, into the subretinal space, and across the retinal pigment epithelium.[75]

Systemic Conditions. Most studies have revealed a positive correlation between *systemic hypertension,* especially the systolic level, and IOP,[9,14,18–20,22,76–78] although at least one study found a significant negative correlation.[21] During cardiopulmonary bypass surgery, reduced ocular perfusion and a slight increase in IOP, possibly resulting from hemodilution, create the potential complication of anterior ischemic optic neuropathy.[79,80] This risk may be minimized by administering mannitol 30 minutes prior to bypass, rather than the standard practice of giving it at the start of the procedure.[81] A slight IOP elevation may persist for the first 2 days after cardiopulmonary bypass surgery.[82] This does not correlate with weight gain or hemodilution and may be associated with postoperative medications.

Systemic hyperthermia has been shown to cause an increased IOP in rabbits[83] and humans.[84] Other systemic factors reported to have a positive correlation with IOP include obesity,[9,22] pulse rate,[20] and hemoglobin concentration.[20,85]

In addition to the possible *hormonal influence* on diurnal fluctuation in IOP, as previously discussed, preliminary evidence suggests that the IOP may increase in response to ACTH, glucocorticoids, and growth hormone, and may decrease in response to progesterone, estrogen, chorionic gonadotropin, and relaxin.[86,87] The IOP has also been reported to be higher in patients with hypothyroidism, and lower in those with hyperthyroidism.[88] Patients with acromegaly were found to have slight IOP elevation, although this was apparently due to the influence of increased central corneal thickness on the tonometric measurement.[89] The IOP does not appear to be influenced by gonadectomy in rabbits[90] or the menstrual cycle in humans,[91,92] although it has been shown to be significantly reduced during pregnancy.[93] Topical antidiuretic hormone (vasopressin) lowers IOP in human eyes, while intravenous administration in rabbits increases the pressure.[94] Intravenous pituitary hormone releasing factors variably influence the IOP in rabbits, with corticotropin releasing factor and luteinizing hormone releasing factor causing a decrease and thyrotropin releasing hormone causing a rise in pressure.[95]

Other systemic disorders associated with abnormal IOP include myotonic dystrophy, in which the IOP is markedly low, apparently as a result of reduced aqueous production.[96] Diabetic patients have been reported to have higher pressures than the rest of the general population,[77,97] while a fall in IOP has been noted during acute hypoglycemia in patients with insulin-dependent diabetes.[98]

Environmental Conditions. Exposure to cold air reduces IOP, apparently as a result of a decrease in episcleral venous pressure.[99] Reduced gravity increases IOP, apparently because of fluid shifts, which may have implications in space travel.[100]

General Anesthesia. General anesthesia is usually associated with a reduction in the IOP,[101] although there are exceptions, such as with trichlorethylene[102] and ketamine,[103–105] which are reported to elevate the ocular pressure. In the following two situations, the ophthalmologist must be particularly concerned about alterations in IOP during general anesthesia.

In *infants* and *children* who are examined under anesthesia for suspicion of congenital glaucoma, the main concern is to avoid the artificial reduction of IOP, as discussed earlier in this chapter, which could mask a pathologic pressure elevation. However, studies with halothane, the anesthetic agent most often used in this situation, are conflicting with regard to the influence on IOP in children, with at least one showing a slight decrease in IOP[16] and others showing no significant difference from pressures recorded in newborns and infants using only topical anesthesia.[106,107] Hypnotics that are used to produce unconsciousness, such as 4-hydroxybutyrate, are also reported to reduce the IOP,[108] and barbiturates and tranquilizers may, in some cases, cause a transient pressure reduction.[105,109]

When operating on an *open eye,* as following penetrating injury or during intraocular surgery, the primary concern is to avoid sudden elevations of IOP that might lead to extrusion of ocular contents. Depolarizing muscle relaxants, such as succinylcholine[110] and suxamethonium,[111] cause a transient rise in IOP, possibly resulting from a combination of extraocular muscle contraction and intraocular vasodilation. Pretreatment with nondepolarizing muscle relaxants, such as *d*-tubocurarine and gallamine,[110,111] or with a subparalytic dose of succinylcholine prior to the full paralyzing dose,[112] has not been proved to prevent IOP elevation during endotracheal intubation. However, pretreatment with diazepam,[113] fazadinium,[114] or atracurium[115] has been reported to eliminate the risk of IOP elevation. It has also been suggested that intramuscular succinylcholine will cause less IOP rise than will intravenous.[116] Tracheal intubation may also cause an IOP rise, and neither intravenous lignocaine[117] nor atracurium[115] has been found to prevent this.

It has been noted that an elevated pCO_2[118,119] causes a rise in IOP, which is not blocked by pretreatment with acetazolamide,[119] while an increased concentration of O_2 is associated with an IOP reduction.[120] Rabbit studies suggest that the latter phenomenon may be due to a decrease in episcleral venous pressure.[121]

Foods and Drugs. The following drugs and other substances have been studied for their effect on the IOP. This list is exclusive of antiglaucoma drugs, which are discussed in Section Three.

Alcohol has been shown to lower the IOP, although more so in patients with glaucoma.[122] In another study, individuals who abstained from liquor had a higher prevalence of ocular hypertensives than did those who drank liquor on a daily basis.[14] The pressure reduction is not associated with a change in facility of aqueous outflow,[122] and it has been suggested that the mechanism may be a combination of suppressed circulating antidiuretic hormone, leading to a reduction of net water movement into the eye, and direct inhibition of aqueous secretion.[123]

Caffeine may cause a slight, transient rise in IOP, although in the levels associated with customary coffee drinking, this does not appear to cause a significant, sustained pressure elevation.[109,124] Herbal tea caused significantly less pressure rise than did regular coffee in glaucoma patients.[124]

A fat-free diet has been shown to reduce IOP, which may be related to a concomitant reduction in plasma prostaglandin levels.[125]

Tobacco smoking may cause a transient rise in the IOP.[126,127] In one study, smoking one cigarette caused an increase in IOP of greater than 5 mm Hg in 37% of open-angle glaucoma patients and in 11% of nonglaucomatous individuals.[127]

Heroin and *marijuana* lower the IOP (the latter is discussed further in Section Three), while *LSD* causes an IOP elevation.[128] *Corticosteroids* may also cause IOP elevation and are discussed in detail in Section Two.

Systemic *vasodilators*, including glyceryl trinitrate (nitroglycerine),[129,130] pentaerythritol tetranitrate,[129] isosorbide dinitrate,[130] becyclan,[130] nicotinic acid,[131] and cyclandelate,[131] are all reported to have no influence on IOP in normal or glaucomatous eyes with open angles. However, one study revealed that nitroglycerin, when administered by perfusion techniques, and isosorbide dinitrate lower the IOP in normal individuals as well as patients with open-angle or angle closure glaucoma.[132] A systemic digitalis preparation, beta-methyldigoxin, has also been shown to cause a decrease in IOP.[133]

Systemic *anticholinergics*, such as atropine,[134,135] propantheline,[136] and pizotifen,[137] have been found to have no influence on IOP in normal or glaucomatous eyes with open anterior chamber angles, especially with short-term therapy. However, topical cyclopentolate will elevate the IOP in some patients with open-angle glaucoma,[134,138] and it has been suggested that these patients may also manifest a slight pressure rise in response to long-term administration of systemic anticholinergics.[135] Drugs that may precipitate angle-closure attacks of glaucoma are discussed in Section Two.

Anticonvulsants (e.g., diphenylhydantoin[109]), amphetamines (e.g., dextroamphetamines[109]), and antihistamines (e.g., cimetidine, a histamine-2 receptor antagonist[139]) have not been found to influence the IOP in eyes with open angles.

Prostaglandins, when administered topically, may either increase or decrease IOP, depending on the dosage used, and they are discussed further in Section Three. In women undergoing prostaglandin-induced abortion, no significant effect on IOP was observed.[140]

TONOMETERS AND TONOMETRY

Classification of Tonometers

All clinical tonometers measure the IOP by relating a deformation of the globe to the force responsible for the deformation. The

a.

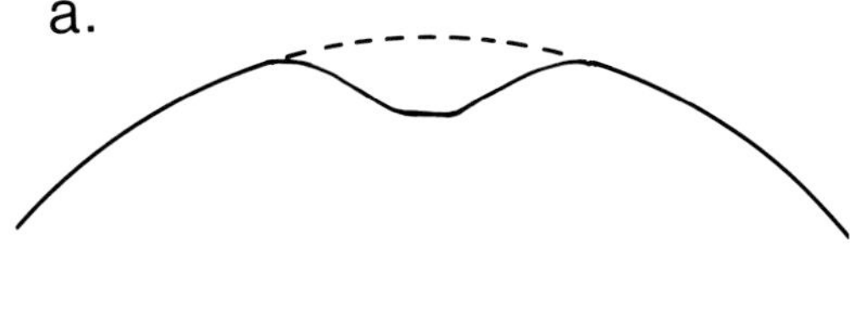

b.

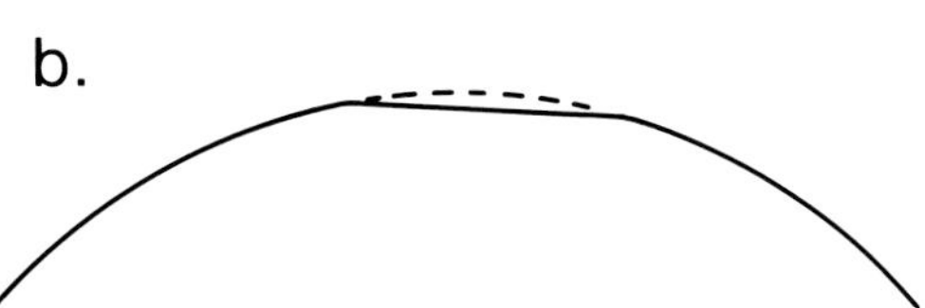

Figure 4.2. Corneal deformation created by (**a.**) indentation tonometers (a truncated cone) and (**b.**) applanation tonometers (simple flattening).

two basic types of tonometers differ according to the shape of the deformation: indentation and applanation (flattening).

Indentation Tonometers

The shape of the deformation with this type of tonometer is a truncated cone (Fig. 4-2*a*). However, the precise shape is variable and unpredictable. In addition, these instruments displace a relatively large intraocular volume. As a result of these characteristics, conversion tables based on empirical data from in vitro and in vivo studies must be used to estimate the IOP. The prototype of this group is the *Schiøtz* tonometer, which was introduced in 1905.

Applanation Tonometers

The shape of the deformation with these tonometers is a simple flattening (Fig. 4.2*b*) and, because the shape is constant, its relationship to the IOP can, in most cases, be derived from mathematical calculations. The applanation tonometers are further differentiated on the basis of the variable that is measured.

Variable Force. This type of tonometer measures the force that is required to applanate (flatten) a standard area of the corneal surface. The prototype is the *Goldmann* applanation tonometer, which was introduced in 1954.

Variable Area. Other applanation tonometers measure the area of the cornea that is flattened by a known force (weight). The prototype in this group is the *Maklakov* tonometer, which was introduced in 1885. However, the division between indentation and applanation tonometers does not correlate entirely with the magnitude of intraocular volume displacement. In the case of Maklakov-type tonometers, the volume displacement is sufficiently large to require the use of conversion tables.

Noncontact Tonometer

A third type of tonometer measures the time required to deform the cornea in response to a standard force (a puff of air).

We will first consider the descriptions and techniques of these various tonometers and then compare their relative values and limitations.

Schiøtz Indentation Tonometry

Description of Tonometer

The body of the tonometer has a footplate, which rests on the cornea. A plunger moves freely (except for the effect of friction) within a shaft in the footplate, and the degree to which it indents the cornea is indicated by the movement of a needle on a scale. A 5.5 gram weight is permanently fixed to the plunger, which can be increased to 7.5, 10, or 15 grams by adding additional weights (Fig. 4.3).

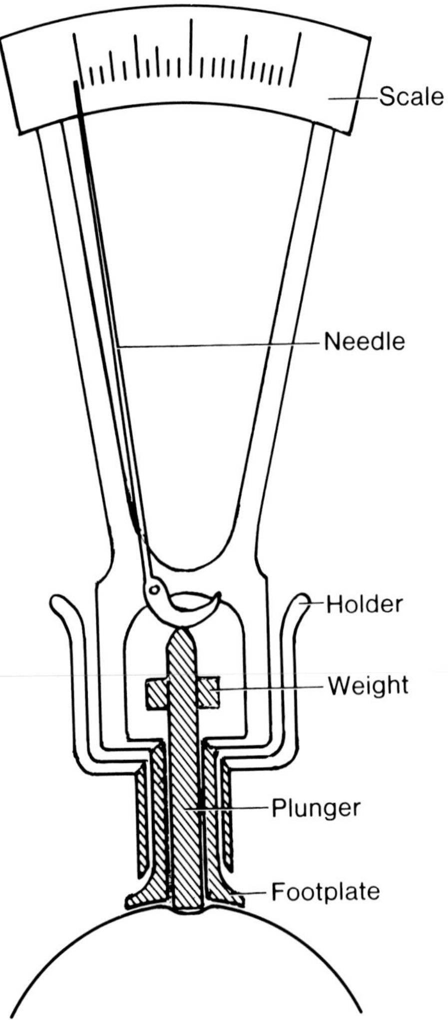

Figure 4.3. Cutaway view showing basic features of Schiøtz-type indentation tonometer.

Basic Concept of Indentation Tonometry

When the plunger indents the cornea, the baseline or resting pressure (P_o) is artificially raised to a new value (P_t). Since the tonometer actually measures P_t, it is necessary to estimate P_o for each scale reading and weight. Schiøtz estimated P_o in experiments in which a manometer was attached to enucleated eyes by a cannula inserted through the optic nerve. A stopcock was placed between the cannula and manometer, and a reservoir was used to adjust the pressure in the eye (Fig. 4.4). He then made two sets of readings. In one set (open manometer), the stopcock was left open when the tonometer was placed on the cornea, which allowed correlation of P_t with the scale reading and weight. In the second set (closed manometer), the desired pressure was introduced in the eye and the stopcock was closed before placing the tonometer on the cornea, thereby allowing correlation of P_o with the scale reading and weight. It was the data from these sets of readings that were used to calibrate the tonometer.

The change in pressure from P_o to P_t is an expression of the resistance an eye offers to the displacement of a volume of fluid (V_c). In the early days of indentation tonometry, the IOP values that were considered to

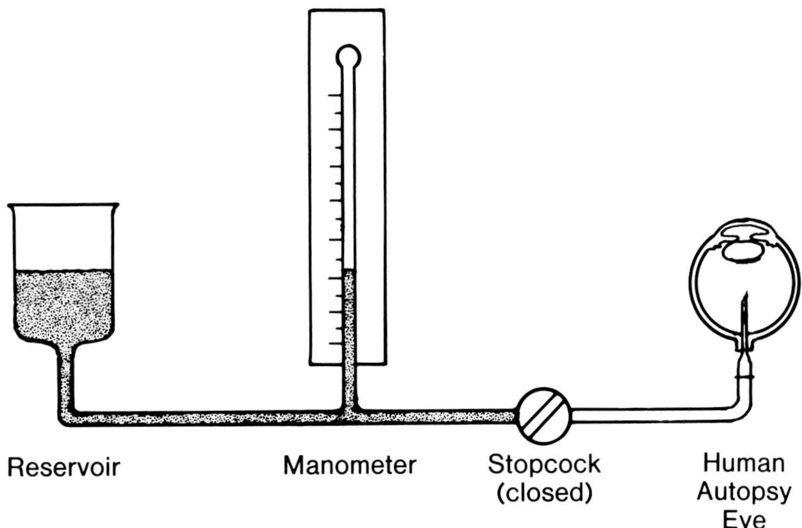

Figure 4.4. Apparatus used in manometric calibration of Schiøtz tonometer.

be normal were considerably higher than today's accepted range, and it was not until Friedenwald's work, beginning in the late 1930s, that indentation tonometry acquired a mathematic basis. Friedenwald[141] developed an empiric formula for the linear relationship between the logarithm of the pressure and the volume change in a given eye. The formula has a single numerical constant, the *coefficient of ocular rigidity* (*K*), which is roughly an expression of the distensibility of the eye. He developed a nomogram for estimating *K* based on two tonometric readings with different weights, and subsequent studies using applanation tonometry with different sized applanating areas have supported the accuracy of his formulations.[142] Based on this formula and additional experiments, Friedenwald[143] calculated an average *K* of 0.0245 and used this to develop a set of conversion tables, referred to as the 1948 tables. He later revised the average *K* to a value of 0.0215,[144] on which he based a new set of tables that became known as the 1955 tables.[145] However, subsequent studies indicate that the 1948 tables agree more closely with measurements by Goldmann applanation tonometry.[146,147]

Technique of Schiøtz Indentation Tonometry

With the patient in a supine position and fixing on a target just overhead, the examiner separates the eyelids and gently rests the tonometer footplate on the anesthetized cornea in a position that allows free vertical movement of the plunger (Fig. 4.5). When the tonometer is properly positioned, the examiner will observe a fine movement of the indicator needle on the scale in response to the ocular pulsations. The scale reading should be taken as the average between the extremes of these excursions. It is customary to start with the fixed 5.5 gram weight. However, if the scale reading is 4 or less, additional weight should be added to the plunger. A conversion table is then used to derive the IOP in millimeters of mercury (mm Hg) from the scale reading and plunger weight. The scale reading, weight, IOP, and conversion table from which the pressure value was derived should all be recorded. For example, a scale reading of 7, using a 5.5 gram weight, which corresponds to an IOP of 12 mm Hg according to the 1955 conversion tables, would be written as 7/5.5 = 12 mm Hg ('55).

Sources of Error with Indentation Tonometry

The accuracy of indentation tonometry depends on the assumption that all eyes respond the same to the external force of indentation, which is not the case. The following are some of the more common variables that introduce potential for error.

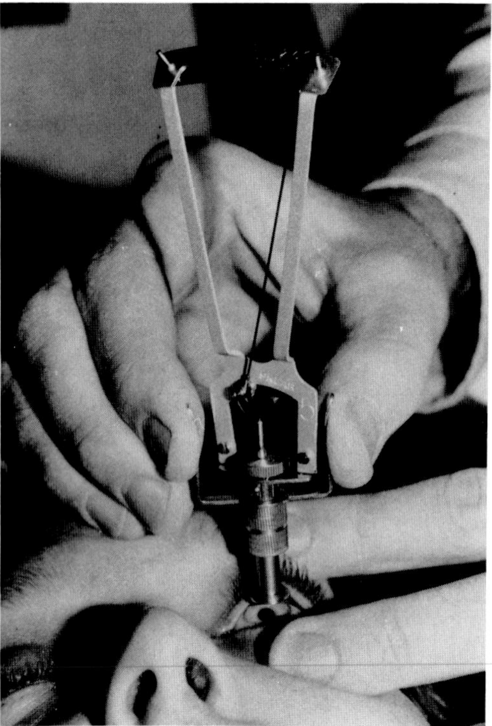

Figure 4.5. Technique of indentation tonometry with Schiøtz tonometer.

Ocular Rigidity. Since conversion tables are based on an "average" coefficient of ocular rigidity (*K*), eyes that deviate significantly from this *K* value will give false IOP measurements. A high *K* will cause a falsely high IOP, while a low *K* will lead to a falsely low reading. Factors that have been associated with abnormally *high ocular rigidity* include high hyperopia,[148] extreme myopia,[141] long-standing glaucoma,[141] age-related macular degeneration,[149] and vasoconstrictor therapy.[141] Conditions associated with a *reduction in K* include high myopia;[148] elevated IOP[150] (which may explain the lower *K* values during water provocative testing); osteogenesis imperfecta;[151] miotic therapy, especially with cholinesterase inhibitors;[148] vasodilator therapy;[141] and retinal detachment surgery utilizing cryopexy,[152] scleral buckling,[153,154] vitrectomy,[154] or intravitreal injection of a compressible gas.[153–155] Keratoconus was once thought to be associated with an abnormally low *K*, but this may be an artifact resulting from the thin cornea, since it is not seen after keratoplasty for this condition.[156] Reports on the relationship of age to ocular rigidity are conflicting.[141,148,157]

The technique for determining *K* is based on the concept of differential tonometry, using two indentation tonometric readings with different weights and Friedenwald's nomogram as previously discussed.[141] It may be more accurate, however, to obtain one reading with a Schiøtz tonometer using a 10 gram weight and the second with an applanation tonometer and to plot these readings on Friedenwald's nomogram.[158] Chandler and Grant[159] suggested that the estimation of ocular rigidity by any method is premature and of little value until more accurate calibrations are achieved. Attempts to represent more accurately the pressure-volume relationship of the corneoscleral coat over a wide range have included a single-parameter ocular rigidity function in which the proportionality constant *K* is insensitive to changes in IOP.[160]

Blood Volume Alteration. The variable expulsion of intraocular blood during indentation tonometry may also influence the IOP measurement.[161]

Corneal Influences. Either a steeper or thicker cornea will cause a greater displacement of fluid during indentation tonometry, which leads to a falsely high IOP reading.[143]

The Moses Effect. This effect on indentation tonometry was discussed under "Tonography" in Chapter 3.

Electronic Indentation Tonometers

Grant combined the concept of Schiøtz tonometry with continuous electronic monitoring of the pressure for use in tonography (discussed in Chapter 3), and similar instruments were subsequently designed, although none are commonly used at this time.

Goldmann Applanation Tonometry

Basic Concept

Goldmann[162] based his concept of tonometry on a modification of the *Maklakov-Fick Law* (also referred to as the *Imbert-Fick Law*).[163] This law states that an external force (*W*) against a sphere equals the pres-

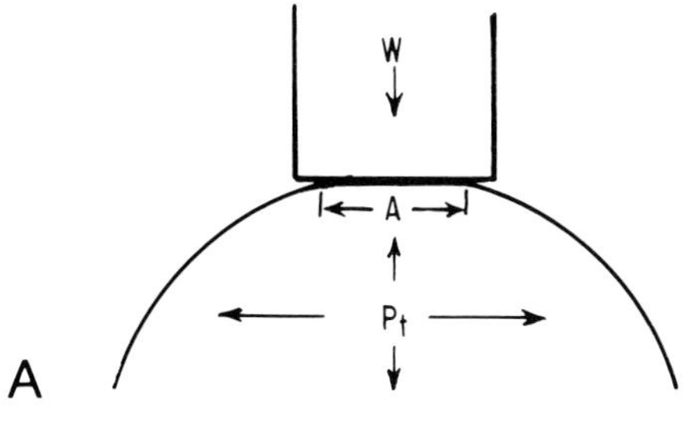

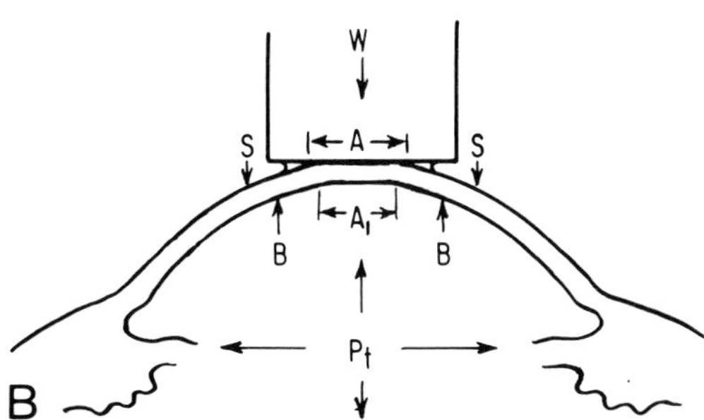

Figure 4.6. A, The Imbert-Fick Law ($W = P_t \times A$); **B,** Modification of Imbert-Fick Law for the cornea ($W + S = P_t \times A_1 + B$).

sure in the sphere (P_t) times the area flattened (applanated) by the external force (A) (Fig. 4.6*A*):

$$W = P_t \times A$$

The validity of the law requires that the sphere is (1) perfectly spherical, (2) dry, (3) perfectly flexible, and (4) infinitely thin. The cornea fails to satisfy any of these requirements, since it is aspherical and wet, and neither perfectly flexible nor infinitely thin. The moisture creates a surface tension (S), while the lack of flexibility requires a force to bend the cornea (B), which is independent of the internal pressure. In addition, since the cornea has a central thickness of approximately 0.55 mm, the outer area of flattening (A) is not the same as the inner area (A_I). Therefore, it was necessary to modify the Imbert-Fick Law in the following manner to account for these characteristics of the cornea (Fig. 4.6*B*):

$$W + S = P_t A_I + B$$

When $A_I = 7.35\ mm^2$, S balances B and $W = P_t$. This internal area of applanation is obtained when the diameter of the external area of corneal applanation is 3.06 mm, which is used in the standard instrument. An external area of 3.53 mm has been reported to be equally acceptable.[164] The volume displacement produced by applanating an area of 3.06 mm is approximately 0.50 mm^3, so that P_t is very close to P_o, and ocular rigidity does not significantly influence the measurement.

Description of Tonometer[165]

The instrument is mounted on a standard slit lamp in such a way that the examiner's view is directed through the center of a plastic biprism, which is used to applanate the cornea. Two beam-splitting prisms within the applanating unit optically convert the circular area of corneal contact into semicircles. The prisms are adjusted so that the inner margins of the semicircles overlap when 3.06 mm of cornea is applanated. In a variation of this design, the prisms are located near the slit lamp objective and the image is doubled and then displaced.[166] The biprism is attached by a rod to a housing, which contains a coil spring and series of levers that are used to adjust the force of the biprism against the cornea (Fig. 4.7).

Technique

The cornea is anesthetized with a topical preparation, and the tear film is stained with sodium fluorescein. With the cornea and biprism illuminated by a cobalt blue light from the slit lamp, the biprism is brought into gentle contact with the apex of the cornea (Fig. 4.8). The fluorescence of the stained tears facilitates visualization of the tear meniscus at the margin of contact between cornea and biprism. The staining may be accomplished by instilling a drop of topical anesthetic and touching a fluorescein-impregnated paper strip to the tears in the lower cul-de-sac. However, a 0.25% solution of sodium fluorescein has been shown to produce the optimum fluorescent semicircles,[167] and commercial solutions are available in combination with topical anesthetics.[168] Studies have shown that the preservative in these commercial preparations imparts a satisfactory degree of resistance to bacterial contamination,[168–170] especially when a pipette-type dispenser is used, al-

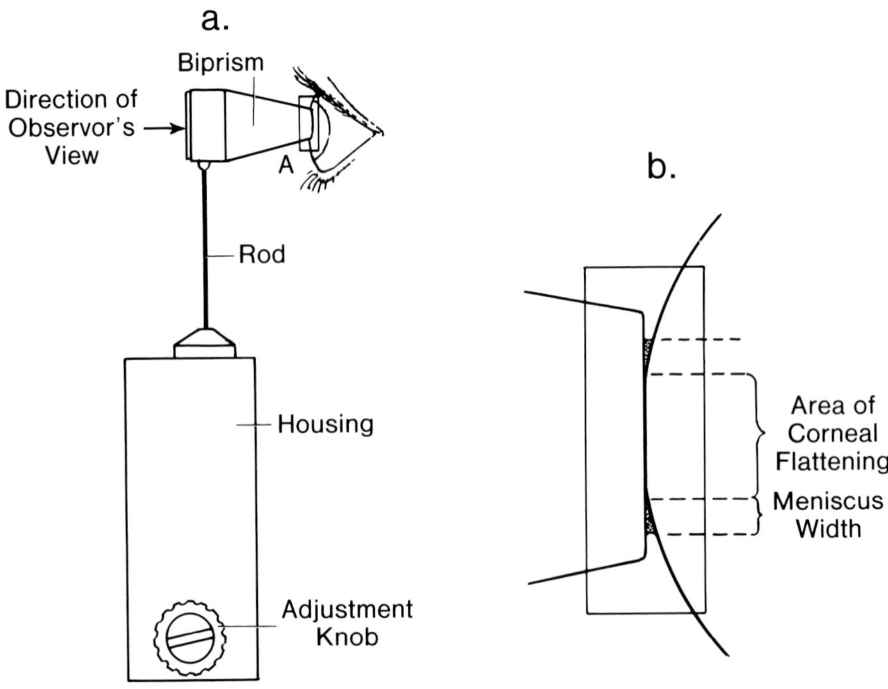

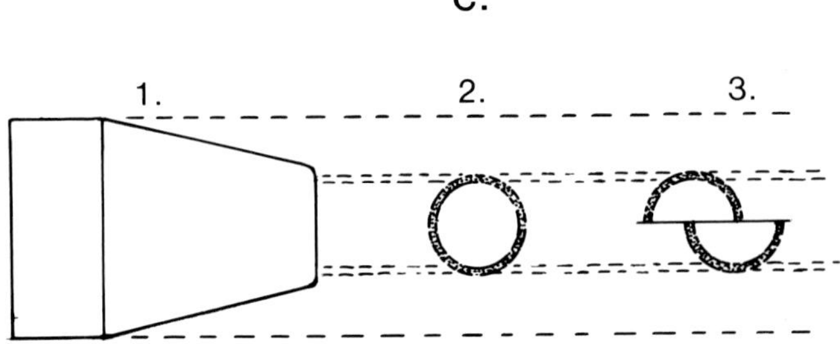

Figure 4.7. Goldmann-type applanation tonometry. **a.** Basic features of tonometer, shown in contact with patient's cornea. **b.** Enlargement shows tear film meniscus created by contact of biprism and cornea. **c.** View through biprism (*1.*) reveals circular meniscus (*2.*), which is converted into semicircles (*3.*) by prisms.

though the cap of a squeeze bottle may be a reservoir for bacterial contamination.[170] Some physicians have believed that Goldmann applanation tonometry could be performed without fluorescein, but this has been shown to give a significant underestimation of the IOP and is not recommended.[171] The fluorescent semicircles are viewed through the biprism, and the force against the cornea is adjusted until the inner edges overlap (Fig. 4.9). As with the indentation tonometer, the influence of the ocular pulsations is seen when the instrument is properly positioned, and the excursions must be averaged to give the desired endpoint. The IOP is then read directly from a scale on the tonometer housing. An electronic applanation tonometer has been described in which the applanation area is electronically defined and the IOP reading is automatically recorded.[172]

Sources of Error with Goldmann Tonometry

The Semicircles. The width of the meniscus may influence the reading slightly,

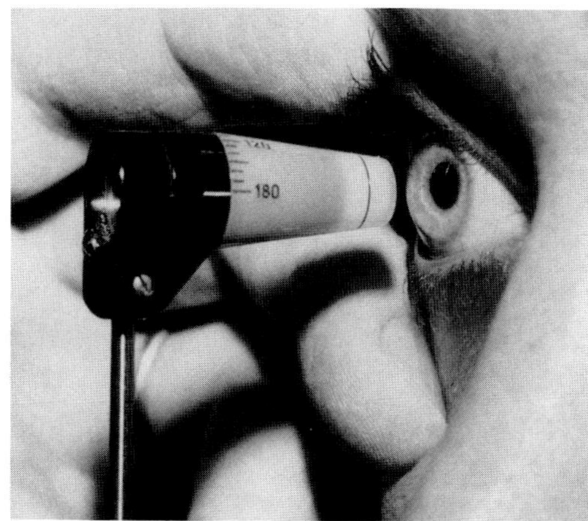

Figure 4.8. Technique of applanation tonometry with Goldmann tonometer.

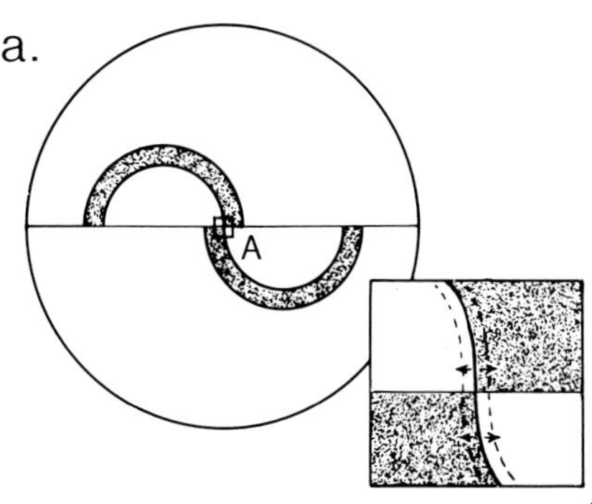

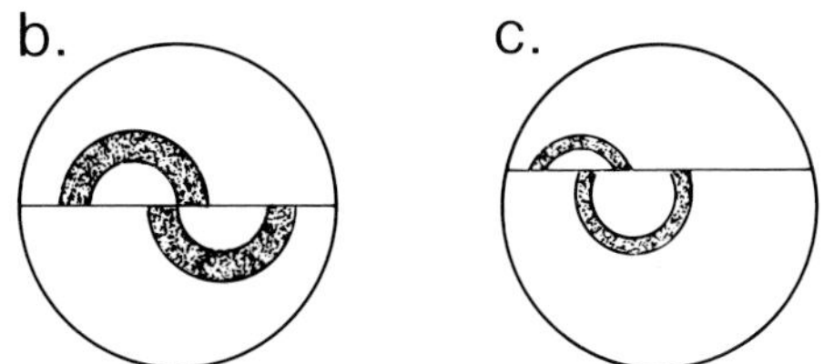

Figure 4.9. Semicircles of Goldmann-type applanation tonometry. **a.** Proper width and position. Enlargement (*A*) depicts excursions of semicircles caused by ocular pulsations. **b.** Semicircles are too wide. **c.** Improper vertical and horizontal alignment.

with wider menisci causing falsely higher pressure estimates.[163] Improper vertical alignment (one semicircle larger than the other) will also lead to a falsely high IOP estimate (Fig. 4.9).[165]

Corneal Variables. The thickness of the cornea has been shown to influence the pressure estimate, with thin corneas producing falsely low readings.[173] A thick cornea causes a falsely high measurement if the thickness is due to increased collagen fibrils,[173,174] whereas low readings occur if the thickness is due to edema.[173] Corneal curvature has also been shown to influence IOP measurements, with an increase of approximately 1 mm Hg for each 3 diopters of increase in corneal power.[175] Marked corneal astigmatism will produce an elliptical area of corneal contact. When the biprism is in the usual orientation, with the mires displaced horizontally, the IOP will be underestimated for with-the-rule and overestimated for against-the-rule astigmatism, with approximately 1 mm Hg of error for every 4 diopters of astigmatism.[176] To minimize this error, the biprism may be rotated until the dividing line between the prisms is 45° to the major axis of the ellipse,[165] or an average may be taken of horizontal and vertical readings.[175] An irregular cornea will also distort the semicircles and interfere with the accuracy of the IOP estimates.[165]

Prolonged Contact. Prolonged contact of the biprism with the cornea leads to corneal injury, as manifested by staining, which makes multiple readings unsatisfactory.[165] In addition, prolonged contact causes an apparent decrease in IOP over a period of minutes.[165] The latter phenomenon is less pronounced in eyes with carotid occlusive disease, suggesting that it may be related to intraocular blood.[177]

Calibration. It is also essential that the Goldmann tonometer be calibrated periodically. Instructions for quick, simple calibration come with the instrument, and this should be performed at least monthly. If the tonometer does not meet calibration specifications, it should be returned to the manufacturer or distributor for correction.

Disinfection of Goldmann (and other) Tonometers

With all tonometers that contact the eye, there is the risk of transmitting infection, such as the adenovirus of epidemic keratoconjunctivitis (EKC) and herpes simplex virus type 1. In addition, there is the potential for transmitting more serious diseases, such as hepatitis and acquired immunodeficiency syndrome (AIDS). Hepatitis B surface antigen DNA polymerase and hepatitis B virus DNA have been found in the tears of a high percentage of hepatitis B carriers,[178,179] and the antigen was detected on the tonometer tip in one-fourth of the patients in one series.[178] Human T cell lymphotrophic virus type III (HTLV-III), the causative agent of AIDS, has been isolated from the tears in 5 of 16 patients with AIDS or AIDS-related complex.[180,181] Although there is no evidence to suggest transmission of HTLV-III by contact with tears, precautions are needed to minimize this possibility as well as the spread of other microbial pathogens that might be present in tears.

A variety of techniques has been described for disinfecting tonometer tips. Adenovirus type 8 was removed or inactivated by soaking the applanation tip for 15 minutes in diluted sodium hypochlorite (1:10 household bleach), 3% hydrogen peroxide, or 70% isopropyl alcohol; or by wiping with alcohol, 1:1000 merthiolate, or dry tissues.[182] Herpes simplex virus type 1 was eliminated by swabbing the applanation tonometer head with 70% isopropyl alcohol.[183] Ten minutes of continuous rinsing in running tap water was reported to remove all detectable hepatitis B surface antigen from contaminated tonometers.[178] Wiping with 3% hydrogen peroxide or 70% isopropyl alcohol swabs completely disinfected tonometer tips contaminated with the human immunodeficiency virus type I of AIDS.[184] Other techniques for preventing spread of infection include disposable film covers for applanation tips[185,186] and sterilization by exposure to ultraviolet light.[187] A disinfectant receptacle has also been described for applanation tonometer heads utilizing a plastic Petri dish with 11-mm holes in the cover.[188]

In August 1988, a Clinical Alert was issued jointly by the American Academy of Ophthalmology, the National Society to Prevent Blindness, and the Contact Lens Association of Ophthalmologists with updated recommendations for ophthalmic practice in relation to AIDS and other infectious diseases.[189] Wiping with an alcohol sponge was considered to be an adequate disinfection procedure for Goldmann-type applanation tips as well as Schiøtz tonometers, digital pneumotonometers, and noncontact tonometers. Alternative measures for disinfecting applanation tips, as previously recommended by the Centers for Disease Control,[190] involve soaking in 1:10 household bleach, 3% hydrogen peroxide, or 70% isopropyl alcohol for 5 minutes. With any technique, it is important to carefully remove the disinfectant from the contact surface before the next use, since both alcohol[191] and hydrogen peroxide[192] have been shown to cause transient corneal defects.

Other Applanation Tonometers with Variable Force

Hand-Held Goldmann-Type Tonometers

Perkins Applanation Tonometer. This instrument uses the same biprism as the Goldmann applanation tonometer. The light source is powered by a battery, and the force is varied manually. A counterbalance makes it possible to use the instrument in either the vertical or horizontal position (Fig. 4.10).[193]

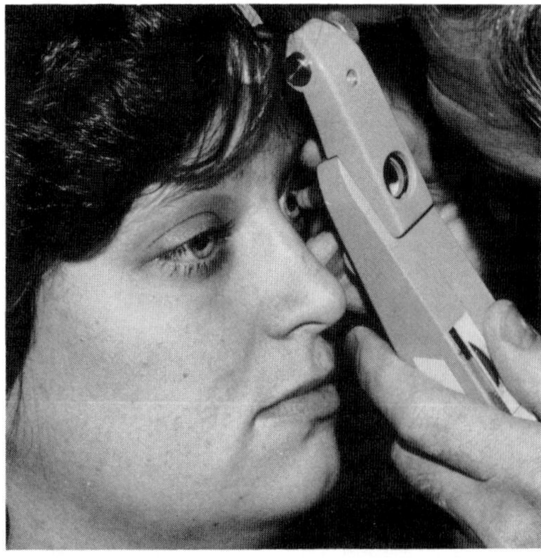

Figure 4.10. Technique of applanation tonometry with Perkins tonometer.

Draeger Applanation Tonometer. This instrument is similar to the Perkins tonometer but uses a different biprism and has an electric motor that varies the force.[194,195]

Mackay-Marg Tonometer

Although the original instrument is no longer available, newer models have been developed that use the same basic principle. Therefore, we will first consider the original unit and then the newer Mackay-Marg-type tonometers.

Basic Concept.[196] The force measured is that which is required to keep the flat plate of a plunger flush with a surrounding sleeve against the pressure of corneal deformation. The effect of corneal rigidity (i.e., the force required to bend the cornea) is transferred to the sleeve, so the plate reads only the IOP.

Description of Instrument.[197] The plate has a diameter of 1.5 mm and is surrounded by a rubber sleeve. The force required to keep the plate flush with the sleeve is electronically monitored and recorded on a paper strip.

Technique.[197] As the instrument tip momentarily touches the cornea, the tracing (representing the force required to keep the plate flush with the sleeve) rises until the applanated area reaches a diameter of 1.5 mm. At this point (the crest), the pressure against the plate represents the IOP plus the force required to bend the cornea. The tracing then falls as the effect of corneal rigidity is transferred to the surrounding sleeve. When a corneal diameter of 3 mm is flattened (the initial trough), the plate is considered to be reading only the IOP. The tracing then rises as a result of artificial elevation of the IOP (Fig. 4.11). Since the tonometer

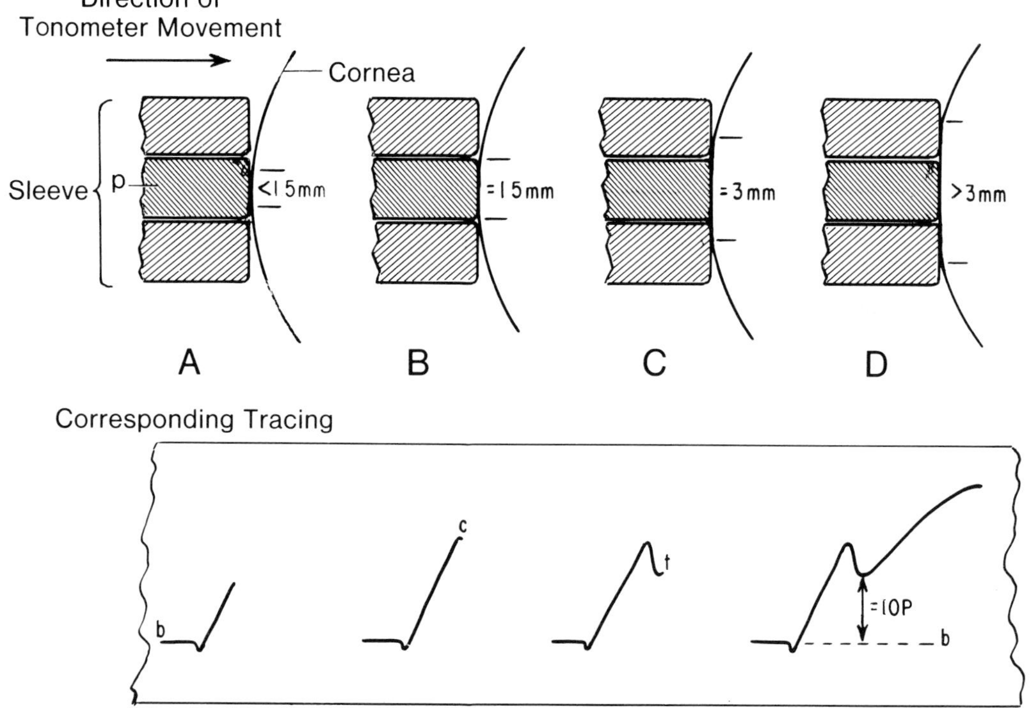

Figure 4.11. Mackay-Marg tonometry (modified from Marg, E, Mackay, RS, Oechsli, R[197]). **A,** As plate (*p*) contacts cornea, tracing begins to rise. **B,** Crest (*c*) is reached when diameter of contact equals that of plate surface (*1.5 mm*). **C,** With further corneal flattening, force of bending cornea is transferred to sleeve, and tracing falls to trough (*t*) when diameter of contact equals 3 mm. **D,** Still further corneal flattening leads to artificial elevation of intraocular pressure (*IOP*). Distance from baseline (*b*) of tracing to trough is read as the IOP.

records IOP instantaneously, several readings should be averaged to compensate for fluctuations resulting from ocular pulsation.

Mackay-Marg-Type Tonometers

The newer models differ from the Mackay-Marg tonometer in having an internal logic program that automatically selects the acceptable measurements and rejects the inappropriate ones. Three or more good IOP readings are averaged and displayed on a digital readout. Among those that have been clinically evaluated are the *CAT 100* applanation tonometer,[198] the *Challenger* digital electronic applanation tonometer (outcome of the redesigned EMT-20),[199] and the *Biotronics* tonometer.[200] None of these has yet been shown to be sufficiently accurate for clinical use.

Tono-Pen. This hand-held Mackay-Marg-type tonometer has a strain gauge that creates an electrical signal as the foot plate flattens the cornea.[201] A built-in single chip microprocessor senses the proper force curves and averages four to 10 readings to give a final digital readout. It also provides the percentage of variability between the lowest and highest acceptable readings from 5 to 20%. The Tono-Pen has had the most extensive clinical evaluation of any Mackay-Marg-type tonometer, although the reported results have been conflicting (these are discussed later in this chapter under "Comparison of Tonometers").

Pneumatic Tonometers (Pneumotonometer)[202,203]

Basic Concept. The concept of this tonometer is similar to that of the Mackay-Marg in that a central sensing device measures the IOP, while the force required to bend the cornea is transferred to a surrounding structure. The sensor in this case, however, is air pressure, rather than an electronically controlled plunger.

Description of Instrument. At one end of a pencil-like holder is a sensing nozzle, which has an outer diameter of 0.25 inch and a central chamber of 2.0 mm. The nozzle is covered with a silastic diaphragm, and pressurized air in the central chamber exhausts at the face of the nozzle between the orifice of the central chamber and the diaphragm.

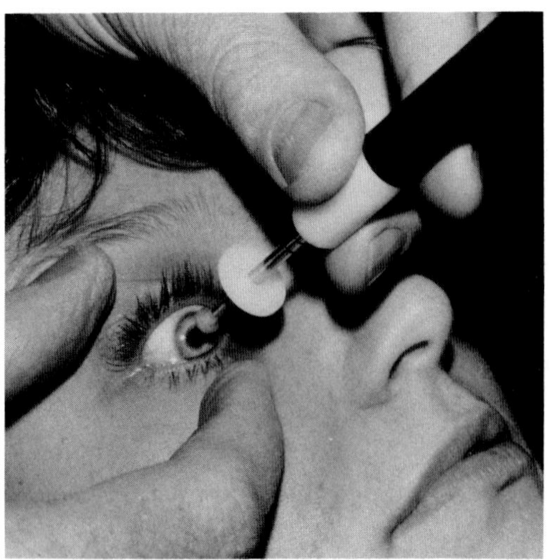

Figure 4.12. Technique of tonometry with pneumatic tonometer.

The air pressure is dependent on the resistance to the exhaust, and a pneumatic-to-electronic transducer converts the air pressure to a recording on a paper strip.

Technique. As the sensing nozzle touches the cornea, the tracing rises as an increasing area of corneal surface comes in contact with the diaphragm (Fig. 4.12). When the area of contact equals that of the central chamber, an initial inflection is recorded, which represents the IOP and the force required to bend the cornea. With further enlargement of the corneal contact, the bending force is transferred to the face of the nozzle and the tracing falls to a trough, which is interpreted as the actual IOP. Still further contact leads to artificial pressure elevation and a second inflection (Fig. 4.13). The instrument can also be used for continuous IOP monitoring.

Maklakov Applanation Tonometry

Basic Concept. Maklakov introduced the concept in which IOP is estimated by measuring the area of cornea that is flattened by a known weight.[204] It is still popular in Russia.

Instrument and Technique.[204,205] A dumbbell-shaped metal cylinder has flat end-plates of polished glass on either end with diameters of 10 mm. A set of four such instruments is available, weighing 5, 7.5, 10, and

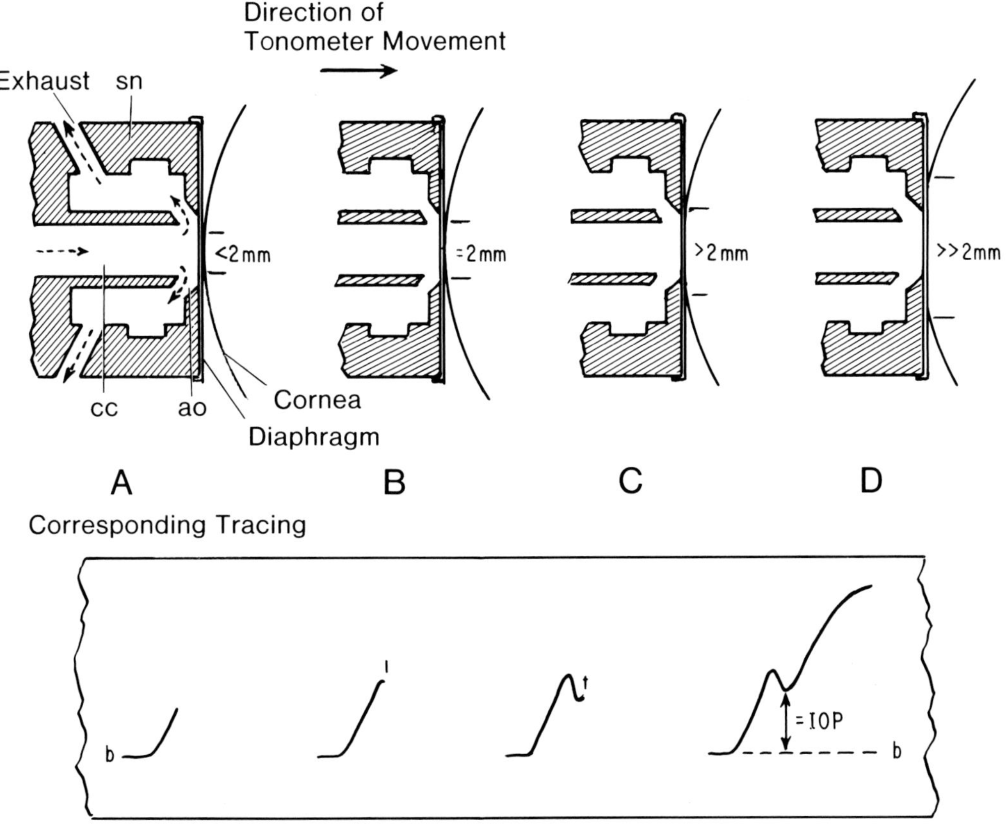

Figure 4.13. Pneumatic tonometry (modified from Durham, DG, Bigliano, RP, Masino, JA[202]). **A,** As sensing nozzle (*sn*) touches cornea, resistance to air flow (*dotted lines*) begins to increase at annular opening (*ao*), with corresponding rise in tracing. **B,** When diameter of corneal contact equals 2 mm, an initial inflection (*i*) is recorded. **C,** With further corneal flattening, force of bending cornea is transferred to face of sensor, and air pressure in central chamber (*cc*) measures IOP, represented by distance from baseline (*b*) to trough (*t*) of tracing. **D,** Further corneal compression by tonometer leads to artificial IOP rise.

15 grams, and a cross-action wire handle is supplied to support the instrument on the cornea. A layer of dye (a suspension of argyrol, glycerin, and water) is applied to either endplate and, with the patient in a supine position and the cornea anesthetized, the instrument is allowed to rest vertically on the cornea for 1 second. This produces a circular white imprint on the endplate, which corresponds to the area of cornea that was flattened. The diameter of the white area is measured with a transparent plastic measuring scale to 0.1 mm, and the IOP is read from a conversion table in the column corresponding to the weight used.

Conversion Tables. Although the volume displacement with Maklakov-type applanation tonometry is less than with indentation tonometry, it is large enough that ocular rigidity must be considered in computing the IOP. Kalfa recognized this problem at approximately the same time that Friedenwald was applying the concept of ocular rigidity to Schiøtz tonometry.[206] He, too, used different weights to estimate the average ocular rigidity of the eyeball, which he called an "elastometric rise." New conversion tables have been developed that provide nomograms for the differential tonometry.[207]

Table 4.2.
Applanation Tonometers with Variable Area

Tonometer	Description/Use
1. Maklakov-Kalfa[204]	1. Prototype
2. Applanometer[208]	2. Ceramic endplates
3. Tonomat[209]	3. Disposable endplates
4. Halberg tonometer[210]	4. Transparent endplate for direct reading: multiple weights
5. Barraquer tonometer[211]	5. Plastic tonometer for use in operating room
6. Ocular Tension Indicator[212]	6. Utilizes Goldmann biprism and standard weight, for screening (measures above or below 21 mm Hg)
7. GlaucoTest[213]	7. Screening tonometer with multiple endplates for selecting different "cut-off" pressures

Other Maklakov-type tonometers are listed in Table 4.2.

Noncontact Tonometer

The noncontact tonometer (NCT) was introduced by Grolman[214] in 1972 and has the unique advantage over other tonometers of not touching the eye, other than with a puff of air. This instrument should not be confused with the pneumatic tonometers, which were discussed previously.

Basic Concept. A puff of room air creates a constant force, which momentarily deforms the cornea. It is difficult to determine the exact nature of the corneal deformation, although it is postulated that the central cornea is flattened at the moment the pressure measurement is made. The time from an internal reference point to the moment of presumed flattening is measured and converted to IOP based on prior comparisons with readings from Goldmann applanation tonometers.

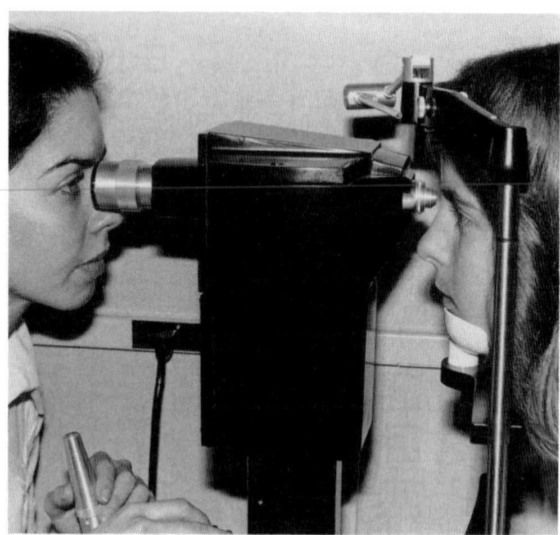

Figure 4.14. Technique of noncontact tonometry. Operator (*left*) aligns target, reflected from cornea of patient (*right*), and triggers air puff with right hand when proper alignment is achieved.

Description of Instrument.[214–216] The original NCT is mounted on a table and consists of three subsystems: (1) An alignment system allows the operator to optically align the patient's cornea in three dimensions (axial, vertical, and lateral); (2) an optoelectronic applanation monitoring system consists of a transmitter, which directs a collimated beam of light at the corneal vertex, and a receiver and detector, which accept only parallel, coaxial rays reflected from the cornea; and (3) a pneumatic system generates a puff of room air, which is directed against the cornea. A newer, hand-held NCT, the *Pulsair* tonometer, is also commercially available.[217,218]

Technique.[214–216] The patient observes an internal target while the operator aligns the cornea by superimposing a reflection of the target from the patient's cornea on a stationary ring (Fig. 4.14). During this time, light from the transmitter is reflected from the undisturbed cornea, which allows only a small number of rays to enter the receiver. When the cornea is properly aligned, the operator depresses a trigger that causes a puff of air to be directed against the cornea. At the moment that the central cornea is flattened, the greatest number of reflected light rays are received, which is recorded as the peak intensity of light detected. The time from an internal reference point to the moment of maximum light detection is converted to IOP and displayed on a digital readout (Fig. 4.15).

The time interval for an average NCT measurement is 1–3 msec (1/500 of the cardiac cycle) and is random with respect to the phase of the cardiac cycle so that the ocular pulse becomes a significant variable (i.e., cannot be averaged as with some tonometers). Furthermore, glaucomatous eyes have a significantly greater range of momentary fluctuations in IOP.[219] The probability that an instantaneous pressure measurement will lie within a given range of mean IOP increases as the number of tonometric measurements, averaged together, increases.[220] For this reason, it is recommended that a minimum of three readings within 3 mm Hg be taken and averaged as the IOP.

Miscellaneous Tonometers

Continuous IOP Monitoring Devices. In the diagnosis and management of glaucoma, there is need for a tonometer that can monitor the IOP continuously for hours, days, or indefinitely without artificially altering the pressure. Preliminary laboratory studies have investigated the feasibility of remote IOP monitoring with telemetric devices. Strain gauges can be used to drive the monitor. The strain gauge can be placed in a contact lens to measure changes in the meridional angle of the corneoscleral junction,[221] or it can be embedded in an encircling scleral band to measure the distention of the globe.[222] Another approach is to use a scleral applanating device attached to a passive radio telemetric pressure transducer.[223,224] An instrument with applanating suction cups has also been devised, which allows bilateral recoding of IOP for up to 1 hour in supine subjects.[225]

Home Tonometry. Another approach to obtaining multiple IOP measurements at various times of day and night (aside from admission to the hospital for tonometry by a physician, nurse, or technician) is to have the measurements made at home. This has been done by teaching a family member to perform Schiøtz tonometry on the relative, although the accuracy of the results is highly variable. A new device, which uses the applanation principle and can be used by the patient without assistance, showed promise in preliminary studies.[36,37,226,227]

Attempts have also been made to estimate the IOP by measuring the duration of contact of a spring driven hammer with the eye (impact tonometer),[228] or the frequency of a vibrating probe in contact with the cornea (Vibra-Tonometer).[229]

Comparison of Tonometers

Comparison with Goldmann Tonometer in Eyes with Regular Corneas

The most precise method for evaluating the accuracy of a tonometer is to compare it with manometric measurements of the cannulated anterior chamber. While this technique is frequently used with animal and autopsy eyes, it has obvious limitations in large scale human studies. The alternative is to compare the tonometer in question against the instrument that previous studies have shown to be the most accurate. In eyes with regular corneas, the Goldmann applanation tonometer is generally accepted as the standard against which other tonometers must be compared. It should be noted, however, that even when two readings are taken on the same eye with Goldmann tonometers within a short time frame, using either one instrument and one examiner[230] or two instruments and two examiners,[231] at least 30% of the paired readings will differ by 2 and 3 mm Hg or more, respectively. Therefore, an error of approximately 2 mm Hg is assumed to be inherent in even the most accurate of pressure measurements.

Schiøtz Tonometer. Studies consistently indicate that the Schiøtz tonometer reads lower than the Goldmann,[232–234] even when the postural influence on IOP is eliminated by performing both measurements in the supine position.[143,235,236] In one study, age was found to be the most important source of variation, with the greatest discrepancies occurring in the fifties and sixties.[237] The magnitude of disagreement be-

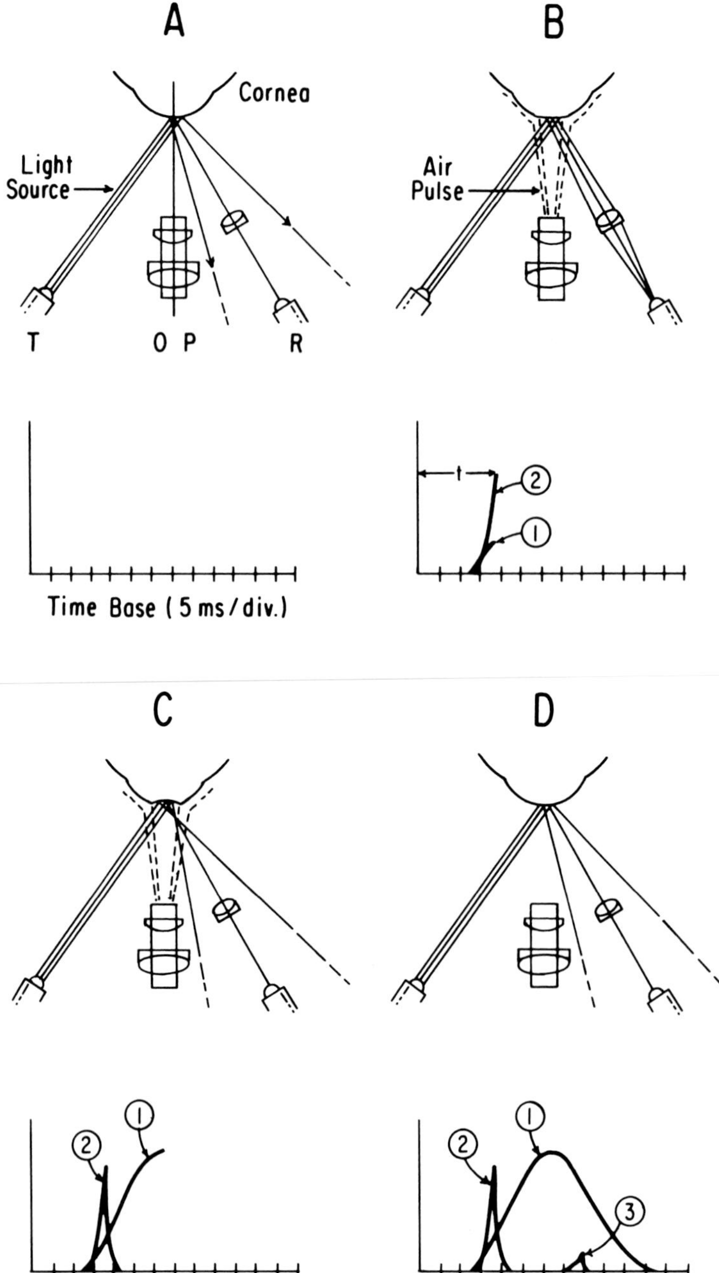

Figure 4.15. Noncontact tonometry (modified from Grolman, B[214]). **A,** Light source from transmitter (*T*) is reflected from undisturbed cornea toward receiver (*R*), while cornea is aligned by optical system (*O*). **B,** Air puff (*1*) from pneumatic system (*P*) deforms cornea, which increases the number of light rays (*2*) received and detected by R. Time (*t*) from internal reference point to moment of maximum light detection (which presumably corresponds to applanation of the cornea) is converted to IOP (based on calibrations with Goldmann applanation tonometer) and displayed on digital readout. **C,** Continued air pulse produces momentary concavity of cornea, causing sharp reduction in light rays received by R. **D,** As cornea returns to undisturbed state, a second moment of applanation causes another light peak (*3*). (Reprinted from Surv Ophthal 24:211, 1980, by permission.)

tween the two tonometers and the influence of ocular rigidity are such that the Schiøtz tonometer is thought to indicate only that the IOP is within a certain range,[143] and it is of limited value even for screening purposes.[233,234,238] The Schiøtz tonometer is particularly unsuitable for situations in which ocular rigidity is known to be significantly altered, such as following retinal detachment surgery[152–154] or in eyes containing compressible gas.[153–155,239]

Perkins Applanation Tonometer. This instrument has compared favorably with the Goldmann tonometer.[240,241] In one study, the difference between readings with the two instruments, expressed as the root mean square difference, was 1.4 mm Hg.[240] This instrument is especially useful in infants and children and is accurate in the horizontal as well as the vertical position. It is, therefore, an excellent tonometer to use in the operating room for examinations under anesthesia, as well as on the ward or wherever a Goldmann applanation tonometer is not available.

Draeger Applanation Tonometer. Comparative studies with Goldmann tonometry have given inconsistent results, with one showing satisfactory agreement,[241] while another found the Draeger instrument to be no better than a properly-used Schiøtz tonometer.[242] Because of its more complex design, the Draeger tonometer is more difficult to use than the Perkins, and patient acceptance tends to be worse.

Mackay-Marg Tonometer. A highly significant correlation was found between IOP readings with the Mackay-Marg and Goldmann tonometers using topical anesthesia for both instruments, with the Mackay-Marg reading systematically higher and the Goldmann systematically lower than their mean results.[243] When the Mackay-Marg was used without anesthesia, the mean IOP was approximately 2 mm Hg higher than that obtained by the same instrument with anesthesia.[243] One study showed significant discrepancies between Mackay-Marg and Goldmann measurements when the former was used by a technician.[244]

Mackay-Marg-Type Tonometers. As previously noted, most of the newer instruments that use the Mackay-Marg principle (e.g., CAT 100, Challenger, EMT-20, and the Biotronics tonometers) have not been found to be sufficiently accurate for clinical use.[198–200] The *Tono-Pen* has compared favorably with manometric readings in human autopsy eyes.[245,246] In clinical comparisons with Goldmann applanation readings, some studies found a good correlation, especially within the normal IOP range,[246–248] although most studies agree that it underestimates Goldmann IOP in the higher range and overestimates in the lower range.[201,247,248] One study found an average absolute deviation of 2.70 mm Hg between paired Goldmann and Tono-Pen readings, with a difference of more than 5 mm Hg in 7% of the readings.[249] In another study, the discrepancy was not sufficiently systematic to allow the application of a correction factor for measurement of diurnal curves.[250]

Pneumatic Tonometers. Comparative studies with one pneumatic tonometer, the pneumatonograph, showed close correlations with Goldmann tonometers,[251,252] even when the pneumatic tonometer was operated by a technician.[234] However, the pneumatonograph read statistically higher,[251,252] and one study of an early model revealed an unsatisfactory correlation.[253] In a laboratory analysis of the pneumatonograph, the investigators found several errors that resulted in compression of the scale readings and an overestimation of the IOP even in the physiologic range.[254] They concluded that the instrument was not suitable for tonography.

Halberg Applanation Tonometer. This instrument compared more favorably with the Goldmann tonometer than did the Schiøtz,[234,255] although it compared less favorably than the pneumatonograph in one study.[234] Its use was considered to be easier to learn than Perkins hand-held tonometry,[256] although medical students in another study preferred and were more accurate with a Schiøtz tonometer.[257]

Glaucotest. Evaluations of this tonometer suggest that it is a good screening instrument,[213] even when used by a technician.[234]

Noncontact Tonometer. In most studies, comparisons with Goldmann applanation tonometers indicate that the NCT is reliable within the normal IOP range, although the reliability is reduced in the higher pressure ranges and is limited by an abnormal cornea or poor fixation.[214–216,258] One study found a close correlation between the mean IOP obtained by the two instruments, but considerable individual patient variation.[259]

The hand-held Pulsair NCT has compared favorably with Goldmann readings in normal and glaucomatous eyes[217] and was effective in identifying ocular hypertension in postoperative eyes.[218] One study, however, revealed an average absolute deviation of 2.49 mm Hg between paired Goldmann and Pulsair readings, with 8% differing by more than 5 mm Hg.[249] Another study showed a strong linear correlation between readings with the two instruments, although the Pulsair tended to read lower at pressures above the normal range.[260]

A significant advantage of the NCT is the elimination of potential hazards associated with all contact tonometers, including (1) abrasion of the cornea, (2) reactions to topical anesthetics, and (3) spread of infection. In addition, the instrument can be used reliably by paramedical personnel and has particular value in mass screening and possibly in studies of topical antiglaucoma drugs. Caution should be advised with abnormal corneas, however, since subepithelial bubbles have been seen after NCT measurements.[261] In addition, there is the remote chance that infection could be spread by contamination of the front surface of the instrument with tear film at the time of air impact, and it should be cleaned after use with an alcohol swab.

Tonometry on Irregular Corneas

The accuracy of Goldmann- and Maklakov-type applanation tonometers and the noncontact tonometers is limited in eyes with irregular corneas. In cases of scarred or edematous corneas, the Mackay-Marg tonometer is generally considered to be the most accurate.[262–264] However, the pneumatic tonometer has also been shown to be useful in eyes with diseased corneas.[264,265] One study using cannulated eye-bank eyes with abnormal corneas showed that the pneumatonograph gave more consistent and objective measurements than did the Mackay-Marg.[266] The Tono-Pen compared favorably with Mackay-Marg tonometry on irregular corneas in one study.[267]

Tonometry over Soft Contact Lenses

It has been claimed that the Mackay-Marg[268] and pneumatonograph[265,269] and Tono-Pen[270,271] can measure the IOP through bandage contact lenses with reasonable accuracy, although soft contact lenses of different powers created a bias with the Tono-Pen.[271] Applanation measurements are said to be affected by the power of the contact lenses with high water content, and correction tables have been developed to compensate for this.[272] An evaluation of NCT readings on eyes with and without soft contact lenses indicated that the power of the lens influenced the difference in IOP between the paired readings, with hyperopic lenses giving the greatest difference.[273]

Tonometry with Gas-Filled Eyes

As previously noted, intraocular gas significantly influences scleral rigidity, rendering indentation tonometry particularly unsatisfactory in such cases. One pneumatic tonometer underestimated Goldmann IOP measurements in eyes with intravitreal gas,[239] while the Tono-Pen was reported to compare favorably with Goldmann readings in eyes following pars plana vitrectomy and gas-fluid exchange.[274] In another study of 50 eyes with irregular corneas following vitrectomy and air/gas-fluid exchange, readings with the Tono-Pen and pneumotonometer were highly correlated, although there was a mean difference of 1.4 mm Hg, with the Tono-Pen usually reading lower.[275] A manometric study with human autopsy eyes indicated that both instruments significantly underestimated the IOP at pressures above 30 mm Hg.[275]

Tonometry in Animals

The Mackay-Marg was found to be more satisfactory than the pneumatonograph for measuring the IOP of canine eyes in one study,[276] while both were highly reliable in another investigation.[277] In primate eyes following epikeratophakia, in which the IOP was controlled with a transducer, the Mackay-Marg gave reliable measurements above 20 mm Hg but had impaired accuracy below this level, while the Goldmann tonometer was accurate over the entire pressure range.[278] Investigators should be cautious of using the pneumatonograph in animals, since it has been calibrated only for human eyes. One study demonstrated calibration of the pneumatonograph for rabbit eyes using open stopcock and closed stopcock methods.[279]

SUMMARY

The distribution of IOP within the general population is almost Gaussian except for a slight skew toward higher pressures. The mean value is approximately 15 mm Hg, and two standard deviations to either side of the mean gives a "normal" range of roughly 10–20 mm Hg. Many factors, in addition to glaucoma, influence the IOP and can be divided into two categories: 1) those that exert a long-term influence, and 2) those that cause short-term fluctuations in the pressure. The former group includes genetics, age, sex, refractive error, and race, while the latter includes time of day, body position, exertion, lid and eye movement, various ocular and systemic conditions, general anesthesia, and some foods and drugs.

Tonometers measure the IOP by relating a deformation of the globe to the force responsible for the deformation. Some tonometers indent the cornea, such as the Schiøtz tonometer, while others flatten or applanate the cornea. Within the latter group, some instruments measure the force required to flatten a standard area, of which the Goldmann tonometer is an example, while others measure the area that is applanated by a standard force. Other instruments, such as the Mackay-Marg and pneumatic tonometers, employ a modified applanation principle with electronic recording of the pressure. Yet another, the noncontact tonometer, deforms the eye with a puff of air and automatically records the IOP.

References

1. Leydhecker, W, Akiyama, K, Neumann, HG: Der intraokulare Druck gesunder menschlicher Augen. Klin Monatsbl Augenheilkd 133:662, 1958.
2. Colton, T, Ederer, F: The distribution of intraocular pressures in the general population. Surv Ophthal 25:123, 1980.
3. Johnson, LV: Tonographic survey. Am J Ophthal 61:680, 1966.
4. Segal, P, Skwierczyńska, J: Mass screening of adults for glaucoma. Ophthalmologica 153:336, 1967.
5. Armaly, MF: On the distribution of applanation pressure. I. Statistical features and the effect of age, sex, and family history of glaucoma. Arch Ophthal 73:11, 1965.
6. Perkins, ES: Glaucoma screening from a public health clinic. Br J Ophthal 1:417, 1965.
7. Loewen, U, Handrup, B, Redeker, A: Results of a glaucoma mass screening program. Klin Monatsbl Augenheilkd 169:754, 1976.
8. Ruprecht, KW, Wulle, KG, Christl, HL: Applanation tonometry within medical diagnostic "check-up" programs. Klin Monatsbl Augenheilkd 172:332, 1978.
9. Shiose, Y, Kawase, Y: A new approach to stratified normal intraocular pressure in a general population. Am J Ophthal 101:714, 1986.
10. David, R, Zangwill, L, Stone, D, Yassur, Y: Epidemiology of intraocular pressure in a population screened for glaucoma. Br J Ophthal 71:766, 1987.
11. Armaly, MF: The genetic determination of ocular pressure in the normal eye. Arch Ophthal 78:187, 1967.
12. Armaly, MF, Monstavicius, BF, Sayegh, RE: Ocular pressure and aqueous outflow facility in siblings. Arch Ophthal 80:354, 1968.
13. Levene, RZ, Workman, PL, Broder, SW, Hirschhorn, K: Heritability of ocular pressure in normal and suspect ranges. Arch Ophthal 84:730, 1970.
14. Seddon, JM, Schwartz, B, Flowerdew, G: Case-control study of ocular hypertension. Arch Ophthal 101:891, 1983.
15. Radtke, ND, Cohan, BE: Intraocular pressure measurement in the newborn. Am J Ophthal 78:501, 1974.
16. Goethals, M, Missotten, L: Intraocular pressure in children up to five years of age. J Pediatr Ophthal Strab 20:49, 1983.
17. Musarella, MA, Morin, JD: Anterior segment and intraocular pressure measurements of the unanesthetized premature infant. Metab Pediatr Syst Ophthal 8:53, 1985.
18. Klein, BE, Klein, R: Intraocular pressure and cardiovascular risk variables. Arch Ophthalmol 99:837, 1981.
19. Hiller, R, Sperduto, RD, Krueger, DE: Race, iris pigmentation, and intraocular pressure. Am J Epidemiol 115:674, 1982.
20. Carel, RS, Korczyn, AD, Rock, M, Goya, I: Association between ocular pressure and certain health parameters. Ophthalmology 91:311, 1984.
21. Schulzer, M, Drance, SM: Intraocular pressure,

systemic blood pressure, and age: a correlation study. Br J Ophthal 71:245, 1987.
22. Shiose, Y: The aging effect on intraocular pressure in an apparently normal population. Arch Ophthal 102:883, 1984.
23. Becker, B: The decline in aqueous secretion and outflow facility with age. Am J Ophthal 46:731, 1958.
24. Gartner, J: Aging changes of the ciliary epithelium border layers and their significance for intraocular pressure. Am J Ophthal 72:1079, 1971.
25. Brubaker, RF, Nagataki, S, Townsend, DJ, Burns, RR, Higgins, RG, Wentworth, W: The effect of age on aqueous humor formation in man. Ophthalmology 88:283, 1981.
26. Tomlinson, A, Phillips, CI: Applanation tension and axial length of the eyeball. Br J Ophthal 54:548, 1970.
27. Deodati, F, Fontan, P, Mouledous, J-M: La tension oculaire du grand myope. Arch D'Ophthalmologie 34:77, 1974.
28. David, R, Zangwill, LM, Tessler, Z, Yassur, Y: The correlation between intraocular pressure and refractive status. Arch Ophthal 103:1812, 1985.
29. Bonomi, L, Mecca, E, Massa F: Intraocular pressure in myopic anisometropia. Internat Ophthal 5:145, 1982.
30. Kass, MA, Zimmerman, TJ, Alton, E, Lemon, L, Becker, B: Intraocular pressure and glaucoma in the Zuni Indians. Arch Ophthal 96:2212, 1978.
31. Katavisto, M: The Diurnal Variations of Ocular Tension in Glaucoma. Acta Ophthalmologica Suppl 78, Copenhagen, 1964.
32. Kitazawa, Y, Horie, T: Diurnal variation of intraocular pressure in primary open-angle glaucoma. Am J Ophthal 79:557, 1975.
33. Newell, FW, Krill, AE: Diurnal tonography in normal and glaucomatous eyes. Trans Am Ophthal Soc 62:349, 1964.
34. Henkind, P, Leitman, M, Weitzman, E: The diurnal curve in man: new observations. Invest Ophthal 12:705, 1973.
35. Smith, J: Diurnal intraocular pressure: correlation to automated perimetry. Ophthalmology 92:858, 1985.
36. Wilensky, JT, Gieser, DK, Mori, MT, et al: Self-tonometry to manage patients with glaucoma and apparently controlled intraocular pressure. Arch Ophthal 105:1072, 1987.
37. Zeimer, RC, Wilensky, JT, Gieser, DK: Presence and rapid decline of early morning intraocular pressure peaks in glaucoma patients. Ophthalmology 97:547, 1990.
38. Boyd, TAS, McLeod, LE: Circadian rhythms of plasma corticoid levels, intraocular pressure and aqueous outflow facility in normal and glaucomatous eyes. Ann NY Acad Sci 117:597, 1964.
39. Rowland, JM, Sawyer, WK, Tittel, J, Ford, CJ: Studies on the circadian rhythm of IOP in rabbits: correlation with aqueous inflow and cAMP content. Curr Eye Res 5:201, 1986.
40. Smith, SD, Gregory, DS: A circadian rhythm of aqueous flow underlies the circadian rhythm of IOP in NZW Rabbits. Invest Ophthal Vis Sci 30:775, 1989.
41. Weitzman, ED, Henkind, P, Leitman, M, Hellman, L: Correlative 24-hour relationships between intraocular pressure and plasma cortisol in normal subjects and patients with glaucoma. Br J Ophthal 59:566, 1975.
42. Kimura, R, Maekawa, N: Effect of orally administered hydrocortisone on the ocular tension in primary open-angle glaucoma subjects. Preliminary report. Acta Ophthalmologica 54:430, 1976.
43. Levi, L, Schwartz, B: Decrease of ocular pressure with oral metyrapone: a double-masked crossover trial. Arch Ophthal 105:777, 1987.
44. Anderson, DR, Grant, WM: The influence of position on intraocular pressure. Invest Ophthal 12:204, 1973.
45. Krieglstein, GK, Brethfeld, V, Collani, EV: Comparative intraocular pressure measurements with position independent hand-applanation tonometers. Graefe's Arch Ophthal 199:101, 1976.
46. Jain, MR, Marmion, VJ: Rapid pneumatic and Mackay-Marg applanation tonometry to evaluate the postural effect on intraocular pressure. Br J Ophthal 60:687, 1976.
47. Kindler-Loosli, C, Schmidt, T: Intraocular pressure after changing the patient's position. Graefe's Arch Ophthal 194:17, 1975.
48. Williams, BI, Peart, WS: Effect of posture on the intraocular pressure of patients with retinal vein obstruction. Br J Ophthal 62:688, 1978.
49. Parsley, J, Powell, RG, Keightley, SJ, Elkington, AR: Postural response of intraocular pressure in chronic open-angle glaucoma following trabeculectomy. Br J Ophthal 71:494, 1987.
50. Tsukahara, S, Sasaki, T: Postural change of IOP in normal persons and in patients with primary wide open-angle glaucoma and low-tension glaucoma. Br J Ophthal 68:389, 1984.
51. Leonard, TJK, Kerr-Muir, MG, Kirkby, GR, Hitchings, RA: Ocular hypertension and posture. Br J Ophthal 67:362, 1983.
52. Williams, BI, Peart, WS, Letley, E: Abnormal intraocular pressure control in systemic hypertension and diabetes mellitus. Br J Ophthal 64:845, 1980.
53. Linder, BJ, Trick, GL, Wolf, ML: Altering body position affects intraocular pressure and visual function. Invest Ophthal Vis Sci 29:1492, 1988.
54. Cook, J, Friberg, TR: Effect of inverted body position on intraocular pressure. Am J Ophthal 98:784, 1984.
55. Friberg, TR, Sanborn, G, Weinreb, RN: Intraocular and episcleral venous pressure increase during inverted posture. Am J Ophthal 103:523, 1987.

56. Biró, I, Botár, Z: On the behavior of intraocular tension in various sport activities. Klin Monatsbl Augenheilkd 140:23, 1962.
57. Lempert, P, Cooper, KH, Culver, JF, Tredici, TJ: The effect of exercise on intraocular pressure. Am J Ophthal 63:1673, 1967.
58. Stewart, RH, LeBlanc, R, Becker, B: Effects of exercise on aqueous dynamics. Am J Ophthal 69:245, 1970.
59. Kypke, W, Hermannspann, U: Glaucoma physical activity and sport. Klin Monatsbl Augenheilkd 164:321, 1974.
60. Shapiro, A, Shoenfeld, Y, Shapiro, Y: The effect of standardised submaximal work load on intraocular pressure. Br J Ophthal 62:679, 1978.
61. Passo, MS, Goldberg, L, Elliot, DL, Van Buskirk, EM: Exercise conditioning and intraocular pressure. Am J Ophthal 103:754, 1987.
62. Shapiro, A, Shapiro, Y, Udassin, R, et al: The effect of salt loading diet on the intraocular pressure. Acta Ophthal 60:35, 1982.
63. Oggel, K, Sommer, G, Neuhann, TH, Hinz, J: Variations of intraocular pressure during Valsalva's maneuver in relation to body position and length of the bulbus in myopia. Graefe's Arch Ophthal 218:51, 1982.
64. Epstein, HM, Fagman, W, Bruce, DL, Abram, A: Intraocular pressure changes during anesthesia for electroshock therapy. Anesthesia and Analgesia 54:479, 1975.
65. Coleman, DJ, Trokel, S: Direct-recorded intraocular pressure variations in a human subject. Arch Ophthal 82:637, 1969.
66. Green, K, Luxenberg, MN: Consequences of eyelid squeezing on intraocular pressure. Am J Ophthal 88:1072, 1979.
67. Moses, RA, Carniglia, PE, Grodzki, WJ Jr, Moses, J: Proptosis and increase of intraocular pressure in voluntary lid fissure widening. Invest Ophthal Vis Sci 25:989, 1984.
68. Losada, F, Wolintz, AH: Bell's palsy: a new ophthalmologic sign. Ann Ophthal 5:1093, 1973.
69. Starrels, ME, Krupin, T, Burde, RM: Bell's palsy and intraocular pressure. Ann Ophthal 7:1067, 1975.
70. Wentworth, WO, Brubaker, RF: Aqueous humor dynamics in a series of patients with third neuron Horner's Syndrome. Am J Ophthal 92:407, 1981.
71. Moses, RA, Lurie, P, Wette, R: Horizontal gaze position effect on intraocular pressure. Invest Ophthal Vis Sci 22:551, 1982.
72. Saunders, RA, Helveston, EM, Ellis, FD: Differential intraocular pressure in strabismus diagnosis. Ophthalmology 87:59, 1981.
73. Raizman, MB, Beck, RW: Sustained increases in intraocular pressure during strabismus surgery. Am J Ophthal 101:308, 1986.
74. Pederson, JE: Experimental retinal detachment: IV. Aqueous humor dynamics in rhegmatogenous detachments. Arch Ophthal 100:1814, 1982.
75. Pederson, JE, Cantrill, HL: Experimental retinal detachment: V. Fluid movement through the retinal hole. Arch Ophthal 102:136, 1984.
76. Bulpitt, CJ, Hodes, C, Everitt, MG: Intraocular pressure and systemic blood pressure in the elderly. Br J Ophthal 59:717, 1975.
77. Leske, MC, Podgor, MJ: Intraocular pressure, cardiovascular risk variables, and visual field defects. Am J Epidemiol 118:280, 1983.
78. Williams, BI, Ledingham, JG: Significance of intraocular pressure measurement in systemic hypertension. Br J Ophthal 68:383, 1984.
79. Levy, NS, Rawitscher, R: The effect of systemic hypotension during cardiopulmonary bypass on intraocular pressure and visual function in humans. Ann Ophthal 9:1547, 1977.
80. Larkin, DFP, Connolly, P, Magner, JB, et al: Intraocular pressure during cardiopulmonary bypass. Br J Ophthal 71:177, 1987.
81. Larkin, DFP, Murphy, R, Magner, JB, Eustace, P: Management of intraocular pressure during cardiopulmonary bypass. Acta Ophthal 65:591, 1988.
82. Deutch, D, Lewis, RA: Intraocular pressure after cardiopulmonary bypass surgery. Am J Ophthal 107:18, 1989.
83. Krupin, T, Bass, J, Oestrich, C, et al: The effect of hyperthermia on aqueous humor dynamics in rabbits. Am J Ophthal 83:561, 1977.
84. Shapiro, A, Shoenfeld, Y, Konikoff, F, et al: The relationship between body temperature and intraocular pressure. Ann Ophthal 13:159, 1981.
85. Broekema, N, van Bijsterveld, OP, de Bos Kuil, RJC: Intraocular pressure during hemodialysis. Ophthalmologica 197:60, 1988.
86. Kass, MA, Sears, ML: Hormonal regulation of intraocular pressure. Surv Ophthal 22:153, 1977.
87. Elman, J, Caprioli, J, Sears, M, et al: Chorionic gonadotropin decreases intraocular pressure and aqueous humor flow in rabbit eyes. Invest Ophthal Vis Sci 28:197, 1987.
88. Aziz, MA: The relationship of I.O.P. to hormonal disturbance. Bull Ophthal Soc Egypt 60:303, 1967.
89. Bramsen, T, Klauber, A, Bierre, P: Central corneal thickness and intraocular tension in patients with acromegaly. Acta Ophthal 58:971, 1980.
90. van den Pol, A, Maul, E, Sears, M: Unilateral gonadectomy does not alter contralateral intraocular pressure in rabbit eyes. Invest Ophthal Vis Sci 16:246, 1977.
91. Feldman, F, Bain, J, Matuk, AR: Daily assessment of ocular and hormonal variables throughout the menstrual cycle. Arch Ophthal 96:1835, 1978.
92. Green, K, Cullen, PM, Phillips, CI: Aqueous hu-

mour turnover and intraocular pressure during menstruation. Br J Ophthal 68:736, 1984.
93. Green, K, Phillips, CI, Cheeks, L, Slagle, T: Aqueous humor flow rate and intraocular pressure during and after pregnancy. Ophthal Res 20:353, 1988.
94. Wallace, I, Moolchandani, J, Krupin, T, et al: Effects of systemic desmopressin on aqueous humor dynamics in rabbits. Invest Ophthal Vis Sci 29:406, 1988.
95. Liu, JHK, Dacus, AC, Bartels, SP: Thyrotropin releasing hormone increases intraocular pressure. Mechanism of action. Invest Ophthal Vis Sci 30:2200, 1989.
96. Walker, SD, Brubaker, RF, Nagataki, S: Hypotony and aqueous humor dynamics in myotonic dystrophy. Invest Ophthal Vis Sci 22:744, 1982.
97. Klein, BEK, Klein, R, Moss, SE: Intraocular pressure in diabetic persons. Ophthalmology 91:1356, 1984.
98. Frier, BM, Hepburn, DA, Fisher, BM, Barrie, T: Fall in intraocular pressure during acute hypoglycaemia in patients with insulin dependent diabetes. Br Med J 294:610, 1987.
99. Ortiz, GJ, Cook, DJ, Yablonski, ME, et al: Effect of cold air on aqueous humor dynamics in humans. Invest Ophthal Vis Sci 29:138, 1988.
100. Wirt, H, Draeger, J: Tonometry in microgravity. Klin Monatsbl Augenheilkd 188:505, 1986.
101. Duncalf, D: Anesthesia and intraocular pressure. Trans Am Acad Ophthal Otol 79:562, 1975.
102. Schreuder, M, Linssen, GH: Intra-ocular pressure and anaesthesia. Direct measurements by needling the anterior chamber in the monkey. Anaesthesia 27:165, 1972.
103. Maddox, TS Jr, Kielar, RA: Comparison of the influence of ketamine and halothane anesthesia on intraocular tensions of nonglaucomatous children. J Ped Ophthal 11:90, 1974.
104. Schutten, WH, Van Horn, DL: The effects of ketamine sedation and ketamine-pentobarbital anesthesia upon the intraocular pressure of the rabbit. Invest Ophthal Vis Sci 16:531, 1977.
105. Erickson-Lamy, KA, Kaufman, PL, McDermott, ML, France, NK: Comparative anesthetic effects on aqueous humor dynamics in the cynomolgus monkey. Arch Ophthal 102:1815, 1984.
106. Ausinsch, B, Graves, SA, Munson, ES, Levy, NS: Intraocular pressures in children during isoflurane and halothane anesthesia. Anesthesiology 42:167, 1975.
107. Dominguez, A, Banos, MS, Alvarez, MG, et al: Intraocular pressure measurement in infants under general anesthesia. Am J Ophthal 78:110, 1974.
108. Wyllie, AM, Beveridge, ME, Smith, I: Intraocular pressure during 4-hydroxy-butyrate narcosis. Br J Ophthal 56:436, 1972.
109. Peczon, JD, Grant, WM: Sedatives, stimulants, and intraocular pressure in glaucoma. Arch Ophthal 72:178, 1964.
110. Meyers, EF, Krupin, T, Johnson, M, Zink, H: Failure of nondepolarizing neuromuscular blockers to inhibit succinylcholine-induced increased intraocular pressure, a controlled study. Anesthesiology 48:149, 1978.
111. Bowen, DJ, McGrand, JC, Hamilton, AG: Intraocular pressures after suxamethonium and endotracheal intubation. Anaesthesia 33:518, 1978.
112. Meyers, EF, Singer, P, Otto, A: A controlled study of the effect of succinylcholine self-taming on intraocular pressure. Anesthesiology 53:72, 1980.
113. Cunningham, AJ, Albert, O, Cameron, J, Watson, AG: The effect of intravenous diazepam on rise of intraocular pressure following succinylcholine. Am J Ophthal 93:536, 1982.
114. Couch, JA, Eltringham, RJ, Magauran, DM: The effect of thiopentone and fazadinium on intraocular pressure. Anaesthesia 34:586, 1979.
115. Murphy, DF, Eustace, P, Unwin, A, Magner, JB: Atracurium and intraocular pressure. Br J Ophthal 69:673, 1985.
116. Goldstein, JH, Gupta, MK, Shah, MD: Comparison of intramuscular and intravenous succinylcholine on intraocular pressure. Ann Ophthal 13:173, 1981.
117. Murphy, DF, Eustace, P, Unwin, A, Magner, JB: Intravenous lignocaine pretreatment to prevent intraocular pressure rise following suxamethonium and tracheal intubation. Br J Ophthal 70:596, 1986.
118. Kielar, RA, Teraslinna, P, Kearney, JT, Barker, D: Effect of changes in PCO_2 on intraocular tension. Invest Ophthal Vis Sci 16:534, 1977.
119. Petounis, AD, Chondreli, S, Vadaluka-Sekioti, A: Effect of hypercapnea and hyperventilation on human intraocular pressure during general anaesthesia following acetazolamide administration. Br J Ophthal 64:422, 1980.
120. Gallin-Cohen, PF, Podos, SM, Yablonski, ME: Oxygen lowers intraocular pressure. Invest Ophthal Vis Sci 19:43, 1980.
121. Yablonski, ME, Gallin, P, Shapiro, D: Effect of oxygen on aqueous humor dynamics in rabbits. Invest Ophthal Vis Sci 26:1781, 1985.
122. Peczon, JD, Grant, WM: Glaucoma, alcohol, and intraocular pressure. Arch Ophthal 73:495, 1965.
123. Houle, RE, Grant, WM: Alcohol, vasopressin, and intraocular pressure. Invest Ophthal 6:145, 1967.
124. Higginbotham, EJ, Kilimanjaro, HA, Wilensky, JT, et al: The effect of caffeine on intraocular pressure in glaucoma patients. Ophthalmology 96:624, 1989.
125. Naveh-Floman, N, Belkin, M: Prostaglandin metabolism and intraocular pressure. Br J Ophthal 71:254, 1987.

126. Shephard, RJ, Ponsford, E, Basu, PK, LaBarre, R: Effects of cigarette smoking on intraocular pressure and vision. Br J Ophthal 62:682, 1978.
127. Mehra, KS, Roy, PN, Khare, BB: Tobacco smoking and glaucoma. Ann Ophthal 8:462, 1976.
128. Green, K: Ocular effects of diacetyl morphine and lysergic acid diethylamide in rabbit. Invest Ophthal 14:325, 1975.
129. Whitworth, CG, Grant, WM: Use of nitrate and nitrite vasodilators by glaucomatous patients. Arch Ophthal 71:492, 1964.
130. Leydhecker, W, Waller, W, Krieglstein, G: The effect of vasodilators on the intraocular pressure. Klin Monatsbl Augenheilkd 164:293, 1974.
131. Peczon, JD, Grant, WM, Lambert, BW: Systemic vasodilators, intraocular pressure, and chamber depth in glaucoma. Am J Ophthal 72:74, 1971.
132. Wizemann, AJS, Wizemann, V: Organic nitrate in glaucoma. Am J Ophthal 90:106, 1980.
133. Hardt, BW, Johnen, R, Fahle, M: The influence of systemic digitalis application on intraocular pressure. Graefe's Arch Ophthal 219:76, 1982.
134. Lazenby, GW, Reed, JW, Grant, WM: Short-term tests of anticholinergic medication in open-angle glaucoma. Arch Ophthal 80:443, 1968.
135. Lazenby, GW, Reed, JW, Grant, WM: Anticholinergic medication in open-angle glaucoma. Long-term tests. Arch Ophthal 84:719, 1970.
136. Hiatt, RL, Fuller, IB, Smith, L, et al: Systemically administered anticholinergic drugs and intraocular pressure. Arch Ophthal 84:735, 1970.
137. Stelzer, R, Wohlzogen, FX: Anticholinergic drugs in open-angle glaucoma. Klin Monatsbl Augenheilkd 177:151, 1980.
138. Valle, O: Effect of cyclopentolate on the aqueous dynamics in incipient or suspected open-angle glaucoma. Acta Ophthalmologica: XXI Meeting of Nordic Ophthalmologists June 13–16, 1973, p. 52.
139. Feldman, F, Cohen, MM: Effect of histamine-2 receptor blockade by cimetidine on intraocular pressure in humans. Am J Ophthal 93:351, 1982.
140. Ober, M, Scharrer, A: Changes in intraocular pressure during prostaglandin-induced abortion. Klin Monatsbl Augenheilkd 180:230, 1982.
141. Friedenwald, JS: Contribution to the theory and practice of tonometry. Am J Ophthal 20:985, 1937.
142. Moses, RA, Tarkkanen, A: Tonometry: the pressure-volume relationship in the intact human eye at low pressures. Am J Ophthal 47:557, 1959.
143. Friedenwald, JS: Some problems in the calibration of tonometers. Am J Ophthal 31:935, 1948.
144. Friedenwald, JS: Tonometer calibration: an attempt to remove discrepancies found in the 1954 calibration scale for Schiøtz tonometers. Trans Am Acad Ophthal Otol 61:108, 1957.
145. Kronfeld, PC: Tonometer calibration empirical validation. The committee on standardization of tonometers. Trans Am Acad Ophthal Otol 61:123, 1957.
146. Anderson, DR, Grant, WM: Re-evaluation of the Schiøtz tonometer calibration. Invest Ophthal 9:430, 1970.
147. Bayard, WL: Comparison of Goldmann applanation and Schiøtz tonometry using 1948 and 1955 conversion scales. Am J Ophthal 69:1007, 1970.
148. Drance, SM: The coefficient of scleral rigidity in normal and glaucomatous eyes. Arch Ophthal 63:668, 1960.
149. Friedman, E, Ivry, M, Ebert, E, et al: Increased scleral rigidity and age-related macular degeneration. Ophthalmology 96:104, 1989.
150. Draeger, J: Die Abhangigkeit des Rigiditatskoeffizienten von der Hohe des intraokularen Druckes. Ophthalmologica 140:55, 1960.
151. Kaiser-Kupfer, MI, McCain, L, Shapiro, JR, et al: Low ocular rigidity in patients with osteogenesis imperfecta. Invest Ophthal Vis Sci 20:807, 1981.
152. Harbin, TS Jr, Laikam, SE, Lipsitt, K, et al: Applanation-Schiøtz disparity after retinal detachment surgery utilizing cryopexy. Ophthalmology 86:1609, 1979.
153. Johnson, MW, Han, DP, Hoffman, KE: The effect of scleral buckling on ocular rigidity. Ophthalmology 97:190, 1990.
154. Simone, JN, Whitacre, MM: The effect of intraocular gas and fluid volumes on intraocular pressure. Ophthalmology 97:238, 1990.
155. Aronowitz, JD, Brubaker, RF: Effect of intraocular gas on intraocular pressure. Arch Ophthal 94:1191, 1976.
156. Foster, CS, Yamamoto, GK: Ocular rigidity in keratoconus. Am J Ophthal 86:802, 1978.
157. Draeger, J: Untersuchungen uber den Rigiditatskoeffizienten. Doc Ophthal 13:431, 1959.
158. Goldmann, H, Schimdt, TH: Der Rigiditatskoeffizient. (Friedenwald). Ophthalmologica 133:330, 1957.
159. Chandler, PA, Grant, WP: Glaucoma, 2nd ed. Lea and Febiger, Philadelphia, 1979, p. 16.
160. van der Werff, TJ: A new single-parameter ocular rigidity function. Am J Ophthal 92:391, 1981.
161. Hetland-Eriksen, J: On tonometry. 2. Pressure recordings by Schiøtz tonometry on enucleated human eyes. Acta Ophthal 44:12, 1966.
162. Goldmann, MH: Un nouveau tonometre a aplanation. Bull Soc Franc Ophthal 67:474, 1954.
163. Goldmann, H, Schmidt, TH: Uber applanationstonometrie. Ophthalmologica 134:221, 1957.
164. Stepanik, J: Tonometry results using a corneal applanation 3.53 mm in diameter. Klin Monatsbl Augenheilkd 184:40, 1984.
165. Moses, RA: The Goldmann applanation tonometer. Am J Ophthal 46:865, 1958.
166. Koester, CJ, Campbell, CJ, Donn, A: Ophthalmic

optical instruments: two recent developments. Jpn J Ophthal 24:1, 1980.
167. Grant, WM: Fluorescein for applanation tonometry. More convenient and uniform application. Am J Ophthal 55:1252, 1963.
168. Quickert, MH: A fluorescein-anesthetic solution for applanation tonometry. Arch Ophthal 77:734, 1967.
169. Stewart, HL: Prolonged antibacterial activity of a fluorescein-anesthetic solution. Arch Ophthal 88:385, 1972.
170. Coad, CT, Osato, MS, Wilhelmus, KR: Bacterial contamination of eyedrop dispensers. Am J Ophthal 98:548, 1984.
171. Roper, DL: Applanation tonometry with and without fluorescein. Am J Ophthal 90:668, 1980.
172. Draeger, J, Hechler, B, Levedag, S, Wirt, H: Automatic measurement of intraocular pressure with an electronic sensor tonometer. Klin Monatsbl Augenheilkd 190:539, 1987.
173. Ehlers, N, Bramsen, T, Sperling, S: Applanation tonometry and central corneal thickness. Acta Ophthal 53:34, 1975.
174. Johnson, M, Kass, MA, Moses, RA, Grodzki, WJ: Increased corneal thickness simulating elevated intraocular pressure. Arch Ophthal 96:664, 1978.
175. Mark, HH: Corneal curvature in applanation tonometry. Am J Ophthal 76:223, 1973.
176. Holladay, JT, Allison, ME, Prager, TC: Goldmann applanation tonometry in patients with regular corneal astigmatism. Am J Ophthal 96:90, 1983.
177. Bynke, H, Wilke, K: Repeated applanation tonometry in carotid occlusive disease. Acta Ophthal 52:125, 1974.
178. Moniz, E, Feldman, F, Newkirk, M, et al: Removal of Hepatitis B surface antigen from a contaminated applanation tonometer. Am J Ophthal 91:522, 1981.
179. Gastaud, P, Baudouin, CH, Ouzan, D: Detection of HBs antigen, DNA polymerase activity, and hepatitis B virus DNA in tears: relevance to hepatitis B transmission by tears. Br J Ophthal 73:333, 1989.
180. Fujikawa, LS, Salahuddin SZ, Palestine AG, et al. Isolation of the human T-lymphotropic virus type III from the tears of a patient with the acquired immunodeficiency syndrome. Lancet 2:529, 1985.
181. Fujikawa, LS, Salahuddin, SZ, Ablashi, D, et al: HTLV-III in the tears of AIDS patients. Ophthalmology 93:1479, 1986.
182. Craven, ER, Butler, SL, McCulley, JP, Luby, JP: Applanation tonometer tip sterilization for adenovirus type 8. Ophthalmology 94:1538, 1987.
183. Ventura, LM, Dix, RD: Viability of herpes simplex virus type 1 on the applanation tonometer. Am J Ophthal 103:48, 1987.
184. Pepose, JS, Linnette, G, Lee, SF, MacRae, S: Disinfection of Goldmann tonometers against human immunodeficiency virus type 1. Arch Ophthal 107:983, 1989.
185. Nardi, M, Bartolomei, MP, Falco, L, Carelli, F: Disposable film cover for the tip of Goldmann's tonometer. Graefe's Arch Ophthal 223:109, 1985.
186. Assia, E, Bartov, E, Blumenthal, M: Disposable parafilm cover for the applanation tonometer. Am J Ophthal 102:397, 1986.
187. Wizemann, A: Modified version of UV sterilizer to disinfect Goldmann tonometer heads, gonioscopes and fundus contact lenses. Klin Monatsbl Augenheilkd 181:40, 1982.
188. Van Buskirk, EM: Disinfectant receptacle for applanation tonometers. Am J Ophthal 104:307, 1987.
189. Am Acad Ophthal: Clinical Alert 2/4, Updated Recommendations for Ophthalmic Practice in Relation to the Human Immunodeficiency Virus. August 1988.
190. Centers for Disease Control: Recommendations for preventing possible transmission of human T-lymphotropic virus type III/lymphadenopathy-associated virus in tears. MMWR 34:533, 1985.
191. Soukiasian, SH, Asdourian, GK, Weiss, JS, Kachadoorian, HA: A complication from alcohol-swabbed tonometer tips. Am J Ophthal 105:424, 1988.
192. Pogrebniak, AE, Sugar, A: Corneal toxicity from hydrogen peroxide-soaked tonometer tips. Arch Ophthal 106:1505, 1988.
193. Perkins, ES: Hand-held applanation tonometer. Br J Ophthal 49:591, 1965.
194. Draeger, J: Simple hand applanation tonometer for use on the seated as well as on the supine patient. Am J Ophthal 62:1208, 1966.
195. Draeger, J: Principle and clinical application of a portable applanation tonometer. Invest Ophthal 6:132, 1967.
196. Mackay, RS, Marg, E: Fast, automatic, electronic tonometers based on an exact theory. Acta Ophthal 37:495, 1959.
197. Marg, E, Mackay, RS, Oechsli, R: Trough height, pressure and flattening in tonometry. Vision Res 1:379, 1962.
198. Blondeau, P: Clinical evaluation of the Dicon CAT 100 applanation tonometer. Am J Ophthal 99:708, 1985.
199. Lim, JI, Ruderman, JM: Comparison of the Challenger digital applanation tonometer and the Goldmann applanation tonometer. Am J Ophthal 102:154, 1986.
200. Miller, K, Sanborn, GE, Jennings, LW: Clinical evaluation of the Cavitron biotronics tonometer. Arch Ophthal 106:1210, 1988.
201. Kao, SF, Lichter, PR, Bergstrom, TJ, et al: Clinical comparison of the Oculab Tono-Pen to the

Goldmann applanation tonometer. Ophthalmology 94:1541, 1987.
202. Durham, DG, Bigliano, RP, Masino, JA: Pneumatic applanation tonometer. Trans Am Acad Ophthal Otol 69:1029, 1965.
203. Langham, ME, McCarthy, E: A rapid pneumatic applanation tonometer. Comparative findings and evaluation. Arch Ophthal 79:389, 1968.
204. Posner, A: An evaluation of the Maklakov applanation tonometer. EENT Monthly 41:377, 1962.
205. Posner, A: Practical problems in the use of the Maklakov tonometer. EENT Monthly 42:82, 1963.
206. Friedenwald, JS: Contribution to the theory and practice of tonometry. II. An analysis of the work of Professor S. Kalfa with the applanation tonometer. Am J Ophthal 22:375, 1939.
207. Schmidt, TFA: Calibration of the Maklakoff tonometer. Am J Ophthal 77:740, 1974.
208. Posner, A: A new portable applanation tonometer. EENT Monthly 43:88, 1964.
209. Posner, A, Inglima, R: The Tonomat applanation tonometer. EENT Monthly 46:996, 1967.
210. Halberg, GP: Hand applanation tonometer. Trans Am Acad Ophthal Otol 72:112, 1968.
211. Barraquer, JI: New applanation tonometer for operating room. Ophthalmologica 153:225, 1967.
212. Jensen, JB: An ocular tension indicator of the applanation type. Acta Ophthal 45:546, 1967.
213. Kaiden, JS, Zimmerman, TJ, Worthen, DM: An evaluation of the GlaucoTest screening tonometer. Arch Ophthal 92:195, 1974.
214. Grolman, B: A new tonometer system. Am J Optom & Arch Am Acad Optom 49:646, 1972.
215. Forbes, M, Pico, G, Grolman, B: A noncontact applanation tonometer description and clinical evaluation. Arch Ophthal 91:134, 1974.
216. Shields, MB: The non-contact tonometer. Its value and limitations. Surv Ophthal 24:211, 1980.
217. Fisher, JH, Watson, PG, Spaeth, G: A new handheld air impulse tonometer. Eye 2:238, 1988.
218. Vernon, SA: Non-contact tonometry in the postoperative eye. Br J Ophthal 73:247, 1989.
219. Piltz, JR, Starita, R, Miron, M, Henkind, P: Momentary fluctuations of intraocular pressure in normal and glaucomatous eyes. Am J Ophthal 99:333, 1985.
220. Moses, RA, Arnzen, RJ: Instantaneous tonometry. Arch Ophthal 101:249, 1983.
221. Greene, ME, Gilman, BG: Intraocular pressure measurement with instrumented contact lenses. Invest Ophthal 13:299, 1974.
222. Wolbarsht, ML, Wortman, J, Schwartz, B, Cook, D: A scleral buckle pressure gauge for continuous monitoring of intraocular pressure. Internat Ophthal 3:11, 1980.
223. Cooper, RL, Beale, DG, Constable, IJ: Passive radiotelemetry of intraocular pressure in vivo: calibration and validation of continual scleral guard-ring applanation transensors in the dog and rabbit. Invest Ophthal Vis Sci 18:930, 1979.
224. Cooper, RL, Beale, DG, Constable, IJ, Grose, GC: Continual monitoring of intraocular pressure: effect of central venous pressure, respiration, and eye movements on continual recordings of intraocular pressure in the rabbit, dog, and man. Br J Ophthal 63:799, 1979.
225. Nissen, OI: Bilateral recording of human intraocular pressure with an improved applanating suction cup tonograph. Acta Ophthal 58:377, 1980.
226. Zeimer, RC, Wilensky, JT, Gieser, DK, et al: Evaluation of a self tonometer for home use. Arch Ophthal 101:1791, 1983.
227. Zeimer, RC, Wilensky, JT, Gieser, DK, et al: Application of a self-tonometer to home tonometry. Arch Ophthal 104:49, 1986.
228. Dekking, HM, Coster, HD: Dynamic tonometry. Ophthalmologica 154:59, 1967.
229. Roth, W, Blake, DG: Vibration tonometry—principles of the vibra-tonometer. J Am Optom Assoc 34:971, 1963.
230. Moses, RA, Liu, CH: Repeated applanation tonometry. Am J Ophthal 66:89, 1968.
231. Phelps, CD, Phelps, GK: Measurement of intraocular pressure: a study of its reproducibility. Graefe's Arch Ophthal 198:39, 1976.
232. Smith, JL, et al.: The incidence of Schiøtz-applanation disparity. Cooperative study. Arch Ophthal 77:305, 1967.
233. Bengtsson, B: Comparison of Schiøtz and Goldmann tonometry in a population. Acta Ophthal 50:445, 1972.
234. Krieglstein, GK: Screening tonometry by technicians. Graefe's Arch Ophthal 194:221, 1975.
235. Armaly, MF, Salamoun, SG: Schiøtz and applanation tonometry. Arch Ophthal 70:603, 1963.
236. Schwartz, JT, Dell'Osso, GG: Comparison of Goldmann and Schiøtz tonometry in a community. Arch Ophthal 75:788, 1966.
237. Bengtsson, B: Some factors affecting the relationship between Schiøtz and Goldmann readings in a population. Acta Ophthal 51:798, 1973.
238. Stepanik, J: Why is the Schiøtz tonometer not suitable for measuring intraocular pressure? Klin Monatsbl Augenheilkd 176:61, 1980.
239. Del Priore, LV, Michels, RG, Nunez, MA, et al: Intraocular pressure measurement after pars plana vitrectomy. Ophthalmology 96:1353, 1989.
240. Dunn, JS, Brubaker, RF: Perkins applanation tonometer clinical and laboratory evaluation. Arch Ophthal 89:149, 1973.
241. Krieglstein, GK, Waller, WK: Goldmann applanation versus hand-applanation and Schiøtz indentation tonometry. Graefe's Arch Ophthal 194:11, 1975.
242. Finlay, RD: Experience with the Draeger applanation tonometer. Trans Ophthal Soc UK 90:887, 1970.

243. Moses, RA, Marg, E, Oechsli, R: Evaluation of the basic validity and clinical usefulness of the Mackay-Marg tonometer. Invest Ophthal 1:78, 1962.
244. Petersen, WC, Schlegel, WA: Mackay-Marg tonometry by technicians. Am J Ophthal 76:933, 1973.
245. Hessemer, V, Rösler, R, Jacobi, KW: Comparison of intraocular pressure measurements with the Oculab Tono-Pen vs manometry in humans shortly after death. Am J Ophthal 105:678, 1988.
246. Boothe, WA, Lee, DA, Panek, WC, Pettit, TH: The Tono-Pen. A manometric and clinical study. Arch Ophthal 106:1214, 1988.
247. Frenkel, REP, Hong, YJ, Shin, DH: Comparison of the Tono-Pen to the Goldmann applanation tonometer. Arch Ophthal 106:750, 1988.
248. Hessemer, V, Rossler, R, Jacobi, KW: Tono-Pen, a new hand-held tonometer: comparison with the Goldmann applanation tonometer. Klin Monatsbl Augenheilkd 193:420, 1988.
249. Armstrong, TA: Evaluation of the Tono-Pen and the Pulsair tonometers. Am J Ophthal 109:716, 1990.
250. Farrar, SM, Miller, KN, Shields, MB, Stoup, CM: An evaluation of the Tono-Pen for the measurement of diurnal intraocular pressure. Am J Ophthal 107:411, 1989.
251. Quigley, HA, Langham, ME: Comparative intraocular pressure measurements with the pneumatonograph and Goldmann tonometer. Am J Ophthal 80:266, 1975.
252. Jain, MR, Marmion, VJ: A clinical evaluation of the applanation pneumatonograph. Br J Ophthal 60:107, 1976.
253. Wuthrich, UW: Postural change and intraocular pressure in glaucomatous eyes. Br J Ophthal 60:111, 1976.
254. Moses, RA, Grodzki, WJ Jr: The pneumatonograph. A laboratory study. Arch Ophthal 97:547, 1979.
255. Francois, J, Vancea, P, Vanderkerckhove, R: Halberg tonometer. An evaluation. Arch Ophthal 86:376, 1971.
256. Zimmerman, TJ, Worthen, DM: A comparison of two hand-applanation tonometers. Arch Ophthal 88:421, 1972.
257. Kaiden, JS, Zimmerman, TJ, Worthen, DM: Hand-held tonometers. An evaluation by medical students. Arch Ophthal 89:110, 1973.
258. Jessen, K, Hoffmann, F: Current standardization of air-pulse tonometers and methods of testing them, taking the non-contact tonometer II as an example. Klin Monatsbl Augenheilkd 183:296, 1983.
259. Derka, H: The American Optical non-contact tonometer and its results compared with the Goldmann applanation tonometer. Klin Monatsbl Augenheilkd 177:634, 1980.
260. Sponsel, WE, Kaufman, PL, Strinden, TI, et al: Evaluation of the Keeler Pulsair non-contact tonometer. Acta Ophthal 67:567, 1989.
261. Insler, MS: Acute corneal bullae produced during noncontact tonometry. Am J Ophthal 101:375, 1986.
262. Kaufman, HE, Wind, CA, Waltman, SR: Validity of Mackay-Marg electronic applanation tonometer in patients with scarred irregular corneas. Am J Ophthal 69:1003, 1970.
263. McMillan, F, Forster, RK: Comparison of MacKay-Marg, Goldmann, and Perkins tonometers in abnormal corneas. Arch Ophthal 93:420, 1975.
264. West, CE, Capella, JA, Kaufman, HE: Measurement of intraocular pressure with a pneumatic applanation tonometer. Am J Ophthal 74:505, 1972.
265. Krieglstein, GK, Waller, WK, Reimers, H, Langham, ME: Intraocular pressure measurements on soft contact lenses. Graefe's Arch Ophthal 199:223, 1976.
266. Richter, RC, Stark, WJ, Cowan, C, Pollack, IP: Tonometry on eyes with abnormal corneas. Glaucoma 2:508, 1980.
267. Rootman, DS, Insler, MS, Thompson, HW, et al: Accuracy and precision of the Tono-Pen in measuring intraocular pressure after keratoplasty and epikeratophakia and in scarred corneas. Arch Ophthal 106:1697, 1988.
268. Meyer, RF, Stanifer, RM, Bobb, KC: MacKay-Marg Tonometry over therapeutic soft contact lenses. Am J Ophthal 86:19, 1978.
269. Rubenstein, JB, Deutsch, TA: Pneumatonometry through bandage contact lenses. Arch Ophthal 103:1660, 1985.
270. Khan, JA, LaGreca, BA: Tono-Pen estimation of intraocular pressure through bandage contact lenses. Am J Ophthal 108:422, 1989.
271. Panek, WC, Boothe, WA, Lee, DA, et al: Intraocular pressure measurement with the Tono-Pen through soft contact lenses. Am J Ophthal 109:62, 1990.
272. Draeger, J: Applanation tonometry on contact lenses with high water content: problems, results, correction factors. Klin Monatsbl Augenheilkd 176:38, 1980.
273. Insler, MS, Robbins, RG: Intraocular pressure by noncontact tonometry with and without soft contact lenses. Arch Ophthal 105:1358, 1987.
274. Hines, MW, Jost, BF, Fogelman, KL: Oculab Tono-Pen, Goldmann applanation tonometery, and pneumatic tonometry for intraocular pressure assessment in gas-filled eyes. Am J Ophthal 106:174, 1988.
275. Lim, JI, Blair, NP, Higginbotham, EJ, et al: Assessment of intraocular pressure in vitrectomized gas-containing eyes. A clinical and manometric comparison of the Tono-Pen to the pneumotonometer. Arch Ophthal 108:684, 1990.

276. Gelatt, KN, Peiffer, RL Jr, Gum, GG, et al: Evaluation of applanation tonometers for the dog eye. Invest Ophthal Vis Sci 16:963, 1977.
277. Gelatt, KN, Gun, GG, Barrie, KP: Tonometry in glaucomatous globes. Invest Ophthal Vis Sci 20:683, 1981.
278. Olson, PF, McDonald, MB, Werblin, TP, Kaufman, HE: Measurement of intraocular pressure after epikeratophakia. Arch Ophthal 101:1111, 1983.
279. Neault, TR, Cooke, D, Brubaker, RF: Modification and calibration of the Bigliano-Webb tonometer for improved accuracy of tonometry in rabbits. Curr Eye Res 8:9, 1989.

Chapter 5

THE OPTIC NERVE HEAD AND PERIPAPILLARY RETINA

The primary consequence of elevated intraocular pressure (IOP) in an eye with glaucoma is progressive atrophy of the optic nerve head. Since it is this pathologic alteration that leads to the irreversible loss of vision, an understanding of glaucomatous optic atrophy is essential in the diagnosis and management of glaucoma.

ANATOMY AND HISTOLOGY

Terminology

Within the context of a discussion on glaucoma, the optic nerve head is defined as the distal portion of the optic nerve that is directly susceptible to elevated IOP. In this sense, the optic nerve head extends from the retinal surface to the myelinated portion of the optic nerve that begins just behind the sclera. The term *optic nerve head* is generally preferred over *optic disc,* since the latter suggests a flat structure without depth. However, the terms *disc* or *papilla* are frequently used when referring to the portion of the optic nerve head that is clinically visible by ophthalmoscopy.

General Description

The optic nerve head is composed of the nerve fibers that originate in the ganglion cell layer of the retina and converge upon the nerve head from all points in the fundus. At the surface of the nerve head, these axons bend acutely to leave the globe through a fenestrated scleral canal, called the *lamina cribrosa*. Within the nerve head, the axons are grouped into approximately 1000 fascicles, or bundles, and are supported by astrogliocytes. There is considerable variation in the size of the optic nerve head. In one study, the diameter varied from 1.18–1.75 mm.[1] Other studies have revealed ranges of 0.85–2.43 mm in the shortest diameter and 1.21–2.86 mm in the longest,[2] or a mean of 1.88 mm vertically and 1.77 horizontally.[3] The disc area may range from 0.68–4.42 mm^2.[2] The diameter of the nerve expands to approximately 3 mm just behind the sclera, where the neurons acquire a myelin sheath. The optic nerve head is also the site of entry and exit of the retinal vessels. This vascular system supplies some branches to the optic nerve head, although the predominant blood supply for the nerve head comes from the ciliary circulation.

Divisions of the Optic Nerve Head

The nerve head may be arbitrarily divided into the following four portions, from anterior to posterior (Fig. 5.1):[4]

Surface Nerve Fiber Layer. The innermost portion of the optic nerve head is composed predominantly of neurons. In the rhesus monkey, this layer is 94% neurons and 5% astrocytes.[5] The axonal bundles acquire progressively more interaxonal glial tissue within the intraocular portion of the nerve head as this structure is followed posteriorly.[5]

Prelaminar Region (also called the anterior portion of the lamina cribrosa[6]). The predominant structures at this level are neurons and astrocytes, with a significant increase in the quantity of astroglial tissue.

Lamina Cribrosa Region. This portion contains fenestrated sheets of scleral connective tissue and occasional elastic fibers. Astrocytes separate the sheets and line the fenestrae,[6] and the fascicles of neurons leave the eye through these openings.

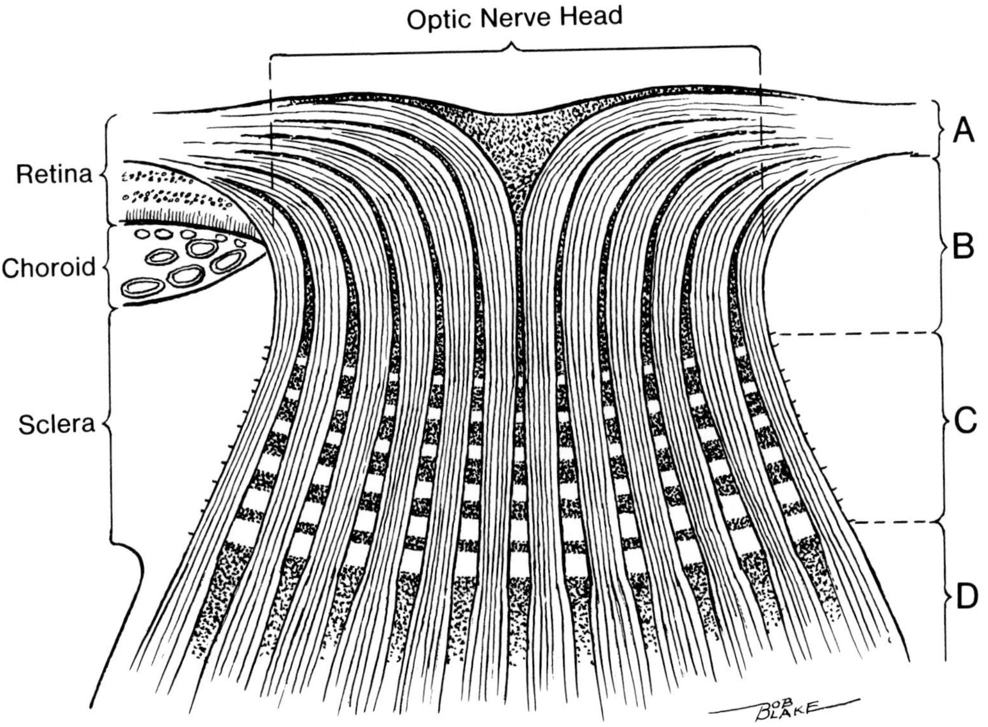

Figure 5.1. Divisions of the optic nerve head: **A,** Surface nerve fiber layer. **B,** Prelaminar region. **C,** Lamina cribrosa region. **D,** Retrolaminar region.

Retrolaminar Region. This area is characterized by a decrease in astrocytes and the acquisition of myelin, which is supplied by obligodendrocytes. The axonal bundles are surrounded by connective tissue septae.

The posterior extent of the retrolaminar region is not clearly defined. An India ink study of monkey eyes showed nonfilling for 3–4 mm behind the lamina cribrosa, when the IOP was elevated.[7] However, a similar study with unlabeled microspheres showed an increased flow in the retrolaminar region close to the lamina even when the pressure was elevated high enough to stop retinal flow.[8]

Vasculature

Arterial Supply. The four divisions of the optic nerve head correlate roughly with a four-part vascular supply (Fig. 5.2):

The surface nerve fiber layer is supplied mainly by arteriolar branches of the central retinal artery, which anastomose with vessels of the prelaminar region[9] and are continuous with the peripapillary retinal and long radial peripapillary capillaries.[4] One or more of the ciliary-derived vessels from the prelaminar region may occasionally enlarge to form cilioretinal arteries.[4]

The prelaminar region is supplied by pre-

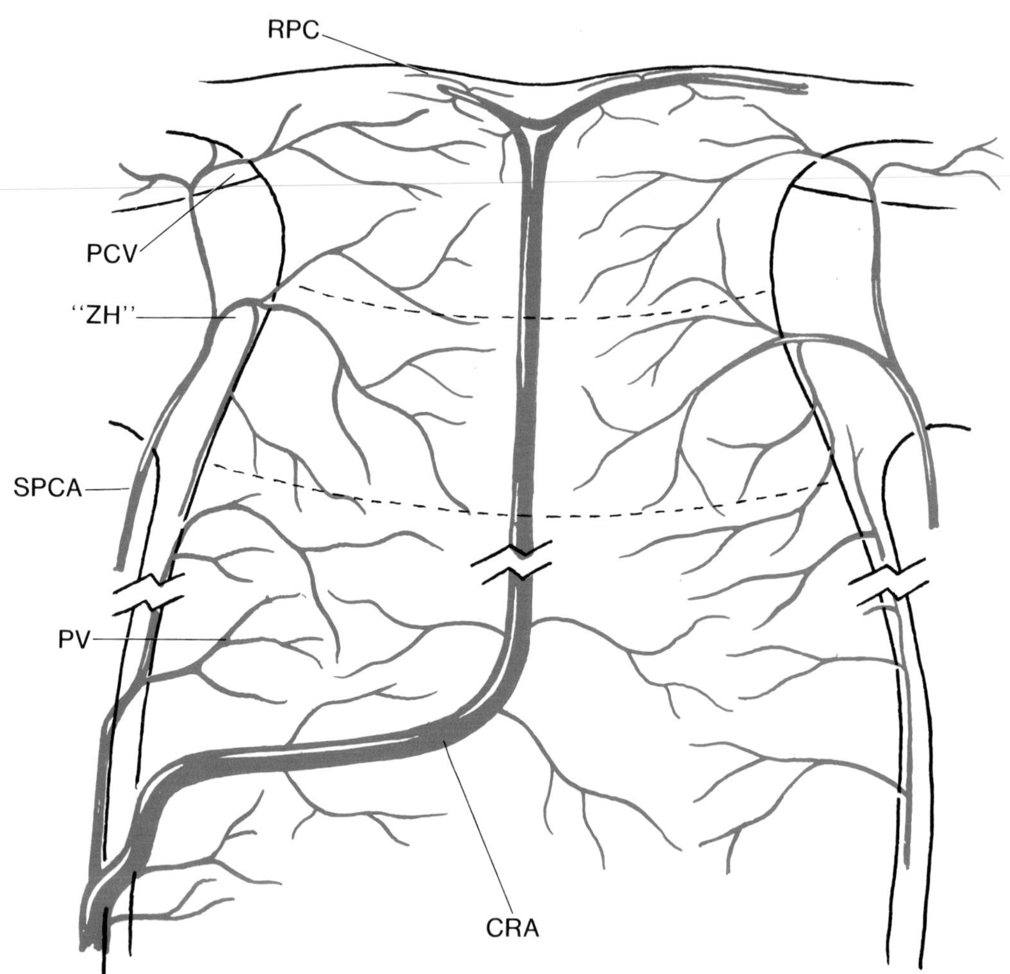

Figure 5.2. Vascular supply of the optic nerve head: central retinal artery (*CRA*); radial peripapillary capillaries (*RPC*); pial vessels (*PV*); short posterior ciliary arteries (*SPCA*); peripapillary choroidal vessels (*PCV*); "circle" of Zinn-Haller (*"ZH"*).

capillaries and capillaries of the short posterior ciliary arteries from direct branches arising from arterioles surrounding the optic nerve or from indirect branches from the peripapillary choroid.[4,9,10]

The lamina cribrosa region is also supplied by vessels that come directly from short posterior ciliary arteries to form a dense plexus in the lamina.[4,9] These arteries also provide an incomplete and inconsistent vascular system around the lamina, called the "circle" of Zinn-Haller.[4,9]

The retrolaminar region is supplied by both the ciliary and retinal circulations, with the former coming from recurrent pial vessels. The central retinal artery provides centripetal branches from the pial system and frequently, but not always, gives off centrifugal vessels.[11] A "central optic nerve artery" has been described as a branch of the ophthalmic artery, supplying the axial portion of the optic nerve.[12] This structure has not been confirmed in subsequent studies but may represent a rare variant of the normal anatomy.[11]

A continuity between small vessels from the retrolaminar region to the retinal surface has been observed,[9] and the optic nerve head microvasculature is said to represent an integral part of the retina-optic nerve vascular system.[10]

Capillaries. Although derived from both the retinal and ciliary circulations, the capillaries of the optic nerve head resemble more closely the features of retinal capillaries than of the choriocapillaris. These characteristics include (1) tight junctions, (2) abundant pericytes, and (c) nonfenestrated endothelium.[10] They do not leak fluorescein and may represent a nerve-blood barrier, supporting the concept of the retina-nerve vasculature as a continuous system with the central nervous system.[9,10] The capillaries become fewer behind the lamina, especially along the margins of the larger vessels.[13]

Venous Drainage. The venous return in the optic nerve head is primarily by the central retinal vein, although some blood enters the choroidal system, thereby establishing another communication between the retina and choroid.[4] Occasionally these communications are enlarged as retinociliary veins, which drain from the retina to the choroidal circulation, or ciliooptic veins, which drain from the choroid to the central retinal vein.[14]

Astroglial Support

Astrocytes provide a continuous layer between the neurons and blood vessels in the optic nerve head.[15] In the rhesus monkey, astrocytes occupy 5% of the nerve fiber layer but increase to 23% of the laminar region, and they then decrease to 11% in the retrolaminar area.[5] The astrocytes are joined by "gap junctions," which resemble tight junctions but have minute gaps between the outer membrane leaflets.[16]

The astroglial tissue also provides a covering for portions of the optic nerve head (Fig. 5.3). The *internal limiting membrane of Elschnig* separates the nerve head from the vitreous and is continuous with the internal limiting membrane of the retina.[15,17–19] The central portion of the internal limiting membrane is referred to as the *central meniscus of Kuhnt*.[18] Ultrastructural studies of the monkey optic nerve head revealed a membrane thickness of 70 nm at the disc margin, which thinned to 50 nm in the midperiphery.[19] Although the central meniscus of Kuhnt is traditionally described as a central thickening of the membrane, the ultrastructural study revealed a thinning to 20 nm.[19] The *intermediary tissue of Kuhnt* separates the nerve from the retina, while the *border tissue of Jacoby* separates the nerve from the choroid.[6,18]

Collagen Support

Lamina Cribrosa. This structure consists of fenestrated sheets of connective tissue and occasional elastic fibers lined by astrocytes[6] and has been shown to have regional differences in human and nonhuman primate eyes. The superior and inferior portions, as compared with the nasal and temporal regions, have larger fenestrae and thinner connective tissue and glial cell support (Fig. 5.4).[20–22] The possible significance of these regional differences to the mechanism of glaucomatous optic atrophy is discussed later in this chapter.

The lamina cribrosa of the human optic nerve head contains a specialized *extracellular matrix* composed of collagen types I through VI, laminin, and fibronectin.[23–25]

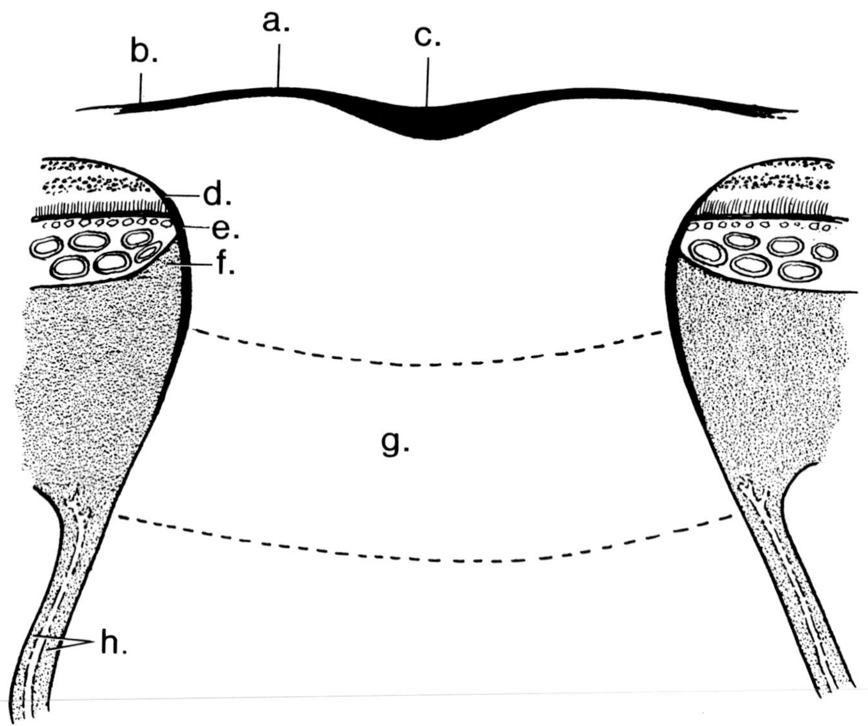

Figure 5.3. Supportive structures of the optic nerve head: internal limiting membrane of Elschnig (*a*); continuous with the internal limiting membrane of the retina (*b*); central meniscus of Kuhnt (*c*); intermediary tissue of Kuhnt (*d*); border tissue of Jacoby (*e*); border tissue of Elschnig (*f*); lamina cribrosa (*g*); meningeal sheaths (*h*).

Studies of young human donors show that the cribriform plates are composed of a core of elastin fibers with a sparse, patchy distribution of collagen type III, coated with collagen type IV and laminin.[26] Cell cultures of human lamina cribrosa revealed two cell types, which appear to synthesize this extracellular matrix.[27] The nature of the extracellular matrix is similar in monkey optic nerve heads.[28,29] Abnormalities of this extracellular matrix in the lamina cribrosa may influence optic nerve function and its susceptibility to glaucomatous damage by elevated IOP.

A rim of connective tissue, the *border tissue of Elschnig,* occasionally extends between the choroid and optic nerve tissues, especially temporally (Fig. 5.3)[18] Posterior to the globe, the optic nerve is surrounded by meningeal sheaths (pia, arachnoid, and dura), which consist of connective tissue lined by meningothelial cells, or mesothelium.[30] Vascularized connective tissue extends from the undersurface of the pia mater to form longitudinal septae, which partially separate the axonal bundles in the intraorbital portion of the optic nerve.[18]

Axons

Retinal Nerve Fiber Layer. As the axons traverse the nerve fiber layer from the ganglion cell bodies to the optic nerve head, they are distributed in a characteristic pattern (Fig. 5.5). Fibers from the temporal periphery originate on either side of a horizontal dividing line, the median raphe, and arch above or below the fovea as the *arcuate nerve fibers,* while those from the central retina, the *papillomacular fibers,* and the nasal fibers take a more direct path to the nerve head. The significance of this anatomy to the visual field defects of glaucoma is discussed in the next chapter. The axons in monkeys and rabbits are grouped into fiber bundles by tissue tunnels composed of

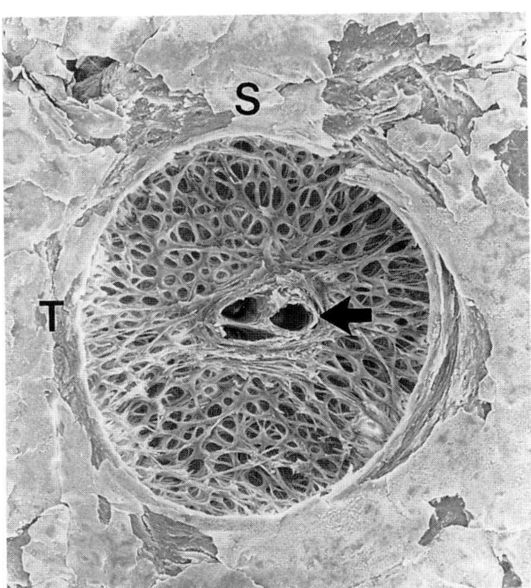

Figure 5.4. Gross anatomic photograph of lamina cribrosa showing central openings for central retinal vessels (*arrow*) and surrounding fenestrae of lamina for passage of axon bundles. Note larger size of fenestrae in superior and inferior quadrants. Superior (*S*), temporal (*T*). (Courtesy of Harry A. Quigley, M.D.)

elongated processes of Müller cells.[31–33] These bundles, especially on the temporal side, become larger as they approach the nerve head, primarily as a result of lateral fusion of bundles,[34] and normally are visible by ophthalmoscopy as retinal striations.[33] The axons within the bundles vary in size, with larger fibers coming from the more peripheral retina.[34] The relative position of the different fiber types within the bundles varies among the monkey species that have been studied.[34]

Axons in Optic Nerve Head. The arcuate nerve fibers occupy the superior and inferior temporal portions of the optic nerve head, with axons from the peripheral retina taking a more peripheral position in the nerve head (Fig. 5.6).[35] The arcuate fibers are the most susceptible to early glaucomatous damage. The papillomacular fibers spread over approximately one-third of the distal optic nerve, primarily inferior temporally where the axonal density is higher.[36,37] They intermingle with extramacular fibers, which may explain the retention of central vision during early glaucomatous optic atrophy.

The mean axonal population in the normal optic nerve head was reported to be 1.2 million, based on a manual count of a small percentage of the total neural area.[38] Using computerized image analysis of sections throughout the nerve, however, lower mean counts of 693,316 in one study[39] and 969,279 in another[37] were reported. All studies agree that there is a large variability of axonal numbers among normal eyes of approximately ±200,000 fibers. The reported mean axonal fiber diameter ranges from 0.65–1.10 μm.[37,39,40] Axons of all sizes are mixed throughout the nerve area, although higher mean diameters appear to be more common in the nasal segment.[37]

Influence of Age

At birth, the optic nerve is small and nearly unmyelinated.[41] Myelination, which proceeds from the brain to the eye during gestation, is largely completed in the retrolaminar region of the optic nerve by the end of the first year of life.[42] The connective tissue of the lamina cribrosa is also incompletely developed at birth, which may account for the greater susceptibility of the infant nerve head to glaucomatous cupping, as well as its potential for reversible cupping.[43] With increasing age, the cores of the cribriform plates enlarge, and there is an increase in the apparent density of collagen types I, III, and IV and elastin.[44] Also with increasing age, there appears to be a progressive loss of axons and a corresponding increase in the cross-sectional area occupied by the leptomeninges and fibrous septae.[37–41] The loss of axons has been estimated at 5000 per year,[37] although a statistically significant relationship between age and mean fiber count has not been shown, possibly because of the large variability in mean total populations.[39] One study suggested a selective loss of large nerve fibers with age,[39] which was not confirmed by others.[37,40]

THE PATHOGENESIS OF GLAUCOMATOUS OPTIC ATROPHY

The Theories

The pathogenesis of glaucomatous optic atrophy has remained a matter of contro-

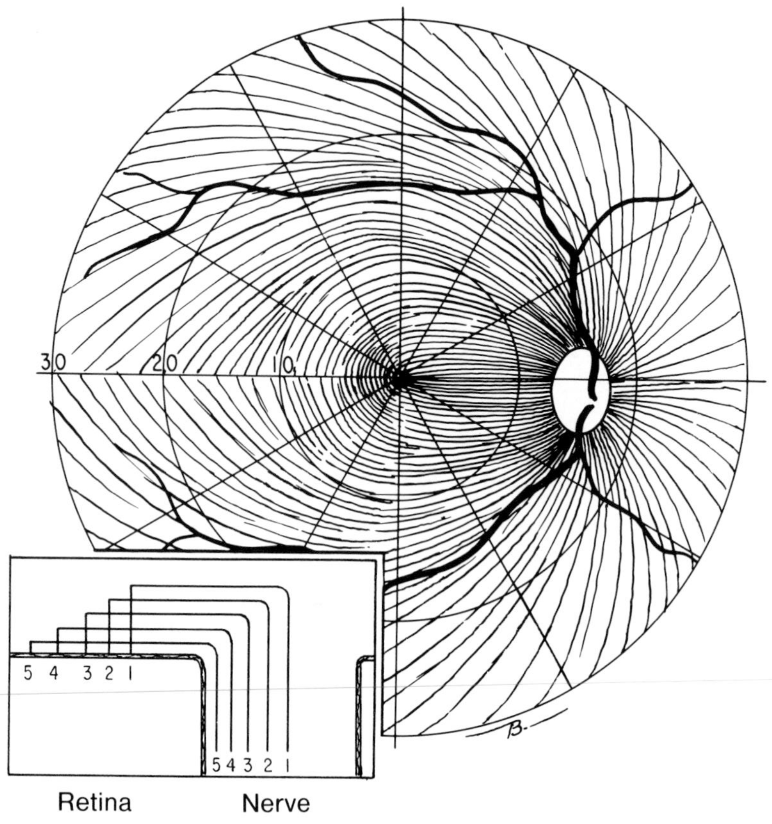

Figure 5.5. Distribution of retinal nerve fibers. Note arching above and below the fovea of fibers temporal to the optic nerve head. Inset depicts cross-sectional arrangement of axons, with fibers originating from peripheral retina running closer to choroid and periphery of optic nerve, while fibers originating nearer to the nerve head are situated closer to the vitreous and occupy a more central portion of the nerve.

versy since the mid-19th century, when two concepts were introduced in the same year. In 1858, Müller[45] proposed that the elevated IOP led to direct compression and death of the neurons (the mechanical theory), while von Jaeger[46] suggested that a vascular abnormality was the underlying cause of the optic atrophy (the vascular theory). In 1892, Schnabel[47] proposed another concept in the pathogenesis of glaucomatous optic atrophy, suggesting that atrophy of neural elements created empty spaces, which pulled the nerve head posteriorly (Schnabel's cavernous atrophy).

Initially, the mechanical theory received the greatest support.[48–50] This concept held sway through the first quarter of the 20th century until LaGrange and Beauvieux[51] popularized the vascular theory in 1925. In general, this belief held that glaucomatous optic atrophy was secondary to ischemia, whether the primary result of the elevated IOP or an unrelated vascular lesion.[52–54] In 1968, however, the role of axoplasmic flow in glaucomatous optic atrophy was introduced,[55] which revived support for the mechanical theory but did not exclude the possible influence of ischemia.

The Evidence

Continued investigation into the pathogenesis of glaucomatous optic atrophy has led to the following bodies of information:

Anatomic and Histopathologic Studies

Histopathologic observations of human eyes with glaucoma provide the most direct

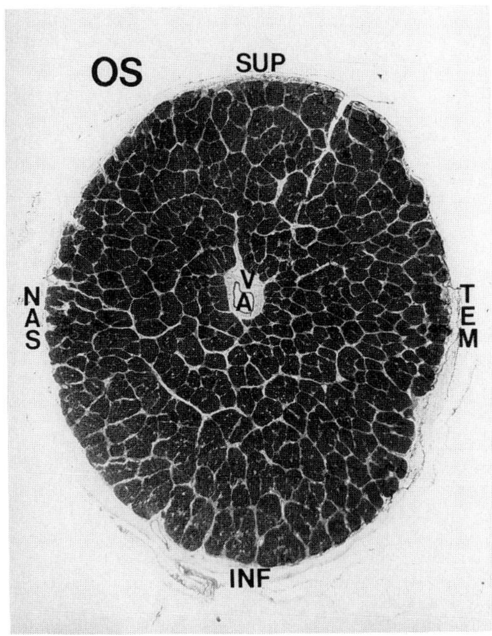

Figure 5.6. Light microscopic view of normal optic nerve head on cross-section with darkly staining axon bundles and intervening glial supportive tissue surrounding openings for central retinal vessels. Superior (*SUP*), temporal (*TEM*), inferior (*INF*), nasal (*NAS*), vein (*V*), artery (*A*). (Courtesy of Harry A. Quigley, M.D.)

method of studying the alterations associated with glaucomatous optic atrophy, although they do not fully explain the mechanisms that caused the damage. One of the limiting factors has been that many of the specimens studied have come from eyes with advanced glaucomatous change, which led to possible misconceptions regarding the early pathogenic features. More recent studies, which have attempted to correlate clinical observations with histopathologic changes in optic nerve heads from eyes with varying stages of glaucoma, appear to clarify many of these points.

Glial Alterations. It was once suggested that loss of astroglial supportive tissue precedes neuronal loss,[56] which was thought to explain the early and reversible cupping in infants.[57] However, subsequent studies have shown that glial cells are not selectively lost in early glaucoma and are actually the only remaining cells after loss of axons in advanced cases.[58,59]

Vascular Alterations. It was also once proposed that loss of small vessels in the optic nerve head accompanies atrophy of axons,[60] and one histologic study suggested a selective loss of retinal radial peripapillary capillaries in eyes with chronic glaucoma.[61] However, subsequent investigations revealed neither a correlation between atrophy of this vascular system and visual field loss[62] nor a major selective loss of optic nerve head capillaries in human eyes with glaucoma.[58,59,63] In animal models of optic atrophy, created by either sustained IOP elevation,[63] sectioning of the optic nerve,[64–66] or photocoagulation of the retinal nerve fiber layer,[67] the resulting disc pallor was not associated with a decrease in the ratio of capillaries to neural tissue, although the caliber of the vessels diminished.[66] Instead, these studies showed a proliferation[65] or reorganization[64,67] of glial tissue, which obscures ophthalmoscopic visualization of the vessels.

Alterations of Lamina Cribrosa. Backward bowing of the lamina cribrosa has long been recognized as a characteristic feature of late glaucomatous optic atrophy,[68,69] as well as an early change in the infant eye with glaucoma.[43] Further study, however, has suggested that alterations in the lamina may actually be a primary event in the pathogenesis of glaucomatous optic atrophy. In enucleated human[70] eyes, acute IOP elevation caused a backward bowing of the lamina, and similar changes were observed in a primate glaucoma model.[71] However, noninvasive measurements of optic nerve head displacement by laser Doppler velocimetry in postmortem glaucomatous eyes suggested a reduction in optic nerve head compliance as the glaucomatous damage progresses.[72] In a histopathologic evaluation of 25 glaucomatous human eyes, compression of successive lamina cribrosa sheets was the earliest detected abnormality, while backward bowing of the entire lamina occurred later and involved primarily the upper and lower poles.[73]

In the early stages of adult glaucoma, the magnitude of backward bowing is not sufficient to explain the ophthalmoscopically observed cupping but may be enough to cause compression of the axons, and it has been suggested that the structure of the lamina cribrosa may be an important determinant in the susceptibility of the optic nerve head to damage from elevated IOP.[58,59] A racial comparison of the relative connective tissue support and regional pore size of the lamina cribrosa did not explain the greater susceptibility of blacks to glaucomatous damage.[74] However, changes in the extracellular matrix may play an important role in the progression of glaucomatous damage and may be a causative agent.[75]

Axonal Alterations. The actual cause of early optic nerve head cupping in glaucoma is loss of axonal tissue.[58,59,76] Experimental models of primate eyes exposed to chronic IOP elevation suggest that the damage is associated with a posterior and lateral displacement of the lamina cribrosa, which compresses the axons.[77] The damage first involves axonal bundles throughout the nerve with somewhat greater involvement of the inferior and superior poles.[73] With continued nerve damage, the susceptibility of the polar zones becomes more prominent (Fig. 5.7).[58,59,73,76] Histologic studies of both monkey[78] and human[79] optic nerves indicate that nerve fibers larger than the normal mean diameter atrophy more rapidly in glaucomatous eyes, although no fiber size is spared from damage. This preferential loss of large fibers appears to be due to a higher proportion of the fibers in the inferior and superior poles, as well as an inherent susceptibility to injury by glaucoma.

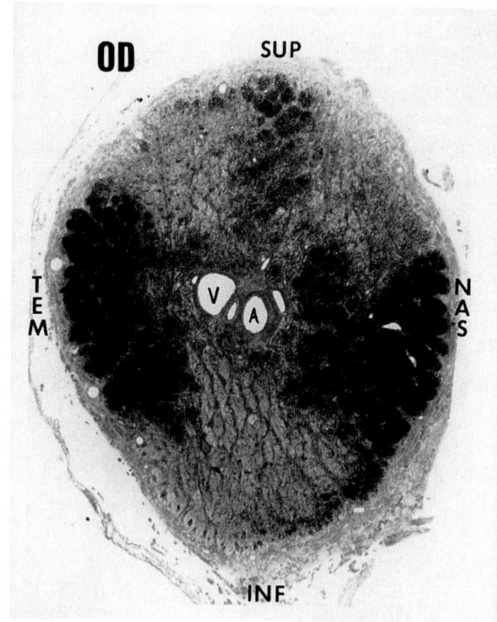

Figure 5.7. Light microscopic cross-sectional view of optic nerve head with glaucomatous atrophy showing loss of axon bundles predominantly in the inferior and superior quadrants (compare with normal nerve head in Figure 5.6). Superior (*SUP*), nasal (*NAS*), inferior (*INF*), temporal (*TEM*), vein (*V*), artery (*A*). (Courtesy of Harry A. Quigley, M.D.)

Studies of Blood Flow

Blood flow in the optic nerve head of cats is relatively high compared with that in more posterior portions of the nerve, and autoregulation appears to compensate for alterations in mean arterial blood pressure.[80] With elevation of IOP, blood flow in the optic nerve head, retina, and choroid of cat eyes is only slightly affected before the pressure is within 25 mm Hg of the mean arterial blood pressure, and flow in the lamina cribrosa is reduced only with extreme pressure elevations, again suggesting autoregulation in the optic nerve head.[81] Another study, however, suggests that the electrical function of ganglion cell axons in cat eyes depends on the perfusion pressure and not on the absolute height of the IOP.[82] Real-time analysis of optic nerve head oxidative metabolism in cats indicates that the metabolic response is dependent on IOP and/or mean arterial pressure and that lowering the IOP can reverse metabolic dysfunction.[83]

Short-term IOP elevation in monkey eyes did not alter optic nerve head blood flow until it exceeded 75 mm Hg, and long-term glaucoma in monkeys had no apparent influence on mean blood flow in the nerve head.[84] A study of oxygen tension in the monkey optic nerve head suggested that autoregulation compensates for changes in perfusion pressure.[85] Blood flow measurements in the optic nerve head of human eyes, using laser Doppler, also demonstrated autoregulatory compensation to reduced perfusion pressure secondary to elevated IOP.[86] A technique of continuously monitoring disc brightness during and after an abrupt artificial elevation of IOP (dynamic provoked circulatory response) showed that the extent to which a glaucomatous eye can adjust to the pressure changes is significantly reduced from that of nonglaucomatous eyes,[87] and it has been suggested that ischemia of the optic nerve head in glaucoma may involve faulty autoregulation.[81,85]

Fluorescein Angiographic Observations

Normal Fluorescein Pattern. The normal fluorescein pattern of the optic nerve head is usually described as having three phases.[4] (1) An initial filling, or preretinal arterial phase, is believed to represent filling of the prelaminar and lamina cribrosa regions by the posterior ciliary arteries. Fluorescein in the retrobulbar vessels may also contribute to this phase.[88] (2) The peak fluorescence, or retinal arteriovenous phase, is primarily due to filling of the dense capillary plexus on the nerve head surface from retinal arterioles. With increasing age, there is a decrease in the filling time of both the retinal and choroidal circulations.[89] (3) A late phase consists of 10–15 minutes of delayed staining of the nerve head, which is probably due to fluorescein in the connective tissue of the lamina cribrosa. Tracer studies in monkeys suggest that the leakage may come from the adjacent choroid.[90]

Artificially Elevated IOP. The effect of artificially elevated IOP on the fluorescein angiographic pattern has provided an understanding of the relative vulnerability of ocular vessels to elevated pressure in the normal and glaucomatous eye. There is a general delay in the entire ocular circulation in response to an elevation of the IOP. The prelaminar portion of the nerve head appears to be the portion of the ocular vascular system that is most vulnerable to elevated pressure in monkeys.[4,91]

Studies regarding the vulnerability of the peripapillary choroid to IOP elevation have provided conflicting results. Fluorescein angiography of monkey eyes has suggested a marked susceptibility of this vascular system to elevated pressure,[4,91] and fluorescein studies of human eyes with glaucoma have shown similar delays in peripapillary choroidal filling.[91–95] The delay appears to be sensitive to elevated IOP,[92] and it has been suggested that this vascular disturbance of the peripapillary choroid contributes to glaucomatous optic atrophy.[94] However, fluorescein angiographic studies of normal human eyes have shown similar delayed or irregular choroidal filling at normal pressures,[96,97] and the peripapillary choroidal capillaries of normal human eyes were relatively resistant to artificial pressure elevations.[98] Furthermore, a fluorescein study of patients with low-tension or chronic simple glaucoma provided no evidence that hypoperfusion of the peripapillary choroid contributed to optic nerve hypoperfusion.[99]

A selective nonfilling of the retinal radial peripapillary capillaries during India ink perfusion has been demonstrated in cats.[100] As previously discussed, however, histopathologic observations are conflicting with regard to alterations of this vascular system in glaucomatous eyes.[61,62] Most studies of monkey[4,91] and normal human eyes[101,102] have shown the choroidal circulation in general to be more vulnerable than that of the retina to elevated IOP, although one study found the two systems to fill at the same level of increased pressure.[103]

Studies of Glaucomatous Eyes. Fluorescein angiographic studies of glaucomatous and nonglaucomatous eyes have revealed two types of filling defects of the optic nerve head: (1) persisting hypoperfusion and (2) transient hypoperfusion.[104,105]

Persisting hypoperfusion, or an absolute filling defect, is more common in eyes with glaucoma, especially low-tension glaucoma, and is said to correlate with visual field loss.[104–106] The characteristics of a filling defect include decreased blood flow, a smaller vascular bed, narrower vessels, and increased permeability of the vessels.[107] The filling defect may be either focal or diffuse. The former is believed to reflect susceptible vasculature with or without elevated IOP and is the typical defect in low-tension glaucoma.[99] Focal defects occur primarily in the inferior and superior poles of the optic nerve head.[104–106,108] In glaucomatous eyes, they are most often seen in the wall of the cup, while in normal eyes they occur more commonly in the floor of the cup.[109] The diffuse defect is thought to represent prolonged pressure elevation.[99]

Patients with ocular hypertension (elevated IOP, but normal optic nerve heads and visual fields) have more filling defects than the normal population, although fewer than in eyes with glaucoma.[106,110] The only other condition reported to give absolute filling defects is sectorial ischemic optic neuropathy.[111] However, the nature of the defect in open-angle glaucoma is believed to be specific, and it has been suggested that fluorescein angiography of the optic nerve head may help to differentiate open-angle glaucoma from other conditions that have similar clinical changes in the optic disc.[111] A correlation between vascular changes of the optic nerve head and visual field loss in glaucoma has not been fully established. However, it has been reported that the development of new visual field defects is associated with changes in the optic nerve head circulation, as determined by fluorescein angiography.[112] Computerized image analysis has been used to objectively quantify fluorescein angiograms of the optic disc and has shown that increases in fluorescein-filling defect areas correlates with glaucomatous progression.[113]

Transient hypoperfusion, or a relative (delayed) filling defect, is seen in the normal population and does not correlate with optic nerve head or visual field changes.[104–106] However, it has been postulated that they may progress to absolute defects, which is believed to provide a sign of impending field loss.[106]

One fluorescein angiographic study revealed fluorescein leakage of the optic nerve head associated with advanced glaucomatous optic atrophy in nine of 150 patients with primary open-angle glaucoma,[114] and staining of the nerve head was seen in 30% of glaucomatous eyes in another fluorescein study.[104,105] Fluorescein angiograms have also been used to study blood flow in glaucomatous eyes, which revealed decreased flow in eyes with elevated IOP and also in two cases of low tension glaucoma.[115]

Observations of Axoplasmic Flow

Physiology of Axoplasmic Flow. Axoplasmic flow, or axonal transport, refers to the movement of material (axoplasm) along the axon of a nerve (the dendrite may also have transport) in a predictable, energy-dependent manner. This movement has been characterized as having fast and slow components, although numerous intermediate rates may also exist.[116] The fast phase moves approximately 410 mm/day in various species and may supply material to synaptic vesicles, the axolemma, and agranular endoplasmic reticulum of the axon, while the slow phase moves at 1–3 mm/day and is believed to subserve growth and maintenance of axons.[116] The flow of axoplasm may be orthograde (from retina to lateral geniculate body) or retrograde (lateral geniculate body to retina).[117]

Experimental Models of Axoplasmic Flow. Animal models (usually in monkeys) have been developed for studying axoplasmic flow by injecting radioactive amino acids, such as tritiated leucine, into the vitreous. The amino acid is incorporated into the protein synthesis of retinal ganglion cells and then moves down the ganglion cell axon into the optic nerve, allowing histologic study of the orthograde movement of radioactively labeled protein.[118] In addition, retrograde flow can be studied by observing the accumulation of certain unlabeled neuronal components, such as mitochondria, by electron microscopy[119] or by injecting tracer elements, such as horseradish peroxidase, into the lateral geniculate body and studying its movement toward the retina.[120] These models can be used to study factors that cause abnormal blockade of axoplasmic flow, which may relate to glaucomatous optic atrophy in the human eye.

Influence of IOP on Axoplasmic Flow. Elevated IOP in monkey eyes causes obstruction of axoplasmic flow at the lamina cribrosa[117,121–126] and the edge of the posterior scleral foramen.[126] The obstruction in general involves both the fast[122,125] and slow[122] phases as well as the orthograde and retrograde components.[117,124,127] In monkey eyes, the obstruction to fast axonal transport preferentially involves the superior, temporal, and inferior portions of the optic nerve head.[128] The height and duration of pressure elevation influence the onset, distribution, and degree of axoplasmic obstruction in the optic nerve head.[125,127,129,130] The mechanism by which elevated IOP leads to obstruction of axoplasmic flow is uncertain, but there are two popular theories: mechanical and vascular.

The mechanical theory suggests that physical alterations in the optic nerve head, such as a misalignment of the fenestrae in the lamina cribrosa as a result of its backbowing, may lead to the axoplasmic flow obstruction.[55,69,125] In support of this hypothesis is the observation that elevated IOP leads to blockage of axonal transport despite an intact nerve head capillary circulation and an elevated arterial pO_2.[117,131] Furthermore, obstruction of axoplasmic flow has also been reported in response to ocular hypotony,[122,124,132] leading some investigators to suggest that a pressure differential across the optic nerve head, whether resulting from a relative increase or decrease in IOP, causes mechanical changes with compression of the axonal bundles.[122,124,132,133]

In conflict with the mechanical theory is the observation that elevated intracranial pressure in monkeys neither caused obstruction of rapid axoplasmic flow nor prevented it in response to elevated IOP despite reduction in the pressure gradient across the lamina.[134] This suggests that more than a simple mechanical or hydrostatic mechanism may be involved with obstruction of axoplasmic flow in response to elevated IOP.[134] Also against the simple mechanical theory are the observations that axon damage is diffuse within bundles, rather than focal as might be expected with a kinking effect,[135] and that the location of transport interruption does not correlate with the cross-section area of fiber bundles, the shape of the laminar pores, or the density of interbundle septa.[136,137]

The vascular theory suggests that ischemic at least plays a role in the obstruction of axoplasmic flow in response to elevated IOP. Interruption of the short posterior ciliary arteries in monkeys has been reported to block both slow[138,139] and fast[140] axoplasmic flow, although it did not cause glaucomatous cupping.[138,139] Central retinal artery occlusion has been associated with obstruction of both rapid orthograde and retrograde axonal transport.[141] Furthermore, accumulation of tracer at the lamina cribrosa was inversely proportional to the perfusion pressure in cat eyes,[142] and IOP-induced blockage of axonal transport was greater in eyes with angiotensin-induced systemic hypertension.[143] It has also been noted in monkey eyes with elevated IOP that leakage from microvasculature of the nerve head was associated with blockage of axonal transport at the lamina cribrosa.[144]

Against a vascular mechanism for pressure-induced obstruction of axoplasmic flow is the observation that ligation of the right common carotid artery in monkeys, which reduced the estimated ophthalmic artery pressure by 10–20 mm Hg below the left side, did not significantly affect the extent to which IOP elevation interrupted axonal transport.[145] When obstruction to retrograde axoplasmic flow was studied in enucleated rat eyes, a direct relationship with IOP was still found despite removing the influence of the blood circulation and the fact that the lamina cribrosa is only a single laminar sheet.[120] It may be, therefore, that factors other than, or in addition to, ischemia and kinking of axons by a multilayered lamina cribrosa are involved in the intraocular pressure-induced obstruction to axoplasmic flow.

Electrophysiologic Studies

When the intraocular tension is elevated artificially in normal human eyes, a significant reduction in the amplitudes of electroretinographic components[146,147] and visual evoked potentials[147] occurs only when the pressure approaches or exceeds the ophthalmic blood pressure. However, the perfusion-pressure amplitude curve of the visual evoked potential in normal eyes showed a kink, suggestive of vascular autoregulation, that was not observed in glaucoma patients,[148] again pointing to a possible deficiency in autoregulation in glaucoma. As previously noted, the electrical function of retinal ganglion cells in cat eyes was found to depend more on perfusion pressure than on the absolute height of the IOP.[82]

Comparison with Nonglaucomatous Disorders

Studies of other ocular disorders provide some indirect insight into the possible mechanism of glaucomatous optic atrophy.

For example, a histopathologic study of severe peripapillary choroidal atrophy revealed a normal optic nerve head, suggesting that the vascular supply of these two structures may be independent.[149] Studies of nonglaucomatous optic atrophy have been used both to support and to refute an ischemic basis for glaucomatous optic atrophy. In patients with *anterior ischemic optic neuropathy,* cupping similar to that seen in glaucoma is observed frequently when the ischemia is due to giant cell arteritis but is less common in nonarteritic cases.[150–152] These observations have led to the suggestion that glaucoma and anterior ischemic optic neuropathy have the same vasogenic basis of optic nerve damage but differ according to the rate of change.[150] It has also been suggested that acute ischemic optic neuropathy may be one of several mechanisms of optic nerve disease in chronic glaucoma.[153] If this is true, the difference in visual field loss suggests that there is also a difference in the nature or distribution of the ischemia.[152] In addition, the pattern of optic nerve fiber loss in nonarteritic anterior ischemic optic neuropathy involves primarily the superior half of the nerve and is unlike that found in glaucoma.[154]

In contrast to the above studies, a review of 170 eyes with nonglaucomatous optic atrophy of various etiologies revealed a small but significant increase in cupping.[155] However, the cups were morphologically different from those seen in glaucoma, which was suggested as evidence against a vascular etiology in glaucomatous cupping. Furthermore, a study of 18 patients with vasogenic shock and poor peripheral tissue perfusion revealed no evidence of glaucomatous optic nerve head or visual field change.[156]

Cavernous atrophy of the optic nerve, as originally described by Schnabel,[47] has been considered to be a form of glaucomatous optic atrophy resulting from severe elevations of IOP. However, this also occurs in patients with normal pressures, in which case it may represent an aging change associated with generalized arteriosclerosis.[157]

The Conclusions

The present evidence suggests that obstruction to axoplasmic flow may be involved in the pathogenesis of glaucomatous optic atrophy. However, it is still not clear as to whether mechanical or vascular factors are primarily responsible for this obstruction, and whether other alterations are also important in the ultimate loss of axons. It may be that all of these factors are involved to some degree or, as Spaeth[104,105] has suggested, that there is more than one mechanism of optic atrophy in eyes with glaucoma. For example, the observed differences in glaucomatous visual field defects between patients with low-tension and high-tension glaucomas have led to the suggestion that ischemia may be the predominant factor in those glaucomas at the lower end of the IOP scale, while a more direct mechanical effect of the pressure may prevail in cases with higher IOP (Fig. 5.8).[158]

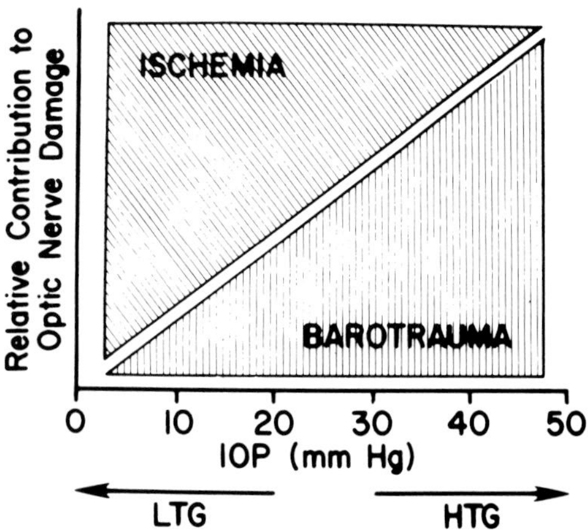

Figure 5.8. Theoretical representation of relative influence exerted by mechanical and vascular forces on the development of glaucomatous optic atrophy at different levels of intraocular pressure. (Reprinted with permission from Caprioli J, Spaeth GL: Am J Ophthal 97:730, 1984.)

CLINICAL APPEARANCE OF GLAUCOMATOUS OPTIC ATROPHY

While investigators continue to study the pathophysiology of glaucomatous optic atrophy, the practicing physician has a responsibility to become thoroughly familiar with the clinical morphology of this condition, since it provides the most reliable early evidence of damage in glaucoma.

Morphology of the Normal Optic Nerve Head

In order to recognize pathologic alterations of the optic nerve head, one must first be familiar with the wide range of normal variations.

General Features

The ophthalmoscopic appearance of the optic nerve head is generally that of a vertical oval, although there is considerable variation in size and shape. Clinical studies have revealed a greater than sixfold difference in the area of normal nerve heads,[159,160] which is consistent with histologic studies cited earlier in this chapter.[1–3] The central portion of the disc usually contains a depression, the *cup,* and an area of *pallor,* which represents a partial or complete absence of axons, with exposure of the lamina cribrosa. While the size and location of cup and pallor are normally the same, it is important to note that this is not always the case, especially in disease states,[161] and these two parameters should not be thought of as being synonymous. The tissue between the cup and disc margins is referred to as the *neural rim.* It represents the location of the bulk of the axons and normally has an orange-red color, because of the associated capillaries. Retinal vessels ride up the nasal wall of the cup, often kinking at the cup margin before crossing the neural rim to the retina (Figs. 5.9 and 5.10).

The Physiologic Cup

Size. The size of the optic nerve head cup, which is commonly described as the horizontal cup/disc ratio (C/D), varies considerably within the normal population, which appears to be explained by the normal variation in disc diameter.[3] Reports of C/D distribution within the general population differ according to examination techniques. When the discs were studied by direct ophthalmoscopy, the distribution was found to be non-Gaussian with most eyes having a C/D of 0.0–0.3 and only 1–2% being 0.7 or greater.[162] However, when stereoscopic views were used, a Gaussian distribution was found, with a mean C/D of 0.4 and approximately 5% with 0.7.[163] In another study, the two techniques of optic nerve head evaluation were compared, and stereoscopic examination with a Hruby lens gave consistently larger C/D estimates, with

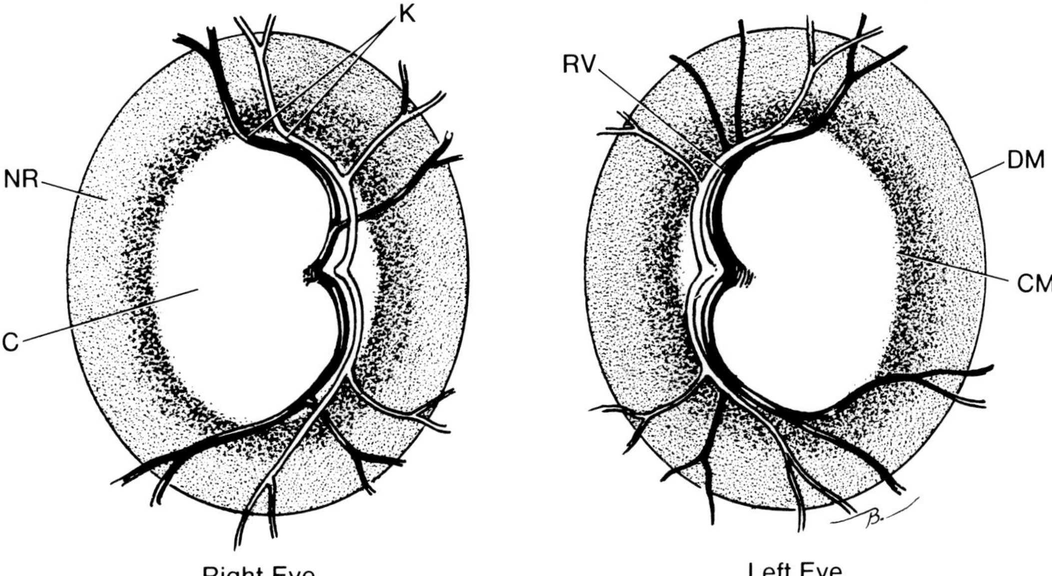

Figure 5.9. Normal optic nerve heads: neural rim (*NR*); disc margin (*DM*); cup margin (*CM*); cup (*C*); retinal vessels (*RV*); kinking of vessels at cup margin (*K*). Note that size of cups is symmetrical between the two eyes and that neural rims are even for 360°.

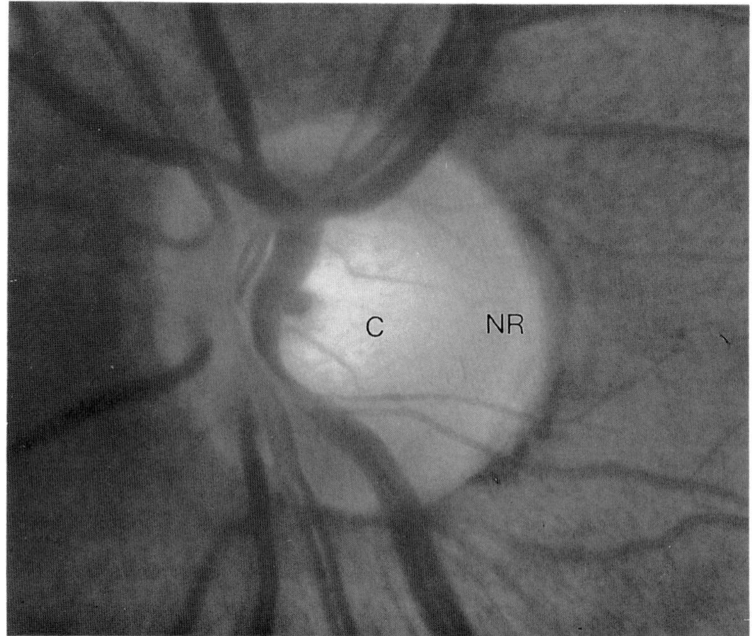

Figure 5.10. Fundus photo of normal optic nerve head. Neural rim (*NR*), cup (*C*).

a mean of 0.38 as compared with 0.25 by direct ophthalmoscopy.[164] These authors noted, however, that the disparity between estimated C/D for the same eye at different times seldom exceeds 0.2, so that the documentation of such a difference over time should be viewed with suspicion.[164] It is also important to note that physiologic cups tend to be symmetrical between the two eyes of the same individual,[162,163,165,166] with a C/D difference of greater than 0.2 between fellow eyes occurring in only 1% of the normal population.[162]

The size of physiologic cups is frequently similar to that of the individual's parents and siblings,[162,167,168] and is believed to be genetically determined on a polygenic, multifactorial basis.[162] The heritability has been estimated at ⅔, with the remaining variance attributed to errors of development.[168] It is helpful, therefore, to examine other members of the family when attempting to distinguish between a large physiologic cup and glaucomatous cupping. The normal C/D does not appear to correlate with a family history of open-angle glaucoma,[162,169] although some studies have suggested a weak correlation with higher IOPs,[163,169–171] abnormal tonographic outflow facilities,[169,170] or highly positive pressure responses to topical corticosteroids.[172]

Some studies have shown no significant correlation between age and the size of the physiologic cup,[160,162,167,169,173] while other investigations suggest that both the cup[163,164,171,174] and pallor[175] do enlarge with increasing age. One study suggests that this change results from a slow but steady increase in the diameter of the optic nerve head with advancing years, without an alteration in the area of the neural rim, the net effect of which is a decrease in the rim breadth and an increase in the cup diameter.[171] However, as previously noted, a progressive loss of axons in the optic nerve has also been observed histologically with increasing age.[37–41] It is important to note that any enlargement of the cup with age is gradual and should not be confused with the more rapid progression of glaucomatous cupping.

Racial differences in optic nerve head parameters have been shown, with blacks having a larger disc and C/D than whites.[176,177] Most studies have found no correlation between cup size and sex,[162,163,167,168] although one investigation revealed larger relative areas of pallor in white males than in white females.[175] Refractive errors do not

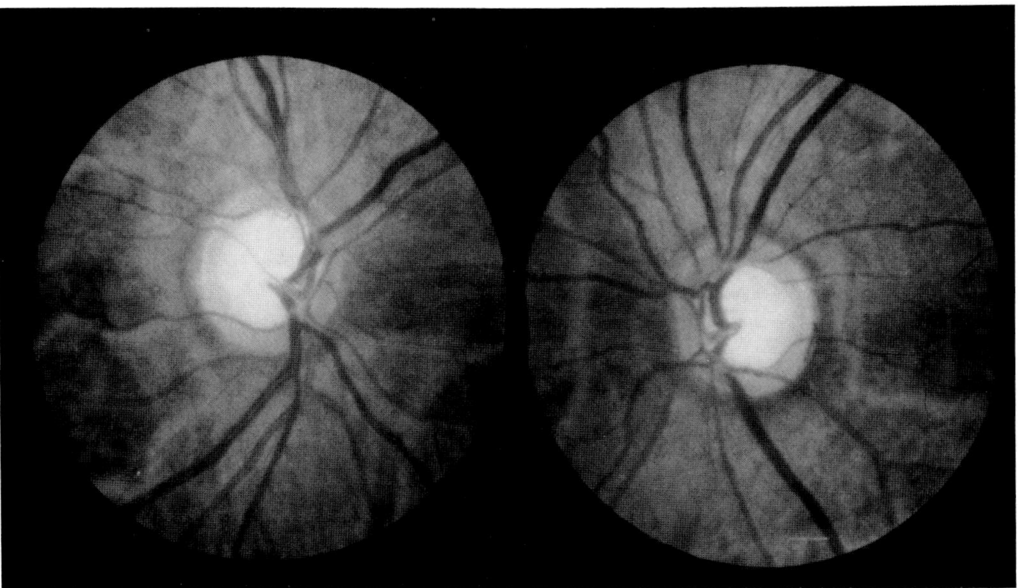

Figure 5.11. Large, physiologic optic nerve head cups, characterized by symmetrical size of cups and intact, even neural rims.

appear to correlate with the diameter of the physiologic cup,[160,162,167,171] although a study of highly myopic eyes (more than 8.00 diopters) revealed a significant correlation between refraction and disc size.[178]

In the differential diagnosis of glaucomatous optic atrophy, it is important to distinguish between a large physiologic cup and glaucomatous enlargement of the cup (Fig. 5.11). One distinguishing feature is symmetry of cup size between right and left eye in the physiologic state, taking into consideration the normal variations as previously discussed. Another helpful feature is the configuration of the cup and neural rim, as well as the appearance of the peripapillary pigmentation and retinal nerve fiber layer (all discussed later in this chapter), which are the same in eyes with either large or normal size physiologic cups.[179] The most important feature, however, is the documentation of progressive cup enlargement, which is highly suggestive of glaucoma.

Shape. The shape of the physiologic cup is roughly correlated with the shape of the disc, which means that the margins of cup and disc tend to run more or less parallel to each other.[180] However, the inferior neural rim is the broadest of the four quadrants, followed by the superior, nasal, and temporal rims.[160] Consequently, the cup has a horizontal oval shape in the majority of normal eyes, so that a vertical C/D greater than the horizontal C/D should be looked upon with suspicion.[160,164] The three-dimensional contour of the cup varies even more than the two-dimensional configuration in normal eyes. In 1899, Elschnig grouped physiologic cups into the following categories on the basis of configuration, and this classification has subsequently been supported by contour mapping of the optic nerve head surface (Fig. 5.12).[181,182]

Type I: Small cup with funnel-shaped walls.
Type II: Temporal, cylindrical (steep-walled) cup.
Type III: Central, trough-shaped cup.
Type IV: Temporal or central cup with a well-developed nasal wall, but a temporal wall that gradually slopes to disc margin. This is particularly common along the inferotemporal margin and can be confused with early glaucomatous cupping.[183]
Type V: Developmental anomalies (discussed later in this chapter).

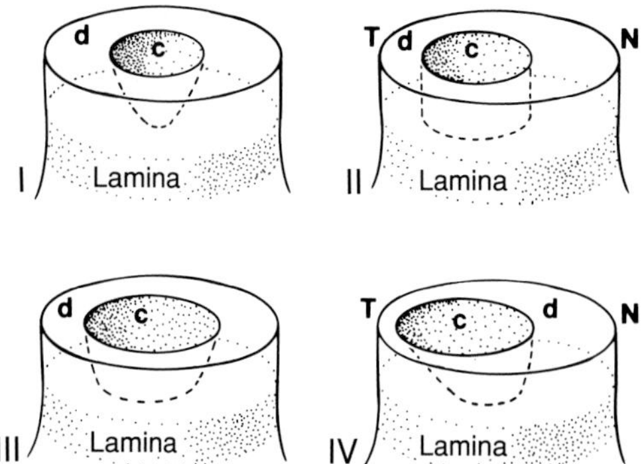

Figure 5.12. Schematic representation of the variation in shape of physiologic cups, based on classification of Elschnig and subsequent contour mapping:[160,161] **I,** small funnel-shaped; **II,** temporal, cylindrical; **III,** central, trough-shaped; **IV,** steep nasal wall with sloping of temporal wall toward disc margin. Disc (*d*), cup (*c*), temporal (*T*), nasal (*N*).

The contour of the cup appears to influence the C/D in that cups with steep margins appear to have larger areas than those with temporal flat slopes.[160]

The Physiologic Neural Rim

By tradition, more is said about the cup than the neural rim of both normal and glaucomatous optic nerve heads. However, it is actually alterations in the neural rim of an eye with glaucoma that lead to changes in the cup as well as to loss of visual field. The C/D is only an indirect measure of the amount of neural tissue in the optic nerve head and may be misleading, since an increasing diameter of the nerve head may be associated with decreasing neural rim width and increasing cup size, despite a stable area of neural tissue.[171,184] It is important, therefore, to pay close attention to the appearance of the neural rim.

As previously noted, the neural rim of the normal optic nerve head is typically broadest in the inferior quadrant, followed by the superior and then the nasal rims, with the temporal rim being the thinnest.[160] Several studies have attempted to correlate the area of the neural rim with that of the disc, and there is general agreement that the two are positively correlated (i.e., larger discs have larger neural rim areas).[160,185–187] However, the contour of the cup influences this correlation, in that the rim area increases by a greater factor with the disc area in discs having cups with flat temporal slopes than in those with circular steep cups.[187] The increase in neural rim area with increasing disc area appears to be due, at least in part, to a greater number of ganglion cell axons.[3]

Several factors can interfere with the interpretation of the neural rim width. *A gray crescent in the optic nerve head* has been described, which typically is slate gray and located in the temporal or inferotemporal periphery of the neural rim.[188] It is more common in black individuals and apparently represents a variation of the normal anatomy. However, mistaking the gray crescent for a peripapillary pigmented crescent could result in the physiologic neural rim being misinterpreted as pathologically thin in that area (Fig. 5.13).

Another source of error in interpreting the neural rim is the *optic nerve head in myopia,* in which the oblique insertion of the nerve may lead to obstruction of the temporal neural rim from ophthalmoscopic view, suggesting pathologic thinning of this tissue (Fig. 5.14). Other features of highly myopic discs that may interfere with interpretation include a larger disc area; a shallower than usual cup, which may mask the deepening of the cup in glaucoma; and a temporal peripapillary crescent, which may be confused with peripapillary pigmentary changes that are seen around some glaucomatous discs.[178]

It has also been observed that patients with diabetes mellitus may have an increase in the neural rim over time, which the authors believed could be due to nerve swelling.[189]

The Physiologic Peripapillary Retina

The Retinal Nerve Fiber Layer. Striations in the retinal nerve fiber layer are normally seen ophthalmoscopically as light reflexes from bundles of nerve fibers.[33,190] They are visible only after the bundles reach a critical thickness and consequently are seen best in the posterior pole and peripapillary regions, especially at the vertical poles of the disc and extending temporally from them.[191] In one large study, the retinal nerve fiber layer was most visible in the in-

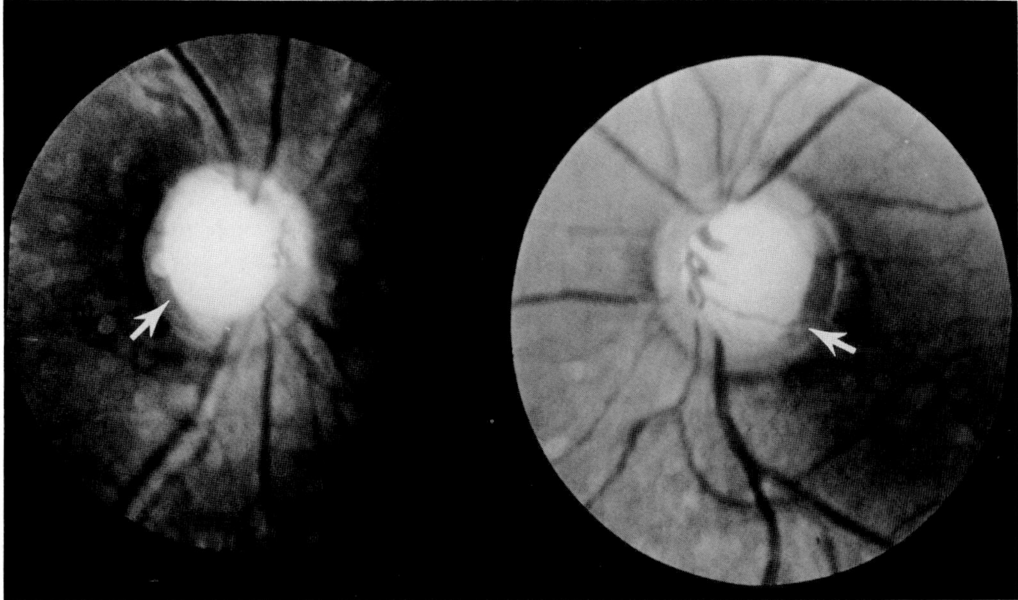

Figure 5.13. Gray crescents in the optic nerve head, obscuring the inferotemporal portions of the neural rims (*arrows*). (Reprinted from Am J Ophthal 89:238, 1980, with permission.)

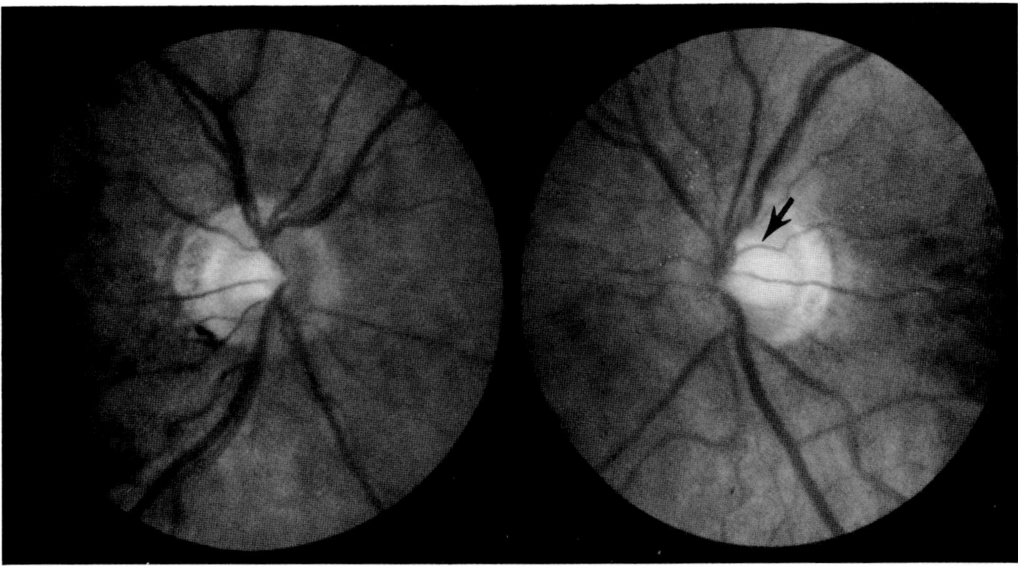

Figure 5.14. Oblique insertion of optic nerve heads in myopic patient obscures visualization of temporal neural rim and creates wide temporal peripapillary crescent, which interferes with distinguishing between physiologic and glaucomatous cupping. In this case, larger cup with baring of circumlinear vessels in left eye (*arrow*) indicates glaucomatous damage.

ferior temporal arcade, followed by the superior temporal arcade, then the temporal macular area, and finally the nasal area.[192] The nerve fiber layer has been noted to decrease with age.[192]

Peripapillary Pigmentary Variations. The normal optic nerve head may be surrounded by zones that vary in width, circumference, and pigmentation. A clinicopathologic study has revealed several clinical configurations with anatomic correlations.[193] A *scleral lip,* which appears commonly as a white rim that marks the disc margin, represents an anterior extension of sclera between the choroid and optic nerve head. A *chorioscleral crescent* is a broader area of more irregular depigmentation, usually associated with a tilted scleral canal, and represents a retraction of retinal pigment epithelium from the disc margin, often associated with a thinning or absence of choroid next to the disc. A peripapillary crescent of increased pigmentation may represent a *malposition of the embryonic fold* with a double layer of retinal pigment epithelium or a double layer of incompletely formed neural retina adjacent to the disc. *Irregular pigmentation* around the disc may also be due to hypopigmented or hyperpigmented retinal pigment epithelium.

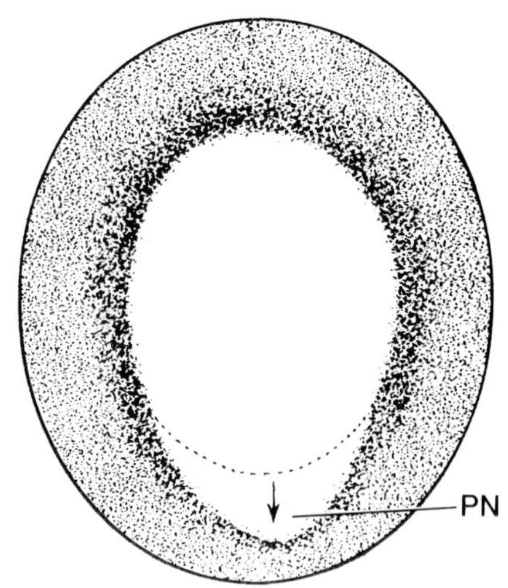

Figure 5.15. Inferior enlargement of cup (*arrow*) from original cup margin (*dotted line*) in glaucomatous optic atrophy, creating a polar notch (*PN*).

Morphology of Glaucomatous Optic Atrophy

The disc changes of glaucoma are typically progressive and asymmetric and present in a variety of characteristic clinical patterns.

Disc Patterns of Glaucomatous Optic Atrophy

As bundles of axons are destroyed in an eye with glaucoma, the neural rim begins to thin in one of several patterns:

Focal Atrophy. Selective loss of neural rim tissue in glaucoma occurs primarily at the inferior and superior poles of the optic nerve head, and to a lesser extent temporally, which leads to enlargement of the cup in a vertical or oblique direction (Fig. 5.15).[194–201] In contrast to the normal optic nerve head, the inferior temporal rim is usually thinner than the superior temporal area, and the quotient of horizontal to vertical C/D is lowered.[201] The mean neural rim area is typically smaller than that of normal discs and is a better parameter than C/D in separating eyes with early glaucoma from normals.[201–203] As previously noted, however, the wide range of neural rim areas in normal eyes even limits the usefulness of this parameter.

The focal atrophy of the neural rim often begins as a small, discrete defect, usually in the inferior temporal quadrant, which has been referred to as *polar notching,*[196,197] *focal notching,*[198] or *pit-like changes.*[199] As the focal defect enlarges and deepens, it may develop a sharp nasal margin, often adjacent to a major retinal vessel, a sign referred to as the *sharpened polar nasal edge.*[196] When the local thinning of neural rim tissue reaches the disc margin (i.e., no visible neural rim remains in that area), a *sharpened rim* is said to be produced.[196] If a retinal vessel crosses the sharpened rim, it will bend sharply at the edge of the disc, creating what has been termed *bayoneting at the disc edge.*[196]

Concentric Atrophy. In contrast to focal atrophy, glaucomatous damage may lead less commonly to enlargement of the cup in concentric circles, which are sometimes horizontal but are more often directed inferior temporally or superior temporally.[197]

Since the loss of neural rim tissue usually begins temporally and then progresses circumferentially toward these poles, this has been called *temporal unfolding*.[196,197] In one study, this generalized expansion of the cup, with retention of its "round" appearance, was the most common form of early glaucomatous damage.[204] Since it is difficult to distinguish this type of glaucomatous cup from a physiologic cup, it is important to compare the cup in the fellow eye for symmetry and to study serial photographs for evidence of progressive change.

A *thinning of the neural rim* may be seen as a crescentic shadow adjacent to the disc margin as the intense beam of a direct ophthalmoscope passes across the neural rim.[205] The histologic explanation for this phenomenon is uncertain but is believed to be associated with early glaucomatous damage,[206] and it should not be confused with the previously discussed gray crescent in the optic nerve head.[188]

Deepening of the Cup. In some cases, the predominant pattern of early glaucomatous optic atrophy is a deepening of the cup, which has been said to occur only when the lamina is not initially exposed.[207] This may produce the picture of *overpass cupping*, in which vessels initially bridge the deepened cup and later collapse into it.[196,197] Exposure of the underlying lamina cribrosa by the deepening cup is often recognized by the gray fenestra of the lamina, which has been referred to as the *laminar dot sign*.[196] In most cases, the lamina cribrosa openings have a dot-like appearance by ophthalmoscopy, although some are more striate, and the latter are said to have a much higher association with glaucomatous visual field defects.[208,209]

Pallor/Cup Discrepancy. In the early stages of glaucomatous optic atrophy, enlargement of the cup may progress ahead of that of the area of pallor. This biphasic pattern differs from other causes of optic atrophy in which the area of pallor is typically larger than the cup.[161] A potential pitfall in interpreting optic nerve head cupping is to look only at the area of pallor and miss the larger area of cupping. The latter can usually be recognized by observing kinking of vessels at the cup margin or by examining the disc with stereoscopic techniques. Although the pallor/cup discrepancy is typical and strongly suggestive of glaucomatous cupping, it may also be seen in normal optic nerve heads.[183]

Pallor/cup discrepancy may occur with diffuse or focal enlargement of the cup. *Saucerization* refers to a pattern of early glaucomatous change in which diffuse, shallow cupping extends to the disc margins with retention of a central pale cup (Figs. 5.16 and 5.17).[210] *Focal saucerization* refers to a more localized shallow, sloping cup, usually in the inferior temporal quadrant.[197] The retention of normal neural rim color in the area of focal saucerization has been called the *tinted hollow*.[196] As the glaucomatous damage progresses, the color is replaced by a grayish hue, termed the *shadow sign*, or by the *laminar dot sign* (Figs. 5.18 and 5.19).[196]

Advanced Glaucomatous Cupping. If the progressive changes of glaucomatous optic atrophy are not arrested by appropriate measures to reduce the IOP, the typical course is eventual loss of all neural rim tissue. The ultimate result is total cupping, which is seen clinically as a white disc with loss of all neural rim tissue and bending of all vessels at the margin of the disc (Fig. 5.20). This has also been called *bean-pot cupping*, because the cross section of a histologic specimen reveals extreme posterior displacement of the lamina cribrosa and undermining of the disc margin (Fig. 5.21).[197,198]

Vascular Signs of Glaucomatous Optic Atrophy

Optic Disc Hemorrhages. Splinter hemorrhages, usually near the margin of the optic nerve head (Figs. 5.22 and 5.23), are a common feature of glaucomatous damage.[211,212] It has been estimated that they occur in at least one-third of all glaucoma patients at some time in the course of their disease.[213] They tend to come and go, so that they may be seen on one visit and gone the next, only to reappear at a later date in the same or new location. The most common location is the inferior quadrant, although they may be seen superiorly or at any other point around the disc margin.

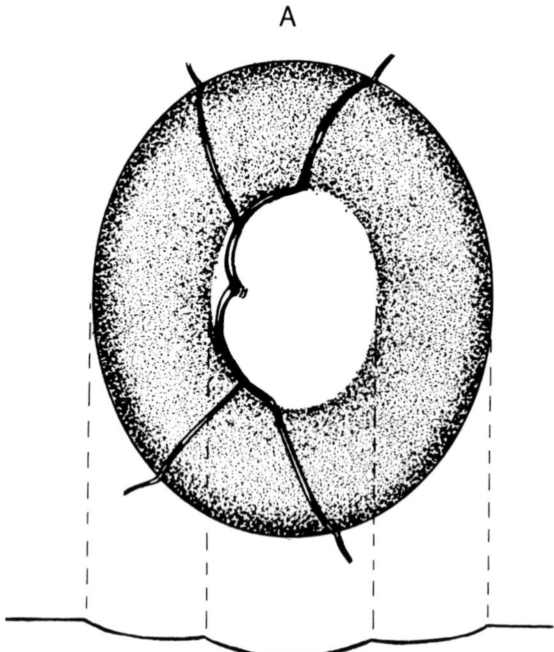

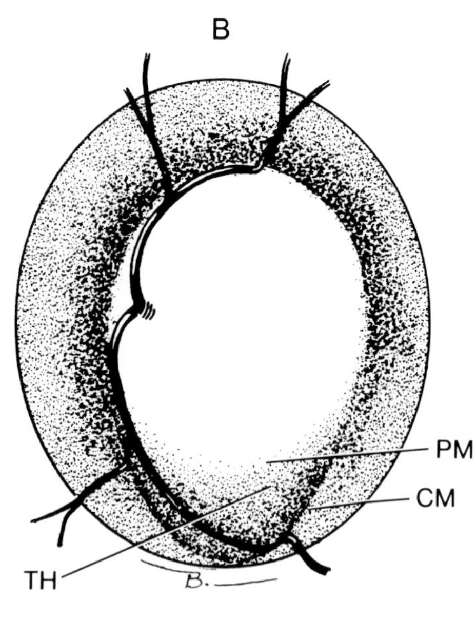

Figure 5.16. Glaucomatous optic atrophy. Pallor/cup discrepancy: **A,** Saucerization with corresponding cross-sectional view. **B,** Focal saucerization with tinted hollow (*TH*) between pallor margin (*PM*) and cup margin (*CM*). Note kinking of vessels in both cases.

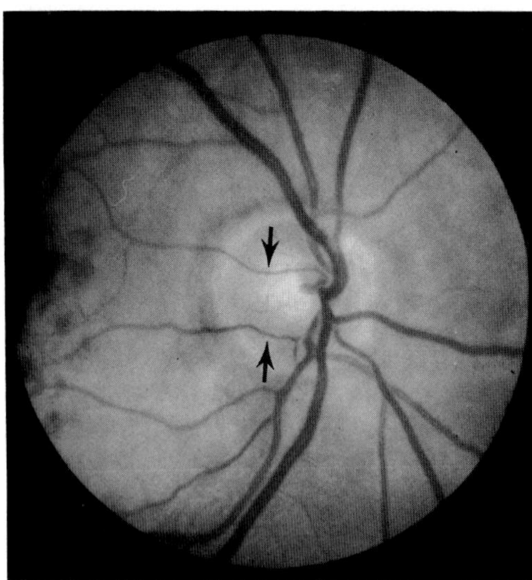

Figure 5.17. Saucerization of optic nerve head, evidenced by gradual sloping of vessels (*arrows*) with kinking at disc margin.

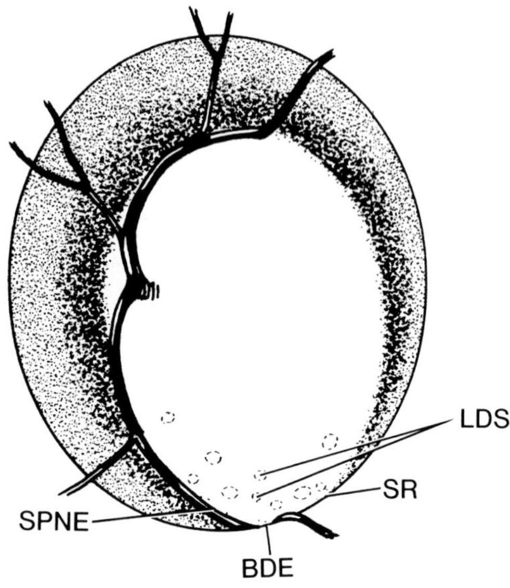

Figure 5.18. Inferior-temporal loss of neural rim in glaucomatous optic atrophy, creating a sharpened rim (*SR*) at the disc margin, a sharpened polar nasal edge (*SPNE*) along the cup margin, bayoneting at the disc edge (*BDE*) where the vessels cross the sharpened rim, and laminar dot sign (*LDS*) resulting from exposure of fenestrae in lamina cribrosa.

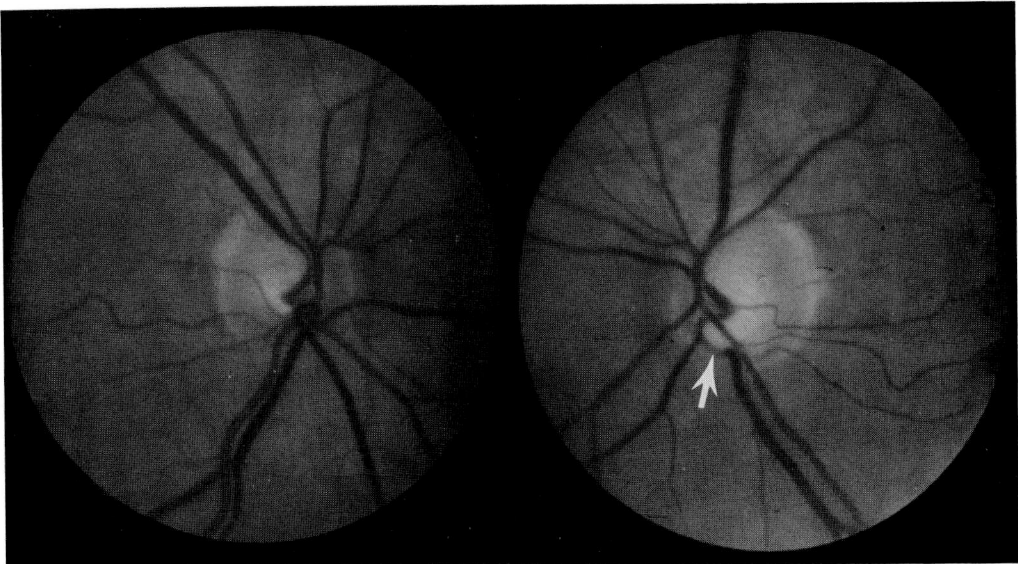

Figure 5.19. Glaucomatous optic atrophy evidenced by a larger left optic nerve head cup, with a sharpened rim and bayoneting of the vessels inferiorly (*arrow*).

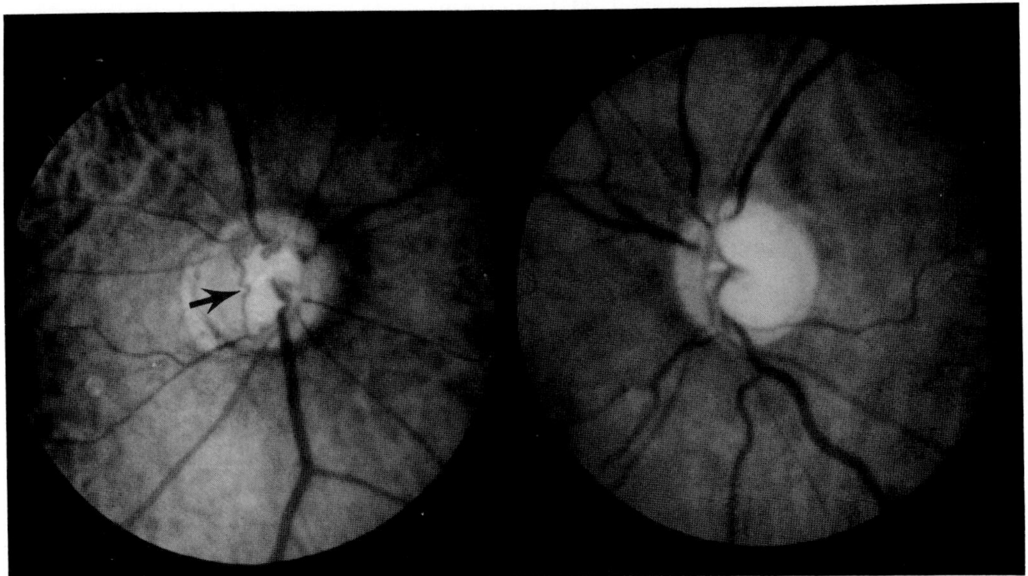

Figure 5.20. Advanced glaucomatous optic atrophy with nearly total cupping of both optic nerve heads and a shunt vessel on the right disc (*arrow*).

While not pathognomonic of glaucoma, disc hemorrhages are a significant finding, since they may be the first sign of glaucomatous damage, often preceding retinal nerve fiber layer defects,[214] notches in the neural rim,[215] and glaucomatous visual field defects.[216,217] They are especially suggestive of glaucoma when associated with high IOP,[218] although disc hemorrhages commonly occur with minimal pressure elevation or in eyes with low-tension glaucoma.[213] They occur more commonly in diabetic patients with glaucoma.[219,220] Although they are not always associated

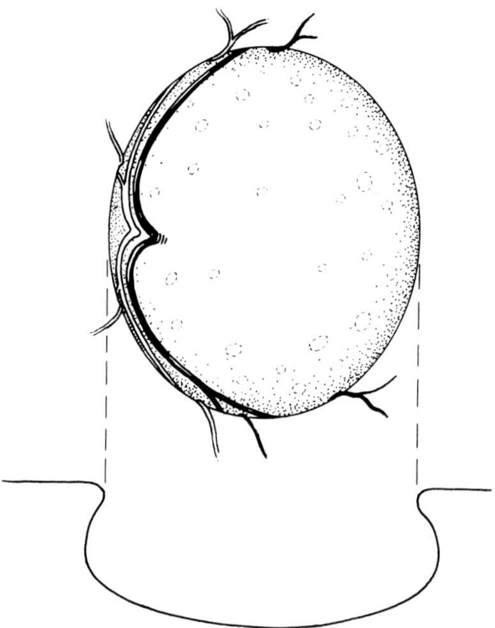

Figure 5.21. Advanced glaucomatous optic atrophy with total (bean-pot) cupping, shown best in cross-sectional view.

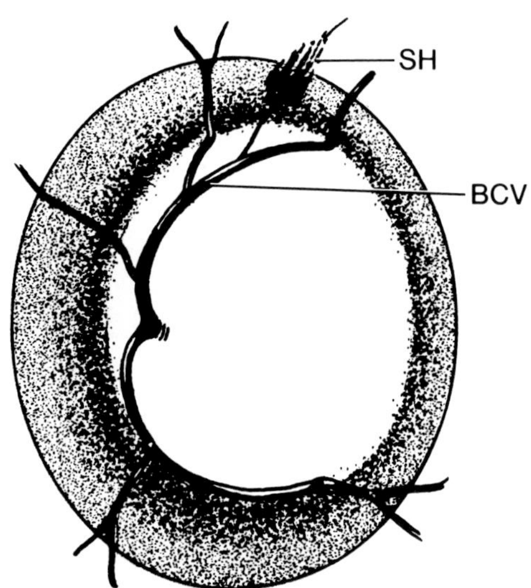

Figure 5.22. Vascular changes in glaucomatous optic atrophy: splinter hemorrhage (*SH*) and baring of circumlinear vessel (*BCV*).

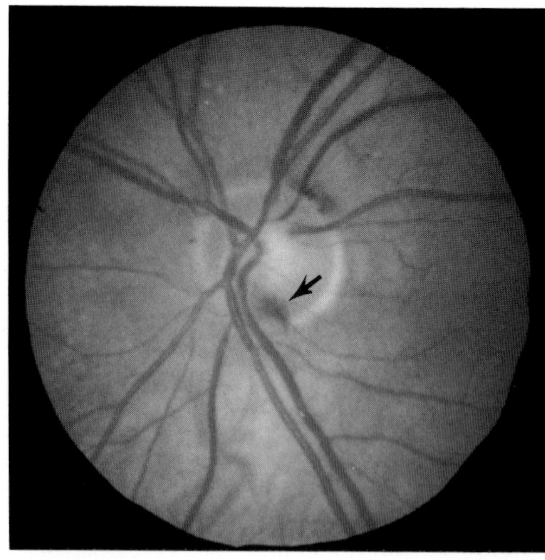

Figure 5.23. Splinter hemorrhage (*arrow*) in glaucomatous optic atrophy.

with an increased rate of disc damage,[220,221] they should probably be viewed as a sign that the glaucoma is out of control.[211,212,218] It has also been noted that a disc hemorrhage in a patient with a symptomatic vitreous detachment may be an early sign of chronic glaucoma.[222]

Tortuosity of Retinal Vessels. Tortuous vessels may be seen on the disc with advanced glaucomatous optic atrophy, and in some cases with only moderate damage. Tortuosity is believed to represent loops of collateral vessels in response to chronic central retinal vessel occlusion.[223] Venovenous anastomoses associated with chronic branch retinal vessel occlusion, as well as the typical picture of acute central retinal vessel occlusion with massive flame hemorrhages, also occur with increased frequency in eyes with chronic glaucoma.[223] Asymptomatic venous stasis changes on the disc, which are seen as enlargement of collateral vessels, have been estimated to occur in 3% of patients with early to moderate glaucoma and may be associated with progression of glaucomatous optic atrophy.[224]

Cilioretinal Arteries. One study of 20 patients with bilateral, symmetrical open-angle glaucoma and unilateral cilioretinal arteries revealed a larger C/D and more visual field damage in the eye with the cilioretinal artery,[225] although another similar study did not support this observation.[226]

Location of Retinal Vessels. The location of retinal vessels in relation to the cup may also have some diagnostic value. The significance of *overpass cupping,* in which vessels bridge a cup that is becoming deeper,[196,197] was previously mentioned. Another vessel sign with some diagnostic value has been called *baring of the circumlinear vessel.*[227,228] In many normal optic nerve heads, one or two vessels may curve to outline a portion of the physiologic cup. With glaucomatous enlargement of the cup, these circumlinear vessels may be "bared" from the margin of the cup (Fig. 5.22). However, this sign may occasionally be seen with nonglaucomatous disorders of the optic nerve,[228] as well as in some individuals with physiologic cups.[229] It was once taught that nasal displacement of the retinal vessels on the optic nerve head was a sign of glaucomatous cupping. However, since these vessels enter and leave the eye along the nasal margin of the cup, their location on the disc is a function of cup size, whether physiologic or glaucomatous, and does not provide a useful diagnostic parameter.[170]

Peripapillary Changes Associated with Glaucomatous Optic Atrophy

Nerve Fiber Bundle Defects. The loss of axonal bundles, which leads to the neural rim changes of glaucomatous optic atrophy, also produces visible defects in the retinal nerve fiber layer. These defects appear as dark stripes of varying width in the peripapillary area, paralleling the normal retinal striations (Fig. 5.24),[230–232] and monkey studies confirm that they are due to loss of axons.[31,233] They often follow disc hemorrhages[214,234] and correlate highly with visual field changes,[230–232] neural rim area,[235] and fluorescein filling defects.[236] Within the high-tension glaucoma population, they also have an increased incidence in high myopes with oblique insertion of the disc.[237]

A problem with retinal nerve fiber layer defects is that they are also seen in many neurologic disorders as well as in ocular hypertensive and normal individuals. However, attention to the appearance of the defects has improved the sensitivity and specificity of this finding. In some eyes, the loss of nerve fibers is diffuse or generalized, while the defects in other cases are localized or slit-like. The diffuse loss is more common in glaucoma patients than in ocular hypertensives[238] but also more common among ocular hypertensives than normotensive individuals.[239] Localized defects are more directly associated with localized visual field loss than is the case with diffuse nerve loss.[240]

Computerized image analysis has been used to measure the height of the juxtapapillary nerve fiber layer, and this has been found to be superior to standard disc parameters in discriminating between normal and glaucomatous eyes.[241]

Peripapillary Depigmentation. Alterations in peripapillary pigmentation are frequently associated with glaucomatous optic atrophy, but are also seen with other conditions, such as myopia and aging changes. As previously noted, several variations of peripapillary pigmentary change may be seen in normal eyes.[193] The scleral lip, or *peripapillary halo,* is a narrow, homogeneous light band at the edge of the disc. The incidence of prominent halos is higher in glaucoma, although the average degree of halos is statistically the same as in nonglaucomatous eyes.[242] A chorioscleral crescent, or *peripapillary atrophy,* is defined as an irregular, variably depigmented area peripheral to the halo. It occurs more frequently and is larger in eyes with glaucomatous damage as compared with normal eyes,[243,244] and it has been observed to enlarge progressively in eyes with glaucoma.[245] There is preliminary evidence that the absence of peripapillary crescents may reduce the risk of glaucomatous damage among ocular hypertensives.[246]

Reversal of Glaucomatous Cupping

It is generally taught that glaucomatous damage of the optic nerve head and visual field is an irreversible process. While this may be true in many cases, especially when associated with actual loss of axons, there are situations in which glaucomatous cupping may be reversible. This is seen most commonly in children with early stages of

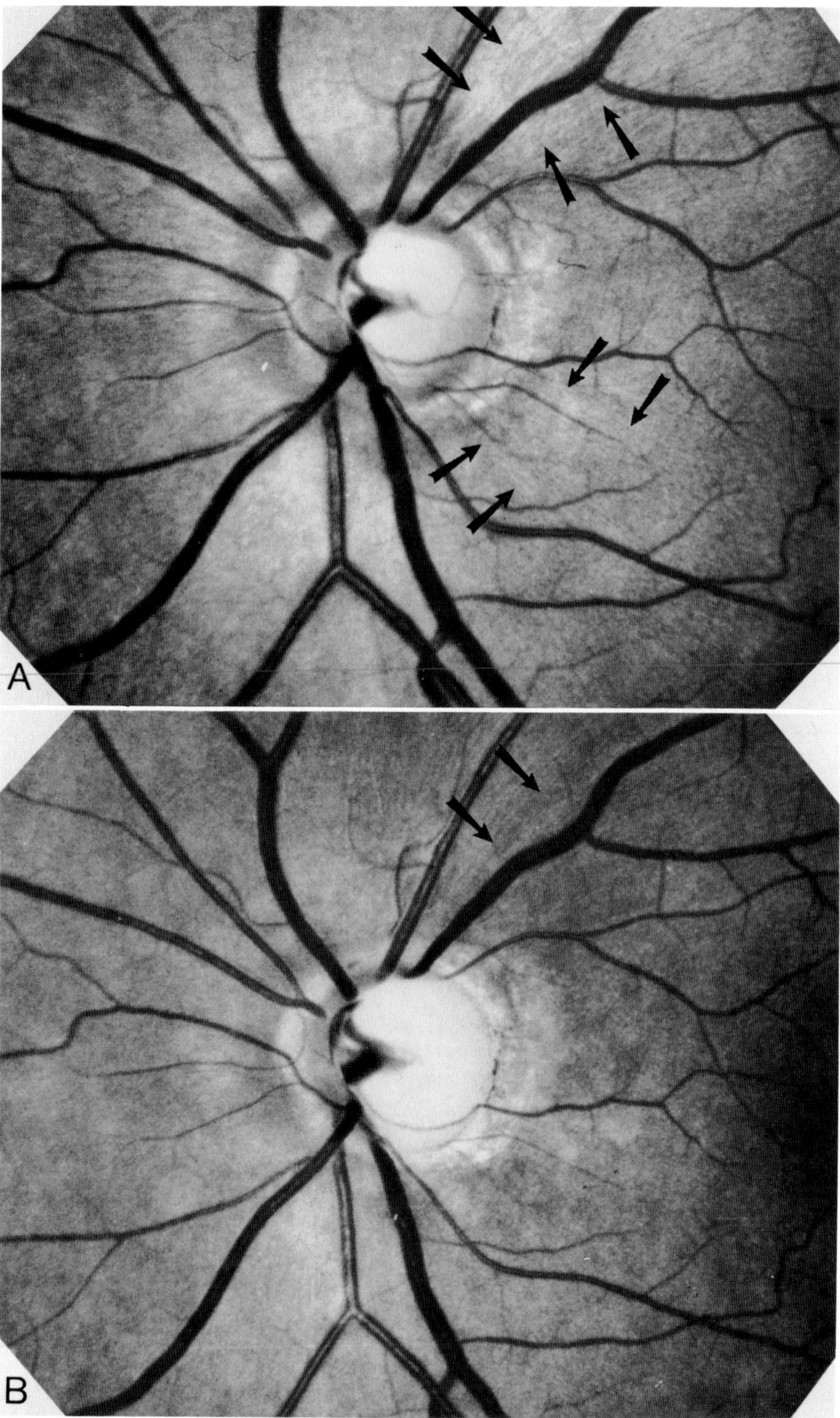

Figure 5.24. Nerve fiber bundle defects of glaucoma. **A,** Normal striations of arcuate nerve fiber bundles, seen best in superior-temporal and inferior-temporal quadrants (*arrows*). **B,** Same eye after extensive glaucomatous damage, showing slit-like defect superiorly (*arrows*) and diffuse loss of nerve fiber bundles inferiorly. (Reprinted with permission from Sommer A, Miller N, Pollack I, Maumenee AE, George T: Arch Ophthal 95:2149, 1977.)

glaucoma, particularly during the first year of life, when the IOP is successfully lowered surgically.[247,248] It has also been reported in adults whose glaucomatous cupping was apparently of recent onset, following a marked reduction in IOP by surgical or medical means.[249–252]

Differential Diagnosis of Glaucomatous Optic Atrophy

Normal variations in the physiologic cup, the neural rim, and the peripapillary retina, as discussed earlier in this chapter, may be confused with the changes of glaucoma. In addition, developmental anomalies and nonglaucomatous optic atrophies may be sources of diagnostic confusion.

Developmental Anomalies

Colobomas of the optic nerve head can simulate glaucomatous cupping. The defect may involve the entire disc, which is enlarged and excavated (Fig. 5.25).[253,254] In some cases, the diagnostic problem is compounded by associated field defects, which may resemble those of glaucoma but are typically not progressive. A variation of optic nerve head colobomas, called the "*morning glory syndrome,*" is characterized by a large funnel-shaped staphylomatous coloboma of the nerve head and peripapillary region with white central tissue, elevated peripapillary pigment disturbance, and multiple radially oriented retinal vessels.[255,256] A high percentage of these patients develop retinal detachments.[257] Yet another optic nerve head anomaly, which may represent an atypical coloboma, is the *congenital pit*.[256] This is a localized, pale depression, usually near the temporal or inferotemporal margin of the disc, although they may be found in any area of the nerve head, and there may be two or even three pits in some eyes.[256] These anomalies may have associated visual disturbance resulting from macular or extramacular serous detachment.[258] Cases have also been reported in which congenital pits were noted to enlarge when observed for many years.[259]

Nonglaucomatous Causes of Acquired Cupping

Studies have shown that ophthalmologists are not always able to distinguish between glaucomatous and nonglaucomatous optic atrophy on the basis of the optic disc appearance alone.[260] Parameters that are most useful in making this differentiation include pallor of the neural rim in nonglaucomatous cases and obliteration of the rim in

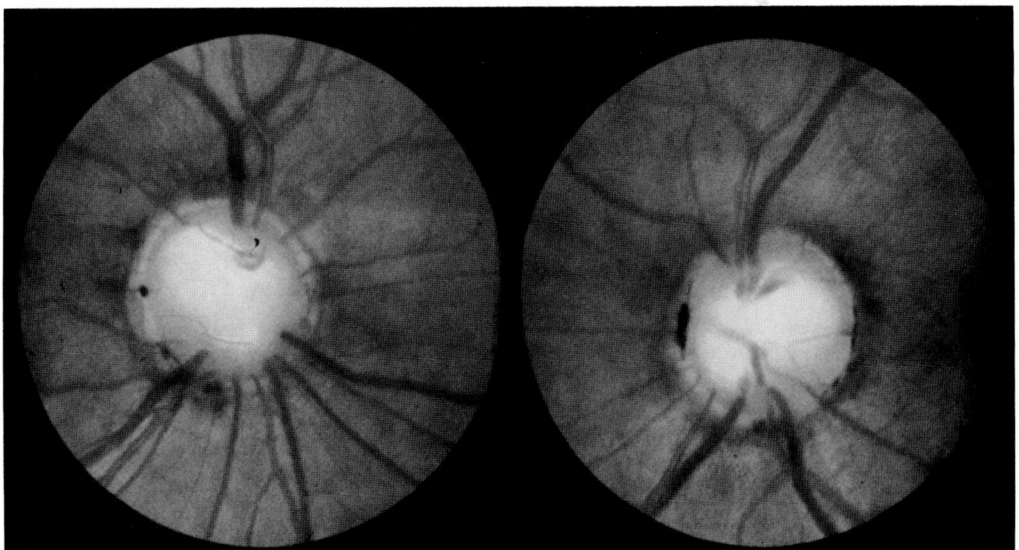

Figure 5.25. Colobomas of the optic nerve head, as an example of developmental anomalies that may be confused with glaucomatous optic atrophy.

glaucoma.[261] Nonglaucomatous conditions that may cause acquired cupping include anterior ischemic optic neuropathy, as previously discussed, especially when the ischemia is due to arteritis.[150–152] A similar entity has been described in which infarction of the optic nerve head caused shallow cupping inferotemporally, associated with arcuate field defects.[262] This differed from glaucoma in that it was not progressive. Acquired cupping may also occur with compressive lesions of the optic nerve, such as an intracranial aneurysm, which was reported to cause cupping indistinguishable from that of early glaucoma.[263] A significant change in C/D was not observed in a series of patients treated with argon or xenon panretinal photocoagulation.[264]

CLINICAL TECHNIQUES FOR EVALUATING THE OPTIC NERVE HEAD

Progressive cupping of the optic nerve head in a patient with glaucoma is the most reliable indicator that the IOP is not being adequately controlled. It is essential, therefore, to evaluate and record the appearance of the nerve head in a way that will accurately reveal subtle glaucomatous changes over the course of follow-up evaluations. In current practice, this involves careful evaluation in the office combined with photographic documentation. In addition, there are newer investigative techniques that may one day provide more precise methods of observation.

Techniques of Office Evaluation and Recording

In the clinical evaluation of the optic nerve head, the direct ophthalmoscope is occasionally useful, especially when looking through a small pupil or evaluating the nerve fiber layer with a red-free filter. A graticule may be incorporated into the ophthalmoscope to aid in evaluating the cup/disc ratio.[265] However, this technique does not permit detection of many of the glaucomatous changes in the nerve head and peripapillary area, and the most useful office approach is to study these structures carefully with stereoscopic methods. The most useful stereoscopic technique is with a slit lamp and an auxiliary fundus lens such as the Goldmann contact lens, or the 90 diopter (Fig. 5.26) or Hruby (Fig. 5.27) noncontact lenses. The Hruby lens is attached to the slit lamp. The 90 diopter lens is hand-held, although a slit-lamp mounting device has also been developed for this lens.[266] Each of these systems provides the advantages of magnification and stereopsis. However, since the lateral and axial magnifications are

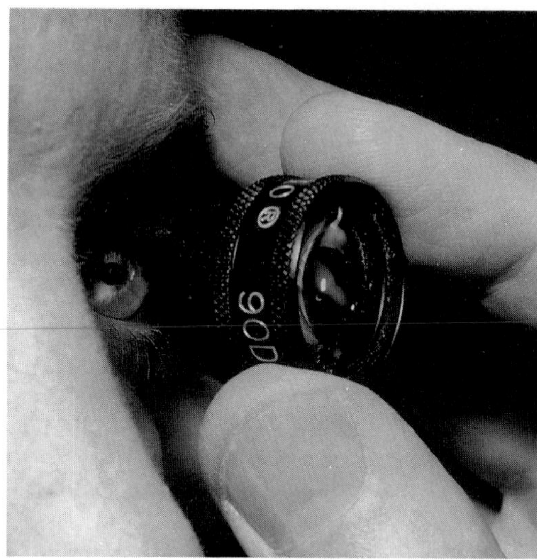

Figure 5.26. 90 diopter lens used with slit lamp for stereoscopic indirect ophthalmoscopic evaluation of optic nerve head.

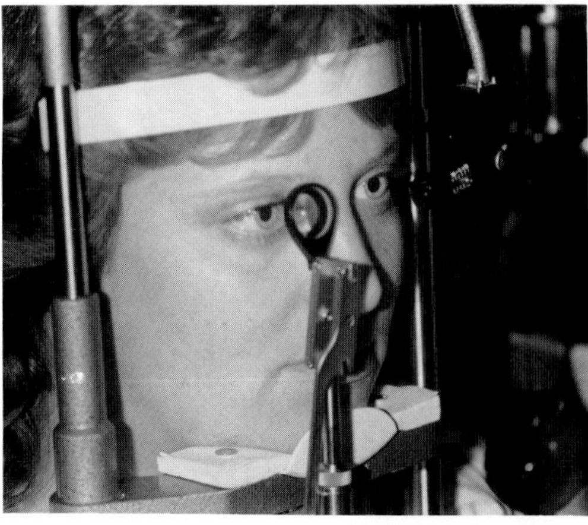

Figure 5.27. Hruby lens attachment to the slit lamp for stereoscopic evaluation of the optic nerve head.

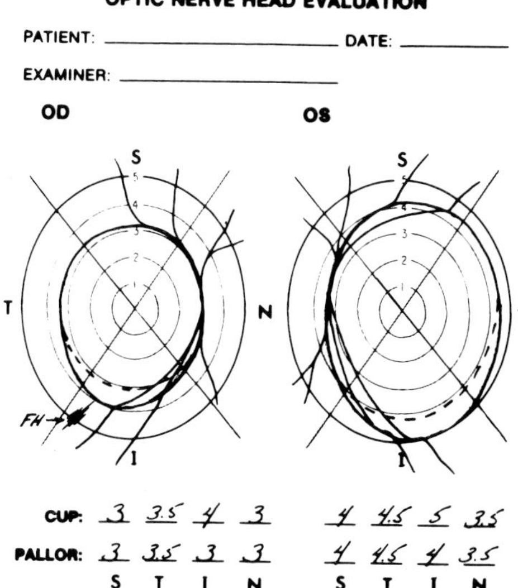

Figure 5.28. Example of optic nerve head drawing, made at time of stereoscopic evaluation of the disc as adjunct to disc photos.

unequal, there is a certain amount of image distortion, with the Goldmann and 90 diopter lenses producing a decrease in apparent depth and the Hruby lens producing a slight increase.[267] Subjective estimates of cup dimensions have been shown to vary greatly, even among expert observers.[268–270] These can be improved by paying attention to the many complex optic nerve head and peripapillary retinal parameters associated with glaucomatous damage.[271] Detailed drawings should be made that include the area of cupping and pallor in all quadrants, the position and kinking of major vessels, splinter hemorrhages, and peripapillary changes (Fig. 5.28). However, no degree of attention to detail is sufficient to detect subtle changes in all cases, and the office evaluation should be considered only as an adjunct to the indispensable use of photographic records.

Photographic and Other Techniques

Two-Dimensional Photos. Whether in color or black-and-white, two-dimensional photos have the advantages of simplicity and lower cost, as compared with stereophotos. In addition, the relative dimensions of the pallor and cup can be measured directly on the photograph.[272,273] Although one study found that monocular and stereoscopic photographs afforded similar levels of accuracy,[274] the former technique is frequently limited by the inability to determine the cup margins precisely. The projections of fine, parallel lines onto the disc have been suggested as a way to improve recognition of the cup contours on both two-dimensional and stereo photographs.[275,276] Techniques have also been developed to electronically scan black-and-white disc photos to obtain an objective measure of the amount of optic disc pallor.[277,278] The main value of two-dimensional photos in the future may be to document the *retinal nerve fiber layer*. Special techniques to enhance the subtle details of this parameter include monochromatic (red-free) filters and high resolution film,[279–282] cross-polarization photography,[283] a wide-angle fundus camera,[284] and a spectral reflectance.[285]

Stereoscopic Photographs. A method that may be more reliable for recording disc cupping, as well as the other aspects of glaucomatous optic atrophy, is the use of color stereophotographs.[161,194] Stereophotographs can be obtained either by taking two photos in sequence on the same film with the use of a sliding carriage adapter (Allen separator),[286] or by taking simultaneous photos with two cameras that use the indirect ophthalmoscopic principle (Donaldson stereoscopic fundus camera),[287,288] or by using a twin-prism separator.[289] These three techniques were compared for reproducibility, and the Donaldson camera was found to be superior.[290] A special viewer has also been developed in which two stereophotographs can be compared simultaneously,[291] and a template has been used for measuring cup and disc dimensions.[292]

Serial Comparisons. *Stereochronoscopy* uses the stereoscopic principle to detect subtle changes in photographs of a disc taken at different times.[293,294] If there has been any progression of the cupping, the disparity in the cup margins of the superimposed photographs will produce a stereoscopic effect. A modification of this concept, referred to as *stereochronometry,* uses a stereoplotter to measure the changes created by the two photos.[295] Other techniques for detecting differences in serial fundus photographs involve analysis of *flicker* while alternately viewing one photograph and then the other,[296] and *electronic subtraction,* in which areas of disparity between the two images will be enhanced.[297]

Colorimetric Measurements. Techniques have also been studied that attempt to detect reduced or changing color intensity of the optic nerve head.[298–300] A photographic technique has also been developed to permit quantitative evaluation of the relative brightness of the illuminated optic nerve head.[301]

Fluorescein Angiography. Studies of the optic nerve head with fluorescein angiography were discussed earlier in this chapter and may one day have practical clinical application in the detection and management of glaucoma.

Ultrasonography. It has been shown that ultrasound can be used to detect glaucomatous cupping of 0.7 cup/disc ratio or greater,[302] and high-resolution contact B-scan echography may one day provide a reliable estimate of the optic cup size in eyes with opaque media.[303]

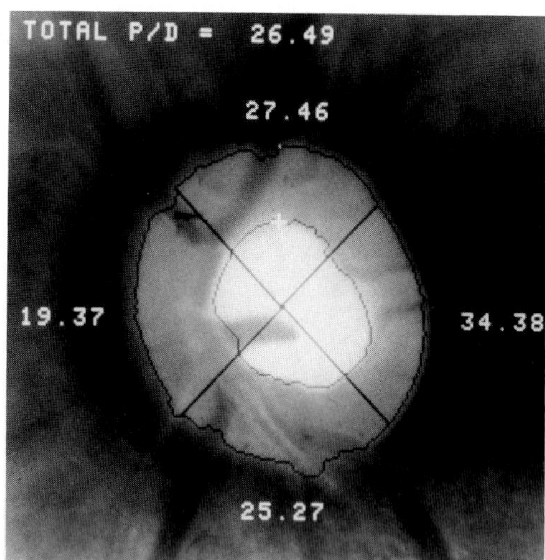

Figure 5.29. Example of automated image analysis. The computer has delineated the optic disc and area of pallor (*black lines*), as well as the disc quadrants. Numbers indicate the percentage of pallor found across the total disc area (*TOTAL P/D*) as well as each of the disc quadrants. (Reprinted with permission from Nagin P, Schwartz B, Nanba K: Ophthalmology 92:243, 1985.)

Computerized Image Analysis of the Optic Nerve Head

The value of even the most sophisticated photographs of the optic nerve head is limited by the need for subjective interpretation of the contour and color patterns of the disc and peripapillary retina. Efforts to refine the assessment of these subtle parameters have included *photogrammetry,* or contour mapping of the optic nerve head,[207,304–308] and *colorimetry,* as previously noted.[298–300] These techniques were initially performed manually, which is very time consuming and, therefore, of limited clinical usefulness. With the advent of computer technology, however, there is now the possibility of applying these concepts to the clinical management of glaucoma.

Instruments

The concept of computerized image analysis of the optic nerve head was pioneered by Dr. Bernard Schwartz, who developed prototypes for analysis of both contour and pallor of the disc (Fig. 5.29).[309,310] Since then, several commercial instruments have been described in the literature, which provide computerized analysis of disc contour and pallor.

The *Rodenstock Optic Nerve Head Analyzer* (ONHA) has undergone the most extensive evaluation (Fig. 5.30).[311–324] Although the ONHA is no longer commercially available, the experience gained through study of this instrument provides the basis for our understanding of computerized image analysis of the optic nerve head and its potential for clinical application as newer instruments and techniques are developed. The instrument measures optic nerve head contour by projecting vertical light stripes on the disc and then obtaining simultaneous stereo video images, which are processed by a microcomputer. Disparity between corresponding points along the light stripes of stereo pairs is used to generate vertical contour lines and a three-dimensional contour map (Fig. 5.31). A pallor map of the disc is generated by obtaining two video images with both red and green wave-

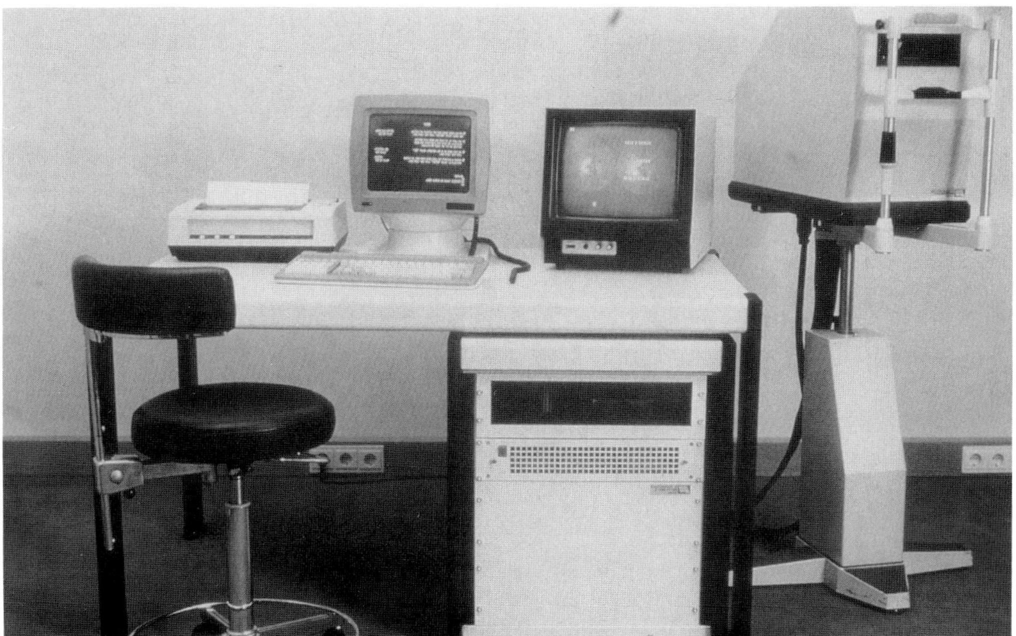

Figure 5.30. Optic Nerve Head Analyzer: *Right,* Video camera for acquisition of simultaneous stereo disc images. *Left,* Microcomputer with screens, keyboard, and printer.

lengths and computing the ratio of color reflectance at various points in the image. The available software provides a limited printout of disc and cup dimensions, which is based on an arbitrary definition of the cup boundary.

Two other instruments, the *Topcon IS 2000* (formerly the PAR IS 2000)[325–328] and the *Humphrey Retinal Analyzer* (RA),[329,330] differ from the ONHA primarily in the method of plotting the three-dimensional topography of the disc and retina. Both instruments can analyze data from either simultaneous stereo images or stereo photographs, and both use the disparity between existing structures in the two images, rather than projected light stripes. The instruments also have more sophisticated software, which provides printouts of actual contour details. In addition, the IS 2000 can be used to monitor positional changes in disc vasculature as a measure of progressive damage.[327]

Other instruments are also currently under investigation. One measures change in disc photos from successive years by localized movement when displayed in rapid sequence on a television monitor.[331] Another focuses a laser beam on the disc and detects reflected light in a confocal detection unit, which produces a tomographic scanning series and allows measurement of three-dimensional structures.[332] Yet another system uses the scatter and reflection of a laser beam from the anterior and posterior surface of the retina to measure thickness.[333]

Evaluation of Instruments

For any of the above instruments to have clinical value, they must first be shown to provide reliable and accurate information. Reliability studies have been performed by obtaining multiple measurements of the same eyes within a short time frame and calculating the variance of intrapatient results. Several such studies have shown that contour measurements by the ONHA have acceptable reliability, especially for cup/disc ratio and neural rim area,[311–315] and comparable results have been reported for the IS 2000[326] and the RA.[329,330] Accuracy of topographic measurements with the ONHA was evaluated with a plastic model eye and was considered clinically acceptable when ap-

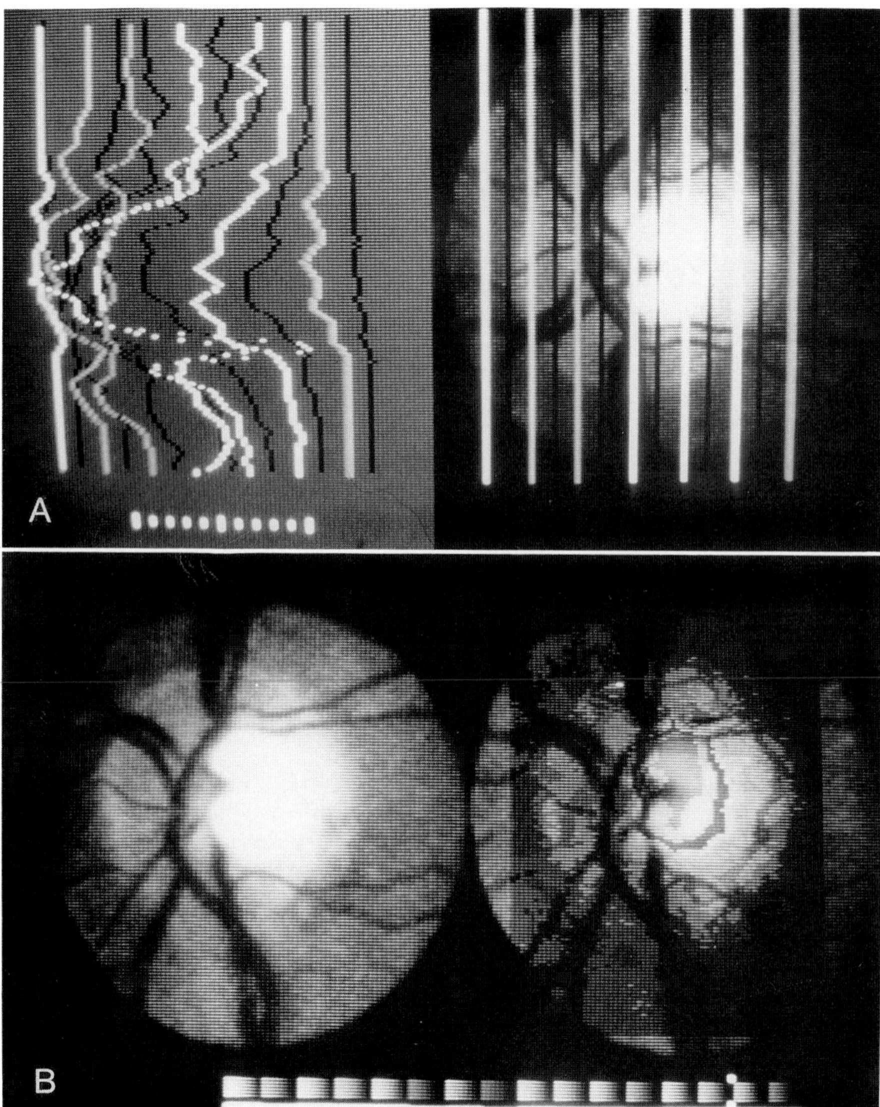

Figure 5.31. Topographic images of optic nerve head obtained with Optic Nerve Head Analyzer: **A,** Vertical contour lines. **B,** Three-dimensional contour map.

propriate correction factors were used.[319] A correlation between computer-generated topographic data and manual analysis of stereoscopic photographs was reported to be highly significant for the ONHA[320,321] and moderate for the IS 2000.[328]

Reliability of pallor measurements has also been studied with the ONHA. Variation was acceptably low by global analysis (distribution of pallor values throughout the image)[316,317] but was inadequate when the area of a specific pallor value within the disc was compared between measurements of the same eye.[318]

Clinical Application of Instruments

Even when an instrument has been shown to provide reliable, accurate data, the information may not be clinically useful. One lesson that has been emphasized through studies of computerized image analysis of the optic nerve head is that current parameters, such as cup/disc ratio and neural rim area, do not adequately describe the complex contour and color patterns of the disc. In addition, the broad range of these values and the overlap between normal and glaucomatous eyes indicate that new parameters are needed to interpret the data generated with new quantitative techniques.[322] It may be that new parameters will be developed to define the overall contour of the disc. On the other hand, it may be that the relative height of the peripapillary nerve fiber layer will prove to be a more useful measure of axonal loss in glaucoma.[323,324] In any case, continued study of computerized image analysis of the optic nerve head promises more sophisticated methods of following changes in the optic nerve head and peripapillary retina in the management of glaucoma.

SUMMARY

The optic nerve head is composed of axons from the retinal ganglion cells, blood vessels, and astroglial and collagen support. The normal optic nerve head has considerable variation in size and surface contour. The pathogenesis of glaucomatous optic atrophy appears to involve obstruction of axoplasmic flow, although it is not clear whether this is a direct mechanical effect of elevated IOP or secondary to vascular changes. Glaucomatous optic atrophy is characterized clinically by a progressive, asymmetric loss of neural rim tissue, which is manifested by an enlargement in the area of cupping and pallor. This most often extends in a focal direction, producing early thinning of the inferior and superior portions of the neural rim. Enlargement of the cup often precedes that of the area of pallor, creating a pallor/cup discrepancy. Other important signs of glaucomatous optic atrophy are disc hemorrhages and peripapillary nerve fiber bundle defects. The differential diagnosis of glaucomatous optic atrophy includes normal variations, developmental anomalies, and nonglaucomatous causes of acquired cupping. Techniques for evaluating the optic nerve head include a careful office examination and photographic documentation, although newer techniques, such as computerized image analysis, are being developed that may one day provide more precise methods of observation.

References

1. Kronfeld, PC: Normal variations of the optic disc as observed by conventional ophthalmoscopy and their anatomic correlations. Trans Am Acad Ophthal Otol 81:214, 1976.
2. Jonas, JB, Gusek, GC, Guggenmoos-Holzmann, I, Naumann, GOH: Size of the optic nerve scleral canal and comparison with intravital determination of optic disc dimensions. Graefe's Arch Ophthal 226:213, 1988.
3. Quigley, HA, Brown, AE, Morrison, JD, Drance, SM: The size and shape of the optic disc in normal human eyes. Arch Ophthal 108:51, 1990.
4. Hayreh, SS: Anatomy and physiology of the optic nerve head. Trans Am Acad Ophthal Otol 78:240, 1974.
5. Minckler, DS, McLean, IW, Tso, MOM: Distribution of axonal and glial elements in the rhesus optic nerve head studied by electron microscopy. Am J Ophthal 82:179, 1976.
6. Anderson, DR: Ultrastructure of human and monkey lamina cribrosa and optic nerve head. Arch Ophthal 82:800, 1969.
7. Hamasaki, DI, Fujino, T: Effect of intraocular pressure on ocular vessels. Arch Ophthal 78:369, 1967.
8. Geijer, C, Bill, A: Effects of raised intraocular pressure on retinal, prelaminar, laminar, and retrolaminar optic nerve blood flow in monkeys. Invest Ophthal Vis Sci 18:1030, 1979.
9. Liebermann, MF, Maumenee, AE, Green, WR: Histologic studies of the vasculature of the anterior optic nerve. Am J Ophthal 82:405, 1976.
10. Anderson, DR, Braverman, S: Reevaluation of the optic disc vasculature. Am J Ophthal 82:165, 1976.
11. Hayreh, SS: The central artery of the retina: its role in the blood supply of the optic nerve. Br J Ophthal 47:651, 1963.
12. Francois, J, Neetens, A: Vascularization of the optic pathway. I. Lamina cribrosa and optic nerve. Br J Ophthal 38:472, 1954.
13. Goder, G: The capillaries of the optic nerve. Am J Ophthal 77:684, 1974.
14. Zaret, CR, Choromokos, EA, Meisler, DM: Cilio-optic vein associated with phakomatosis. Ophthalmology 87:330, 1980.
15. Anderson, DR, Hoyt, WF, Hogan, MJ: The fine structure of the astroglia in the human optic nerve and optic nerve head. Trans Am Ophthal Soc 65:275, 1967.
16. Quigley, HA: Gap junctions between optic nerve head astrocytes. Invest Ophthal Vis Sci 16:582, 1977.

17. Anderson, DR: Ultrastructure of the optic nerve head. Arch Ophthal 83:63, 1970.
18. Anderson, DR, Hoyt, WF: Ultrastructure of intraorbital portion of human and monkey optic nerve. Arch Ophthal 82:506, 1969.
19. Heegaard, S, Jensen, OA, Prause, JU: Structure of the vitread face of the monkey optic disc (*Macacca mulatta*). Graefe's Arch Ophthal 226:377, 1988.
20. Quigley, HA, Addicks, EM: Regional differences in the structure of the lamina cribrosa and their relation to glaucomatous optic nerve damage. Arch Ophthal 99:137, 1981.
21. Radius, RL, Gonzales, M: Anatomy of the lamina cribrosa in human eyes. Arch Ophthal 99:2159, 1981.
22. Radius, RL: Regional specificity in anatomy at the lamina cribrosa. Arch Ophthal 99:478, 1981.
23. Hernandez, MR, Igoe, F, Neufeld, AH: Extracellular matrix of the human optic nerve head. Am J Ophthal 102:139, 1986.
24. Rehnberg, M, Ammitzboll, T, Tengroth, B: Collagen distribution in the lamina cribrosa and the trabecular meshwork of the human eye. Br J Ophthal 71:886, 1987.
25. Goldbaum, MH, Jeng, S, Logemann, R, Weinreb, RN: The extracellular matrix of the human optic nerve. Arch Ophthal 107:1225, 1989.
26. Hernandez, MR, Luo, XX, Igoe, F, Neufeld, AH: Extracellular matrix of the human lamina cribrosa. Am J Ophthal 104:567, 1987.
27. Hernandez, MR, Igoe, F, Neufeld, AH: Cell culture of the human lamina cribrosa. Invest Ophthal Vis Sci 29:78, 1988.
28. Morrison, JC, Jerdan, JA, L'Hernault, NL, Quigley, HA: The extracellular matrix composition of the monkey optic nerve head. Invest Ophthal Vis Sci 29:1141, 1988.
29. Morrison, JC, L'Hernault, NL, Jerdan, JA, Quigley, HA: Ultrastructural location of extracellular matrix components in the optic nerve head. Arch Ophthal 107:123, 1989.
30. Anderson, DR: Ultrastructure of meningeal sheaths. Normal human and monkey optic nerves. Arch Ophthal 82:659, 1969.
31. Radius, RL, Anderson, DR: The histology of retinal nerve fiber layer bundles and bundle defects. Arch Ophthal 97:948, 1979.
32. Radius, RL, Anderson, DR: The course of axons through the retina and optic nerve head. Arch Ophthal 97:1154, 1979.
33. Radius, RL, de Bruin, J: Anatomy of the retinal nerve fiber layer. Invest Ophthal Vis Sci 21:745, 1981.
34. Ogden, TE: Nerve fiber layer of the primate retina: morphometric analysis. Invest Ophthal Vis Sci 25:19, 1984.
35. Minckler, DS: The organization of nerve fiber bundles in the primate optic nerve head. Arch Ophthal 98:1630, 1980.
36. Hoyt, WF, Luis, O: Visual fiber anatomy in the infrageniculate pathway of the primate. Arch Ophthal 68:94, 1962.
37. Mikelberg, FS, Drance, SM, Schulzer, M, et al: The normal human optic nerve. Ophthalmology 96:1325, 1989.
38. Balazsi, AG, Rootman, J, Drance, SM, et al: The effect of age on the nerve fiber population of the human optic nerve. Am J Ophthal 97:760, 1984.
39. Repka, MX, Quigley, HA: The effect of age on normal human optic nerve fiber number and diameter. Ophthalmology 96:26, 1989.
40. Johnson, BM, Miao, M, Sadun, AA: Age-related decline of human optic nerve axon populations. Age 10:5, 1987.
41. Dolman, CL, McCormick, AQ, Drance, SM: Aging of the optic nerve. Arch Ophthal 98:2053, 1980.
42. Magoon, EH, Robb, RM: Development of myelin in human optic nerve and tract: a light and electron microscopic study. Arch Ophthal 99:655, 1981.
43. Quigley, HA: The pathogenesis of reversible cupping in congenital glaucoma. Am J Ophthal 84:358, 1977.
44. Hernandez, MR, Luo, XX, Andrzejewska, W, Neufeld, AH: Age-related changes in the extracellular matrix of the human optic nerve head. Am J Ophthal 107:476, 1989.
45. Müller, H: Anatomische Beitrage zur Ophthalmologie: Ueber Nervean-Veranderungen an der Eintrittsstelle des Schnerven. Arch Ophthal 4:1, 1858.
46. von Jaeger, E: Ueber Glaucom und seine Heilung durch Iridectomie. Z Ges der Aertze zu Wien 14:465, 484, 1858.
47. Schnabel, J: Das glaucomatose Sehnervenleiden. Archiv fur Augenheilkunde XXIV:18, 1892.
48. Laker, C: Ein experimenteller Beitrag zur Lehre von der glaukomatosen Excavation. Klin Monatsbl Augenheilkd 24:187, 1886.
49. Schreiber, L: Ueber Degeneration der Netzhaut naut experimentellen und pathologisch-anatomischen Untersuchungen. Graefe's Arch Ophthal 64:237, 1906.
50. Fuchs, E: Ueber die Lamina cribrosa. Graefe's Arch Ophthal 91:435, 1916.
51. LaGrange, F, Beauvieux, J: Anatomie de l'excavation glaucomateuse. Arch Ophthal (Paris) 42:129, 1925.
52. Duke-Elder, S: Fundamental concepts in glaucoma. Arch Ophthal 42:538, 1949.
53. Gafner, F, Goldmann, H: Experimentelle Untersuchungen uber den Zusammenhang von Augendrucksteigerung und Gesichtsfeldschadigung. Ophthalmologica 130:357, 1955.

54. Duke-Elder, S: The problems of simple glaucoma. Trans Ophthal Soc UK 82:307, 1962.
55. Lampert, PW, Vogel, MH, Zimmerman, LE: Pathology of the optic nerve in experimental acute glaucoma. Electron microscopic studies. Invest Ophthal 7:199, 1968.
56. Shaffer, RN: The role of the astroglial cells in glaucomatous disc cupping. Doc Ophthal 26:516, 1969.
57. Shaffer, RN, Hetherington, J Jr: The glaucomatous disc in infants. A suggested hypothesis for disc cupping. Trans Am Acad Ophthal Otol 73:929, 1969.
58. Quigley, HA, Green, WR: The histology of human glaucoma cupping and optic nerve damage: clinicopathologic correlation in 21 eyes. Ophthalmology 86:1803, 1979.
59. Quigley, HA, Addicks, EM, Green, WR, Maumenee, AE: Optic nerve damage in human glaucoma. II. The site of injury and susceptibility to damage. Arch Ophthal 99:635, 1981.
60. Schwartz, B: Cupping and pallor of the optic disc. Arch Ophthal 89:272, 1973.
61. Kornzweig, AL, Eliasoph, I, Feldstein, M: Selective atrophy of the radial peripapillary capillaries in chronic glaucoma. Arch Ophthal 80:696, 1968.
62. Daicker, B: Selective atrophy of the radial peripapillary capillaries and visual field defects in glaucoma. Graefe's Arch Ophthal 195:27, 1975.
63. Quigley, HA, Hohman, RM, Addicks, EM, Green, WR: Blood vessels of the glaucomatous optic disc in experimental primate and human eyes. Invest Ophthal Vis Sci 25:918, 1984.
64. Quigley, HA, Hohman, RM, Addicks, EM: Quantitative study of optic nerve head capillaries in experimental optic disc pallor. Am J Ophthal 93:689, 1982.
65. Quigley, HA, Anderson, DR: The histologic basis of optic disk pallor in experimental optic atrophy. Am J Ophthal 83:709, 1977.
66. Henkind, P, Bellhorn, R, Rabkin, M, Murphy, ME: Optic nerve transection in cats. II. Effect on vessels of optic nerve head and lamina cribrosa. Invest Ophthal Vis Sci 16:442, 1977.
67. Radius, RL, Anderson, DR: The mechanism of disc pallor in experimental optic atrophy. A fluorescein angiographic study. Arch Ophthal 97:532, 1979.
68. Hayreh, SS: Pathogenesis of cupping of the optic disc. Br J Ophthal 58:863, 1974.
69. Emery, JM, Landis, D, Paton, D, et al: The lamina cribrosa in normal and glaucomatous human eyes. Trans Am Acad Ophthal Otol 78:290, 1974.
70. Levy, NS, Crapps, EE: Displacement of optic nerve head in response to short-term intraocular pressure elevation in human eyes. Arch Ophthal 102:782, 1984.
71. Radius, RL, Pederson, JE: Laser-induced primate glaucoma. II. Histopathology. Arch Ophthal 102:1693, 1984.
72. Zeimer, RC, Ogura, Y: The relation between glaucomatous damage and optic nerve head mechanical compliance. Arch Ophthal 107:1232, 1989.
73. Quigley, HA, Hohman, RM, Addicks, EM, et al: Morphologic changes in the lamina cribrosa correlated with neural loss in open-angle glaucoma. Am J Ophthal 95:673, 1983.
74. Dandona, L, Quigley, HA, Brown, AE, Enger, C: Quantitative regional structure of the normal human lamina cribrosa. A racial comparison. Arch Ophthal 108:393, 1990.
75. Hernandez, MR, Andrzejewska, WM, Neufeld, AH: Changes in the extracellular matrix of the human optic nerve head in primary open-angle glaucoma. Am J Ophthal 109:180, 1990.
76. Vrabee, F: Glaucomatous cupping of the human optic disk. A neuro-histologic study. Graefe's Arch Ophthal 198:223, 1976.
77. Quigley, HA, Addicks, EM: Chronic experimental glaucoma in primates. II. Effect of extended intraocular pressure elevation on optic nerve head and axonal transport. Invest Ophthal Vis Sci 19:137, 1980.
78. Quigley, HA, Sanchez, RM, Dunkelberger, GR, et al: Chronic glaucoma selectively damages large optic nerve fibers. Invest Ophthal Vis Sci 23:913, 1987.
79. Quigley, HA, Dundelberger, GR, Green, WR: Chronic human glaucoma causing selectively greater loss of large optic nerve fibers. Ophthalmology 95:357, 1988.
80. Weinstein, JM, Duckrow, RB, Beard, D, Brennant, RW: Regional optic nerve blood flow and its autoregulation. Invest Ophthal Vis Sci 24:1559, 1983.
81. Sossi, N, Anderson, DR: Effect of elevated intraocular pressure on blood flow. Occurrence in cat optic nerve head studied with Iodoantipyrine I 125. Arch Ophthal 101:98, 1983.
82. Grehn, F, Prost, M: Function of retinal nerve fibers depends on perfusion pressure: neurophysiologic investigations during acute intraocular pressure elevation. Invest Ophthal Vis Sci 24:347, 1983.
83. Novack, RL, Stefansson, E, Hatchell, DL: Intraocular pressure effects on optic nerve-head oxidative metabolism measured in vivo. Graefe's Arch Ophthal 228:128, 1990.
84. Quigley, HA, Hohman, RM, Sanchez, R, Addicks, EM: Optic nerve head blood flow in chronic experimental glaucoma. Arch Ophthal 103:956, 1985.
85. Ernest, JT: Pathogenesis of glaucomatous optic nerve disease. Trans Am Ophthal Soc LXXIII:366, 1975.
86. Riva, CE, Grunwald, JE, Sinclair, SH: Laser

doppler measurement of relative blood velocity in the human optic nerve head. Invest Ophthal Vis Sci 22:241, 1982.
87. Robert, Y, Steiner, D, Hendrickson, P: Papillary circulation dynamics in glaucoma. Graefe's Arch Ophthal 227:436, 1989.
88. Ernest, JT, Archer, D: Fluorescein angiography of the optic disk. Am J Ophthal 75:973, 1973.
89. Schwartz, B, Kern, J: Age, increased ocular and blood pressures, and retinal and disc fluorescein angiogram. Arch Ophthal 93:1980, 1980.
90. Tso, MOM, Shih, C-Y, McLean, IW: Is there a blood-brain barrier at the optic nerve head? Arch Ophthal 93:815, 1975.
91. Hayreh, SS: Optic disc changes in glaucoma. Br J Ophthal 56:175, 1972.
92. Rosen, ES, Boyd, TAS: New method of assessing choroidal ischemia in open-angle glaucoma and ocular hypertension. Am J Ophthal 70:912, 1970.
93. Raitta, C, Sarmela, T: Fluorescein angiography of the optic disc and the peripapillary area in chronic glaucoma. Acta Ophthal 48:303, 1970.
94. Blumenthal, M, Best, M, Galin, MA, Toyofuku, H: Peripapillary choroidal circulation in glaucoma. Arch Ophthal 86:31, 1971.
95. Hayreh, SS: The pathogenesis of optic nerve lesions in glaucoma. Trans Am Acad Ophthal Otol 81:197, 1976.
96. Oosterhuis, JA, Boen-Tan, TN: Choroidal fluorescence in the normal human eye. Ophthalmologica 162:246, 1971.
97. Evans, PY, Shimizu, K, Limaye, S, et al: Fluorescein cineangiography of the optic nerve head. Trans Am Acad Ophthal Otol 77:260, 1973.
98. Best, M, Toyofuke, H: Ocular hemodynamics during induced ocular hypertension in man. Am J Ophthal 74:932, 1972.
99. Hitchings, RA, Spaeth, GL: Fluorescein angiography in chronic simple and low-tension glaucoma. Br J Ophthal 61:126, 1977.
100. Alterman, M, Henkind, P: Radial peripapillary capillaries of the retina. II. Possible role in Bjerrum scotoma. Br J Ophthal 52:26, 1968.
101. Blumenthal, M, Gitter, KA, Best, M, Galin, MA: Fluorescein angiography during induced ocular hypertension in man. Am J Ophthal 69:39, 1970.
102. Blumenthal, M, Best, M, Galin, MA, Gitter, KA: Ocular circulation: analysis of the effect of induced ocular hypertension on retinal and choroidal blood flow in man. Am J Ophthal 71:819, 1971.
103. Archer, DB, Ernest, JT, Krill, AE: Retinal, choroidal, and papillary circulations under conditions of induced ocular hypertension. Am J Ophthal 73:834, 1972.
104. Spaeth, GL: Fluorescein angiography: its contributions towards understanding the mechanisms of visual loss in glaucoma. Trans Am Ophthal Soc LXXIII:491, 1975.
105. Spaeth, GL: The Pathogenesis of Nerve Damage in Glaucoma: Contributions of Fluorescein Angiography. Grune & Stratton, New York, 1977.
106. Schwartz, B, Rieser, JC, Fishbein, SL: Fluorescein angiographic defects of the optic disc in glaucoma. Arch Ophthal 95:1961, 1977.
107. Sonty, S, Schwartz, B: Two-point fluorophotometry in the evaluation of glaucomatous optic disc. Arch Ophthal 98:1422, 1980.
108. Fishbein, SL, Schwartz, B: Optic disc in glaucoma. Topography and extent of fluorescein filling defects. Arch Ophthal 95:1975, 1977.
109. Adam, G, Schwartz, B: Increased fluorescein filling defects in the wall of the optic disc cup in glaucoma. Arch Ophthal 98:1590, 1980.
110. Loebl, M, Schwartz, B: Fluorescein angiographic defects of the optic disc in ocular hypertension. Arch Ophthal 95:1980, 1977.
111. Talusan, E, Schwartz, B: Specificity of fluorescein angiographic defects of the optic disc in glaucoma. Arch Ophthal 95:2166, 1977.
112. Talusan, ED, Schwartz, B, Wilcox, LM Jr: Fluorescein angiography of the optic disc. A longitudinal follow-up study. Arch Ophthal 98:1579, 1980.
113. Tuulonen, A, Nagin, P, Schwartz, B, Wu, D-C: Increase of pallor and fluorescein-filling defects of the optic disc in the followup of ocular hypertensives measured by computerized image analysis. Ophthalmology 94:558, 1987.
114. Tsukahara, S: Hyperpermeable disc capillaries in glaucoma. Adv Ophthal 35:65, 1978.
115. Moses, RA: Intraocular blood flow from analysis of angiograms. Invest Ophthal Vis Sci 24:354, 1983.
116. Minckler, DS, Tso, MOM: A light microscopic, autoradiographic study of axoplasmic transport in the normal rhesus optic nerve head. Am J Ophthal 82:1, 1976.
117. Minckler, DS, Bunt, AH, Johanson, GW: Orthograde and retrograde axoplasmic transport during acute ocular hypertension in the monkey. Invest Ophthal Vis Sci 16:426, 1977.
118. Taylor, AC, Weiss, P: Demonstration of axonal flow by the movement of tritium-labeled protein in mature optic nerve fibers. Proc Natl Acad Sci USA 54:1521, 1965.
119. Weiss, P, Pillai, A: Convection and fate of mitochondria in nerve fibers: axonal flow as vehicle. Proc Natl Acad Sci USA 54:48, 1965.
120. Johansson, J-O: Inhibition of retrograde axoplasmic transport in rat optic nerve by increased IOP in vitro. Invest Ophthal Vis Sci 24:1552, 1983.
121. Anderson, DR, Hendrickson, A: Effect of intraocular pressure on rapid axoplasmic transport in monkey optic nerve. Invest Ophthal 13:771, 1974.
122. Minckler, DS, Tso, MOM, Zimmerman, LE: A light microscopic, autoradiographic study of axoplasmic transport in the optic nerve head during ocular hypotony, increased intraocular pressure, and papilledema. Am J Ophthal 82:741, 1976.

123. Quigley, HA, Anderson, DR: The dynamics and location of axonal transport blockade by acute intraocular pressure elevation in primate optic nerve. Invest Ophthal 15:606, 1976.
124. Minckler, DS, Bunt, AH, Klock, IB: Radioautographic and cytochemical ultrastructural studies of axoplasmic transport in the monkey optic nerve head. Invest Ophthal Vis Sci 17:33, 1978.
125. Quigley, HA, Guy, J, Anderson, DR: Blockage of rapid axonal transport. Effect of intraocular pressure elevation in primate optic nerve. Arch Ophthal 97:525, 1979.
126. Sakugawa, M, Chihara, E: Blockage at two points of axonal transport in glaucomatous eyes. Graefe's Arch Ophthal 223:214, 1985.
127. Radius, RL, Anderson, DR: Reversibility of optic nerve damage in primate eyes subjected to intraocular pressure above systolic blood pressure. Br J Ophthal 65:661, 1981.
128. Radius, RL: Distribution of pressure-induced fast axonal transport abnormalities in primate optic nerve. Arch Ophthal 99:1253, 1981.
129. Quigley, HA, Anderson, DR: Distribution of axonal transport blockade by acute intraocular pressure elevation in the primate optic nerve head. Invest Ophthal Vis Sci 16:640, 1977.
130. Gaasterland, D, Tanishima, T, Kuwabara, T: Axoplasmic flow during chronic experimental glaucoma. I. Light and electron microscopic studies of the monkey optic nerve head during development of glaucomatous cupping. Invest Ophthal Vis Sci 17:838, 1978.
131. Quigley, HA, Flower, RW, Addicks, EM, McLeod, DS: The mechanism of optic nerve damage in experimental acute intraocular pressure elevation. Invest Ophthal Vis Sci 19:505, 1980.
132. Minckler, DS, Bunt, AH: Axoplasmic transport in ocular hypotony and papilledema in the monkey. Arch Ophthal 95:1430, 1977.
133. Tso, MOM: Axoplasmic transport in papilledema and glaucoma. Trans Am Acad Ophthal Otol 83:771, 1977.
134. Anderson, DR, Hendrickson, AE: Failure of increased intracranial pressure to affect rapid axonal transport at the optic nerve head. Invest Ophthal Vis Sci 16:423, 1977.
135. Radius, RL, Anderson, DR: Rapid axonal transport in primate optic nerve. Distribution of pressure-induced interruption. Arch Ophthal 99:650, 1981.
136. Radius, RL, Bade, B: Axonal transport interruption and anatomy at the lamina cribrosa. Arch Ophthal 100:1661, 1982.
137. Radius, RL: Pressure-induced fast axonal transport abnormalities and the anatomy at the lamina cribrosa in primate eyes. Invest Ophthal Vis Sci 24:343, 1983.
138. Levy, NS, Adams, CK: Slow axonal protein transport and visual function following retinal and optic nerve ischemia. Invest Ophthal 14:91, 1975.
139. Levy, NS: The effect of interruption of the short posterior ciliary arteries on slow axoplasmic transport and histology within the optic nerve of the rhesus monkey. Invest Ophthal 15:495, 1976.
140. Radius, RL: Optic nerve fast axonal transport abnormalities in primates. Occurrence after short posterior ciliary artery occlusion. Arch Ophthal 98:2018, 1980.
141. Radius, RL, Anderson, DR: Morphology of axonal transport abnormalities in primate eyes. Br J Ophthal 65:767, 1981.
142. Radius, RL, Bade, B: Pressure-induced optic nerve axonal transport interruption in cat eyes. Arch Ophthal 99:2163, 1981.
143. Sossi, N, Anderson, DR: Blockage of axonal transport in optic nerve induced by elevation of intraocular pressure. Effect of arterial hypertension induced by Angiotensin I. Arch Ophthal 101:94, 1983.
144. Radius, RL, Anderson, DR: Breakdown of the normal optic nerve head blood-brain barrier following acute elevation of intraocular pressure in experimental animals. Invest Ophthal Vis Sci 19:244, 1980.
145. Radius, RL, Schwartz, EL, Anderson, DR: Failure of unilateral carotid artery ligation to affect pressure-induced interruption of rapid axonal transport in primate optic nerves. Invest Ophthal Vis Sci 19:153, 1980.
146. Sipperley, J, Anderson, DR, Hamasaki, D: Short-term effect of intraocular pressure elevation on the human electroretinogram. Arch Ophthal 90:358, 1973.
147. Bartl, G: The electroretinogram and the visual evoked potential in normal and glaucomatous eyes. Graefe's Arch Ophthal 207:243, 1978.
148. Pillunat, LE, Stodtmeister, R, Wilmanns, I, Christ, TH: Autoregulation of ocular blood flow during changes in intraocular pressure. Preliminary results. Graefe's Arch Ophthal 223:219, 1985.
149. Weiter, J, Fine, BS: A histologic study of regional choroidal dystrophy. Am J Ophthal 83:741, 1977.
150. Hayreh, SS: Anterior Ischemic Optic Neuropathy. Springer-Verlag, New York, 1975.
151. Quigley, H, Anderson, DR: Cupping of the optic disc in ischemic optic neuropathy. Trans Am Acad Ophthal Otol 83:755, 1977.
152. Sebag, J, Thomas, JV, Epstein, DL, Grant, WM: Optic disc cupping in arteritic anterior ischemic optic neuropathy resembles glaucomatous cupping. Ophthalmology 93:357, 1986.
153. Hitchings, RA: The optic disc in glaucoma, III: Diffuse optic disc pallor with raised intraocular pressure. Br J Ophthal 62:670, 1978.
154. Quigley, HA, Miller, NR, Green, WR: The pat-

tern of optic nerve fiber loss in anterior ischemic optic neuropathy. Am J Ophthal 100:769, 1985.
155. Radius, RL, Maumenee, AE: Optic atrophy and glaucomatous cupping. Am J Ophthal 85:145, 1978.
156. Jampol, LM, Board, RJ, Maumenee, AE: Systemic hypotension and glaucomatous changes. Am J Ophthal 85:154, 1978.
157. Brownstein, S, Font, RL, Zimmerman, LE, Murphy, SB: Nonglaucomatous cavernous degeneration of the optic nerve. Report of two cases. Arch Ophthal 98:345, 1980.
158. Caprioli, J, Spaeth, GL: Comparison of visual field defects in the low-tension glaucomas with those in the high-tension glaucomas. Am J Ophthal 97:730, 1984.
159. Jonas, JB, Gusek, GC, Guggenmoos-Holzmann, I, Naumann, GOH: Variability of the real dimensions of normal human optic discs. Graefe's Arch Ophthal 226:332, 1988.
160. Jonas, JB, Gusek, GC, Naumann GOH: Optic disc, cup and neuroretinal rim size, configuration and correlations in normal eyes. Invest Ophthal Vis Sci 29:1151, 1988.
161. Schwartz, B: Cupping and pallor of the optic disc. Arch Ophthal 89:272, 1973.
162. Armaly, MF: Genetic determination of cup/disc ratio of the optic nerve. Arch Ophthal 78:35, 1967.
163. Schwartz, JT, Reuling, FH, Garrison, RJ: Acquired cupping of the optic nerve head in normotensive eyes. Br J Ophthal 59:216, 1975.
164. Carpel, EF, Engstrom, PF: The normal cup-disk ratio. Am J Ophthal 91:588, 1981.
165. Fishman, RS: Optic disc asymmetry. A sign of ocular hypertension. Arch Ophthal 84:590, 1970.
166. Holm, OC, Becker, B, Asseff, CF, Podos, SM: Volume of the optic disk cup. Am J Ophthal 73:876, 1972.
167. Hollows, FC, McGuiness, R: The size of the optic cup. Trans Ophthal Soc Aust NZ 19:33, 1966.
168. Bengtsson, B: The inheritance and development of cup and disc diameters. Acta Ophthal 58:733, 1980.
169. Armaly, MF, Sayegh, RE: The cup/disc ratio. The findings of tonometry and tonography in the normal eye. Arch Ophthal 82:191, 1969.
170. Armaly, MF: The optic cup in the normal eye. I. Cup width, depth, vessel displacement, ocular tension and outflow facility. Am J Ophthal 68:401, 1969.
171. Bengtsson, B: The alteration and asymmetry of cup and disc diameters. Acta Ophthal 58:726, 1980.
172. Becker, B: Cup/disk ratio and topical corticosteroid testing. Am J Ophthal 70:681, 1970.
173. Snydacker, D: The normal optic disc. Ophthalmoscopic and photographic studies. Am J Ophthal 58:958, 1964.
174. Schwartz, B: Optic disc changes in ocular hypertension. Surv Ophthal 25:148, 1980.
175. Schwartz, B, Reinstein, NM, Lieberman, DM: Pallor of the optic disc. Quantitative photographic evaluation. Arch Ophthal 89:278, 1973.
176. Beck, RW, Messner, DK, Musch, DC, et al: Is there a racial difference in physiologic cup size? Ophthalmology 92:873, 1985.
177. Chi, T, Ritch, R, Stickler, D, et al: Racial differences in optic nerve head parameters. Arch Ophthal 107:836, 1989.
178. Jonas, JB, Gusek, GC, Naumann, GOH: Optic disc morphometry in high myopia. Graefe's Arch Ophthal 226:587, 1988.
179. Jonas, JB, Zach, F-M, Gusek, GC, Naumann, GOH: Pseudoglaucomatous physiologic large cups. Am J Ophthal 107:137, 1989.
180. Tomlinson, A, Phillips, CI: Ovalness of the optic cup and disc in the normal eye. Br J Ophthal 58:543, 1974.
181. Portney, GL: Qualitative parameters of the normal optic nerve head. Am J Ophthal 76:655, 1973.
182. Portney, GL: Photogrammetric categorical analysis of the optic nerve head. Trans Am Acad Ophthal Otol 78:275, 1974.
183. Shields, MB: Problems in recognizing non-glaucomatous optic nerve head cupping. Perspect Ophthal 2:129, 1978.
184. Balazsi, AG, Drance, SM, Schulzer, M, Douglas, GR: Neuroretinal rim area in suspected glaucoma and early chronic open-angle glaucoma. Correlation with parameters of visual function. Arch Ophthal 102:1011, 1984.
185. Caprioli, J, Miller, JM: Optic disc rim area is related to disc size in normal subjects. Arch Ophthal 105:1683, 1987.
186. Britton, RJ, Drance, SM, Schulzer, M, et al: The area of the neuroretinal rim of the optic nerve in normal eyes. Am J Ophthal 103:497, 1987.
187. Jonas, JB, Gusek, GC, Guggenmoos-Holzmann, I, Naumann, GOH: Correlations of the neuroretinal rim area with ocular and general parameters in normal eyes. Ophthal Res 20:298, 1988.
188. Shields, MB: Gray crescent in the optic nerve head. Am J Ophthal 89:238, 1980.
189. Klein, BEK, Moss, SE, Klein, R, et al: Neuroretinal rim area in diabetes mellitus. Invest Ophthal Vis Sci 31:805, 1990.
190. Radius, RL: Thickness of the retinal nerve fiber layer in primate eyes. Arch Ophthal 100:807, 1982.
191. Quigley, HA, Addicks, EM: Quantitative studies of retinal nerve fiber layer defects. Arch Ophthal 100:807, 1982.
192. Jonas, JB, Nguyen, NX, Naumann, GOH: The retinal nerve fiber layer in normal eyes. Ophthalmology 96:627, 1989.
193. Fantes, FE, Anderson, DR: Clinical histologic

correlation of human peripapillary anatomy. Ophthalmology 96:20, 1989.

194. Kirsch, RE, Anderson, DR: Clinical recognition of glaucomatous cupping. Am J Ophthal 75:442, 1973.
195. Weisman, RL, Asseff, DF, Phelps, CD, et al: Vertical elongation of the optic cup in glaucoma. Trans Am Acad Ophthal Otol 77:157, 1973.
196. Read, RM, Spaeth, GL: The practical clinical appraisal of the optic disc in glaucoma: the natural history of cup progression and some specific disc-field correlations. Trans Am Acad Ophthal Otol 78:255, 1974.
197. Spaeth, GL, Hitchings, RA, Sivalingam, E: The optic disc in glaucoma: pathogenetic correlation of five patterns of cupping in chronic open-angle glaucoma. Trans Am Acad Ophthal Otol 81:217, 1976.
198. Hitchings, RA, Spaeth, GL: The optic disc in glaucoma. I: Classification. Br J Ophthal 60:778, 1976.
199. Radius, RL, Maumenee, AE, Green, WR: Pit-like changes of the optic nerve head in open-angle glaucoma. Br J Ophthal 62:389, 1978.
200. Betz, PH, Camps, F, Collignon-Brach, J, et al: Biometric study of the disc cup in open-angle glaucoma. Graefe's Arch Ophthal 218:70, 1982.
201. Jonas, JB, Gusek, GC, Naumann, GOH: Optic disc morphometry in chronic primary open-angle glaucoma: I. Morphometric intrapapillary characteristics. Graefe's Arch Ophthal 226:522, 1988.
202. Airaksinen, PJ, Drance, SM, Schulzer, M: Neuroretinal rim area in early glaucoma. Am J Ophthal 99:1, 1985.
203. Drance, SM, Balazsi, G: The neuro-retinal rim area in early glaucoma. Klin Monatsbl Augenheilkd 184:271, 1984.
204. Pederson, JE, Anderson, DR: The mode of progressive disc cupping in ocular hypertension and glaucoma. Arch Ophthal 98:490, 1980.
205. Cher, I, Robinson, LP: "Thinning" of the neural rim of the optic nerve-head. An altered state, providing a new ophthalmoscopic sign associated with characteristics of glaucoma. Trans Ophthal Soc U K 93:213, 1973.
206. Cher, I, Robinson, LP: Thinning of the neural rim: a simple new sign on the optic disc related to glaucoma—statistical considerations. Aust J Ophthal 2:27, 1974.
207. Portney, GL: Photogrammetric analysis of the three-dimensional geometry of normal and glaucomatous optic cups. Trans Am Acad Ophthal Otol 81:239, 1976.
208. Susanna, R Jr: The lamina cribrosa and visual field defects in open-angle glaucoma. Can J Ophthal 18:124, 1983.
209. Miller, KM, Quigley, HA: The clinical appearance of the lamina cribrosa as a function of the extent of glaucomatous optic nerve damage. Ophthalmology 95:135, 1988.
210. Chandler, PA, Grant, WM: Glaucoma, 2nd ed. Lea and Febiger, Philadelphia, 1977.
211. Drance, SM, Fairclough, M, Butler, DM, Kottler, MS: The importance of disc hemorrhage in the prognosis of chronic open angle glaucoma. Arch Ophthal 95:226, 1977.
212. Susanna, R, Drance, SM, Douglas, GR: Disc hemorrhages in patients with elevated intraocular pressure. Occurrence with and without field changes. Arch Ophthal 97:284, 1979.
213. Gloster, J: Incidence of optic disc hemorrhages in chronic simple glaucoma and ocular hypertension. Br J Ophthal 65:452, 1981.
214. Airaksinen, PJ, Mustonen, E, Alanko, HI: Optic disc hemorrhages precede retinal nerve fiber layer defects in ocular hypertension. Acta Ophthal (Copenh) 59:627, 1981.
215. Bengtsson, B, Holmin, C, Krakau, CET: Disc hemorrhage and glaucoma. Acta Ophthal 59:1, 1981.
216. Shihab, ZM, Lee, P-F, Hay, P: The significance of disc hemorrhage in open-angle glaucoma. Ophthalmology 89:211, 1982.
217. Bengtsson, B: Characteristics of manifest glaucoma at early stages. Graefe's Arch Ophthal 227:241, 1989.
218. Diehl, DLC, Quigley, HA, Miller, NR, et al: Prevalence and significance of optic disc hemorrhage in a longitudinal study of glaucoma. Arch Ophthal 108:545, 1990.
219. Poinoosawmy, D, Gloster, J, Nagasubramanian, S, Hitchings, RA: Association between optic disc haemorrhages in glaucoma and abnormal glucose tolerance. Br J Ophthal 70:599, 1986.
220. Tuulonen, A, Takamoto, T, Wu, D-C, Schwartz, B: Optic disc cupping and pallor measurements of patients with a disk hemorrhage. Am J Ophthal 103:505, 1987.
221. Heijl, A: Frequent disc photography and computerized perimetry in eyes with optic disc haemorrhage. Acta Ophthal 64:274, 1986.
222. Bengtsson, B: Chronic glaucoma and symptomatic vitreous detachment. Acta Ophthal 64:152, 1986.
223. Hitchings, RA, Spaeth, GL: Chronic retinal vein occlusion in glaucoma. Br J Ophthal 60:694, 1976.
224. Tuulonen, A: Asymptomatic miniocclusions of the optic disc veins in glaucoma. Arch Ophthal 107:1475, 1989.
225. Shihab, ZM, Beebe, WE, Wentlandt, T: Possible significance of cilioretinal arteries in open-angle glaucoma. Ophthalmology 92:880, 1985.
226. Lindenmuth, KA, Skuta, GL, Musch, DC, Bueche, M: Significance of cilioretinal arteries in primary open angle glaucoma. Arch Ophthal 106:1691, 1988.
227. Herschler, J, Osher, RH: Baring of the circumlin-

ear vessel. An early sign of optic nerve damage. Arch Ophthal 98:865, 1980.
228. Osher, RH, Herschler, J: The significance of baring of the circumlinear vessel. A prospective study. Arch Ophthal 99:817, 1981.
229. Sutton, GE, Motolko, MA, Phelps, CD: Baring of a circumlinear vessel in glaucoma. Arch Ophthal 101:739, 1983.
230. Sommer, A, Miller, NR, Pollack, I, et al: The nerve fiber layer in the diagnosis of glaucoma. Arch Ophthal 95:2149, 1977.
231. Sommer, A, Pollack, I, Maumenee, AE: Optic disc parameters and onset of glaucomatous field loss. II. Static screening criteria. Arch Ophthal 97:1449, 1979.
232. Quigley, HA, Miller, NR, George, T: Clinical evaluation of nerve fiber layer atrophy as an indicator of glaucomatous optic nerve damage. Arch Ophthal 98:1564, 1980.
233. Iwata, K, Kurosawa, A, Sawaguchi, S: Wedge-shaped retinal nerve fiber layer defects in experimental glaucoma: preliminary report. Graefe's Arch Ophthal 223:184, 1985.
234. Airaksinen, PJ, Tuulonen, A: Early glaucoma changes in patients with and without optic disc hemorrhage. Acta Ophthal 62:197, 1984.
235. Airaksinen, PJ, Drance, SM: Neuroretinal rim area and retinal nerve fiber layer in glaucoma. Arch Ophthal 103:203, 1985.
236. Nanba, K, Schwartz, B: Nerve fiber layer and optic disc fluorescein defects in glaucoma and ocular hypertension. Ophthalmology 95:1227, 1988.
237. Chihara, E, Sawada, A: Atypical nerve fiber layer defects in high myopes with high-tension glaucoma. Arch Ophthal 108:228, 1990.
238. Airaksinen, PJ, Drance, SM, Douglas, GR, et al: Diffuse and localized nerve fiber loss in glaucoma. Am J Ophthal 98:566, 1984.
239. Sommer, A, Quigley, HA, Robin, AL, et al: Evaluation of nerve fiber layer assessment. Arch Ophthal 102:1766, 1984.
240. Airaksinen, PJ, Drance, SM, Douglas, GR, et al: Visual field and retinal nerve fiber layer comparisons in glaucoma. Arch Ophthal 103:205, 1985.
241. Caprioli, J: The contour of the juxtapapillary nerve fiber layer in glaucoma. Ophthalmology 97:358, 1990.
242. Wilensky, JT, Kolker, AE: Peripapillary changes in glaucoma. Am J Ophthal 81:341, 1976.
243. Jonas, JB, Naumann, OH: Parapapillary chorioretinal atrophy in normal and glaucoma eyes. II. Correlations. Invest Ophthal Vis Sci 30:919, 1989.
244. Buus, DR, Anderson, DR: Peripapillary crescents and halos in normal-tension glaucoma and ocular hypertension. Ophthalmology 96:16, 1989.
245. Rockwood, EJ, Anderson, DR: Acquired peripapillary changes and progression in glaucoma. Graefe's Arch Ophthal 226:510, 1988.
246. Kasner, O, Feuer, WJ, Anderson, DR: Possibly reduced prevalence of peripapillary crescents in ocular hypertension. Can J Ophthal 24:211, 1989.
247. Kessing, SV, Gregersen E: Distended disk in early stages of congenital glaucoma. Acta Ophthal 55:431, 1977.
248. Quigley, HA: Childhood glaucoma. Results with trabeculotomy and study of reversible cupping. Ophthalmology 89:219, 1982.
249. Pederson, JE, Herschler, J: Reversal of glaucomatous cupping in adults. Arch Ophthal 100:426, 1982.
250. Schwartz, B, Takamoto, T, Nagin, P: Measurements of reversibility of optic disc cupping and pallor in ocular hypertension and glaucoma. Ophthalmology 92:1396, 1985.
251. Greenidge, KC, Spaeth, GL, Traverso, CE: Change in appearance of the optic disc associated with lowering of intraocular pressure. Ophthalmology 92:897, 1985.
252. Katz, LJ, Spaeth, GL, Cantor, LB, et al: Reversible optic disk cupping and visual field improvement in adults with glaucoma. Am J Ophthal 107:485, 1989.
253. Jensen, PE, Kalina, RE: Congenital anomalies of the optic disk. Am J Ophthal 82:27, 1976.
254. Pagon, RA: Ocular coloboma. Surv Ophthal 25:223, 1981.
255. Kindler, P: Morning glory syndrome: unusual congenital optic disk anomaly. Am J Ophthal 69:376, 1970.
256. Apple, DJ, Rabb, MF, Walsh, PM: Congenital anomalies of the optic disc. Surv Ophthal 27:3, 1982.
257. Haik, BG, Greenstein, SH, Smith, ME, et al: Retinal detachment in the morning glory anomaly. Ophthalmology 91:1638, 1984.
258. Brown, GC, Shields, JA, Goldberg, RE: Congenital pits of the optic nerve head. II. Clinical studies in humans. Ophthalmology 87:51, 1980.
259. Theodossiadis, G: Evolution of congenital pit of the optic disk with macular detachment in photocoagulated and nonphotocoagulated eyes. Am J Ophthal 84:620, 1977.
260. Trobe, JD, Glaser, JS, Cassady, J, et al: Optic atrophy. Differential diagnosis by fundus observation alone. Arch Ophthal 98:1040, 1980.
261. Trobe, JD, Glaser, JS, Cassady, J, et al: Nonglaucomatous excavation of the optic disc. Arch Ophthal 98:1046, 1980.
262. Lichter, PR, Henderson, JW: Optic nerve infarction. Am J Ophthal 85:302, 1978.
263. Portney, GL, Roth, AM: Optic cupping caused by an intracranial aneurysm. Am J Ophthal 84:98, 1977.
264. Johns, KJ, Leonard-Martin, T, Feman, SS: The

effect of panretinal photocoagulation on optic nerve cupping. Ophthalmology 96:211, 1989.
265. Romano, JH: Graticule incorporated into an ophthalmoscope for the clinical evaluation of the cup/disc ratio. Br J Ophthal 67:214, 1983.
266. Rosenwasser, GOD, Tiedeman, JS: A stable slit lamp mounting device for 90 D lens use in non-contact ophthalmoscopy. Ophthalmic Surg 17:525, 1986.
267. Repka, MX, Uozato, H, Guyton, DL: Depth distortion during slitlamp biomicroscopy of the fundus. Ophthalmology 93(S):47, 1986.
268. Shaffer, RN, Ridgway, WL, Brown, R, Kramer, SG: The use of diagrams to record changes in glaucomatous disks. Am J Ophthal 80:460, 1975.
269. Lichter, PR: Variability of expert observers in evaluating the optic disc. Trans Am Ophthal Soc LXXIV:532, 1976.
270. Schwartz, JT: Methodologic differences and measurement of cup-disc ratio. An epidemiologic assessment. Arch Ophthal 94:1101, 1976.
271. Tielsch, JM, Katz, J, Quigley, HA, et al: Intraobserver and interobserver agreement in measurement of optic disc characteristics. Ophthalmology 95:350, 1988.
272. Gloster, J, Parry, DG: Use of photographs for measuring cupping in the optic disc. Br J Ophthal 58:850, 1974.
273. Hitchings, RA, Genio, C, Anderton, S, Clark, P: An optic disc grid: its evaluation in reproducibility studies on the cup/disc ratio. Br J Ophthal 67:356, 1983.
274. Sharma, NK, Hitchings, RA: A comparison of monocular and 'stereoscopic' photographs of the optic disc in the identification of glaucomatous visual field defects. Br J Ophthal 67:677, 1983.
275. Cohan, BE: Multiple-slit illumination of the optic disc. Arch Ophthal 96:497, 1978.
276. Kennedy, SJ, Schwartz, B, Takamoto, T, Eu, JKT: Interference fringe scale for absolute ocular fundus measurement. Invest Ophthal Vis Sci 24:169, 1983.
277. Schwartz, B, Kern, J: Scanning microdensitometry of optic disc pallor in glaucoma. Arch Ophthal 95:2159, 1977.
278. Rosenthal, AR, Falconer, DG, Barrett, P: Digital measurement of pallor-disc ratio. Arch Ophthal 98:2027, 1980.
279. Frisen, L: Photography of the retinal nerve fibre layer: an optimised procedure. Br J Ophthal 64:641, 1980.
280. Sommer, A, D'Anna, SA, Kues, HA, George, T: High-resolution photography of the retinal nerve fiber layer. Am J Ophthal 96:535, 1983.
281. Airaksinen, PJ, Nieminen, H: Retinal nerve fiber layer photography in glaucoma. Ophthalmology 92:877, 1985.
282. Peli, E, Hedges, TR III, McInnes, T, et al: Nerve fiber layer photography. A comparative study. Acta Ophthal 65:71, 1987.
283. Sommer, A, Kues, HA, D'Anna, SA, et al: Cross-polarization photography of the nerve fiber layer. Arch Ophthal 102:864, 1984.
284. Airaksinen, PJ, Nieminen, H, Mustonen, E: Retinal nerve fibre layer photography with a wide angle fundus camera. Acta Ophthal 60:362, 1982.
285. Knighton, RW, Jacobson, SG, Kemp, CM: The spectral reflectance of the nerve fiber layer of the macaque retina. Invest Ophthal Vis Sci 30:2393, 1989.
286. Allen, L: Stereoscopic fundus photography with the new instant positive print films. Am J Ophthal 57:539, 1964.
287. Donaldson, DD: A new camera for stereoscopic fundus photography. Arch Ophthal 73:253, 1965.
288. Donaldson, DD, Prescott, R, Kennedy, S: Simultaneous stereoscopic fundus camera incorporating a single optical axis. Invest Ophthal Vis Sci 19:289, 1980.
289. Saheb, NE, Drance, SM, Nelson, A: The use of photogrammetry in evaluating the cup of the optic nervehead for a study in chronic simple glaucoma. Can J Ophthal 7:466, 1972.
290. Rosenthal, AR, Kottler, MS, Donaldson, DD, Falconer, DG: Comparative reproducibility of the digital photogrammetric procedure utilizing three methods of stereophotography. Invest Ophthal Vis Sci 16:54, 1977.
291. Donaldson, DD, Grant, WM: Stereoscopic comparator with primary use for optic discs. Arch Ophthal 96:503, 1978.
292. Klein, BEK, Magli, YL, Richie, KA, et al: Quantitation of optic disc cupping. Ophthalmology 92:1654, 1985.
293. Schirmer, KE, Kratky, V: Stereochronoscopy of the optic disc with stereoscopic cameras. Arch Ophthal 98:1647, 1980.
294. Goldmann, H, Lotmar, W, Zulauf, M: Quantitative studies in stereochronoscopy (Sc): application to the disc in glaucoma. II. Statistical evaluation. Graefe's Arch Ophthal 222:82, 1984.
295. Takamoto, T, Schwartz, B: Stereochronometry: Quantitative measurement of optic disc cup changes. Invest Ophthal Vis Sci 26:1445, 1985.
296. Heijl, A, Bengtsson, B: Diagnosis of early glaucoma with flicker comparisons of serial disc photographs. Invest Ophthal Vis Sci 30:2376, 1989.
297. Alanko, H, Jaanio, E, Airaksinen, PJ, Nieminen, H: Demonstration of glaucomatous optic disc changes by electronic subtraction. Acta Ophthal 58:14, 1980.
298. Gloster, J: The colour of the optic disc. Doc Ophthal 26:155, 1969.
299. Davies, EWG: Quantitative assessment of colour of the optic disc by a photographic method. Exp Eye Res 9:106, 1970.
300. Berkowitz, JS, Balter, S: Colorimetric measure-

ment of the optic disk. Am J Ophthal 69:385, 1970.
301. Hendrickson, P, Robert, Y, Stockli, HP: Principles of photometry of the papilla. Arch Ophthal 102:1704, 1984.
302. Cohen, JS, Stone, RD, Hetherington, J Jr, Bullock, J: Glaucomatous cupping of the optic disk by ultrasonography. Am J Ophthal 82:24, 1976.
303. Darnley-Fisch, DA, Byrne, SF, Hughes, JR, et al: Contact B-scan echography in the assessment of optic nerve cupping. Am J Ophthal 109:55, 1990.
304. Kottler, MS, Rosenthal, AR, Falconer, DG: Analog vs. digital photogrammetry for optic cup analysis. Invest Ophthal 15:651, 1976.
305. Krohn, MA, Keltner, JL, Johnson, CA: Comparison of photographic techniques and films used in stereophotogrammetry of the optic disk. Am J Ophthal 88:859, 1979.
306. Schirmer, KE: Simplified photogrammetry of the optic disc. Arch Ophthal 94:1997, 1976.
307. Rosenthal, AR, Falconer, DG, Pieper, I: Photogrammetry experiments with a model eye. Br J Ophthal 64:881, 1980.
308. Johnson, CA, Keltner, JL, Krohn, MA, Portney, GL: Photogrammetry of the optic disc in glaucoma and ocular hypertension with simultaneous stereo photography. Invest Ophthal Vis Sci 18:1252, 1979.
309. Schwartz, B: New techniques for the examination of the optic disc and their clinical application. Trans Am Acad Ophthal Otol 81:227, 1976.
310. Nagin, P, Schwartz, B: Detection of increased pallor over time. Computerized image analysis in untreated ocular hypertension. Ophthalmology 91:252, 1984.
311. Mikelberg, FS, Douglas, GR, Schulzer, M, et al: Reliability of optic disk topographic measurements recorded with a video-ophthalmograph. Am J Ophthal 98:98, 1984.
312. Caprioli, J, Klingbeil, U, Sears, M, Pope, B: Reproducibility of optic disc measurements with computerized analysis of stereoscopic video images. Arch Ophthal 104:1035, 1986.
313. Shields, MB, Martone: JF, Shelton, AR, et al: Reproducibility of topographic measurements with the Optic Nerve Head Analyzer. Am J Ophthal 104:581, 1987.
314. Tomita, G, Goto, Y, Yamada, T, Kitazawa, Y: Reliability of optic measurement with computerized stereoscopic video image analyzer. Acta Soc Ophthal Jpn 90:1317, 1986.
315. Bishop, KI, Werner, EB, Krupin, T, et al: Variability and reproducibility of optic disk topographic measurements with the Rodenstock optic nerve head analyzer. Am J Ophthal 106:696, 1988.
316. Miller, JM, Caprioli, J: Videographic quantification of optic disc pallor. Invest Ophthal Vis Sci 29:320, 1988.
317. Mikelberg, FS, Douglas, GR, Drance, SM, et al: Reproducibility of computerized pallor measurements obtained with the Rodenstock disk analyzer. Graefe's Arch Ophthal 226:269, 1988.
318. Miller, KN, Shields, MB, Ollie, AR: Reproducibility of pallor measurements with the Optic Nerve Head Analyzer. Graefe's Arch Ophthal 227:562, 1989.
319. Shields, MB, Tiedeman, JS, Miller, KN, et al: Accuracy of topographic measurements with the Optic Nerve Head Analyzer. Am J Ophthal 107:273, 1989.
320. Mikelberg, FS, Airaksinen, PJ, Douglas, GR, et al: The correlation between optic disk topography measured by the video-ophthalmograph (Rodenstock Analyzer) and clinical measurement. Am J Ophthal 100:417, 1985.
321. Mikelberg, FS, Douglas, GR, Schulzer, M, et al: The correlation between cup-disk ratio, neuroretinal rim area, and optic disk area measured by the video-ophthalmograph (Rodenstock Analyzer) and clinical measurement. Am J Ophthal 101:7, 1986.
322. Caprioli, J, Miller, JM: Videographic measurements of optic nerve topography in glaucoma. Invest Ophthal Vis Sci 29:1294, 1988.
323. Caprioli, J, Miller, JM: Measurement of relative nerve fiber layer surface height in glaucoma. Ophthalmology 96:633, 1989.
324. Caprioli, J, Ortiz-Colberg, R, Miller, JM, Tressler, C: Measurements of peripapillary nerve fiber layer contour in glaucoma. Am J Ophthal 108:404, 1989.
325. Varma, R, Spaeth, GL: The PAR IS 2000: a new system for retinal digital image analysis. Ophthal Surg 19:183, 1988.
326. Varma, R, Steinmann, WC, Spaeth, GL, Wilson, RP: Variability in digital analysis of optic disc topography. Graefe's Arch Ophthal 226:435, 1988.
327. Varma, R, Spaeth, GL, Hanau, C, et al: Positional changes in the vasculature of the optic disk in glaucoma. Am J Ophthal 104:457, 1987.
328. Varma, R, Spaeth, GL, Steinmann, WC, Katz, LJ: Agreement between clinicians and an image analyzer in estimating cup-to-disc ratios. Arch Ophthal 107:526, 1989.
329. Dandona, L, Quigley, HA, Jampel, HD: Reliability of optic nerve head topographic measurements with computerized image analysis. Am J Ophthal 108:414, 1989.
330. Dandona, L, Quigley, HA, Jampel, HD: Variabil-

ity of depth measurements of the optic nerve head and peripapillary retina with computerized image analysis. Arch Ophthal 107:1786, 1989.

331. Algazi, VR, Keltner, JL, Johnson, CA: Computer analysis of the optic cup in glaucoma. Invest Ophthal Vis Sci 26:1759, 1985.

332. Kruse, FE, Burk, ROW, Volcker, H-E, et al: Reproducibility of topographic measurements of the optic nerve head with laser tomographic scanning. Ophthalmology 96:1320, 1989.

333. Zeimer, RC, Mori, MT, Khoobehi, B: Feasibility test of a new method to measure retinal thickness noninvasively. Invest Ophthal Vis Sci 30:2099, 1989.

Chapter 6

VISUAL FUNCTION IN GLAUCOMA

Advances in the technology of visual field testing are changing our clinical perception of normal and abnormal fields of vision. For example, the familiar two-dimensional presentation of concentric lines around the point of fixation is giving way to three-dimensional displays in symbols and numeric values. It is important to keep in mind, however, that the normal field of vision and the changes created by glaucoma are just the same as when Bjerrum discovered the arcuate scotoma using the back of his consulting-room door as a background for his field testing nearly 100 years ago. We will begin this chapter, therefore, by considering the normal field of vision and how it is altered by glaucomatous damage and then review the instruments and techniques by which these parameters can be measured. The limited scope of this chapter provides only an overview of the subject, and the reader is referred to the several excellent textbooks on perimetry for further details.[1–6]

THE NORMAL VISUAL FIELD

A helpful way to begin the study of visual fields and the methods by which they are measured is to consider Traquair's classic analogy of "an island of vision surrounded by a sea of blindness" (Fig. 6.1). This three-dimensional concept can be reduced to quantitative values by plotting lines (isopters) at various levels around the island, or by measuring the height (sensitivity) at different points within the island of vision.

Boundaries. The shoreline of the island corresponds to the peripheral limits of the visual field, which normally measure, with maximum target stimulation, approximately 60° above and nasal, 70–75° below, and 100–110° temporal to fixation.[2] Therefore, the typical configuration of the normal visual field is a horizontal oval, often with a shallow inferonasal depression (Fig. 6.1). The shape is usually of greater diagnostic significance than the absolute size of the visual field, since the latter is influenced by many physiologic variables.

Contour. The peaks and valleys on the island correspond to areas of increased or decreased vision within the peripheral limits of the visual field. These contours can be mapped by recording the relative visual sensitivities at specific points in the field of vision, or by using test objects with reduced stimulus value to plot smaller isopters within the absolute boundaries. The area of maximum visual acuity in the normal field is at the point of fixation, corresponding to the foveola of the retina, and appears as a smoothly rising peak surrounded by a high plateau.[7] The visual sensitivity then tapers down more gradually until it again falls abruptly at the peripheral limits.

Blind Spot. Within the boundaries of the normal visual field is a deep depression, or blind spot, which corresponds to the region of the optic nerve head. It is located approximately 15° temporal to fixation and has two portions: (1) an absolute scotoma, and (2) a relative scotoma.[8] The absolute scotoma corresponds to the actual optic nerve head and is seen as a vertical oval. Since there are

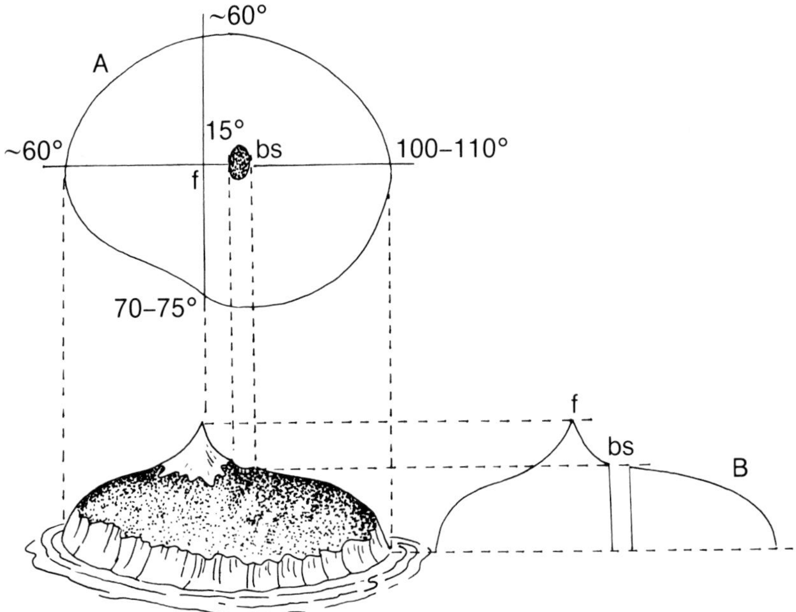

Figure 6.1. The normal visual field is depicted as Traquair's "island of vision surrounded by a sea of blindness," with projections showing the peripheral limits (*A*) and the profile (*B*). Fixation (*f*) corresponds to the foveola of the retina, and the blind spot (*bs*), to the optic nerve head. The approximate dimensions of the absolute peripheral boundary of the visual field and the location of the blind spot are shown (*A*).

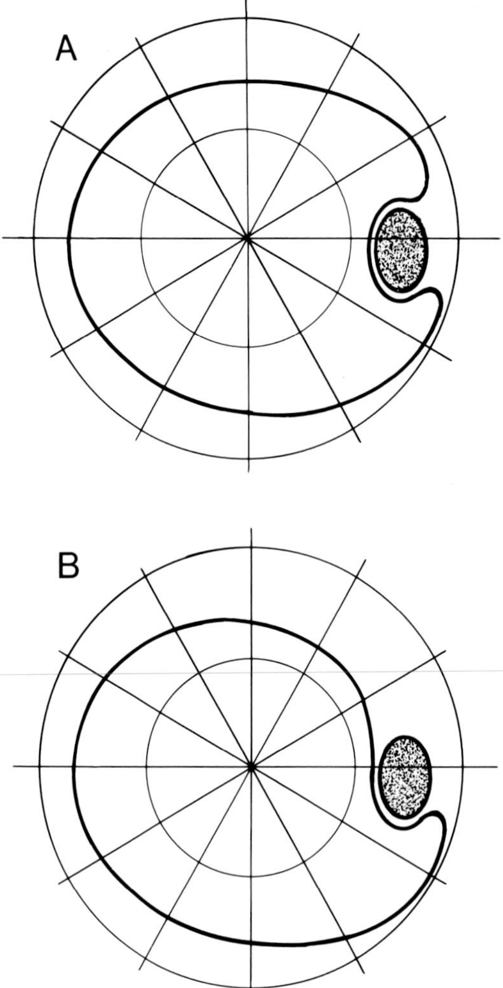

Figure 6.2. False baring (**A**) and true baring (**B**) of the blind spot.

no photoreceptors in the nerve head, this portion of the blind spot is independent of the test object stimulus value. The relative scotoma surrounds the absolute portion and corresponds to peripapillary retina, which has reduced visual sensitivity, especially inferiorly and superiorly. This portion of the blind spot is dependent on the stimulus value and varies with different testing methods. If the temporal margin of the relative blind spot comes close to the corresponding isopter, the two boundaries may artifactually become confluent, creating *false baring of the blind spot*. In addition, because the reduced sensitivity of the peripapillary retina is greater in the upper and lower poles, test objects with small stimulus value may cause vertical elongation of the blind spot, which can break through the isopter causing *true baring of the blind spot* (Fig. 6.2).

GLAUCOMATOUS INFLUENCES ON VISUAL FUNCTION

The increased sensitivity with which newer instruments allow evaluation of vision is changing our understanding of the natural history of progressive visual field loss in glaucoma. While central vision is typically one of the last regions to be totally lost, studies have shown mild reduction in this portion of the visual field even in the early stages of glaucoma.[9–11] The mechanism for this is uncertain, although evidence has been provided for abnormal autoregulation of macular retinal blood flow in open-angle glaucoma,[12] and blue field entoptic testing showed a correlation between reduced leukocyte velocity of the macular retinal microvasculature and reduced visual function in glaucoma.[13] In addition, while defects related to loss of retinal nerve fiber bundles are the most characteristic visual field changes induced by glaucoma, we are now finding that these alterations may be preceded by diffuse depression of retinal sensitivity, which can be demonstrated by a variety of psychophysical tests.

Generalized Depression of the Visual Field

The diffuse reduction in visual threshold appears to be one of the earliest detectable alterations in the visual field of a patient with glaucoma,[9] although one study suggested that this impression may be caused by multiple local defects.[14] In any case, the diagnostic value of this phenomenon is limited by its nonspecific nature, although it should still be looked for and noted in the course of visual field testing and analysis. In the future, these observations may acquire greater diagnostic significance as more sensitive techniques of measurement are developed, and as our knowledge of glaucomatous and nonglaucomatous visual field changes expands.

Concentric Contraction. Generalized reduction in the visual field may become manifest as a decrease in sensitivity for specific retinal locations or as a concentric constriction of the visual field, both of which have been noted to precede other detectable glaucomatous field defects in many patients.[15,16] Isopter contraction, as an early field defect of glaucoma, is often more marked in the nasal field, which has been called "crowding of the peripheral nasal isopters."[17] However, since generalized isopter contraction is produced by many factors, it has limited diagnostic value.[18]

Enlargement of the Blind Spot. Enlargement of the blind spot, due to depression of peripapillary retinal sensitivity, is also considered to be an early glaucomatous field change. However, it may be seen with other optic nerve or retinal disorders and can be produced in normal individuals with threshold targets, so that it is not a pathognomonic sign of glaucoma.[18]

Angioscotomata. Angioscotomata are long, branching scotomas above and below the blind spot, which are presumed to result from shadows created by the large retinal vessels. This finding is thought to represent an early glaucomatous field defect,[19] although it is technically difficult to demonstrate and not highly diagnostic.

Other Measures of Generalized Visual Impairment in Glaucoma

In addition to the diffuse reduction in retinal sensitivity that can be demonstrated by visual field changes in early glaucoma, there are other psychophysical tests that support the concept that a generalized decrease in visual function may be the earliest visual change in glaucoma.

Color Vision

Reduced sensitivity to colors has been described in various forms of glaucoma and may precede any detectable loss of peripheral or central vision by standard acuity or visual field testing. Most studies agree that the color vision deficit is associated primarily with blue-sensitive pathways.[10,20–29] This is consistent with the observation that blue signals travel in larger diameter axons, which are more susceptible than small fibers to increased intraocular pressure (IOP).[30] Blue cones contribute little to the sensation of brightness or to visual acuity, which may explain why standard visual acuity tests, perimetry, or contrast sensitivity studies might miss such a color vision loss. The visual dysfunction is significantly more common in high-tension glaucoma as compared with low-tension glaucoma[27] and is strongly related to higher IOP levels,[28] suggesting that the damage is pressure induced.

It is not clear whether the loss of color vision and the visual field changes associated with nerve fiber bundle loss share the same mechanism. Ocular hypertensives with yellow-blue and blue-green defects were found to have diffuse early changes in visual field sensitivity[23] as well as an increased chance of developing glaucomatous visual field loss as compared with similar patients without these color vision disturbances.[20] The same color abnormalities in patients with early glaucoma correlated significantly with diffuse retinal nerve fiber loss.[29] However, no significant correlation between color vision scores and visual field performance was found among ocular hypertensives when age correction was applied to the color variable,[31] and another study revealed no clear association between early glaucomatous cupping and color vision anomalies.[24]

The clinical usefulness of color vision testing in the early detection of glaucoma is limited by a lack of sensitivity and specificity. In most reported studies, the color vision testing was performed with the Farnsworth-Munsell 100-hue test, dichotomous (D-15) tests, or variants of these, all of which are laborious and of questionable precision. One test that was found to discriminate more effectively between patients with glaucomatous damage and the normal population employs a computer-driven color television system in which the patient must recognize flickering color contrasts by the sensation of flashing on the screen.[32] Specificity is limited by the fact that the tritan deficit is also the one most frequently seen with age-related changes. When study populations were matched for age and lens density, however, color vision loss in glaucoma was still attributable in part to the disease process.[33]

Contrast Sensitivity

Subtle loss of both central and peripheral vision can be demonstrated in some patients with glaucoma, prior to detectable visual field changes with standard techniques, by measuring the amount of contrast required for a patient to discriminate between adjacent visual stimuli.

Spatial Contrast Sensitivity. Sinewave gratings of parallel light and dark bands (Arden gratings), in which the patient must detect the striped pattern at various levels of contrast and spatial frequencies, have had the most extensive evaluation within this group of psychophysical tests.[34] Impaired contrast sensitivity by this testing method has been reported among glaucoma patients.[34–40] In some studies, the impairment correlates with visual field[36–38] and optic nerve head[38] damage, and it has been suggested that it may be the most sensitive method of measuring visual loss in glaucoma patients.[40] However, the overlap with other causes of reduced spatial contrast sensitivity, including age, create high false-negative and false-positive rates.[38,39,41–43] Spatial contrast sensitivity has been shown to decrease in normal subjects after 50 years of age, and small age-corrected reductions in glaucoma patients were found only in those under 50.[44] This influence of age on spatial contrast sensitivity appears to be independent of the crystalline lens.[45]

The original Arden gratings were limited by the subjectivity of the required responses.[46,47] A modification, in which the patient must indicate the orientation of the gratings, is reported to minimize the latter limitation.[47] The two testing methods most commonly used are microprocessor-controlled video displays and photographically reproduced grating patterns, both of which have been shown to give good approximations of the spatial contrast sensitivity function.[48]

Sinewave gratings and laser interference fringes have also been used as stimuli in visual field testing, which may allow detection of peripheral defects, especially with gratings of low spatial frequency, before they can be found with conventional targets.[49–51] Low-contrast letter charts have also been developed and are reported to correlate well with the results of sinewave gratings and reveal visual loss that is not detected with the standard Snellen chart.[52]

Temporal Contrast Sensitivity. Temporal contrast sensitivity, in which the patient must detect a visual stimulus flickering at various frequencies, provides another measure of contrast sensitivity. The stimulus may be presented either as a homogeneous flickering field (flicker fusion frequency)[2] or as a counterphase flickering grating of low spatial frequency (spatiotemporal contrast sensitivity).[44,53] Glaucoma patients may have reduced function with either method, although the latter appears to be a more sensitive test.[53,54] In one study, spatiotemporal contrast sensitivity was tested in four retinal quadrants and was found to be more useful in detecting glaucoma than spatial contrast sensitivity testing of the central retina, although age influence again limited the usefulness of the test to those under 50.[44] There is also a question as to whether temporal contrast sensitivity loss among ocular hypertensives represents early glaucomatous damage or a transient influence of raised IOP. One study suggested that either mechanism may be found within subsets of this population.[55]

Several techniques have been evaluated to improve contrast sensitivity testing. One study suggested that the determination of a ratio between spatial contrast sensitivity and flicker sensitivity is a more precise measure of visual pathology than the absolute value of either test.[56] Another test of temporal contrast sensitivity, in which the patient must discriminate two rapidly successive pulses of light from a single pulse, is reported to be highly sensitive and specific in separating glaucomatous from normal eyes.[57]

Electrophysiologic Studies

The measures of visual function described above are all dependent on the patient's subjective response. Work is also being done in this area on alternative objective methods.

Electroretinography. Electroretinograms (ERG) evoked by reversing checkerboard or grating patterns (*pattern ERG*) are sensitive to retinal ganglion cell and optic nerve dysfunction and have reduced amplitudes in glaucoma patients.[58–65] This appears in the early stages of glaucoma[66,67] and in some ocular hypertensives,[68–70] especially those at higher risk of developing glaucoma.[68] The reduction in ocular hypertensives does not correlate with IOP or cup/disc ratio,[69] nor precisely with color vision deficits,[70] suggesting a complementary role for this test in detecting glaucoma. Decreased amplitude and an increase in peak latency also correlate with increasing age,[63] paralleling the estimated normal loss of ganglion cells. Indeed, reduction in pattern ERG was directly related to histologically defined optic nerve damage in a monkey model.[71]

The electroretinogram evoked by a flash of light (*flash ERG*) is affected more by outer retinal elements and is not typically abnormal in glaucoma. Acute IOP elevation in cats, however, caused a reduction in both pattern and flash ERG, proportional to the reduction in perfusion pressure and irrespective of the absolute IOP, suggesting a vascular mechanism to which the ganglion cells are less likely to recover.[72] Glaucoma patients in one study had reduced ERG amplitudes in response to a flickering stimulus (*flicker ERG*).[65]

Visual Evoked Potentials. Visual evoked potentials (VEP) may also be abnormal in patients with chronic[21,58,62,73–75] or acute glaucoma,[76] although this is more variable than the pattern ERG response.[61,71] However, larger diameter axons, which are preferentially damaged in glaucoma, correlate with fast, transiently responding retinal ganglion cells, and a reduced response to high-frequency flicker VEP (above 13 Hz) correlated with the degree of glaucomatous damage.[77]

Glaucoma patients were also found in one study to have increased baseline values with *electro-oculography*.[78]

Miscellaneous Tests

Dark adaptation, tested with chromatic stimuli, has been reported to be abnormal in populations of ocular hypertensives.[79] *Dichoptic testing,* in which one-half of a test object is presented to one eye, and the other half to the fellow eye, as an aid to determining the location of a defect in the visual pathway, was found in preliminary studies to give abnormal responses in patients with open-angle glaucoma.[80] A *relative afferent pupillary defect* offers yet another measure of visual pathway disturbance in glaucoma.[81] It has been shown to be proportional to the amount of visual field loss[82–84] and may precede detectable field loss by static automated perimetry.[84] When pupillary status, such as marked miosis, prevents determination of relative afferent pupillary defect, it has been shown that *brightness comparison testing,* in which the patient is asked to judge whether the same light source is brighter with one eye or the other through closed lids, correctly predicts the presence of a relative afferent pupillary defect in 92% of glaucoma patients.[85] In another study, 86% of glaucoma patients had a significant disparity in brightness discrimination between the two eyes.[86]

Nerve Fiber Bundle Defects

While the measures of generalized reduction in visual function, as considered above, may one day be important in the early detection of glaucoma, they are too inconsistent and nonspecific at the present time to be of highly significant clinical value. Focal defects resulting from loss or impairment of retinal nerve fiber bundles are more specific for glaucoma and constitute the most definitive early evidence of visual field loss from these disorders. The nature of the nerve fiber bundle defects relates to the retinal topography of these fibers, as discussed in Chapter 5.

Scatter

Before considering the specific forms of visual field loss associated with nerve fiber bundle defects, it is important to note that discrete scotomas may be preceded by variable threshold responses to repeated testing in the same area.[87–90] This has been referred to as scatter, fluctuation, or localized minor disturbances. The phenomenon has been studied with the *differential light threshold,* which is defined as the light stimulus that can be recognized above background with a probability of 50% in a given retinal location.[91] Studies with this technique show that patients with glaucoma have substantially greater scatter during one examination (*short-term fluctuation*), as well as from one test to another (*long-term fluctuation*).[91–94] While scatter is not a definitive sign of glaucomatous visual field damage, it should be looked upon with suspicion as an early warning sign of impending absolute field loss.

Arcuate Defects

The arcuate, or Bjerrum (pronounced "Bee yer′ um"), area within the visual field arches above and below fixation from the blind spot to the median raphe, corresponding to the arcuate retinal nerve fibers (Fig. 6.3*a*). The nasal extreme of the arcuate area along the median raphe may come within 1° of fixation and extends nasally for 10–20°.[95,96] Early visual loss in glaucoma commonly occurs within this arcuate area, especially in the superior half, which correlates with the predilection of the inferior and superior temporal poles of the optic nerve head for early glaucomatous damage.[95–97] As field defects develop within the arcuate area, they most often appear first as one or more localized defects, or *paracentral scotomas* (Fig. 6.3*b*). The typical pattern of progression of glaucomatous visual field defects is for a shallow paracentral depression to become denser and larger,[98] eventually forming a central absolute defect, surrounded by a relative scotoma.[89,99,100] Occasionally, the early arcuate defect may connect with the blind spot and taper to a point in a slightly curved course, which has been referred to as a *Seidel scotoma* (Fig. 6.3*c*). As the isolated defects enlarge and coalesce, they form an arching scotoma that eventually fills the entire arcuate area from the blind spot to the median raphe, which is called an *arcuate* or *Bjerrum scotoma* (Fig. 6.3*d*). With further progression, a double arcuate (or ring) scotoma will develop (Fig. 6.3*e*). The rate of visual field loss correlates with the size of the scotoma, in that the larger the scotoma, the more rapidly it is likely to enlarge.[101]

Differential Diagnosis of Arcuate Scotomas

Although the arcuate defect is probably the most reliable early form of glaucomatous field loss, it is not pathognomonic, and the following additional causes must be considered, especially when the field and disc changes do not seem to correlate: chorioretinal lesions, optic nerve head lesions, anterior optic nerve lesions, and posterior lesions of the visual pathway (Table 6.1)[95,96,102]

Nasal Steps (Fig. 6.3*e*)

The loss of retinal nerve fibers rarely proceeds at the same rate in the upper and lower portions of an eye. Consequently, a step-like defect is frequently created where the nerve fibers meet along the median raphe. Since the superior field is involved somewhat more frequently than the inferior portion in the early stages of glaucoma, the nasal step more often results from a greater defect above the horizontal midline, which is referred to as a superior nasal step. However, inferior nasal steps are not uncommon. Nasal steps are also distinguished by their central or peripheral location.[103] A *central nasal step* is created at the nasal termination of unequal double arcuate scotomata. Unequal contraction of the peripheral isopters resulting from loss of corresponding bundles of peripheral arcuate nerve fibers produces a defect that has been called the *peripheral nasal step of Ronne*. It may begin as an isolated scotoma in the nasal periphery.[104] The shape of the peripheral nasal step differs according to its distance from fixation and is not necessarily found in all isopters.[99,100]

Vertical Step (Fig. 6.3*f*)

A stepwise defect along the vertical midline, referred to as a vertical step or hemianopic offset, is a less common feature of glaucomatous field loss, although it has been reported to occur in up to 20% of cases.[105] The mechanism of this field defect is not fully understood, although it may relate to a segregation within the optic nerve head of axons from either side of the vertical midline.[105] The defect more often appears on the nasal side of the vertical midline. However, studies of normal subjects have also revealed greater sensitivity temporal to the hemianopic border, and it has been suggested that a small peripheral step at the

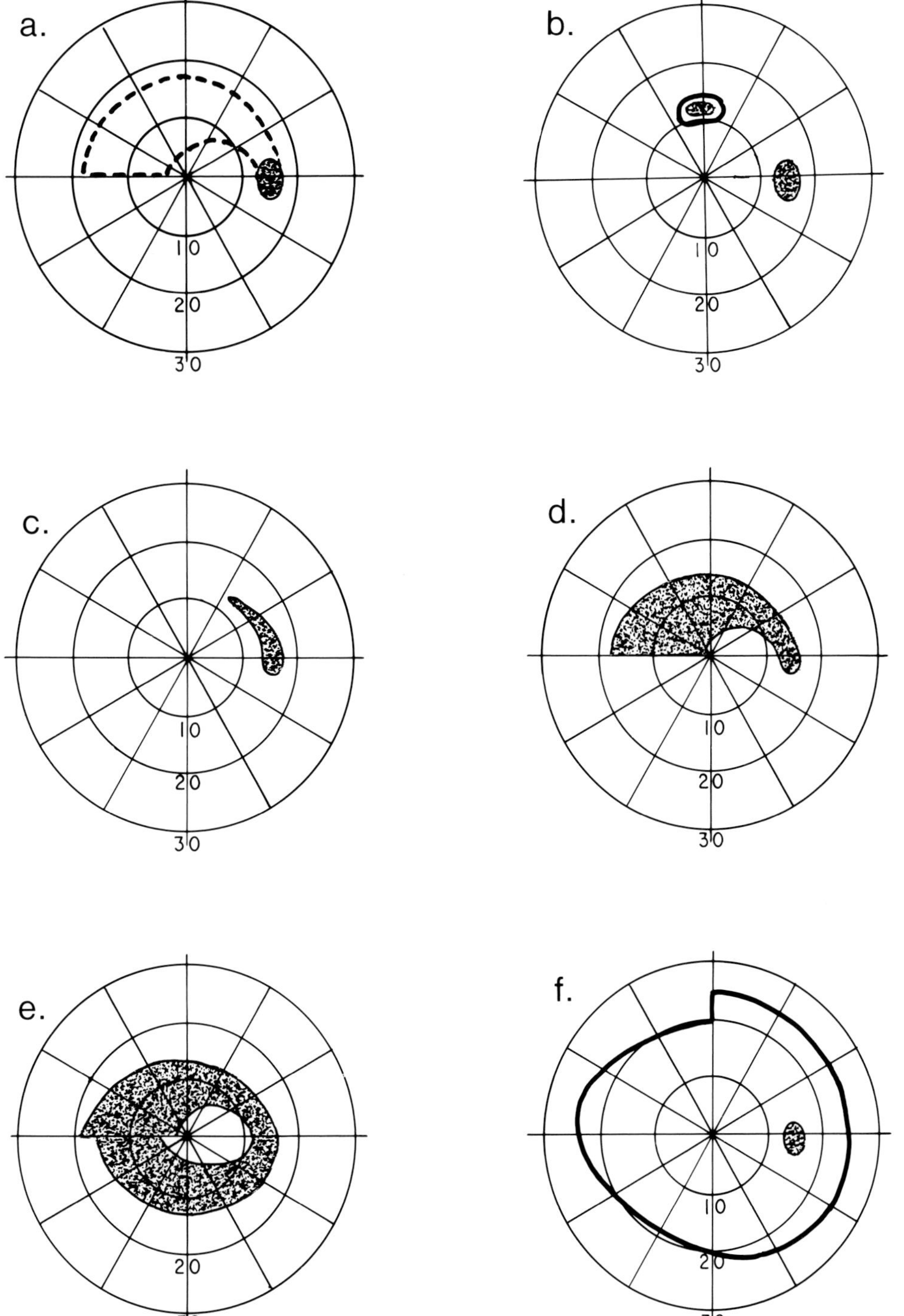

Figure 6.3. Arcuate nerve fiber bundle defects. **a,** The arcuate (or Bjerrum) area is shown within the dotted lines. **b,** Superior paracentral scotoma, with central absolute defect surrounded by a relative scotoma. **c,** Seidel scotoma. **d,** Complete arcuate (Bjerrum) scotoma. **e,** Double arcuate (ring) scotoma with superior central nasal step. **f,** Vertical step (or hemianopic offset).

Table 6.1.
Differential Diagnosis of Arcuate Scotomas[a]

A. Chorioretinal lesions
  1. Juxtapapillary choroiditis and retinochoroiditis
  2. Myopia with peripapillary atrophy
  3. Retinal pigment epithelium and photoreceptor degeneration
  4. Retinal artery occlusions
B. Optic nerve head lesions
  1. Drusen
  2. Retinal artery plaques
  3. Chronic papilledema
  4. Papillitis
  5. Colobomas (including optic nerve pit)
C. Anterior optic nerve lesions
  1. Carotid and ophthalmic artery occlusion
  2. Ischemic infarct
  3. Cerebral arteritis
  4. Retrobulbar neuritis
  5. Electric shock
  6. Exophthalmos
D. Posterior lesions of the visual pathway
  1. Pituitary adenoma
  2. Opticochiasmatic arachnoiditis
  3. Meningiomas of the dorsum sella or optic foramen
  4. Progressive external ophthalmoplegia
  5. Pseudotumor cerebri

[a] Modified from Harrington.[102]

vertical midline should arouse suspicion of glaucoma only if the defect is located temporally.[106,107] In addition, the presence of a hemianopic field defect should always arouse suspicion of a neurologic lesion, especially when the disc and field changes do not appear to correspond.

Temporal Sector Defect

Since the retinal nerve fibers nasal to the optic nerve head converge on the disc by a direct route, a lesion involving these fiber bundles produces a sector defect temporal to the blind spot.[99,100] This defect usually appears later in the course of glaucomatous field loss.[108]

The Value of Peripheral Field Testing

Defects along the peripheral boundaries of the visual field, as described above (i.e., peripheral nasal steps, vertical steps, and temporal sector defects), are most often found in association with scotomas in the arcuate area, although in some patients with early glaucomatous visual field loss, they may be the only detectable abnormality.[103,104,109,110] With automated static perimetry (discussed later in this chapter), it has become common practice to measure only the central 24–30° of the visual field, because of the increased time requirement with this technique. The question arises, therefore, as to how much information is being missed by ignoring the more peripheral portions of the field. In the presence of paracentral scotomas, peripheral isopters do not appear to add significant information regarding the progression of visual field damage.[111] In the initial diagnosis, however, a peripheral field defect, usually a nasal step, may be the only abnormality detected by automated perimetry in 3–11% of patients, depending on the testing method.[112–115] To be clinically useful, the time required to obtain this information must not add excessively to the overall testing time, and further study is needed to determine whether this can be achieved with newer programs for automated perimetry.

Advanced Glaucomatous Field Defects

The natural history of progressive glaucomatous field loss is eventual development of complete double arcuate scotomas with extension to the peripheral limits in all areas except those located temporally. This results in a *central island* and a *temporal island* of vision in advanced glaucoma. With continued damage, these islands of vision progressively diminish in size until the tiny central island is totally extinguished, which may occur abruptly. Glaucoma surgery appears to accelerate the loss of the small central island in some patients, possibly because of the sudden change in IOP, although the frequency with which this surgical complication occurs is not large enough to constitute a contraindication to surgery in these patients.[116] The temporal island of vision is more resistant and may persist long after central vision is lost. However, it, too, will eventually be destroyed if the IOP is not controlled, leaving the patient with no light perception.

Visual Field Changes in Low-Tension Glaucoma

The nature of visual field defects may be influenced by the level of the IOP, although the reports are somewhat conflicting. One study of open-angle glaucoma patients with early visual field loss showed that those with diffuse depression had higher pressures than those with localized defects.[117] In addition, open-angle glaucoma patients whose IOP has never exceeded approximately 21 mm Hg, commonly referred to as low-tension glaucoma, have been found in some studies to have scotomas with steeper slopes, greater depth, and closer proximity to fixation than did chronic glaucoma patients with higher IOP.[118,119] Others, however, found no significant difference between these two groups when the same degree of optic nerve damage was present.[120,121]

Visual Field Changes with Acute Pressure Elevation

The preceding discussions have dealt with field changes that are associated primarily with chronic forms of glaucoma. When the IOP elevation is sudden and marked, as in acute angle-closure glaucoma, a variety of associated field changes has been reported, including general depression, early loss of central vision, arcuate scotomata, and enlargement of the blind spot.[122] After the acute attack is brought under control, the fields will return to normal in some patients, while others may have reduced color vision, generalized decreased sensitivity, or constriction of isopters, especially superiorly.[123]

When the IOP is elevated artificially, either by compression of the globe[124–126] or administration of topical steroids,[127–130] typical glaucomatous field defects[124–129] or constriction of central isopters[130] occur in some eyes. The changes are reversible when the IOP returns to normal.[128,129] This response to artificial pressure elevation is said to occur more commonly in glaucoma patients,[124,125] especially those with low-tension glaucoma,[122] although one study found no significant difference between glaucoma and nonglaucoma patients.[126]

Reversibility of Glaucomatous Field Defects

Although visual field loss from glaucoma has traditionally been considered irreversible, it has been reported that both central visual acuity and the field of vision may improve if the IOP is reduced in the early stages of the disease.[131–134] Other investigators, however, were unable to demonstrate reversibility following pressure reduction achieved by argon laser trabeculoplasty.[135,136] These conflicting findings may indicate that a critical level of pressure reduction and/or intervention at a critical time in the disease process is needed to achieve reversal of field loss.

Correlation Between Optic Nerve Head and Visual Field Defects

In most patients with glaucoma, clinically recognizable disc changes precede detectable field loss,[137] and the presence or absence of glaucomatous field defects can usually, but not always, be predicted from the appearance of the optic nerve head.[137–142] Quigley and co-workers[143] correlated axon loss in the optic nerve head with visual field defects and not only confirmed that nerve fiber loss occurs prior to reproducible field defects in some patients with elevated IOP, but that the extent of axonal loss is usually much greater than the corresponding visual field change. With standard manual perimetric techniques, up to 35% of the fibers may be gone in an eye with a normal field while more than half the fibers may be lost by the time reproducible early field defects are found, and 10% or fewer axons may remain by the stage of severe field loss. When correlating retinal ganglion cell atrophy with automated perimetry in glaucoma patients, a 20% loss of cells, especially large ganglion cells, in the central 30° of the retina correlated with a 5-dB sensitivity loss (discussed later in this chapter), a 40% loss corresponded with a 10-dB decrease, and some ganglion cells remained in areas with 0-dB sensitivity.[144]

The nature of optic nerve head cupping can also be used to predict the type (in addition to the presence) of field loss. Extensive or focal absence of neural rim tissue, especially at the inferior or superior poles, is the most reliable indicator of visual field disturbance[138,145–147] and is usually associated with a field defect in the corresponding arcuate area. In some cases, field loss may occur before the pallor reaches the disc margin,[145] and unusual cases have been reported with field damage despite round, symmetric cups.[138]

The ability to predict impending glaucomatous visual field loss by the appearance of the optic nerve head is less accurate than correlating disc damage with established field loss. No single parameter or combination of parameters in glaucomatous optic atrophy has been found to be totally satisfactory for this purpose. The parameters that correlate best with visual field loss are magnification-corrected measurements of neuroretinal rim area[148–151] and defects in the retinal nerve fiber layer.[152–156] Diffuse structural changes in the optic nerve head or retinal nerve fiber layer are more often associated with diffuse depression of visual function, while localized changes correlate more with localized visual field changes.[155] In some cases, the early field loss associated with retinal nerve fiber layer defects can be detected with automatic perimetry when it has been missed with manual perimetry.[157,158]

The correlation between optic nerve head and visual field defects in glaucoma is close enough to prompt a search for other underlying disease processes, such as neurologic disorders, if a correlation is not found. Nevertheless, the absence of a perfect correlation indicates that both disc and field examinations are essential in managing the glaucoma patient.[159] In general, optic nerve head and retinal nerve fiber layer changes have their greatest value in the early stages of glaucoma, while progressive visual field loss becomes the more useful guide to therapy in advanced cases.[137,160]

TECHNIQUES AND INSTRUMENTS FOR MEASURING THE FIELD OF VISION

Basic Principles

Just as a cartographer maps the boundaries and topography of an island, so the perimetrist can measure both the peripheral limits of a visual field and the relative visual acuity of areas within those limits. This may be accomplished by using kinetic and/or static techniques with instruments that are either manually operated or computer assisted (automatic).

Kinetic Techniques

This method involves moving the test object from a nonseeing to a seeing area and recording the point at which it is first seen in relation to fixation (Fig. 6.4*A*). The procedure documents the boundaries of the visual field, for both the absolute limits as well as areas of relative differences in visual acuity within the field (Fig. 6.5). As previously noted, the boundaries, or contour lines, are called *isopters*. The size and shape of a particular isopter depends, in part, on the stimulus value of the corresponding test object.

Static Techniques

This approach involves the presentation of stationary test objects using either suprathreshold or threshold presentations. *Suprathreshold static presentation* is an "on-off" technique in which a test object that is just above the anticipated threshold for the

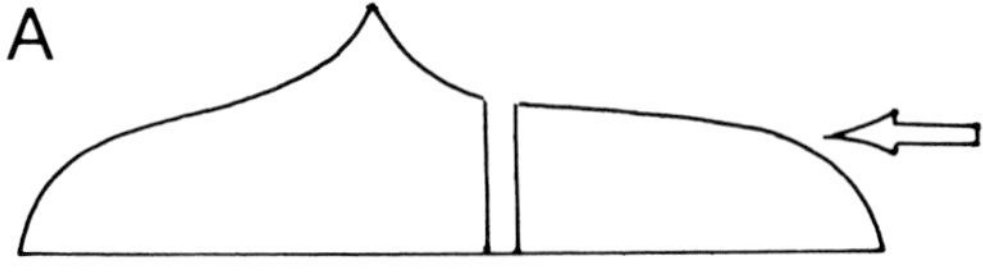

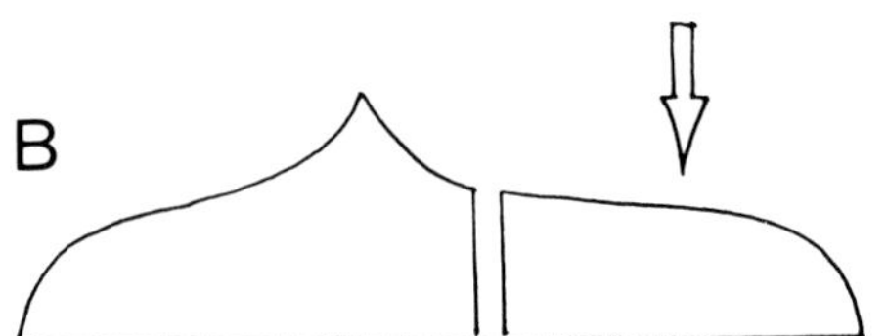

Figure 6.4. Standard techniques for measuring the visual field. In kinetic technique (**A**), test object moves from nonseeing to seeing area. Static technique (**B**) measures sensitivity of retina at a given point.

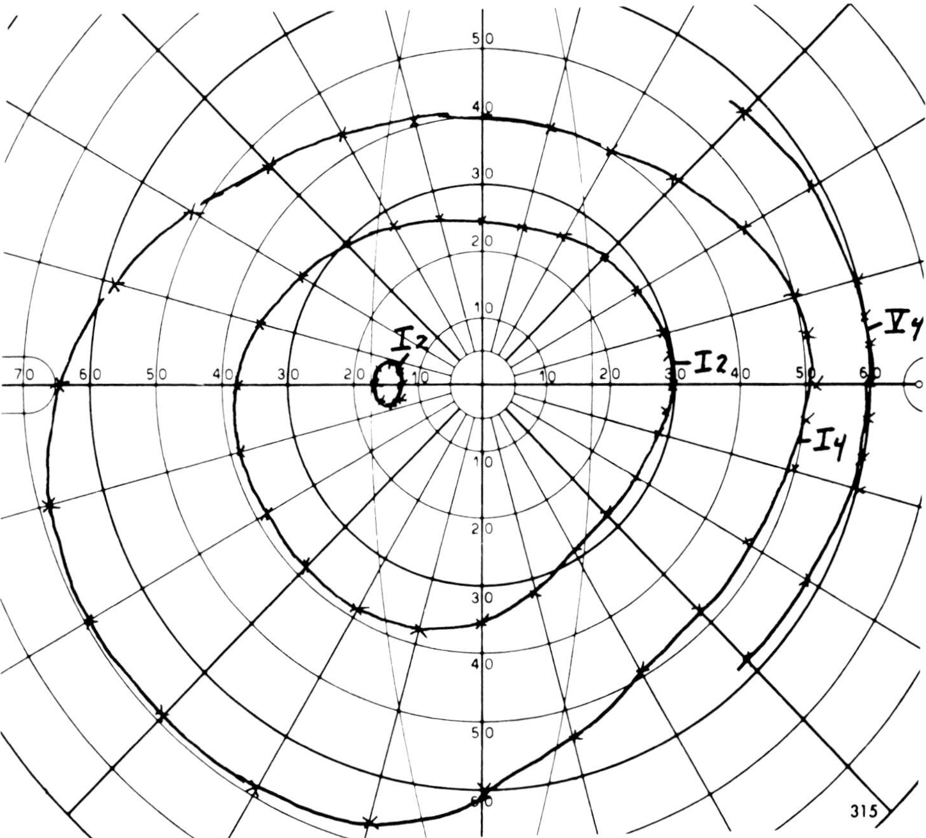

Figure 6.5. Example of manual kinetic perimetry, showing two complete isopters (I_2 and I_4) and third partial isopter (V_4) in nasal periphery, with blind spot measured by I_2 target.

corresponding portion of the visual field is presented momentarily, and the points at which the patient fails to recognize the target are noted. It is a way of "spot checking" for areas of relative or absolute blindness, usually within the central visual field. *Threshold static (profile) perimetry* measures the relative intensity thresholds for the visual acuity of individual retinal points within the field of vision. The technique involves gradually increasing the target light from subthreshold intensity and recording the level at which the patient first indicates recognition of the target (Fig. 6.4*B*), or decreasing it from a suprathreshold level and recording the lowest stimulus value seen. The points tested can be along one meridian, either radiating from fixation or along a circular line around a fixed point from fixation, and displayed on a flat abscissa or a circular chart (Fig. 6.6).[2] The more common technique with automated perimetry, however, is to test retinal points distributed throughout a portion of the visual field and record the visual thresholds as symbols or numeric values (Fig. 6.7, *A* and *B*).

Threshold static perimetry has been shown to be more sensitive than kinetic perimetry in detecting glaucomatous field loss.[161] In one study of patients with open-angle glaucoma, a defect was found in one-third of the cases with static circular perimetry that was missed by kinetic perimetry.[162]

Test Objects

The standard target for both kinetic and static perimetry is a white disc, the stimulus value of which can be adjusted by varying the target size and/or luminosity relative to that of the background. In normal subjects,

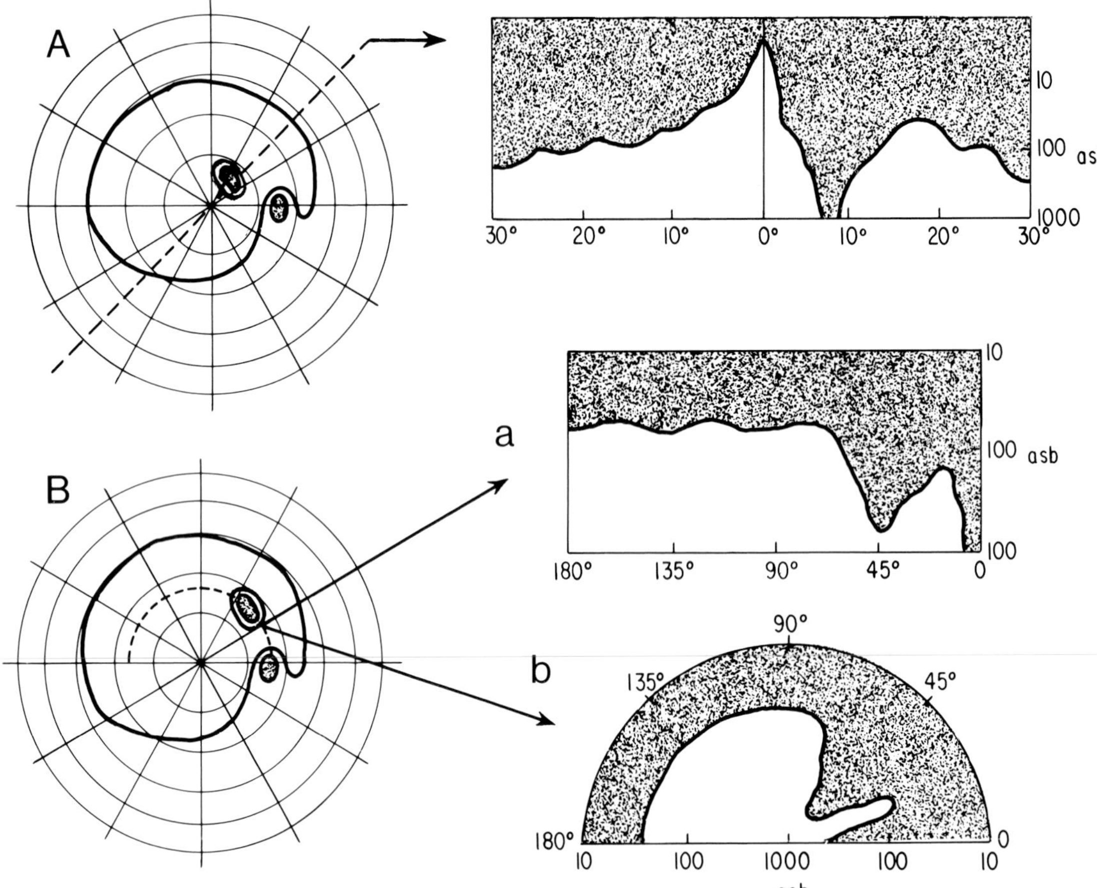

Figure 6.6. Threshold static (profile) perimetry. **A,** Meridian static perimetry. **B,** Circular static perimetry on flat abscissa (**a**) and circular chart (**b**). The dotted lines indicate the cuts through the fields that are being displayed in profile.

the mean retinal sensitivity has been shown to increase with the increasing size of the test object.[163] The following modifications in the test object have also been evaluated in an effort to increase the sensitivity of the testing procedure.

Color stimuli, as compared with white targets, may influence the visual field results in one of two ways. With targets that reflect light, as used with tangent screen testing, color targets have less luminance and a lower stimulus value than white. More significantly, if the luminance is kept constant and the color saturation is varied, the stimulus value might be more sensitive to specific color vision defects, as in some patients with glaucoma.[164] Some studies have suggested that such a technique can reveal field defects that are larger than those obtained with conventional luminance perimetry,[165,166] although others have found color targets to be no more sensitive than white ones in detecting glaucomatous defects.[167–169] One study suggested that a blue target on a yellow background might be more sensitive for detection of incipient glaucomatous damage, but not for manifest field loss.[166]

Another modification of test objects, as previously mentioned, has been the use of *contrast sensitivity,* such as sinewave gratings of low spatial frequency and laser interference fringes, in an effort to increase sensitivity to peripheral defects.[49–51] Different target *shapes and patterns,* which the patient must distinguish, are also reported to

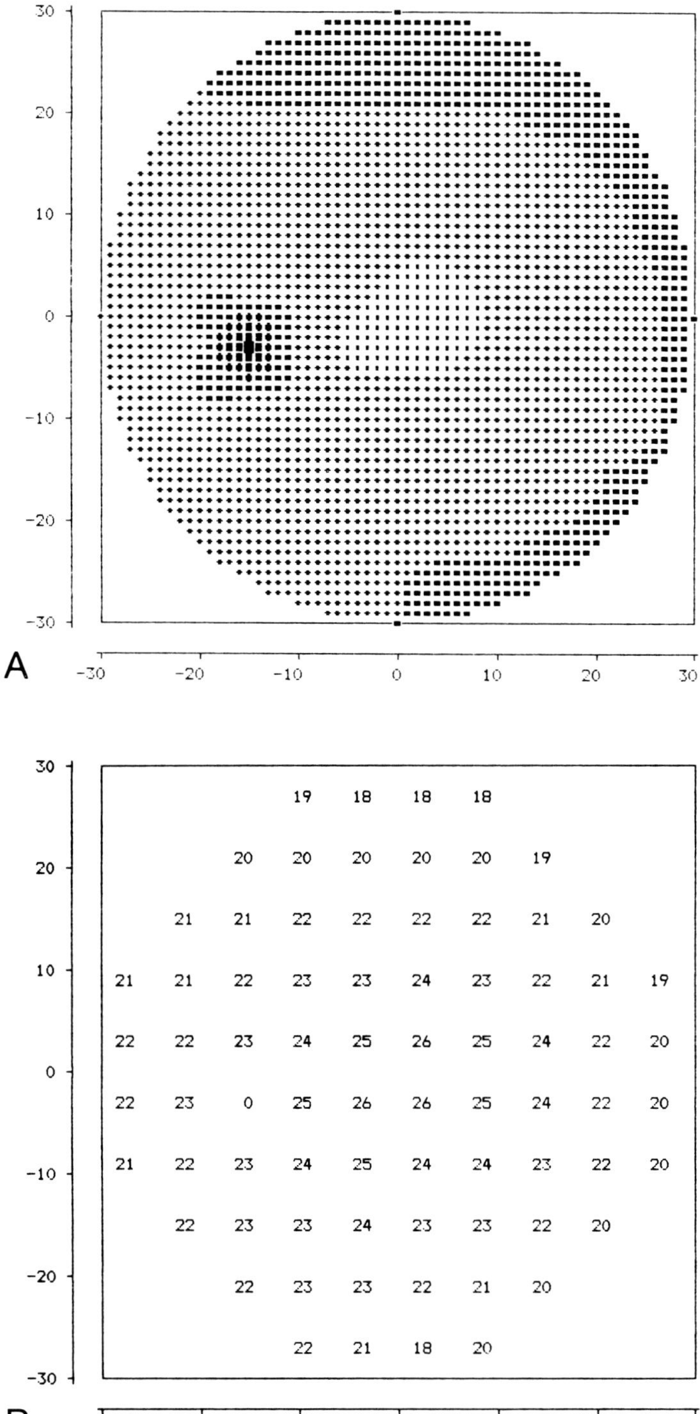

Figure 6.7. Examples of threshold static (computer assisted) perimetry. Retinal sensitivity is measured at points throughout a portion of the visual field (central 30° in this example). Results can be displayed with symbols (**A**) and/or in numerical values (**B**).

be of particular value in detecting optic nerve disease.[170,171] All of these target modifications, however, are still under investigation, and the standard at the present time remains the white stimulus of varying size and luminosity.

Presentation of Test Object

To minimize the patient's anticipation of when or where the next test object will appear, the presentation should be random, rather than following a predictable pattern, and the time between stimuli should be varied slightly. To avoid patient anxiety when testing in a nonseeing area, the examination should return periodically to a previously seen area. For kinetic targets, a stimulus velocity of 4°/sec appears to be optimal for all targets in the central and peripheral visual field.[172] The test object should always be moved from a nonseeing to a seeing area (i.e., from the periphery toward fixation) when outlining an isopter and from the center of the blind spot or a scotoma. Suprathreshold static targets should be presented for a consistent duration of time, usually ½ to 1 second, and test objects should be just above threshold for the area being tested.

Background Illumination

Background illumination for manual perimetric techniques has traditionally been mesopic to stimulate both rods and cones. The adapting field luminances currently used in static and kinetic perimetry range from photopic to mesopic (4 to 31.5 apostilbs), although the optimum luminance has yet to be established. One study suggested that the lower levels of background illumination may allow minor reductions in light transmission by the ocular media to produce significant changes in the recorded threshold sensitivity.[173] In a comparison of scotopic and photopic fields, localized scotomas in glaucoma patients were of equal depth, but diffuse scotopic defects significantly exceeded the photopic, suggesting that not all ganglion cell types are equally susceptible to glaucomatous damage.[174]

With bowl perimeters, photometric adjustment should be made with the patient in place, since facial coloring affects luminosity. The most important principle regarding illumination is to keep both target and background constant and reproducible from one examination to the next.

Physiologic Factors That Influence Visual Fields

The following factors should be compensated for, if possible, or otherwise should be considered when interpreting the fields.

Clarity of Ocular Media. *Cataracts,* especially if associated with miosis, can cause or exaggerate central or peripheral field defects, which could be mistaken for the development or progression of glaucomatous field loss. Even minimal light scattering, as may be caused by an early cataract that has a relatively insignificant effect on visual acuity, may influence threshold measurements.[175] As previously noted, this effect may be greater with lower levels of background illumination.[173] In a study of 90 eyes with open-angle glaucoma and cataracts, 41% had reversal of a partial or complete scotoma after cataract extraction.[176] Nuclear cataracts depress central perimetric sensitivity more than peripheral with both large and small targets, while nonnuclear cataracts influence central sensitivity more for small targets and peripheral sensitivity for large targets.[177] Attempts have been made to correlate visual field damage with lens opacity[178] and visual acuity[179] to aid clinicians in determining the significance of field change in patients with glaucoma and cataracts. Reduced clarity of the ocular media from other causes, such as a corneal disturbance, a cloudy posterior lens capsule after cataract surgery, or vitreous opacities, may also affect the visual fields. Applanation tonometry prior to automated static threshold perimetry was found in one study to have no detrimental effect on the visual field results.[180]

Pupil Size. *Miosis* alone may depress central and peripheral threshold sensitivities and exaggerate field defects,[181] even after correction of induced myopia.[182] One study used neutral density filters to reduce the retinal illumination the equivalent of halving the pupillary diameter, which reduced the mean threshold with two automated perimeters by 1.1–1.7 dB.[183] For this reason, the pupil size should be recorded with each field, and the influence of miosis should be considered when a field change is detected. Mydriasis has less influence on the visual field, although pupillary dilation with tropicamide 1% in healthy subjects on no ocular medication was shown in one study to significantly reduce threshold sensitivity with automated perimetry.[184]

Refractive Errors. Refractive errors primarily influence the central field. Myopia does not require correction when using a 300 mm perimeter, unless the refractive error exceeds 3 diopters. Posterior staphylomas can create areas of relative myopia, called *refraction scotomas,* that may be confused with glaucomatous field defects, but they can usually be eliminated with an appropriate refractive correction. *Hyperopia* has a greater influence on perimetric results, especially for the central field, and even small refractive errors can significantly alter threshold sensitivity.[185–187] Age tables are available to aid in determining the appropriate correction for presbyopia. A contact lens provides the best correction for the aphakic eye, although spectacle correction can be used for the central 25–30° with no correction for the peripheral field. Astigmatism should be corrected unless the cylinder is less than 1 diopter, in which case it can be included as the spherical equivalent.

Age. Increasing age is also associated with a reduction in retinal threshold sensitivity. This effect starts as early as 20 years of age, progresses linearly throughout life, and involves the peripheral and superior areas more than the pericentric and inferior portions of the field.[184,189] This age-related visual field sensitivity appears to be primarily due to neural loss rather than preretinal factors.[190]

Psychologic Factors That Influence Visual Fields

The patient's understanding of the test and his or her alertness, concentration, fixation, and cooperation all influence the results of visual field testing.[191] A learning effect with automated perimetry may influence the results of a patient's first or second field, suggesting that an initial field that does not agree with the clinical findings should be repeated.[192–194] Another study found that moderate alcohol ingestion did not influence differential light sensitivity as tested by automated perimetry.[195] With manual perimetry, the skill of the perimetrist will, of course, significantly influence the visual field results.[196]

Manual Perimetry

Tangent Screens

The tangent screen is a flat square of black felt or flannel with a central white fixation target on which 30° of the visual field can be studied. The test should be performed in mesopic lighting of approximately 7 footcandles with the patient seated either 1 or 2 meters from the screen. Both kinetic and suprathreshold static techniques can be used with the tangent screen. With the kinetic approach, the examiner moves a test object from the periphery toward fixation until the patient indicates recognition of the target. The procedure is repeated at various intervals around fixation until the isopter has been mapped. The stimulus value of the test objects can be changed by varying the size and/or color. The corresponding isopter is designated by the ratio of target diameter to the distance between patient and target, with both expressed in millimeters, e.g., "2/1000 white" for a 2 mm white test object at 1 meter (when the color is not indicated it is understood to be white).

Suprathreshold static perimetry can be performed by turning the disc-shaped test object from the black to the white side or by using a self-illuminating target with an on-off switch. Specific locations at which the patient fails to see the target are then evaluated further with kinetic techniques.

The tangent screen has the advantages of low cost and simplicity of operation. However, reproducibility of the fields, which is essential in managing patients with glaucoma, is limited by variations in background lighting and stimulus value of the targets and by difficulty in monitoring fixation. Furthermore, it does not include the peripheral field, where early glaucomatous defects may appear.

Arc and Bowl Perimeters

With these instruments, both the central and peripheral fields of vision can be exam-

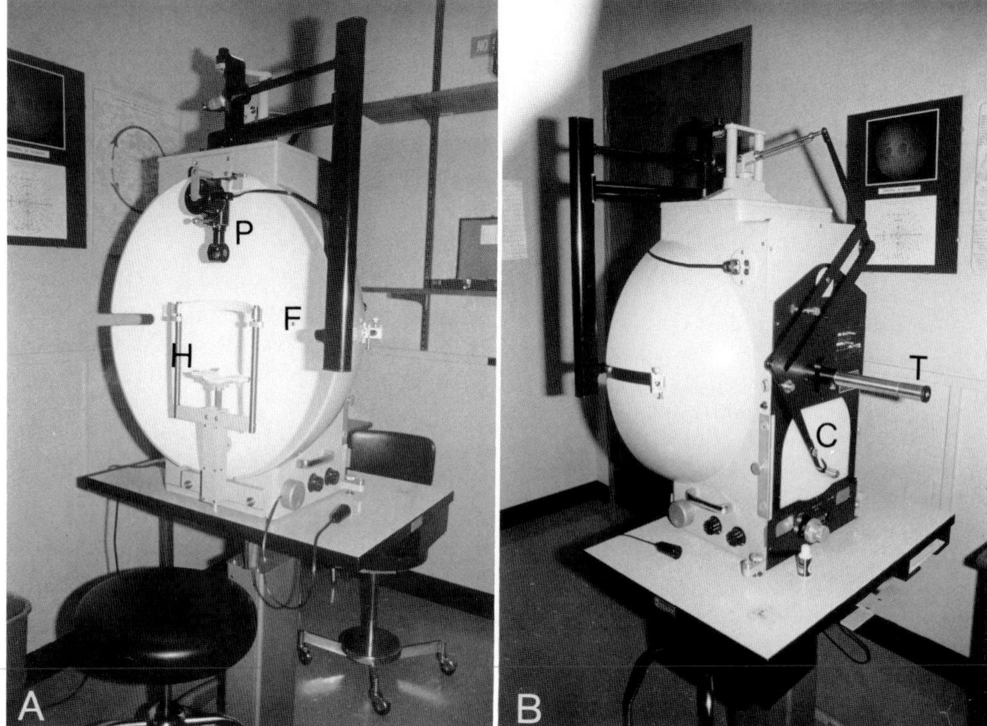

Figure 6.8. Goldmann manual perimeter: **A,** Patient's side, showing headrest (*H*), fixation target (*F*), and projection device for test objects (*P*). **B,** Operator's side, showing telescope for fixation monitoring (*T*) and visual field chart (*C*) for locating and recording position of test objects.

ined. The screen of the perimeter may be either a curved ribbon of metal (arc perimeter), or bowl-shaped. The latter is preferable for glaucoma examinations, and the prototype is the *Goldmann perimeter* (Fig. 6.8).[197] Other similar instruments have been compared with the Goldmann unit, with variable results.[198] The bowl of the Goldmann perimeter has a radius of 300 mm and extends 95° to each side of fixation. The target is projected onto the bowl, and the stimulus value of the test object can be varied in several ways: by changing the (1) size, (2) intensity, or (3) light transmission. The latter variable merely provides finer intensity adjustment for the stimulus. Arbitrary designations for each value variable are usually printed on the visual field chart, with 0-V for size, 1–4 for intensity, and a–e for transmission. An isopter, therefore, might be designated as "I2e," which indicates a test object size of ¼ mm², an intensity of 10 millilamberts, and 100% transmission of the light source. The patient's fixation can be monitored by the examiner through a telescope in the center of the bowl.

The Goldmann perimeter can be used for both kinetic and static visual field testing. Other perimeters have been designed exclusively for the measurement of static threshold (profile) fields. The prototype instrument in the latter group is the *Tübingen perimeter,* which consists of a bowl-type screen and stationary test objects with variable light intensity.[199]

Specific Techniques for Manual Perimetry

Within the context of glaucoma detection and management, visual field testing has two basic aspects: (1) screening techniques to detect the presence of glaucomatous field loss, and (2) in-depth techniques to determine more accurately the extent of the damage and to follow the fields for evidence of progressive change.

Screening Techniques. Armaly[200] developed a method of visual field screening for glaucoma that was modified by Drance and associates,[201–203] and it is commonly referred to as *selective perimetry* or the Armaly-Drance technique. The basic concept is to test those areas in the visual field that have the highest probability of showing glaucomatous defects. The technique uses a Goldmann-type perimeter with suprathreshold static perimetry to test for central field defects and both suprathreshold static and kinetic perimetry to examine the peripheral field, with emphasis on the nasal and temporal periphery (Fig. 6.9). An evaluation of the technique in 106 normal individuals and 49 with glaucomatous defects revealed a high sensitivity and specificity,

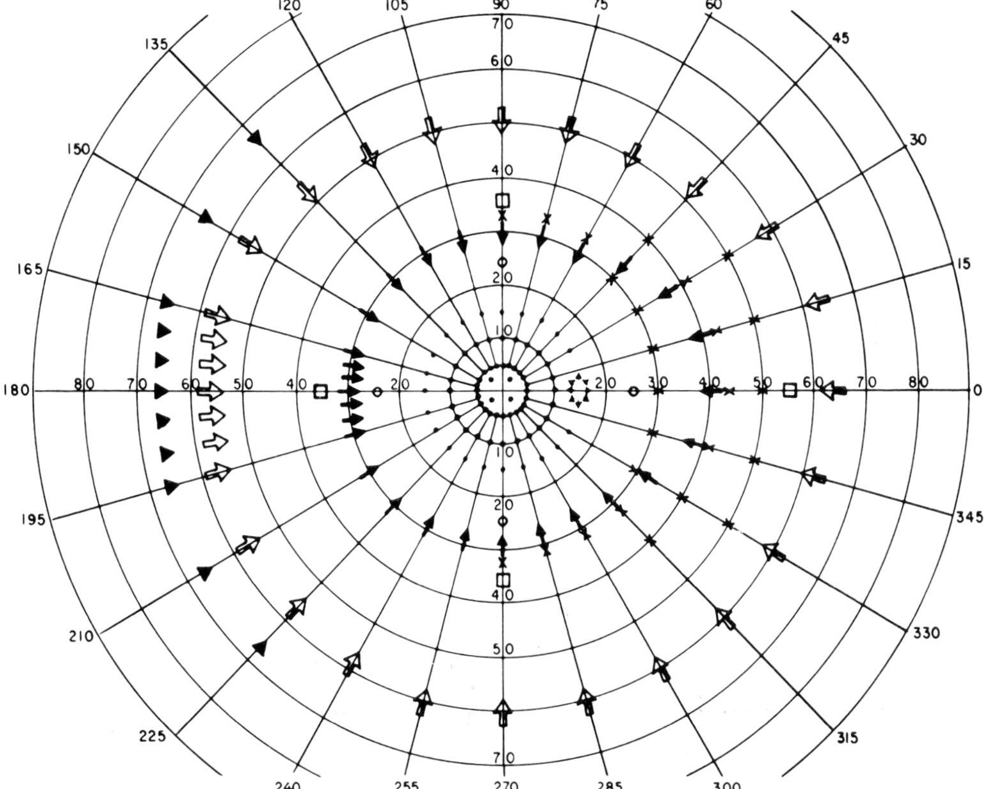

Figure 6.9. Screening technique with Goldmann-type perimeter (modification of Armaly-Drance selective perimetry). (1) The central threshold target is determined as the smallest diameter and lowest intensity that can be visualized at any of the four threshold sites (*open circles*). (2) The central threshold target is presented by static technique in each quadrant 5° from fixation (*solid circles*) to familiarize the patient with the testing procedure. (3) The blind spot is outlined with kinetic checks of the central threshold target at eight cardinal points (*small arrowheads*). (4) Isopter boundaries of the central threshold target are plotted every 5° for 15° above and below the nasal horizontal meridian and every 15° along the rest of the circumference (*solid arrows*). (5) Spots are checked with the central threshold target along points 5, 10, and 15° from fixation (*solid circles*). (6) The peripheral threshold target is determined at threshold site (*open squares*). (7) Isopter boundaries of the peripheral threshold target are determined as in step 4 (*open arrows*). (8) Spots are checked with the peripheral threshold target in the temporal periphery (*X*). (9) The nasal peripheral isopter is plotted with the 4e target 45° above and below the horizontal meridian (*large arrowheads*). A refractive correction is used with central threshold target but not with the peripheral threshold or V_4e targets. (Reprinted with permission from de Oliveira-Rassi M, Shields MB: Am J Ophthal 94:4, 1982.)

which made it suitable for clinical and survey screening.[201,203] An additional modification is to use the V4e isopter nasally to rule out crowding of the peripheral nasal isopters.[17] Another technique for use with Goldmann-type perimeters uses three suprathreshold targets within three concentric zones from fixation in accordance with the normal physiologic sensitivity gradient.[204] Other investigators have developed protocols to significantly reduce the number of test points without sacrificing sensitivity or specificity by concentrating the testing in those portions of the field where a defect is most likely to be found.[205,206]

In-Depth Techniques. When a glaucomatous field defect is suspected by use of a screening technique, the physician has two choices. The patient can be asked to return another day either for a repeat screening field or an in-depth study. In many cases, however, it is more practical to proceed with the in-depth test at the time the defect is detected. The conversion from a screening to an in-depth field study is facilitated with the Armaly-Drance technique, since both are performed on a Goldmann-type perimeter with identical or similar target settings. The principle of in-depth field testing is to map out the size and shape of all scotomas as well as complete isopters, using both the central threshold target and two or more additional targets of greater stimulus value (Fig. 6.10). Profile static perimetry is also of value in studying areas of known loss for the depth and shape of the scotoma and for subtle evidence of progressive damage in serial fields.

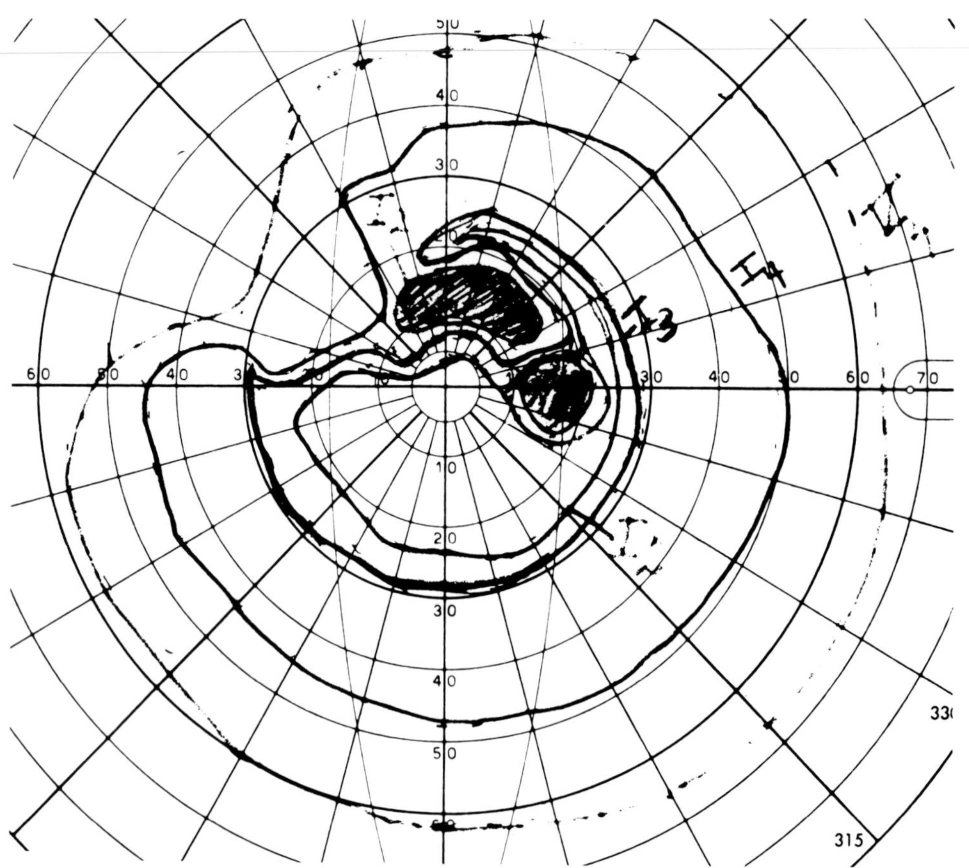

Figure 6.10. In-depth technique with Goldmann-type perimeter in which a superior arcuate scotoma and nasal step have been plotted with four targets (I_2, I_3, I_4, and V_4).

Recording and Scoring Manual Visual Field Data

The complex nature of visual field data makes it difficult to reduce the information to simple descriptions or numbers. Therefore, storage of the data in raw form (i.e., as transferred directly from the testing screen) is usually the most practical means of record keeping. However, methods for conversion of visual fields from kinetic and static perimeter charts to computer use, for area calculations, graphic display, and storage in the patient's data base, have been described.[207,208] When it is necessary to estimate the percent of functional visual field loss, a system is available (the Esterman grids), in which the field is divided into 100 blocks of varying size according to functional value, with each representing 1%.[209–211] The system has been adopted by the AMA as a standard for rating visual field disability.[212] Grids are available for scoring the tangent screen,[209] perimeter,[210] or the binocular field.[211] In patients with severe visual loss from glaucoma, the binocular Esterman score of data generated by an automated perimeter correlated well with combined monocular visual field results.[213]

Automated Perimetry

Why Automation?

The introduction of automation represents the latest step in the historic evolution of visual field technology. The first era of perimetry, which began in the mid-19th century with the work of von Graefe, was characterized by tangent screens and arc perimeters. A major limitation of these instruments was lack of standardization of the test objects and the background as well as patient fixation. These needs were addressed in the era of standardization, which began in the middle of this century with the contributions of Goldmann. The main problem that remained, however, was the subjectivity of both the patient and perimetrist. While the former limitation is one with which we must continue to cope, the influence of the perimetrist has been eliminated to variable degrees with the advent of the era of automation, which began in the 1970s.

By reducing the influence of the perimetrist, automated perimetry improves the uniformity and reproducibility of visual fields. In addition, the use of computers has provided new capabilities that are not possible with manual perimetry, including random presentation of targets, estimations of patient reliability, and statistical evaluation of data at many levels. It must be noted, however, that while automated perimetry is more accurate and informative, it is neither faster nor cheaper than manual perimetry.

Classification of Automated Perimeters[214]

Semiautomatic Perimeters. With these instruments, the perimetrist is still involved in a portion of the actual field testing, such as presenting the stimuli, making decisions, and recording data. These instruments are used primarily as *rapid screening devices* to aid in the detection of glaucoma.

The *Harrington-Flocks screener* uses the flash presentation of multiple dot patterns, and the patient is asked to indicate the number of dots seen.[215] The device was found to be reliable in a study of 1500 screening tests.[216] The *Friedmann visual field analyzer* is a similar instrument, which involves the static presentation of single or multiple test objects that can be varied in intensity.[217,218] Studies have also demonstrated the reliability of this device for mass screening programs.[219] It was found to be at least as sensitive as careful manual perimetry with the Goldmann perimeter in detecting early glaucomatous visual field defects,[220] and may even be of value in following the progression of glaucomatous damage, although it is limited by the fact that it only measures the central 25°.[221] It is also limited by the fact that normal subjects often miss stimuli in the extreme superior periphery and arcuate regions,[222] although it may be possible to overcome this by comparing each field response score with scores from normal and abnormal populations.[223]

More recently, *television* has been used for mass screening of visual fields by employing a modification of the Harrington-Flocks multiple dot pattern technique.[224] A television screen, personal computer, and thermal printer have also been used to develop a low-cost automated field analyzer.[225] The value of these methods has yet to be established.

Fully Automatic Perimeters. With these instruments, the perimetrist is replaced by a computer and has no influence on the visual field results, aside from the important aspects of ensuring that the patient understands the testing procedure, is comfortably positioned at the perimeter, and complies with the requirements of the test. The remainder of this chapter deals with this class of computerized perimeters.

Instrumentation

Since the introduction of computerized perimeters in the 1970s, a wide variety of models has been designed. Many of these are no longer commercially available, while most of the others represent modifications of the originals.

Automated perimeters have two main components: the perimetric unit and the control unit. The perimetric unit in most systems uses a bowl-type screen, similar to that of the Goldmann manual perimeter.

Static Targets. Static targets are used in all cases, although additional kinetic targets have been evaluated in some units.[114,115] The targets may either be projected onto the bowl or illuminated from light-emitting diodes (LEDs) or fiberoptics in the perimetric bowl. The former has the advantage of unlimited presentation locations on the screen, while the latter two have fixed positions in the bowl. In addition, the LEDs are recessed in dark cavities, which may allow perception by the most sensitive retinal areas of a stimulus that is of lower intensity than the background light.[226,227] This "dark hole phenomenon" is associated with increased variability in retesting the threshold.[226,227] Projected targets also have the advantage of allowing for change in size to alter the stimulus values. In practice, the size is usually kept constant, although it has been shown that larger targets may permit the measurement of visual function in areas that had been considered absolute scotomas with standard-sized stimuli.[228] With all target systems, the patient is provided with a device to indicate when a target is seen, which is recorded by the computer.

Fixation. Patient fixation is monitored in a variety of ways depending on the sophistication of the instrument. Some use a telescope, similar to the Goldmann manual perimeter, while others allow the operator to observe the patient's eye on a television screen. Automatic fixation monitoring is also incorporated into most units, either by periodically retesting the patient's response in the previously determined blind spot or by monitoring a light reflex from the patient's cornea. With the latter, the computer can be programmed to stop the test whenever fixation is lost.

Control Unit. The control unit provides interaction between the operator and computer through a dialogue screen and either a keyboard or light pen. The computer within the control unit reads a program diskette or chip and controls and monitors instrumentation function according to that program, evaluates patient's response, and computes data. The control unit also contains a printer, which provides a hard copy of the data in symbols or numeric values. Computers in the more sophisticated units also store data and can perform statistical analyses of the data in relation to programmed normal data or against previous fields of the same patient.

Testing Strategies

All fully automated perimeters take advantage of computer capabilities by using *random presentation* of the static targets to avoid patient anticipation of the next presentation sites. In addition, an *adaptive technique* is employed, in which stimuli are presented according to the presumed normal retinal threshold contour (i.e., the relative *differential light thresholds* throughout the visual field) based on either age-corrected normal data or the patient's response to preliminary spot tests (Fig. 6.11). This approach, in comparison with the presentation of a constant stimulus value throughout a portion of the field, as with many manual techniques, improves the balance between sensitivity (the ability to detect defects) and specificity (the ability to detect normal areas). Fully automated perimeters differ at this point as to whether they are limited to

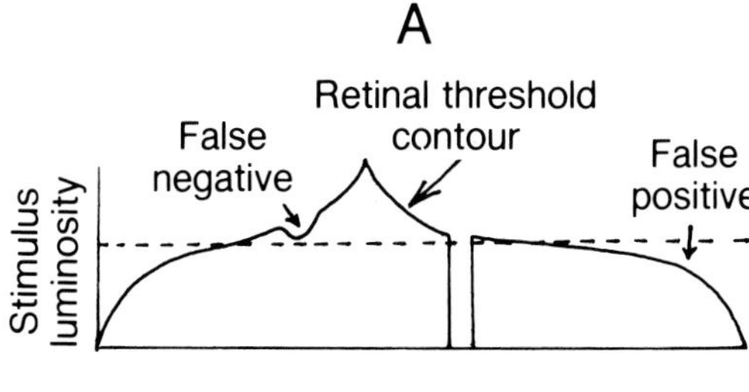

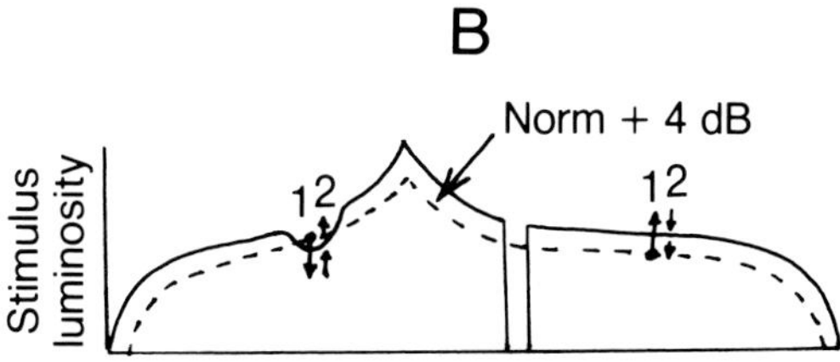

Figure 6.11. Adaptive strategy used in automated static perimetry. **A,** When a constant luminosity is presented throughout a portion of the visual field, true defects near fixation may be missed (*false negative*), while more peripheral normal areas may be read as abnormal (*false positive*). **B,** The adaptive strategy minimizes this by changing the stimulus value according to the retinal threshold contour. With full threshold programs, the retinal threshold is crossed by increasing or decreasing the stimulus value (*1*) and is then crossed a second time with smaller increments of change in luminosity (*2*).

suprathreshold measurements or are also capable of full thresholding.

Suprathreshold Static Perimeters. With these instruments, a stimulus is presented with a value that is slightly above the anticipated normal for the corresponding retinal location. Some instruments simply indicate whether or not the target was seen, while others will present a second, high-intensity target in nonseeing areas to distinguish between relative and absolute defects. In either case, however, these instruments are limited to screening functions, since they do not provide sufficient information about the depth or contour of a field defect to be used either as a baseline study or for following the patient during therapy. With the continued advances in automated perimetry, these instruments are becoming largely replaced by full threshold static perimeters.

Threshold Static Perimeters. These instruments are capable of a variety of testing strategies, in addition to suprathreshold screening. The most commonly used programs measure the retinal threshold at 70–80 points within the central 24–30°. A suprathreshold target is first presented, and the luminosity is then gradually increased or decreased until the patient's threshold is crossed (i.e., the target comes into or goes out of view, respectively). The threshold is then crossed a second time with smaller increments of changes in luminosity to refine the threshold determination. Many programs will continuously adjust subsequent stimulus values according to prior measurements (e.g., the level is increased when testing near a known scotoma on the basis of optimized algorithms). Special programs have been evaluated that automatically increase the density of test locations around defective areas, although the value of this approach has yet to be established.[229,230] Other programs are designed to reduce testing time either by adjusting the initial target values according to previous fields by the same patient or by thresholding only locations that are missed with the suprathreshold target. In one study that compared the latter techniques with a full-threshold program, the abbreviated strategy took only one-third as much time but provided a different diagnostic result in 18 of 104 eyes.[231]

Variability and Reliability. Several strategies are used to document variability and reliability of test results. With most full-thresholding programs, a percentage of random locations is retested to determine the reproducibility at those points (referred to as *short-term fluctuation* and expressed as the square root of the variance). It has also been shown that short-term fluctuation can be estimated from grids of single threshold determinations,[232] which can be used to shorten the testing time. The patient's general reliability is assessed with a series of *false positives* (responding when no target is presented) and *false negatives* (failing to respond where a stimulus was previously seen), as well as the frequency of *fixation losses* during the test. Several evaluations of a perimeter that monitors fixation by periodic checks of the blind spot (Humphrey Field Analyzer) revealed a high percentage of tests that were considered unreliable because patients exceeded the established criterion for fixation loss.[233–235]

Test Patterns. A broad menu of test patterns is available with most instruments. The most commonly used are limited to the central 24–30° with a 6° separation between test locations. The 6° grid will miss the physiologic blind, and presumably small glaucomatous defects, in a high percentage of cases, and it has been suggested that tighter grids should be used, especially in the central 10–28°.[236–238] Special programs are available to study smaller portions of the field with tighter grids. Programs are also available to study the peripheral field beyond 30° either in the nasal quadrant or for 360°. The peripheral studies can be performed alone or in conjunction with a central field program and usually have wider target separation. Static testing of the peripheral nasal field has been shown to provide valuable additional information in detecting glaucomatous defects.[239] Automated kinetic measurement of the peripheral field, especially nasally, was also found to provide useful information, in addition to that obtained from central testing, in many patients.[114,115]

Printout. The computer printout records the threshold for each retinal point tested, which theoretically is the target that is just bright enough to be seen 50% of the time at that location. The absolute luminous intensity is measured in *apostilbs* but is expressed in logarithmic units referred to as *decibels* (dB), which provides a more linear relationship between visual perception and a change in light intensity. A decibel is 0.1 log-unit, so that a 10-dB decrease represents a 10-fold stimulus increase, while a 20-dB decline represents a 100-fold stimulus increase. Log-units and decibels are relative and are not the same for all instruments. The printout may show the retinal threshold contour in decibels or in a grayscale or other symbols, with each symbol representing a decibel range (Fig. 6.12). The numeric printout may also show the difference between the test results and the age-corrected nor-

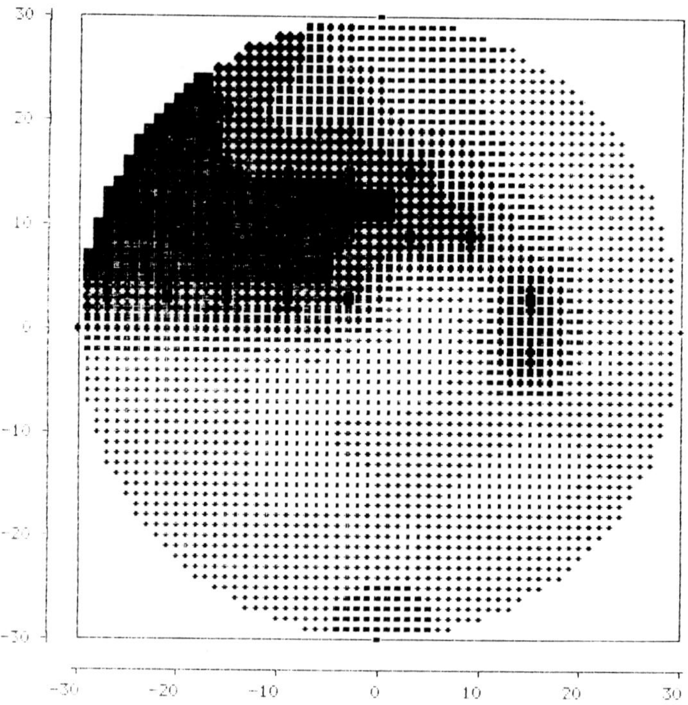

Figure 6.12. Computer printout of visual field measured by automated static technique showing superior arcuate scotoma and nasal step. (Same patient as in Fig. 6.10).

mal, and a graphic method has been devised to show the development of visual field defects by superimposing two to four grayscale printouts and displaying changing areas as stripes.[240]

Interpreting the Results

Computerized visual field printouts can be read by the clinician in much the same manner as with manual perimetric charts (i.e., looking primarily for nerve fiber layer defects such as paracentral and arcuate scotomas, and nasal steps). In addition, static threshold data can be analyzed mathematically, which may allow detection of more subtle visual field abnormalities. The statistical techniques used in this approach are referred to as *visual field indices*.

Indices. An average of all threshold values is called *mean sensitivity,* while the average difference between each threshold value and the age-corrected normal is referred to as *mean defect* (or mean deviation). These indices primarily reflect diffuse changes. One way to detect localized defects is to calculate the number of threshold values that deviate significantly from the age-corrected normal, which is called *loss variance* (or pattern standard deviation). *Corrected loss variance* (or corrected pattern standard deviation) takes into account the *short-term fluctuation,* as previously discussed. These indices for localized loss are insensitive to the location of the defects. For example, three abnormal locations could either be randomly distributed or clustered. Since the latter is clinically more significant, techniques were developed, referred to as *spatial correlation* (or cluster analysis), to detect clustered defects.[241] The clinical significance of a defect can be evaluated further with *probability maps,* which display the field results in terms of the frequency with which the measured findings are seen in a normal population.[242,243] It has also been shown that comparing sums of threshold values in corresponding areas of the superior and inferior hemispheres is useful in detecting glaucomatous field loss.[244,245]

Threshold Variability. There is a certain degree of short-term fluctuation in the retinal threshold sensitivity profile (or hill of vision) among normal individuals, especially in the midperiphery and superior quadrant.[246–248] In addition, each normal person will show some variation from test to test, which is referred to as *long-term fluctuation*.[248] Both of these normal variations must be taken into account when attempting to interpret the significance of visual field data. Furthermore, the likelihood of increased variability in glaucomatous visual fields must also be taken into consideration. Average total long-term fluctuation in clinically stable glaucoma patients is similar to that in normals.[249] However, long-term fluctuation can be considerable in field areas with moderate loss of sensitivity.[250] In addition, short-term fluctuation is increased around both physiologic[251] and glaucomatous[252] scotomas. Short-term and long-term fluctuations are greater among older patients,[253] and short-term fluctuation is often greatest in the patient's first automated field test, indicating the influence of experience.[254] In one study, a change in mean sensitivity of approximately 5–7 dB between two successive fields was needed to have 95% confidence that the trend would be confirmed by the third field.[255] The difference between right and left eyes of a patient may also be useful in detecting early glaucomatous visual field loss.[256,257]

Trend Analysis. Statistical models are available with some automated perimeters to help the clinician determine the significance of visual field indices and variability. Those that have received the most reported investigation are the *Delta program* with the Octopus perimeter[258] and the *STATPAC* with the Humphrey Field Analyzer.[259] Although most statistical models provide better agreement than experienced clinical observers with regard to significant change over time, there is no generally accepted technique for this purpose at the present time.[260] One study, which compared the results of a threshold program on the Octopus perimeter to those from manual perimetry, demonstrated that indices used currently may not be clinically reliable in the assessment of changes in the visual field.[261] As Anderson[1] has proposed, the interpretation of automated visual field data should include simple observation, statistics, and common sense.

Comparison of Specific Automated Perimeters

Suprathreshold Static Perimeters. As previously noted, most instruments that are limited to suprathreshold measurements have now been replaced by models with full thresholding capabilities, although they may still have value as screening devices. The *Fieldmaster 101 and 200,* which use fiberoptic light sources in a bowl perimeter, received the most reported evaluation. These models compared favorably with manual perimetry using Goldmann or Tübingen perimeters, and were considered to have great potential as quantitative visual field screening devices.[262–266] More recently, the *Henson CFS2000* screening program has been shown to have good predictive power.[267]

Threshold Perimeters. The first of these instruments to receive extensive study was the *Octopus 201* and subsequent models *2000 and 500* (Fig. 6.13). With each unit, stimuli are projected onto a bowl, and fixation is monitored by both the corneal light reflex method and a television view of the patient's eye. The models differ primarily according to computer capabilities. These automated perimeters have compared favorably with manual perimetry done with Goldmann and Tübingen perimeters and can frequently detect field loss missed with the Goldmann perimeter.[268–270]

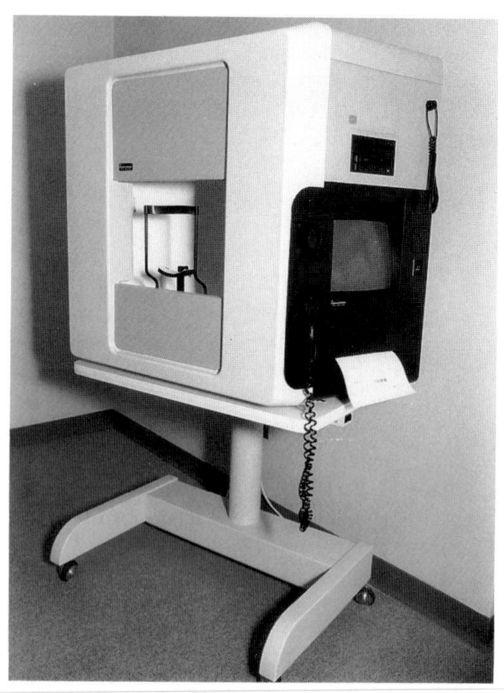

Figure 6.14. Humphrey Field Analyzer.

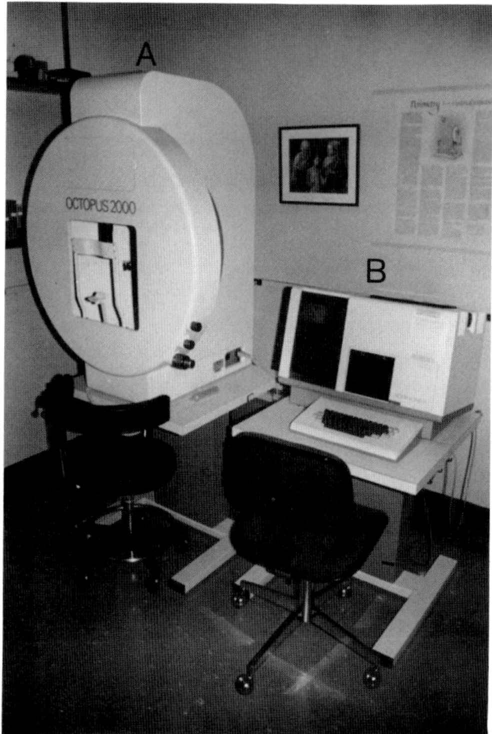

Figure 6.13. Octopus 2000R automated static perimeter, showing perimetric unit (*A*) and control unit (*B*).

The *Humphrey Field Analyzer* also uses projected stimuli with strategies similar to the Octopus, except for fixation monitoring by periodic blind spot checks (Fig. 6.14). It is currently the most commonly used automated perimeter. It has also compared favorably with manual perimetry on the Goldmann perimeter, often detecting defects that the latter missed.[271] In one study, however, patients preferred the Goldmann perimeter, while the technician favored the Humphrey.[272] The Octopus and Humphrey units have been compared in several studies. In one study, both short-term and long-term fluctuations were greater with the Octopus.[273] In another study, both automated perimeters identified slightly more defects by meridional threshold testing than the Tübingen manual perimeter.[274]

The *Fieldmaster 300* (Squid) is another projection perimeter. Examples of LED perimeters include the *Dicon 2000, Fieldmaster 50,* and *DigiLab 350.* In a comparative study of these four instruments along with the Octopus and Humphrey, no device was clearly superior and all had some degree of long-term variability.[275,276] Patients preferred the Octopus, Squid, and Fieldmaster 50, while technicians were most impressed with the Humphrey and Squid.[275] Projection perimeters made it easier to perform cross-comparisons of test results.[275] In another study, however, threshold equivalence between the Octopus, Humphrey, and Dicon units was such that the prediction when converting from one instrument to another was only 10% less reliable than with two examinations on the same instrument.[277] The *Competer* is another LED perimeter that has compared favorably with manual perimeters[278–280] and the Octopus.[281,282]

SUMMARY

The normal visual field may be depicted as a three-dimensional contour, representing areas of relative retinal sensitivity and characterized by a peak at the point of fixation, an absolute depression corresponding to the optic nerve head (blind spot), and a sloping of the remaining areas to the boundaries of the field. Early glaucomatous damage may produce a generalized depression of this contour, which can be demonstrated with several psychophysical tests. The more specific visual field changes of glaucoma, however, are localized defects that correspond to loss of retinal nerve fiber bundles and include paracentral and arcuate scotomas above and below fixation and step-like defects along the nasal midline (nasal step). Instruments that are used to measure the field of vision (perimeters) may have kinetic and/or static targets, which can be controlled manually or automatically. The targets are presented against a background that is either flat (tangent screen) or bowl-shaped, with the latter units providing more reliable measurements. Automated perimeters may be semiautomatic or fully automatic, and comparative studies indicate that computer-assisted static perimeters are more sensitive than manual perimeters in detecting glaucomatous visual field loss.

References

1. Anderson, DR: Perimetry With and Without Automation, 2nd ed. CV Mosby, St. Louis, 1987.
2. Harrington, DO: The Visual Fields. A Textbook and Atlas of Clinical Perimetry, 5th ed. CV Mosby, St. Louis, 1981.
3. Drance, SM, Anderson, DR: Automatic perimetry. In: Glaucoma. A Practical Guide. Grune and Stratton, Orlando, 1985.
4. Tate, GW Jr, Lynn, JR: Principles of Quantitative Perimetry: Testing and Interpreting the Visual Field. Grune and Stratton, New York, 1977.
5. Reed, H, Drance, SM: The Essentials of Perimetry Static and Kinetic, 2nd ed. Oxford University Press, London, 1972.
6. Whalen, WR, Spaeth, GL: Computerized Visual Fields. What They Are and How to Use Them. Slack Inc, Thorofare, NJ, 1985.
7. Hart, WM, Burde, RM: Three-dimensional topography of the central visual field. Sparing of foveal sensitivity in macular disease. Ophthalmology 90:1028, 1983.
8. Armaly, MF: The size and location of the normal blind spot. Arch Ophthal 81:192, 1969.
9. Anctil, J-L, Anderson, DR: Early foveal involvement and generalized depression of the visual field in glaucoma. Arch Ophthal 102:363, 1984.
10. Stamper, RL: The effect of glaucoma on central visual function. Trans Am Ophthal Soc 82:792, 1984.
11. Pickett, JE, Terry, SA, O'Connor, PS, O'Hara, M: Early loss of central visual acuity in glaucoma. Ophthalmology 92:891, 1985.
12. Grunwald, JE, Riva, CE, Stone, RA, et al: Retinal autoregulation in open-angle glaucoma. Ophthalmology 91:1690, 1984.
13. Sponsel, WE, DePaul, KL, Kaufman, PL: Correlation of visual function and retinal leukocyte velocity in glaucoma. Am J Ophthal 109:49, 1990.
14. Langerhorst, CT, Van den Berg, TJ, Greve EL: Is there general reduction of sensitivity in glaucoma? Internat Ophthal 13:31, 1989.
15. Hart, WM, Yablonski, M, Kass, MA, Becker, B: Quantitative visual field and optic disc correlates early in glaucoma. Arch Ophthal 96:2209, 1978.
16. Flammer, J, Eppler, E, Niesel, P: Quantitative perimetry in the glaucoma patient without local visual field defects. Graefe's Arch Ophthal 219:92, 1982.
17. de Oliveira-Rassi, M, Shields, MB: Crowding of the peripheral nasal isopters in glaucoma. Am J Ophthal 94:4, 1982.

18. Drance, SM: The early field defects in glaucoma. Invest Ophthal 8:84, 1969.
19. Colenbrander, MC: The early diagnosis of glaucoma. Ophthalmologica 162:276, 1971.
20. Drance, SM, Lakowski, R, Schulzer, M, Douglas, GR: Acquired color vision changes in glaucoma. Use of 100-hue test and Pickford anomaloscope as predictors of glaucomatous field change. Arch Ophthal 99:829, 1981.
21. Motolko, M, Drance, SM, Douglas, GR: The early psychophysical disturbances in chronic open-angle glaucoma. A study of visual functions with asymmetric disc cupping. Arch Ophthal 100:1632, 1982.
22. Adams, AJ, Rodic, R, Husted, R, Stamper, R: Spectral sensitivity and color discrimination changes in glaucoma and glaucoma-suspect patients. Invest Ophthal Vis Sci 23:516, 1982.
23. Flammer, J, Drance, SM: Correlation between color vision scores and quantitative perimetry in suspected glaucoma. Arch Ophthal 102:38, 1984.
24. Hamill, TR, Post, RB, Johnson, CA, Keltner, JL: Correlation of color vision deficits and observable changes in the optic disc in a population of ocular hypertensives. Arch Ophthal 102:1637, 1984.
25. Heron, G, Adams, AJ, Husted, R: Central visual fields for short wavelength sensitive pathways in glaucoma and ocular hypertension. Invest Ophthal Vis Sci 29:64, 1988.
26. Adams, AJ, Heron, G, Husted, R: Clinical measures of central vision function in glaucoma and ocular hypertension. Arch Ophthal 105:782, 1987.
27. Yamazaki, Y, Lakowski, R, Drance, SM: A comparison of the blue color mechanism in high- and low-tension glaucoma. Ophthalmology 96:12, 1989.
28. Yamazaki, Y, Drance, SM, Lakowski, R, Schulzer, M: Correlation between color vision and highest intraocular pressure in glaucoma patients. Am J Ophthal 106:397, 1988.
29. Airaksinen, PJ, Lakowski, R, Drance, SM, Price, M: Color vision and retinal nerve fiber layer in early glaucoma. Am J Ophthal 101:208, 1986.
30. Quigley, HA, Sanchez, RM, Dunkelberg, GR, L'Hernault, NL, Baginski, TA: Chronic glaucoma selectively damages large optic nerve fibers. Invest Ophthal Vis Sci 28:913, 1987.
31. Breton, ME, Krupin, T: Age covariance between 100-hue color scores and quantitative perimetry in primary open angle glaucoma. Arch Ophthal 105:642, 1987.
32. Gündüz, K, Arden, GB, Perry, S, et al: Color vision defects in ocular hypertension and glaucoma: quantification with a computer-driven color television system. Arch Ophthal 106:929, 1988.
33. Sample, PA, Boynton, RM, Weinreb, RN: Isolating the color vision loss in primary open-angle glaucoma. Am J Ophthal 106:686, 1988.
34. Arden, GB, Jacobson, JJ: A simple grating test for contrast sensitivity: preliminary results indicate value in screening for glaucoma. Invest Ophthal Vis Sci 17:23, 1978.
35. Strasser, B, Haddad, R, Keibl, L: Arden test for early glaucomatous damage. Klin Monatsbl Augenheilkd 178:136, 1981.
36. Lundh, BL, Lennerstrand, G: Eccentric contrast sensitivity loss in glaucoma. Acta Ophthal 59:21, 1981.
37. Motolko, MA, Phelps, CD: Contrast sensitivity in asymmetric glaucoma. Internat Ophthal 7:45, 1984.
38. Hitchings, RA, Powell, DJ, Arden, GB, Carter, RM: Contrast sensitivity gratings in glaucoma family screening. Br J Ophthal 65:515, 1981.
39. Stamper, RL, Hsu-Winges, C, Sopher, M: Arden contrast sensitivity testing in glaucoma. Arch Ophthal 100:947, 1982.
40. Ross, JE, Bron, AJ, Clarke, DD: Contrast sensitivity and visual disability in chronic simple glaucoma. Br J Ophthal 68:821, 1984.
41. Sokol, S, Domar, A, Moskowitz, A: Utility of the Arden grating test in glaucoma screening: high false-positive rate in normals over 50 years of age. Invest Ophthal Vis Sci 19:1529, 1980.
42. Hyvarin, L, Rovamo, J, Laurinen, P, et al: Contrast sensitivity in monocular glaucoma. Acta Ophthal 61:742, 1983.
43. Lundh, BL: Central contrast sensitivity tests in the detection of early glaucoma. Acta Ophthal 63:481, 1985.
44. Korth, M, Horn, F, Storck, B, Jonas, JB: Spatial and spatiotemporal contrast sensitivity of normal and glaucoma eyes. Graefe's Arch Ophthal 227:428, 1989.
45. Owsley, C, Gardner, T, Sekuler, R, Lieberman, H: Role of the crystalline lens in the spatial vision loss of the elderly. Invest Ophthal Vis Sci 26:1165, 1985.
46. Higgins, KE, Jaffe, MJ, Coletta, NJ, et al: Spatial contrast sensitivity. Importance of controlling the patient's visibility criterion. Arch Ophthal 102:1035, 1984.
47. Vaegan, F, Halliday, BL: A forced-choice test improves clinical contrast sensitivity testing. Br J Ophthal 66:477, 1982.
48. Tweten, S, Wall, M, Schwartz, BD: A comparison of three clinical methods of spatial contrast-sensitivity testing in normal subjects. Graefe's Arch Ophthal 228:24, 1990.
49. Regan, D, Beverley, KI: Visual fields described by contrast sensitivity, by acuity, and by relative sensitivity to different orientations. Invest Ophthal Vis Sci 24:754, 1983.
50. Neima, D, LeBlanc, R, Regan, D: Visual field

defects in ocular hypertension and glaucoma. Arch Ophthal 102:1042, 1984.
51. Phelps, CD: Acuity perimetry and glaucoma. Trans Am Ophthal Soc LXXXII:753, 1984.
52. Regan, D, Neima, D: Low-contrast letter charts as a test of visual function. Ophthalmology 90:1192, 1983.
53. Atkin, A, Bodis-Wollner, I, Wolkstein, M, et al: Abnormalities of central contrast sensitivity in glaucoma. Am J Ophthal 88:205, 1979.
54. Tyler, CW: Specific deficits of flicker sensitivity in glaucoma and ocular hypertension. Invest Ophthal Vis Sci 20:204, 1981.
55. Tytla, ME, Trope, GE, Buncic, JR: Flicker sensitivity in treated ocular hypertension. Ophthalmology 97:36, 1990.
56. Regan, D, Neima, D: Balance between pattern and flicker sensitivities in the visual fields of ophthalmological patients. Br J Ophthal 68:310, 1984.
57. Stelmach, LB, Drance, SM, Di Lollo, V: Two-pulse temporal resolution in patients with glaucoma, suspected glaucoma, and in normal observers. Am J Ophthal 102:617, 1986.
58. Bobak, P, Bodis-Wollner, I, Harnois, C, et al: Pattern electroretinograms and visual-evoked potentials in glaucoma and multiple sclerosis. Am J Ophthal 96:72, 1983.
59. Wanger, P, Persson, HE: Pattern-reversal electroretinograms in unilateral glaucoma. Invest Ophthal Vis Sci 24:749, 1983.
60. Papst, N, Bopp, M, Schnaudigel, OE: Flash and pattern electroretinograms in advanced glaucoma. Klin Monatsbl Augenheilkd 184:199, 1984.
61. Papst, N, Bopp, M, Schnaudigel, OE: Pattern of electroretinogram and visually evoked cortical potentials in glaucoma. Graefe's Arch Ophthal 222:29, 1984.
62. Price, MJ, Drance, SM, Price M, et al: The pattern of electroretinogram and visual-evoked potential in glaucoma. Graefe's Arch Ophthal 226:542, 1988.
63. Korth, M, Horn, F, Storck, B, Jonas, J: The pattern-evoked electroretinogram (PERG): age-related alterations and changes in glaucoma. Graefe's Arch Ophthal 227:123, 1989.
64. Watanabe, I, Iijima H, Tsukahara, S: The pattern electroretinogram in glaucoma: an evaluation by relative amplitude from the Bjerrum area. Br J Ophthal 73:131, 1989.
65. Odom, JV, Feghali, JG, Jin, J-C, Weinstein, GW: Visual function deficits in glaucoma. Electroretinogram pattern and luminance nonlinearities. Arch Ophthal 108:222, 1990.
66. Wanger, P, Persson, HE: Pattern-reversal electroretinograms and high-pass resolution perimetry in suspected or early glaucoma. Ophthalmology 94:1098, 1987.
67. Weinstein, GW, Arden, GB, Hitchings, RA, et al: The pattern electroretinogram (PERG) in ocular hypertension and glaucoma. Arch Ophthal 106:923, 1988.
68. Trick, GL: PRRP abnormalities in glaucoma and ocular hypertension. Invest Ophthal Vis Sci 27:1730, 1986.
69. Trick, GL, Bickler-Bluth, M, Cooper, DG, et al: Pattern reversal electroretinogram (PRERG) abnormalities in ocular hypertension: correlation with glaucoma risk factors. Curr Eye Res 7:201, 1988.
70. Trick, GL, Nesher, R, Cooper, DG, et al: Dissociation of visual deficits in ocular hypertension. Invest Ophthal Vis Sci 29:1486, 1988.
71. Johnson, MA, Drum, BA, Quigley, HA, et al: Pattern-evoked potentials and optic nerve fiber loss in monocular laser-induced glaucoma. Invest Ophthal Vis Sci 30:897, 1989.
72. Siliprandi, R, Bucci, MG, Canella R, Carmignoto, G: Flash and pattern electroretinograms during and after acute intraocular pressure elevation in cats. Invest Ophthal Vis Sci 29:558, 1988.
73. Cappin, JM, Nissim, S: Visual evoked responses in the assessment of field defects in glaucoma. Arch Ophthal 93:9, 1975.
74. Towle, VL, Moskowitz, A, Sokol, S, Schwartz, B: The visual evoked potential in glaucoma and ocular hypertension: effects of check size, field size, and stimulation rate. Invest Ophthal Vis Sci 24:175, 1983.
75. Howe, JW, Mitchell, KW: The objective assessment of contrast sensitivity function by electrophysiological means. Br J Ophthal 68:626, 1984.
76. Mitchell, KW, Wood, CM, Howe, JW, et al: The visual evoked potential in acute primary angle closure glaucoma. Br J Ophthal 73:448, 1989.
77. Schmeisser, ET, Smith, TJ: High-frequency flicker visual-evoked potential losses in glaucoma. Ophthalmology 96:620, 1989.
78. Saraux, H, Grall, Y, Keller, J, et al: Electro-oculography and the glaucomatous eye. J Fr Ophthal 5:243, 1982.
79. Goldthwaite, D, Lakowski, R, Drance, SM: A study of dark adaptation in ocular hypertensives. Can J Ophthal 11:55, 1976.
80. Enoch, JM: Quantitative layer-by-layer perimetry. Invest Ophthal Vis Sci 17:208, 1978.
81. Kohn, AN, Moss, AP, Podos, SM: Relative afferent pupillary defects in glaucoma without characteristic field loss. Arch Ophthal 97:294, 1979.
82. Thompson, HS, Montague, P, Cox, TA, Corbett, JJ: The relationship between visual acuity, pupillary defect, and visual field loss. Am J Ophthal 93:681, 1982.
83. Brown, RH, Zilis, JD, Lynch, MG, Sanborn, GE: The afferent pupillary defect in asymmetric glaucoma. Arch Ophthal 105:1540, 1987.
84. Johnson, LN, Hill, RA, Bartholomew, MJ: Correlation of afferent pupillary defect with visual

field loss on automated perimetry. Ophthalmology 95:1649, 1988.
85. Browning, DJ, Buckley, EG: Reliability of brightness comparison testing in predicting afferent pupillary defects. Arch Ophthal 106:341, 1988.
86. Teoh, SL, Allan, D, Dutton, GN, Foulds, WS: Brightness discrimination and contrast sensitivity in chronic glaucoma—a clinical study. Br J Ophthal 74:215, 1990.
87. Werner, EB, Drance, SM: Early visual field disturbances in glaucoma. Arch Ophthal 95:1173, 1977.
88. Werner, EB, Saheb, N, Thomas, D: Variability of static visual threshold responses in patients with elevated IOPs. Arch Ophthal 100:1627, 1982.
89. Hart, WM Jr, Becker, B: The onset and evolution of glaucomatous visual field defects. Ophthalmology 89:268, 1982.
90. Sturmer, J, Gloor, B, Tobler, HJ: How glaucomatous visual fields manifest themselves in reality. Klin Monatsbl Augenheilkd 184:390, 1984.
91. Flammer, J, Drance, SM, Zulauf, M: Differential light threshold. Short- and long-term fluctuation in patients with glaucoma, normal controls, and patients with suspected glaucoma. Arch Ophthal 102:704, 1984.
92. Heijl, A, Drance, SM: Changes in differential threshold in patients with glaucoma during prolonged perimetry. Br J Ophthal 67:512, 1983.
93. Flammer, J, Drance, SM, Fankhause, F, Augustiny, L: Differential light threshold in automated static perimetry. Factors influencing short-term fluctuation. Arch Ophthal 102:876, 1984.
94. Flammer, J, Drance, SM, Schulzer, M: Covariates of the long-term fluctuation of the differential light threshold. Arch Ophthal 102:880, 1984.
95. Harrington, DO: The Bjerrum scotoma. Trans Am Ophthal Soc 62:324, 1964.
96. Harrington, DO: The Bjerrum scotoma. Am J Ophthal 59:646, 1965.
97. Gramer, E, Gerlach, R, Krieglstein, GK, Leydhecker, W: Topography of early visual field defects in computerized perimetry. Klin Monatsbl Augenheilkd 180:515, 1982.
98. Mikelberg, FS, Drance, SM: The mode of progression of visual field defects in glaucoma. Am J Ophthal 98:443, 1984.
99. Drance, SM: The glaucomatous visual field. Br J Ophthal 56:186, 1972.
100. Drance, SM: The glaucomatous visual field. Invest Ophthal 11:85, 1972.
101. Mikelberg, FS, Schulzer, M, Drance, SM, Lau, W: The rate of progression of scotomas in glaucoma. Am J Ophthal 101:1, 1986.
102. Harrington, DO: Differential diagnosis of the arcuate scotoma. Invest Ophthal 8:96, 1969.
103. LeBlanc, RP, Becker, B: Peripheral nasal field defects. Am J Ophthal 72:415, 1971.
104. Werner, EB, Beraskow, J: Peripheral nasal field defects in glaucoma. Ophthalmology 86:1875, 1979.
105. Lynn, JR: Correlation of pathogenesis, anatomy, and patterns of visual loss in glaucoma. In: Symposium on Glaucoma. CV Mosby, St. Louis, 1975, p. 151.
106. Damgaard-Jensen, L: Vertical steps in isopters at the hemiopic border—in normal and glaucomatous eyes. Acta Ophthal 55:111, 1977.
107. Damgaaard-Jensen, L: Demonstration of peripheral hemiopic border steps by static perimetry. Acta Ophthal 55:815, 1977.
108. Brais, P, Drance, SM: The temporal field in chronic simple glaucoma. Arch Ophthal 88:518, 1976.
109. Armaly, MF: Visual field defects in early open angle glaucoma. Trans Am Ophthal Soc 69:147, 1971.
110. Armaly, MF: Selective perimetry for glaucomatous defects in ocular hypertension. Arch Ophthal 87:518, 1972.
111. Schulzer, M, Mikelberg, FS, Drance, SM: A study of the value of the central and peripheral isoptres in assessing visual field progression in the presence of paracentral scotoma measurements. Br J Ophthal 71:422, 1987.
112. Mills, RP: Usefulness of peripheral testing in automated screening perimetry. Proc 6th Int Vis Field Symp, Heijl, A, Greve, EL, eds. Junk Publ, Dordrecht, The Netherlands, 1985, p. 207.
113. Caprioli, J, Spaeth, GL: Static threshold examination of the peripheral nasal visual field in glaucoma. Arch Ophthal 103:1150, 1985.
114. Stewart, WC, Shields, MB, Ollie, AR: Peripheral visual field testing by automated kinetic perimetry in glaucoma. Arch Ophthal 106:202, 1988.
115. Miller, KN, Shields, MB, Ollie, AR: Automated kinetic perimetry with two peripheral isopters in glaucoma. Arch Ophthal 107:1316, 1989.
116. Lichter, RR, Ravin, JG: Risks of sudden visual loss after glaucoma surgery. Am J Ophthal 78:1009, 1974.
117. Caprioli, J, Sears, M, Miller, JM: Patterns of early visual field loss in open-angle glaucoma. Am J Ophthal 103:512, 1987.
118. Hitchings, RA, Anderton, SA: A comparative study of visual field defects seen in patients with low-tension glaucoma and chronic simple glaucoma. Br J Ophthal 67:818, 1983.
119. Caprioli, J, Spaeth, GL: Comparison of visual field defects in the low-tension glaucomas with those in the high-tension glaucomas. Am J Ophthal 97:730, 1984.
120. Drance, SM: The visual field of low tension glaucoma and shock-induced optic neuropathy. Arch Ophthal 95:1359, 1977.
121. Motolko, M, Drance, SM, Douglas, GR: Visual field defects in low-tension glaucoma. Comparison of defects in low-tension glaucoma and

chronic open angle glaucoma. Arch Ophthal 100:1074, 1982.
122. Radius, RL, Maumenee, AE: Visual field changes following acute elevation of intraocular pressure. Trans Am Acad Ophthal Otol 83:61, 1977.
123. McNaught, EI, Rennie, A, McClure, E, Chisholm, IA: Pattern of visual damage after acute angle-closure glaucoma. Trans Ophthal Soc U K 94:406, 1974.
124. Drance, SM: Studies in the susceptibility of the eye to raised intraocular pressure. Arch Ophthal 68:478, 1962.
125. Tsamparlakis, JC: Effects of transient induced elevation of the intraocular pressure on the visual field. Br J Ophthal 48:237, 1964.
126. Scott, AB, Morris, A: Visual field changes produced by artificially elevated intraocular pressure. Am J Ophthal 63:308, 1967.
127. Armaly, MF: Effect of corticosteroids on intraocular pressure and fluid dynamics. III. Changes in visual function and pupil size during topical dexamethasone application. Arch Ophthal 71:636, 1964.
128. Kolker, AE, Becker, B, Mills, DW: Intraocular pressure and visual fields: effects of corticosteroids. Arch Ophthal 72:772, 1964.
129. LeBlanc, RP, Stewart, RH, Becker, B: Corticosteroid provocative testing. Invest Ophthal 9:946, 1970.
130. Hart, Wm Jr, Becker, B: Visual field changes in ocular hypertension. A computer-based analysis. Arch Ophthal 95:1176, 1977.
131. Armaly, MF: The visual field defect and ocular pressure level in open angle glaucoma. Invest Ophthal 8:105, 1969.
132. Heilmann, K: On the reversibility of visual field defects in glaucomas. Trans Am Acad Ophthal Otol 78:304, 1974.
133. Flammer, J, Drance, SM: Reversibility of a glaucomatous visual field defect after acetazolamide therapy. Can J Ophthal 18:139, 1983.
134. Katz, LJ, Spaeth, GL, Cantor, LB, et al: Reversible optic disk cupping and visual field improvement in adults with glaucoma. Am J Ophthal 107:485, 1989.
135. Heijl, A, Bengtsson, B: The short-term effect of laser trabeculoplasty on the glaucomatous visual field. A prospective study using computerized perimetry. Acta Ophthal 62:705, 1984.
136. Holmin, C, Krakau, CET: Trabeculoplasty and visual field decay: a follow-up study using computerized perimetry. Curr Eye Res 3:1101, 1984.
137. Drance, SM: The disc and the field in glaucoma. Ophthalmology 85:209, 1978.
138. Hoskins, HD Jr, Gelber, EC: Optic disk topography and visual field defects in patients with increased intraocular pressure. Am J Ophthal 80:284, 1975.
139. Shutt, HKR, Boyd, TAS, Salter, AB: The relationship of visual fields, optic disc appearances and age in non-glaucomatous and glaucomatous eyes. Can J Ophthal 2:83, 1967.
140. Drance, SM: Correlation between optic disc changes and visual field defects in chronic open-angle glaucoma. Trans Am Acad Ophthal Otol 81:224, 1976.
141. Holmin, C: Optic disc evaluation versus the visual field in chronic glaucoma. Acta Ophthal 60:275, 1982.
142. Hitchings, RA, Spaeth, GL: The optic disc in glaucoma. II: Correlation of the appearance of the optic disc with the visual field. Br J Ophthal 61:107, 1977.
143. Quigley, HA, Addicks, EM, Green, WR: Optic nerve damage in human glaucoma. III. Quantitative correlation of nerve fiber loss and visual field defect in glaucoma, ischemic neuropathy, papilledema, and toxic neuropathy. Arch Ophthal 100:135, 1982.
144. Quigley, HA, Dunkelberger, GR, Green, WR: Retinal ganglion cell atrophy correlated with automated perimetry in human eyes with glaucoma. Am J Ophthal 107:453, 1989.
145. Read, RM, Spaeth, GL: The practical clinical appraisal of the optic disc in glaucoma: the natural history of cup progression and some specific disc-field correlations. Trans Am Acad Ophthal Otol 78:255, 1974.
146. Gloster, J: Quantitative relationship between cupping of the optic disc and visual field loss in chronic simple glaucoma. Br J Ophthal 62:665, 1978.
147. Hitchings, RA, Anderton, S: Identification of glaucomatous visual field defects from examination of monocular photographs of the optic disc. Br J Ophthal 67:822, 1983.
148. Airaksinen, JP, Drance, SM, Douglas, GR, Schulzer, M: Neuroretinal rim areas and visual field indices in glaucoma. Am J Ophthal 99:107, 1985.
149. Guthauser, U, Flammer, J, Niesel, P: The relationship between the visual field and the optic nerve head in glaucomas. Graefe's Arch Ophthal 225:129, 1987.
150. Caprioli, J, Miller, JM: Correlation of structure and function in glaucoma: quantitative measurements of disc and field. Ophthalmology 95:723, 1988.
151. Jonas, JB, Gusek, GC, Naumann, GOH: Optic disc morphometry in chronic primary open-angle glaucoma. II. Correlation of the intrapapillary morphometric data to visual field indices. Graefe's Arch Ophthal 226:531, 1988.
152. Sommer, A, Miller, NR, Pollack, I, et al: The nerve fiber layer in the diagnosis of glaucoma. Arch Ophthal 95:2149, 1977.
153. Sommer, A, Pollack, I, Maumenee, AE: Optic

disc parameters and onset of glaucomatous field loss. II. Static screening criteria. Arch Ophthal 97:1449, 1979.
154. Airaksinen, PJ, Drance, SM, Douglas, GR, et al: Visual field and retinal nerve fiber layer comparisons in glaucoma. Arch Ophthal 103:205, 1985.
155. Drance, SM, Airaksinen, PJ, Price, M, et al: The correlation of functional and structural measurements in glaucoma patients and normal subjects. Am J Ophthal 102:612, 1986.
156. Okada, K, Minato, T, Miyaji, S: A method for contrasting control visual fields in the Humphrey Field Analyzer and Monochromatic turned-over fundus photographs. Ophthalmology (Japan) 30:925, 1988.
157. Airaksinen, PJ, Heijl, A: Visual field and retinal nerve fibre layer in early glaucoma after optic disc haemorrhage. Acta Ophthal 61:186, 1983.
158. Katz, J, Sommer, A: Similarities between the visual fields of ocular hypertensive and normal eyes. Arch Ophthal 104:1648, 1986.
159. Armaly, MF: The correlation between appearance of the optic cup and visual function. Trans Am Acad Ophthal Otol 73:898, 1969.
160. Funk, J, Bornscheuer, C, Grehn, F: Neuroretinal rim area and visual field in glaucoma. Graefe's Arch Ophthal 226:431, 1988.
161. Portney, GL, Krohn, MA: The limitations of kinetic perimetry in early scotoma detection. Ophthalmology 85:287, 1978.
162. Ourgaud, M: Static circular perimetry in open-angle glaucoma. J Fr Ophthal 5:387, 1982.
163. Choplin, NT, Sherwood, MB, Spaeth, GL: The effect of stimulus size on the measured threshold values in automated perimetry. Ophthalmology 97:371, 1990.
164. Hart, WM Jr, Hartz, RK, Hagen, RW, Clark, KW: Color contrast perimetry. Invest Ophthal Vis Sci 25:400, 1984.
165. Hart, WM Jr, Gordon, MO: Color perimetry of glaucomatous visual field defects. Ophthalmology 91:338, 1984.
166. Hart, WM Jr, Silverman, SE, Trick, GL, et al: Glaucomatous visual field damage. Luminance and color-contrast sensitivities. Invest Ophthal Vis Sci 31:359, 1990.
167. Logan, N, Anderson, DR: Detecting early glaucomatous visual field changes with a blue stimulus. Am J Ophthal 95:432, 1983.
168. Mindel, JS, Safir, A, Schare, PW: Visual field testing with red targets. Arch Ophthal 101:927, 1983.
169. Hart, WM Jr, Burde, RM: Color contrast perimetry: the spatial distribution of color defects in optic nerve and retinal diseases. Ophthalmology 92:768, 1985.
170. Johnson, CA, Keltner, JL, Balestrery, FG: Acuity profile perimetry. Description of technique and preliminary clinical trials. Arch Ophthal 97:684, 1979.
171. Drum, BA, Severns, M, O'Leary, DK, et al: Selective loss of pattern discrimination in early glaucoma. Applied Optics 28:1135, 1989.
172. Johnson, CA, Keltner, JL: Optimal rates of movement for kinetic perimetry. Arch Ophthal 105:73, 1987.
173. Klewin, KM, Radius, RL: Background illumination and automated perimetry. Arch Ophthal 104:395, 1986.
174. Drum, B, Armaly, MF, Huppert, W: Scotopic sensitivity loss in glaucoma. Arch Ophthal 104:712, 1986.
175. Heuer, DK, Anderson, DR, Knighton, RW, et al: The influence of simulated light scattering on automated perimetric threshold measurements. Arch Ophthal 106:1247, 1988.
176. Bigger, JF, Becker, B: Cataracts and open-angle glaucoma. The effect of cataract extraction on visual fields. Am J Ophthal 71:335, 1971.
177. Wood, JM, Wild, JM, Smerdon, DL, Crews, SJ: Alterations in the shape of the automated perimetric profile arising from cataract. Graefe's Arch Ophthal 227:157, 1989.
178. Guthauser, U, Flammer, J: Quantifying visual field damage caused by cataract. Am J Ophthal 106:480, 1988.
179. Radius, RL: Perimetry in cataract patients. Arch Ophthal 96:1574, 1978.
180. Ruben, JB, Lewis, RA, Johnson, CA, Adams, C: The effect of Goldmann applanation tonometry on automated static threshold perimetry. Ophthalmology 95:267, 1988.
181. Lindenmuth, KA, Skuta, GL, Rabbani, R, Musch, DC: Effects of pupillary constriction on automated perimetry in normal eyes. Ophthalmology 96:1298, 1989.
182. McCluskey, DJ, Douglas, JP, O'Connor, PS, et al: The effect of pilocarpine on the visual field in normals. Ophthalmology 93:843, 1986.
183. Heuer, DK, Anderson, DR, Feuer, WJ, Gressel, MG: The influence of decreased retinal illumination on automated perimetric threshold measurements. Am J Ophthal 108:643, 1989.
184. Lindenmuth, KA, Skuta, GL, Rabbani, R, et al: Effects of pupillary dilation on automated perimetry in normal patients. Ophthalmology 97:367, 1990.
185. Weinreb, RN, Perlman, JP: The effect of refractive correction on automated perimetric thresholds. Am J Ophthal 101:706, 1986.
186. Goldstick, BJ, Weinreb, RN: The effect of refractive error on automated global analysis program G-1. Am J Ophthal 104:229, 1987.
187. Heuer, DK, Anderson, DR, Feuer, WJ, Gressel, MG: The influence of refraction accuracy on automated perimetric threshold measurements. Ophthalmology 94:1550, 1987.

188. Haas, A, Flammer, J, Schneider, U: Influence of age on the visual fields of normal subjects. Am J Ophthal 101:199, 1986.
189. Jaffe, GJ, Alvarado, JA, Juster, RP: Age-related changes of the normal visual field. Arch Ophthal 104:1021, 1986.
190. Johnson, CA, Adams, AJ, Lewis, RA: Evidence for a neural basis of age-related visual field loss in normal observers. Invest Ophthal Vis Sci 30:2056, 1989.
191. Drance, SM, Berry, V, Hughes, A: Studies in the reproducibility of visual field areas in normal and glaucomatous subjects. Can J Ophthal I:14, 1966.
192. Heijl, A, Lindgren, G, Olsson, J: The effect of perimetric experience in normal subjects. Arch Ophthal 107:81, 1989.
193. Werner, EB, Krupin, T, Adelson, A, Feitl, ME: Effect of patient experience on the results of automated perimetry in glaucoma suspect patients. Ophthalmology 97:44, 1990.
194. Wild, JM, Dengler-Harles, M, Searle, AET, et al: The influence of the learning effect on automated perimetry in patients with suspected glaucoma. Acta Ophthal 67:537, 1989.
195. Zulauf, M, Flammer, J, Signer, C: The influence of alcohol on the outcome of automated static perimetry. Graefe's Arch Ophthal 224:525, 1986.
196. Trobe, JD, Acosta, PC, Shuster, JJ, Krischer, JP: An evaluation of the accuracy of community-based perimetry. Am J Ophthal 90:654, 1980.
197. Goldmann, H: Ein selbstregistrierendes Projektionskugelperimeter. Ophthalmologica 109:71, 1945.
198. Portney, GL, Hanible, JE: A comparison of four projection perimeters. Am J Ophthal 81:678, 1976.
199. Harms, H: Entwicklungsmoglichkeiten der Perimetrie. Graefe's Arch Ophthal 150:28, 1950.
200. Armaly, MF: Ocular pressure and visual fields. A ten-year follow-up study. Arch Ophthal 81:25, 1969.
201. Rock, WJ, Drance, SM, Morgan, RW: A modification of the Armaly visual field screening technique for glaucoma. Can J Ophthal 6:283, 1971.
202. Drance, SM, Brais, P, Fairclough, M, Bryett, J: A screening method for temporal visual defects in chronic simple glaucoma. Can J Ophthal 7:428, 1972.
203. Rock, WJ, Drance, SM, Morgan, RW: Visual field screening in glaucoma. An evaluation of the Armaly technique for screening glaucomatous visual fields. Arch Ophthal 89:287, 1973.
204. Fischer, RW: Supraliminal pattern perimetry with the Goldmann perimeter. Klin Monatsbl Augenheilkd 185:204, 1984.
205. Rabin, S, Kolesar, P, Podos, SM, Wilensky, JT: A visual field screening protocol for glaucoma. Am J Ophthal 92:530, 1981.
206. Stepanik, J: Diagnosis of glaucoma with the Goldmann perimeter. Klin Monatsbl Augenheilkd 183:330, 1983.
207. Hart, WM, Jr: Computer processing of visual data. II. Automated pattern analysis of glaucomatous visual fields. Arch Ophthal 99:133, 1981.
208. Weleber, RG, Tobler, WR: Computerized quantitative analysis of kinetic visual fields. Am J Ophthal 101:461, 1986.
209. Esterman, B: Grid for scoring visual fields. I. Tangent screen. Arch Ophthal 77:780, 1967.
210. Esterman, B: Grid for scoring visual fields. II. Perimeter. Arch Ophthal 79:400, 1968.
211. Esterman, B: Functional scoring of the binocular field. Ophthalmology 89:1226, 1982.
212. American Medical Association Guides to the Evaluation of Permanent Impairment, 2nd ed. American Medical Association, Chicago, 1984, p. 141.
213. Mills, RP, Drance, SM: Esterman disability rating in severe glaucoma. Ophthalmology 93:371, 1986.
214. Portney, GL, Krohn, MA: Automated perimetry: background, instruments and methods. Surv Ophthal 22:271, 1978.
215. Harrington, DO, Flocks, M: Multiple pattern method of visual field examination. J Am Med Assoc 157:645, 1955.
216. Roberts, W: The multiple-pattern tachystoscopic visual field screener in glaucoma. Arch Ophthal 58:244, 1957.
217. Friedman, A: The assessment of the efficacy of glaucoma control by static perimetry, or 'point' analysis of clinical visual thresholds. Trans Ophthal Soc UK 82:381, 1962.
218. Friedman, AI: Serial analysis of changes in visual field defects, employing a new instrument, to determine the activity of diseases involving the visual pathways. Ophthalmologica 152:1, 1966.
219. Greve, EL, Verduin, WM: Mass visual field investigation in 1834 persons with supposedly normal eyes. Graefe's Arch Ophthal 183:286, 1972.
220. Batko, KA, Anctil, J-L, Anderson, DR: Detecting glaucomatous damage with the Friedmann analyzer compared with the Goldmann perimeter and evaluation of stereoscopic photographs of the optic disk. Am J Ophthal 95:435, 1983.
221. Hicks, BC, Anderson, DR: Quantitation of glaucomatous visual field defects with the Mark II Friedmann analyzer. Am J Ophthal 95:692, 1983.
222. Henson, DB, Dix, SM, Oborne, AC: Evaluation of the Friedmann visual field analyser Mark II. Part 1. Results from a normal population. Br J Ophthal 68:458, 1984.
223. Henson, DB, Dix, SM: Evaluation of the Friedmann visual field analyser Mark II. Part 2. Results from a population with induced visual field defects. Br J Ophthal 68:463, 1984.
224. Flocks, M, Rosenthal, AR, Hopkins, JL: Mass

visual screening via television. Ophthalmology 85:1141, 1978.
225. Accornero, N, Berardelli, A, Cruccu, G, Manfredi, M: Computerized video screen perimetry. Arch Ophthal 102:40, 1984.
226. Britt, JM, Mills, RP: The black hole effect in perimetry. Invest Ophthal Vis Sci 29:795, 1988.
227. Desjardins, D, Anderson, DR: Threshold variability with an automated LED perimeter. Invest Ophthal Vis Sci 29:915, 1988.
228. Wilensky, JT, Mermelstein, JR, Siegel, HG: The use of different-sized stimuli in automated perimetry. Am J Ophthal 101:710, 1986.
229. Fankhauser, F, Funkhouser, A, Kwasniewska, S: Evaluating the applications of the spatially adaptive program (SAPRO) in clinical perimetry: Part I. Ophthal Surg 17:338, 1986.
230. Asman, P, Britt, JM, Mills, RP, Heijl, A: Evaluation of adaptive spatial enhancement in suprathreshold visual field screening. Ophthalmology 95:1656, 1988.
231. Stewart, WC, Shields, MB, Ollie, AR: Full threshold versus quantification of defects for visual field testing in glaucoma. Graefe's Arch Ophthal 227:51, 1989.
232. Schulzer, M, Mills, RP, Hopp, RH, et al: Estimation of the short-term fluctuation from a single determination of the visual field. Invest Ophthal Vis Sci 31:730, 1990.
233. Katz, J, Sommer, A: Reliability indexes of automated perimetric tests. Arch Ophthal 106:1252, 1988.
234. Bickler-Bluth, M, Trick, GL, Kolker, AE, Cooper, DG: Assessing the utility of reliability indices for automated visual fields: testing ocular hypertensives. Ophthalmology 96:616, 1989.
235. Nelson-Quigg, JM, Twelker, JD, Johnson, CA: Response properties of normal observers and patients during automated perimetry. Arch Ophthal 107:1612, 1989.
236. King, D, Drance, SM, Douglas, GR, Wijsman K: The detection of paracentral scotomas with varying grids in computed perimetry. Arch Ophthal 104:524, 1986.
237. Weber, J, Dobek, K: What is the most suitable grid for computer perimetry in glaucoma patients? Ophthalmologica 192:88, 1986.
238. Gramer, E, Althaus, G, Leydhecker, W: The importance of grid density in automatic perimetry. A clinical study. Z Prakt Augenheilkd 7:197, 1986.
239. Seamone, C, LeBlanc, R, Rubillowicz, M, et al: The value of indices in the central and peripheral visual fields for the detection of glaucoma. Am J Ophthal 106:180, 1988.
240. Weber, J, Krieglstein, GK, Papoulis, C: Use of graphic analysis of topographical trends (GATT) for perimetric follow-up of glaucoma. Klin Monatsbl Augenheilkd 195:319, 1989.
241. Chauhan, BC, Drance, SM, Lai, C: A cluster analysis for threshold perimetry. Graefe's Arch Ophthal 227:216, 1989.
242. Heijl, A, Lindgren, G, Olsson, J, Asman, P: Visual field interpretation with empiric probability maps. Arch Ophthal 107:204, 1989.
243. Heijl, A, Asman, P: A clinical study of perimetric probability maps. Arch Ophthal 107:199, 1989.
244. Duggan, C, Sommer, A, Auer, C, Burkhard, K: Automated differential threshold perimetry for detecting glaucomatous visual field loss. Am J Ophthal 100:420, 1985.
245. Sommer, A, Enger, C, Witt, K: Screening for glaucomatous visual field loss with automated threshold perimetry. Am J Ophthal 103:681, 1987.
246. Jacobs, NA, Patterson, IH: Variability of the hill of vision and its significance in automated perimetry. Br J Ophthal 69:824, 1985.
247. Katz, J, Sommer, A: Asymmetry and variation in the normal hill of vision. Arch Ophthal 104:65, 1986.
248. Heijl, A, Lindgren, G, Olsson, J: Normal variability of static perimetric threshold values across the central visual field. Arch Ophthal 105:1544, 1987.
249. Werner, EB, Petrig, B, Krupin, T, Bishop, KI: Variability of automated visual fields in clinically stable glaucoma patients. Invest Ophthal Vis Sci 30:1083, 1989.
250. Heijl, A, Lindgren, A, Lindgren, G: Test-retest variability in glaucomatous visual fields. Am J Ophthal 108:130, 1989.
251. Haefliger, IO, Flammer, J: Increase of the short-term fluctuation of the differential light threshold around a physiologic scotoma. Am J Ophthal 107:417, 1989.
252. Diestelhorst, M, Kullenberg, C, Krieglstein, GK: Short-term fluctuation of retinal sensitivity at the borders of glaucomatous field defects. Klin Monatsbl Augenheilkd 191:439, 1987.
253. Katz, J, Sommer, A: A longitudinal study of the age-adjusted variability of automated visual fields. Arch Ophthal 105:1083, 1987.
254. Werner, EB, Adelson, A, Krupin, T: Effect of patient experience on the results of automated perimetry in clinically stable glaucoma patients. Ophthalmology 95:764, 1988.
255. Hoskins, HD, Magee, SD, Drake, MV, Kidd, MN: Confidence intervals for change in automated visual fields. Br J Ophthal 72:591, 1988.
256. Brenton, RS, Phelps, CD, Rojas, P, Woolson, RF: Interocular differences of the visual field in normal subjects. Invest Ophthal Vis Sci 27:799, 1986.
257. Feuer, WJ, Anderson, DR: Static threshold asymmetry in early glaucomatous visual field loss. Ophthalmology 96:1285, 1989.
258. Hills, JF, Johnson, CA: Evaluation of the t test as a method of detecting visual field changes. Ophthalmology 95:261, 1988.

259. Enger, C, Sommer, A: Recognizing glaucomatous field loss with the Humphrey STATPAC. Arch Ophthal 105:1355, 1987.
260. Werner, EB, Bishop, KI, Koelle, J, et al: A comparison of experienced clinical observers and statistical tests in detection of progressive visual field loss in glaucoma using automated perimetry. Arch Ophthal 106:619, 1988.
261. Chauhan, BC, Drance, SM, Douglas, GR: The use of visual field indices in detecting changes in the visual field in glaucoma. Invest Ophthal Vis Sci 31:512, 1990.
262. Keltner, JL, Johnson, CA, Balestrery, FG: Suprathreshold static perimetry. Initial clinical trials with the Fieldmaster automated perimeter. Arch Ophthal 97:260, 1979.
263. Johnson, CA, Keltner, JL: Automated suprathreshold static perimetry. Am J Ophthal 89:731, 1980.
264. Bobrow, JC, Drews, RC: Clinical experience with the Fieldmaster perimeter. Am J Ophthal 93:238, 1982.
265. Keltner, JL, Johnson, CA: Effectiveness of automated perimetry in following glaucomatous visual field progression. Ophthalmology 89:247, 1982.
266. Krieglstein, GK, Glaab, E, Gramer, E: The Fieldmaster-200 computer perimeter: a comparative, controlled clinical study of its sensitivity and specificity in glaucomatous field defects. Klin Monatsbl Augenheilkd 179:340, 1981.
267. Vernon, SA, Henry, DJ, Jones, SJ: Calculating the predictive power of the Henson field screener in a population at risk of glaucomatous field loss. Br J Ophthal 74:220, 1990.
268. Li, SG, Spaeth, GL, Scimeca, HA, et al: Clinical experiences with the use of an automated perimeter (Octopus) in the diagnosis and management of patients with glaucoma and neurologic diseases. Ophthalmology 86:1302, 1979.
269. Schmied, U: Automatic (Octopus) and manual (Goldmann) perimetry in glaucoma. Graefe's Arch Ophthal 213:239, 1980.
270. Wilensky, JT, Joondeph, BC: Variation in visual field measurements with an automated perimeter. Am J Ophthal 97:328, 1984.
271. Beck, RW, Bergstrom, TJ, Lichter, PR: A clinical comparison of visual field testing with a new automated perimeter, the Humphrey Field Analyzer, and the Goldmann perimeter. Ophthalmology 92:77, 1985.
272. Trope, GE, Britton, R: A comparison of Goldmann and Humphrey automated perimetry in patients with glaucoma. Br J Ophthal 71:489, 1987.
273. Brenton, RS, Argus, WA: Fluctuations on the Humphrey and Octopus perimeters. Invest Ophthal Vis Sci 28:767, 1987.
274. Mills, RP, Hopp, RH, Drance, SM: Comparison of quantitative testing with the Octopus, Humphrey, and Tübingen perimeters. Am J Ophthal 102:496, 1986.
275. Keltner, JL, Johnson, CA, Lewis, RA: Quantitative office perimetry. Ophthalmology 92:862, 1985.
276. Lewis, RA, Johnson CA, Keltner, JL, Labermeier, PK: Variability of quantitative automated perimetry in normal observers. Ophthalmology 93:878, 1986.
277. Anderson, DR, Feuer, WJ, Alward, WLM, Skuta, GL: Threshold equivalence between perimeters. Am J Ophthal 107:493, 1989.
278. Heijl, A, Drance, SM, Douglas, GR: Automatic perimetry (COMPETER). Ability to detect early glaucomatous field defects. Arch Ophthal 98:1560, 1980.
279. Heijl, A, Drance, SM: Computerized profile perimetry in glaucoma. Arch Ophthal 98:2199, 1980.
280. Gramer, E, Proll, M, Krieglstein, GK: Reproducibility of central visual field testing using kinetic or computerized static perimetry. Klin Monatsbl Augenheilkd 176:374, 1980.
281. Gramer, E, Gerlach, R, Krieglstein, GK: The sensitivity of the Competer® computer perimeter for detecting early glaucomatous field defects. Klin Monatsbl Augenheilkd 180:203, 1982.
282. Heijl, A, Drance, SM: A clinical comparison of three computerized automatic perimeters in the detection of glaucoma defects. Arch Ophthal 99:832, 1981.

Chapter 7

GLAUCOMA SCREENING

GLAUCOMA SCREENING

The basic features of glaucoma that have been considered in this section (intraocular pressure (IOP), optic nerve head and peripapillary retina, and visual function) constitute not only the common denominators for this group of disorders but also the main parameters by which they are detected and followed during therapy. In Section Two, we will consider how these parameters relate to specific clinical forms of glaucoma. It may be helpful, however, to first take a broader look at how these basic features can be used in various screening programs for the early detection of glaucoma.

Since the blindness of glaucoma can only be prevented by early recognition and proper treatment of the disorder, it is essential that mechanisms for early detection be available. Some forms of glaucoma are associated with symptoms that may cause the patient to seek medical care in the early stages of the disorder. In the vast majority of cases, however, there are no early warning signs. It is for these types of glaucoma, which include chronic forms of both primary and secondary glaucomas, that screening mechanisms are needed. The following discussion pertains to these conditions.

The Problems of Mass Screening

For any screening program to be effective, it must be both sensitive and specific. *Sensitivity* is the ability to identify screenees who truly have the disease, and it is expressed as the percentage screening positive of the total number of confirmed cases (i.e., a screening level with high sensitivity has few false negatives). *Specificity* is the ability to give a negative finding when the screenee is truly free of the disease, and it is expressed as the percentage screening negative of those who do not have the disorder (i.e., a screening level with high specificity has few false positives).[1,2]

In the past, most glaucoma screening programs have been limited to the use of tonometry, which has only a fair sensitivity of 50–70% and a poor specificity of 10–30%.[3,4] As a result, when the referral criterion is based on a single IOP measurement, a large percentage of the population who do not have glaucoma will be required to undergo costly follow-up evaluations, while a smaller but clinically more significant group of individuals who do have glaucoma will be told that they are free of the disease. This has led most investigators of glaucoma detection programs to believe that screening with tonometry alone is not warranted. The critical need for early detection remains, however, and continued study has shown that adding one or more additional diagnostic parameters, such as evaluation of the optic nerve head or visual field, as well as targeting high risk populations significantly improves both the sensitivity and specificity of the screening program. Other problems with mass screening for glaucoma include the location of the screening program and the mechanisms of follow-up. In the remainder of this chapter, we will consider how the efficiency of glaucoma detection programs may be improved by directing attention to each of these areas.

The Screening Tests

IOP Measurement

The Tonometer. The efficiency of a screening program is greatly influenced by the reliability of the tonometer that is used.[5] For example, the Schiøtz tonometer reads significantly lower than the Goldmann applanation tonometer, which increases the chance of missing patients who actually have glaucoma. Furthermore, the effect of ocular rigidity on Schiøtz tonometry makes it difficult to simply adjust the screening level for this instrument. The Perkins applanation tonometer, because of its accuracy and portability, is a useful instrument for mass screening,[6,7] but it requires a highly skilled operator. The noncontact tonometer (NCT) can be operated with considerable accuracy by paramedical personnel with minimal training and eliminates the risk of corneal abrasion, spread of infection, and reactions to topical anesthetics.[8] These advantages make the NCT particularly useful in mass screening programs, although the cost of the instrument remains a problem in many communities. Less expensive instruments that may have value in glaucoma screening include the Halberg applanation tonometer[9] the GlaucoTest,[10,11] and the Tono-Pen,[12] each of which was considered in Chapter 4.

The Referral Level. The main problem with IOP as a screening parameter is the overlap of the distributions in nonglaucoma and glaucoma populations, so that a simple "cut-off" pressure level between these two groups does not exist (Fig. 7.1). The optimum referral level is one that minimizes false negatives without significantly sacrificing specificity. This level is generally set at 21 mm Hg, although some investigators have used a cut-off as high as 24 mm Hg.[13] One group used a two-phase approach in which a pressure greater than 18 mm Hg with the NCT was the basis for a second

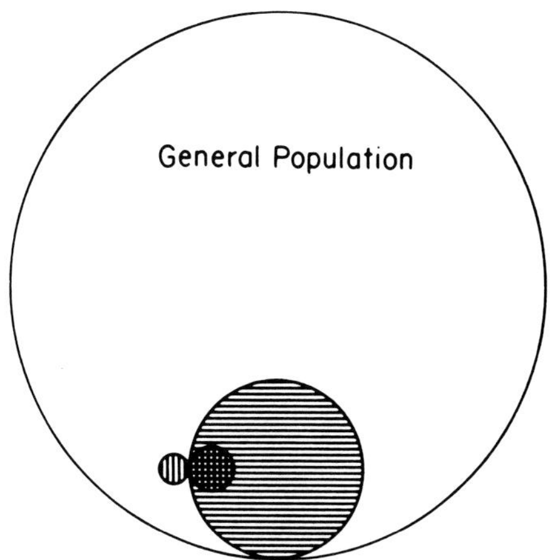

Figure 7.1. Schematic representation of problem with tonometry alone for glaucoma screening. A significant percentage of most general populations will have intraocular pressures above 21 mm Hg. Only a small percentage of the latter group, however, will have glaucomatous field loss, and almost an equal number of individuals with pressures below 21 mm Hg will also have glaucomatous field loss. (Reprinted with permission from Sommer A: Epidemiology and Statistics for the Ophthalmologist, New York, Oxford, Oxford University Press, 1980.)

measurement by a physician with applanation tonometry, in which case 21 mm Hg was the criterion for referral.[14] However, since no pressure level provides a satisfactory balance between sensitivity and specificity, IOP screening may actually be counterproductive unless it is combined with one or more additional tests.

Optic Nerve Head and Peripapillary Retinal Evaluation

Relative Value of Tonometry and Ophthalmoscopy. Studies have been conducted to determine whether IOP measurement or evaluation of the optic nerve head is more useful in the early detection of glaucoma. In one trial of 11,660 subjects, 57 cases of glaucoma with field loss (0.49%) were detected, using a combination of tonometry and ophthalmoscopy.[14] Of these 57 cases, tonometry alone would have detected 28 and ophthalmoscopy alone would have identified 39, but 10 cases would have been missed without the combination of both tests. In other words, IOP screening alone would have missed half of the patients with glaucoma, while disc screening alone would have overlooked nearly one-third of the cases. Most of the cases missed by ophthalmoscopy were early glaucoma with minor field change, while those overlooked by tonometry were more advanced with extensive field loss. Another study was conducted in a health care setting by a nonophthalmologist physician trained in the use of the NCT and the recognition of suspicious discs.[13] Of 770 screenees, 2.5% were referred for elevated IOP alone, 8.7% for abnormal discs, and 2.1% for a combination of both. These studies support the growing impression that optic nerve head screening is more practical and efficient than tonometry. However, because of the difficulty in visualizing and interpreting some discs[15] as well as those cases with high pressure prior to nerve damage, the combination of both tests is essential for the early detection of glaucoma.

Methods of Disc Evaluation. A practical limitation of optic nerve head screening is the need for a trained physician to interpret the findings. In the office of an ophthalmologist or nonophthalmologist physician, this can be accomplished by means of the techniques discussed in Chapter 5. In a mass screening program, however, the use of dilation and the need for a physician create problems. One solution has been to take photographs with a nonmydriatic fundus camera and to send these to an appropriate center for detailed study.[14] The criteria that are considered for referral should include pallor and cup (area, asymmetry, vertical bias, and rim notching), nerve fiber bundle defect, and disc hemorrhage.[13,14] With the continuing advances in technology, it may one day be possible to have automatic analysis of photographs of the optic nerve head.[13]

Visual Function Tests

Since progressive loss of visual function is the ultimate result in all forms of glaucoma, visual function screening tests may offer the most sensitive and specific method of detecting established cases. The main limitation, however, is that most standard techniques for measuring the field of vision, which is currently the most commonly used psychophysical test of visual function in glaucoma, are too time consuming to be practical for mass screening programs. Manual and automated techniques are being developed for visual field screening, which, it is hoped, will reduce the time requirement to an acceptable level, without significantly reducing sensitivity and specificity. Many of these were considered in Chapter 6. The most promising concept is to combine automated perimetry with threshold-related testing of selected points in the field of vision that are more likely to contain early glaucomatous damage.[16–18] These approaches are still limited, however, by the relatively high cost of the instruments, and less expensive, manual techniques are also being developed,[19] which may be a reasonable alternative in some parts of the world. In addition, newer psychophysical tests, such as color vision and contrast sensitivity techniques, may eventually become sufficiently sophisticated to be useful as a rapid means of assessing visual function in the early detection of glaucoma.[20]

High-Risk Populations

The Public Health Service suggests that any medical screening program must detect at least 2% pathology in the general population to be considered a cost-effective measure.[16] Most statistics on the overall prevalence of glaucoma indicate that this group of disorders would not meet the criterion. To become cost-effective, therefore, glaucoma screening programs must be directed at the high-risk segment of a population. With regard to primary open-angle glaucoma, which is the most common target disorder in glaucoma screening programs, the leading risk factors are increasing age, black race, first-degree relatives with glaucoma, high myopia, and vascular disease, including diabetes mellitus.[13] Since several of these factors will be more prevalent in health care settings than in the general population, the screening site becomes another important variable in the success of a glaucoma detection program.

The Screening Site

Community Programs. A commonly used site in the past has been community-based mass public screening clinics (service organization-sponsored programs, health fairs, etc.). However, studies have shown these to be the least efficient form of glaucoma screening, because they provide a low detection rate[13,21] and an inadequate means of ensuring that positive screenees follow through with a proper medical examination.[22] The latter is probably due to the fact that mass screening programs are usually conducted on a periodic basis by volunteers with lack of adequate mechanisms for follow-up. The main value of community programs for the early detection of glaucoma appears to be the public awareness they create for the danger of glaucoma.

Health Care Setting. The preferred alternative to community-based detection programs is the use of health care facilities, for which several options exist.[1,13,14,22] One approach is in-house screening in industrial settings, using *employee health clinics*. In one study, this was found to have the highest follow-up rate,[22] and it provides the potential for excellent screening if it is used properly with physician supervision, although it is limited to those individuals who are in a position to take advantage of it. For the remaining majority of most populations, other health care settings must be considered. *Public health departments* offer a logical setting for glaucoma detection programs as part of multiphasic health testing services.[14] A study in North Carolina has supported the feasibility of such a program, but also indicated the need for better methods of insuring that positive screenees follow-up with an adequate medical examination.[22] Therefore, the remaining, and best, method for the early detection of glaucoma is the *physician's office*. While some large ophthalmology groups may be able to provide effective screening programs within their clinic setting, this is not feasible in most communities. The alternative is to encourage nonophthalmologist physicians (e.g., family physicians, internists, etc.) to include glaucoma screening as part of their routine physical examination.[1,13] Ophthalmologists can probably be most effective in detecting glaucoma in their community by working with their colleagues in other fields of medicine with regard to recognizing suspicious discs, using tonometry, and being aware of the risk factors for glaucoma.

Follow-Up

As noted above, an essential criterion for the success of any detection program is the percentage of positive screenees who follow through with an adequate medical examination. In addition, it is important to periodically evaluate the efficiency of a screening program with regard to the sensitivity and specificity of the detection methods. Both require continuing communication with the ophthalmologist to whom the positive screenees are referred, as well as periodic recall of the negative screenees. As previously discussed, the health care setting again provides the most effective means for achieving this follow-up. However, this cannot be accomplished without careful attention to data collection, storage, and retrieval of data. With the rapid expansion of computer technology in medicine, this will undoubtedly assume an increasingly important role in this aspect of glaucoma detection.

Legal Implications

A detailed appraisal of mass screening for glaucoma (limited to tonometry) concluded that it is legally permissible since the potential benefit (i.e., detection of a sight-threatening disease) outweighs the potential hazards, such as rare ocular injury, the emotional trauma of a false positive test, and the risk of false negative testing.[23] The same report also concluded that full disclosure to the potential screenee of all possible hazards of the test is not required.

SUMMARY

Early detection and treatment of glaucoma is necessary to prevent visual loss.

The lack of early warning signs with most forms of glaucoma necessitates the use of screening programs to detect the disease in its initial stages. Tonometry is neither sufficiently sensitive nor specific enough to be used alone as the screening test. The use of one or more additional studies, especially the evaluation of the optic nerve head or visual field, as well as the use of risk factors for glaucoma, significantly improves both sensitivity and specificity. Other important factors to consider in developing a glaucoma screening program include the screening site and the methods of follow-up.

References

1. Pollack, IP: The challenge of glaucoma screening. Surv Ophthal 13:4, 1968.
2. Packer, H, Deutsch, AR, Deweese, MW, et al: Efficiency of screening tests for glaucoma. JAMA 192:693, 1965.
3. Kahn, JA, Leibowitz, HM, Ganley, JP, et al: The Framingham eye study, outline and major prevalence findings. Am J Epidemiol 106:17, 1977.
4. Armaly, MF: Lessons to be learned from the collaborative glaucoma study. Surv Ophthal 25:139, 1980.
5. Schwartz, JT: Vagary in tonometric screening. Am J Ophthal 64:50, 1967.
6. Dunn, JS, Brubaker, RF: Perkins applanation tonometer. Clinical and laboratory evaluation. Arch Ophthal 89:149, 1973.
7. Krieglstein, GK, Waller, WK: Goldmann applanation versus hand-applanation and Schiøtz indentation tonometry. Graefe's Arch Ophthal 194:11, 1975.
8. Shields, MB: The non-contact tonometer. Its value and limitations. Surv Ophthal 24:211, 1980.
9. Zimmerman, TJ, Worthen, DM: A comparison of two hand-applanation tonometers. Arch Ophthal 88:421, 1972.
10. Kaiden, JS, Zimmerman, TJ, Worthen, DM: An evaluation of the GlaucoTest screening tonometer. Arch Ophthal 92:195, 1974.
11. Krieglstein, GK: Screening tonometry by technicians. Graefe's Arch Ophthal 194:221, 1975.
12. Boothe, WA, Lee, DA, Panek, WC, Pettit, TH: The Tono-Pen. A manometric and clinical study. Arch Ophthal 106:1214, 1988.
13. Levi, L, Schwartz, B: Glaucoma screening in the health care setting. Surv Ophthal 28:164, 1983.
14. Shiose, Y, Komuro, K, Itoh, T, et al: New system for mass screening of glaucoma, as part of automated multiphasic health testing services. Jpn J Ophthal 25:160, 1981.
15. Bechetoille, A, Aouchiche, M, Hartani, D: The study of Touggourt, a proposition for the large scale discovery of chronic glaucoma by examination of the optic disc. J Fr Ophthal 3:495, 1980.
16. Keltner, JL, Johnson, CA: Screening for visual field abnormalities with automated perimetry. Surv Ophthal 28:175, 1983.
17. Kosoko, O, Sommer, A, Auer, C: Screening with automated perimetry using a threshold-related three-level algorithm. Ophthalmology 93:882, 1986.
18. Henson, DB, Bryson, H: Clinical results with the Henson-Hamblin CFS 2000. Doc Ophthal Proc Series 49, 7th Internatl Vis Field Symp, Amsterdam, 233, 1987.
19. Damato, BE: Oculokinetic perimetry: a simple visual field test for use in the community. Br J Ophthal 69:927, 1985.
20. Sponsel, WE: Tonometry in question: can visual screening tests play a more decisive role in glaucoma and management? Surv Ophthal (suppl) 33:291, 1989.
21. Berwick, DM: Screening in health fairs. A critical review of benefits, risks, and costs. JAMA 254:1492, 1985.
22. McPherson, SD Jr: The challenge and responsibilities of a community approach to glaucoma control. The Sightsaving Review 50:15, 1980.
23. Franklin, MA: Medical mass screening programs: a legal appraisal. Cornell Law Quarterly 47:205, 1962.

Section Two

The Clinical Forms of Glaucoma

Chapter 8

CLASSIFICATION OF THE GLAUCOMAS

CLASSIFICATION SYSTEMS

In Section One, we considered the common parameters shared by the many forms of glaucoma, which include the intraocular pressure (IOP) and the influence of elevated pressure on the optic nerve head and visual field. In Section Two, we will look at the specific clinical and histopathologic features that characterize the individual glaucomas. The present chapter provides a brief introduction to the clinical forms of glaucoma within the context of classification systems for these disorders.

There are several systems by which the glaucomas may be classified. The two most commonly used are based on (1) *etiology,* i.e., the underlying disorder that leads to an alteration in aqueous humor dynamics; and (2) *mechanism,* i.e., the specific alteration in the anterior chamber angle that leads to a rise in IOP.

Classification Based on Etiology

The glaucomas may first be divided on the basis of primary and secondary forms. The concept of "primary" and "secondary" glaucoma is obviously artificial, since all of the glaucomas are secondary to some abnormality. The use of these terms in this text, however, relates to any apparent underlying disorder responsible for the alteration in aqueous humor dynamics. *Primary glaucomas* are not consistently associated with obvious systemic or other ocular disorders that might account for this alteration. They are typically bilateral and are generally believed to have a genetic basis. *Secondary glaucomas* are characterized by associated ocular or systemic abnormalities that appear to be responsible for the alteration in aqueous humor dynamics. They may be either unilateral or bilateral and inherited or acquired.

A third group of glaucomas, which is occasionally distinguished from the primary and secondary categories, is the *developmental glaucomas,* in which a developmental abnormality of the anterior chamber angle is responsible for increased resistance to aqueous outflow. One condition within this group is called primary congenital glaucoma, because systemic or other ocular abnormalities are not consistently present. The other forms of developmental glaucoma have additional ocular and systemic anomalies. These developmental glaucomas, with or without associated anomalies, are usually detected during childhood. In addition to these two classes of childhood glaucomas, children are also subject to a variety of nondevelopmental secondary glaucomas.

A classification of the glaucomas based on etiology is presented in Table 8.1, and this system will be used for the organization of chapters in the present section. Many of these conditions have more than one mechanism of IOP elevation, depending on the stage of the disorder. For example, patients with neovascular glaucoma will have an open-angle mechanism during the early stages of their disease, which may eventually progress to an angle-closure mechanism. It may be helpful, therefore, to first consider a classification of the various mechanisms of glaucomas, before studying the individual disorders according to their etiology.

Classification Based on Mechanism

With possible rare exceptions, the elevated IOP in all forms of glaucoma is due

Table 8.1.
A Classification of the Glaucomas Based on Etiology

A. Primary glaucomas
   1. Primary open-angle glaucoma
   2. Primary angle-closure glaucoma
B. Developmental glaucomas
   1. Primary congenital glaucoma
   2. Developmental glaucomas with associated anomalies
C. Secondary glaucomas
   1. Glaucomas associated with primary disorders of the corneal endothelium
   2. Glaucomas associated with disorders of the iris
   3. Glaucomas associated with disorders of the lens
   4. Glaucomas associated with disorders of the retina, vitreous, and choroid
   5. Glaucomas associated with elevated episcleral venous pressure
   6. Glaucomas associated with intraocular tumors
   7. Glaucomas associated with ocular inflammation
   8. Steroid-induced glaucoma
   9. Glaucomas associated with intraocular hemorrhage
   10. Glaucomas associated with ocular trauma
   11. Glaucomas following ocular surgery

to increased resistance to aqueous outflow. The various mechanisms of outflow obstruction can first be divided into *open-angle* and *angle-closure* forms (Table 8.2), a concept introduced by Barkan in 1938.[1]

Open-Angle Glaucomas

As the name implies, these forms of glaucoma occur in eyes with open anterior chamber angles (Fig. 8.1). The mechanism of increased resistance to aqueous outflow in these cases is a direct alteration in the structures involved with aqueous drainage, which may have either a primary, secondary, or developmental etiology.

Primary Open-Angle Glaucoma. In this condition, the actual alteration responsible for the increased resistance to aqueous outflow is uncertain, but the many theories are reviewed in Chapter 9.

Secondary Open-Angle Glaucomas. Among these disorders, several mechanisms of outflow obstruction may be seen (Fig. 8.2). In the *pretrabecular* mechanisms, aqueous outflow is prevented by various types of membranes across the inner surface of the trabecular meshwork in an otherwise open anterior chamber angle. In the *trabecular* forms, the obstruction to aqueous outflow results from alterations within the trabecular meshwork, caused either by the accumulation of material, such as cells, pigment granules, fibrin, etc., or by structural alterations in the trabeculae, such as edema or fibrosis. The *posttrabecular* types of secondary open-angle glaucoma are due to aqueous outflow obstruction distal to the trabecular meshwork, either in Schlemm's canal, the scleral outlet channels, or the episcleral veins.

Developmental Open-Angle Glaucomas. In some forms of developmental glaucoma, the anterior chamber angle is

Table 8.2.
A Classification of the Glaucomas Based on Mechanism

I. Open-angle glaucomas
   A. Primary open-angle glaucomas
   B. Secondary open-angle glaucomas
      1. Pretrabecular forms (membranes)
      2. Trabecular forms
         a. Accumulation of material
         b. Structural alterations
      3. Posttrabecular forms
   C. Developmental open-angle glaucomas
      1. Primary congenital glaucoma
      2. Developmental glaucomas with associated anomalies
II. Angle-closure glaucomas
   A. Primary angle-closure glaucoma
   B. Secondary angle-closure glaucomas
      1. Anterior forms ("pulling" mechanism)
      2. Posterior forms ("pushing" mechanism)
         a. With pupillary block
         b. Without pupillary block
   C. Developmental angle-closure glaucomas

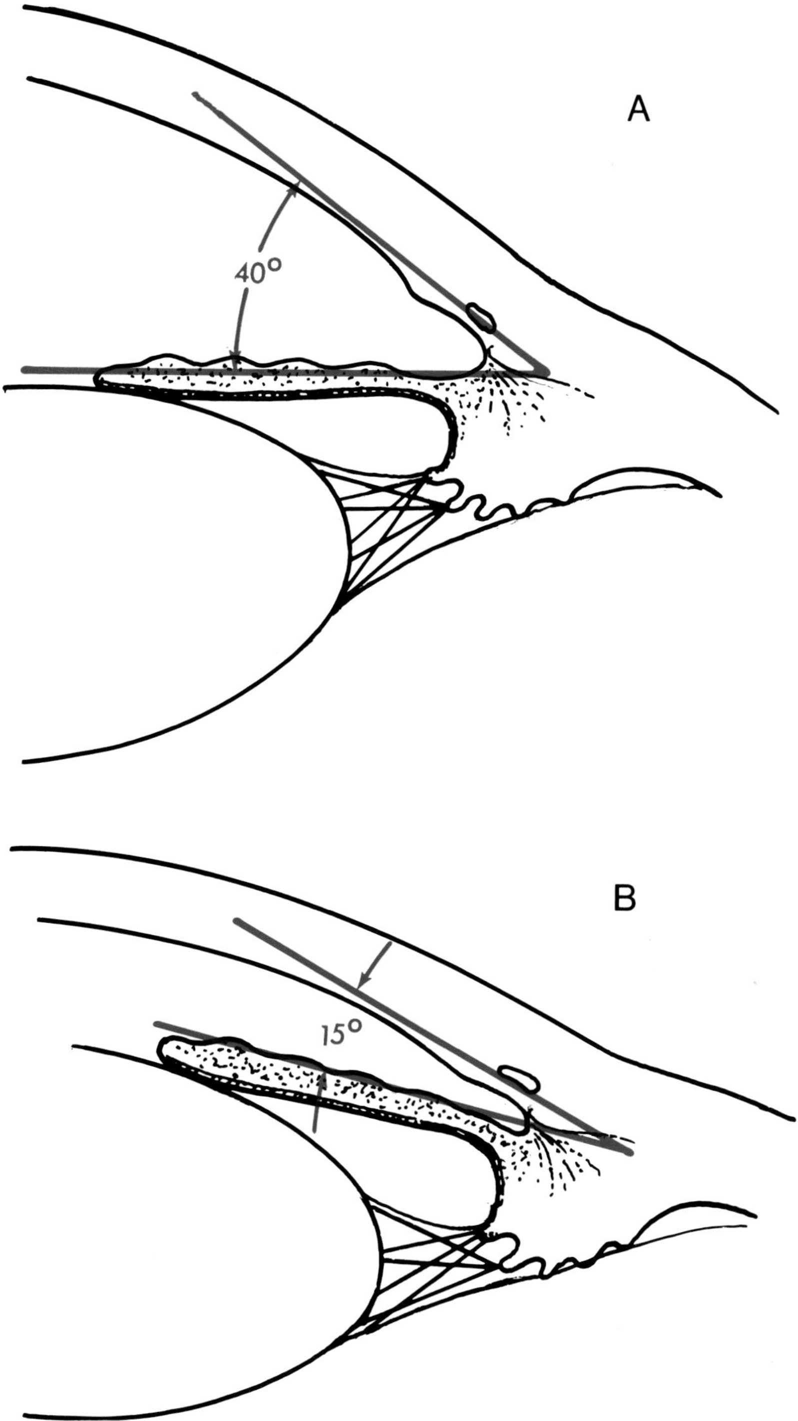

Figure 8.1. The angle of the anterior chamber (*red lines*) is formed by the cornea and iris: **A,** the typical configuration in open-angle forms of glaucoma. **B,** the narrow angle that typically precedes most forms of angle-closure glaucoma.

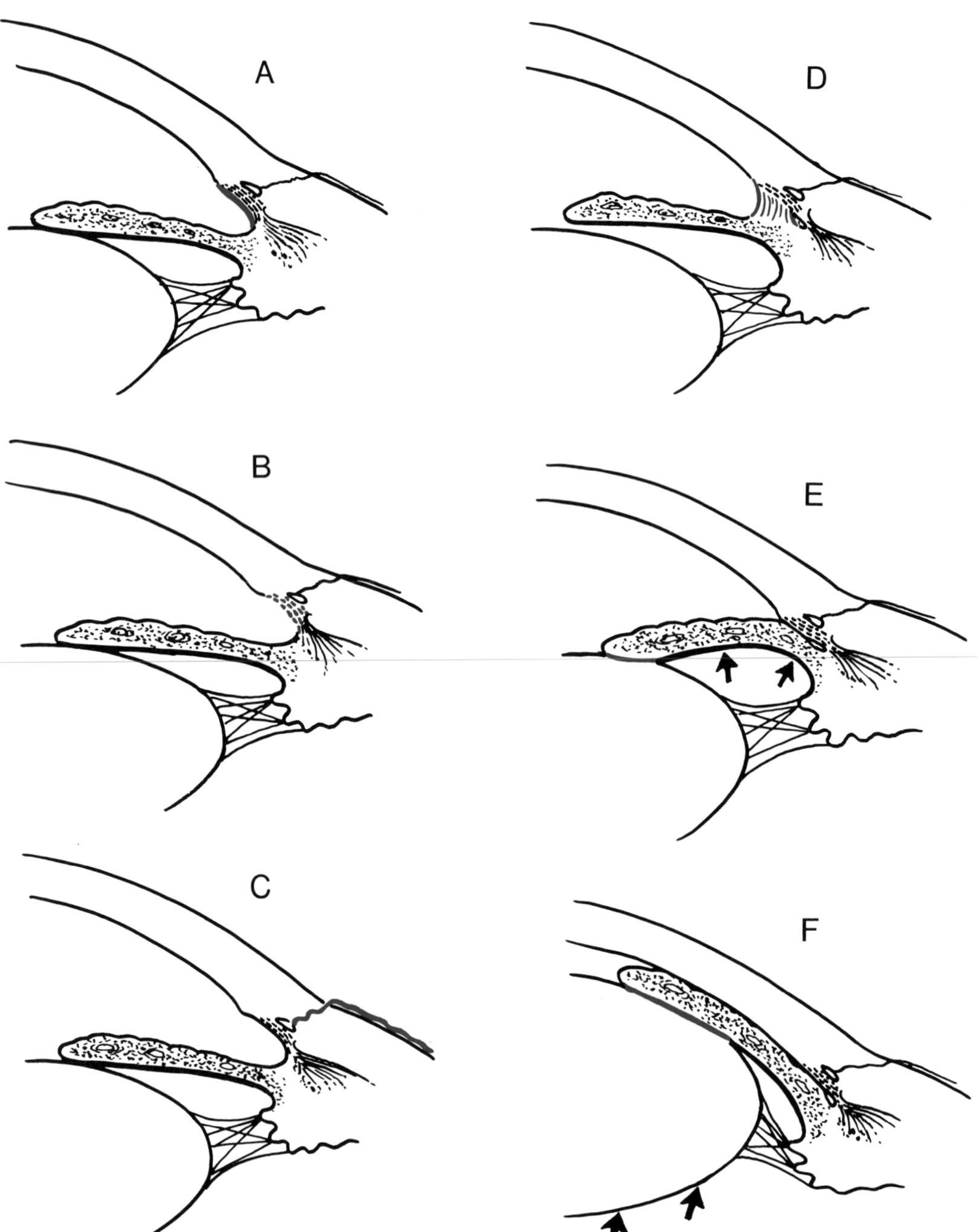

Figure 8.2. Basic mechanisms of secondary glaucomas (the site of obstruction to aqueous outflow is shown in red). Open-angle forms of secondary glaucoma may be of the pretrabecular (**A**), trabecular (**B**), or posttrabecular type (**C**). Angle-closure forms of secondary glaucoma may be of the anterior "pulling" type (**D**) or of the posterior "pushing" type. The latter may occur with (**E**) or without (**F**) pupillary block (*arrows* indicate location of force pushing lens-iris or vitreous-iris diaphragm forward).

open, but there is increased resistance to aqueous outflow. The mechanism in these cases may be either incomplete development of the aqueous outflow system or secondary alterations in these tissues resulting from developmental anomalies of adjacent structures.

Angle-Closure Glaucomas

In these forms of glaucoma, the anterior chamber is shallow and aqueous outflow is blocked by the root of the iris, which lies in apposition to the trabecular meshwork (Fig. 8.1). The aqueous drainage system may be otherwise normal, although concomitant damage to these structures may also be present. As with the open-angle glaucomas, the underlying etiology may be either primary, secondary, or developmental.

Primary Angle-Closure Glaucoma. The factors leading to closure of the anterior chamber angle in this disorder, which are only partly understood, are considered in Chapter 10.

Secondary Angle-Closure Glaucomas. Within this group of glaucomas, a number of conditions have been recognized, which may either pull or push the peripheral iris into the anterior chamber angle (Fig. 8.2). In the *anterior forms* of secondary angle-closure glaucoma, the peripheral iris is pulled into apposition with the trabecular meshwork by the contracture of structures in the anterior chamber angle, such as membranes or inflammatory precipitates. In the *posterior forms* of secondary angle-closure glaucoma, the iris is pushed into the anterior chamber angle by increased pressure behind the iris. These conditions may be further divided into those with and without pupillary block. In the former cases, the peripheral iris bows forward as a result of increased resistance to flow from the posterior to the anterior chamber, which may result from a slight forward shift in the lens-iris diaphragm or from synechiae between the iris and lens. In the posterior forms without pupillary block, there is a forward shift of the lens-iris or vitreous-iris diaphragm resulting from posterior space-occupying changes such as a tumor, hemorrhage, ciliary body congestion, or choridal detachment.

Developmental Angle-Closure Glaucomas. In these forms of glaucoma, the closed angle is a result of either incomplete development of the anterior chamber angle or a secondary closure of the angle due to anomalies of adjacent ocular structures.

SUMMARY

Two methods of classifying the many clinical forms of glaucoma are (1) etiologic and (2) mechanical. The former is based on the underlying disorder that leads to an alteration in aqueous humor dynamics, which may be primary, secondary, or developmental. The mechanical classification is based on the alteration in the anterior chamber angle, which results from the underlying abnormality and leads to the elevated IOP. The latter classification is first divided into open-angle and angle-closure forms of glaucoma, which are then subdivided according to the underlying etiology and specific structural alteration.

References

1. Barkan, O: Glaucoma: classification, causes, and surgical control. Results of microgonioscopic research. Am J Ophthal 21:1099, 1938.

Chapter 9

PRIMARY OPEN-ANGLE GLAUCOMA

TERMINOLOGY

There is general agreement that *primary open-angle glaucoma* (POAG), in its typical form, is defined by the following three criteria: (1) an intraocular pressure (IOP) consistently above 21 mm Hg in at least one eye; (2) an open, normal appearing anterior chamber angle with no apparent ocular or systemic abnormality that might account for the elevated IOP; and (3) typical glaucomatous visual field and/or optic nerve head damage, as described in Chapters 6 and 5, respectively. Synonymous terms that also appear in the literature include *open-angle glaucoma, chronic open-angle glaucoma, chronic simple glaucoma,* and *open-angle glaucoma with damage*.

The Significance of IOP

The commonly used IOP level of 21 mm Hg is based on the concept that two standard deviations above the mean within a Gaussian distribution represents the upper limit of "normal" for that biological parameter. However, since the distribution of IOP in the general population is skewed to the right, or higher pressures, this principle provides only a rough approximation of the normal limits. What is even more important, many eyes will not develop glaucomatous optic atrophy or visual field loss, at least not for long periods of time, despite IOP well above 21 mm Hg, while others will suffer progressive glaucomatous damage at pressures that are never recorded to exceed this level. These latter observations have brought into question the role of IOP in the mechanism of POAG. While there is convincing evidence that IOP is a causative factor, there is also evidence that other causative factors figure into the formula for glaucomatous damage,[1] which would appear to explain the lack of absolute correlation between IOP and the development of POAG. In any case, this discrepancy between IOP level and glaucomatous damage has led to the use of additional terms (and confusion) within the general category of POAG.

Ocular Hypertension

Patients who have the first two criteria for POAG (i.e., an IOP above 21 mm Hg for which there is no apparent cause) but who have normal optic nerve heads and visual fields are commonly said to have *ocular hypertension*.[2,3] Other authors, however, point out disadvantages of this term. Some believe that it does not connote the potential seriousness of the situation (i.e., that a certain percentage of these patients eventually will develop glaucomatous damage) and may lead to a false sense of security on the part of both patient and physician. Furthermore, it is hard to know whether the terminology should arbitrarily be changed to "glaucoma" when the IOP reaches a level at which treatment for pressure alone is believed to be indicated. Chandler and Grant[4] prefer the term *early open-angle glaucoma without damage* for this condition, while Shaffer[5] suggests *glaucoma suspect*. The latter term may also include other risk factors for glaucoma, such as suspicious optic nerve heads. Whatever term one chooses to use for this condition, the most important point is that both physician and patient must be fully aware of its potential consequences. Later in this chapter, we will consider the management of such patients.

Low-Tension Glaucoma

At the other end of the spectrum with regard to susceptibility to IOP are those patients with open, normal appearing anterior chamber angles, who have glaucomatous optic nerve head and visual field damage despite pressures that have never been documented above 21 mm Hg. These patients have traditionally been said to have *low-tension glaucoma*. More recently some authors have used the alternative term *normal-tension glaucoma,* since the IOP is usually "normal" or "high normal" and rarely "low normal." Some believe that low-tension glaucoma is a variant of POAG,[6–8] while others believe that the mechanism of optic atrophy in the two conditions is different.[9–10] Although a number of differences between the two disorders have been described, which are considered later in this chapter, an overlap of findings makes it difficult to clearly separate all of these patients into one category or the other.

It may well be that POAG represents a spectrum of disorders in which several causative factors, of which IOP is one, have varying degrees of influence. For example, one group of investigators has described two subgroups of POAG.[11] The first of these, which they refer to as *senile sclerotic glaucoma,* is seen in the elderly, with relatively low IOP and normal anterior chamber angles; while the second, *high tension glaucoma,* occurs in a younger age group with high IOP and signs of developmental abnormalities of the angle. The two groups are also distinguished by the nature of the optic atrophy, and the appearance of the peripapillary retina and the choroid. In another study, a population of POAG patients revealed two statistically distinct groups: a smaller group with evidence of vasospastic abnormalities and a high correlation between mean deviation index of visual field severity and the highest IOP; and a larger group with evidence of coagulation and biochemical abnormalities but no correlation between the field index and highest IOP.[12] In any case, until a better understanding of the similarities and differences between the various conditions included in the category of POAG becomes available, we will continue to consider them collectively within the present chapter.

EPIDEMIOLOGY

Frequency Among the Glaucomas

Primary open-angle glaucoma is clearly the most common single form of glaucoma, although it is difficult to precisely establish the ratio of individuals with this disorder to the total number of patients with all forms of glaucoma. In one survey of 4231 individuals between the ages of 40 and 75 years, 39 glaucoma patients were detected, of whom 13 (i.e., one-third of the glaucoma population, or 0.28% of the general population) had

POAG.[13] This figure, however, may differ considerably from one population to the next.

Prevalence Within General Populations

Several large surveys have been conducted to determine the number of patients with ocular hypertension and POAG (or glaucoma in general) within a population at a given time.[13–18] The prevalence of glaucoma is less than 1% in most studies, although reports vary considerably according to the population being studied, the diagnostic criteria, and the screening techniques. However, most surveys show that the prevalence of ocular hypertension is considerably higher than that of glaucoma, even when all forms of glaucoma are included, which some investigators take as evidence that elevated IOP does not invariably lead to glaucoma.[19]

Incidence Among Ocular Hypertensives

Numerous studies have been conducted to determine the rate of occurrence of POAG within populations of untreated ocular hypertensives (Table 9.1).[20–30] Most studies spanned an observation period of 5–10 years, during which time the incidence of patients developing glaucomatous field loss was roughly 1% per year. However, there are large differences in the results of these studies, which suggest variable degrees of susceptibility among populations of ocular hypertensives. It should also be kept in mind that "normotensive" individuals may develop glaucoma. In some cases this may represent low-tension glaucoma, while other patients may initially have IOPs below 21 mm Hg but later have a rise in pressure and develop POAG.[29,30]

Natural History of Field Loss in POAG

Leydhecker[31] studied the distribution of IOP and glaucomatous visual field loss in a large population survey. When persons with pressures higher than 20 mm Hg and those with definite glaucomatous field defects were plotted against their age, the two slopes were parallel and separated horizontally by 18 years, which led to the notion that 10–20 years may elapse between the onset of ocular hypertension and the development of visual field loss. This concept may be subject to considerable error, however, since the study did not show that the same individuals with elevated pressures were the ones who subsequently developed field loss. Lichter and Shaffer[32] found that field loss in a population of 378 ocular hypertensives, observed for a period averaging 12¾ years, occurred earlier than Leydhecker suggested, despite the fact that most were being treated during this time. Furthermore, once field loss has occurred, further damage tends to progress more rapidly than in the fellow undamaged eye exposed to the same IOP,[33] which appears to reflect

Table 9.1.
Incidence of Primary Open-Angle Glaucoma Among Ocular Hypertensives

Investigator(s)	No. Ocular Hypertensives (Patients)	Observation Period (Years)	No. Developed Open-Angle Glaucoma (Patients)
Perkins[20,30]	124	5–7	4 (3.2%)
Walker[21]	109	11	11 (11%)
Wilensky, et al.[22]	50	avg. 6	3 (6%)
Norskov[23]	68	5	0
Linner[24]	92	10	0
Kitazawa, et al.[25]	75	avg. 9.5	7 (9.3%)
David, et al.[26]	61	avg. 3.3 range 1–11	10 (16.4%)
Hart, et al.[27]	92	5	33 (35%)
Armaly, et al.[29]	5886	13	(1.7%)
Lundberg, et al.[28]	41	20	14 (34%)

the increased susceptibility of the damaged eye.[34]

RISK FACTORS

Primary open-angle glaucoma has no associated symptoms or other warning signs prior to the development of advanced visual field loss. It is for this reason that glaucoma screening programs, as discussed in Chapter 7, are needed for the early detection of this disorder. Such programs must use the following risk factors, which are commonly associated with the disease, to identify those segments of the population requiring the closest attention. In addition, once a patient has been found to have persistent IOP elevation (the most significant risk factor) but no apparent optic nerve head or visual field damage, the physician must consider the additional risk factors in trying to decide which of these individuals require closer observation or the initiation of therapy before definite damage. These risk factors can be considered in two categories: (1) the general features of patients with POAG, and (2) the clinical features that are detected during the basic glaucoma examination.

General Features of Patients

Age. All studies agree that the prevalence of primary open-angle glaucoma increases with the age of the population being considered.[17,35–38] It is unusual for the disorder to reach the clinical stage before the age of 40, and most cases are seen after age 65. For example, in one general population survey of 3000 individuals, the prevalence of POAG and low-tension glaucoma by age group was 0.22% among 40–49 year olds, 0.10% for 50–59, 0.57% for 60–69, 2.81% for 70–79, and 14.29% for patients 80+ years of age.[35] Age, therefore, becomes an increasingly significant risk factor with each decade.

It is important to emphasize, however, that POAG is by no means limited to those over 40 years of age. In one study, 25% of glaucoma patients 10–35 years old had this form of glaucoma.[39] Another study of 13 POAG patients under 40 years of age, four of whom were in their teens, emphasized the unusual severity of the disease in younger patients and stressed the need for applanation tonometry in all individuals old enough to permit the study.[40]

Race. Several studies have shown that POAG is more prevalent, develops at an earlier age, and is more severe in blacks as compared with whites.[41–45] In one large population survey of Jamaicans, the prevalence of the disease was approximately 1.4%,[43] while 81.6% of 140 patients with open-angle glaucoma in another study were black, compared with a 48.7% prevalence of blacks from a random sample of the same population.[44] Furthermore, nonwhites are said to have 7–8 times more blindness from glaucoma than whites.[45] In another study, 25 black and 47 white ocular hypertensives were followed for 1–12 years, during which time glaucomatous damage developed in 18.1% of the former and 5.4% of the latter group.[43] One possible explanation for this racial difference in susceptibility to elevated IOP might be the high incidence of sickle cell anemia among blacks, increasing the potential for optic nerve head ischemia. However, this theory was not supported in a study that found sickle trait in only 2 of 40 blacks undergoing filtering surgery for POAG.[46] Another possible explanation for the increased susceptibility in blacks is the observation in one study of larger physiologic cup-disc ratios as compared with whites.[47]

Sex. The prognostic significance of sex is less clear than that of age and race, although several studies suggest a higher prevalence among men.[14,15,17,48,49]

Diabetes Mellitus. The prevalence of POAG and ocular hypertension is several times higher in the diabetic population than in the general population, according to most surveys.[49–52] In addition, the prevalence of diabetes or a positive glucose tolerance test is higher in patients with POAG[51,53] or a high IOP response to topical steroids.[51,54]

Other Endocrine Disorders. One study suggested that POAG patients have an increased prevalence of various thyroid disorders,[55] while another investigation revealed low normal protein-bound iodine and radioactive iodine uptake.[56] However, baseline thyroxine, thyrotropin (TSH), and triiodothyronine (T_3) resin uptake levels in patients with POAG did not differ from normal values.[57] Other endocrine disorders have not been associated with POAG but may influence the IOP and, therefore, should be considered in the diagnosis and management of glaucoma. For example, elevated IOP has occurred in patients with Cushing's syndrome, with normalization of pressure after treatment of the systemic disease.[58,59] One study showed that relatives of such patients were often positive topical steroid responders (discussed later in this chapter) and suggested this as the mechanism of the pressure rise.[59] Pituitary dysfunction may be associated with instability of IOP[60] and aqueous humor dynamics,[61] and elevated estrogen or progesterone may lower the pressure,[62] while male hormones may raise it.[63]

Cardiovascular and Hematologic Abnormalities. These systemic disorders are particularly common among patients with low-tension glaucoma, which is discussed later in this chapter. The association of these abnormalities is less clear among patients with the high pressure form of POAG. Some investigators found an association with hemodynamic crisis and low diastolic ophthalmic artery pressure or diastolic blood pressure.[49,64–66] However, other studies showed an association with increased systemic blood pressure,[67,68] and yet others revealed no significant deviation from the general population.[69,70] While most patients do not suffer optic nerve damage following a sudden loss in blood pressure, there is evidence that this may increase the risk of further nerve damage among glaucoma patients.[71] These individuals should be followed closely for evidence of changes in the optic nerve head or visual field during situations such as the adjustment of medication for systemic hypertension or general surgery. A plasma lipid profile was not found to be helpful in identifying open-angle glaucoma patients.[72]

Family History. A family history of POAG is generally considered to be a significant prognostic indicator. Primary open-angle glaucoma is believed to have a genetic basis. Although the exact hereditary mode is unknown, indirect evidence suggests that it is most likely polygenetic or multifactorial. Of more immediate concern to the clinician, however, is the increased prevalence of POAG among close relatives of glaucoma patients, which ranges from 5–19% according to two reports.[73,74] In a 10–12-year follow-up of 101 patients with a family history of POAG, 3% developed glaucoma and another 6% became glaucoma suspects.[75] Another survey revealed a family history of glaucoma in 50% of patients with open-angle glaucoma.[76] A preliminary study also suggested an association between open-angle glaucoma in caucasians and the rhesus D(+) blood group.[77]

Clinical Features

Intraocular Pressure. As previously noted, an elevated IOP is only a risk factor for the development of POAG, although it is a causative risk factor and most studies agree that it is the most important single prognostic risk factor. The degree of risk for developing glaucomatous damage is related to the level of IOP. One study of 307 patients revealed the following prevalence of optic nerve head damage in each pressure group:[78]

IOP (mm Hg)	*Percent with Nerve Damage*
25–29	7
30–34	14
35–39	52
40–44	61
45–49	73
50–54	83
55–59	83
>60	70

A fluctuation in the IOP is also important and may have more prognostic value than an individual pressure reading.[68] In one study, ocular hypertensives whose pressures increased with time had a greater risk of developing glaucomatous damage.[79] In another study, 15% of ocular hypertensive patients had an IOP rise of 5–9 mm Hg when going from the sitting to the supine position, suggesting the value of measuring the pressure in this position when evaluating such individuals.[80] Despite the importance of IOP as a risk factor in most forms of glaucoma, it must be emphasized, as discussed in Chapter 7, that this parameter will not always be abnormal, especially with single measurements. In one population survey, 8 of 15 newly diagnosed cases had pressures below 20.5 mm Hg.[81]

Optic Nerve Head. The second most significant risk factor for the development of POAG is the size of the physiologic cup before glaucomatous damage occurs. Although Armaly[82] found that the cup/disc ratio was not related to a family history of POAG, Chandler and Grant[83] observed that a wide, deep physiologic cup tolerates increased IOP poorly and the tendency is toward enlargement and total cupping. This concept was supported by a study in which 27 of 102 ocular hypertensives who developed field loss during a 5-year observation period had significantly larger vertical cup/disc ratios than those who did not develop field loss.[84] In another study, eyes that were falsely suspected of having field loss on the basis of the optic nerve head appearance had a high incidence of subsequent field loss.[85] Eyes with the combination of IOP consistently above 28 mm Hg and cup/disc ratios of 0.5 or greater are at such a high risk of developing glaucomatous damage that therapy should probably be started.[84]

The greatest diagnostic value of observing the optic nerve head comes when the first definite evidence of progressive glaucomatous damage is detected.[86] A helpful early finding is defects in the retinal nerve fiber layer, which may be found in association with glaucomatous optic atrophy before apparent changes are seen in the nerve head.[87] These features were considered in detail in Chapter 5, and the importance of close observation for these changes in glaucoma suspects is reemphasized.

Myopia. There is an increased prevalence of POAG among myopes,[88] as well as an increased frequency of myopia among patients who have POAG, ocular hypertension, and low-tension glaucoma.[89] Of particular clinical significance is the observation that myopic eyes are more susceptible to the effects of elevated IOP. Of 10 patients who developed glaucomatous field defects during observation for raised IOP, six were myopic (less than -1.00 diopter), three were emmetropes ($+1.00$ to -1.00 diopters), and one was hyperopic (more than $+1.00$ diopter).[89] Surprisingly, however, once IOP has been lowered by means of therapy, the visual fields of myopic eyes improve more often and worsen less often than those of nonmyopic eyes, which may relate to the increased susceptibility of the latter group to risk factors that are independent of IOP, such as low ophthalmic artery pressure.[90]

Cornea. The cornea is typically normal in POAG. In one study, patients with cornea guttata were reported to frequently have abnormal tonographic values,[91] and preliminary specular microscopic studies of patients with chronic glaucoma suggested abnormal corneal endothelium.[92] However, a subsequent study comparing individuals with normal IOP, untreated ocular hypertension, treated ocular hypertension, or POAG revealed no significant difference in the central corneal endothelial density or central corneal thickness.[93]

Gonioscopy. By traditional definition, the anterior chamber angle in eyes with POAG is open and grossly normal, as described in Chapter 3. Preliminary studies, however, suggest that these patients may have more iris processes, a higher insertion of the iris root, more trabecular meshwork pigmentation,[94] and a greater than normal degree of segmentation in the pigmentation of the meshwork.[95]

Visual Abnormalities. Central visual acuity, as measured by standard clinical tests, typically remains normal until peripheral visual field loss is advanced and is, therefore, of no value in the early detection of POAG. However, preliminary evidence suggests that more subtle abnormalities in vision, such as contrast sensitivity and color vision (discussed in Chapter 6), may one day be useful as risk factors in diagnosing POAG prior to the development of typical visual field loss. There is also evidence that motion perception, as measured with a dynamic random dot display, is abnormal in POAG and may be detected before apparent optic nerve damage.[96] Once typical glaucomatous damage to the visual field has been documented in one eye, the diagnosis of glaucoma is usually established, and there is a high incidence of subsequent field loss in the fellow eye. The latter was reported to be 29% in 31 patients followed for 3–7 years,[97] and 25% in 104 individuals after 5 years of follow-up in another series.[98]

LOW-TENSION GLAUCOMA

As noted earlier in this chapter, there are those who consider low-tension glaucoma to be clearly distinguishable from the high-tension form of POAG. There is, in fact, considerable evidence, which is considered in this section, that the two entities differ in several ways beyond only the IOP levels. However, reports are conflicting and it is difficult to draw a clear division between the two conditions. It may be that POAG is a spectrum of disorders, in which elevated IOP is the most influential causative factor at one end, while other factors that influence glaucomatous optic atrophy predominate at the other end. In any case, we will now consider some of the clinical differences between low-tension glaucoma and the high-tension form of POAG and the mechanisms that might be responsible for these differences.

Clinical Differences From High-Tension POAG

Optic Nerve Head. The neural rim has been found by some to be significantly thinner in low-tension patients, especially inferiorly and inferotemporally, than in high-tension patients with comparable total visual field loss.[99,100] Other studies, however, have revealed less striking differences. In one study, the discs were similar, although cupping in low-tension glaucoma was broadly sloping, resulting in less disc volume alteration.[101] In another study, the only significant difference in disc appearance was an increased prevalence in the high-tension group of an "hourglass pattern" to the lamina cribrosa, in which thick connective tissue bundles crossed horizontally between 3 and 9 o'clock, with thinner bundles and larger pores above and below.[102] While this finding was not so striking as to allow segregation of the two forms of POAG on that basis alone, it was believed to suggest that the architecture of the lamina may be a causative factor in low-tension glaucoma. Yet another study found that optic disc hemorrhages were more prevalent in the low-tension group, raising the possibility of vascular disease as another causative factor in these patients.[103] In the latter study, the low-tension eyes could be divided into those that frequently develop recurrent disc hemorrhages and those that rarely bleed, providing more evidence for multiple causative factors in low-tension glaucoma.

Visual Fields. Differences have also been reported in the nature of visual field loss between low-tension and high-tension POAG patients with comparable optic nerve damage. In general, low-tension glaucoma patients appear to have deeper, more localized scotomata,[100,104,105] although one study found no significant difference in the depth or slopes of the scotomata.[106] There are also conflicting reports regarding the proximity of scotomata to fixation between the two groups, which may relate to the testing methods.[106,107] One study found a significantly greater rate of progressive visual field loss in low-tension glaucoma,[108] and another revealed a difference in the pattern of the progression, with the high-tension patients initially increasing mainly in area and later in depth, while the increases in area and depth remained in constant proportion in low-tension glaucoma patients.[109]

Possible Mechanisms of Low-Tension Glaucoma

Influence of Intraocular Pressure. Although low-tension glaucoma, by definition, is distinguished from the high-tension form of POAG by an IOP that is never recorded to exceed 21 mm Hg, the pressures do tend to be higher and to have wider diurnal variations than those in the normal population.[110] Furthermore, in low-tension patients with asymmetric IOP, the visual field loss is typically worse in the eye with the higher pressure.[111,112] These observations suggest that slightly elevated IOP is a causative factor in low-tension glaucoma, although other factors are also involved.

Other Causative Factors. As noted earlier in this section, additional causative factors may relate to the architecture of the lamina cribrosa[102] and the vascular perfusion of the optic nerve head.[103] Drance and co-workers[6,7] described two forms of low-tension glaucoma: (1) a *nonprogressive form,* which is usually associated with a transient episode of vascular shock; and (2) a *progressive form,* which is believed to result from chronic vascular insufficiency of the optic nerve head. A variety of cardiovascular and hematologic abnormalities have been described, which might account for both forms,[113] and Hayreh[114] has suggested that low-tension glaucoma differs from anterior ischemic optic neuropathy only in that the latter is a more acute process. Reported associated findings include hemodynamic crises[6,7] and reduced diastolic ophthalmodynamometry levels[6,113] and ocular pulse amplitudes,[115] while reports of alterations in systemic blood pressure are conflicting.[6,9,67,113] Visual evoked responses during stepwise artificially increased IOP were significantly different between patients with low-tension and high-tension POAG, suggesting a lack of autoregulation of optic nerve head circulation in the former group.[116] Patients with low-tension glaucoma have also been found to have an increased frequency of headaches with or without migraine features[117] and an abnormally reduced blood flow in the fingers in response to exposure to cold.[118] The latter observations suggest the possibility of vasospastic events in the mechanism of low-tension glaucoma, with therapeutic implications that are discussed at the end of this chapter.

Hematologic abnormalities that have been reported to be associated with low-tension glaucoma include increased blood and plasma viscosity[119] and hypercoagulability (e.g., increased platelet adhesiveness and euglobulin lysis time).[6,112] Other studies, however, have revealed no statistically significant abnormalities in coagulation tests[120,121] or in vascular or rheologic profiles.[121] Hypercholesterolemia has also been reported to be higher among patients with low-tension glaucoma.[122]

Whatever factors may have a causative role in low-tension glaucoma, it is likely that they have a genetic basis, with one reported family having an autosomal dominant mode.[123]

Differential Diagnosis of Low-Tension Glaucoma

The differential diagnosis of low-tension glaucoma should include wide diurnal IOP fluctuations, in which high pressures are occurring at times when they are not being recorded. Other patients may have once had high pressures that caused damage but that have since spontaneously normalized. One example of this is pigmentary glaucoma, in which the IOP often improves with increasing age.[124] Another situation to distinguish from low-tension glaucoma is the individual with advanced optic atrophy and visual field loss, in which even high normal pressures often cause further progressive damage. It is also important to rule out nonglaucomatous causes of disc and field changes, as discussed in Chapters 5 and 6.

ADJUNCTIVE TESTS

Numerous tests have been studied in an attempt to find additional prognostic indicators of POAG. Although none of these has yet been clearly proved to be of clinical value, the physician should be familiar with some of the more frequently discussed adjunctive tests.

Tonography

The details of this procedure and its limitations as a clinical tool in the diagnosis of POAG were discussed in Chapter 3.

Water Provocative Test

Drinking a large quantity of water in a short period of time will generally lead to a rise in the IOP. Based on the theory that glaucomatous eyes have a greater pressure response to water drinking, a "provocative" test was developed for the early detection of POAG.

Procedure. After an 8-hour fast, the test begins with baseline applanation tonometric readings. Indentation tonometry is unsatisfactory, since water drinking reduces ocular rigidity.[125] The patient is then instructed to drink approximately 1 liter of tap water, following which applanation tonometry is performed every 15 minutes for 1 hour. The maximum IOP rise usually occurs in 15–30 minutes and returns to the initial level after approximately 60 minutes in both normal and glaucomatous eyes.[126] A rise of 8 mm Hg is generally considered to be a significant response. It has also been suggested that performing tonography after a water drinking test has additional diagnostic value.[127,128]

Mechanism. The mechanism of IOP rise after water drinking is uncertain. One theory is that reduced serum osmolality might cause increased aqueous inflow, although studies have revealed an inconsistent correlation between the IOP and serum osmolality.[129,130] Tonographic studies have shown reduced aqueous outflow facility in human[131–133] and rabbit[134] eyes, and a suggestion of increased aqueous production has been observed in monkeys.[135]

Clinical value. Kronfeld[133] found that the combined water drinking test and tonography gave statistically significant lowering of aqueous outflow facility in 35 ocular hypertensives. However, the response was too small to be clinically significant for the individual patient. He concluded that the two tests in this situation added little to the information provided by tonometry. Two additional studies suggest that the water provocative test has no diagnostic value, since 22% false positives and 48% false negatives were found in one series,[136] while the other group had 24% false negatives.[137]

Dilation Provocative Tests

These tests are used primarily in eyes suspected of having potentially occludable anterior chamber angles, which are discussed in the next chapter. However, cycloplegics and mydriatics have also been studied with regard to their influence on open-angle forms of glaucoma. Although these studies have not yet provided clinically useful diagnostic tests for POAG, it is important to understand how different eyes respond to these drugs, especially when interpreting a mydriatic provocative test for angle-closure glaucoma.

Cycloplegic Effect. *Strong topical cycloplegics,* such as 1% cyclopentolate, 1% atropine, 5% homatropine, or 0.25% scopolamine, have been shown to cause a significant IOP rise (greater than 6 mm Hg) in many eyes with POAG.[138] Oral atropine did not influence IOP with short-term administration in POAG patients,[139] although some had a pressure rise after 1 week of medication.[140] A pressure response to topical cycloplegics may also occur in eyes with angle-closure glaucoma when an uncontrolled pressure persists despite a patent iridectomy[141] and in nonglaucomatous eyes after several weeks of topical dexamethasone.[142] Primary open-angle glaucoma eyes are more likely to have this pressure rise if they are being treated with miotics,[143] and the mechanism of the pressure response to strong cycloplegics is believed to include inhibition of the miotic effect and direct inhibitory action on the ciliary muscle.[143,144]

A *weak cycloplegic,* such as 1% tropicamide, may also cause a pressure rise in some patients with open-angle glaucoma, especially when on miotic therapy, suggesting that the mechanism is competition with the miotic.[145,146] In one study, this did not correlate with the early IOP response after argon laser trabeculoplasty.[146]

Mydriatic Effect. The mydriatic action of cycloplegic-mydriatic agents, or a mydriatic such as phenylephrine, is also believed to cause elevated IOP in some eyes with open anterior chamber angles.[147–151] This occurs only when there is an associated shower of pigment in the anterior chamber, and the mechanism is thought to be temporary obstruction of the trabecular meshwork by pigment granules. This occurs predominantly in eyes with the exfoliation syndrome or pigmentary glaucoma but may also occur in some cases of POAG with heavy pigmentation in the anterior chamber angle.[147–151] In one case of POAG, the postdilation pressure rise was permanent, and histopathology of the trabeculectomy specimens suggested that this was due to a breakdown of the endothelium covering the trabecular beams.[151]

Therapeutic Trials

Based on a theory that eyes with POAG respond to antiglaucoma drugs with a greater IOP response than is the case with nonglaucomatous eyes, the following attempts have been made to develop prognostic tests.

Epinephrine Test. There is evidence that patients with POAG may be particularly sensitive to epinephrine.[152] Such individuals reportedly have a greater IOP drop and more frequent cardiac arrhythmias in response to topical epinephrine than do patients with secondary glaucoma.[152] It has been theorized that the mechanism of this increased responsiveness is an epinephrine-stimulated rise in intraocular cyclic adenosine monophosphate to which the POAG patient may be unusually sensitive.[153,154] Based on this apparent sensitivity to epinephrine, a test was devised in which 1–2% epinephrine twice daily was administered, and a pressure drop of more than 5 mm Hg over a 1–7-day period was considered a "response."[155] (A subsequent study indicated that the pressure drop 4 hours after a single dose could also be used as the indicator of response.[156]) In a 5–10-year follow-up of 80 ocular hypertensives, 85% of those who developed field loss were positive responders, while only 28% without field loss had shown the positive response.[155] However, in another study the positive response was found in 53% of 32 ocular hypertensives and 56% of 18 open-angle glaucoma patients with field loss.[157] Further study is needed, therefore, to confirm the prognostic value of this test.

Other Therapeutic Trials. Other tests that have been suggested include the *pilocarpine test,* in which an IOP drop of more than 4 mm Hg at the peak of the diurnal curve, in response to pilocarpine therapy, is thought to suggest glaucoma.[158] The *acetazolamide test* is used to estimate the coefficient of aqueous outflow facility based on applanation IOP measurements after the drug is given intravenously.[159] Neither of these tests, however, has confirmed clinical value.

Uniocular Therapeutic Trial. While the value of the therapeutic trials discussed above awaits further study, an entirely different concept of therapeutic trials has clinical value today. Administration of a topical antiglaucoma drug to one eye (using the other as a control) is a valuable clinical adjunct in helping to decide whether or not to institute medical therapy in ocular hypertensives, as well as in establishing the efficacy of a particular medical regimen. The purpose of this trial is simply to determine the effectiveness in reducing IOP and the side effects that can be expected from that medication.[160] It has been suggested that this information can be obtained, at least in part, during a 4-hour office trial with 2% pilocarpine.[161]

Topical Steroid Response

In the next section of this chapter, we will consider the influence of corticosteroids in the mechanism of POAG. The tendency of these patients, as well as a certain percentage of the general population, to respond to topical steroid therapy with an IOP rise has also been evaluated as a predictive test for POAG. Of 788 normotensives or ocular hypertensives, treated with 0.1% dexamethasone four times daily for 6 weeks and followed for a minimum of 5 years, glaucomatous visual field loss developed in 31% of high responders (IOP greater than 31 mm Hg during the steroid administration), 3.4% of intermediate responders (20–30 mm Hg), and in no low responders (less than 20 mm Hg).[162] However, the predictive value of this test was not as good as that of a multivariate analysis of the risk factors discussed earlier in this chapter.

IOP Effect on Visual Function

The influence of transient, artificially-induced IOP elevation on the visual field helps to identify which eyes are more susceptible to raised pressure[163] and may provide a possible approach to the early identification of POAG patients.[164] Using the reverse approach, a reduction in the vertical diameter of the blind spot has been correlated with declining IOP following oral antiglaucoma medication to establish the pressure level that the eye can tolerate.[165] However, long-term investigations are needed to establish the value of these tests as prognostic indicators.

Other Reported Tests

It was once suggested that populations of POAG patients have significantly more nontasters of phenylthiourea[166] or phenylthiocarbamide, although this was not confirmed in a subsequent study.[167] It was also reported that patients with POAG have a higher prevalence of the histocompatibility (HLA) antigens HLA-B12 and HLA-B7,[168] although numerous studies have subsequently shown no significant correlation between HLA antigens and glaucoma.[169–178]

THEORIES OF MECHANISM

As with virtually all forms of glaucoma, elevation of the IOP in POAG is due to obstruction of aqueous outflow. However, the precise mechanism(s) of outflow obstruction in this condition has not been fully explained, despite the fact that it has been studied more than in any other type of glaucoma. The following data from these studies provide only suggestions of what the final answer may hold.

Histopathologic Observations

The most likely source for the eventual explanation of aqueous outflow obstruction in POAG lies in the study of histopathologic material. However, the interpretation of these findings must take into consideration additional influences, such as age, the secondary effects of prolonged IOP elevation, the alterations that medical and surgical treatment of the glaucoma might have induced, and artifacts created by tissue processing.

Trabecular Meshwork. Grant[179] demonstrated that the largest proportion of resistance to aqueous outflow in enucleated human eyes could be eliminated by incising the trabecular meshwork. Whether this tissue is the actual site of abnormal resistance in POAG has not been determined, but the following observations have been reported.

Collagen of the trabecular beams is fragmented, with thickening of the glass membrane, increased curly collagen, diffuse nodular proliferation of extracellular long-spacing collagen, coiling of fiber bundles, and changes in orientation and osmophilia of the fibers.[180–183] However, similar changes are seen in association with aging, and one study found that the changes correlated more closely with age than with reduction in outflow facility,[184] while another revealed no statistical difference in mean collagen levels of the meshwork between eyes with POAG and age-matched normal eyes.[185] It has been suggested that the changes in POAG may represent an exaggeration of the normal aging process.[186]

Endothelial cells lining the trabeculae appear to be more active than in normotensive eyes[181–183] and are reported to show proliferation with foamy degeneration and basement membrane thickening.[180,182] The cellularity of the trabecular meshwork in eyes with POAG is lower than in nonglaucomatous eyes, but the rate of decline with age is similar in the two groups.[187] A reduced frequency of actin filaments (contractile proteins) in trabecular endothelium has also been demonstrated in eyes with POAG.[188]

Intertrabecular spaces, as might be anticipated from the general thickening of the trabeculae, are narrowed.[182,185] In addition, they may contain red blood cells, pigment, and dense amorphous material.[182] It has also been reported that glycosaminoglycans are more abundant in the meshwork of human eyes with POAG.[183,189] A scanning electron microscopic study of 10 trabeculectomy specimens revealed an unknown substance coating the meshwork that was believed to be sufficient to obstruct aqueous outflow,[190] although this finding has not been confirmed by other investigators.[191–193] Perfusion of cationized ferritin in enucleated eyes of POAG patients suggests that the outflow obstruction is segmental.[194]

Juxtacanilicular connective tissue just beneath the inner wall endothelium of Schlemm's canal has been noted by several observers to contain a layer of amorphous, osmophilic material.[183,184,195–198] This has been described as moderately electron-dense, nonfibrillar material[184] with characteristics of basement membrane and curly collagen[197] and cytochemical properties of chondroitin sulfate protein complex.[184] However, the concentration of electron-dense materials, while significantly higher than that of normal controls, is not believed to be enough to account for the outflow reduction characteristic of POAG.[198] Matrix vesicles, representing extracellular lysosomes,[199] a sheath material from subendothelial elastic-like fibers,[200] and the extracellular glycoprotein fibronectin,[201] have also been found in abnormal amounts in the juxtacanalicular tissue of eyes with POAG. These patients also differ from the normal population in collagen binding of plasma fibronectin.[202] Giant vacuoles, as described in Chapter 2, are found in the inner wall endothelium of Schlemm's canal in normal eyes and are thought to be related to aqueous transport. In eyes with POAG, the giant vacuoles have been found in most studies to be decreased or absent.[168,169,182,183,197,203,204]

Schlemm's Canal. A collapse of Schlemm's canal will also increase resistance to aqueous outflow and has been proposed as the mechanism of outflow obstruction in POAG.[205–206] The collapse represents a bulge of trabecular meshwork into the canal, which might result from alterations in the meshwork and/or relaxation of the ciliary muscle. In support of this theory, some histopathologic studies have revealed a narrowed Schlemm's canal with adhesions between the inner and outer walls.[182,183,205] A mathematical model of Schlemm's canal, however, tentatively suggests that resistance to aqueous outflow is in the inner wall of the canal and is not caused by a weakening of the trabecular meshwork with a resultant collapse of Schlemm's canal alone.[207]

Intrascleral Channels. Alterations of the intrascleral outflow channels could also be a mechanism of increased resistance to aqueous outflow in POAG. Histopathologic observations have revealed attenuation of the channels, which may be due to a swelling of glycosaminoglycans in the adjacent sclera.[180] Krasnov[208] has suggested that intrascleral blockage may be the mechanism of outflow obstruction in approximately half of the eyes with POAG. However, this theory was not supported by a study in which removal of tissue overlying Schlemm's canal did not improve outflow facility until the canal was actually entered.[205]

Influence of Aqueous Humor

There is also the possibility that abnormal constituents of the aqueous humor may adversely affect the outflow structures to increase resistance to outflow. In one study, the relative concentration of a protein doublet was significantly different in the aqueous of POAG patients as compared with controls.[209]

Corticosteroid Sensitivity

As previously noted, there is evidence that patients with POAG are unusually sensitive to corticosteroids and that this steroid sensitivity may be related to the abnormal resistance to aqueous outflow. We will consider first the evidence for the increased sensitivity and then look at theories of how this may influence outflow.

Topical Corticosteroid Response. It has been well documented that chronic corticosteroid therapy, especially with topical administration, leads to elevated IOP in many individuals. In a small percentage of the general population, the magnitude of this pressure rise is sufficient to cause a severe form of secondary glaucoma, which is considered in Chapter 20. The present discussion is limited to prospective studies of topical steroid response in various populations.

General population studies have been performed in which a potent topical corticosteroid, such as 0.1% betamethasone or 0.1% dexamethasone, was given 3–4 times daily for 3–6 weeks. These studies all agree that a significant number of individuals will respond with variable degrees of IOP elevation. The studies differ considerably, however, with regard to many important aspects of this pressure response. For example, the distribution of pressure responses in the general population was found in some studies to be trimodal, with approximately two-thirds having a low response (usually defined as a rise of less than 5 mm Hg), one-third showing an intermediate response (6–15 mm Hg rise), and 4–5% having a rise greater than 15 mm Hg.[210–212] Another study, however, could not confirm the trimodal concept,[213] and when the topical corticosteroid test was repeated in the same population, individuals did not always give the same response each time.[214]

Primary open-angle glaucoma populations have been shown to have a greater number of individuals with a high IOP response to topical corticosteroids. The actual reported percentage of high responders, however, varies according to the criteria used to define this group.[210–212] Reports also differ as to whether ocular hypertensives do[215] or do not[216] have a greater incidence of high responders than the general population. In one study, a significant number of ocular hypertensives with high responses were reported to have reversible glaucomatous field defects.[217] Another study suggested that high corticosteroid responders, whether ocular normotensive or hypertensive at the time of testing, have an increased chance of developing glaucomatous damage.[218] As previously discussed, however, the topical corticosteroid response was not found to be a useful prognostic indicator for POAG in one long-term study.[162]

Eyes that have sustained an attack of *angle-closure glaucoma* also have a high percentage of topical steroids responders,[219] although those at risk of angle closure[219] or that have undergone prophylactic peripheral iridectomies[220] do not differ from the general population. It has also been shown that topical corticosteroid responsiveness among insulin-dependent diabetics does not correlate with the rate of development of diabetic retinopathy.[221]

Inheritance of the topical corticosteroid response and how this may relate to POAG have been matters of particular controversy. Becker[210,222] postulated an autosomal recessive mode for the corticosteroid response and suggested that the gene is either closely related or identical to that for POAG, which he believed had an autosomal recessive inheritance. Armaly[212] agreed that the two conditions might be genetically related but proposed a polygenetic inheritance for POAG with the gene for the topical corticosteroid response being one of the genes involved. Results of additional studies were consistent with a genetic basis for the topical corticosteroid response but could confirm neither the recessive mode[223] nor even a relationship to glaucoma.[216] Still other investigators could not even substantiate that the corticosteroid response was entirely genetic. A twin heritability study of monozygotic and like-sex dizygotic twins revealed a low estimate of heritability that did not support a predominant role of inheritance in the response to corticosteroids, and it suggested that nongenetic factors play the major role.[213,224–226] In further support of the nongenetic concept of topical corticosteroid response, eyes with unilateral angle-closure glaucoma[227] or angle recession[228] responded to topical corticosteroids with a higher pressure rise in the involved eye than the fellow eye, which had not suffered angle closure or trauma. These observations suggest that topical corticosteroid responsiveness, at least in some individuals, may be acquired.

Plasma Cortisol Studies. Some investigators believe that studies of plasma cortisol provide additional evidence that patients with POAG may be unusually sensitive to corticosteroids. The results of these studies, however, are again conflicting. Higher than normal plasma cortisol levels[229] as well as percent plasma free cortisol (not bound to plasma proteins) of total plasma cortisol[230] have been demonstrated in POAG patients. Other investigators, however, were unable to confirm the association of elevated plasma cortisol and POAG.[231,232] One study suggested that an elevated plasma cortisol level is closely related to the IOP at the time of cortisol sampling.[233]

Plasma cortisol suppression has also been suggested to be abnormal in patients with POAG. This test consists of measuring plasma cortisol before and after the oral administration of dexamethasone. The normal response is a reduction in plasma cortisol of 35% or more approximately 9 hours after administration of the corticosteroid, as a result of suppression of trophic hormones. The reported results of plasma cortisol suppression in POAG patients are conflicting, in that some investigators have found less than normal suppression,[229,234] which did not appear to be genetically determined,[235] while other investigators found no significant difference from nonglaucomatous individuals.[231,236] Pretreatment with diphenylhydantoin (Dilantin) normally prevents plasma cortisol suppression, presumably by enhancing liver enzyme degradation of the dexamethasone before it suppresses the release of trophic hormones from the pituitary. However, in 89% of POAG patients, diphenylhydantoin did not prevent the plasma cortisol suppression.[231] This observation did not appear to be due to an alteration in liver enzyme degradation of dexamethasone,[237] but rather to an increased sensitivity to lower levels of circulating steroids.[238] The corticosteroid sensitivity in POAG patients appears to be relatively specific, since oral dexamethasone does not have an abnormal effect on baseline thyroid function tests or thyroid stimulating hormone suppression in these individuals.[239] However, a study of cultured skin fibroblast sensitivity to corticosteroids suggested that a generalized cellular hypersensitivity to glucocorticoids is not intrinsic to POAG.[240] These authors postulated that environmental alterations and/or endogenous factors may influence steroid responses.

The relationship of topical corticosteroid response to plasma cortisol suppression has also been investigated, and a correlation between high topical corticosteroid responders and reduced plasma cortisol suppression has been reported.[236,241,242] In addition, approximately half of the high topical corticosteroid responders from a general population study had plasma cortisol suppression despite pretreatment with diphenylhydantoin.[231] The latter individuals also more closely resembled POAG patients on the basis of other parameters, such as a larger cup/disc ratio and an abnormal glucose tolerance test.[231] However, a five-year prospective study failed to show that plasma cortisol suppression can predict the development of POAG among high topical steroid responders.[243]

Lymphocyte Transformation Inhibition. Another source of evidence for increased corticosteroid sensitivity in patients with POAG comes from studies of lymphocyte transformation inhibition, although reports continue to be conflicting. Lymphocytes from peripheral blood can be transformed from the usual state of relative metabolic inactivity to a metabolically active state by mitogenic agents such as phytohemagglutinin. The degree of transformation can be measured by the uptake of tritiated thymidine into DNA. Corticosteroids inhibit the lymphocyte transformation, and the degree of inhibition can be taken as a measure of sensitivity to corticosteroids. Using this model, some studies have revealed increased corticosteroid sensitivity among patients with POAG,[244,245] while other investigators have been unable to confirm these findings.[246–248] The effect of ouabain on lymphocyte transformation is normal in POAG patients and high topical corticosteroid responders, suggesting that steroid sensitivity, if it exists, is specific and not the general vulnerability of "sick cells."[249]

Relationship of IOP to Corticosteroid Sensitivity. If patients with POAG are unusually sensitive to corticosteroids, by what mechanism(s) might this lead to elevated IOP? Furthermore, does this mechanism(s) only function in response to exogenously administered corticosteroids, or do normal circulating corticosteroids also adversely influence the IOP in POAG patients? Attempts to answer these question include the following theories.

Hypothalamic-pituitary-adrenal axis theory. It has been suggested that an abnormal response of the hypothalamic-pituitary-adrenal axis in POAG patients, and possibly in other forms of glaucoma, may be related to alterations in aqueous humor dynamics in response to corticosteroids.[242,250]

Cyclic-adenosine monophosphate theory. It may be that corticosteroids influence the IOP by altering cyclic-adenosine monophosphate (cyclic-AMP). Corticosteroids have a permissive effect on the beta-adrenergic stimulation of adenyl cyclase, the enzyme responsible for the synthesis of cyclic-AMP.[251] How this relates to aqueous humor dynamics is uncertain, although POAG patients and high topical steroid responders appear to be unusually sensitive to cyclic-AMP. Evidence for this increased sensitivity has been observed in studies of lymphocyte transformation, as previously described, which is normally inhibited by cyclic-AMP. Theophylline inhibits the enzyme phosphodiesterase, which destroys cyclic-AMP, and POAG patients reportedly require less theophylline than control subjects to stimulate inhibition of lymphocyte transformation.[252]

Glycosaminoglycans theory. It has also been proposed that IOP elevation associated with corticosteroid sensitivity may be related to glycosaminoglycans in the trabecular meshwork.[253] When polymerized, glycosaminoglycans become hydrated, swell, and obstruct aqueous outflow. Catabolic enzymes, released from lysosomes in the trabecular cells, depolymerize the glycosaminoglycans. Corticosteroids stabilize the lysosome membrane, preventing release of these enzymes, thereby increasing the polymerized form of glycosaminoglycans and the resistance to aqueous outflow.

Phagocytosis theory. Yet another possible effect of steroids on IOP may be related to the phagocytic activity of endothelial cells lining the trabecular meshwork. As discussed in Chapter 2, these cells are normally phagocytic, and it may be that they function to "clean" the aqueous of debris before it reaches the inner wall endothelium of Schlemm's canal. Failure to do so might result in a build-up of material that could account for the amorphous layer in the juxtacanalicular connective tissue, as previously described. Corticosteroids suppress phagocytosis, and it may be that the trabecular endothelium in POAG patients is unusually sensitive even to endogenous corticosteroids.[254] Cells cultured from trabecular meshwork of patients with POAG have been found to have abnormal metabolism of cortisol.[255]

Immunologic Studies

Increased gamma globulin[256] and plasma cells[257] in the trabecular meshwork of eyes with POAG have been reported, and a high percentage of patients with this disease were found in one study to have positive antinuclear antibodies reactions.[258] These reports suggested a possible immunologic mechanism in the pathogenesis of POAG. However, subsequent assays for specific immunoglobulins in the trabecular meshwork of eyes with POAG revealed no difference from nonglaucomatous eyes.[259–261] In addition, further evaluation of antinuclear antibodies in patients with POAG,[262,263] as well as Clq-binding immune complexes, collagen antibodies, anti-nDNA-antibodies,[263] and cell-mediated immunity, as indicated by leukocyte migration inhibition in vitro,[264] have all failed to show any significant difference from the nonglaucoma population. The absence of a correlation between HLA antigens and POAG was discussed earlier in this chapter. At the present time, therefore, the bulk of the evidence is against an immunogenic mechanism in POAG.

MANAGEMENT

The following discussion is limited to the principles of deciding when to begin treatment and what basic type of therapy to use. The details of the drugs and surgical procedures are considered in Section Three.

When to Treat

In the typical case of POAG with established visual field and/or optic nerve head damage, treatment to reduce the IOP is clearly indicated whatever the pressure may be. The importance of elevated IOP as a causative factor of POAG and the importance of reducing the pressure in the management of the disease have been clinically established.[265,266] However, in the case of ocular hypertension with normal optic nerve heads and visual fields, the appropriate course is less clear. As discussed earlier in this chapter, not all such patients appear destined to develop glaucomatous damage, and there is no way of predicting with certainty which ones will go on to manifest the full picture of POAG. Prospective studies have indicated that elevated IOP, abnormalities of the optic nerve head, black race, advancing age, myopia, a family history of glaucoma, and cardiovascular disorders are significant risk factors for the development of this disorder.[22,267,268] However, no single risk factor or group of factors has yet been shown to predict the future development of glaucomatous damage with reasonable accuracy.[269]

For lack of a precise indicator of future glaucomatous damage, it has been customary practice that patients with moderate IOP elevations be followed without treatment, but with periodic visual field and optic nerve head examinations. However, of two randomized, prospective studies of ocular hypertension, one randomizing patients[270] and the other right and left eyes[271,272] between timolol therapy and no treatment, both found that the treated eyes had a more favorable course with regard to glaucomatous damage. Most ophthalmologists will initiate therapy at a certain IOP level despite normal discs and fields, based on the belief that, beyond that particular pressure, the increased risk of developing glaucomatous damage is sufficient to justify therapeutic intervention. Goldmann[273] began medical therapy at 25 mm Hg, while Chandler and Grant[83] suggested 30 mm Hg as a guideline for initiating treatment in the absence of apparent damage. Clearly, any arbitrary pressure level should be adjusted for each patient on the basis of that individual's risk factors. In addition to the risk factors for POAG, other patients for whom the initiation of therapy at lower pressure levels might be considered include those who are at risk for central retinal vein occlusion, as well as individuals who are one-eyed, who are more likely to return for follow-up if they are being treated, who desire treatment, or in whom visual fields or disc evaluation is not possible. In doubtful cases, a uniocular trial of therapy, as discussed earlier in this chapter, may be helpful, since a good pressure reduction with minimal side effects might argue in favor of continuing the therapy in both eyes.

How to Treat

Once the decision has been made to begin treatment, the next questions are what form of therapy should be used and what should be the guidelines for successful therapy?

Medical Therapy. Primary open-angle glaucoma has traditionally been thought of as a medical disease, in that laser and incisional surgery are usually reserved for cases that cannot be controlled with medication. The basic principle of medical therapy is to use the least amount of medicine that will control the glaucoma with the fewest side effects. To this end, it is customary to begin with a low dose of topical medication and to increase the concentration and/or advance to combinations of drugs until the desired pressure level is reached. It is good practice to treat only one eye initially in symmetric cases, so the fellow eye can be used as a control in determining the efficacy of therapy. The question of which drug to use first depends on the ocular and systemic status of each individual patient, as well as the physician's personal preference. The relative advantages and disadvantages of the various antiglaucoma drugs are considered in Section Three. One study showed that a significant IOP reduction was usually associated with any initial medication, whereas the pressure did not change significantly with a change to a stronger medication or combined medical therapy.[274] It is important, therefore, to carefully document the efficacy and patient tolerance of any new medication that is added.

Although IOP reduction has been shown to be important in preventing visual loss in glaucoma,[265,266] it is not possible to predict what pressure level will be adequate to prevent progressive glaucomatous damage in each individual case. In general, a pressure below 20 mm Hg is recommended in eyes with early damage, while a pressure below 18 mm Hg appears to be desirable for advanced cases.[275] Patients with marked visual field loss tend to experience further loss at a greatly accelerated rate,[276] and these individuals may require pressures in the mid- to low teens.[277] However, at least one study has shown a poor correlation between IOP reduction and progressive visual field loss,[278] and the main guide to therapy should be the appearance of the optic nerve heads and visual fields. Progressive change in the latter parameters demands further pressure reduction regardless of what the pressure level may be. In fact, it has been shown that the appearance of the disc and field may improve with IOP reduction,[279–281] and it has been suggested that improvement in these parameters, rather than merely arrested progression, is necessary to establish with certainty that the glaucoma is controlled.[279,280]

If the IOP begins to rise after long-term treatment with a particular medical regimen, the explanation may either be progression of the disease or a loss of responsiveness to the medication. Before increasing the concentration or adding other drugs, therefore, it is best to first test the second possibility by temporarily discontinuing the current medication (one drug at a time). If the pressure does not go up significantly with this trial of discontinuation, it suggests that the drug has lost part or all of its effectiveness, and it is probably best to change to a different medication. In some cases, it is possible to return to the first drug after several months or years with renewed effectiveness of that medication.

Tolerance and Compliance with Medical Therapy. Surgical intervention is usually indicated whenever there is progressive glaucomatous damage despite "maximum tolerable medical therapy." In some cases, this may mean that all available forms of antiglaucoma drugs in their highest concentrations are being used. Other cases of medical failure may result from inability to use one or more medications because of drug intolerances, while others may be related to poor compliance with the recommended therapy. In one study, 11 of 40 randomly selected POAG patients failed to comply with their medical therapy,[282] while 42% of patients in another study missed at least some of their medications.[283] Patients more often miss doses during the middle of the day and are more compliant with twice daily medication than when the drug is prescribed three or four times each day.[283] Reported factors related to poor compliance include male gender, no other medical disease present, glaucoma not ranked most troubling when other disorders were present, side effects with medication, and failure to relate glaucoma to blindness.[282]

Surgical Intervention. When the glaucoma is uncontrolled medically, laser trabeculoplasty is usually the first surgical procedure of choice, followed by incisional surgical intervention when necessary. Trabeculectomy, or other forms of glaucoma filtering surgery, are usually the preferred incisional surgical techniques for POAG.

In advanced cases with total cupping of the disc and a small, central field, it is no longer possible to use progressive disc and field change as a guide to laser or incisional surgical intervention, and reliance must be placed on the IOP. As noted above, these eyes probably require pressures in the mid- to low teens.

Loss of central vision may occur after glaucoma surgery as well as during medical therapy. Kolker[275] found this to occur with equal frequency with these two modalities of treatment, while other investigators suggest that surgery is associated with less field loss.[284] When progressive field loss does occur despite low pressure levels following surgery, it is frequently due to vascular insufficiency of the optic nerve head.[285]

Early Surgery. Although incisional surgical intervention is traditionally withheld until medical and laser therapy have proved to be inadequate, recent studies are beginning to suggest that earlier filtering surgery may be desirable. At question is the balance between the side effects and risk of inadequate IOP control with medical therapy and the potential complications of filtering surgery. In one study of 52 POAG patients assigned to either medical therapy or filtering surgery and followed for up to 17.5 years, the early surgery group had less visual field loss but more rapid deterioration of visual acuity caused by cataracts.[286] In another study of 99 POAG patients, in whom one eye was randomly assigned either to medical therapy or a trabeculectomy as the initial therapy, early surgery was associated with a lower mean IOP (15 mm Hg vs 20.8 mm Hg, respectively) and better protection of the visual field.[287] These authors concluded that the risk of delaying surgery is significantly greater than that of performing trabeculectomy as primary treatment. Yet a third study of 168 POAG patients compared medical therapy, laser trabeculoplasty, and filtering surgery and found that the latter gave the greatest IOP reduction, while the former gave the least.[288] Clearly, there is a need for further evaluation of early surgery in the management of POAG.

Treatment of Low-Tension Glaucoma

Damage to the optic nerve head and visual field may progress even at low normal pressures in this condition. Indeed, there is no firm evidence that treating the IOP improves the prognosis. Nevertheless, most clinicians try to keep the pressure as low as possible with medication or with laser or incisional surgery. Although filtering surgery did not help in one reported series,[289] other surgeons have found that it may prevent progressive damage.[15,251,290,291] The most important aspect of management may be the treatment of any cardiovascular abnormality (e.g., gastrointestinal lesions, anemia, congestive heart failure, transient ischemic attacks, and cardiac arrhythmias) to ensure maximum perfusion of the optic nerve head.[9] Ultimately, the treatment of choice in low-tension glaucoma may prove to be therapy that directly improves the function of the optic nerve head. A pilot study of 25 low-tension glaucoma patients suggested that long-term oral therapy with nifedipine, a calcium channel blocker, may protect the visual field in these patients, possibly by relieving the effect of vasospasm on the nerve head.[292] Further work in this area is clearly indicated.

SUMMARY

Primary open-angle glaucoma is the most common form of glaucoma. It has a familial tendency and is more prevalent with increasing age, black race, myopia, and certain systemic diseases, such as diabetes and cardiovascular abnormalities. It is typically asymptomatic until advanced visual field loss occurs and is characterized by an open, normal-appearing anterior chamber angle. By definition, the IOP is consistently above 21 mm Hg, although there is a clinical variation in which disc and field changes develop despite pressures that never reach this level (low-tension glaucoma). Other patients have pressure elevation without glaucomatous damage, and no test has yet been developed to predict which of these individuals have POAG. The precise mechanism of increased resistance to aqueous outflow in this condition remains unclear, although it is most likely related to subtle alterations in the trabecular meshwork and/or Schlemm's canal. Initial treatment in nearly all cases is topical and oral medication. When progressive damage continues, despite maximum tolerable medical therapy, laser trabeculoplasty is usually indicated, followed by glaucoma filtering surgery if necessary.

References

1. Anderson, DR: Glaucoma: the damage caused by pressure. Am J Ophthal 108:485, 1989.
2. Kolker, AE, Becker, B: 'Ocular hypertension' vs open-angle glaucoma: a different view. Arch Ophthal 95:586, 1977.
3. Phelps, CD: Ocular hypertension: to treat or not to treat? Arch Ophthal 95:588, 1977.
4. Chandler, PA, Grant, WM: 'Ocular hypertension' vs open-angle glaucoma. Arch Ophthal 95:585, 1977.
5. Shaffer, R: 'Glaucoma suspect' or 'ocular hypertension'? Arch Ophthal 95:588, 1977.
6. Drance, SM, Sweeney, VP, Morgan, RW, Feldman, F: Studies of factors involved in the production of low tension glaucoma. Arch Ophthal 89:457, 1973.
7. Drance, SM, Morgan, RW, Sweeney, VP: Shock-induced optic neuropathy. A cause of nonprogressive glaucoma. N Engl J Med 288:392, 1973.
8. Lewis, RA, Hayreh, SS, Phelps, CD: Optic disk and visual field correlations in primary open-angle and low-tension glaucoma. Am J Ophthal 96:148, 1983.
9. Chumbley, LC, Brubaker, RF: Low-tension glaucoma. Am J Ophthal 81:761, 1976.
10. Caprioli, J, Spaeth, GL: Comparison of visual field defects in the low-tension glaucomas with those in the high-tension glaucomas. Am J Ophthal 97:730, 1984.
11. Geijssen, HC, Greve, EL: The spectrum of primary open angle glaucoma I: Senile sclerotic glaucoma versus high tension glaucoma. Ophthal Surg 18:207, 1987.
12. Schulzer, M, Drance, SM, Carter, CJ, et al: Biostatistical evidence for two distinct chronic open angle glaucoma populations. Br J Ophthal 74:196, 1990.
13. Hollows, FC, Graham, PA: Intra-ocular pressure, glaucoma, and glaucoma suspects in a defined population. Br J Ophthal 50:570, 1966.
14. Segal, P, Skwierczynska, J: Mass screening of adults for glaucoma. Ophthalmologica 153:336, 1967.
15. Kahn, HA, Leibowitz, HM, Ganley, JP, Kini, MM, Colton, T, Nickerson, RS, Dawber, TR: The Framingham eye study. I. Outline and major prevalence findings. Am J Epidemiol 106:17, 1977.
16. Leske, MC, Rosenthal, J: Epidemiologic aspects of open-angle glaucoma. Am J Epidemiol 109:250, 1979.
17. Bjornsson, G: The primary glaucoma in Iceland. Epidemiological studies. Acta Ophthal 91 (suppl):89, 1967.
18. Popvic, V: The glaucoma population in Gothenburg. Acta Ophthal 60:745, 1982.
19. Graham, PA: Epidemiology of simple glaucoma and ocular hypertension. Br J Ophthal 56:223, 1972.
20. Perkins, ES: The Bedford glaucoma survey. I. Long-term follow-up of borderline cases. Br J Ophthal 57:179, 1973.
21. Walker, WM: Ocular hypertension. Follow-up of 109 cases from 1963 to 1974. Trans Ophthal Soc UK 94:525, 1974.
22. Wilensky, JT, Podos, SM, Becker, B: Prognostic indicators in ocular hypertension. Arch Ophthal 91:200, 1974.
23. Norskov, K: Routine tonometry in ophthalmic practice. II. Five-year follow-up. Acta Ophthal 48:873, 1970.
24. Linner, E: Ocular hypertension. I. The clinical course during ten years without therapy. Aqueous humour dynamics. Acta Ophthal 54:707, 1976.
25. Kitazawa, Y, Horie, T, Aoki, S, et al: Untreated ocular hypertension. A long-term prospective study. Arch Ophthal 95:1180, 1977.
26. David, R, Livingston, DG, Luntz, MH: Ocular hypertension—a long-term follow-up of treated and untreated patients. Br J Ophthal 61:668, 1977.
27. Hart, WM Jr, Yablonski, M, Kass, MA, Becker, B: Multivariate analysis of the risk of glaucomatous visual field loss. Arch Ophthal 97:1455, 1979.
28. Lundberg, L, Wettrell, K, Linner, E: Ocular hy-

pertension. A prospective twenty-year follow-up study. Acta Ophthal 65:705, 1987.

29. Armaly, MF: Ocular pressure and visual fields. A ten-year follow-up study. Arch Ophthal 81:25, 1969.
30. Perkins, ES: The Bedford glaucoma survey. II. Rescreening of normal population. Br J Ophthal 57:186, 1973.
31. Leydhecker, W: Zur verbreitung des glaucoma simplex in der scheinbar gesunden, augenarztlich nicht behandelten bevolkerung. Doc Ophthal 13:359, 1959.
32. Lichter, PR, Shaffer, RN: Ocular hypertension and glaucoma. Trans Pacific Coast Oto-Ophthal Soc 54:63, 1973.
33. Harbin, TS Jr, Podos, SM, Kolker, AE, Becker, B: Visual field progression in open-angle glaucoma patients presenting with monocular field loss. Trans Am Acad Ophthal Otol 81:253, 1976.
34. Grant, WM, Burke, JF Jr: Why do some people go blind from glaucoma? Ophthalmology 89:991, 1982.
35. Wright, JE: The Bedford glaucoma survey. In: Glaucoma Symposium, Hunt, J, ed. E & S Livingston, Ltd, Edinburgh 1966, p. 12.
36. Martinez, GS, Campbell, AJ, Reinken, J, Allan, BC: Prevalence of ocular disease in a population study of subjects 65 years old and older. Am J Ophthal 94:181, 1982.
37. Podgor, MJ, Leske, MC, Ederer, F: Incidence estimates for lens changes, macular changes, open-angle glaucoma and diabetic retinopathy. Am J Epidemiol 118:206, 1983.
38. Whitmore, WG: Eye disease in a geriatric nursing home population. Ophthalmology 96:393, 1989.
39. Goldwyn, R, Waltman, SR, Becker, B: Primary open-angle glaucoma in adolescents and young adults. Arch Ophthal 84:579, 1970.
40. Mandell, AI, Elfervig, J: Open-angle glaucoma in patients under forty years of age. Pers Ophthal 1:215, 1977.
41. Wilensky, JT, Gandhi, N, Pan, T: Racial influences in open-angle glaucoma. Ann Ophthal 10:1398, 1978.
42. David, R, Livingston, D, Luntz, MH: Ocular hypertension: a comparative follow-up of black and white patients. Br J Ophthal 62:676, 1978.
43. Wallace, J, Lovell, HG: Glaucoma and intraocular pressure in Jamaica. Am J Ophthal 67:93, 1969.
44. Martin, MJ, Sommer, A, Gold, EB, Diamond, EL: Race and primary open-angle glaucoma. Am J Ophthal 99:383, 1985.
45. Hiller, R, Kahn, HA: Blindness from glaucoma. Am J Ophthal 80:62, 1975.
46. Schwartz, AL, Helfgott, MA: The incidence of sickle trait in blacks requiring filtering surgery. Ann Ophthal 9:957, 1977.
47. Beck, RW, Messner, DK, Musch, DC, et al: Is there a racial difference in physiologic cup size? Ophthalmology 92:873, 1985.
48. Kahn, HA, Milton, RC: Alternative definitions of open-angle glaucoma. Effect on prevalence and associations in the Framingham Eye Study. Arch Ophthal 98:2172, 1980.
49. Richler, M, Werner, EB, Thomas, D: Risk factors for progression of visual field defects in medically treated patients with glaucoma. Can J Ophthal 17:245, 1982.
50. Armstrong, JR, Daily, RK, Dobson, HL, Girard, LJ: The incidence of glaucoma in diabetes mellitus. A comparison with the incidence of glaucoma in the general population. Am J Ophthal 50:55, 1960.
51. Becker, B: Diabetes mellitus and primary open-angle glaucoma. Am J Ophthal 71:1, 1971.
52. Vesti, N: The prevalence of glaucoma and ocular hypertension in type 1 and 2 diabetes mellitus. An epidemiological study of diabetes mellitus on the island of Falster, Denmark. Acta Ophthal 61:662, 1983.
53. Marre, E, Marre, M: A contribution to glaucoma in the presence of diabetes mellitus. Klin Monatsbl Augenheilkd 153:396, 1968.
54. Armaly, MF: Dexamethasone ocular hypertension and eosinopenia, and glucose tolerance test. Arch Ophthal 78:193, 1967.
55. McLenachan, J, Davies, DM: Glaucoma and the thyroid. Br J Ophthal 49:441, 1965.
56. Becker, B, Kolker, AE, Ballin, N: Thyroid function and glaucoma. Am J Ophthal 61:997, 1966.
57. Krupin, T, Jacobs, LS, Podos, SM, Becker, B: Thyroid function and the intraocular pressure response to topical corticosteroids. Am J Ophthal 83:643, 1977.
58. Neuner, HP, Dardenne, U: Ocular changes in the Cushing syndrome. Klin Monatsbl Augenheilkd 152:570, 1968.
59. Haas, JS, Nootens, RH: Glaucoma secondary to benign adrenal adenoma. Am J Ophthal 78:497, 1974.
60. Abdel-Aziz, M, Labib, MA: The relationship of the intraocular pressure and the hormonal disturbance. Part II—The pituitary gland. Bull Ophthal Soc Egypt 62:61, 1969.
61. Caygill, WM: Aqueous humor dynamics following pituitary irradiation in diabetic patients with retinopathy. Am J Ophthal 71:826, 1971.
62. Treister, G, Mannor, S: Intraocular pressure and outflow facility. Effect of estrogen and combined estrogen-progestin treatment in normal human eyes. Arch Ophthal 83:311, 1970.
63. Abdel-Aziz, M, Labib, MA: The relationship of the intra-ocular pressure to hormonal disturbance. Part IV. The gonads. Bull Ophthal Soc Egypt 62:83, 1969.
64. Morgan, RW, Drance, SM: Chronic open-angle

glaucoma and ocular hypertension. An epidemiological study. Br J Ophthal 59:211, 1975.
65. Drance, SM, Schulzer, M, Thomas, B, Douglas, GR: Multivariate analysis in glaucoma. Use of discriminant analysis in predicting glaucomatous visual field damage. Arch Ophthal 99:1019, 1981.
66. Feldman, F, Sweeney, VP, Drance, SM: Cerebro-vascular studies in chronic simple glaucoma. Can J Ophthal 4:358, 1969.
67. Leighton, DA, Phillips, CI: Systemic blood pressure in open-angle glaucoma, low tension glaucoma, and the normal eye. Br J Ophthal 56:447, 1972.
68. Nagin, P, Schwartz, B: Detection of increased pallor over time. Computerized image analysis in untreated ocular hypertension. Ophthalmology 91:252, 1984.
69. Kahn, HA, Leibowitz, HM, Ganley, JP, et al: The Framingham eye study. II. Association of ophthalmic pathology with single variables previously measured in the Framingham Heart Study. Am J Epidemiol 106:33, 1977.
70. Bengtsson, B: Findings associated with glaucomatous visual field defects. Acta Ophthal 58:20, 1980.
71. Said, A, Labib, MAM, Abboud, I, Hegazi, A: The relationship between systemic hypertension and chronic simple glaucoma. Bull Ophthal Soc Egypt 60:71, 1967.
72. Chisholm, IA, Stead, S: Plasma lipid patterns in patients with suspected glaucoma. Can J Ophthal 23:164, 1988.
73. Perkins, ES: Family studies in glaucoma. Br J Ophthal 58:529, 1974.
74. Kolker, AE: Glaucoma family study. Ten-year follow-up (preliminary report). Israel J Med Sci 8:1357, 1972.
75. Rosenthal, AR, Perkins, ES: Family studies in glaucoma. Br J Ophthal 69:664, 1985.
76. Shin, DH, Becker, B, Kolker, AE: Family history in primary open-angle glaucoma. Arch Ophthal 95:598, 1977.
77. David, R, Jenkins, T: Genetic markers in glaucoma. Br J Ophthal 64:227, 1980.
78. Pohjanpelto, PEJ, Plava, J: Ocular hypertension and glaucomatous optic nerve damage. Acta Ophthal 52:194, 1974.
79. Schwartz, B, Talusan, AG: Spontaneous trends in ocular pressure in untreated ocular hypertension. Arch Ophthal 98:105, 1980.
80. Leonard, TJK, Kerr-Muir, MG, Kirkby, GR, Hitchings, RA: Ocular hypertension and posture. Br J Ophthal 67:362, 1983.
81. Bengtsson, B: The prevalence of glaucoma. Br J Ophthal 65:46, 1981.
82. Armaly, MF: Genetic determination of cup/disc ratio of the optic nerve. Arch Ophthal 78:35, 1967.
83. Chandler, PA, Grant, WM: Lectures on Glaucoma. Lea & Febiger, Philadelphia, 1965, p. 13.
84. Yablonski, ME, Zimmerman, TJ, Kass, MA, Becker, B: Prognostic significance of optic disk cupping in ocular hypertensive patients. Am J Ophthal 89:585, 1980.
85. Susanna, R, Drance, SM: Use of discriminant analysis. I. Prediction of visual field defects from features of the glaucoma disc. Arch Ophthal 96:1568, 1978.
86. Hitchings, RA, Wheeler, CA: The optic disc in glaucoma. IV: Optic disc evaluation in the ocular hypertensive patient. Br J Ophthal 64:232, 1980.
87. Sommer, A, Miller, NR, Pollack, I, et al: The nerve fiber layer in the diagnosis of glaucoma. Arch Ophthal 95:2149, 1977.
88. Daubs, JG, Crick, RP: Effect of refractive error on the risk of ocular hypertension and open angle glaucoma. Trans Ophthal Soc UK 101:121, 1981.
89. Perkins, ES, Phelps, CD: Open angle glaucoma, ocular hypertension, low-tension glaucoma, and refraction. Arch Ophthal 100:1464, 1982.
90. Phelps, CD: Effect of myopia on prognosis in treated primary open-angle glaucoma. Am J Ophthal 93:622, 1982.
91. Buxton, JN, Preston, RW, Riechers, R, Guilbault, N: Tonography in cornea guttata. A preliminary report. Arch Ophthal 77:602, 1967.
92. Hiles, DA, Biglan, AW, Fetherolf, EC: Central corneal endothelial cell counts in children. Am Intra-Ocular Implant Soc J V:292, 1979.
93. Korey, M, Gieser, D, Kass, MA, et al: Central corneal endothelial cell density and central corneal thickness in ocular hypertension and primary open-angle glaucoma. Am J Ophthal 94:610, 1982.
94. Kimura, R, Levene, RZ: Gonioscopic differences between primary open-angle glaucoma and normal subjects over 40 years of age. Am J Ophthal 80:56, 1975.
95. Campbell, DG, Boys-Smith, JW, Woods, WD: Variation of pigmentation and segmentation of pigmentation in primary open angle glaucoma. Invest Ophthal Vis Sci (suppl) 25:122, 1984.
96. Silverman, SE, Trick, GL, Hart, WM, Jr: Motion perception is abnormal in primary open-angle glaucoma and ocular hypertension. Invest Ophthal Vis Sci 31:722, 1990.
97. Kass, MA, Kolker, AE, Becker, B: Prognostic factors in glaucomatous visual field loss. Arch Ophthal 94:1274, 1976.
98. Susanna, R, Drance, SM, Douglas, GR: The visual prognosis of the fellow eye in uniocular chronic open-angle glaucoma. Br J Ophthal 62:327, 1978.
99. Caprioli, J, Spaeth, GL: Comparison of the optic nerve head in high- and low-tension glaucoma. Arch Ophthal 103:1145, 1985.
100. Gramer, E, Althaus, G, Leydhecker, W: Localization and depth of glaucomatous visual field defects in relation to the size of the neuroretinal rim area of the disk in low-tension glaucoma, glau-

coma simplex, and pigmentary glaucoma. Clinical study with the Octopus 201 perimeter and the optic nerve head analyzer. Klin Monatsbl Augenheilkd 189:190, 1986.

101. Fazio, P, Krupin, T, Feitl, ME, et al: Optic disc topography in patients with low-tension and primary open angle glaucoma. Arch Ophthal 108:705, 1990.
102. Miller, KM, Quigley, HA: Comparison of optic disc features in low-tension and typical open-angle glaucoma. Ophthalmic Surg 18:882, 1987.
103. Kitazawa, Y, Shirato, S, Yamamoto, T: Optic disc hemorrhage in low-tension glaucoma. Ophthalmology 93:853, 1986.
104. Drance, SM, Douglas, GR, Airaksinen, PJ, et al: Diffuse visual field loss in chronic open-angle and low-tension glaucoma. Am J Ophthal 104:577, 1987.
105. Chauhan, BC, Drance, SM, Douglas, GR, Johnson, CA: Visual field damage in normal-tension and high-tension glaucoma. Am J Ophthal 108:636, 1989.
106. King, D, Drance, SM, Douglas, G, et al: Comparison of visual field defects in normal-tension glaucoma and high-tension glaucoma. Am J Ophthal 101:204, 1986.
107. Caprioli, J, Spaeth GL: Comparison of visual field defects in the low-tension glaucomas with those in the high-tension glaucomas. Am J Ophthal 97:730, 1984.
108. Gliklich, RE, Steinmann, WC, Spaeth, GL: Visual field change in low-tension glaucoma over a five-year follow-up. Ophthalmology 96:316, 1989.
109. Gramer, E, Althaus, G: Quantification and progression of visual field damage in low-tension, primary open angle, and pigmentary glaucoma. Klin Monatsbl Augenheilkd 191:184, 1987.
110. Gramer, E, Leydhecker, W: Glaucoma without elevated IOP: a clinical study. Klin Monatsbl Augenheilkd 186:262, 1985.
111. Cartwright, MJ, Anderson, DR: Correlation of asymmetric damage with asymmetric intraocular pressure in normal-tension glaucoma (low-tension glaucoma). Arch Ophthal 106:898, 1988.
112. Crichton, A, Drance, SM, Douglas, GR, Schulzer, M: Unequal intraocular pressure and its relation to asymmetric visual field defects in low-tension glaucoma. Ophthalmology 96:1312, 1989.
113. Goldberg, I, Hollows, FC, Kass, MA, Becker, B: Systemic factors in patients with low-tension glaucoma. Br J Ophthal 65:56, 1981.
114. Hayreh, SS: Anterior Ischemic Optic Neuropathy. Springer-Verlag, New York, 1975, p. 22.
115. Perkins, ES, Phelps, CD: Ocular pulse amplitudes in low-tension glaucoma. Klin Monatsbl Augenheilkd 184:303, 1984.
116. Pillunat, LE, Stodtmeister, R, Wilmanns, I: Pressure compliance of the optic nerve head in low tension glaucoma. Br J Ophthal 71:181, 1987.
117. Phelps, CD, Corbett, JJ: Migraine and low-tension glaucoma: a case-control study. Invest Ophthal Vis Sci 26:1105, 1985.
118. Drance, SM, Douglas, GR, Wijsman, K, et al: Response of blood flow to warm and cold in normal and low-tension glaucoma patients. Am J Ophthal 105:35, 1988.
119. Klaver, JHJ, Greve, EL, Goslinga, H, et al: Blood and plasma viscosity measurements in patients with glaucoma. Br J Ophthal 69:765, 1985.
120. Joist, JH, Lichtenfeld, P, Mandell, AI, Kolker, AE: Platelet function, blood coagulability, and fibrinolysis in patients with low tension glaucoma. Arch Ophthal 94:1893, 1976.
121. Carter, CJ, Brooks, DE, Doyle, DL, Drance, SM: Investigations into a vascular etiology for low-tension glaucoma. Ophthalmology 97:49, 1990.
122. Winder, AF: Circulating lipoprotein and blood glucose levels in association with low-tension and chronic simple glaucoma. Br J Ophthal 61:641, 1977.
123. Bennett, SR, Alward, WLM, Folberg, R: An autosomal dominant form of low-tension glaucoma. Am J Ophthal 108:238, 1989.
124. Ritch, R: Nonprogressive low-tension glaucoma with pigmentary dispersion. Am J Ophthal 94:190, 1982.
125. Vucicevic, ZM, Ralston, J, Burns, WP, Gaffney, HP: Influence of the water drinking test on scleral rigidity. Arch Ophthal 82:761, 1969.
126. Armaly, MF: Water-drinking test. I. Characteristics of the ocular pressure response and the effect of age. Arch Ophthal 83:169, 1970.
127. Becker, B, Christensen, RE: Water-drinking and tonography in the diagnosis of glaucoma. Arch Ophthal 56:321, 1956.
128. Becker, B: Tonography in the diagnosis of simple (open angle) glaucoma. Trans Am Acad Ophthal Otol 65:156, 1961.
129. Spaeth, GL: The water drinking test. Indications that factors other than osmotic considerations are involved. Arch Ophthal 77:50, 1967.
130. Kimura, R: Clinical studies on glaucoma. Report III. The diagnostic significance of the water-drinking test. Acta Soc Ophthal Jpn 71:2133, 1967.
131. Ballin, N, Becker, B: Provocative testing for primary open-angle glaucoma in "senior citizens." Invest Ophthal 6:126, 1967.
132. Armaly, MF, Sayegh, RE: Water-drinking test. II. The effect of age on tonometric and tonographic measures. Arch Ophthal 83:176, 1970.
133. Kronfeld, PC: Water drinking and outflow facility. Invest Ophthal 14:49, 1975.
134. Thorpe, RM, Kolker, AE: A tonographic study of water loading in rabbits. Arch Ophthal 77:238, 1967.

135. Casey, WJ: Intraocular pressure and facility in monkeys after water drinking. A study in the Cynomolgus monkey, *Macaca irus*. Arch Ophthal 74:841, 1965.
136. Roth, JA: Inadequate diagnostic value of the water-drinking test. Br J Ophthal 58:55, 1974.
137. Rasmussen, KE, Jørgensen, HA: Diagnostic value of the water-drinking test in early detection of simple glaucoma. Acta Ophthal 54:160, 1976.
138. Harris, LS: Cycloplegic-induced intraocular pressure elevations. A study of normal and open-angle glaucomatous eyes. Arch Ophthal 79:242, 1968.
139. Lazenby, GW, Reed, JW, Grant, WM: Short-term tests of anticholinergic medication in open-angle glaucoma. Arch Ophthal 80:443, 1968.
140. Lazenby, GW, Reed, JW, Grant, WM: Anticholinergic medication in open-angle glaucoma. Long-term tests. Arch Ophthal 84:719, 1970.
141. Harris, LS, Galin, MA: Cycloplegic provocative testing. Arch Ophthal 81:356, 1969.
142. Harris, LS, Galin, MA, Mittag, TW: Cycloplegic provocative testing after topical administration of steroids. Arch Ophthal 86:12, 1971.
143. Harris, LS, Galin, MA: Cycloplegic provocative testing. Effect of miotic therapy. Arch Ophthal 81:544, 1969.
144. Bárány, E, Christensen, RE: Cycloplegia and outflow resistance in normal human and monkey eyes and in primary open-angle glaucoma. Arch Ophthal 77:757, 1967.
145. Portney, GL, Purcell, TW: The influence of tropicamide on intraocular pressure. Ann Ophthal 7:31, 1975.
146. Shaw, BR, Lewis, RA: Intraocular pressure elevation after pupillary dilation in open angle glaucoma. Arch Ophthal 104:1185, 1986.
147. Kristensen, P: Mydriasis-induced pigment liberation in the anterior chamber associated with acute rise in intraocular pressure in open-angle glaucoma. Acta Ophthal 43:714, 1965.
148. Kristensen, P: Pigment liberation test in open-angle glaucoma. Acta Ophthal 46:586, 1968.
149. Valle, O: The cyclopentolate provocative test in suspected or untreated open-angle glaucoma. III. The significance of pigment for the result of the cyclopentolate provocative test in suspected or untreated open-angle glaucoma. Acta Ophthal 54:654, 1976.
150. Mapstone, R: Pigment release. Br J Ophthal 65:258, 1981.
151. Haddad, R, Strasser, G, Heilig, P, Jurecka, W: Decompensation of chronic open-angle glaucoma following mydriasis-induced pigmentary dispersion into the aqueous humour: a light and electron microscopic study. Br J Ophthal 65:252, 1981.
152. Becker, B, Montgomery, SW, Kass, MA, Shin, DH: Increased ocular and systemic responsiveness to epinephrine in primary open-angle glaucoma. Arch Ophthal 95:789, 1977.
153. Shin, DH, Kass, MA, Becker, B: Intraocular pressure response to topical epinephrine and HLA-B12. Arch Ophthal 96:1012, 1978.
154. Palmberg, PF, Hajek, S, Cooper, D, Becker, B: Increased cellular responsiveness to epinephrine in primary open-angle glaucoma. Arch Ophthal 95:855, 1977.
155. Becker, B, Shin, DH: Response to topical epinephrine. A practical prognostic test in patients with ocular hypertension. Arch Ophthal 94:2057, 1976.
156. Kass, MA, Becker, B: A simplified test of epinephrine responsiveness. Arch Ophthal 96:999, 1978.
157. Drance, SM, Saheb, NE, Schulzer, M: Response to topical epinephrine in chronic open-angle glaucoma. Arch Ophthal 96:1001, 1978.
158. Hollwich, F: The pilocarpine-test for the early diagnosis of glaucoma. Klin Monatsbl Augenheilkd 163:115, 1973.
159. Nissen, OI, Kjer, P, Olsen, L: A comparison between an acetazolamide test and weight tonography in pathological and apathological circulation of the aqueous humor. Invest Ophthal 15:844, 1976.
160. Drance, SM: The uniocular therapeutic trial in the management of elevated intraocular pressure. Surv Ophthal 25:203, 1980.
161. Rothkoff, L, Biedner, B, Biger, Y, Blumenthal, M: A proposed pilocarpine therapeutic test. Arch Ophthal 96:1380, 1978.
162. Lewis, JM, Priddy, T, Judd, J, et al: Intraocular pressure response to topical dexamethasone as a predictor for the development of primary open-angle glaucoma. Am J Ophthal 106:607, 1988.
163. Drance, SM: Studies in the susceptibility of the eye to raised intraocular pressure. Arch Ophthal 68:478, 1962.
164. Goldmann, H: Open-angle glaucoma. Br J Ophthal 56:242, 1972.
165. Wodowosow, AM, Boriskina, MG, Kotjeljnikowa, OF: Further observations concerning the campimetric method of measuring individually tolerated intraocular pressure in glaucoma. Klin Monatsbl Augenheilkd 180:135, 1982.
166. Becker, B, Morton, WR: Phenylthiourea taste testing and glaucoma. Arch Ophthal 72:323, 1964.
167. Kalmus, H, Lewkonia, I: Relation between some forms of glaucoma and phenylthiocarbamide tasting. Br J Ophthal 57:503, 1973.
168. Shin, DH, Becker, B, Waltman, SR, et al: The prevalence of HLA-B12 and HLA-B7 antigens in primary open-angle glaucoma. Arch Ophthal 95:224, 1977.
169. Ritch, R, Podos, SM, Henley, W, et al: Lack of association of histocompatibility antigens with

primary open-angle glaucoma. Arch Ophthal 96:2204, 1978.

170. Shaw, JF, Levene, RZ, Sowell, JG: The incidence of HLA antigens in black primary open-angle glaucoma patients. Am J Ophthal 86:501, 1978.

171. Damgaard-Jensen, L, Kissmeyer-Nielsen, F: HLA histocompatibility antigens in open-angle glaucoma. Acta Ophthal 56:384, 1978.

172. Scharf, J, Gideoni, O, Zonis, S, Barzilai, A: Histocompatibility antigens (HLA) and open-angle glaucoma. Ann Ophthal 10:914, 1978.

173. David, R, Maier, G, Baumgarten, I, Abrahams, C: HLA antigens in glaucoma and ocular hypertension. Br J Ophthal 63:293, 1979.

174. Rosenthal, AR, Payne, R: Association of HLA antigens and primary open-angle glaucoma. Am J Ophthal 88:479, 1979.

175. Ticho, U, Cohen, T, Brautbar, C: Absence of association between HLA antigens and primary open-angle glaucoma in Israel. Israel J Med Sci 15:124, 1979.

176. Kass, MA, Palmberg, P, Becker, B, Miller, JP: Histocompatibility antigens and primary open-angle glaucoma. A reassessment. Arch Ophthal 96:2207, 1978.

177. Olivius, E, Polland, W: Histocompatibility (HLA) antigens in capsular glaucoma and simplex glaucoma. Acta Ophthal 58:406, 1980.

178. Slagsvold, JE, Nordhagen, R: The HLA system in primary open-angle glaucoma and in patients with pseudoexfoliation of the lens capsule (exfoliation or fibrillopathia epitheliocapsularis). Acta Ophthal 58:188, 1980.

179. Grant, WM: Further studies on facility of flow through the trabecular meshwork. Arch Ophthal 60:523, 1958.

180. Ashton, N: The exit pathway of the aqueous. Trans Ophthal Soc UK 80:397, 1960.

181. Speakman, JS, Leeson, TS: Site of obstruction to aqueous outflow in chronic simple glaucoma. Br J Ophthal 46:321, 1962.

182. Zatulina, NI: Electron-microscopy of trabecular tissue in far-advanced stage of simple open-angle glaucoma. Oftal Z 28:117, 1973.

183. Li, Y, Yi, Y: Histochemical and electron microscopic studies of the trabecular meshwork in primary open-angle glaucoma. Eye Science 1:17, 1985.

184. Segawa, K: Electron microscopic changes of the trabecular tissue in primary open-angle glaucoma. Ann Ophthal 11:49, 1979.

185. Finkelstein, I, Trope, GE, Basu, PK, et al: Quantitative analysis of collagen content and amino acids in trabecular meshwork. Br J Ophthal 74:280, 1990.

186. Fine, BS, Yanoff, M, Stone, RA: A clinicopathologic study of four cases of primary open-angle glaucoma compared to normal eyes. Am J Ophthal 91:88, 1981.

187. Alvarado, J, Murphy, C, Juster, R: Trabecular meshwork cellularity in primary open-angle glaucoma and nonglaucomatous normals. Ophthalmology 91:564, 1984.

188. Tripathi, RC, Tripathi, BJ: Contractile protein alteration in trabecular endothelium in primary open-angle glaucoma. Exp Eye Res 31:721, 1981.

189. Armaly, MF, Wang, Y: Demonstration of acid mucopolysaccharides in the trabecular meshwork of the Rhesus monkey. Invest Ophthal 14:507, 1975.

190. Chaudhry, HA, Dueker, DK, Simmons, RJ, et al: Scanning electron microscopy of trabeculectomy specimens in open-angle glaucoma. Am J Ophthal 88:78, 1979.

191. Maglio, M, McMahon, C, Hoskins, D, Alvarado, J: Potential artifacts in scanning electron microscopy of the trabecular meshwork in glaucoma. Am J Ophthal 90:645, 1980.

192. Quigley, HA, Addicks, EM: Scanning electron microscopy of trabeculectomy specimens from eyes with open-angle glaucoma. Am J Ophthal 90:854, 1980.

193. Gieser, DK, Tanenbaum, M, Smith, ME, et al: Amorphous coating in open-angle glaucoma. Am J Ophthal 92:130, 1981.

194. de Kater, AW, Melamed, S, Epstein, DL: Patterns of aqueous human outflow in glaucomatous and nonglaucomatous human eyes. A tracer study using cationized ferritin. Arch Ophthal 107:572, 1989.

195. Rohen, JW: Fine structural changes in the trabecular meshwork of the human eye in different forms of glaucoma. Klin Monatsbl Augenheilkd 163:401, 1973.

196. Zimmerman, LE: The outflow problem in normal and pathologic eyes. Trans Am Acad Ophthal Otol 70:767, 1966.

197. Rodrigues, MM, Spaeth, GL, Sivalingam, E, Weinreb, S: Value of trabeculectomy specimens in glaucoma. Ophthal Surg 9:29, 1978.

198. Alvarado, JA, Yun, AJ, Murphy, CG: Juxtacanalicular tissue in primary open angle glaucoma and in nonglaucomatous normals. Arch Ophthal 104:1517, 1986.

199. Rohen, JW: Presence of matrix vesicles in the trabecular meshwork of glaucomatous eyes. Graefe's Arch Ophthal 218:171, 1982.

200. Rohen, JW: Why is intraocular pressure elevated in chronic simple glaucoma? Ophthalmology 90:758, 1983.

201. Babizhayev, MA, Brodskaya, MW: Fibronectin detection in drainage outflow system of human eyes in ageing and progression of open-angle glaucoma. Mech Ageing Dev 47:145, 1989.

202. Worthen, DM, Cleveland, PH, Slight, JR, Abare, J: Selective binding affinity of human plasma fi-

bronectin for the collagens I-IV. Invest Ophthal Vis Sci 26:1740, 1985.
203. Tripathi, RC: Ultrastructure of the trabecular wall of Schlemm's canal. (A study of normotensive and chronic simple glaucomatous eyes.) Trans Ophthal Soc UK 89:449, 1969.
204. Tripathi, RC: Ultrastructure of Schlemm's canal in relation to aqueous outflow. Exp Eye Res 7:335, 1968.
205. Nesterov, AP, Batmanov, YE: Trabecular wall of Schlemm's canal in the early stage of primary open-angle glaucoma. Am J Ophthal 78:639, 1974.
206. Moses, RA, Grodski, WJ Jr, Etheridge, EL, Wilson, CD: Schlemm's canal: The effect of intraocular pressure. Invest Ophthal Vis Sci 20:61, 1981.
207. Johnson, MC, Kamm, RD: The role of Schlemm's canal in aqueous outflow from the human eye. Invest Ophthal Vis Sci 24:320, 1983.
208. Krasnov, MM: Sinusotomy. Foundations, results, prospects. Trans Am Acad Ophthal Otol 76:368, 1972.
209. Herschler, J, Litin, BS: Biochemical abnormalities in the aqueous in chronic open-angle glaucoma. Ophthalmic Surg 18:792, 1987.
210. Becker, B, Hahn, KA: Topical corticosteroids and heredity in primary open-angle glaucoma. Am J Ophthal 57:543, 1964.
211. Armaly, MF: The heritable nature of dexamethasone-induced ocular hypertension. Arch Ophthal 75:32, 1966.
212. Armaly, MF: Inheritance of dexamethasone hypertension and glaucoma. Arch Ophthal 77:747, 1967.
213. Schwartz, JT, Reuling, FH, Feinleib, M, et al: Twin study on ocular pressure after topical dexamethasone. 1. Frequency distribution of pressure response. Am J Ophthal 76:126, 1973.
214. Palmberg, PF, Mandell, A, Wilensky, JT, et al: The reproducibility of the intraocular pressure response to dexamethasone. Am J Ophthal 80:844, 1975.
215. Dean, GO Jr, Deutsch, AR, Hiatt, RL: The effect of dexamethasone on borderline ocular hypertension. Ann Ophthal 7:193, 1975.
216. Levene, R, Wigdor, A, Edelstein, A, Baum, J: Topical corticosteroid in normal patients and glaucoma suspects. Arch Ophthal 77:593, 1967.
217. LeBlanc, RP, Stewart, RH, Becker, B: Corticosteroid provocative testing. Invest Ophthal 9:946, 1970.
218. Kitazawa, Y, Horie, T: The prognosis of corticosteroid-responsive individuals. Arch Ophthal 99:819, 1981.
219. Akingbehin, AO: Corticosteroid-induced ocular hypertension. I. Prevalence in closed-angle glaucoma. Br J Ophthal 66:536, 1982.
220. Kitazawa, Y: Primary angle-closure glaucoma. Corticosteroid responsiveness. Arch Ophthal 84:724, 1970.
221. Krupin, T, Schoch, LH, Cooper, D, Becker, B: Lack of correlation between ocular hypertensive response to topical corticosteroids and progression of retinopathy in insulin-dependent diabetes mellitus. Am J Ophthal 96:52, 1983.
222. Becker, B: The genetic problem of chronic simple glaucoma. Ann Ophthal 3:351, 1971.
223. Francois, J, Heintz-De Bree, C, Tripathi, RC: The cortisone test and the heredity of primary open-angle glaucoma. Am J Ophthal 62:844, 1966.
224. Schwartz, JT, Reuling, FH, Feinleib, M, et al: Twin heritability study of the effect of corticosteroids on intraocular pressure. J Med Genet 9:137, 1972.
225. Schwartz, JT, Reuling, FH Jr, Feinleib, M, et al: Twin heritability study of the corticosteroid response. Trans Am Acad Ophthal Otol 77:126, 1973.
226. Schwartz, JT, Reuling, FH, Feinleib, M, et al: Twin study on ocular pressure following topically applied dexamethasone. II. Inheritance of variation in pressure response. Arch Ophthal 90:281, 1973.
227. Akingbehin, AO: Corticosteroid-induced ocular hypertension. II. An acquired form. Br J Ophthal 66:541, 1982.
228. Spaeth, GL: Traumatic hyphema, angle recession, dexamethasone hypertension, and glaucoma. Arch Ophthal 78:714, 1967.
229. Schwartz, B, Levene, RZ: Plasma cortisol differences between normal and glaucomatous patients. Before and after dexamethasone suppression. Arch Ophthal 87:369, 1972.
230. Schwartz B, McCarty, G, Rosner, B: Increased plasma free cortisol in ocular hypertension and open angle glaucoma. Arch Ophthal 105:1060, 1987.
231. Krupin, T, Podos, SM, Becker, B: Effect of diphenylhydantoin on dexamethasone suppression of plasma cortisol in primary open-angle glaucoma. Am J Ophthal 71:997, 1971.
232. Meredig, WE, Puelhorn, G, Jentzen, F, Hartmann, F: The plasmacortisol-level in patients suffering from glaucoma. Graefe's Arch Ophthal 213:215, 1980.
233. Schwartz, B, Seddon, JM: Increased plasma cortisol levels in ocular hypertension. Arch Ophthal 99:1791, 1981.
234. Rosenberg, S, Levene, R: Suppression of plasma cortisol in normal and glaucomatous patients. Arch Ophthal 92:6, 1974.
235. Levene, RZ, Schwartz, B, Workman, PL: Heritability of plasma cortisol. Arch Ophthal 87:389, 1972.
236. Becker, B, Ramsey, CK: Plasma cortisol and the intraocular pressure response to topical corticosteroids. Am J Ophthal 69:999, 1970.

237. Podos, SM, Becker, B, Beaty, C, Cooper, DG: Diphenylhydantoin and cortisol metabolism in glaucoma. Am J Ophthal 74:498, 1972.
238. Becker, B, Podos, SM, Asseff, CF, Cooper, DG: Plasma cortisol suppression in glaucoma. Am J Ophthal 75:73, 1973.
239. Krupin, T, Jacobs, LS, Podos, SM, Becker, B: Thyroid function and the intraocular pressure response to topical corticosteroids. Am J Ophthal 83:643, 1977.
240. Polansky, J, Palmberg, P, Matulich, D, et al: Cellular sensitivity to glucocorticoids in patients with POAG. Steroid receptors and responses in cultured skin fibroblasts. Invest Ophthal Vis Sci 26:805, 1985.
241. Levene, RZ, Schwartz, B: Depression of plasma cortisol and the steroid ocular pressure response. Arch Ophthal 80:461, 1968.
242. Schwartz, B: Hypothalamic-pituitary-adrenal axis and steroid glaucoma. Klin Monatsbl Augenheilkd 161:280, 1972.
243. Kass, MA, Krupin, T, Becker, B: Plasma cortisol suppression test used to predict the development of primary open-angle glaucoma. Am J Ophthal 82:496, 1976.
244. Bigger, JF, Palmberg, PF, Becker, B: Increased cellular sensitivity to glucocorticoids in primary open-angle glaucoma. Invest Ophthal 11:832, 1972.
245. Foon, KA, Yuen, K, Ballintine, EF, Rosenstreich, DL: Analysis of the systemic corticosteroid sensitivity of patients with primary open-angle glaucoma. Am J Ophthal 83:167, 1977.
246. BenEzra, D, Ticho, U, Sachs, U: Lymphocyte sensitivity to glucocorticoids. Am J Ophthal 82:866, 1976.
247. Sowell, JC, Levene, RZ, Bloom, J, Bernstein, M: Primary open-angle glaucoma and sensitivity to corticosteroids in vitro. Am J Ophthal 84:715, 1977.
248. McCarty, G, Schwartz, B, Miller, K: Absence of lymphocyte glucocorticoid hypersensitivity in primary open-angle glaucoma. Arch Ophthal 99:1258, 1981.
249. Palmberg, PF, Rachlin, D, Becker, B: Differential sensitivity at the cellular level in primary open-angle glaucoma: prednisolone and ouabain. Invest Ophthal 15:403, 1976.
250. Schwartz, B, Golden, MA, Wiznia, RA, Miller, SA: Differences of adrenal stress control mechanisms in subjects with glaucoma and normal subjects. Effect of vasopressin and pyrogen. Arch Ophthal 99:1770, 1981.
251. Kass, MA, Shin, DH, Becker, B: The ocular hypotensive effect of epinephrine in high and low corticosteroid responders. Invest Ophthal 16:530, 1977.
252. Zink, HA, Palmberg, PF, Bigger, JF: Increased sensitivity to theophylline associated with primary open-angle glaucoma. Invest Ophthal 12:603, 1973.
253. Francois, J, Victoria-Troncoso, V: Mucopolysaccharides and pathogenesis of cortisone glaucoma. Klin Monatsbl Augenheilkd 165:5, 1974.
254. Bill, A: The drainage of aqueous humor. Invest Ophthal 14:1, 1975.
255. Southren, AL, Gordon, GG, Munnangi, PR, et al: Altered cortisol metabolism in cells cultured from trabecular meshwork specimens obtained from patients with primary open-angle glaucoma. Invest Ophthal Vis Sci 24:1413, 1983.
256. Becker, B, Keates, EU, Coleman, SL: Gammaglobulin in the trabecular meshwork of glaucomatous eyes. Arch Ophthal 68:643, 1962.
257. Becker, B, Unger, H-H, Coleman, SL, Keates, EU: Plasma cells and gamma-globulin in trabecular meshwork of eyes with primary open-angle glaucoma. Arch Ophthal 70:38, 1963.
258. Waltman, SR, Yarian, D: Antinuclear antibodies in open-angle glaucoma. Invest Ophthal 13:695, 1974.
259. Shields, MB, McCoy, RC, Shelburne, JD: Immunofluorescent studies on the trabecular meshwork in open-angle glaucoma. Invest Ophthal 15:1014, 1976.
260. Rodrigues, MM, Katz, SI, Foidart, JM, Spaeth, GL: Collagen, Factor VIII antigen, and immunoglobulins in the human aqueous drainage channels. Ophthalmology 87:337, 1980.
261. Radda, TM, Gnad, HC, Aberer, W: The questionable immunopathogenesis of primary open-angle glaucoma. Klin Monatsbl Augenheilkd 181:388, 1982.
262. Felberg, NT, Leon, SA, Gasparini, J, Spaeth, GL: A comparison of antinuclear antibodies and DNA-binding antibodies in chronic open-angle glaucoma. Invest Ophthal Vis Sci 16:757, 1977.
263. Radda, TM, Menzel, J, Drobec, P, Aberer, W: Immunological investigation in primary open angle glaucoma. Graefe's Arch Ophthal 218:55, 1982.
264. Henley, WL, Okas, S, Leopold, IH: Cellular immunity in chronic ophthalmic disorders. 4. Leukocyte migration inhibition in diseases associated with glaucoma. Am J Ophthal 76:60, 1973.
265. Quigley, HA, Maumenee, AE: Long-term follow-up of treated open-angle glaucoma. Am J Ophthal 87:519, 1979.
266. Vogel, R, Crick, RP, Newson, RB, et al: Association between intraocular pressure and loss of visual field in chronic simple glaucoma. Br J Ophthal 74:3, 1990.
267. Drance, SM, Schulzer, M, Douglas, GR, Sweeney, VP: Use of discriminant analysis. II. Identification of persons with glaucomatous visual field defects. Arch Ophthal 96:1571, 1978.
268. Kass, MA, Hart, WM Jr, Gordon, M, Miller, JP: Risk factors favoring the development of glauco-

matous visual field loss in ocular hypertension. Surv Ophthal 25:155, 1980.

269. Armaly, MF, Krueger, DE, Maunder, L, et al: Biostatistical analysis of the collaborative glaucoma study. I. Summary report of the risk factors for glaucomatous visual-field defects. Arch Ophthal 98:2163, 1980.
270. Epstein, DL, Krug, JH, Jr, Hertzmark, E, et al: A long-term clinical trial of timolol therapy versus no treatment in the management of glaucoma suspects. Ophthalmology 96:1460, 1989.
271. Kass, MA, Gordon, MO, Hoff, MR, et al: Topical timolol administration reduces the incidence of glaucomatous damage in ocular hypertensive individuals. Arch Ophthal 107:1590, 1989.
272. Kass, MA: Timolol treatment prevents or delays glaucomatous visual field loss in individuals with ocular hypertension: a five-year, randomized, double-masked, clinical trial. Tr Am Ophthal Soc 87:598, 1989.
273. Goldmann, H: An analysis of some concepts concerning chronic simple glaucoma. Am J Ophthal 80:409, 1975.
274. Begg, IS, Cottle, RW, Collaborative Glaucoma Study Group: Epidemiological approach to open-angle glaucoma: 1. Control of intraocular pressure. Report of the Canadian Ocular Adverse Drug Reaction Registry Program. Can J Ophthal 23:273, 1988.
275. Kolker, AE: Visual prognosis in advanced glaucoma: a comparison of medical and surgical therapy for retention of vision in 101 eyes with advanced glaucoma. Trans Am Ophthal Soc 75:539, 1977.
276. Wilson, R, Walker, AM, Dueker, DK, Crick, RP: Risk factors for rate of progression of glaucomatous visual field loss. A computer-based analysis. Arch Ophthal 100:737, 1982.
277. Odberg, T: Visual field prognosis in advanced glaucoma. Acta Ophthal 65 (suppl) 182:27, 1987.
278. Schulzer, M, Mikelberg, FS, Drance, SM: Some observations on the relation between intraocular pressure reduction and the progression of glaucomatous visual loss. Br J Ophthal 71:486, 1987.
279. Spaeth, GL: Control of glaucoma: a new definition. Ophthal Surg 14:303, 1983.
280. Spaeth, GL, Fellman, RL, Starita, RL, et al: A new management system for glaucoma based on improvement of the appearance of the optic disc or visual field. Trans Am Ophthal Soc 83:268, 1985.
281. Shin, DH, Bielik, M, Hong, YJ, et al: Reversal of glaucomatous optic disc cupping in adult patients. Arch Ophthal 115:1599, 1989.
282. Bloch, S, Rosenthal, AR, Friedman, L, Caldarolla, P: Patient compliance in glaucoma. Br J Ophthal 61:531, 1977.
283. MacKean, JM, Elkington, AR: Compliance with treatment of patients with chronic open-angle glaucoma. Br J Ophthal 67:46, 1983.
284. Smith, RJH: Medical versus surgical therapy in glaucoma simplex. Br J Ophthal 56:277, 1972.
285. Werner, EB, Drance, SM: Progression of glaucomatous field defects despite successful filtration. Can J Ophthal 12:275, 1977.
286. Smith, RJH: The enigma of primary open angle glaucoma. Trans Ophthal Soc UK 105:618, 1986.
287. Jay, JL, Murray, SB: Early trabeculectomy versus conventional management in primary open angle glaucoma. Br J Ophthal 72:881, 1988.
288. Migdal, C, Hitchings, R: Control of chronic simple glaucoma with primary medical, surgical and laser treatment. Trans Ophthal Soc UK 105:653, 1986.
289. Bloomfield, S: The results of surgery for low-tension glaucoma. Am J Ophthal 36:1067, 1953.
290. Sugar, HS: Low tension glaucoma: a practical approach. Ann Ophthal 11:1155, 1979.
291. Abedin, S, Simmons, RJ, Grant, WM: Progressive low-tension glaucoma. Treatment to stop glaucomatous cupping and field loss when these progress despite normal intraocular pressure. Ophthalmology 89:1, 1982.
292. Kitazawa, Y, Shirai, H, Go, FJ: The effect of Ca^{2+}-antagonist on visual field in low-tension glaucoma. Graefe's Arch Ophthal 227:408, 1989.

Chapter 10

PRIMARY ANGLE-CLOSURE GLAUCOMA

Terminology

Several forms of primary angle-closure glaucoma (PACG) have been recognized on the basis of clinical presentation and mechanism of angle closure. A variety of terms have been applied to these entities, which has led to some confusion regarding nomenclature. The following classification of PACG will be used in this chapter and provides a brief introduction to the subject. Details of mechanism and clinical appearance will be considered later in the chapter.

Pupillary Block Glaucoma

In this category of PACG, the initiating event is believed to be a functional block between the pupillary portion of the iris and the anterior lens surface,[1] which is associated with mid-dilation of the pupil.[2] This functional block causes a build-up of aqueous in the posterior chamber, leading to a forward shift of the peripheral iris and closure of the anterior chamber angle (Fig. 10.1).[1–3] Three forms of pupillary block glaucoma may be distinguished on the basis of symptoms and clinical findings:

Acute Angle-Closure Glaucoma. In this form of pupillary block glaucoma, the symptoms are sudden and severe, with marked pain, blurred vision, and a red eye. The condition was once referred to as congestive glaucoma.[4]

Subacute Angle-Closure Glaucoma. This clinical entity is believed to have the same pupillary block mechanism as the acute form, but symptoms are either mild or absent.[5] The condition has also been called intermittent, prodromal, or subclinical,[6] and was probably once lumped with the "noncongestive" glaucomas.[4] However, the latter term also included open-angle glaucoma and has been largely abandoned since Barkan[4] classified the glaucomas on the basis of an open or closed anterior chamber angle. Patients with subacute angle-closure glaucoma may have repeated subacute or subclinical attacks before finally having an acute attack or developing peripheral anterior synechiae with chronic pressure elevation.[5]

Chronic Angle-Closure Glaucoma. In this condition, portions of the anterior chamber angle are permanently closed by

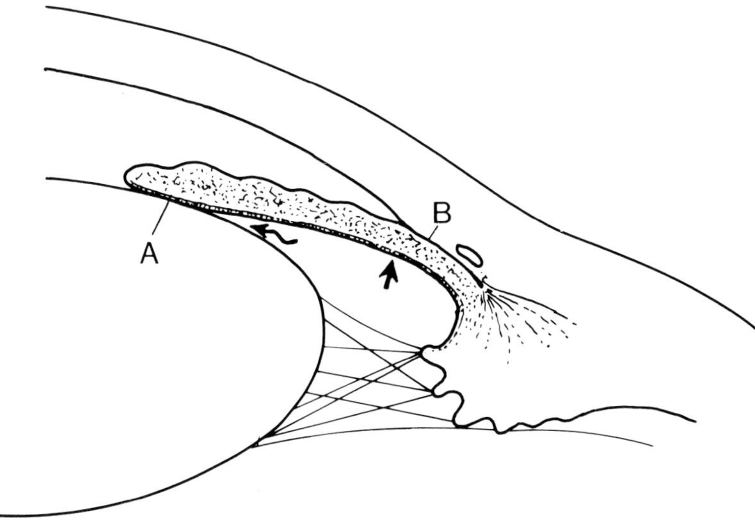

Figure 10.1. Pupillary block glaucoma. A functional block between the lens and iris (*A*) leads to increased pressure in the posterior chamber (*arrows*) with forward shift of the peripheral iris and closure of the anterior chamber angle (*B*).

peripheral anterior synechiae, and the intraocular pressure (IOP) is chronically elevated.[6,7] The synechial closure may result from a prolonged acute attack or repeated subacute attacks of angle-closure glaucoma. A variation of this condition has been called shortening of the angle,[8] or creeping angle-closure glaucoma.[9]

Plateau Iris

In a very small percentage of patients with PACG, the mechanism appears to be an abnormal anatomic configuration of the anterior chamber angle, which leads to occlusion of the trabecular meshwork by peripheral iris in association with dilation of the pupil.[10,11] This situation differs from pupillary block glaucoma in that closure of the anterior chamber angle apparently is due to an infolding of iris into the angle in association with pupillary dilation, but without a significant pupillary block component (Fig. 10.2). The condition has been divided into the *plateau iris configuration* and *plateau iris syndrome*,[12] which are explained later in this chapter.

Combined Mechanism Glaucoma

In some eyes there appears to be both an open-angle and an angle-closure mechanism to the glaucoma. The diagnosis is usually made after a primary acute angle-closure glaucoma attack in which the IOP remains elevated after a peripheral iridectomy, despite an open, normal-appearing angle. In one study this was seen in 6 of 267 (2.2%) eyes that underwent peripheral iridectomy for presumed angle-closure glaucoma.[13]

Epidemiology

In most populations, PACG is considerably less common than primary open-angle glaucoma, although a precise ratio between the two conditions has not been clearly established. However, there is a reversal in the ratio of primary angle-closure and open-angle glaucoma among Canadian,[14] Alaskan,[15] and Greenland[16,17] Eskimos, with the former disorder occurring in approximately 0.5% of the general population and in 2–3% of those over 40 years of age, with a predilection for women. This prevalence of PACG may be due to a smaller corneal diameter and anterior chamber depth, and a thicker, more anteriorly placed lens among these individuals.[18–20]

Studies of the anterior chamber angle in general populations provide an impression of the prevalence of those at risk of developing angle-closure glaucoma. In two large

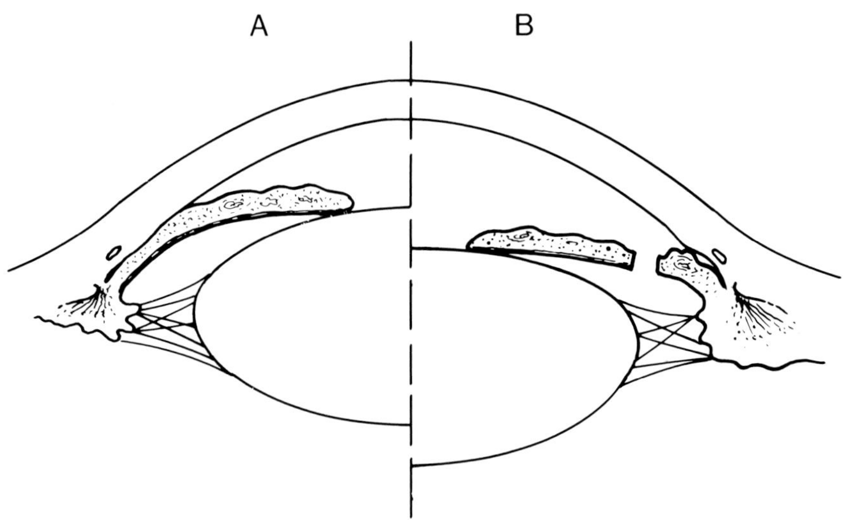

Figure 10.2. Pupillary block glaucoma (*A*) contrasted with the plateau iris syndrome (*B*). In the latter situation, note the relatively deeper central anterior chamber, the flat iris plane, patent iridectomy, and bunching up of peripheral iris in the anterior chamber angle.

studies, 5–6% of those screened had suspicious anterior chamber angles, but only 0.64–1.1% were considered to have critically narrow angles.[21,22]

CLINICAL FEATURES

The diagnosis of PACG has several facets. During the course of every ocular examination, the physician must consider general risk factors in the medical history and look for anatomic features that might predispose to angle-closure. When suspicious findings are noted, provocative tests are sometimes used to determine the potential for angle-closure glaucoma. In other situations, the patient may present with signs and symptoms suggestive of angle-closure glaucoma, and the correct diagnosis will depend on an understanding of the symptoms, predisposing circumstances, and physical findings of the disease, as well as the differential diagnosis. These various aspects of diagnosing potential or manifest PACG will now be considered.

Risk Factors: General Features of Patients

The following factors influence the configuration of the anterior chamber angle and the risk of developing PACG.

Age. The depth and volume of the anterior chamber diminish with age,[23] which may result from a thickening and forward displacement of the lens.[24] Consequently, the percentage of individuals with critically narrow angles is higher in older age groups. The prevalence of PACG also increases with age, although it may peak earlier in life than with primary open-angle glaucoma. One study found a bimodal peak, with the first at ages 53–58 years and the second at 63–70 years.[24] However, it can occur at any age, including rare cases in childhood.[25]

Race. Primary angle-closure glaucoma is less common among blacks and is more often of the chronic form when it does occur in that race.[26–28] The explanation for this difference is uncertain. One study suggested it might be due to a thinner average lens thickness,[27] although another investigation revealed the anterior chamber depth in Nigerian blacks to be equivalent to that of whites.[29] It has also been suggested that the weaker response to mydriatics observed among African blacks could indicate that darker irides are less able to exert the force that may lead to pupillary block.[30] Angle-closure glaucoma also has a reduced prevalence among American Indians and is often secondary to a swollen lens when it does occur in this group.[28] As previously noted, the relative prevalence of PACG among the primary glaucomas is increased in various populations of Eskimos.[14–20]

Sex. There is a statistically significant predominance of *females* in populations with PACG, which is thought to be due to the shallower anterior chamber among women in general.[14–16,23,29,31]

Refractive Error. The depth and volume of the anterior chamber are also related to the degree of ametropia, with smaller dimensions in *hyperopes*.[23] However, the presence of myopia does not eliminate the possibility of angle-closure glaucoma, since rare cases have been reported in such patients.[32]

Family History. The potential for PACG is generally believed to be inherited. In one study, 20% of 95 relatives of angle-closure glaucoma patients were believed to have potentially occludable angles.[33] However, aside from a few reported families in which many members developed angle-closure glaucoma, the family history is not very useful in predicting a future angle-closure attack.[34]

HLA antigens were studied in 35 angle-closure glaucoma patients, and no correlation was found.[35]

Systemic Disorders. One study has shown an inverse correlation between type 2 diabetes or an abnormal glucose tolerance test and the anterior chamber depth.[36] The same authors have suggested an increased prevalence of denervation supersensitivity to autonomic agonists in angle closure glaucoma.[37]

Risk Factors: Findings During Routine Examination

The following observations during the course of a routine ocular examination will help to establish the potential for angle closure.

Intraocular Pressure

Unless the patient has angle closure at the time of the examination, the IOP will usually be normal. One study, however, found a larger than normal amplitude in the diurnal IOP curve, which the authors believed might have prognostic value.[38] Tonography also characteristically reveals normal outflow facility before or between attacks, unless synechial damage has begun to develop.[2]

Evaluation of Peripheral Anterior Chamber

Photogrammetric studies of all forms of angle-closure glaucoma have revealed anterior chamber depths, volumes, and diameters that are smaller than those of matched controls.[39] Anterior chamber depth and volume have also been shown to have diurnal variation, with lower values in the evening,[40] although a correlation with this and the diurnal IOP variation, noted above, is not clear. In any case, the most important step in the diagnosis of either potential or manifest angle-closure glaucoma is to evaluate the anterior chamber depth and especially the configuration of the anterior chamber angle. While this is best accomplished by gonioscopy, there are preliminary screening measures that may be useful in some situations, as well as techniques of quantifying the anterior chamber depth.

Penlight Examination. For situations in which a slit lamp and goniolens are not available, the anterior chamber depth can be estimated with oblique penlight illumination across the surface of the iris. With the light coming from the temporal side of the eye, a relatively flat iris will be illuminated on both the temporal and nasal side of the pupil, while an iris that is bowed forward will have a shadow on the nasal side (Fig. 10.3).[41]

Slit-Lamp Examination. The central anterior chamber depth may be estimated during examination with the slit lamp, and techniques for quantitating this parameter have been proposed.[42–44] However, the anterior chamber depth has been shown to have a weak correlation with the angle width,[45] and the parameter of greater diagnostic value within the context of angle-closure glaucoma is the depth of the peripheral anterior chamber. van Herick and co-workers[46] developed a technique for making this estimation with the slit lamp by comparing the peripheral anterior chamber depth to the

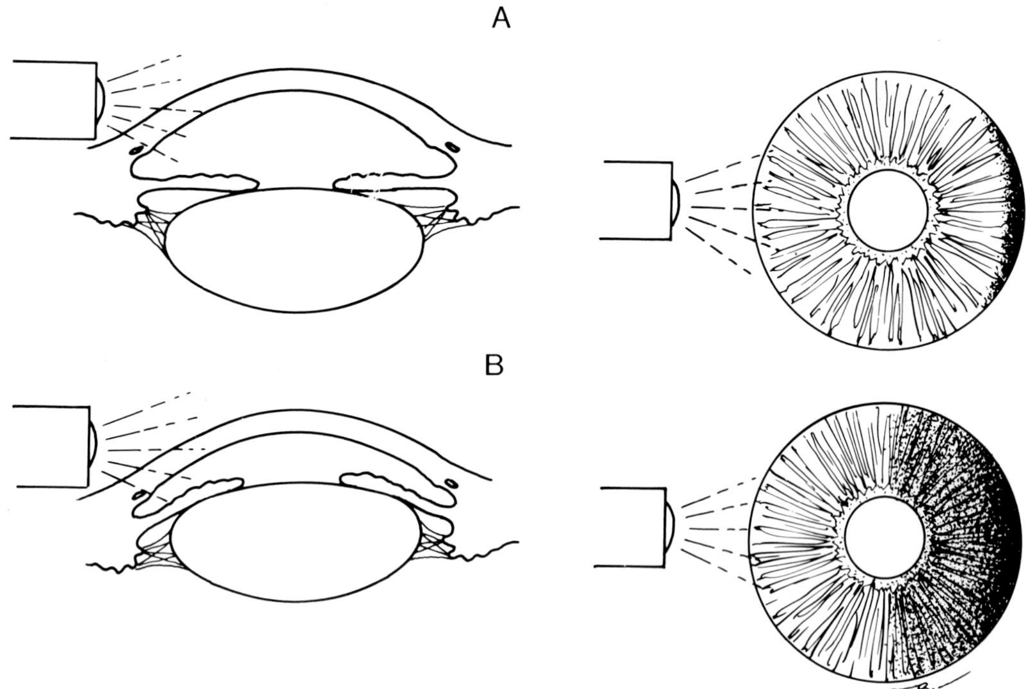

Figure 10.3. Oblique flashlight illumination as a screening measure for estimating the anterior chamber depth. **A,** With a deep chamber, nearly the entire iris is illuminated. **B,** When the iris is bowed forward, only the proximal portion is illuminated, and a shadow is seen in the distal half.

thickness of the adjacent cornea (Figs. 10.4 and 10.5). When the depth is less than ¼ the corneal thickness, the anterior chamber angle may be dangerously narrow.[46]

Gonioscopy. Whenever the peripheral anterior chamber depth is believed to be shallow (van Herick slit lamp Grade 1 or 2), careful gonioscopic examination of the angle is required. Numerous grading systems have been suggested in an attempt to correlate gonioscopic appearance with the potential for angle-closure. Scheie[47] proposed a system based on the extent of the *anterior chamber angle structures* that can be visualized (Fig. 10.6). He noted a high risk of angle closure in eyes with Grade III or IV angles. Shaffer[48] suggested using the *angular width* of the angle recess as the criterion for grading the angle and attempted to correlate this with the potential for angle-closure (Fig. 10.7).

Other authors believe that no single criterion fully describes the anterior chamber angle. Becker[49] proposed combining an estimation of the anterior chamber angle width and the height of the iris insertion, while Spaeth[22] suggested an evaluation of three variables: (1) angular width of the angle recess; (2) configuration of the peripheral iris; and (3) apparent insertion of the iris root (Fig. 10.8). Whatever system the clinician prefers to use to document the appearance of the anterior chamber angle, it is important to pay close attention to these three aspects of the angle. Additional features of the angle should also be studied and documented, such as peripheral anterior synechiae and abnormalities in pigmentation. It was noted in one study that patients with narrow angles may have a predominance of trabecular meshwork pigmentation in the superior quadrant, rather than the more common inferior location, which the authors believed might be due to a rubbing between the peripheral iris and the meshwork.[50]

Newer Techniques. Efforts to quantify more accurately the anterior chamber depth and related dimensions include the use of ultrasonography and newer photographic

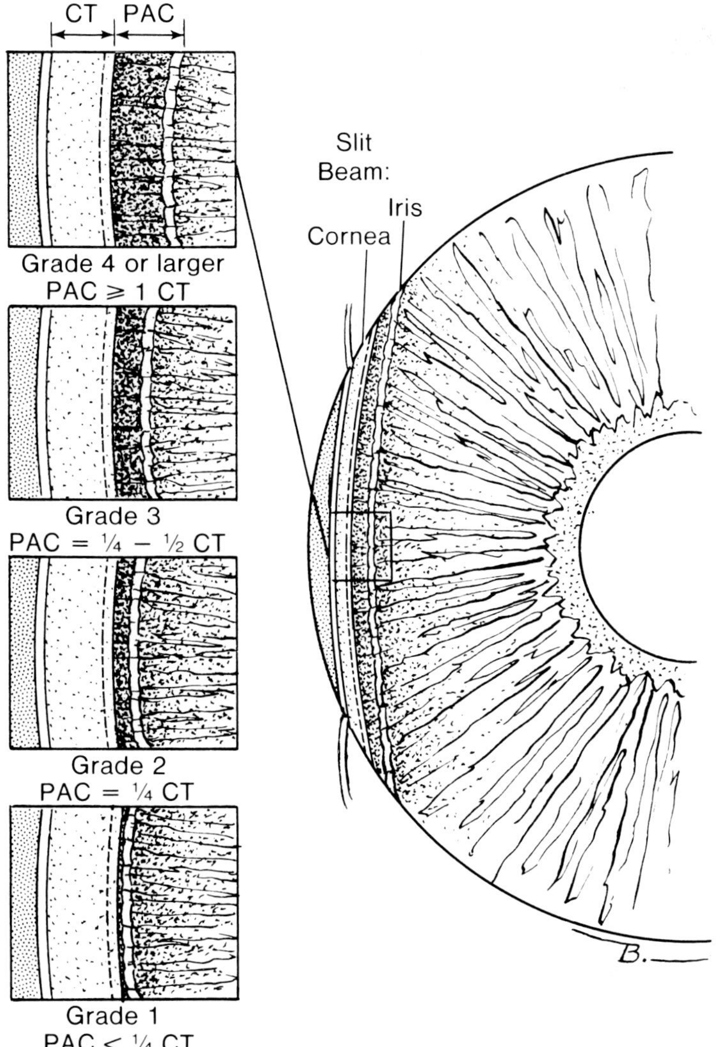

Figure 10.4. Slit-lamp technique of van Herick et al.[46] for estimating the depth of the peripheral anterior chamber (*PAC*) by comparing it with the adjacent corneal thickness (*CT*).

techniques. It has been suggested that the biometric calculation of the lens thickness/axial length ratio can be used as a prognostic indicator of PACG.[51,52] New photographic techniques include photogrammetry[39,40] and other methods[53,54] to document more accurately the configuration of the anterior chamber angle. The clinical value of all of these newer techniques, however, awaits further study.

Provocative Tests

Having decided that a patient has suspiciously narrow anterior chamber angles, the physician is now faced with a difficult decision. If it could be predicted that the patient would one day have an attack of angle-closure glaucoma, the appropriate course in most cases would be prophylactic peripheral iridotomies. The results of one study suggest that optic nerve damage occurs in the early time period after IOP rise, supporting the value of detection and surgery prior to an attack.[55] However, it is not always possible to predict with certainty, on the basis of the anterior chamber angle appearance, which eyes will eventually suffer a glaucomatous attack.

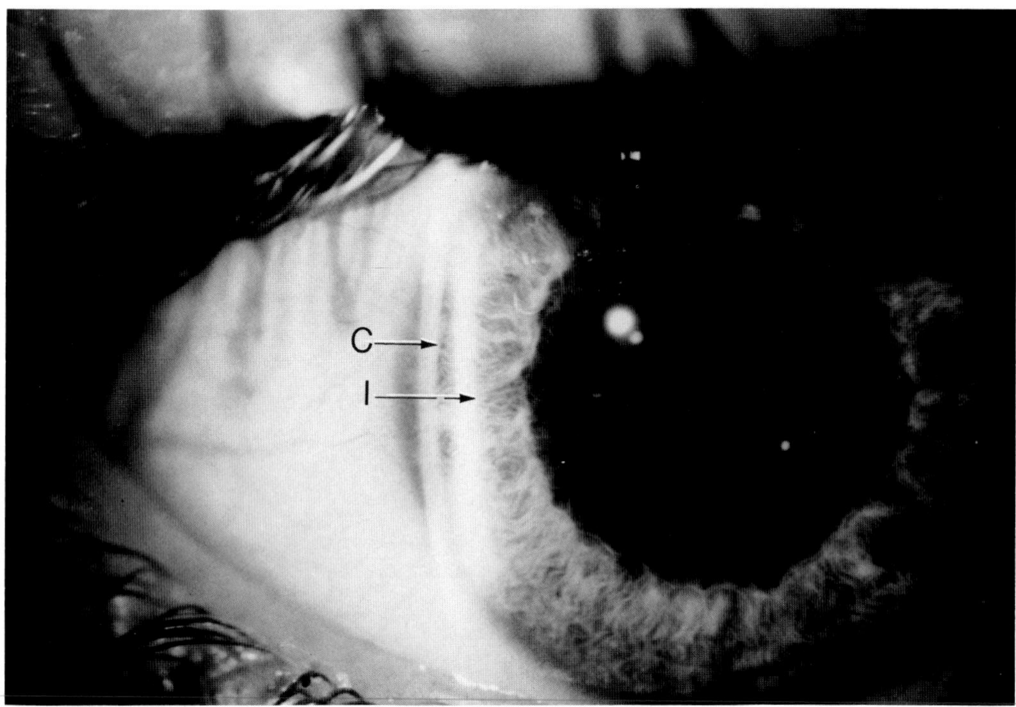

Figure 10.5. Slit-lamp photograph of van Herick technique for estimation of peripheral anterior chamber depth showing slit beam on cornea (*C*) and iris (*I*).

Some surgeons use provocative tests when attempting to identify those patients for whom treatment should be recommended. A variety of such tests have been designed to precipitate an angle-closure attack, with the rationale that it is better for this to occur in the physician's office, where it can be treated promptly, than in a situation where it might go unrecognized or where medical attention might not be readily available. It is important that a provocative test be as physiologic as possible in an effort to create a situation that might occur under natural circumstances.

Mydriatic Provocative Tests

A short-acting topical mydriatic (e.g., 0.5% tropicamide) is instilled, and a rise in IOP of 8 mm Hg or more is considered to be a positive test. However, gonioscopic confirmation of angle closure is essential, since mydriatics and cycloplegics can also cause pressure rises in eyes with open anterior chamber angles, as discussed in Chapter 9.

Dark Room Provocative Test

Mydriasis is induced by placing the patient in a dark room for 60–90 minutes. It is important that the patient remain awake during this time to avoid the miosis of sleep. A positive test again is taken as a pressure rise of 8 mm Hg or more with gonioscopic confirmation of angle closure. Exposure to light should be kept to a minimum during the post-dark room studies to avoid reversing the pressure-inducing mechanism.[56] It has also been reported that using a 30% decrease in the tonographic facility of outflow as an additional parameter increased the positive yield from 30 to 67%.[57]

Prone Provocative Test

The patient is placed in a prone position for 60 minutes, and a pressure rise of 8 mm Hg or more is taken as a positive response.[58] The mechanism of angle closure with this test is uncertain, but it is apparently not related to mydriasis.[59] One theory holds that angle closure during prone provocative test-

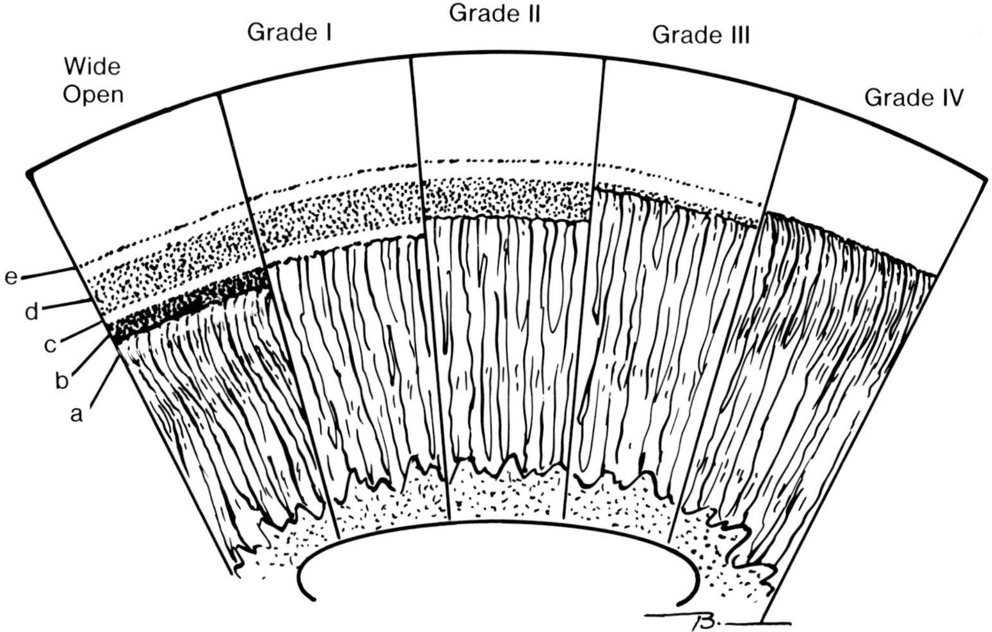

Figure 10.6. Scheie's[47] gonioscopic classification of the anterior chamber angle, based on the extent of visible angle structures: **a,** root of the iris; **b,** ciliary body band; **c,** scleral spur; **d,** trabecular meshwork; and **e,** Schwalbe's line.

CLASSIFICATION	GONIOSCOPIC APPEARANCE
Wide open	All structures visible
Grade I narrow	Hard to see over iris root into recess
Grade II narrow	Ciliary body band obscured
Grade III narrow	Posterior trabeculum obscured
Grade IV narrow (closed)	Only Schwalbe's line visible

ing is due to pupillary block associated with a slight forward shift of the lens, although in one study no significant shallowing of the anterior chamber could be demonstrated in patients with positive prone provocative tests.[60]

The prone provocative test was compared with the mydriatic and dark room tests in 76 angle-closure glaucoma eyes and was found to yield 71% positive responses before peripheral iridectomy and 6.5% after surgery, in contrast to 58% and 1.4%, respectively, for the mydriatic test, and 48% and 6.5% with the dark room test.[61] In another study of 19 patients with a diagnosis of narrow angle glaucoma, the percentage of positive provocative tests was approximately 50% with either the prone or dark room test alone, compared with 11% and 16% with phenylephrine or cyclopentolate mydriatic provocative testing, respectively.[59] When a combined prone and dark room test was performed on the same patient, the yield was almost 90% positives.[59]

Pilocarpine/Phenylephrine Test[62–65]

Two percent pilocarpine and 10% phenylephrine are instilled simultaneously every minute for three applications to achieve a mid-dilated pupil. If this does not achieve a positive response (IOP rise greater than 8 mm Hg) in 2 hours, the test is repeated. If the second test is also negative after 90 minutes, it is terminated with 0.5% thymoxamine, and a mydriatic provocative test with 0.5% tropicamide is performed on another day. In a study of 119 high-risk patients, 74 had positive responses with the initial pilocarpine/phenylephrine test, while nine more had positive responses to tropicamide, and only one of the remaining 36 developed an-

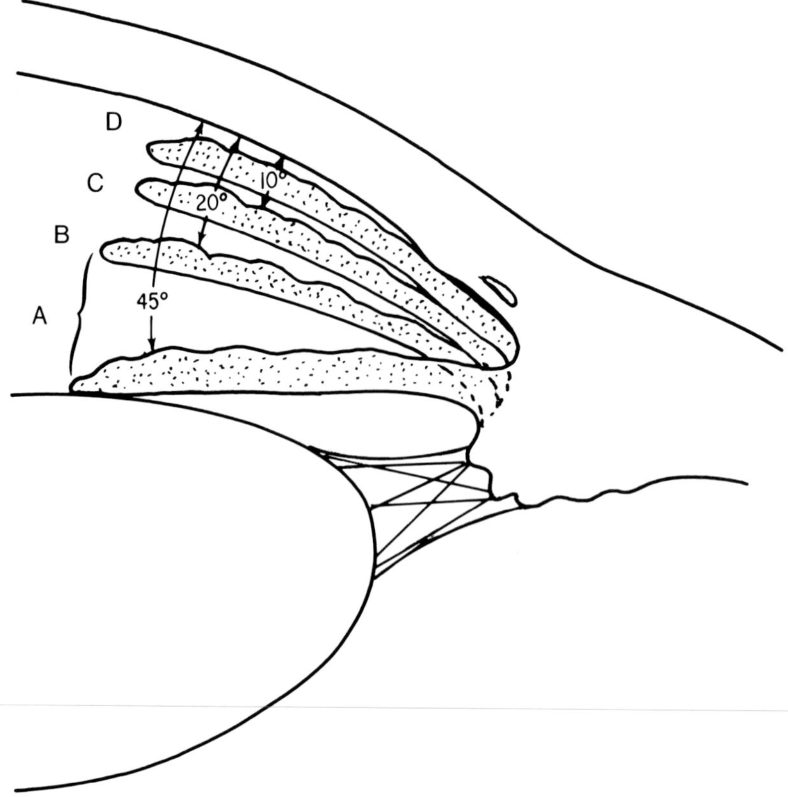

Figure 10.7. Shaffer's[48] gonioscopic classification of the anterior chamber angle, based on the angular width of the angle recess:

ANGULAR WIDTH	CLINICAL INTERPRETATION
A, Wide open (20–45°)	Closure improbable
B, Moderately narrow (10–20°)	Closure possible
C, Extremely narrow (<10°)	Closure probable
D, Partly or totally closed	Closure present

gle-closure glaucoma during a follow-up that averaged 3 years.[62]

Other Approaches

Another provocative test uses annular compression with a 16 mm suction cup to produce forward shift of the lens-iris diaphragm.[66] Still other physicians believe that no currently available provocative test is suitable and stress instead the importance of an accurate history and physical examination as the best guide to management.[67]

Precipitating Factors

In an eye that is anatomically predisposed to develop angle-closure, the following factors may precipitate an attack.

Factors that Produce Mydriasis

Dim Illumination. A common history for the development of PACG is the onset of an acute attack when the patient is in a dark room, such as a theater or restaurant. It has been reported that the incidence of angle-closure increases in the winter and autumn.[31,68] In one study, however, there was a direct association with hours of sunshine and an inverse association with cloud amount, which the authors thought might be related to the contrast between day and evening levels of illumination.[68]

Emotional Stress. Occasionally an acute angle-closure attack will follow severe emotional stress. It may be that this is related to the mydriasis of increased sympathetic

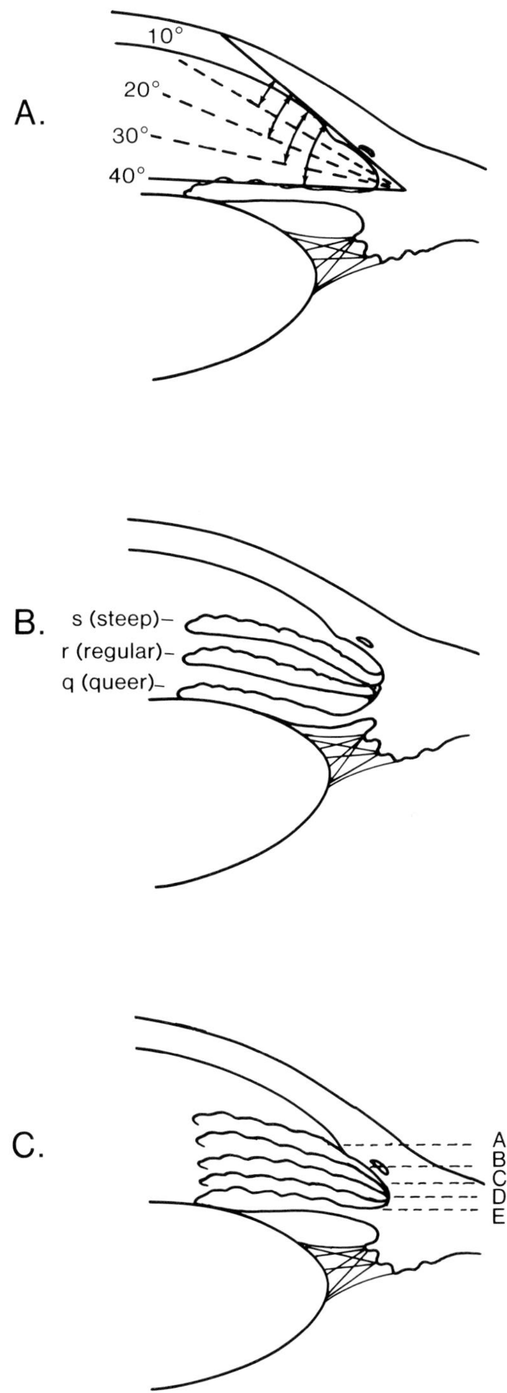

Figure 10.8. Spaeth's[22] gonioscopic classification of the anterior chamber angle, based on three variables: **A,** angular width of the angle recess; **B,** configuration of the peripheral iris; and **C,** apparent insertion of the iris root.

tone, although the exact mechanism is not fully understood.

Drugs. Mydriatics may also precipitate a primary angle-closure attack in an anatomically predisposed eye.

Anticholinergics (e.g., atropine, cyclopentolate, tropicamide, etc.) create a particularly high risk when administered topically.[69] In one study, 0.5% cyclopentolate precipitated attacks in 9 of 21 (43%) high-risk eyes, while 0.5% tropicamide did the same in 19 of 58 (33%) eyes.[70] Systemic atropine and other mydriatics can also create a hazard, especially when large doses are used along with spinal or general anesthesia during surgery.[71] It has been suggested that high-risk eyes should be protected with topical pilocarpine before, during, and after surgery.[72] However, miosis can also precipitate angle-closure attacks, and an alternative approach to managing the high-risk eye is close observation during the postoperative period, or prophylactic peripheral iridotomy, depending on the degree of risk. Other systemic drugs with weaker anticholinergic properties (e.g., antihistaminic, antiparkinsonism, antipsychotic, and gastrointestinal spasmolytic drugs) also present a risk proportional to the pupillary effect.[70] Botulinum toxin, used in the treatment of strabismus and blepharospasm, inhibits acetylcholine release with subsequent mydriasis and has been reported to cause acute angle-closure glaucoma.[73]

Adrenergics, such as topical epinephrine, may precipitate an angle-closure attack in the predisposed eye. Phenylephrine can also precipitate an attack, although it was found to be safer than cyclopentolate or tropicamide for dilating high-risk eyes.[71] In addition, systemic drugs with adrenergic properties (e.g., vasoconstrictors, central nervous system stimulants, appetite depressants, bronchodilators, and hallucinogenic agents) may present a risk in the predisposed eye.[69]

Factors that Produce Miosis

As previously noted, miotic therapy may occasionally lead to an acute attack of PACG. This has also been observed following the miosis induced by reading or bright lights. Possible mechanisms include (1) an increase in the relative pupillary block as a result of a wider zone of contact between iris and lens, and (2) relaxation of the lens zonules, allowing a forward shift of the iris-lens diaphragm. With strong miotics, such as the cholinesterase inhibitors (e.g., diisopropyl fluorophosphate and echothiophate iodide), the mechanism of angle-closure may be either the miosis or congestion of the uveal tract. Chandler[2] favored the former theory, since he noted that an acute rise in IOP following the use of a miotic did not occur in an eye with a peripheral iridecomy.

Vasodilators were once believed to create a risk of precipitating angle-closure attacks, but this subsequently has been disproved.[69]

Symptoms of Angle-Closure Attack

Primary angle-closure glaucoma, in marked contrast to primary open-angle glaucoma, is characterized by profound symptoms, although the severity of these symptoms depends on the stage of the disease.

Subacute Angle-Closure Glaucoma

This form of the disease may have no recognizable symptoms. In other cases, the patient may notice a dull ache behind the eye and/or slight blurring of vision. A symptom that is especially typical of the subacute attack is colored halos around lights. This is believed to result from an alteration in the cornea, which causes it to act as a diffraction grating, producing a blue-green central and yellow-red peripheral halo. These symptoms, which more often occur at night after the patient has been in a dark room, will often spontaneously clear by the following morning, presumably due to the miosis of sleep.

Acute Angle-Closure Glaucoma

This condition is characterized by pain, redness, and blurred vision. The pain is typically a severe, deep ache, which follows the trigeminal distribution and may be associated with nausea, vomiting, bradycardia, and profuse sweating. The conjunctival hyperemia is marked and usually consists of both a ciliary flush and peripheral conjunctival congestion. The blurred vision, which is also typically marked, may be due to stretching of the corneal lamellae initially and later to edema of the cornea, as well as a direct effect of the IOP on the optic nerve head. Occasionally, the corneal decompensation may persist, requiring penetrating keratoplasty.[74]

Chronic Angle-Closure Glaucoma

This form of PACG is typically asymptomatic until advanced visual field loss develops, although the patient may give a history suggestive of one or more episodes of subacute or acute angle-closure glaucoma.

Clinical Findings During an Acute Attack

The patient who presents during an acute attack of PACG will typically have marked IOP elevation in the range of 40–60 mm Hg or more, with a profound reduction in central visual acuity. The following additional findings will help to confirm the diagnosis.

External Examination. Characteristic findings include the previously noted conjunctival hyperemia, as well as a cloudy cornea and an irregular (usually vertically oval), mid-dilated, fixed pupil (Fig. 10.9). The pupillary change is thought to result from paralysis of the sphincter, which is apparently due to a reduction in circulation induced by the elevated IOP[75–77] and possibly to degeneration of the ciliary ganglion.[78]

Slit-Lamp Examination. This step of the evaluation confirms the presence of the corneal edema, which frequently must be cleared by topical application of glycerin before the anterior chamber can be studied. The corneal edema usually clears after the pressure is normalized as previously noted, although this is not always the case.[74] Specular microscopic examination has revealed significant corneal endothelial cell loss in these cases, which correlates with the duration of IOP elevation,[79] visual field loss, a large cup-disc ratio, and previous intraocular surgery.[80]

The anterior chamber is shallow but typically is formed centrally with anterior bowing of the midperipheral iris, often making contact with peripheral cornea. Aqueous

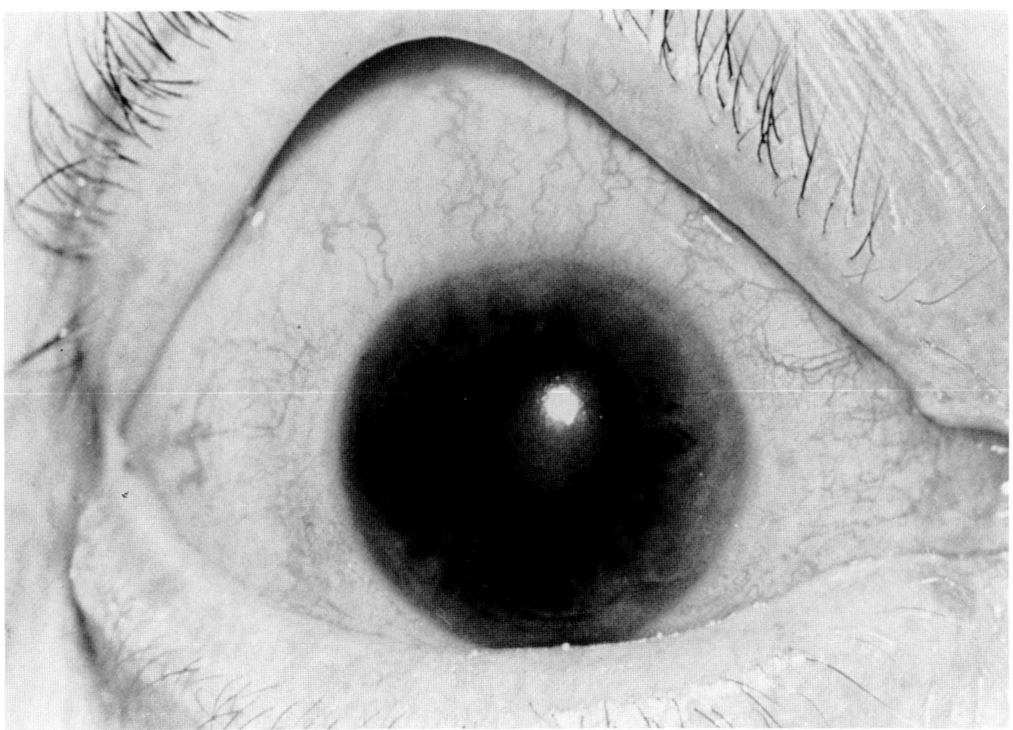

Figure 10.9. External appearance of eye during attack of acute angle-closure glaucoma, showing diffuse conjunctival hyperemia, cloudy cornea, and irregular, mid-dilated pupil. (Courtesy of H. Saul Sugar, M.D.)

flare may be present. Other findings may include pigment dispersion, sector atrophy of the iris, and glaukomflecken, which are irregular white opacities in the anterior portion of the lens (Fig. 10.10).

Gonioscopy. It is essential to confirm the diagnosis of PACG by demonstrating a closed anterior chamber angle. If gonioscopy is not possible because of persistent corneal edema, gonioscopy of the fellow eye may provide useful information if it reveals an extremely narrow angle. In a study of 10 eyes with angle-closure glaucoma, the Koeppe lens was thought to be more reliable than the Goldmann three-mirror or Zeiss four-mirror lenses in determining whether the angle was open or closed, because it caused no artifactual widening of the angle and allowed the best view over a convex iris.[81] Peripheral anterior synechiae may also be present, and the techniques and importance of making this determination are discussed later in this chapter under "Management."

Fundus Examination. The optic nerve head may be hyperemic and edematous in the early stages of the attack. Monkeys exposed to high IOPs usually developed congestion of the optic nerve head within 12–15 hours, which persisted for 4–5 days.[82] The disc then became pale, and glaucomatous cupping was observed after 9–10 days. In a study of human eyes with a history of angle-closure glaucoma, pallor without cupping was seen in eyes following acute attacks, while both pallor and cupping occurred in chronic cases.[83] Central retinal vein occlusion may also occur during acute angle-closure glaucoma.[84]

Visual Fields. As discussed in Chapter 6, visual field changes associated with acute elevation of IOP most often show nonspecific constriction. In one study of 25 patients with acute angle-closure glaucoma that had been surgically corrected, the most common field defect was constriction of the upper field,[85] while another revealed nerve

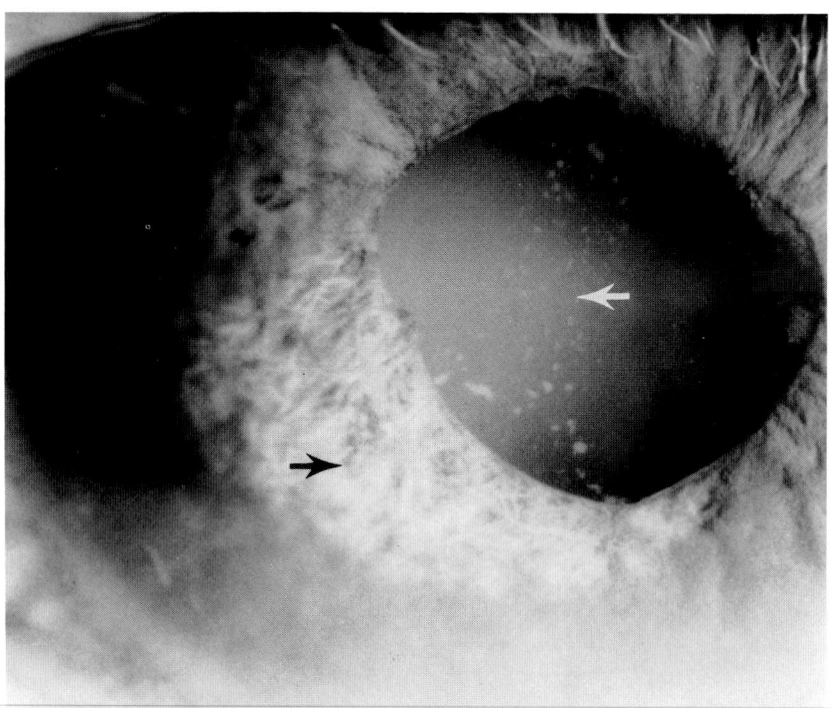

Figure 10.10. Slit-lamp photograph of eye after acute angle-closure glaucoma attack, showing glaukomflecken (*white arrow*) and sector iris atrophy (*black arrow*).

fiber bundle defects in 7 of 18 acute and 9 of 11 chronic cases.[83]

THEORIES OF MECHANISM

Relative Pupillary Block

As noted earlier in this chapter, the most common mechanism leading to PACG appears to be increased resistance to aqueous flow from the posterior to the anterior chamber between the iris and lens. This concept was suggested by Curran[1] and Banziger[3] in the early 1920s, and advanced by the teachings of Chandler,[2] who noted that an eye with a shallow anterior chamber has a wider zone of contact between the surfaces of the iris and lens. He postulated that the musculature of the iris exerts a backward pressure against the lens that increases the resistance to flow of aqueous into the anterior chamber. This increases the pressure in the posterior chamber, causing the thin peripheral iris to bulge into the anterior chamber angle. It has been suggested on the basis of gonioscopic studies that the angle closure occurs in two stages, with the first being iridocorneal contact anterior to the trabecular meshwork, followed by apposition of the iris to the meshwork as the pressure rises.[86,87] Considerable clinical evidence strongly favors the basic concept of pupillary block, the most convincing of which is the excellent response to peripheral iridotomy, which presumably works by circumventing the block (Fig. 10.11).[2]

Anatomic Factors Predisposing to Pupillary Block. Several anatomic aspects of the eye combine to produce a shallow anterior chamber. These include a thicker, more anteriorly placed lens, a smaller diameter and shorter posterior curvature of the cornea, and a shorter axial length of the globe.[88–94] As previously noted, the lens thickness/axial length ratio appears to correlate best with the predisposition to angle closure.[51,52] It has also been shown that the anterior chamber depth is not a static dimension but can undergo rapid, transient change.[95]

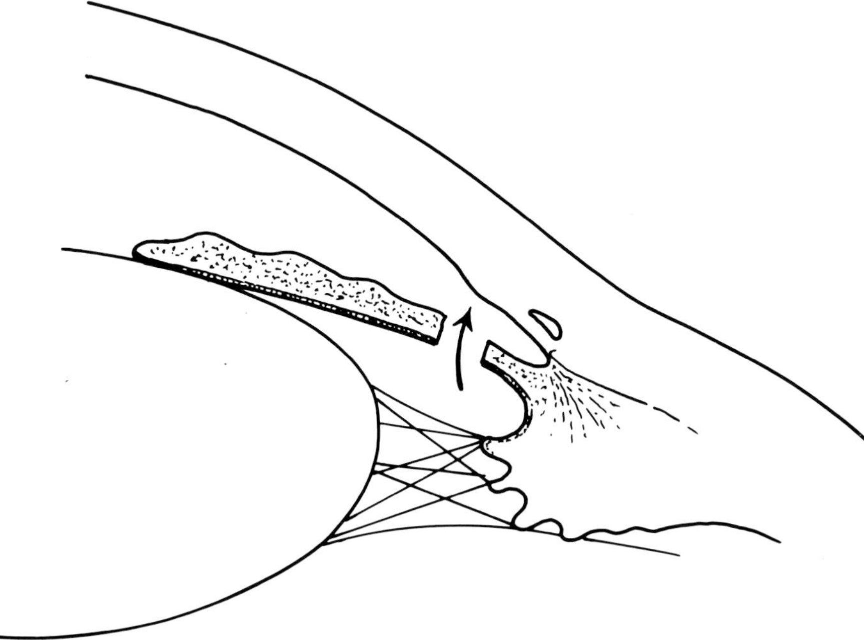

Figure 10.11. The strongest evidence in support of the pupillary block mechanism of angle-closure glaucoma is the excellent response to peripheral iridotomy, which circumvents the block (*arrow*).

Relatives of patients with PACG have been noted to have a more anterior insertion of the iris into the ciliary body, a narrower angular approach to the recess of the anterior chamber angle, and a more anterior peripheral convexity of the iris as compared with average eyes in the general population.[22] All of the above parameters are variably influenced by hyperopia, increasing age, and genetics.

Another factor predisposing to a pupillary block mechanism may be a forward displacement to the lens due to loose zonules, which is made worse by miotic therapy and relieved with cycloplegia.[96]

The Significance of Pupillary Dilation. Chandler[2] emphasized that a mid-dilated pupil of 3.5–6 mm is the critical degree of dilation that seems to bring on the acute attack. He believed that this might be due to continued pupillary block combined with sufficient relaxation of peripheral iris to allow its forward displacement into the anterior chamber. Mapstone[97] proposed a mathematic model to explain the influence of a mid-dilated pupil, in which the combined pupil-blocking forces of the dilator and sphincter muscles and the stretching force of the iris were greatest with the iris in the mid-dilated position. Factors that may precipitate an angle-closure attack by dilating the pupil were discussed earlier in this chapter.

Plateau Iris

A second basic mechanism leading to PACG appears to result from an abnormal anatomic configuration of the anterior chamber angle. It is far less common than the pupillary block mechanism and is usually recognized only after a peripheral iridotomy for presumed pupillary block glaucoma has failed. Two variations of plateau iris have been described.[12]

Plateau Iris Configuration. This diagnosis is made preoperatively based on the gonioscopic findings of a closed anterior chamber angle, but a flat iris plane (as opposed to the forward bowing of peripheral iris with the pupillary block mechanism) and a more normal central anterior chamber depth. Relative pupillary block plays a significant role in this situation, and most of these cases are cured by peripheral iridotomy.

Plateau Iris Syndrome. This constitutes a small percentage of eyes with the plateau iris configuration and represents the true plateau iris mechanism. The peripheral iris bunches up in the anterior chamber angle when the pupil is dilated, presumably due in part to an anterior insertion of the iris (Fig. 10.2). This diagnosis is made postoperatively when angle closure recurs with pupillary dilation despite a patent iridotomy and deep central anterior chamber. These cases are treated with pilocarpine.

Chronic Angle-Closure Glaucoma

Peripheral anterior synechiae may eventually develop with prolonged or recurrent acute or subacute attacks, leading to chronic angle-closure glaucoma. In addition, a more insidious form has been recognized in which the angle slowly closes from the periphery toward Schwalbe's line.[6–9] The synechial closure usually begins superiorly, where the angle is normally narrowest, and progresses inferiorly.[7] This condition has been referred to as shortening of the angle[8] or creeping angle closure.[9] These cases are frequently cured by peripheral iridotomy if detected early enough but occasionally require filtering surgery.

DIFFERENTIAL DIAGNOSIS

The sudden onset of pain, redness, and blurred vision, which characterizes the acute PACG attack, may also be seen with other forms of glaucoma, creating a differential diagnostic problem.

Open-Angle Glaucomas

Open-angle glaucomas may occasionally present as an acute attack, especially when secondary to events such as inflammation, hemorrhage, or rubeosis iridis. These cases are usually readily distinguished from PACG on the basis of the gonioscopic appearance and associated findings. However, in the eye with an elevated IOP and a narrow anterior chamber angle, it may be difficult to distinguish between PACG and primary open-angle glaucoma with narrow angles. A *thymoxamine test* has been suggested for this situation.[98] Thymoxamine is an alpha-adrenergic blocker, which produces miosis by relaxing the dilator muscle without affecting the ciliary musculature. Topical thymoxamine 0.5% can often open a narrow or appositionally-closed angle but will not alter the IOP in an eye with open-angle glaucoma. Unfortunately, however, thymoxamine is not commercially available in the United States. An alternative approach in distinguishing between these two conditions is to perform a laser iridotomy, which will relieve the pressure elevation in a pure angle-closure case, while additional measures will be required if an open-angle component is present.

Secondary Angle-Closure Glaucomas

Secondary angle-closure glaucomas may present even more difficult diagnostic problems, especially when the initiating event is posterior to the lens-iris diaphragm, where early detection can be difficult. The following are some of the ocular disorders that may lead to secondary angle closure (the details of these conditions will be considered in subsequent chapters):

1. Central retinal vein occlusion (Chapter 16).
2. Ciliary body swelling, inflammation, or cysts (Chapters 18, 19).
3. Ciliary block (malignant) glaucoma (Chapter 23).
4. Posterior segment tumors (Chapter 18).
5. Contracting retrolental tissue (Chapter 16).
6. Scleral buckling procedures and panretinal photocoagulation (Chapter 23).
7. Nanophthalmos (Chapter 16).
8. Corneal thickening (Chapter 13).

MANAGEMENT

The details regarding drugs and surgical procedures used in the treatment of PACG are considered in Section Three. The present discussion is limited to the general approach and basic concepts of management.

Medical Therapy

Although the vast majority of eyes with PACG are managed surgically, it is desirable to first bring the glaucoma under medical control. In the case of an acute attack, this constitutes a medical emergency and should be approached in two stages: (1) reduce the IOP, and (2) relieve the angle closure.

Reduction of IOP. Miotic therapy is frequently ineffective when the IOP is high, presumably because of pressure-induced ischemia of the iris, which leads to paralysis of the sphincter muscle.[75–77] For this reason, the first line of defense is to administer drugs that will promptly lower the IOP. *Carbonic anhydrase inhibitors* (e.g., acetazolamide 500 mg intramuscularly, intravenously, or orally) and/or a topical *beta-adrenergic blocker* will, in many cases, lower the pressure sufficiently to allow effective miotic therapy.[99,100] *Hyperosmotics* are often used in conjunction with these drugs. They may be given orally as glycerol or isosorbide or, if the patient is too nauseated to tolerate oral medication, may be given intravenously as mannitol or urea.

Relief of Angle-Closure. Once the IOP has been reduced, a miotic is instilled to break the pupillary block and open the anterior chamber angle. A single drop of *pilocarpine* approximately 3 hours after administration of acetazolamide or timolol has been reported to effectively break the angle-closure attack.[99,100] This is also safer than copious use of pilocarpine, since it reduces the chances of drug toxicity. The concentration of pilocarpine does not appear to be important in this situation, and a low dosage of 1–2% is preferable. Thymoxamine has theoretic advantages over pilocarpine, since the mechanism of miosis is relaxation of the dilator muscle, which permits its use during high pressures and reduces the posterior vector force caused by sphincter contracture.[101,102] However, others have not found thymoxamine alone to be effective in the treatment of angle-closure glaucoma.[103] Strong miotics, such as eserine and echothiophate iodide, are generally contraindicated in acute angle-closure glaucoma, since they may aggravate the situation by producing vascular congestion or increasing the pupillary block.

Surgical Management

Once the IOP has been brought under control medically (or all efforts at medical control have been exhausted), the surgeon is then faced with two decisions: (1) when to operate, and (2) what procedure to use.

When to Operate. In the uncommon event that the elevated pressure cannot be controlled medically, Chandler and Grant[104] advise considering surgery within the next few hours, especially if vision is failing. However, the risks of incisional surgery are considerably higher under these circumstances. Indentation of the central cornea for several 30-second intervals, using a blunt instrument such as a cotton-tipped applicator, may lower the IOP before surgery and occasionally break the attack by forcing aqueous from the central to the peripheral anterior chamber (Fig. 10.12).[105] With the advent of laser surgery, however, the safest approach to medically unresponsive cases is to proceed with laser iridotomy. When an iridotomy cannot be achieved, as is occasionally the case when corneal edema is present, laser pupilloplasty or peripheral iridoplasty may break the attack.[106,107] Once the attack is broken and the cornea has cleared, a laser iridotomy should then be formed.

If the IOP does respond to medical therapy, the eye should be reexamined gonioscopically to determine the mechanism of the pressure reduction. An open anterior chamber angle without corneal indentation by the goniolens suggests that the angle-closure attack has been broken. In this situation, there is less urgency as to when surgical intervention should be performed. In the days of incisional surgical iridectomy, some surgeons preferred to wait a day or two until the eye was quieter. With laser iridotomy, however, there is no advantage in waiting unless marked iritis or corneal edema is present. In one long-term study of 116 cases, delay in treatment had a detrimental effect on the final outcome.[108] If the gonioscopy reveals that the angle is still closed, despite medical lowering of the IOP, it may be that the pressure reduction is due to the carbonic anhydrase inhibitor, beta-blocker, and hyperosmotic and that the angle-closure has not actually been relieved. Since the high pressure may recur as the effects of these medications begin to wear off, there is all the more urgency in proceeding promptly with the laser iridotomy.

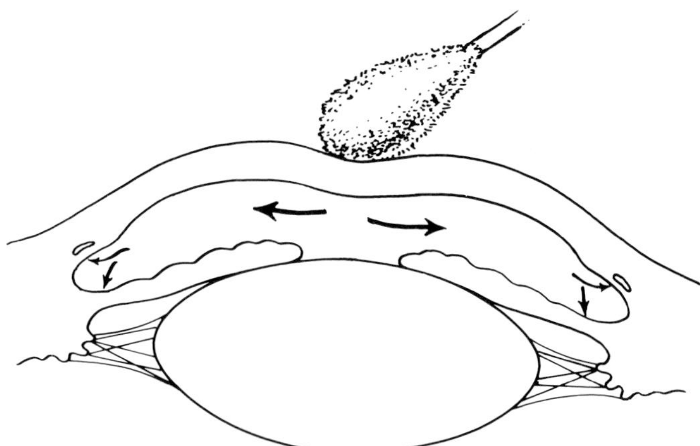

Figure 10.12. Corneal indentation with a soft instrument, such as a cotton-tipped applicator, may lower the intraocular pressure during a primary angle-closure attack by forcing aqueous from the central to the peripheral anterior chamber (*arrows*), thereby temporarily opening the chamber angle and reestablishing aqueous outflow.[105]

What Operation to Use. The eye with PACG typically responds well to a peripheral iridotomy, and the initial procedure of choice in nearly every case is a laser iridotomy. However, follow-up studies indicate that approximately 25% of eyes treated with an iridotomy alone will eventually require medication to control chronic pressure elevation and some will need filtering surgery.[13,109–111] This is related to the amount of permanent damage to the anterior chamber angle, which sometimes correlates with the extent of gonioscopically visible peripheral anterior synechiae.

Chamber deepening procedures have been devised in an attempt to quantitate the degree of synechiae in eyes with angle-closure glaucoma. Forbes[112,113] described an office procedure (*compressive gonioscopy*) in which the degree of synechial closure is determined by indenting the central cornea with a Zeiss four-mirror gonioprism. This forces aqueous into the peripheral portion of the anterior chamber, which deepens it and facilitates visualization of the angle (Fig. 10.13). Similar approaches have been used at the time of incisional surgery. Chandler and Simmons[114] suggested deepening the anterior chamber with saline to study the angle with a Koeppe goniolens before proceeding with the surgery, while Shaffer[115] performed the same maneuver after making an iridectomy. Other factors that are said to be helpful in determining when filtering surgery will be necessary are a poor tonographic facility of outflow[116] and visual field loss,[117] while some have found that the duration of the attack does not appear to be a reliable indicator.[117,118]

The advent of laser iridotomy has provided an alternative approach to determining which eyes may require filtering surgery. Even if compressive gonioscopy reveals partial synechial closure of the anterior chamber angle, it is best to proceed first with the laser iridotomy, since this has been shown to control the pressure in many cases of chronic angle-closure glaucoma.[119] If the iridotomy does not restore a normal IOP, the eye is then treated with medication or filtering surgery if required. Caution must be taken when performing filtering surgery (as well as an incisional surgical iridectomy) on eyes with angle-closure glaucoma due to the increased risk of malignant (ciliary block) glaucoma (discussed in Chapter 23).[120] Care must also be taken with the prolonged use of topical corticosteroids following laser or incisional surgery in these patients, since a high percentage will have steroid-induced IOP elevation after an attack of angle-closure glaucoma.[121,122]

A prophylactic peripheral iridotomy is generally recommended for the fellow eye following an attack of PACG. Several large studies have shown that approximately

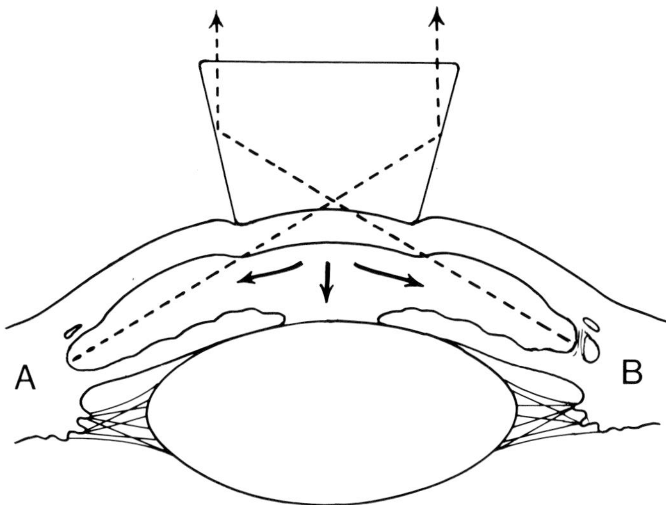

Figure 10.13. Compressive gonioscopy with a Zeiss four-mirror gonioprism deepens the peripheral anterior chamber by displacing aqueous from the central portion of the chamber (*arrows*). This facilitates gonioscopic examination of the anterior chamber angle before surgery by helping to distinguish between appositional (*A*) and synechial (*B*) closure of the angle.[112,113]

50–75% of the patients who develop PACG in one eye will have an attack in the fellow, unoperated eye within 5–10 years despite miotic prophylaxis,[123–128] whereas such an attack is rare after an iridectomy.[126,129,130] Since the attack in the fellow eye usually occurs in the first year after the initial event,[131] often during hospitalization or within one month of discharge for the first attack,[132] the prophylactic procedure should be done promptly. Rare exceptions include a deeper anterior chamber in the fellow eye as a result of anisometropia or a dislocated lens. Some surgeons have suggested that fellow eyes with negative provocative tests might be followed closely without surgery.[131,133] However, with the relative safety of laser iridotomy, a prophylactic procedure in all high-risk fellow eyes appears to be prudent.

Extracapsular cataract extraction with posterior chamber intraocular lens implantation has also been shown to be effective surgical therapy for PACG.[134] This, of course, should be limited to eyes with a significant cataract, should include an iridectomy, and is best suited for chronic cases.

SUMMARY

Primary angle-closure glaucoma is much less common than primary open-angle glaucoma in most populations. A predisposing factor is a narrow anterior chamber angle, which has a familial tendency and is associated with increasing age and hyperopia. An angle-closure attack may be precipitated in a predisposed individual by factors that induce mydriasis, such as dim illumination, emotional stress, and drugs. The most common mechanism of PACG is pupillary block, in which aqueous flow from the posterior to the anterior chamber is obstructed by a functional block between the lens and iris. The clinical presentation may be that of an acute attack with severe pain, marked conjunctival hyperemia, a cloudy cornea, and profound visual loss, or that of a subacute attack with a dull ache, slight blurring of vision, and colored halos around lights. Still other cases may be chronic and typically asymptomatic. Treatment usually begins with medical therapy to lower the IOP and relieve the angle closure, followed by a peripheral iridotomy to prevent future attacks.

References

1. Curran, EJ: A new operation for glaucoma involving a new principle in the aetiology and treat-

ment of chronic primary glaucoma. Arch Ophthal 49:131, 1920.
2. Chandler, PA: Narrow-angle glaucoma. Arch Ophthal 47:695, 1952.
3. Banziger, TH: The mechanism of acute glaucoma and the explanation for the effectiveness of iridectomy for the same. Ber Deutsch Ophthal Ges 43:43, 1922.
4. Barkan, O: Glaucoma: classification, causes, and surgical control. Results of microgonioscopic research. Am J Ophthal 21:1099, 1938.
5. Chandler, PA, Trotter, RR: Angle-closure glaucoma. Subacute types. Arch Ophthal 53:305, 1955.
6. Pollack, IP: Chronic angle-closure glaucoma. Diagnosis and treatment in patients with angles that appear open. Arch Ophthal 85:676, 1971.
7. Bhargava, SK, Leighton, DA, Phillips, CI: Early angle-closure glaucoma. Distribution of iridotrabecular contact and response to pilocarpine. Arch Ophthal 89:369, 1973.
8. Gorin, G: Shortening of the angle of the anterior chamber in angle-closure glaucoma. Am J Ophthal 49:141, 1960.
9. Lowe, RF: Primary creeping angle-closure glaucoma. Br J Ophthal 48:544, 1964.
10. Tornquist, R: Angle-closure glaucoma in an eye with a plateau type of iris. Acta Ophthal 36:413, 1958.
11. Shaffer, RN: Gonioscopy, ophthalmoscopy, and perimetry. Trans Am Acad Ophthal Otol 64:112, 1960.
12. Wand, M, Grant, WM, Simmons, RJ, Hutchinson, BT: Plateau iris syndrome. Trans Am Acad Ophthal Otol 83:122, 1977.
13. Hyams, SW, Keroub, C, Pokotilo, E: Mixed glaucoma. Br J Ophthal 61:105, 1977.
14. Drance, SM: Angle closure glaucoma among Canadian Eskimos. Can J Ophthal 8:252, 1973.
15. Arkell, SM, Lightman, DA, Sommer, A, et al: The prevalence of glaucoma among Eskimos of Northwest Alaska. Arch Ophthal 105:482, 1987.
16. Clemmesen, V, Alsbirk, PH: Primary angle-closure glaucoma (a.c.g.) in Greenland. Acta Ophthal 49:47, 1971.
17. Alsbirk, PH: Early detection of primary angle-closure glaucoma. Limbal and axial chamber depth screening in a high risk population (Greenland Eskimos). Acta Ophthal 66:556, 1988.
18. Drance, SM, Morgan, RW, Bryett, J, et al: Anterior chamber depth and gonioscopic findings among the Eskimos and Indians of the Canadian arctic. Can J Ophthal 8:255, 1973.
19. Alsbirk, PH: Corneal diameter in Greenland Eskimos. Acta Ophthal 53:635, 1975.
20. Alsbirk, PH: Anterior chamber depth, genes and environment. A population study among long-term Greenland Eskimo immigrants in Copenhagen. Acta Ophthal 60:223, 1982.
21. Kolker, A, Hetherington, J Jr: Becker-Shaffer's Diagnosis and Therapy of the Glaucomas, 4th ed. CV Mosby, St. Louis, 1976, p. 183.
22. Spaeth, GL: The normal development of the human anterior chamber angle: A new system of descriptive grading. Trans Ophthal Soc UK XCI:709, 1971.
23. Fontana, ST, Brubaker, RF: Volume and depth of the anterior chamber in the normal aging human eye. Arch Ophthal 98:1803, 1980.
24. Markowitz, SN, Morin, JD: Angle-closure glaucoma: relation between lens thickness, anterior chamber depth and age. Can J Ophthal 19:300, 1984.
25. Appleby, RS Jr, Kinder, RSL: Bilateral angle-closure glaucoma in a 14-year-old boy. Arch Ophthal 86:449, 1971.
26. Alper, MG, Laubach, JL: Primary angle-closure glaucoma in the American Negro. Arch Ophthal 79:663, 1968.
27. Clemmesen, V, Luntz, MH: Lens thickness and angle-closure glaucoma. A comparative oculometric study in South African Negroes and Danes. Acta Ophthal 54:193, 1976.
28. Wilensky, J: Racial influences in glaucoma. Ann Ophthal 9:1545, 1977.
29. Olurin, O: Anterior chamber depths of Nigerians. Ann Ophthal 9:315, 1977.
30. Emiru, VP: Response to mydriatics in the African. Br J Ophthal 55:538, 1971.
31. Teikari, J, Raivio, I, Nurminen, M: Incidence of acute glaucoma in Finland from 1973 to 1982. Graefe's Arch Ophthal 225:357, 1987.
32. Hagan, JC III, Lederer, CM Jr: Primary angle closure glaucoma in a myopic kinship. Arch Ophthal 103:363, 1985.
33. Spaeth, GL: Gonioscopy: uses old and new. The inheritance of occludable angles. Ophthalmology 85:222, 1978.
34. Lichter, PR, Anderson, DR, ed: Discussions on Glaucoma. Grune and Stratton, New York, 1977, p. 139.
35. Gieser, DK, Wilensky, JT: HLA antigens and acute angle-closure glaucoma. Am J Ophthal 88:232, 1979.
36. Mapstone, R, Clark, CV: Prevalence of diabetes in glaucoma. Br Med J 291:93, 1985.
37. Mapstone, R, Clark, CV: The prevalence of autonomic neuropathy in glaucoma. Trans Ophthal Soc UK 104:265, 1985.
38. Shapiro, A, Zauberman, H: Diurnal changes of the intraocular pressure of patients with angle-closure glaucoma. Br J Ophthal 63:225, 1979.
39. Lee, DA, Brubaker, RF, Ilstrup, DM: Anterior chamber dimensions in patients with narrow angles and angle-closure glaucoma. Arch Ophthal 102:46, 1984.
40. Mapstone, R, Clark, CV: Diurnal variation in the

dimensions of the anterior chamber. Arch Ophthal 103:1485, 1985.
41. Vargas, E, Drance, SM: Anterior chamber depth in angle-closure glaucoma. Clinical methods of depth determination in people with and without the disease. Arch Ophthal 90:438, 1973.
42. Smith, RJH: A new method of estimating the depth of the anterior chamber. Br J Ophthal 63:215, 1979.
43. Jacobs, IH: Anterior chamber depth measurement using the slit-lamp microscope. Am J Ophthal 88:236, 1979.
44. Douthwaite, WA, Spence, D: Slit-lamp measurement of the anterior chamber depth. Br J Ophthal 70:205, 1986.
45. Makabe, R: Comparative studies of the anterior chamber angle width by ultrasonography and gonioscopy. Klin Monatsbl Augenheilkd 194:6, 1989.
46. van Herick, W, Shaffer, RN, Schwartz, A: Estimation of width of angle of anterior chamber. Incidence and significance of the narrow angle. Am J Ophthal 68:626, 1969.
47. Scheie, HG: Width and pigmentation of the angle of the anterior chamber. A system of grading by gonioscopy. Arch Ophthal 58:510, 1957.
48. Shaffer, RN: Symposium: primary glaucomas. III. Gonioscopy, ophthalmoscopy and perimetry. Trans Am Acad Ophthal Otol 62:112, 1960.
49. Becker, S: Clinical Gonioscopy—A Test and Stereoscopic Atlas. CV Mosby, St. Louis, 1972.
50. Desjardins, D, Parrish, RK II: Inversion of anterior chamber pigment as a possible prognostic sign in narrow angles. Am J Ophthal 100:480, 1985.
51. Markowitz, SN, Morin, JD: The clinical course in primary angle-closure glaucoma: A reassessment. Can J Ophthal 21:130, 1986.
52. Panek, WC, Christensen, RE, Lee, DA, et al: Biometric variables in patients with occludable anterior chamber angles. Am J Ophthal 110:185, 1990.
53. Richards, DW, Russell, SR, Anderson, DR: A method for improved biometry of the anterior chamber with a Scheimpflug technique. Invest Ophthal Vis Sci 29:1826, 1988.
54. Kondo, T, Miura, M: A method of measuring pupil-blocking force in the human eye. Graefe's Arch Ophthal 225:361, 1987.
55. Hillman, JS: Acute closed-angle glaucoma: an investigation into the effect of delay in treatment. Br J Ophthal 63:817, 1979.
56. Gloster, J, Poinoosawmy, D: Changes in intraocular pressure during and after the dark-room test. Br J Ophthal 57:170, 1973.
57. Foulds, WS: Observations on the facility of aqueous outflow in closed-angle glaucoma. Br J Ophthal 43:613, 1959.
58. Hyams, SW, Friedman, BZ, Neumann, E: Elevated intraocular pressure in the prone position. A new provocative test for angle-closure glaucoma. Am J Ophthal 66:661, 1968.
59. Harris, LS, Galin, MA: Prone provocative testing for narrow angle glaucoma. Arch Ophthal 87:493, 1972.
60. Neumann, E, Hyams, SW: Gonioscopy and anterior chamber depth in the prone-position provocative test for angle-closure glaucoma. Ophthalmologica 167:9, 1973.
61. Friedman, Z, Neumann, E: Comparison of prone-position, dark-room, and mydriatic tests for angle-closure glaucoma before and after peripheral iridectomy. Am J Ophthal 74:24, 1972.
62. Mapstone, R: Provocative tests in closed-angle glaucoma. Br J Ophthal 60:115, 1976.
63. Mapstone, R: Normal response to pilocarpine and phenylephrine. Br J Ophthal 61:510, 1977.
64. Mapstone, R: Outflow changes in positive provocative tests. Br J Ophthal 61:634, 1977.
65. Mapstone, R: Partial angle closure. Br J Ophthal 61:525, 1977.
66. Nesterov, AP, Kiselev, GA, Devlikamova, ER: New compression tests in glaucoma. II. Posterior annular compression test. Acta Ophthal 51:749, 1973.
67. Lowe, RF: Primary angle-closure glaucoma. A review of provocative tests. Br J Ophthal 51:727, 1967.
68. Hillman, JS, Turner, JDC: Association between acute glaucoma and the weather and sunspot activity. Br J Ophthal 61:512, 1977.
69. Grant, WM: Ocular complications of drugs. Glaucoma. J Am Med Assn 207:2089, 1969.
70. Mapstone, R: Dilating dangerous pupils. Br J Ophthal 61:517, 1977.
71. Fazio, DT, Bateman, JB, Christensen, RE: Acute angle-closure glaucoma associated with surgical anesthesia. Arch Ophthal 103:360, 1985.
72. Schwartz, H, Apt, L: Mydriatic effect of anticholinergic drugs used during reversal of nondepolarizing muscle relaxants. Am J Ophthal 88:609, 1979.
73. Corridan, P, Nightingale, S, Mashoudi, N, Williams, AC: Acute angle-closure glaucoma following botulinum toxin injection for blepharospasm. Br J Ophthal 74:309, 1990.
74. Krontz, DP, Wood, TO: Corneal decompensation following acute angle-closure glaucoma. Ophthal Surg 19:334, 1988.
75. Charles, ST, Hamasaki, DI: The effect of intraocular pressure on the pupil size. Arch Ophthal 83:729, 1970.
76. Rutkowski, PC, Thompson, HS: Mydriasis and increased intraocular pressure. I. Pupillographic studies. Arch Ophthal 87:21, 1972.
77. Anderson, DR, Davis, EB: Sensitivities of ocular tissues to acute pressure-induced ischemia. Arch Ophthal 93:267, 1975.

78. Kapoor, S, Sood, M: Glaucoma-induced changes in the ciliary ganglion. Br J Ophthal 59:573, 1975.
79. Bigar, F, Witmer, R: Corneal endothelial changes in primary acute angle-closure glaucoma. Ophthalmology 89:596, 1982.
80. Markowitz, SN, Morin, JD: The endothelium in primary angle-closure glaucoma. Am J Ophthal 98:103, 1984.
81. Campbell, DG: A comparison of diagnostic techniques in angle-closure glaucoma. Am J Ophthal 88:197, 1979.
82. Zimmerman, LE, de Venecia, G, Hamasaki, DI: Pathology of the optic nerve in experimental acute glaucoma. Invest Ophthal 6:109, 1967.
83. Douglas, GR, Drance, SM, Schulzer, M: The visual field and nerve head in angle-closure glaucoma. A comparison of the effects of acute and chronic angle closure. Arch Ophthal 93:409, 1975.
84. Sonty, S, Schwartz, B: Vascular accidents in acute angle closure glaucoma. Ophthalmology 88:225, 1981.
85. McNaught, EI, Rennie, A, McClure, E, Chisholm, IA: Pattern of visual damage after acute angle-closure glaucoma. Trans Ophthal Soc UK 94:406, 1974.
86. Mapstone, R: One gonioscopic fallacy. Br J Ophthal 63:221, 1979.
87. Mapstone, R: The mechanism and clinical significance of angle closure. Glaucoma 2:249, 1980.
88. Tornquist, R: Corneal radius in primary acute glaucoma. Br J Ophthal 41:421, 1957.
89. Lowe, RF: Causes of shallow anterior chamber in primary angle-closure glaucoma. Ultrasonic biometry of normal and angle-closure glaucoma eyes. Am J Ophthal 67:87, 1969.
90. Phillips, CI: Aetiology of angle-closure glaucoma. Br J Ophthal 56:248, 1972.
91. Lowe, RF, Clark, BAJ: Posterior corneal curvature. Correlations in normal eyes and in eyes involved with primary angle-closure glaucoma. Br J Ophthal 57:464, 1973.
92. Tomlinson, A, Leighton, DA: Ocular dimensions in the heredity of angle-closure glaucoma. Br J Ophthal 57:475, 1973.
93. Kerman, BM, Christensen, RE, Foos, RY: Angle-closure glaucoma: a clinicopathologic correlation. Am J Ophthal 76:887, 1973.
94. Markowitz, SN, Morin, JD: The ratio of lens thickness to axial length for biometric standardization in angle-closure glaucoma. Am J Ophthal 99:400, 1985.
95. Mapstone, R: Acute shallowing of the anterior chamber. Br J Ophthal 65:446, 1981.
96. Campbell, David G. (personal communication).
97. Mapstone, R: Mechanics of pupil block. Br J Ophthal 52:19, 1968.
98. Wand, M, Grant, WM: Thymoxamine test. Differentiating angle-closure glaucoma from open-angle glaucoma with narrow angles. Arch Ophthal 96:1009, 1978.
99. Ganias, F, Mapstone, R: Miotics in closed-angle glaucoma. Br J Ophthal 59:205, 1975.
100. Airaksinen, PJ, Saari, KM, Tiainen, TJ, Jaanio, E-AT: Management of acute closed-angle glaucoma with miotics and timolol. Br J Ophthal 63:822, 1979.
101. Rutkowski, PC, Fernandez, JL, Galin, MA, Halasa, AH: Alpha-adrenergic receptor blockade in the treatment of angle-closure glaucoma. Trans Am Acad Ophthal Otol 77:137, 1973.
102. Halasa, AH, Rutkowski, PC: Thymoxamine therapy for angle-closure glaucoma. Arch Ophthal 90:177, 1973.
103. Wand, M, Grant, WM: Thymoxamine hydrochloride: an alpha-adrenergic blocker. Surv Ophthal 25:75, 1980.
104. Chandler, PA, Grant, WM: Glaucoma, 2nd ed. Lea & Febiger, Philadelphia, 1979, p. 140.
105. Anderson, DR: Corneal indentation to relieve acute angle-closure glaucoma. Am J Ophthal 88:1091, 1979.
106. Ritch, R: Argon laser treatment for medically unresponsive attacks of angle-closure glaucoma. Am J Ophthal 94:197, 1982.
107. Shin, DH: Argon laser treatment for relief of medically unresponsive angle-closure glaucoma attacks. Am J Ophthal 94:821, 1982.
108. David, R, Tessler, Z, Yassur, Y: Long-term outcome of primary acute angle-closure glaucoma. Br J Ophthal 69:261, 1985.
109. Krupin, T, Mitchell, KB, Johnson, MF, Becker, B: The long-term effects of iridectomy for primary acute angle-closure glaucoma. Am J Ophthal 86:506, 1978.
110. Playfair, TJ, Watson, PG: Management of acute primary angle-closure glaucoma: a long-term follow-up of the results of peripheral iridectomy used as an initial procedure. Br J Ophthal 63:17, 1979.
111. Romano, JH, Hitchings, RA, Pooinasawmy, D: Role of Nd:YAG peripheral iridectomy in the management of ocular hypertension with a narrow angle. Ophthal Surg 19:814, 1988.
112. Forbes, M: Gonioscopy with corneal indentation. A method for distinguishing between appositional closure and synechial closure. Arch Ophthal 76:488, 1966.
113. Forbes, M: Indentation gonioscopy and efficacy of iridectomy in angle-closure glaucoma. Trans Am Ophthal Soc LXXII:488, 1974.
114. Chandler, PA, Simmons, RJ: Anterior chamber deepening for gonioscopy at time of surgery. Arch Ophthal 74:177, 1965.
115. Shaffer, RN: Operating room gonioscopy in angle closure glaucoma surgery. Trans Am Ophthal Soc 55:59, 1957.
116. Williams, DJ, Gills, JP Jr, Hall, GA: Results of

233 peripheral iridectomies for narrow-angle glaucoma. Am J Ophthal 65:548, 1968.

117. Playfair, TJ, Watson, PG: Management of chronic or intermittent primary angle-closure glaucoma: a long-term follow-up of the results of peripheral iridectomy used as an initial procedure. Br J Ophthal 63:23, 1979.
118. Murphy, MB, Spaeth, GL: Iridectomy in primary angle-closure glaucoma. Classification and differential diagnosis of glaucoma associated with narrowness of the angle. Arch Ophthal 91:114, 1974.
119. Gieser, DK, Wilensky, JT: Laser iridectomy in the management of chronic angle-closure glaucoma. Am J Ophthal 98:446, 1984.
120. Eltz, H, Gloor, B: Trabeculectomy in cases of angle closure glaucoma—successes and failures. Klin Monatsbl Augenheilkd 177:556, 1980.
121. Akingbehin, AO: Corticosteroid-induced ocular hypertension. I. Prevalence in closed-angle glaucoma. Br J Ophthal 66:536, 1982.
122. Akingbehin, AO: Corticosteroid-induced ocular hypertension. II. An acquired form. Br J Ophthal 66:541, 1982.
123. Lowe, RF: Acute angle-closure glaucoma. The second eye: an analysis of 200 cases. Br J Ophthal 46:641, 1962.
124. Benedikt, O: Prophylactic iridectomy in the partner eye after angle closure glaucoma. Klin Monatsbl Augenheilkd 156:80, 1970.
125. Ritzinger, I, Benedikt, O, Dirisamer, F: Surgical or conservative prophylaxis of the partner eye after primary acute angle block glaucoma. Klin Monatsbl Augenheilkd 164:645, 1974.
126. Wollensak, J, Ehrhorn, J: Angle block glaucoma and prophylactic iridectomy in the eye without symptoms. Klin Monatsbl Augenheilkd 167:791, 1975.
127. Imre, GY, Bogi, J: The fellow eye in acute angle-closure glaucoma. Klin Monatsbl Augenheilkd 169:264, 1976.
128. Snow, JT: Value of prophylactic peripheral iridectomy on the second eye in angle-closure glaucoma. Trans Ophthal Soc UK 97:189, 1977.
129. Lowe, RF: Primary angle-closure glaucoma. A review 5 years after bilateral surgery. Br J Ophthal 57:457, 1973.
130. Imre, G, Bogi, J: Results of prophylactic iridectomy. Klin Monatsbl Augenheilkd 181:409, 1982.
131. Mapstone, R: The fellow eye. Br J Ophthal 65:410, 1981.
132. Edwards, RS: Behaviour of the fellow eye in acute angle-closure glaucoma. Br J Ophthal 66:576, 1982.
133. Hyams, SW, Friedman, Z, Keroub, C: Fellow eye in angle-closure glaucoma. Br J Ophthal 59:207, 1975.
134. Greve, EL: Primary angle closure glaucoma: Extracapsular extraction or filtering procedure? Int Ophthal 12:157, 1988.

Chapter 11

PRIMARY CONGENITAL GLAUCOMA

I. Terminology
   A. Classification of childhood glaucomas
   B. Classification of primary congenital glaucomas
II. General features
   A. Frequency
   B. Age of onset
   C. Heredity
   D. Race
III. Clinical features
   A. History
   B. External exam
   C. Tonometry
   D. Slit-lamp examination
   E. Gonioscopy
   F. Funduscopy
IV. Etiology
   A. Normal development of the anterior ocular segment
   B. Theories of abnormal development in primary congenital glaucoma
V. Differential diagnosis
   A. Excessive tearing
   B. Corneal disorders
   C. Other glaucomas of childhood
VI. Management
   A. Medical therapy
   B. Surgery
   C. Postoperative care

TERMINOLOGY

Classification of Childhood Glaucomas

As noted in Chapter 8, the glaucomas of childhood may be classified into three groups: 1) *primary congenital glaucoma,* in which a developmental abnormality of the anterior chamber angle leads to obstruction of aqueous outflow without a consistent association with other ocular or systemic developmental anomalies; 2) *developmental glaucomas with associated anomalies,* in which a developmental abnormality is responsible for the glaucoma, but in which additional ocular and systemic anomalies are typically present; and 3) *secondary glaucomas in childhood,* in which the mechanism of obstruction of outflow is acquired from other events, such as inflammation or neoplasia, rather than a primary developmental anomaly of the angle. In one study of 63 cases of glaucoma in childhood, the relative proportions of these three groups were 22.2%, 46%, and 31.8%, respectively.[1]

Primary congenital glaucoma is the subject of this chapter, while developmental glaucomas with associated anomalies are considered in Chapter 12. Since children are subject to many of the same secondary glaucomas as adults, these glaucomas are discussed together in the subsequent chapters on secondary glaucomas, with special attention to those situations that are unique to children.

Classification of Primary Congenital Glaucomas

The term *primary congenital glaucoma* or *primary congenital open-angle glaucoma*[2] may relate to a group of disorders, and other names that have been used for this group refer primarily to the age of onset or clinical appearance. *Primary infantile glaucoma* is a term that is often applied to those cases that appear during the first few years of life.[3] This form of congenital glaucoma has also been called "buphthalmos" (cow's eye) or "hydrophthalmia," referring to the enlargement of the eye that may occur with this condition. However, the latter names should not be used as synonyms for primary infantile glaucoma, since enlargement of the globe may also be seen with other childhood glaucomas. When primary congenital glaucoma appears later in childhood or early adulthood, it is sometimes referred to as *juvenile glaucoma*.[4] Three years of age is generally taken as the division between infantile and juvenile glaucoma, because it is at approximately this age that the eye no longer expands in response to elevated intraocular pressure (IOP).[2,4] Others prefer a broader definition for juvenile glaucoma that includes all forms of primary open-angle glaucoma that are diagnosed between the ages of 10 and 35 years.[5]

GENERAL FEATURES

Frequency

As noted above, primary congenital glaucoma was found to occur in 22.2% of all childhood glaucomas in one study.[1] In another survey, it accounted for approximately 70% of the congenital glaucomas.[6] However, it occurs much less frequently than the primary glaucomas that are seen in adults, and it has been estimated that the average ophthalmic practice will have only one case of primary congenital glaucoma every 5 years.[3]

Age of Onset

Primary congenital glaucoma is usually diagnosed at birth or shortly thereafter, and most cases are recognized in the first year of life. As previously noted, these cases are often referred to as *primary infantile glaucoma*. However, the condition may become apparent at any time throughout childhood or even during young adulthood (juvenile glaucoma).

Heredity

Although it is generally believed that primary congenital glaucoma has a genetic basis, reports vary as to the precise mode of inheritance. An autosomal recessive mode with incomplete or variable penetrance has been suspected,[3] although more recent studies suggest that most cases are caused by multifactorial inheritance.[7,8] In studies of identical twins, congenital glaucoma was usually present in both siblings,[7,9] although only one member was afflicted in one pair of monozygotic twins,[10] suggesting that nongenetic factors may also be involved. An incomplete form of the disease has also been observed in a child whose sibling had the typical findings of primary congenital glaucoma.[11] Chromosal abnormalities have been reported with various congenital glaucomas, although only rarely do these patients have the typical clinical findings of primary congenital glaucoma.[12]

Reports are conflicting as to whether parents of children with primary congenital glaucoma have an increased prevalence of abnormal anterior chamber angles or topical corticosteroid responses.[13,14] No statistically significant differences in HLA histocompatibility antigens were found in one study of patients with primary congenital glaucoma as compared with controls.[15]

Race

In one study of juvenile glaucoma that used the liberal definition of all primary open-angle glaucomas diagnosed between the ages of 10 and 35 years, blacks tended to present at younger ages than whites and had a higher proportion with glaucomatous damage.[5]

CLINICAL FEATURES

Primary congenital glaucoma is typically bilateral, although a significant IOP elevation may occur in only one eye in 25–30% of the cases. The following ocular features, with the possible exception of gonioscopic findings, are not unique to primary congenital glaucoma but may be a part of any childhood glaucoma during the first few years of life.

History

There is a classic triad of manifestations, any one of which should arouse suspicion of glaucoma in an infant or young child: (1) *epiphora* (excessive tearing); 2) *photophobia* (hypersensitivity to light), which is due to corneal edema and is manifested by the child's hiding his or her face in bright lighting, or even in ordinary lighting in severe cases; and (3) *blepharospasm* (squeezing the eyelids), which may be another manifestation of the photophobia.

External Examination

Corneal Diameter. The average horizontal corneal diameter at birth is normally 10.5 mm.[3,16] In a study of premature infants, the mean corneal diameter was 8.2 mm.[17] Distention of the globe in response to elevated IOP (*buphthalmos*) leads to enlargement of the cornea, especially at the corneoscleral junction, and a diameter of more than 12 mm in the first year of life is highly suspicious. Grossly, this is more obvious in asymmetric cases (Fig. 11.1). In one study, corneal diameter was found to be a more reliable guide than axial length in the assessment of congenital glaucoma.[16]

Corneal Edema. Initially, this may be a direct result of the elevated IOP, producing a corneal haze that clears with normalization of the pressure. In more advanced cases, a dense opacification of the corneal stroma may persist despite reduction of the IOP (Fig. 11.2). One study suggests that the latter may result from reduced aqueous production with poor corneal nutrition.[18]

Refractive Error

The enlargement of the globe with elevated IOP during the first 3 years of life creates a *myopic shift* in the refractive error, which may lead to amblyopia if significantly asymmetric. Myopia is also commonly associated with juvenile glaucoma,[5] although it is not clear how often the glaucoma or the myopia was the primary event.

Tonometry

Any of the aforementioned findings demands a thorough examination to rule out congenital glaucoma. Since the pressure is often measured during general anesthesia, the possible influence of the anesthesia on

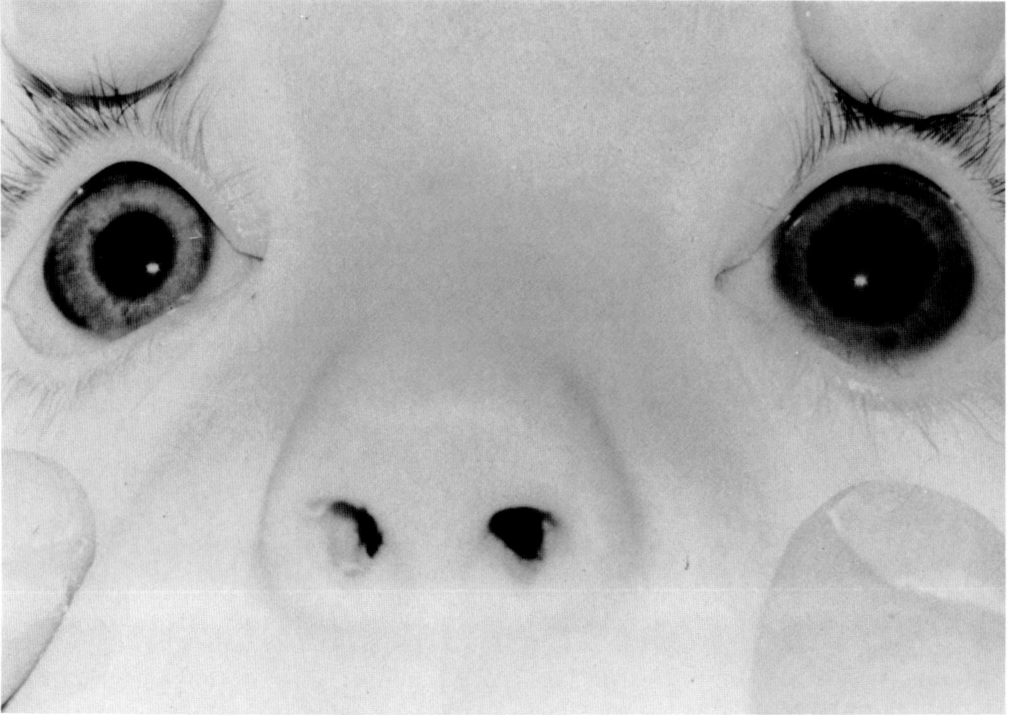

Figure 11.1. Infant with primary congenital glaucoma showing buphthalmos and corneal clouding, both of which are more marked in the left eye.

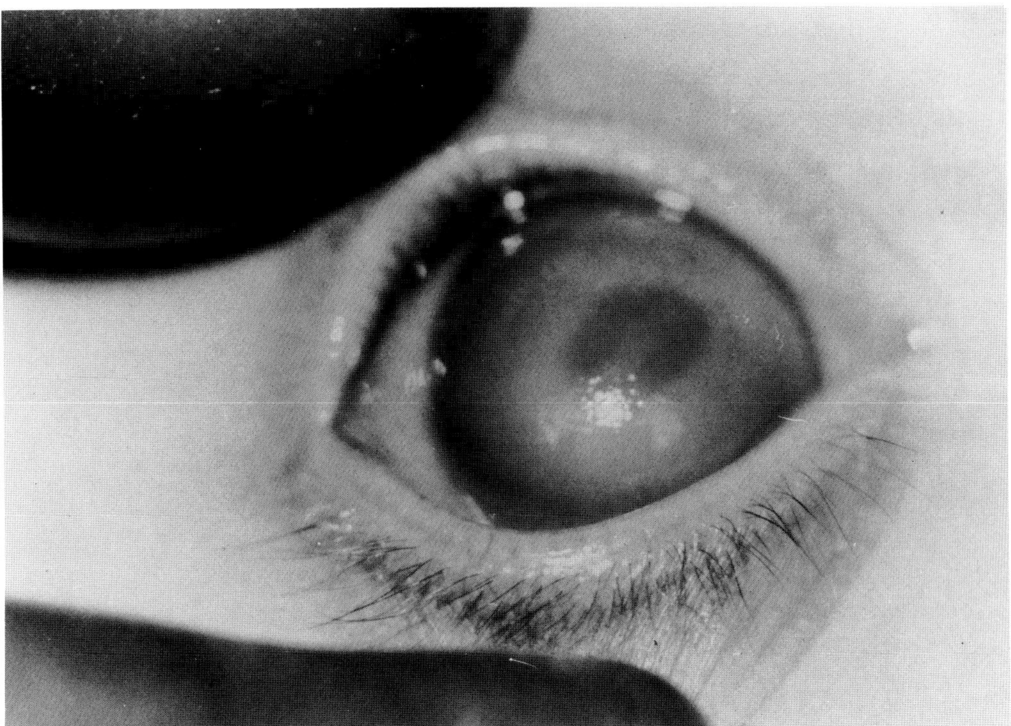

Figure 11.2. Dense corneal opacity of newborn with primary congenital glaucoma.

IOP (see Chapter 4) must be considered. The normal pressure in an infant under halothane anesthesia is said to be approximately 9–10 mm Hg,[19,20] and a pressure of 20 mm Hg or more should arouse suspicion.[19] It has also been reported that children can be successfully examined under chloral hydrate sedation and, using this approach, the pressures by Mackay-Marg tonometry in 17 nonglaucomatous eyes ranged from 11–17 mm Hg.[21] However, the most reliable method of measuring the IOP is probably with the child awake, if cooperation permits, and the Perkins tonometer has been found to be particularly suitable in this situation.[22] In one study, the mean IOP in unanesthetized newborns was 11.4 ± 2.4 mm Hg,[23] although another study of premature infants, measured with a Perkins tonometer without anesthesia, gave a mean pressure of 18 mm Hg.[17]

Slit-Lamp Examination

This portion of the examination is best performed with a portable slit lamp, with or without general anesthesia. A common finding in the cornea is tears in Descemet's membrane (*Haab's striae*), which may be single or multiple and are characteristically oriented horizontally or concentrically to the limbus (Fig. 11.3). They are typically associated with corneal edema in the early phases of the glaucoma. However, as the IOP is normalized and the tears are repaired by endothelial overgrowth, the edema may clear but the linear opacities will persist. Specular microscopy has shown that these patients also have a significantly reduced corneal endothelial cell count.[24]

The anterior chamber is characteristically deep, especially when distention of the globe is present. The iris is typically normal, although it may have stromal hypoplasia with loss of the crypts.

Gonioscopy

Evaluation of the anterior chamber angle is essential for the accurate diagnosis of primary congenital glaucoma. The instruments and techniques of gonioscopy were discussed in Chapter 3. In performing gonioscopy on infants and children under anes-

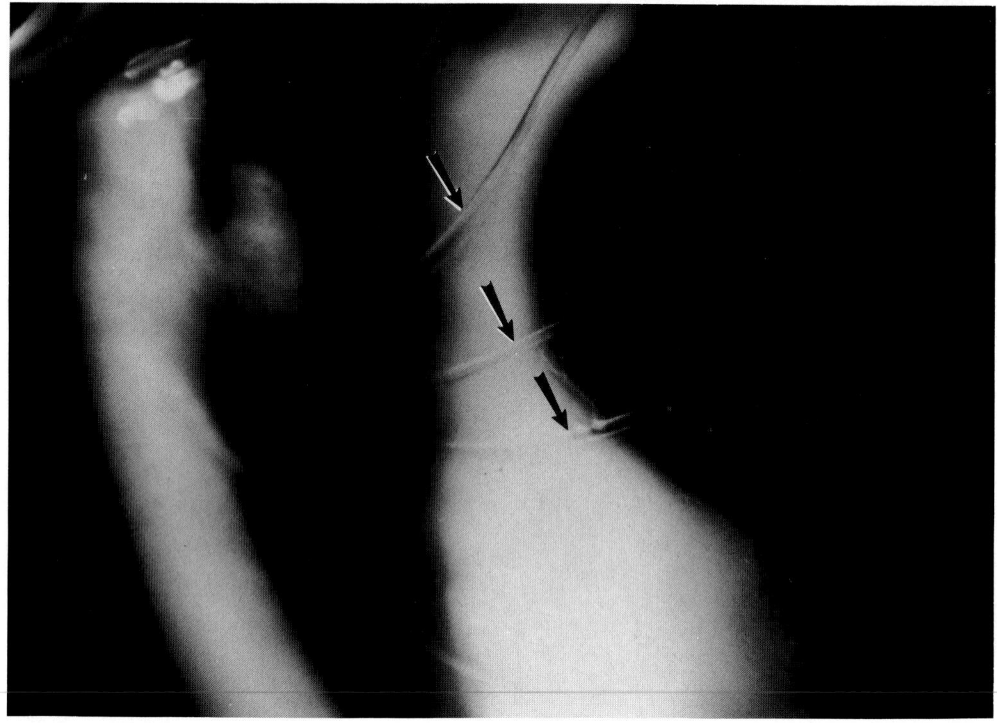

Figure 11.3. Slit-lamp appearance of tears in Descemet's membrane, or Haab's striae (*arrows*), in patient with primary congenital glaucoma.

thesia, an infant Koeppe goniolens is recommended.

The normal anterior chamber angle in childhood differs significantly from that of adults, and the ophthalmologist must be familiar with these differences in order to recognize the abnormal state. The most characteristic feature of the child's anterior chamber angle is the trabecular meshwork, which has the appearance of a smooth, homogeneous membrane, extending from peripheral iris to Schwalbe's line, during the first year of life. It becomes coarser and more pigmented with the passing years. In addition, the peripheral iris in the young child tends to be thinner and flatter.[2]

In primary congenital glaucoma, the typical gonioscopic appearance is an open angle, with a high insertion of the iris root, which forms a scalloped line (Fig. 11.4). Abnormal tissue, with a glistening appearance, may be seen in the angle and appears to pull the peripheral iris anteriorly. Although the angle is usually avascular, loops of vessels from the major arterial circle may be seen above the iris root, which has been called the "Loch Ness monster phenomenon."[25] In addition, the peripheral iris may be covered by a fine, fluffy tissue that has been referred to as "Lister's morning mist."[25]

The clinical features of primary congenital glaucoma seem to merge with other forms of developmental glaucoma. A gonioscopic assessment of more than 100 eyes with developmental glaucoma revealed a spectrum ranging from the common form described above, through a more cicatrized, vascularized condition, to the gross anomalies of the Axenfeld-Rieger syndrome,[26] which is discussed in the next chapter.

Funduscopy

Evaluation of the optic nerve head is one of the most important methods for diagnosing congenital glaucoma, as well as for following the response to therapy. This is usually done with the child anesthetized or sedated, often with an undilated pupil, in which case visualization of the disc may be

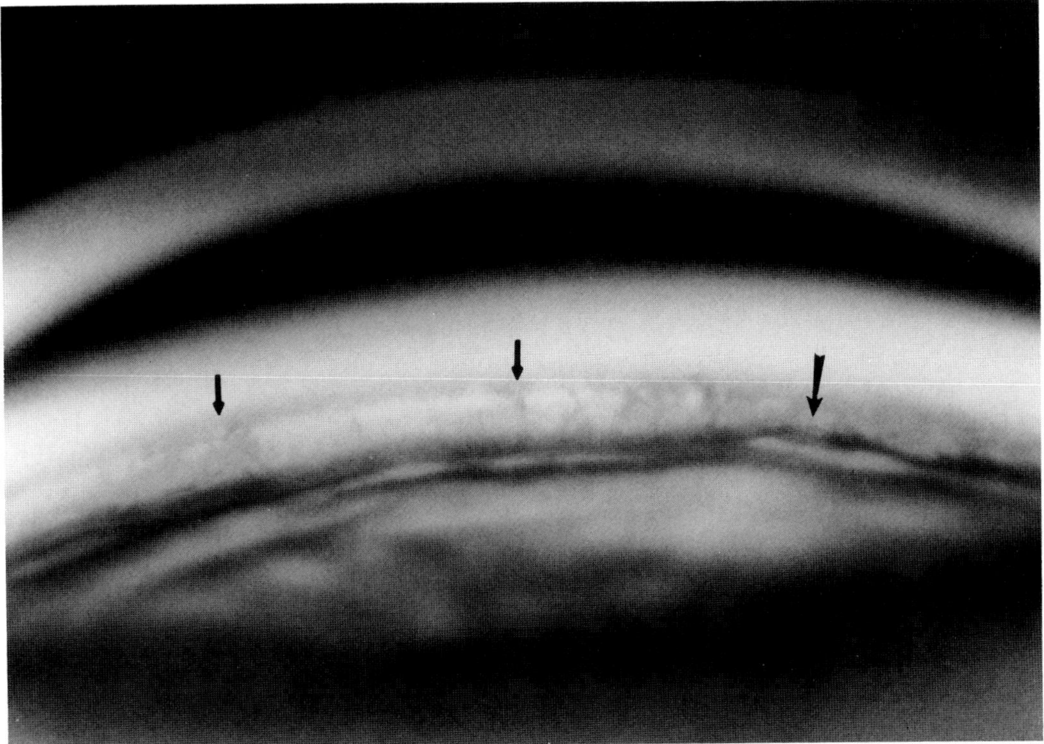

Figure 11.4. Gonioscopic appearance of patient with juvenile glaucoma showing high insertion of iris (*large arrow*) and numerous iris processes (*small arrows*).

facilitated by using a direct ophthalmoscope with a Koeppe lens on the cornea (Fig. 11.5).

The optic nerve head in normal newborns is typically pink but may have slight pallor, and a small physiologic cup is usually present.[27] The morphology of glaucomatous optic atrophy in childhood resembles that seen in adult eyes, with a preferential loss of neural tissue in the vertical poles.[28] A child's eye does differ from that of the adult, however, in that the scleral canal in children enlarges in response to elevated IOP, especially in the horizontal meridian, causing further enlargement of the cup in addition to that resulting from the actual loss of neural tissue.[28]

Cupping of the optic nerve head proceeds more rapidly in infants than in adults and is more likely to be reversible if the pressure is lowered early enough.[29–32] This appears to be due to incomplete development of connective tissue in the lamina cribrosa, which allows compression or posterior movement of the optic disc tissue in response to elevated IOP, with an elastic return to normal when the pressure is lowered.[30]

Visual Fields

When tested after the child becomes old enough for a reliable study, the visual fields are identical to those in adult-onset glaucoma, with an initial predilection for the arcuate areas.[28]

Visual Acuity

Good vision may be achieved if the IOP is controlled before optic atrophy occurs. Occasionally, however, the acuity is poor despite adequate pressure control. In some cases this is due to optic nerve damage, corneal clouding, or irregular astigmatism.[28,33] Other children may have normal-appearing optic nerve heads and clear media but develop amblyopia from anisometropia or strabismus.[34] Retinal detachment is also an occasional cause of poor visual results.[35]

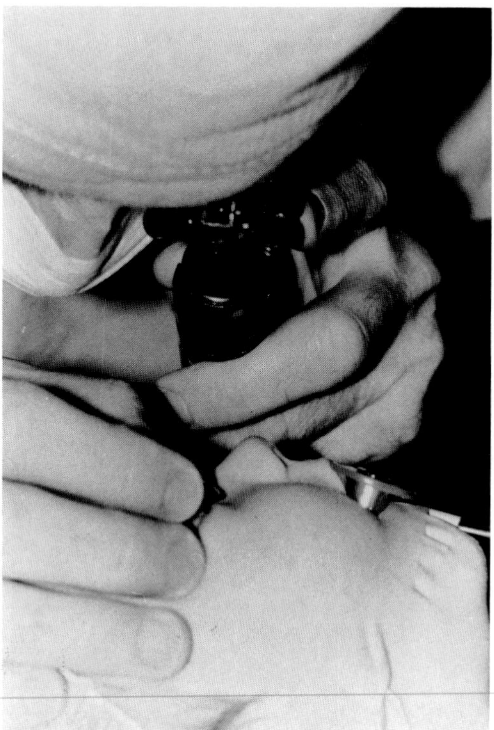

Figure 11.5. Fundus examination with direct ophthalmoscope through infant Koeppe lens during examination under anesthesia of infant with suspected glaucoma.

Ultrasonography

It has been suggested that ultrasonography may be helpful in documenting progression of infantile glaucoma by recording changes in the axial length of the globe.[36,37] It has also been reported that the axial length may decrease up to 0.8 mm following surgical reduction of the IOP.[37] As previously noted, however, a comparison of corneal diameter and axial length showed the former to be a more reliable guide in the assessment of congenital glaucoma.[16]

ETIOLOGY

Normal Development of the Anterior Ocular Segment

A basic understanding of the normal development of the anterior ocular segment is necessary before considering the theories of mechanism for primary congenital glaucoma or for any of the developmental glaucomas with associated anomalies.

General Development

The lens vesicle begins to develop as an invagination of surface ectoderm during the 3rd week of gestation and separates from the latter structure by the 6th week.[38] At this time, the optic cup, which arises from neural ectoderm, has reached the periphery of the lens, and a triangular mass of undifferentiated cells overrides the rim of the cup and surrounds the anterior periphery of the lens. From this tissue mass will arise portions of the cornea, iris, and the anterior chamber angle structures.

Neural Crest Cell Contribution

It was traditionally taught that the undifferentiated cell mass, referred to above, is derived from mesoderm. However, more recent studies indicate that the tissue is of cranial neural crest cell origin. Johnston and co-workers[39] studied orofacial development in chick embryos by transplanting labeled neural crest or mesodermal cells into unlabeled host embryos. The donor tissue was either material labeled with tritiated thymidine or material from the Japanese quail. Cells from the latter bird are characterized by condensed chromatin in the center of the nucleus, in contrast to a more diffuse chromatin pattern in chick cells. Using these models, it was determined that corneal endothelium and stroma, iris, ciliary body, and sclera are of neural crest origin, except for the associated vascular endothelium, which is derived from mesodermal mesenchyme. Tripathi and Tripathi[40] subsequently provided support for the concept that human trabecular meshwork is also of neural crest origin by showing immunohistochemical evidence of neuronal-specific enolase, an enzyme that is normally confined to neurons and cells of the neuroendocrine system, in the cells of the anterior region of the meshwork and those of the inner uveal beams.

Development of Cornea and Iris

From the mass of undifferentiated cells, three waves of tissue come forward between the surface ectoderm and lens. The first of these layers differentiates into the primordial corneal endothelium by the 8th week and subsequently produces Descemet's membrane, while the second wave grows between the corneal endothelium and epithelium to produce the stroma of the cornea.[41,42] The third wave insinuates between the primordia of the cornea and the lens and gives rise to the pupillary membrane and the stroma of the iris. In later months, the pigment epithelial layer of the iris develops from neural ectoderm.

Development of Anterior Chamber Angle

The aqueous outflow structures in the anterior chamber angle appear to arise from the same mesenchymal mass of neural crest cell origin. However, the precise details of this development are not fully understood. Theories have included atrophy[38] or resorption[43] (progressive disappearance of portions of fetal tissue), cleavage[44] (separation of two preexisting tissue layers as a result of differential growth rates), and rarefaction[45] (mechanical distention resulting from growth of the anterior ocular segment). However, more recent work suggests that none of these concepts is completely correct.

Anderson[46] studied 40 normal fetal and infant eyes by light and electron microscopy and found that the anterior surface of the iris at 5 months gestation inserts at the edge of the corneal endothelium, covering the cells that are destined to become trabecular meshwork. This appears to be what Worst[25] called the fetal pectinate ligament, separating the corneoscleral meshwork primordium from the anterior chamber angle. Anderson noted a posterior repositioning of the anterior uveal structures in relation to the cornea and sclera in progressively older tissue specimens, presumably as a result of the differential growth rates. At birth, the insertion of the iris and ciliary body is near the level of the scleral spur, and the posterior migration of these structures continues for approximately the first year of life.

There is some difference of interpretation regarding the innermost layer of the trabecular meshwork primordium as it is uncovered by the posteriorly receding iris. Anderson[46] believed that the smooth surface represents multilayered mesenchymal tissue, which begins to cavitate by the 7th fetal month. However, others have suggested that a true endothelial layer covers the meshwork during gestation. Hansson and Jerndal[47] studied human fetal eyes by scanning electron microscopy and described a single layer of endothelium, continuous with that of the cornea, extending over the primitive anterior chamber angle and iridopupillary structures, creating a closed cavity at the beginning of the 5th fetal month. Worst[25] observed a similar sheet of flat endothelial cells on the pupillary membrane and believed that the disappearance of this layer progresses centrifugally toward the anterior chamber angle.

Hansson and Jerndal[47] noted that the anterior chamber angle portion of the endothelial layer begins to flatten, with loss of clear-cut cell borders, by the 7th fetal month. During the final weeks of gestation and the first weeks after birth, the endothelial layer undergoes fenestration with migration of cells into the underlying uveal meshwork. Van Buskirk[48] also observed intact endothelium completely lining the anterior chamber angle by the second gestational trimester in macaque monkey eyes studied by scanning electron microscopy. He noted that fenestration and gradual retraction of this tissue occurs in the third trimester and progresses in a posterior-to-anterior direction. McMenamin,[49] however, in a scanning electron microscopic study of 32 human fetal eyes, found that the endothelial layer in the iridocorneal angle was perforated by discrete intercellular gaps by 12–14 weeks and that the gaps between the inner uveal trabecular endothelial cells were sufficiently developed by 18–20 weeks to allow a route of communication between the fetal anterior chamber and primitive trabecular tissue.

Studies of glycoconjugates, complex carbohydrates on the cell surface, in the aqueous outflow pathways of mice suggest that they are important in the morphogenesis of the corneoscleral angle and provide some required signals for the differentiation of cells in the trabecular meshwork.[50,51]

The above observations have been combined into a concept of anterior chamber angle development, depicted in Figure 11.6 A–D.[52]

Theories of Abnormal Development in Primary Congenital Glaucoma

Although it is generally agreed that the IOP elevation in primary congenital glaucoma is due to an abnormal development of the anterior chamber angle that leads to obstruction of aqueous outflow, there is no universal agreement as to the nature of the developmental alteration. Theories of mechanism parallel the basic concepts regarding the normal development of the anterior chamber angle, most of which are no longer accepted as being entirely correct. We will first review the major theories that have been proposed in the past and then consider how they fit with our current understanding of the developmental abnormality of primary congenital glaucoma.

Mann[53] postulated that incomplete atrophy of anterior chamber mesoderm resulted in retention of abnormal tissue that blocked aqueous outflow. Barkan[43] suggested that incomplete resorption of the mesodermal cells by adjacent tissue led to the formation of a membrane across the anterior chamber angle. This ''membrane'' became known as *Barkan's membrane,* although its existence has not been proved histologically. Electron microscopic studies by Anderson[46,54] revealed no membrane, despite the appearance of such as structure by gonioscopy and the dissecting microscope. Allen, Burian, and Braley[44] postulated that incomplete cleavage of mesoderm in the anterior chamber angle results in the congenital defect, although the cleavage theory for normal development has not been proved.

Worst[25] proposed a combined theory, which included elements of the atrophy and resorption concepts but rejected the cleavage theory. He suggested that incomplete development of the scleral spur leads to a high insertion of the longitudinal portion of the ciliary muscle on the trabeculum. In addition, he believed that a single layer of endothelial cells covers the anterior chamber angle during gestation and that its abnormal retention in primary congenital glaucoma constitutes Barkan's membrane. Maumenee[55,56] also observed an abnormal anterior insertion of the ciliary musculature into the trabecular meshwork and reasoned that this might compress the scleral spur forward and externally, thus narrowing Schlemm's canal. Anderson[46] and others[57] provided further histopathologic support for the high insertion of the anterior uvea into the trabecular meshwork, suggesting that this is due to a developmental arrest in the normal migration of the uvea across the meshwork in the third trimester of gestation. Maumenee[56] also noted the absence of Schlemm's canal in some histopathologic specimens and suggested that this might be a cause of aqueous outflow obstruction in congenital glaucoma, although Anderson[54] believes that this may be a secondary change.

Smelser and Ozanics[45] explained primary congenital glaucoma as a failure of anterior chamber angle mesoderm to become properly rearranged into the normal trabecular meshwork. Subsequent light and electron microscopic studies favor this theory by showing structural changes of the uveal meshwork[54,58–62] and, in some cases of both infantile and juvenile glaucoma, a thick layer of amorphous material beneath the internal endothelium of Schlemm's canal.[60–62] Kupfer and associates[63,64] emphasized the contribution of the cranial neural crest cells in the development of the anterior chamber angle and suggested that abnormal development of structures derived from these cells may result in the defects of the various forms of congenital glaucoma.

In summary, primary congenital glaucoma appears to result from a developmental arrest of anterior chamber angle tissue derived from neural crest cells, leading to aqueous outflow obstruction by one or more of several mechanisms. The high insertion of ciliary body and iris into the posterior portion of the trabecular meshwork may compress the trabecular beams. In addition, there may be primary developmental defects at various levels of the meshwork and, in some cases, of Schlemm's canal. However, a true membrane over the meshwork does not appear to be a feature of this disorder.

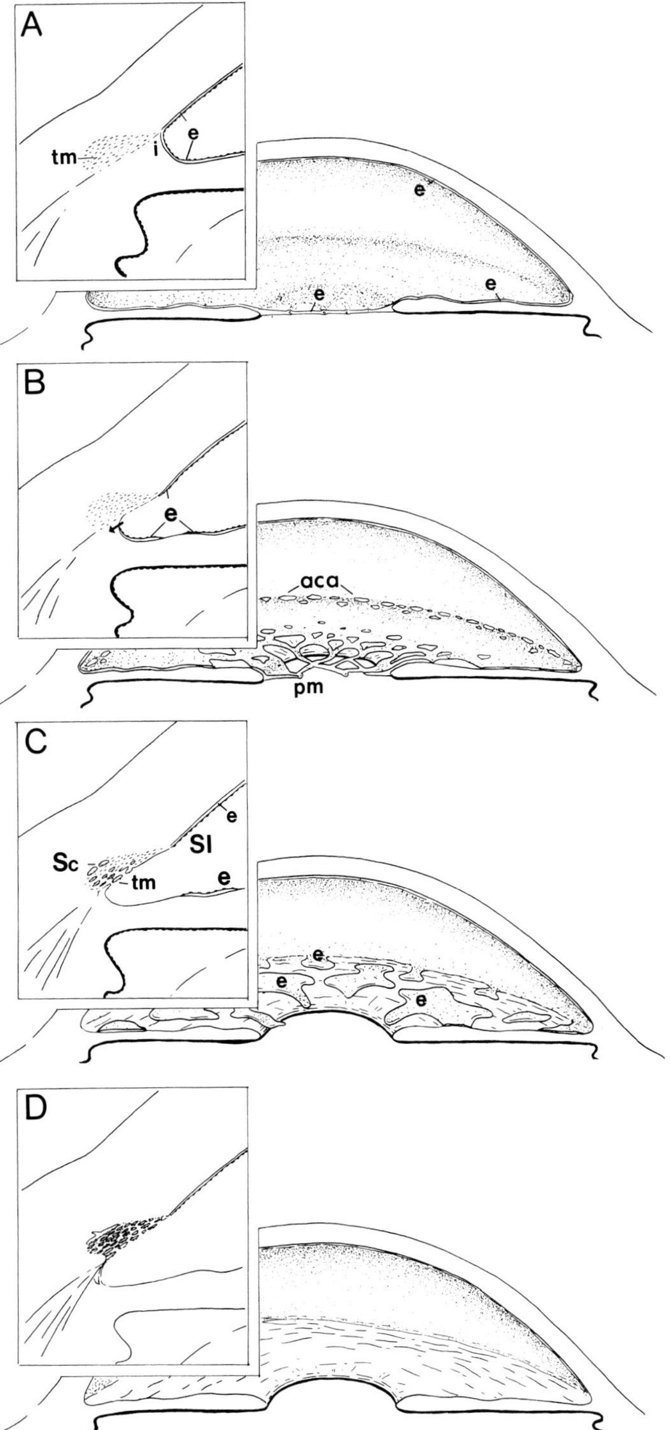

Figure 11.6. A concept of anterior chamber angle development (insets show cross-sectional views of chamber angle). **A,** At 5 months gestation, a continuous layer of endothelium (*e*) creates a closed cavity of the anterior chamber, and the anterior surface of the iris (*i*) inserts in front of the primordial trabecular meshwork (*tm*). **B,** During the third trimester, the endothelial layer progressively disappears from the pupillary membrane (*pm*) and iris and cavitates over the anterior chamber angle (*aca*), possibly becoming incorporated into the trabecular meshwork. At the same time, the peripheral uveal tissue begins to slide posteriorly in relation to the chamber angle structures (*arrow*). **C,** Development of the trabecular lamellae and intertrabecular spaces begins in the inner, posterior aspect of the primordial tissue and progresses toward Schlemm's canal (*Sc*) and Schwalbe's line (*Sl*). **D,** The normal anterior chamber angle is not fully developed until 1 year of life. (Reprinted from Trans Am Ophthal Soc 81:736, 1983, with permission.)

DIFFERENTIAL DIAGNOSIS

Some of the clinical features of primary congenital glaucoma are also found in other conditions, and these must be considered in the differential diagnosis.

Excessive Tearing

In the infant, excessive tearing is most commonly caused by obstruction of the lacrimal drainage system. The epiphora of nasolacrimal duct obstruction is distinguished from that of infantile-onset glaucoma in that the former condition is usually associated with fullness of the lacrimal sac and often has purulent discharge. In addition, the epiphora of infantile glaucoma is frequently associated with photophobia and blepharospasm, although these three findings can also result from a variety of external ocular disorders.

Corneal Disorders

Large corneas may represent congenital megalocornea without glaucoma or an enlarged globe resulting from high myopia. However, infantile-onset glaucoma also typically causes progressive myopia secondary to enlargement of the globe.

Tears in Descemet's membrane may result from birth trauma.[65] These tears are usually vertical or oblique, in contrast to those of congenital glaucoma (Haab's striae), which tend to be horizontal to or concentric with the limbus. The tears in Descemet's membrane may also be confused with band-like structures in posterior polymorphous dystrophy[66] and posterior corneal vesicles.[67] Haab's striae may be distinguished from these disorders by thin, smooth areas between thickened, curled edges, in contrast to central thickening in the latter conditions.[66]

Corneal opacification in infancy may be associated with a variety of disorders:[68] (1) developmental anomalies (Peters' anomaly and sclerocornea); (2) dystrophies (congenital hereditary corneal dystrophy and posterior polymorphous dystrophy); (3) choristomas (dermoid and dermis-like choristoma); (4) edema resulting from birth trauma; (5) intrauterine inflammation (congenital syphilis and rubella); and (6) inborn errors of metabolism (mucopolysaccharidoses and cystinosis).

Other Glaucomas of Childhood

The differential diagnosis of primary congenital glaucoma should also include developmental glaucomas with associated anomalies, as well as the childhood glaucomas secondary to systemic or other ocular disorders, all of which are discussed in subsequent chapters.

MANAGEMENT

Medical Therapy

Primary congenital glaucoma is almost always managed surgically, with medical therapy used only as a temporizing measure before surgery or when surgical intervention has repeatedly failed. In general, the same basic principles of medical therapy apply to the treatment of primary congenital glaucoma as to the adult glaucomas. One possible exception is the use of miotics, which may paradoxically raise the IOP by collapse of the trabecular meshwork because of the high insertion of uveal tissue into the posterior meshwork. Dosages for children and special precautions are discussed in Section Three.

Surgery

The primary surgical techniques are designed to eliminate the resistance to aqueous outflow created by the structural abnormalities in the anterior chamber angle. At present this is accomplished with incisional surgery, using either an internal (goniotomy) or external (trabeculotomy) approach, although pulsed lasers may one day become effective for this purpose. The present discussion is limited to the concepts of management, while details of the operative procedures are considered in Section Three.

Goniotomy. Barkan[69,70] described a technique in which abnormal tissue (originally believed to be Barkan's membrane) is incised under direct visualization with the aid of a goniolens. It is now believed that the incision is not through a membrane, but rather through the inner portion of the trabecular meshwork. This presumably relieves the compressive traction of the anterior uvea on the meshwork and eliminates any resistance imposed by incompletely developed inner meshwork.

Trabeculotomy. Harms and Dannheim[71] described a technique in which Schlemm's canal is identified by external dissection, and the trabecular meshwork is incised by passing a probe into the canal and then rotating it into the anterior chamber. One advantage of this procedure is that it can be performed in eyes with cloudy corneas, which is not the case with goniotomy. While some surgeons employ the technique only in cases with corneal opacification or when multiple goniotomies have failed, others prefer it as the initial procedure in primary congenital glaucoma.

Both goniotomy and trabeculotomy have their advocates, and reported success rates vary considerably, with neither procedure having clear-cut superiority. A more detailed comparison of the two operations is presented in Section Three. With both procedures, success is related to the severity and duration of the glaucoma. The worst prognosis occurs in infants with elevated pressures and cloudy corneas at birth. The most favorable outcome is seen in infants operated on between the 2nd and 8th month of life, and the surgery then becomes less effective with increasing age.[72]

Other Glaucoma Procedures. When multiple goniotomies and/or trabeculotomies have failed, the surgeon usually resorts to a filtering procedure, such as a trabeculectomy. Some surgeons prefer a full-thickness technique, such as thermal sclerostomy,[73] which may have a better chance of pressure control but may also be associated with a higher risk of postoperative complications. A combined trabeculectomy/trabeculotomy may also be used when repeated surgery is required. In some desperate situations, in which all else has failed, a cyclodestructive procedure may be useful. In one small series of cases with marked buphthalmos and congenitally opaque corneas, cyclocryotherapy led to both normalization of IOP and a reduction in corneal diameter, allowing subsequent successful penetrating keratoplasty.[74]

Penetrating Keratoplasty. Corneal cloudiness may persist following normalization of the IOP, leading to the need for penetrating keratoplasty. These patients typically do not do well, with only 25% of eyes achieving 20/40 or better vision in one series.[75] The most common postoperative complications are IOP elevation and graft failure. While significant visual improvement can be achieved with penetrating keratoplasty,[74] it is suggested that it be reserved for patients with severe visual disability whose glaucoma is well controlled.[75]

Postoperative Care

The follow-up care of patients with primary congenital glaucoma has several important facets. In the early postoperative period, close observation is required regarding success of the glaucoma procedure. Corneal edema may persist for weeks after successful reduction of IOP and is, therefore, an unreliable indicator of early success, while changes in the optic nerve head provide the most important indicator of the course of the disease.[34] The IOP is also a significant factor in postoperative visual capacity, with substantially better vision among those whose pressures remain no higher than 19 mm Hg.[72]

Even when the pressure is well controlled, however, a significant number of children never achieve good vision. In two large studies, approximately half of the patients had visual acuities of less than 20/50.[72,76] As previously noted, this reduction may result from persistent corneal changes, occasionally requiring penetrating keratoplasty. However, a high percentage of patients suffer amblyopia from the induced anisometropia, and it is critical that this be diagnosed early and managed appropriately.

Finally, the patient and family must understand that pressure elevation can recur at any age in individuals with primary congenital glaucoma, and these patients must be followed throughout their life.

SUMMARY

Primary congenital glaucoma is one of several childhood glaucomas, characterized by a developmental abnormality of the anterior chamber angle without consistently associated systemic or other ocular anomalies. The condition is believed to have a genetic basis, is usually diagnosed during the first year of life, and is most often bilateral. Characteristic clinical features include epiphora, photophobia, blepharospasm, and an enlarged, cloudy cornea. The normal development of the anterior chamber angle primarily involves tissues of cranial neural crest cell origin, and incomplete development is believed to be the mechanism of primary congenital glaucoma. The differential diagnosis must include other causes of epiphora and corneal abnormalities, as well as the additional forms of glaucoma in childhood. Primary congenital glaucoma is usually managed surgically with either a goniotomy or trabeculotomy, although attention must also be given to the amblyopia, which is a common sequela of this disorder.

References

1. Barsoum-Homsy, M, Chevrette, L: Incidence and prognosis of childhood glaucoma. A study of 63 cases. Opthalmology 93:1323, 1986.
2. Walton, DS: Primary congenital open-angle glaucoma. In: Glaucoma, Chandler, PA, Grant, WM. Lea and Febiger, Philadelphia, 1979, p. 329.
3. Shaffer, RN, Weiss, DI: Congenital and Pediatric Glaucomas. CV Mosby, St. Louis, 1970, p. 37.
4. Kwitko, ML: Glaucomas in Infants and Children. Appleton-Century-Crofts, New York, 1973, p. 185.
5. Lotufo, D, Ritch, R, Szmyd, L, Burris, JE: Juvenile glaucoma, race, and refraction. JAMA 261:249, 1989.
6. Azuma, I: A survey on the congenital glaucoma. Klin Monatsbl Augenheilkd 184:287, 1984.
7. Merin, S, Morin, D: Heredity of congenital glaucoma. Br J Ophthal 56:414, 1972.
8. Demenais, F, Elston, RC, Bonaiti, C, et al: Segregation analysis of congenital glaucoma. Approach by two different models. Am J Hum Genet 33:300, 1981.
9. Rasmussen, DH, Ellis, PP: Congenital glaucoma in identical twins. Arch Ophthal 84:827, 1970.
10. Fried, K, Sachs, R, Krakowsky, D: Congenital glaucoma in only one of identical twins. Ophthalmologica 174:185, 1977.
11. Pollack, A, Oliver, M: Congenital glaucoma and incomplete congenital glaucoma in two siblings. Acta Ophthal 62:359, 1984.
12. Katsushima, H, Kii, T, Soma, K, et al: Primary congenital glaucoma in a patient with trisomy 2q (q33→qter) and monosomy 9p (p24→pter). Arch Ophthal 105:323, 1987.
13. Kaufman, PL, Kolker, AE: Ocular findings and corticosteroid responsiveness in parents of children with primary infantile glaucoma. Invest Ophthal 14:46, 1975.
14. Jerndal, T, Munkby, M: Corticosteroid response in dominant congenital glaucoma. Acta Ophthal 56:373, 1978.
15. Hvidberg, A, Kessing, SvV, Svejgaard, A: HLA histocompatibility antigens in primary congenital glaucoma. Glaucoma 1:134, 1979.
16. Kiskis, AA, Markowitz, SN, Morin, JD: Corneal diameter and axial length in congenital glaucoma. Can J Ophthal 20:93, 1985.
17. Musarella, MA, Morin, JD: Anterior segment and intraocular pressure measurements of the unanesthetized premature infant. Metab Pediatr Syst Ophthal 8:53, 1985.
18. Imre, G, Bogi, J: Corneal edema in young glaucoma patients. Klin Monatsbl Augenheilkd 179:465, 1981.
19. Dominquez, A, Banos, MS, Alvarez, MG, et al: Intraocular pressure measurement in infants under general anesthesia. Am J Ophthal 78:110, 1974.
20. Grote, P: Augeninnendruckmessungen bei Kleinkindern ohne Glaukam in Halothanmaskennarkose. Ophthalmologica 171:202, 1975.
21. Judisch, GF, Anderson, S, Bell, WE: Chloral hydrate sedation as a substitute for examination under anesthesia in pediatric ophthalmology. Am J Ophthal 89:560, 1980.
22. Van Buskirk, EM, Plamer, EA: Office assessment of young children for glaucoma. Ann Ophthal 11:1749, 1979.
23. Radtke, ND, Cohen, BF: Intraocular pressure measurement in the newborn. Am J Ophthal 78:501, 1974.
24. Wenzel, M, Krippendorff, U, Hunold, W, Reim, M: Endothelial cell damage in congenital and juvenile glaucoma. Klin Monatsbl Augenheilkd 195:344, 1989.
25. Worst, JGF: The Pathogenesis of Congenital Glaucoma. An Embryological and Goniosurgical Study. Charles C. Thomas, Springfield, Ill., 1966.
26. Luntz, MH: Congenital, infantile, and juvenile glaucoma. Ophthalmology 86:793, 1979.
27. Khodadoust, AA, Ziai, M, Biggs, SL: Optic disc in normal newborns. Am J Ophthal 66:502, 1968.
28. Robin, AL, Quigley, HA, Pollack, IP, et al: An analysis of visual acuity, visual fields, and disk cupping in childhood glaucoma. Am J Ophthal 88:847, 1979.
29. Shaffer, RN, Hetherington, J Jr: The glaucomatous disc in infants. A suggested hypothesis for disc cupping. Trans Am Acad Ophthal Otol 73:929, 1969.
30. Quigley, HA: The pathogenesis of reversible cup-

ping in congenital glaucoma. Am J Ophthal 84:358, 1977.
31. Robin, AL, Quigley, HA: Transient reversible cupping in juvenile-onset glaucoma. Am J Ophthal 88:580, 1979.
32. Quigley, HA: Childhood glaucoma. Results with trabeculotomy and study of reversible cupping. Ophthalmology 89:219, 1982.
33. Morin, JD, Bryars, JH: Causes of loss of vision in congenital glaucoma. Arch Ophthal 93:1575, 1980.
34. Rice, NSC: Management of infantile glaucoma. Br J Ophthal 56:294, 1972.
35. Cooling, RJ, Rice, NSC, McLeod, D: Retinal detachment in congenital glaucoma. Br J Ophthal 64:417, 1980.
36. Sampaolesi, R, Caruso, R: Ocular echometry in the diagnosis of congenital glaucoma. Arch Ophthal 100:574, 1982.
37. Tarkkanen, A, Uusitalo, R, Mianowicz, J: Ultrasonographic biometry in congenital glaucoma. Acta Ophthal 61:618, 1983.
38. Mann, IC: The Development of the Human Eye, 3rd ed. Grune and Stratton, London, 1964.
39. Johnston, MC, Noden, DM, Hazelton, RD, et al: Origins of avian ocular and periocular tissues. Exp Eye Res 29:27, 1979.
40. Tripathi, BJ, Tripathi, RC: Neural crest origin of human trabecular meshwork and its implications for the pathogenesis of glaucoma. Am J Ophthal 107:583, 1989.
41. Wulle, KG: Electron microscopy of the fetal development of the corneal endothelium and Descemet's membrane of the human eye. Invest Ophthal 11:397, 1972.
42. Hay, ED: Development of the vertebrate cornea. Internat Rev Cytol 63:263, 1980.
43. Barkan, O: Pathogenesis of congenital glaucoma. Gonioscopic and anatomic observation of the angle of the anterior chamber in the normal eye and in congenital glaucoma. Am J Ophthal 40:1, 1955.
44. Allen, L, Burian, HM, Braley, AE: A new concept of the development of the anterior chamber angle. Its relationship to developmental glaucoma and other structural anomalies. Arch Ophthal 53:783, 1955.
45. Smelser, GK, Ozanics, V: The development of the trabecular meshwork in primate eyes. Am J Ophthal 71:366, 1971.
46. Anderson, DR: The development of the trabecular meshwork and its abnormality in primary infantile glaucoma. Trans Am Ophthal Soc 79:458, 1981.
47. Hansson, H-A, Jerndal, T: Scanning electron microscopic studies on the development of the iridocorneal angle in human eyes. Invest Ophthal 10:252, 1971.
48. Van Buskirk, EM: Clinical implications of iridocorneal angle development. Ophthalmology 88:361, 1981.
49. McMenamin, PG: Human fetal iridocorneal angle: a light and scanning electron microscopic study. Br J Ophthal 73:871, 1989.
50. Beauchamp, GR, Lubeck, D, Knepper, PA: Glycoconjugates, cellular differentiation, and congenital glaucoma. J Ped Ophthal Strab 22:149, 1985.
51. Vaden Hoek, TL, Goossens, W, Knepper, PA: Fluorescence-labeled lectins, glycoconjungates, and the development of the mouse AOP. Invest Ophthal Vis Sci 28:451, 1987.
52. Shields, MB: Axenfeld-Rieger syndrome. A theory of mechanism and distinctions from the iridocorneal endothelial syndrome. Trans Am Ophthal Soc 81:736, 1983.
53. Mann, IC: Development of the Human Eye. Cambridge University Press, Cambridge, England, 1928.
54. Anderson, DR: Pathology of the glaucomas. Br J Ophthal 56:146, 1972.
55. Maumenee, AE: The pathogenesis of congenital glaucoma. A new theory. Am J Ophthal 47:827, 1959.
56. Maumenee, AE: Further observations on the pathogenesis of congenital glaucoma. Am J Ophthal 55:1163, 1963.
57. Wright, JD Jr, Robb, RM, Dueker, DK, Boger, WP III: Congenital glaucoma unresponsive to conventional therapy: a clinicopathological case presentation. J Ped Ophthal Strab 20:172, 1983.
58. Sampaolesi, R, Argento, C: Scanning electron microscopy of the trabecular meshwork in normal and glaucomatous eyes. Invest Ophthal Vis Sci 16:302, 1977.
59. Maul, E, Strozzi, L, Munoz, C, Reyes, C: The outflow pathway in congenital glaucoma. Am J Ophthal 89:667, 1980.
60. Rodrigues, MM, Spaeth, GL, Weinreb, S: Juvenile glaucoma associated with goniodysgenesis. Am J Ophthal 81:786, 1976.
61. Tawara, A, Inomata, H: Developmental immaturity of the trabecular meshwork in congenital glaucoma. Am J Ophthal 92:508, 1981.
62. Tawara, A, Inomata, H: Developmental immaturity of the trabecular meshwork in juvenile glaucoma. Am J Ophthal 98:82, 1984.
63. Kupfer, C, Ross, K: The development of outflow facility in human eyes. Invest Ophthal 10:513, 1971.
64. Kupfer, C, Kaiser-Kupfer, MI: Observations on the development of the anterior chamber angle with reference to the pathogenesis of congenital glaucomas. Am J Ophthal 88:424, 1979.
65. Angell, LK, Robb, RM, Berson, FG: Visual prognosis in patients with ruptures in Descemet's membrane due to forceps injuries. Arch Ophthal 99:2137, 1981.
66. Cibis, GW, Tripathi, RC: The differential diagnosis of Descemet's tears (Haab's Striae) and poste-

rior polymorphous dystrophy bands. A clinicopathologic study. Ophthalmology 89:614, 1982.
67. Pardos, GJ, Krachmer, JH, Mannis, MJ: Posterior corneal vesicles. Arch Ophthal 99:1573, 1981.
68. Ching, FC: Corneal opacification in infancy. Med Coll Virginia Quarterly 8:230, 1972.
69. Barkan, O: Operation for congenital glaucoma. Am J Ophthal 25:552, 1942.
70. Barkan, O: Goniotomy for the relief of congenital glaucoma. Br J Ophthal 32:701, 1948.
71. Harms, H, Dannheim, R: Trabeculotomy results and problems. In: Microsurgery in Glaucoma, Mackenson, G, ed. Basel, S Karger, 1970, p. 121.
72. Dannheim, R, Haas, H: Visual acuity and intraocular pressure after surgery in congenital glaucoma. Klin Monatsbl Augenheilkd 177:296, 1980.
73. Cadera, W, Pachtman, MA, Cantor, LB, et al: Congenital glaucoma with corneal cloudiness treated by thermal sclerostomy. Can J Ophthal 20:98, 1985.
74. Frucht-Pery, J, Feldman, ST, Brown, SI: Transplantation of congenitally opaque corneas from eyes with exaggerated buphthalmos. Am J Ophthal 107:655, 1989.
75. Huang, SCM, Soong, HK, Benz, RM, et al: Problems associated with penetrating keratoplasty for corneal edema in congenital glaucoma. Ophthal Surg 20:399, 1989.
76. Morgan, KS, Black, B, Ellis, FD, Helveston, EM: Treatment of congenital glaucoma. Am J Ophthal 92:799, 1981.

Chapter 12

DEVELOPMENTAL GLAUCOMAS WITH ASSOCIATED ANOMALIES

The glaucomas considered in this chapter all have, as the mechanism of aqueous outflow obstruction, a developmental abnormality of the anterior chamber angle. Unlike primary congenital glaucoma, however, these conditions have additional ocular and systemic anomalies that help to characterize each clinical entity.

General Terminology

Considerable discussion and confusion have surrounded the lumping, splitting, and classifying of this large number of disorders. Based on the observation that most of the ocular and facial structures involved in these developmental disorders are of neural crest origin,[1,2] the term *neurocristopathies* has been used as a unifying concept for diseases arising from neural crest maldevelopment.[3,4] Hoskins and associates[5] have advocated a shift away from eponyms and syndrome names for individual disorders toward an emphasis on descriptive terminology. Noting that the trabecular meshwork, iris, and cornea are the three major structures involved in these conditions, they suggested the terms "trabeculodysgenesis," "iridodysgenesis," and "corneodysgenesis," or combinations thereof, as a system of classifying the developmental defects.

While there is value in categorizing disorders on the basis of anatomic descriptions and mechanisms, the overlapping of manifestations and limited understanding of disease mechanisms make it difficult to apply such a system in all cases of developmental glaucomas with associated anomalies. For this reason, traditional eponyms and syndrome names will be retained, with some suggested modifications, for purposes of discussion in this chapter.

AXENFELD-RIEGER SYNDROME

Terminology

In 1920, Axenfeld[6] described a patient with a white line in the posterior aspect of the cornea, near the limbus, and tissue strands extending from peripheral iris to this prominent line. Beginning in the mid-1930s, Rieger[7–9] reported cases with similar anterior segment anomalies but with additional changes in the iris, including corectopia, atrophy, and hole formation. It was also discovered that some of these patients had associated systemic developmental defects, especially of the teeth and facial bones.[10,11] Axenfeld[6] referred to his case as "posterior embryotoxon of the cornea," while Rieger[9] used the term "mesodermal dysgenesis of the cornea and iris." In current nomenclature, these conditions are commonly designated by three eponyms: (1) *Axenfeld's anomaly* (limited to peripheral anterior segment defects); (2) *Rieger's anomaly* (peripheral abnormalities with additional changes in the iris); and (3) *Rieger's syndrome* (ocular anomalies plus systemic developmental defects).

The similarity of anterior chamber angle abnormalities in Axenfeld's anomaly and Rieger's anomaly and syndrome has led most investigators to agree that these three arbitrary categories represent a spectrum of developmental disorders.[12–15] Furthermore, the overlap of ocular and systemic anomalies is such that the traditional classification is difficult to apply in all cases. Various collective terms have been applied to this spectrum of disorders, such as "anterior chamber cleavage syndrome"[13] and "mesodermal dysgenesis of the cornea and iris."[9] As noted in Chapter 11, however, the theories of normal development on which these names are based are no longer believed to be correct. In addition, the former collective term included the central ocular defects of Peters' anomaly, which is discussed later in this chapter. While some patients may have the combined defects of Axenfeld's or Rieger's anomaly and Peters' anomaly, the association is rare and the mechanisms of the two disorders, in most cases, are different.

More recently, the term *Axenfeld-Rieger* (A-R) *syndrome* has been used for all clinical variations within this spectrum of developmental disorders.[15,16] This name retains reference to the original eponyms and is not dependent on any theory of normal development, understanding of which is still incomplete, nor does it require arbitrary subclassification of the clinical variations.

General Features

All patients with the A-R syndrome, irrespective of ocular manifestations, share the same general features: (1) a bilateral, developmental disorder of the eyes; (2) a frequent family history of the disorder, with an autosomal dominant mode of inheritance; (3) no sex predilection; (4) frequent systemic developmental defects; and (5) a high incidence of secondary glaucoma. The age at which the A-R syndrome is diagnosed ranges from birth to adulthood, with most cases becoming recognized during infancy or childhood. The diagnosis may result from discovery of an abnormal iris or other ocular anomaly, signs of congenital glaucoma, reduced vision in older patients, or systemic anomalies. Other cases are diagnosed during a routine examination, which may have been prompted by a family history of the disorder.

Ocular Features

Ocular defects in the A-R syndrome are typically bilateral. The structures most commonly involved are the peripheral cornea, anterior chamber angle, and iris.

Cornea

The characteristic abnormality of the cornea is a *prominent, anteriorly displaced Schwalbe's line*. This appears on slit-lamp examination as a white line on the posterior cornea near the limbus. In some cases, the line is incomplete, usually limited to the temporal quadrant (Fig. 12.1), while in other patients it may be seen for 360° (Fig. 12.2). In some cases, the prominent line can be seen only by gonioscopy, while rare cases with other ocular and systemic features of the A-R syndrome may have grossly normal Schwalbe's lines.[17]

It is not uncommon for an individual to have a prominent Schwalbe's line with no

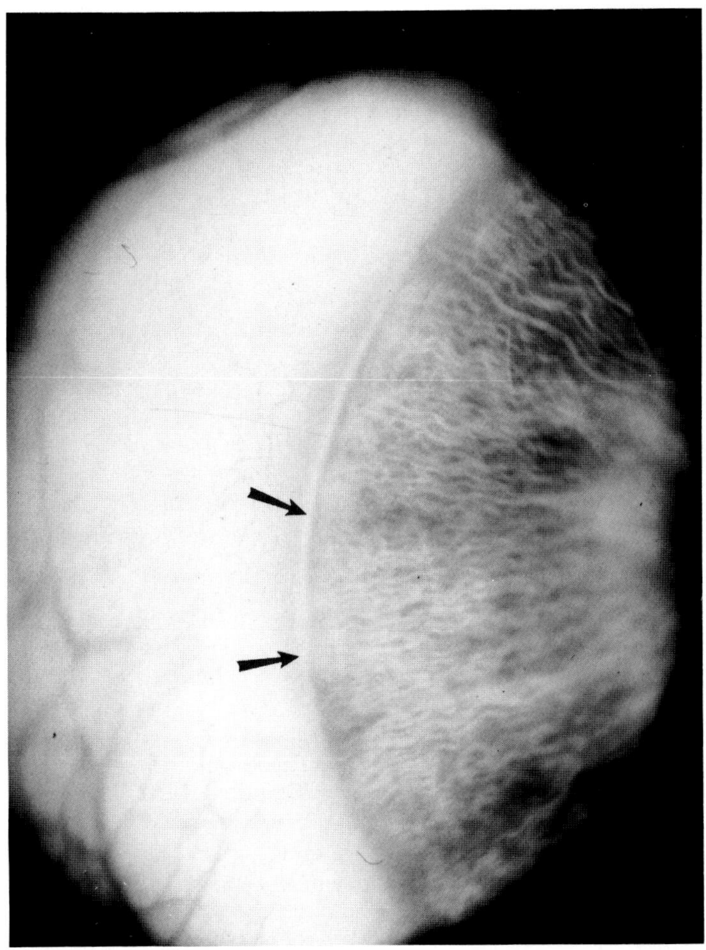

Figure 12.1. Prominent, anteriorly displaced Schwalbe's line (posterior embryotoxon) in temporal quadrant (*arrows*). (Reprinted from The Secondary Glaucomas, ed. Ritch R, Shields MB, Chapter 2, St. Louis, The CV Mosby Co., 1982, with permission.)

other evidence of the A-R syndrome. This isolated defect is often referred to as *posterior embryotoxon*, the term originally used by Axenfeld,[6] and reportedly occurs in 8%[12] to 15%[18] of the general population. It may represent a forme fruste of the A-R syndrome but is not included in this spectrum of anomalies, since it is neither associated with an increased incidence of secondary glaucoma nor with systemic anomalies. A prominent Schwalbe's line may rarely be associated with other disorders, including primary congenital glaucoma[19] and the iridocorneal endothelial syndrome.[20]

The cornea is otherwise normal in the typical case of the A-R syndrome, with the exception of occasional patients with variation in the overall size (megalocornea or, less often, microcornea) or shape of the cornea.[12] Congenital opacities of the central cornea have also been observed in a few cases. The corneal endothelium is typically normal. By specular microscopy, the cells have distinct margins, although mild to moderate variation in the size and shape is commonly observed, especially in older patients and in those with long-standing glaucoma or previous intraocular surgery.[15]

Anterior Chamber Angle

Gonioscopic examination typically reveals a prominent Schwalbe's line, although

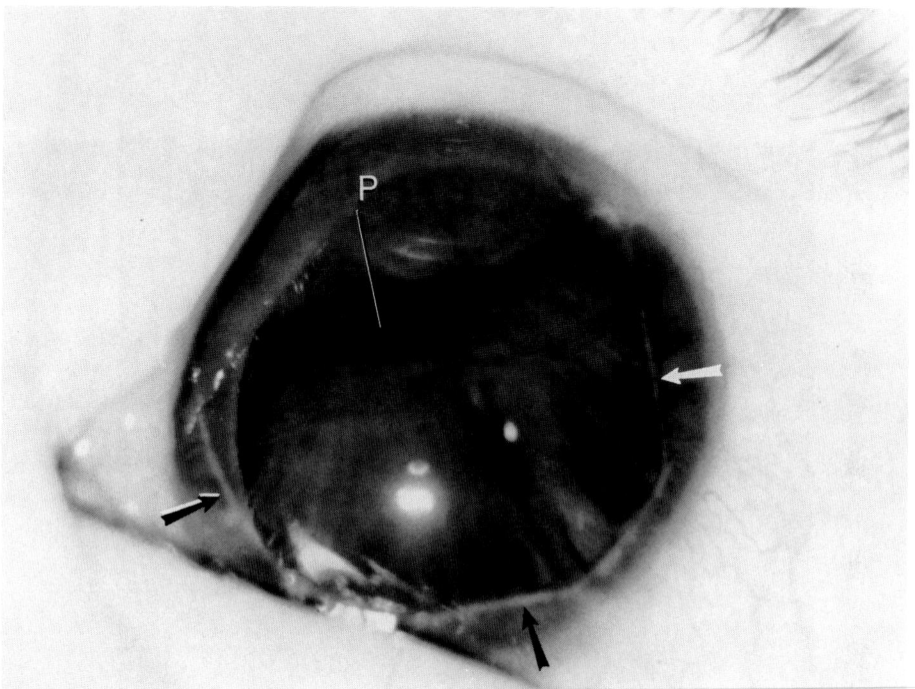

Figure 12.2. Prominent, anteriorly displaced Schwalbe's line in all quadrants (*arrows*) with pupillary distortion (*P*) in patient with Axenfeld-Rieger syndrome. (Reprinted from The Secondary Glaucomas, ed. Ritch R, Shields MB, Chapter 2, St. Louis, The CV Mosby Co., 1982, with permission.)

there is considerable variation among patients in the extent to which Schwalbe's line is enlarged and anteriorly displaced. In occasional cases, the line is suspended from the cornea in some areas by a thin membrane.[15,21] Tissue strands bridge the anterior chamber angle from the peripheral iris to the prominent ridge (Fig. 12.3). These *iridocorneal adhesions* are typically similar in color and texture to the adjacent iris. The strands range in size from threadlike structures to broad bands extending for nearly 15° of the circumference. In some eyes, only one to two tissue strands are seen, while others have several per quadrant. Beyond the tissue strands, the anterior chamber angle is open and the trabecular meshwork is visible, but the scleral spur is typically obscured by peripheral iris, which inserts into the posterior portion of the meshwork.[12,15,18]

Iris

Aside from the peripheral abnormalities, the iris is normal in some eyes with the A-R syndrome. In other cases, defects of the iris range from mild stromal thinning to marked atrophy with hole formation, corectopia, and ectropion uveae (Fig. 12.4). When corectopia is present, the pupil is usually displaced toward a prominent peripheral tissue strand, which is often visible by slit-lamp biomicroscopy. The atrophy and hole formation typically occur in the quadrant away from the direction of the corectopia.

In a small number of patients with the A-R syndrome, abnormalities of the central iris have been observed to progress.[15,22–24] This is more often seen during the first years of life but may also occur in older patients. The progressive changes usually consist of displacement or distortion of the pupil and occasional thinning or hole formation of the iris. Abnormalities of the peripheral iris or anterior chamber angle do not appear to progress after birth, except for occasional thickening of iridocorneal tissue strands.[15]

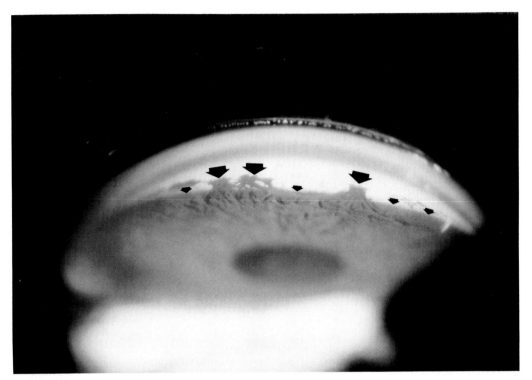

Figure 12.3. Gonioscopic appearance of patient with Axenfeld-Rieger syndrome showing tissue strands extending from peripheral iris to prominent Schwalbe's line (*large arrows*) and high insertion of iris into trabecular meshwork (*small arrows*). (Reprinted from Trans Am Ophthal Soc 81:736, 1983, with permission.)

Additional Ocular Abnormalities

Many additional ocular abnormalities have been reported in one or more cases or pedigrees. While none of these occurs with sufficient frequency to be included as a typical feature of the A-R syndrome and may actually represent a separate entity, there is the impression that these patients are subject to a wide range of ocular anomalies.[12,15] Reported abnormalities include strabismus, limbal dermoids, corneal pannus,[25] cataracts,[26] congenital ectropion uveae,[27] congenital pupillary-iris-lens membrane,[28] peripheral spoke-like transillumination defects of the iris, retinal detachment,[29] macular degeneration, chorioretinal colobomas, choroidal hypoplasia, and hypoplasia of the optic nerve heads.[12,15]

Glaucoma

Slightly more than half of the patients with the A-R syndrome develop glaucoma. This may become manifest during infancy, although it more commonly appears in childhood or young adulthood. The extent of the iris defects and iridiocorneal strands does not correlate precisely with the presence or severity of the glaucoma. On the other hand, the high insertion of peripheral iris into the trabecular meshwork, which is present to some degree in all cases, appears to be more pronounced in those eyes with glaucoma.[15]

Systemic Features

The systemic anomalies most commonly associated with the A-R syndrome are developmental defects of the teeth and facial bones. The dental abnormalities include a reduction in crown size (microdontia), a decreased but evenly spaced number of teeth (hypodontia), and a focal absence of teeth (oligodontia or anodontia) (Fig. 12.5).[10,11,30] The teeth most commonly missing are ante-

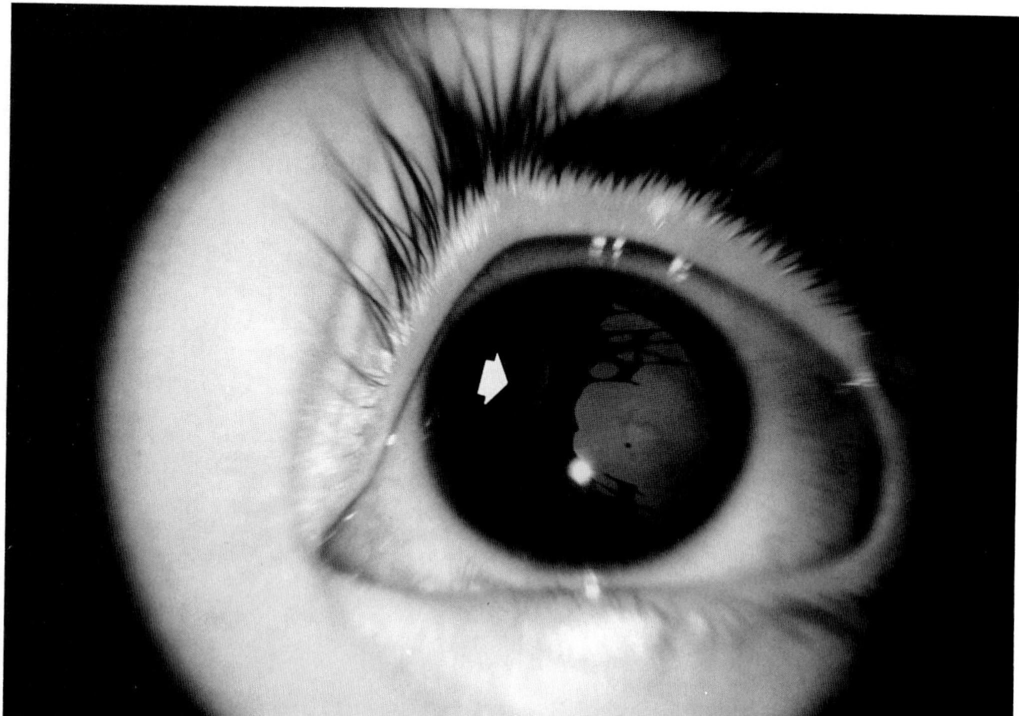

Figure 12.4. Advanced iris changes in patient with Axenfeld-Rieger syndrome showing small, markedly displaced pupil (*arrow*) and large iris hole in opposite quadrants. (Reprinted from Trans Am Ophthal Soc 81:736, 1983, with permission.)

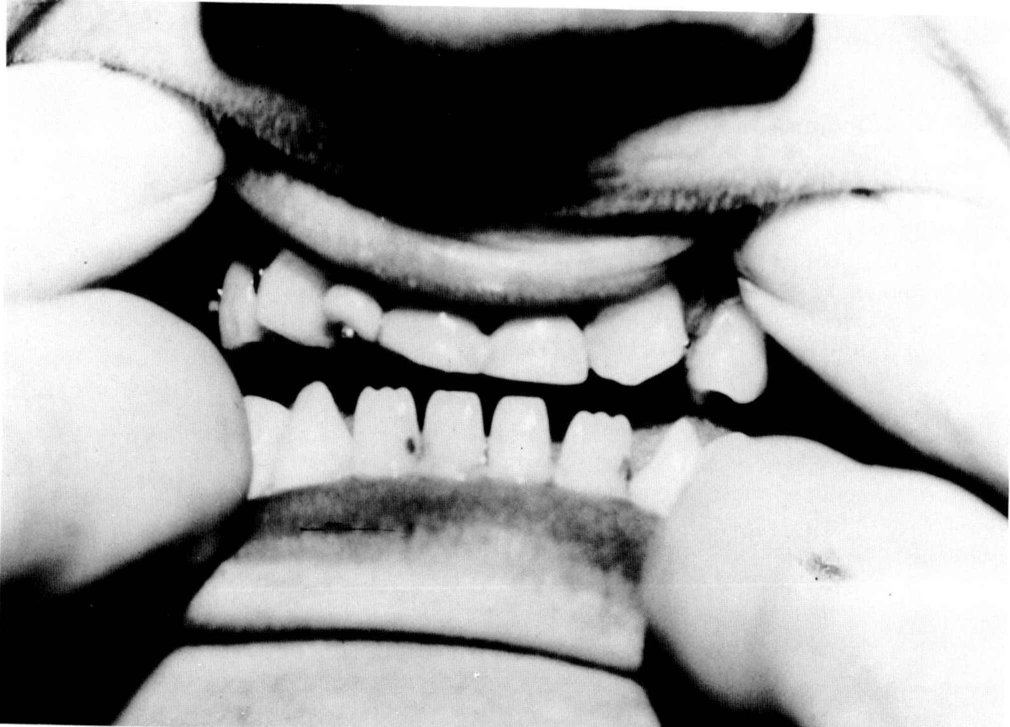

Figure 12.5. Patient with Axenfeld-Rieger syndrome demonstrating typical dental anomaly of microdontia (reduction in crown size of teeth). (Reprinted from The Secondary Glaucomas, ed. Ritch R, Shields MB, Chapter 2, St. Louis, The CV Mosby Co., 1982, with permission.)

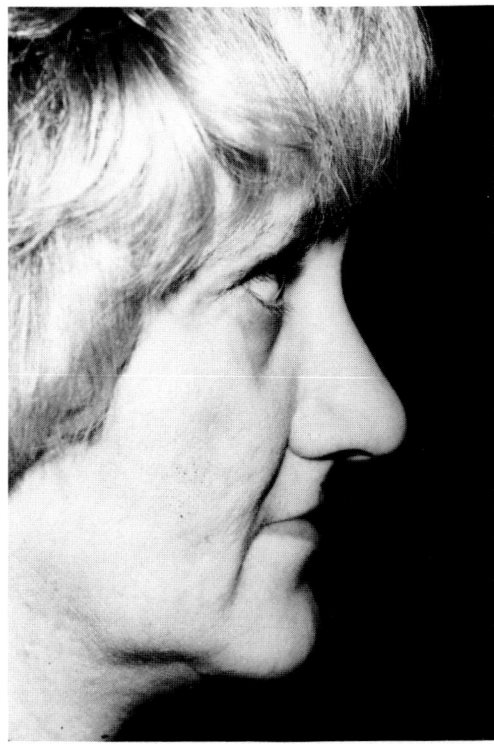

Figure 12.6. Patient with Axenfeld-Rieger syndrome demonstrating characteristic facial configuration of midface flattening (upper lip and cheek) and protruding lower lip. (Reprinted from The Secondary Glaucomas, ed. Ritch R, Shields MB, Chapter 2, St. Louis, The CV Mosby Co., 1982, with permission.)

rior maxillary primary and permanent central incisors. Facial anomalies include maxillary hypoplasia with flattening of the midface and a receding upper lip and prominent lower lip, especially in association with dental hypoplasia (Fig. 12.6). Hypertelorism, telecanthus, a broad flat nose, micrognathia, and mandibular prognathism have also been described.[12,25]

Anomalies in the region of the pituitary gland are a less common, but more serious, finding associated with the A-R syndrome. A primary empty sella syndrome has been documented in several patients,[15,31] and one case of congenital parasellar arachnoid cyst has been reported.[15] Growth hormone deficiency and short stature have also been described in association with the entity.[32,33] Other abnormalities reported in association with the A-R syndrome include redundant periumbilical skin and hypospadias,[34] oculocutaneous albinism,[35] heart defects, middle ear deafness, mental deficiency, and a variety of neurologic and dermatologic disorders.[12]

Histopathologic Features

The central cornea is typically normal, while the peripheral cornea has the characteristic prominent, anteriorly displaced Schwalbe's line. The latter structure is composed of dense collagen and ground substance covered by a monolayer of spindle-shaped cells with a basement membrane (Fig. 12.7).[15,18,21] The peripheral iris is attached in some areas to the corneoscleral junction by tissue strands, which usually connect with the prominent Schwalbe's line. Occasionally, however, the adhesions insert either anterior or posterior to Schwalbe's line or on both sides of the ridge.[15] The strands consist of either iridic stroma, a membrane composed of a monolayer of spindle-shaped cells and/or a basement membrane-like layer, or both.

A membrane, similar to that seen in association with the iridocorneal tissue strands, has also been observed on the iris, usually on the portion toward which the pupil is distorted.[12,15,36,37] In the quadrants away from the direction of pupillary displacement, the stroma of the iris is often thin or absent, exposing pigment epithelium that may also contain holes.

The iris peripheral to the iridocorneal adhesions inserts into the posterior aspect of the trabecular meshwork (Fig. 12.8). The meshwork may be composed of a scant number of attenuated lamellae, which extend from beneath peripheral iris to the prominent Schwalbe's line and are often compressed, especially in the outer layers. Transmission electron microscopic study suggests that the apparent compression may be due to incomplete development of the trabecular meshwork.[15] Schlemm's canal is either rudimentary or absent.

Theories of Mechanism

Based on clinical and histopathologic observations and the current concepts of normal anterior segment development, as discussed in Chapter 11, a developmental ar-

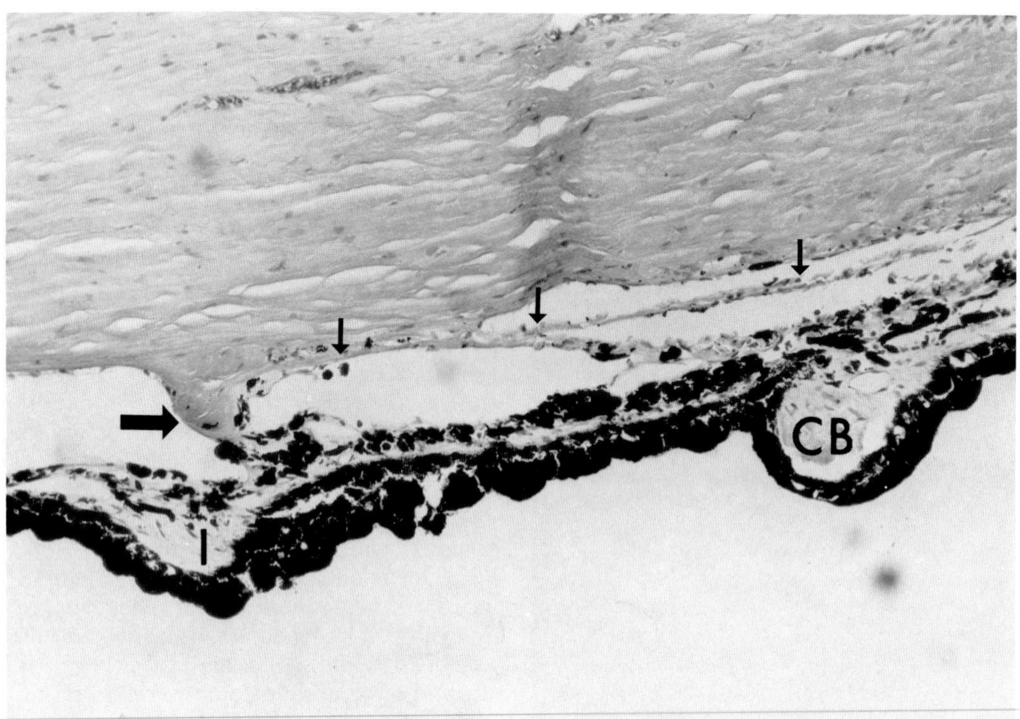

Figure 12.7. Light microscopic view of eye with Axenfeld-Rieger syndrome showing prominent, anteriorly displaced Schwalbe's line (*large arrow*) attached to iris (*I*) by tissue strand. Scant, attenuated trabecular lamellae (*small arrows*) extend to Schwalbe's line and attach to peripheral iris; anterior portion of ciliary body (*CB*). (Hematoxylin-eosin; original magnification, ×150). (Reprinted from Trans Am Ophthal Soc 81:736, 1983, with permission.)

rest, late in gestation, of certain anterior segment structures derived from neural crest cells has been postulated as the mechanism of the A-R syndrome.[15] This leads to the abnormal retention of the primordial endothelial layer on portions of the iris and anterior chamber angle, and alterations in the aqueous outflow structures (Fig. 12.9). The retained endothelium with associated basement membrane is believed to create the iridocorneal strands, while contraction of this tissue layer on the iris leads to the iridic changes, which sometimes continue to progress after birth. The developmental arrest also accounts for the high insertion of anterior uvea into the posterior trabecular meshwork, similar to the alterations seen in primary congenital glaucoma, and results in the incomplete maturation of the trabecular meshwork and Schlemm's canal. The latter defects are believed to be responsible for the associated glaucoma.

The neural crest cells also give rise to most of the mesenchyme related to the forebrain and pituitary gland, bones and cartilages of the upper face, and dental papillae.[3,4] This could explain the developmental anomalies involving the pituitary gland, the facial bones, and the teeth. Other defects, however, such as those of the umbilicus and genitourinary system, are more difficult to associate with a primary defect of cranial neural crest cells.

As previously noted, the disorder is believed to have a genetic basis with an autosomal dominant pattern of inheritance. Cases with chromosomal abnormalities have also been reported.[38,39]

Differential Diagnosis

Iridocorneal Endothelial (ICE) Syndrome

The iris and anterior chamber angle abnormalities in this spectrum of disease (dis-

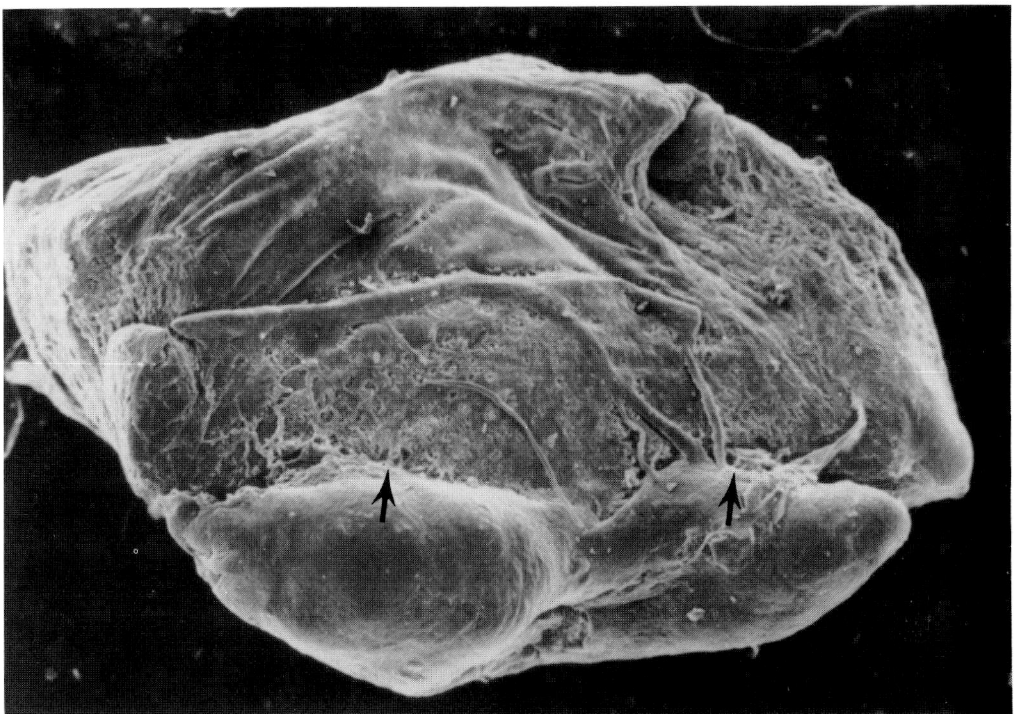

Figure 12.8. Scanning electron microscopic view of trabeculectomy specimen from patient with Axenfeld-Rieger syndrome showing high insertion of iris into trabecular meshwork (*arrows*). (Reprinted from Surv Ophthal 29:387, 1985, with permission.)

cussed in Chapter 13) resemble those of A-R syndrome both clinically and histopathologically. This has led some investigators to suggest that the two syndromes are parts of a common spectrum of disorders.[36,37,40] However, clinical features that distinguish the ICE syndrome include corneal endothelial abnormalities, unilaterality, absence of family history, and onset in young adulthood. Both conditions are characterized histopathologically by a membrane over the angle and iris, which is associated with many of the alterations in each disorder. However, while the membrane in the A-R syndrome represents a primordial remnant, that of the ICE syndrome is due to a proliferation from the abnormal corneal endothelium.

Posterior Polymorphous Dystrophy

One variation of this developmental disorder of the corneal endothelium (discussed in Chapter 13) has changes of the iris and anterior chamber angle similar to those of the A-R syndrome. However, the differentiation can be made on the basis of the typical corneal endothelial abnormality.

Peters' Anomaly

This spectrum of disorders (discussed next in the present chapter) involves the central portion of the cornea, iris, and lens. Similar changes have been reported in association with the peripheral defects of the A-R syndrome, and the two conditions were once included in a single category of developmental disorders.[13,14] However, this association is rare, and the mechanisms for the two groups of developmental disorders are distinctly different.

Aniridia

The rudimentary iris and anterior chamber abnormalities with associated glaucoma in this developmental disorder (discussed later in this chapter) may, in some cases, lead to confusion with the A-R syndrome.

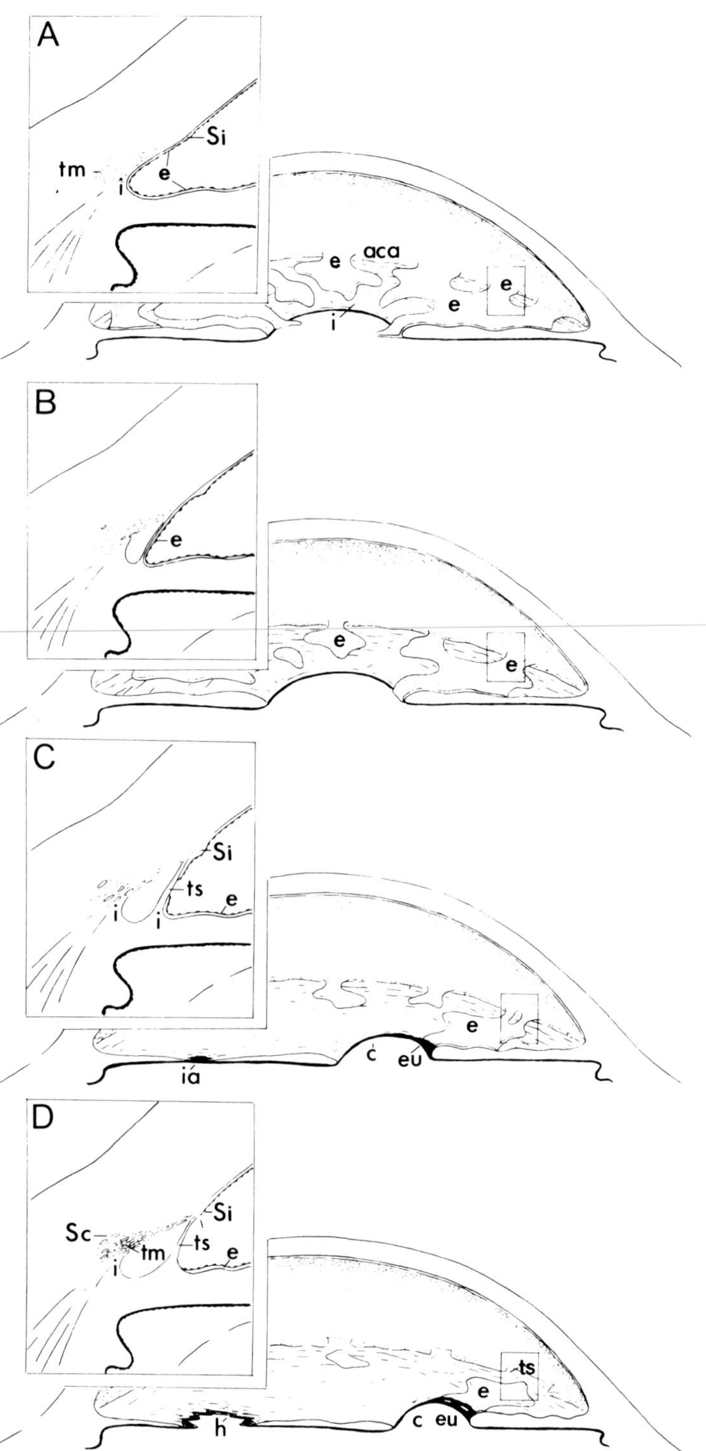

Figure 12.9. Theory of mechanism for ocular abnormalities of Axenfeld-Rieger syndrome (insets show cross-sectional views of anterior chamber angle corresponding to area within rectangle): *A*, Partial retention of primordial endothelium (*e*) on iris (*i*) and anterior chamber angle (*aca*); incomplete posterior recession of peripheral uvea from trabecular meshwork (*tm*); abnormal differentiation between corneal and chamber angle endothelium with prominent, anteriorly displaced Schwalbe's line (*Si*); *B*, Development of tissue strands from retained endothelium crossing anterior chamber angle; *C*, Contraction of retained endothelium with iris changes of corectopia (*c*), ectropion uvea (*eu*) and iris atrophy (*ia*), which may continue after birth; tissue strand (*ts*); *D*, Incomplete development of trabecular meshwork and Schlemm's canal (*Sc*); continued traction on iris, with possible secondary ischemia, leads to hole formation (*h*). (Reprinted from Trans Am Ophthal Soc 81:736, 1983, with permission.)

Congenital Iris Hypoplasia

Patients may have congenital hypoplasia of the iris without the anterior chamber angle defects of the A-R syndrome or any other ocular abnormality.[41] Iris hypoplasia has also been reported in association with juvenile-onset glaucoma with autosomal dominant inheritance.[42]

Oculodentodigital Dysplasia

The dental anomalies in this condition are similar to those seen in the A-R syndrome. In addition, these patients may occasionally have mild stromal hypoplasia of the iris,[12] anterior chamber angle defects, microphthalmia, and glaucoma.[43]

Ectopia Lentis et Pupillae

This autosomal recessive condition is characterized by bilateral displacement of the lens and pupil,[44] with the two structures typically going in opposite directions. The corectopia in this disorder may resemble that of the A-R syndrome, but the absence of anterior chamber angle defects is a differential feature.

Congenital Ectropion Uveae

This condition has been described as a rare, nonprogressive anomaly characterized by the presence of pigment epithelium on the stroma of the iris.[45,46] It may be an isolated finding or may appear in association with systemic anomalies, including neurofibromatosis, facial hemiatrophy, and the Prader-Willi syndrome.[45] Glaucoma is present in a high percentage of cases, and the ectropion uvea may be confused with that found in some patients with the A-R syndrome.

As discussed under "Additional Ocular Abnormalities," patients with the A-R syndrome may have a wide variety of ocular and systemic developmental abnormalities, and it is hard to know which of these patients have a variation of the A-R syndrome and which should be considered to have a separate entity.

Management

The primary concern regarding the management of ocular defects in a patient with the A-R syndrome is detection and control of the associated glaucoma. Intraocular pressure (IOP) elevation most often develops between childhood and early adulthood, but it may appear in infancy or, in rare cases, not until the elderly years.[15] Therefore, patients with the A-R syndrome must be followed for suspicion of glaucoma throughout their life.

With the exception of infantile cases, medical therapy should usually be tried before surgical intervention is recommended. Pilocarpine and other miotics are often ineffective, and drugs that reduce aqueous production, such as beta blockers and carbonic anhydrase inhibitors, are most likely to be beneficial. Surgical options include goniotomy, trabeculotomy, and trabeculectomy. The first two have been used in infantile cases with limited success. Trabeculectomy is the surgical procedure of choice for most patients with glaucoma secondary to the A-R syndrome.

While laser surgery has not been found effective in managing the glaucoma in the A-R syndrome, it has been reported that the Nd:YAG laser can be used to lyse iridocorneal adhesions to minimize corectopia when it is impairing vision.[47]

PETERS' ANOMALY

In 1897, von Hippel[48] reported a case of buphthalmos with bilateral central corneal opacities and adhesions from these defects to the iris. Peters, beginning in 1906,[49] described similar patients with what has become generally known as Peters' anomaly.

General Features

The condition is present at birth and is usually bilateral. Most cases are sporadic, although there are reported cases of autosomal recessive inheritance and, less commonly, autosomal dominant transmission.[50] Chromosomal defects have also been described.[51–53] It typically occurs in the absence of additional abnormalities, although rare associations with various systemic and other ocular anomalies have been reported.[54,55] Because of the varied genetic and nongenetic patterns and the spectrum of ocular and systemic abnormalities, it has been suggested that Peters' anomaly is a morphologic finding rather than a distinct entity.[54]

Clinicopathologic Features

The hallmark of Peters' anomaly is a central defect in Descemet's membrane and corneal endothelium with thinning and opacification of the corresponding area of corneal stroma (Fig. 12.10).[56–59] Adhesions may extend from the borders of this defect to the central iris. Bowman's membrane may also be absent centrally.[58,59] Immunohistochemical studies of the cornea suggest that extracellular matrix elements such as fibronectin may be important in the pathogenesis of Peters' anomaly.[60]

The disorder has been subdivided into the following three groups (Fig. 12.11), each of which may have more than one pathogenic mechanism.[57]

Not Associated with Keratolenticular Contact or Cataract. In these cases, the defect in Descemet's membrane may represent primary failure of corneal endothelial development.[58] However, rare cases may be secondary to intrauterine inflammation,[61] which was originally postulated by von Hippel[48] and gave rise to the term "von Hippel's internal corneal ulcer."

Associated with Keratolenticular Contact or Cataract. Most histopathologic studies of this variation suggest that the lens developed normally and was then secondarily pushed forward against the cornea by one of several mechanisms, causing the loss of Descemet's membrane (Fig. 12.12).[57,58] It is also possible that some cases may result from incomplete separation of the lens vesicle from surface ectoderm.

Associated with Axenfeld-Rieger Syndrome. This rare association was discussed earlier in this chapter.

Associated Glaucoma

Approximately half of the patients with Peters' anomaly will develop glaucoma, which is frequently present at birth. The

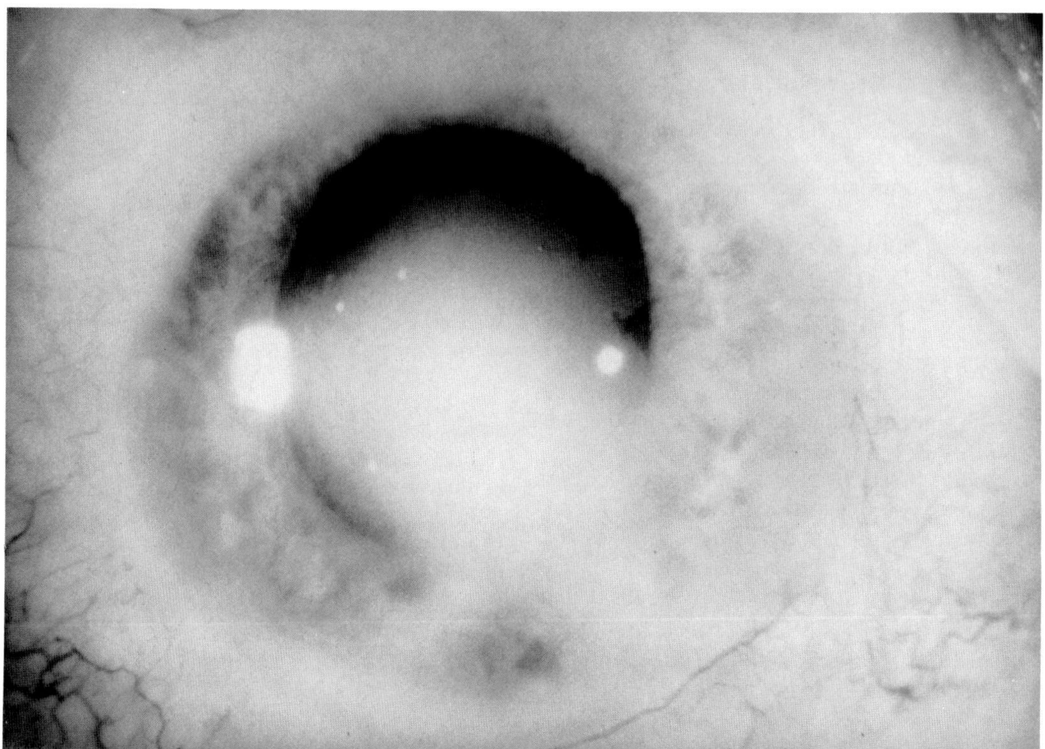

Figure 12.10. External appearance of patient with Peters' anomaly showing central corneal opacity. (Courtesy of George O. Waring, M.D.).

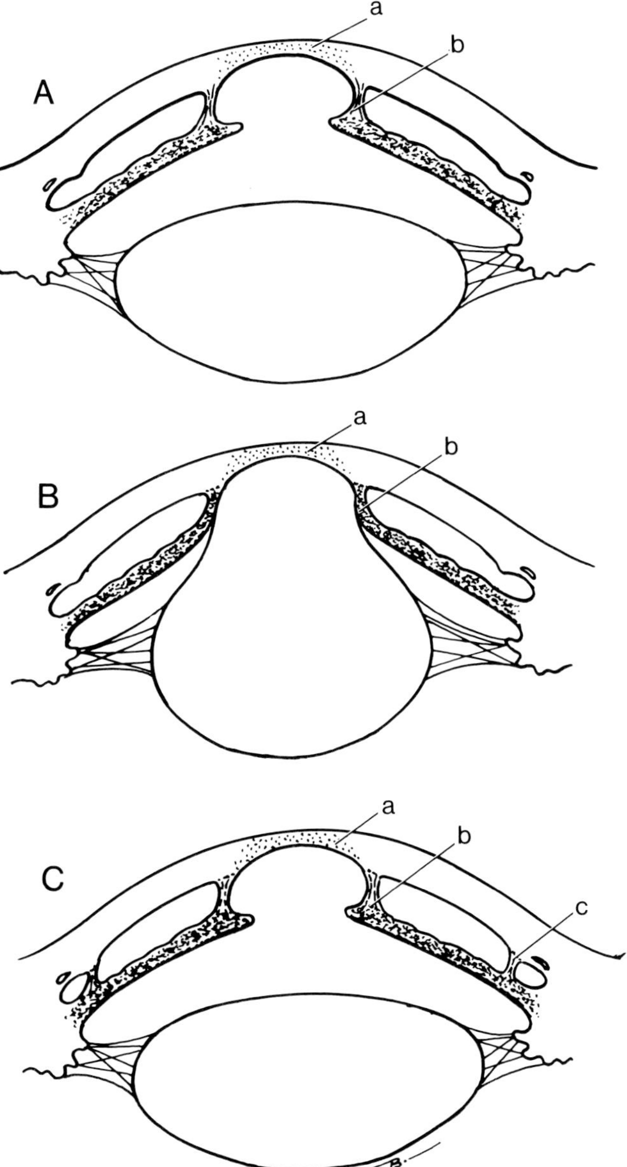

Figure 12.11. Peters' anomaly with central corneal defect (*a*) and adhesions (*b*) from corneal defect to central iris, showing three forms according to Townsend, et al:[57] *A*, Without keratolenticular contact or cataract; *B*, with keratolenticular contact or cataract; or *C*, with peripheral defects of Axenfeld-Rieger syndrome (*c*).

mechanism of the glaucoma is uncertain, since the anterior chamber angle is usually grossly normal by clinical examination. Histopathologic studies have revealed peripheral anterior synechiae in some cases,[57] while ultrastructural studies of two young patients with Peters' anomaly and open angles revealed changes in the trabecular meshwork that are characteristic of aging.[62,63] In cases of Peters' anomaly associated with the anterior chamber angle abnormalities of the Axenfeld-Rieger syndrome, the mechanism of glaucoma is presumably the same as in the latter condition, as discussed earlier in this chapter.

Differential Diagnosis

Other Causes of Central Corneal Opacities in Infants

The corneal clouding of Peters' anomaly must be distinguished from that of primary congenital glaucoma, birth trauma, the mucopolysaccharidoses, and congenital hered-

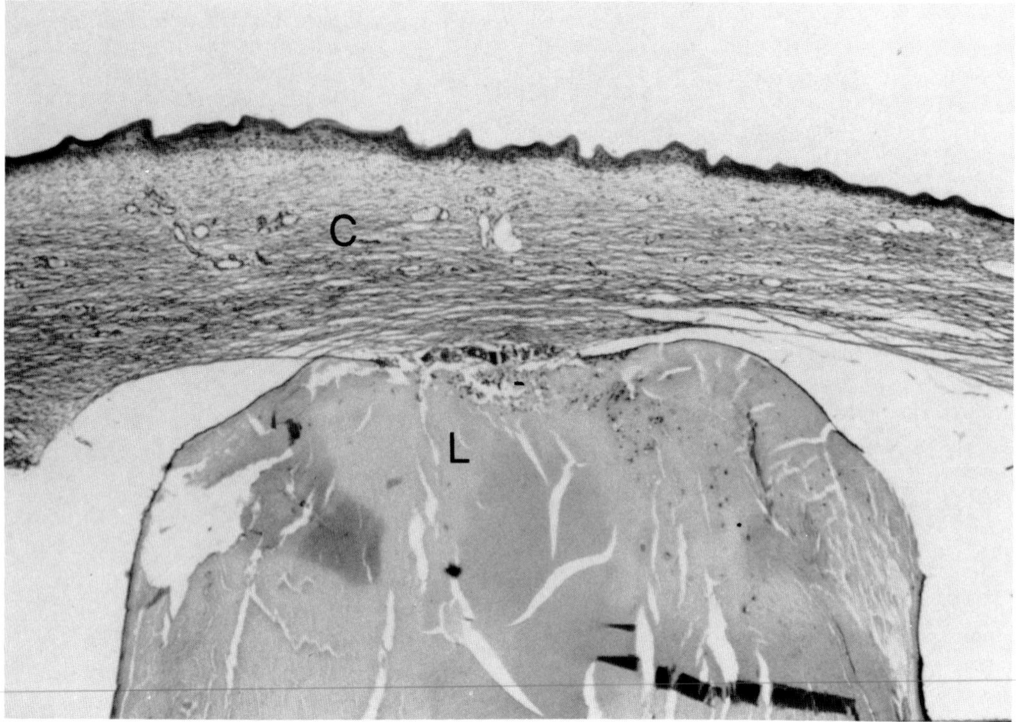

Figure 12.12. Light microscopic view of eye with Peters' anomaly showing central defect of posterior cornea (*C*) in contact with lens (*L*). (Courtesy of George O. Waring, M.D.)

itary corneal dystrophy. Several of the mucopolysaccharidoses have been associated with glaucoma and are discussed later in this chapter, and one case of congenital glaucoma and iris hypoplasia has been reported in association with congenital hereditary corneal dystrophy.[64]

Posterior Keratoconus

This rare disorder is characterized by a thinning of the central corneal stroma, with excessive curvature of the posterior corneal surface and variable overlying stromal haze.[14,65] An ultrastructural study revealed a multilaminar Descemet's membrane with abnormal anterior banding and localized posterior excrescences.[66] Glaucoma is rarely associated with posterior keratoconus.[14]

Congenital Corneal Leukomas and Staphylomas

These cases represent the more severe forms of central dysgenesis of the anterior ocular segment and are frequently associated with glaucoma.[12]

Management

All infants and children with cloudy corneas must be examined carefully for the possibility of associated glaucoma. The glaucoma usually requires surgical intervention, and a trabeculectomy may offer the best chance of success. Penetrating keratoplasty is also frequently necessary.

ANIRIDIA

General Features

Aniridia is a bilateral developmental disorder, characterized by the congenital absence of a normal iris. However, the name *aniridia* is a misnomer, since the iris is only partly absent, with a rudimentary stump of variable width. Aniridia is associated with multiple ocular defects, some of which are present at birth, while others may develop later in childhood or early adulthood. In addition, some cases of aniridia may be associated systemic abnormalities.

Four phenotypes of aniridia have been identified on the basis of associated ocular and systemic abnormalities:[67] (1) associated with foveal hypoplasia, nystagmus, corneal pannus, glaucoma, and reduced vision; (2) predominant iris changes and normal visual acuity; (3) associated with Wilms' tumor (the *aniridia-Wilms' tumor syndrome*) or other genitourinary anomalies; and (4) associated with mental retardation.

Most cases are inherited by autosomal dominant transmission, although sporadic cases also occur. The latter patients frequently have the associated Wilms' tumor, and a deletion of the short arm of chromosome 11 has been identified in some of these cases.[68–71] Other patients, especially those with mental retardation, have an autosomal recessive mode of inheritance.[72]

Clinicopathologic Features

Iris

In some cases, the iris is so rudimentary that it can be seen only by gonioscopy (Fig. 12.13), while other eyes may have enough peripheral iris to be visible by external and slit-lamp examination (Fig. 12.14).

Cornea

In a high percentage of cases, a corneal pannus and opacity begin in the peripheral cornea in early life and advance toward the center of the cornea with increasing age. Microcornea[73,74] and keratolenticular adhesions[75] have also been reported.

Lens

Localized congenital opacities are common but usually insignificant. However, progressive cataracts may lead to significant visual impairment by approximately the third decade of life. The lens may also be subluxed,[73] or congenitally absent or reabsorbed.[74,76]

Foveal Hypoplasia

This is a frequent finding and presumably accounts for the characteristic poor visual

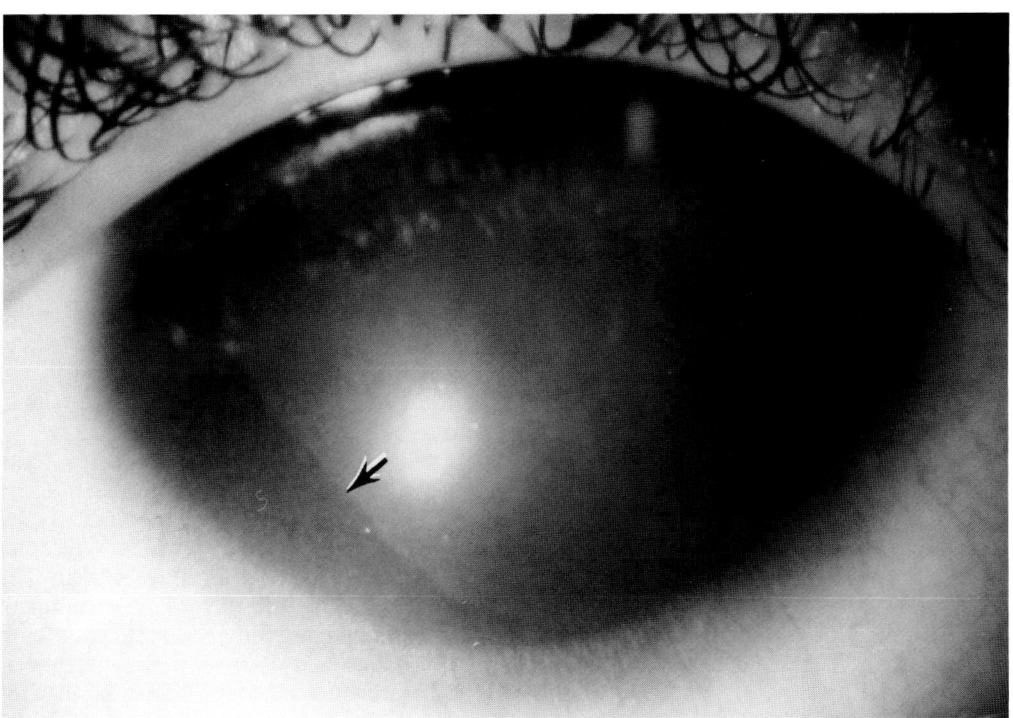

Figure 12.13. Slit-lamp view of patient with aniridia in which no iris is visible, revealing equator of lens (*arrow*).

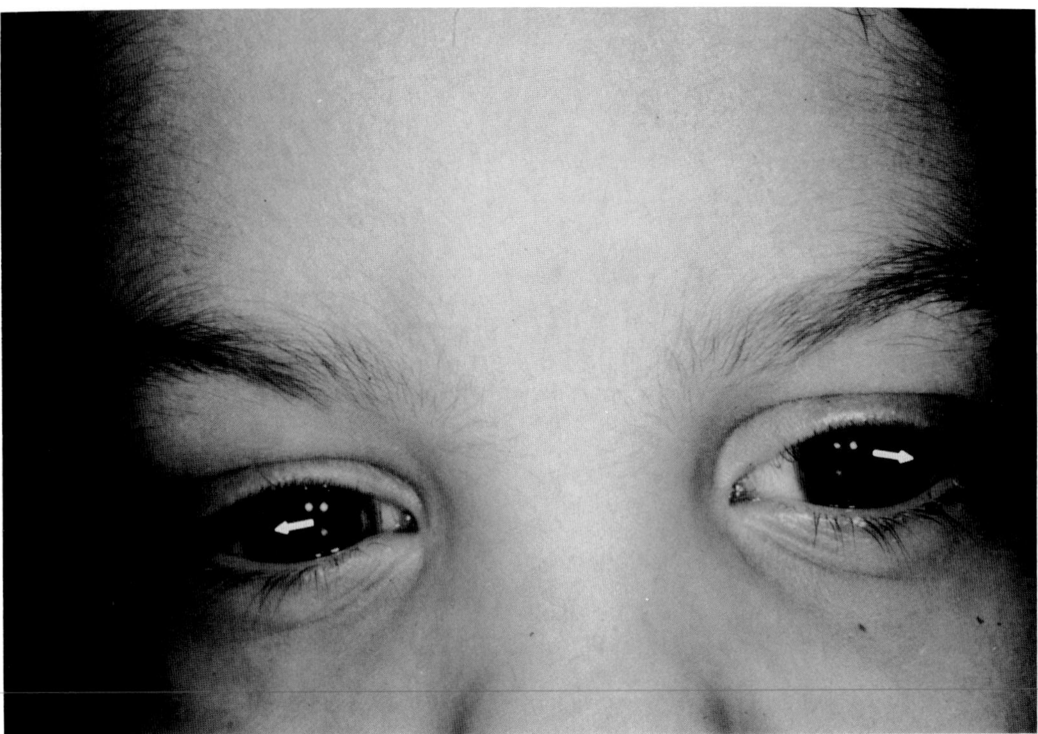

Figure 12.14. External view of patient with aniridia in which rudimentary, peripheral iris is visible in both eyes (*arrows*).

acuity and nystagmus of aniridia. However, in three infants with sporadic aniridia and nystagmus, normal electroretinograms suggested that the poor visual function was not a result of gross retinal anomalies.[77] It was thought that the absence of a pupillary effect caused the visual impairment, although some aniridic patients have reasonably good vision and no nystagmus despite significant hypoplasia of the iris.[67]

Other Ocular and Systemic Defects

Aniridia has also been reported in association with choroidal colobomas, persistent pupillary membranes,[78] sclerocornea and the Hallermann-Streiff syndrome,[69] small optic nerve heads, strabismus, and ptosis.[76,79] The association with Marfan's syndrome, cervical ribs, and dental anomalies in one patient has also been reported.[80]

Associated Glaucoma

Glaucoma occurs in 50–75% of patients with aniridia but usually does not appear before late childhood or adolescence.[81] The development of the glaucoma appears to correlate with the gonioscopic appearance of the anterior chamber angle. In infancy, the angle is usually open and unobstructed, although some eyes may have strands of tissue with occasional fine blood vessels extending from the iris root to the trabecular meshwork or higher.[81] Some patients have congenital anomalies in the filtration angle, which appears to be more common in patients with chromosomal defects and may lead to glaucoma early in life.[70]

During the first 5–15 years of life, many eyes with aniridia will undergo progressive change in the anterior chamber angle as the rudimentary stump of iris comes to lie over the trabecular meshwork (Fig. 12.15). The progressive obstruction of the anterior chamber angle may be due to contracture of the tissue strands between the peripheral iris and angle wall (Fig. 12.16).[81] In eyes with mild IOP elevation, the obstruction to aqueous outflow may be limited to the superior quadrant, while in eyes with more ad-

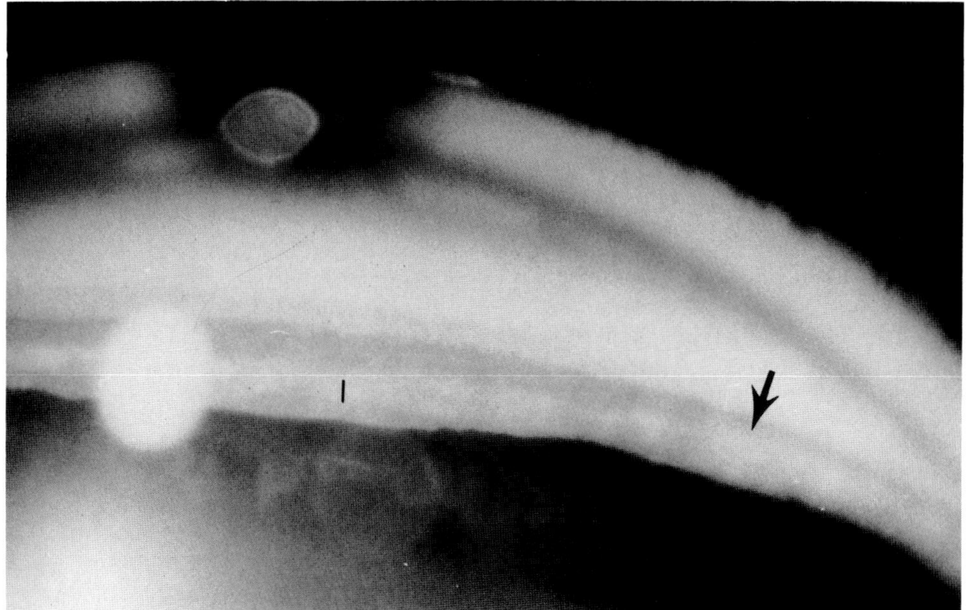

Figure 12.15. Gonioscopic view of patient with aniridia and glaucoma showing rudimentary, peripheral iris (*I*), a portion of which has been drawn up toward the trabecular meshwork (*arrow*).

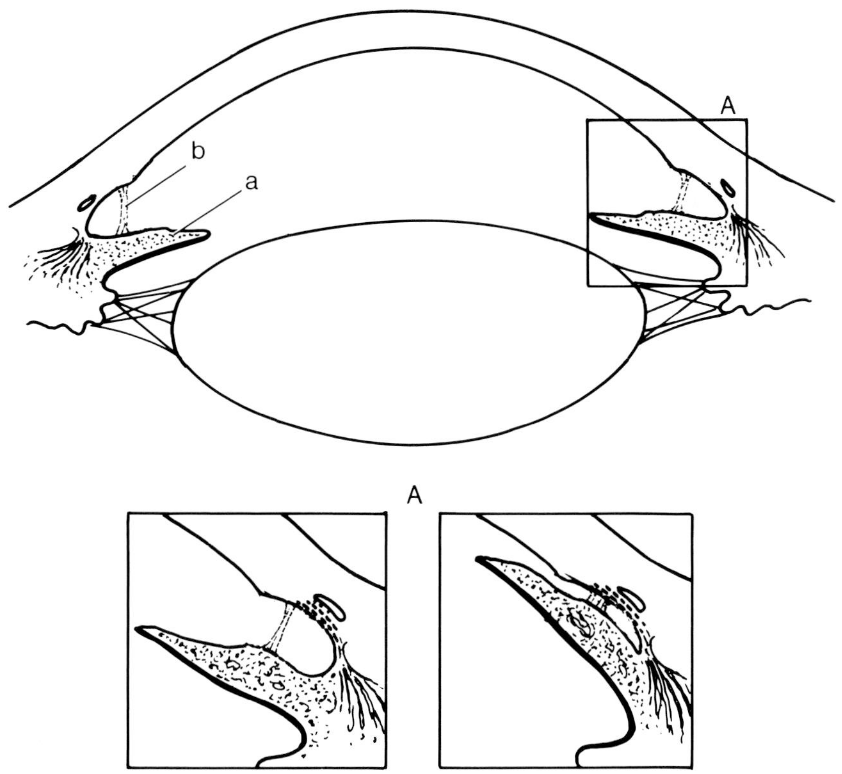

Figure 12.16. Aniridia with rudimentary iris (*a*) and fine tissue strands (*b*) extending across the anterior chamber angle. Insets (*A*) show theory of progressive angle closure by contracture of tissue strands.

vanced glaucoma, the iris stroma covers most of the trabecular meshwork.

Management of the Glaucoma

Conventional medical therapy may control the IOP initially but eventually proves to be inadequate in most cases. Filtering surgery is usually the procedure of choice, although it is often unsuccessful, especially in children. Cyclocryotherapy or cyclophotocoagulation may have lasting benefit in some cases. Goniotomy is of no value in advanced cases, but preliminary experience suggests that early goniotomy to separate the strands between the iris and the trabecular meshwork may prevent the development of glaucoma.[81,82]

OTHER SYNDROMES WITH ASSOCIATED GLAUCOMA

In addition to the disorders already considered in this chapter, glaucoma may be a feature of many other congenital syndromes. The present discussion is limited to those syndromes that represent multiple-system, developmental anomalies.

Lowe's (Oculocerebrorenal) Syndrome

Lowe's syndrome is a sex-linked disorder characterized by mental retardation, renal rickets, aminoaciduria, hypotonia, acidemia, and irritability. The two principal ocular abnormalities are cataracts, which are usually bilateral and occur in nearly all cases, and glaucoma, which is seen in approximately two-thirds of the patients. Other ocular findings include microphthalmia, strabismus, nystagmus, miosis, and iris atrophy. Female carriers may be identified by cortical lens opacities and genetic studies.[83]

The mechanism of the glaucoma is related to faulty development of the filtration angle. Gonioscopy reveals only minor anatomic defects, including poor visualization of the scleral spur and a narrow ciliary body band. Goniotomy may be beneficial in some cases.

Chromosomal Anomalies

Trisomy 21 (Down's Syndrome)

This condition is characterized by mental retardation and a typical facies. Ocular findings include epicanthus, blepharitis, nystagmus, strabismus, light-colored and spotted irides, keratoconus, cataracts, and congenital glaucoma.[84] The glaucoma usually appears in infancy, with the typical findings of infantile glaucoma.[85]

Trisomy D (13–15) Syndrome

The principal systemic features include mental retardation, deafness, heart disease, and motor seizures. The condition is usually not compatible with life, although milder forms have been reported.[86] Ocular findings include microphthalmia, coloboma with cartilage, congenital cataracts, retinal dysplasia, hyperplastic primary vitreous, and dysembryogeneses of the anterior chamber angle.[87] Glaucoma may be present as a result of several of these developmental defects.

Trisomy 18 (Edwards' Syndrome)

The ocular histopathologic findings in one infant included an anterior position of the iris obstructing the anterior chamber angle.[88]

Turners' Syndrome (XO)

These patients are typically short-statured, postadolescent females with sexual infantilism and multiple systemic anomalies. Ocular findings include ptosis, epicanthus, cataract, strabismus, blue sclera, corneal nebulae, and color blindness.[89] Developmental glaucoma is rarely associated.

Stickler's Syndrome

Stickler's syndrome, or hereditary progressive arthro-ophthalmopathy, is an autosomal dominant connective tissue dysplasia, characterized by ocular, orofacial, and generalized skeletal abnormalities.[90] The *Pierre-Robin anomaly* of mandibular hypoplasia, glossoptosis, and cleft palate may be seen in some patients. The most common ocular manifestations are high myopia, open-angle glaucoma, cataracts, vitreoretinal degeneration, and retinal detachment.[91,92] In one study of 39 patients from 12 families, 10% had ocular hypertension, which may be associated with numerous iris processes, suggestive of a developmental abnormality of the angle.[92] Neovascular glaucoma has also been reported in association with Stickler's syndrome.[93] The open-angle glaucoma usually can be controlled medically, although miotics should be avoided if possible, because of the potential for retinal detachment.

Zellweger's Syndrome

Zellweger's syndrome, or the cerebrohepatorenal syndrome, is a multisystem congenital disorder characterized by central nervous system abnormalities, hepatic interstitial fibrosis, and renal cysts. Ocular findings include nystagmus, corneal clouding, cataracts, retinal vascular and pigmentary abnormalities, optic nerve head lesions, and congenital glaucoma.[94] Iridocorneal adhesions may be the mechanism of the glaucoma.[95]

Hallermann-Streiff Syndrome

Micrognathia and dwarfism in this condition may be associated with ocular findings, including cataracts and microphthalmos. Glaucoma may also be present as a result of absorption of lens material or associated aniridia.[69]

Rubenstein-Taybi (broad-thumb) Syndrome

These individuals have mental and motor retardation and typical congenital skeletal deformities with characteristically large thumbs and first toes. Ocular findings include bushy brows, hypertelorism, epicanthus, antimongoloid slant of eyelids, and hyperopia. Infantile or juvenile glaucoma has also been observed in several patients.[96–98]

Oculodentodigital Dysplasia

The systemic features of this disorder are hypoplastic dental enamel, microdontia, bilateral syndactyly, and a characteristic thin nose. Multiple ocular anomalies have been described, including glaucoma. There are probably several mechanisms of glaucoma in this syndrome, with reported cases of mild developmental abnormalities of the anterior chamber angle,[43] gonioscopic changes resembling infantile glaucoma,[99] and one case of chronic angle closure glaucoma associated with bilateral microcornea.[100]

Mucopolysaccharidoses

The prototype, *Hurler's syndrome,* is an autosomal recessive disease with central nervous system, skeletal, and visceral abnormalities. The typical ocular finding is corneal clouding. Glaucoma has also been reported in Hurler's syndrome and was believed to result from mucopolysaccharide-containing cells in the aqueous outflow system.[101] In a 3-year-old child with Hurler's syndrome and open-angle glaucoma, the IOP returned to normal after bone marrow transplantation.[102] Patients with mucopolysaccharidosis type VI, the *Maroteaux-Lamy syndrome,* may have acute or chronic angle closure glaucoma, which appears to be associated more with increased thickness of the peripheral cornea than with pupillary block.[103] Glaucoma, apparently with open angles, was also described in two siblings with mucopolysaccharidosis type IV, the *Marquio syndrome.*[104]

Cystinosis

This is a rare autosomal recessive metabolic disorder characterized by widespread accumulation of cystine crystals in ocular and nonocular tissues. A case of pupillary-block glaucoma was reported in one patient, which was thought to be due to the cystine accumulation in the iris stroma.[105]

Prader-Willi Syndrome

This condition is characterized by muscular hypotonia, hypogonadism, obesity, and mental retardation, and is frequently caused by an abnormality of chromosome 15. Ocular findings include oculocutaneous albinism[106] and congenital ectropion uveae, which may be associated with open-angle glaucoma.[45] One patient with Prader-Willi syndrome, congenital ectropion uvea, and glaucoma had factor XI deficiency and the suggestion of a primary hypothalamic defect.[107]

Waardenburg's Syndrome

This autosomal dominant disorder is characterized by lateral displacement of the medial canthi, hyperplasia of the medial brows, a prominent, broad root of the nose, sectoral or complete iris heterochromia, congenital deafness, and a white forelock.[108,109] It is thought to represent a defect of neural crest-derived tissues. Open-angle glaucoma is an uncommon finding, although it was present in one of Waardenburg's original cases, and may be due to a developmental abnormality of neural crest-derived tissues in the angle.[109]

Cockayne's Syndrome

This autosomal recessive disorder is characterized by dwarfism and a "birdlike" facies. Ocular manifestations include "salt-and-pepper" retinopathy, cataracts, corneal ulcers or opacities, nystagmus, hypoplastic irides and irregular pupils. While glaucoma has not been associated, the histopathologic examination of one case revealed a high insertion of the anterior uvea into the posterior aspect of the trabecular meshwork,[110] similar to that seen in primary congenital glaucoma and the Axenfeld-Rieger syndrome.

Fetal Alcohol Syndrome

This condition presumably results from a teratogenic effect of alcohol during a critical period of gestation, possibly influenced by a genetic background. The anterior ocular segment may be involved, with developmental abnormalities resembling those of the Axenfeld-Rieger syndrome and Peters' anomaly.[111] Mouse studies suggest that the ocular abnormalities result from an acute insult to the optic primordia during a specific period that corresponds to the 3rd week after fertilization in the human.[112]

SUMMARY

Several conditions are characterized by glaucoma due to developmental defects of the anterior chamber angle with additional ocular and systemic abnormalities. These disorders are typically bilateral and are usually diagnosed at birth or in early childhood, and most are believed to have a genetic basis. One such condition, the Axenfeld-Rieger syndrome, is a spectrum of disorders in which the ocular anomalies include a prominent Schwalbe's line, tissue strands across the anterior chamber angle, and variable degrees of iris distortion, while systemic defects most often involve the teeth and facial bones. Peters' anomaly also has variable clinical manifestations with alterations primarily of the central cornea, iris, and lens. In aniridia, the hallmark is a rudimentary stump of peripheral iris, although there may be additional ocular abnormalities of the cornea, lens, or fovea, as well as systemic disorders including Wilms' tumor and mental retardation. A large number of other syndromes with ocular and systemic abnormalities may occasionally be accompanied by developmental glaucoma.

References

1. LeDourain, N: The neural crest in the neck and other parts of the body. Birth Defects 11:19, 1975.
2. Johnston, MC, Norden, DM, Hazelton, RD, et al: Origins of avian ocular and periocular tissues. Exp Eye Res 29:27, 1979.
3. Bolande, RP: The neurocristopathies: a unifying concept of disease arising in neural crest maldevelopment. Human Pathol 5:279, 1974.
4. Beauchamp, GR, Knepper, PA: Role of the neural crest in anterior segment development and disease. J Ped Ophthal Strab 21:209, 1984.
5. Hoskins, HD, Shaffer, RN, Hetherington, J: Anatomical classification of the developmental glaucomas. Arch Ophthal 102:1331, 1984.
6. Axenfeld, TH: Embryotoxon corneae posterius. Ber Deutsch Ophthal Ges 42:301, 1920.
7. Rieger, H: Demonstration von zwei: Fallen von Verlagerung and Schlitzform der Pupille mit Hypoplasie des Irisvorderblattes an beiden Augen einer 10- und 25-jahrigen Patientin. Z Augenheilkd 84:98, 1934.
8. Rieger, H: Beitrage zur Kenntnis seltener Missbildungen der Iris. II. Uber Hypoplasie des Irisvorderblattes mit Verlagerung and Entrundungder Pupille. Graefe's Arch Ophthal 133:602, 1935.
9. Rieger, H: Dysgenesis mesodermalis Corneae et Iridis. Z Augenheilkd 86:333, 1935.
10. Mathis, H: Zahnunterzahl und Missbildungen der Iris. Z Stomatol 34:895, 1936.

11. Rieger, H: Erbfragen in der Augenheilkunde. Graefe's Arch Ophthal 143:277, 1941.
12. Alkemade, PPH: Dysgenesis Mesodermalis of the Iris and the Cornea. Charles C. Thomas, Assen, Netherlands, 1969.
13. Reese, AB, Ellsworth, RM: The anterior chamber cleavage syndrome. Arch Ophthal 75:307, 1966.
14. Waring, GO III, Rodrigues, MM, Laibson, PR: Anterior chamber cleavage syndrome. A stepladder classification. Surv Ophthal 20:3, 1975.
15. Shields, MB: Axenfeld-Rieger syndrome. A theory of mechanism and distinctions from the iridocorneal endothelial syndrome. Trans Am Ophthal Soc 81:736, 1983.
16. Shields, MB, Buckley, E, Klintworth, GK, Thresher, R: Axenfeld-Rieger syndrome. A spectrum of developmental disorders. Surv Ophthal 29:387, 1985.
17. Chisholm, IA, Chudley, AE: Autosomal dominant iridogoniodysgenesis with associated somatic anomalies: four-generation family with Rieger's syndrome. Br J Ophthal 67:529, 1983.
18. Burian, HM, Braley, AE, Allen, L: External and gonioscopic visibility of the ring of Schwalbe and the trabecular zone. An interpretation of the posterior corneal embryotoxon and the so-called congenital hyaline membranes on the posterior corneal surface. Trans Am Ophthal Soc 51:389, 1955.
19. Maumenee, AE: Further observations on the pathogenesis of congenital glaucoma. Am J Ophthal 55:1163, 1963.
20. Shields, MB, Campbell, DG, Simmons, RF: The essential iris atrophies. Am J Ophthal 85:749, 1978.
21. Wolter, JR, Sandall, GS, Fralick, FB: Mesodermal dysgenesis of anterior eye: with a partially separated posterior embryotoxon. J Ped Ophthal 4:41, 1967.
22. Cross, HE, Maumenee, AE: Progressive spontaneous dissolution of the iris. Surv Ophthal 18:186, 1973.
23. Judisch, GF, Phelps, CD, Hanson, J: Rieger's syndrome. A case report with a 15-year follow-up. Arch Ophthal 97:2120, 1979.
24. Gregor, Z, Hitchings, RA: Rieger's anomaly: a 42-year follow-up. Br J Ophthal 64:56, 1980.
25. Piper, HF, Schwinger, E, Von Domarus, H: Dysplasia of the limbus corneae, the mesodermal iris layer, and the facial skeleton in one family. Klin Monatsbl Augenheilkd 186:287, 1985.
26. Henkind, P, Friedman, AH: Iridogoniodysgenesis with cataract. Am J Ophthal 72:949, 1971.
27. Dowling, JL, Albert, DM, Nelson, LB, Walton, DS: Primary glaucoma associated with iridotrabecular dysgenesis and ectropion uveae. Ophthalmology 92:912, 1985.
28. Cibis, GW, Waeltermann, JM, Hurst, E, et al: Congenital pupillary-iris-lens membrane with goniodysgenesis (a new entity). Ophthalmology 93:847, 1986.
29. Spallone, A: Retinal detachment in Axenfeld-Rieger syndrome. Br J Ophthal 73:559, 1989.
30. Wesley, RK, Baker, JD, Golnick, AL: Rieger's syndrome: (oligodontia and primary mesodermal dysgenesis of the iris) clinical features and report of an isolated case. J Ped Ophthal Strab 15:67, 1978.
31. Kleinman, RE, Kazarian, EL, Raptopoulos, V, Braverman, LE: Primary empty sella and Rieger's anomaly of the anterior chamber of the eye: a familial syndrome. N Engl J Med 304:90, 1981.
32. Feingold, M, Shiere, F, Fogels, HR, Donaldson, D: Rieger's syndrome. Pediatrics 44:564, 1969.
33. Sadeghi-Nejad, A, Senior, B: Autosomal dominant transmission of isolated growth hormone deficiency in iris-dental dysplasia (Rieger's syndrome). J Ped 85:644, 1974.
34. Jorgenson, RJ, Levin, LS, Cross, HE, et al: The Rieger syndrome. Am J Med Genet 2:307, 1978.
35. Lubin, JR: Oculocutaneous albinism associated with corneal mesodermal dysgenesis. Am J Ophthal 91:347, 1981.
36. Pau, H: Fortschreitende Atrophie des Irisstromas mit Lochbildung und Proliferation des Hornhautendothels. Klin Monatsbl Augenheilkd 147:894, 1965.
37. Troeber, R, Rochels, R: Histological findings in dysgenesis mesodermalis iridis et corneae Rieger. Graefe's Arch Ophthal 213:169, 1980.
38. Ferguson, JG Jr, Hicks, EL: Rieger's anomaly and glaucoma associated with partial trisomy 16q. Arch Ophthal 105:323, 1987.
39. Stathacopoulos, RA, Bateman, JB, Sparkes, RS, Hepler, RS: The Rieger syndrome and a chromosome 13 deletion: J Ped Ophthal Strab 24:198, 1987.
40. Kupfer, C, Kaiser-Kupfer, MI, Datiles, M, McCain, L: The contralateral eye in the iridocorneal endothelial (ICE) syndrome. Ophthalmology 90:1343, 1983.
41. Rubel, E: Angeborene Hypoplasie bzw. Aplasie des Irisvorderblattes. Klin Monatsbl Augenheilkd 51:174, 1913.
42. Jerndal, T: Goniodysgenesis and hereditary juvenile glaucoma. Acta Ophthal Suppl 107:1, 1970.
43. Judisch, GF, Martin-Casals, A, Hanson, JW, Olin, WH: Oculodentodigital dysplasia. Four new reports and a literature review. Arch Ophthal 97:878, 1979.
44. Cross, HE: Ectopia lentis et pupillae. Am J Ophthal 88:381, 1979.
45. Ritch, R, Forbes, M, Hetherington, J Jr, et al: Congenital ectropion uveae with glaucoma. Ophthalmology 91:326, 1984.
46. Gramer, E, Krieglstein, GK: Infantile glaucoma

in unilateral uveal ectropion. Graefe's Arch Ophthal 211:215, 1979.
47. Chang, JSM, Jr, Lee, DA, Christensen, RE: Neodymium:YAG laser lysis of iridocorneal adhesions in mesodermal dysgenesis. Am J Ophthal 108:598, 1989.
48. von Hippel, E: Ueber Hydrophthalmus congenitus nebst Bemerkungen uber die Verfarbung der Cornea durch Blutfarbstoff. Pathologisch-anatomische Untersuchung. Graefe's Arch Ophthal 44:539, 1897.
49. Peters, A: Ueber angeborene Defektbildung der Descemetschen Membran. Klin Monatsbl Augenheilkd 44:27, 1906.
50. DeRespinis, PA, Wagner, RS: Peters' anomaly in a father and son. Am J Ophthal 104:545, 1987.
51. Bateman, JB, Maumenee, IH, Sparkes, RS: Peters' anomaly associated with partial deletion of the long arm of chromosome 11. Am J Ophthal 97:11, 1984.
52. Cibis, GW, Waeltermann, J, Harris, DJ: Peters' anomaly in association with ring 21 chromosomal abnormality. Am J Ophthal 100:733, 1985.
53. Azuma, I: Peters' anomaly associated with glaucoma and chromosomal abnormality. Folia Ophthal Jap 35:1869, 1984.
54. Kivlin, JD, Fineman, RM, Crandall, AS, Olson, RJ: Peters' anomaly as a consequence of genetic and nongenetic syndromes. Arch Ophthal 104:61, 1986.
55. Van Schooneveld, MJ, Delleman, JW, Beemer, FA, Bleeker-Wagemakers, EM: Peters'-plus: a new syndrome. Ophthal Ped Gen 4:141, 1984.
56. Townsend, WM: Congenital corneal leukomas. 1. Central defect in Descemet's membrane. Am J Ophthal 77:80, 1974.
57. Townsend, WM, Font, RL, Zimmerman, LE: Congenital corneal leukomas. 2. Histopathologic findings in 19 eyes with central defect in Descemet's membrane. Am J Ophthal 77:192, 1974.
58. Stone, DL, Kenyon, KR, Green, WR, Ryan, SJ: Congenital central corneal leukoma (Peters' anomaly). Am J Ophthal 81:173, 1976.
59. Nakanishi, I, Brown, SI: The histopathology and ultrastructure of congenital, central corneal opacity (Peters' anomaly). Am J Ophthal 72:801, 1971.
60. Lee, C-F, Yue, BYJT, Robin, J, et al: Immunohistochemical studies of Peters' anomaly. Ophthalmology 96:958, 1989.
61. Polack, FM, Graue, EL: Scanning electron microscopy of congenital corneal leukomas (Peters' anomaly). Am J Ophthal 88:169, 1979.
62. Kupfer, C, Kuwabara, T, Stark, WJ: The histopathology of Peters' anomaly. Am J Ophthal 80:653, 1975.
63. Heath, DH, Shields, MB: Glaucoma and Peters' anomaly. A clinicopathologic case report. Graefe's Arch Ophthal (in press).
64. Pedersen, OO, Rushood, A, Olsen EG: Anterior mesenchymal dysgenesis of the eye. Congenital hereditary endothelial dystrophy and congenital glaucoma. Acta Ophthal 67:470, 1989.
65. Wolter, JR, Haney, WP: Histopathology of keratoconus posticus circumscriptus. Arch Ophthal 69:357, 1963.
66. Krachmer, JH, Rodrigues, MM: Posterior keratoconus. Arch Ophthal 96:1867, 1978.
67. Elsas, FJ, Maumenee, IH, Kenyon, KR, Yoder, F: Familial aniridia with preserved ocular function. Am J Ophthal 83:718, 1977.
68. Hittner, HM, Riccardi, VM, Franke, U: Aniridia caused by a heritable chromosome 11 deletion. Ophthalmology 86:1173, 1979.
69. Schanzlin, DJ, Goldberg, DB, Brown, SI: Hallermann-Streiff syndrome associated with sclerocornea, aniridia, and a chromosomal abnormality. Am J Ophthal 90:411, 1980.
70. Margo, CE: Congenital aniridia: a histopathologic study of the anterior segment in children. J Ped Ophthal Strab 20:192, 1983.
71. Bateman, JB, Sparkes, MC, Sparkes, RS: Aniridia: enzyme studies in an 11p− chromosomal deletion. Invest Ophthal Vis Sci 25:612, 1984.
72. Gillespie, FD: Aniridia, cerebellar ataxia, and oligophrenia in siblings. Arch Ophthal 73:338, 1965.
73. David, R, MacBeath, L, Jeenkins, T: Aniridia associated with microcornea and subluxated lenses. Br J Ophthal 62:118, 1978.
74. Yamamoto, Y, Hayasaka, S, Setogawa, T: Family with aniridia, microcornea, and spontaneously reabsorbed cataract. Arch Ophthal 106:502, 1988.
75. Beauchamp, GR: Anterior segment dysgenesis, keratolenticular adhesion and aniridia. J Ped Ophthal Strab 17:55, 1980.
76. Shields, MB, Reed, JW: Aniridia and congenital ptosis. Ann Ophthal 7:203, 1975.
77. Harnois, C, Boisjoly, HM, Jotterand, V: Sporadic aniridia and Wilms' tumor: visual function evaluation of three cases. Graefe's Arch Ophthal 227:244, 1989.
78. Hamming, N, Wilensky, J: Persistent pupillary membrane associated with aniridia. Am J Ophthal 86:118, 1978.
79. Bergamini, L, Ferraris, F, Gandiglio, G, Inghirami, L: Su di una singolare sindrome neuro-oftalmologica congenita e familiare (ptosi palpebrale, aniridia, cataratta, nistagomo, subatrofia ottica). Rivista Oto-Neuro-Oftalmologica XLI:81, 1966.
80. Sachdev, MS, Sood, NN, Kumar, H, Ghose, S: Bilateral aniridia with Marfan's syndrome and dental anomalies—a new association. Jpn J Ophthal 30:360, 1986.
81. Grant, WM, Walton, DS: Progressive changes in the angle in congenital aniridia with development of glaucoma. Am J Ophthal 78:842, 1974.
82. Walton, DS: Aniridic glaucoma: the results of gonio-surgery to prevent and treat this problem. Tr Am Ophthal Soc 84:59, 1986.

83. Wadelius, C, Fagerholm, P, Pettersson, U, Anneren, G: Lowe oculocerebrorenal syndrome. DNA-based linkage of the gene to Xq24–q26, using tightly linked flanking markers and the correlation to lens examination in carrier diagnosis. Am J Hum Genet 44:241, 1989.
84. Shapiro, MB, France, TD: The ocular features of Down's syndrome. Am J Ophthal 99:659, 1985.
85. Traboulsi, EI, Levine, E, Mets, MB, et al: Infantile glaucoma in Down's syndrome (Trisomy 21). Am J Ophthal 105:389, 1988.
86. Lichter, PR, Schmickel, RD: Posterior vortex vein and congenital glaucoma in a patient with trisomy 13 syndrome. Am J Ophthal 80:939, 1975.
87. Hoepner, J, Yanoff, M: Ocular anomalies in trisomy 13–15: an analysis of 13 eyes with two new findings. Am J Ophthal 74:729, 1972.
88. Mayer, UM, Grosse, KP, Schwanitz, G: Ophthalmologic findings in trisomy 18. Graefe's Arch Ophthal 218:46, 1982.
89. Lessell, S, Forbes, AP: Eye signs in Turner's syndrome. Arch Ophthal 76:211, 1966.
90. Stickler, GB, Belau, PG, Farrell, FJ, et al: Hereditary progressive arthro-ophthalmopathy. Mayo Clin Proc 40:433, 1965.
91. Blair, NP, Albert, DM, Liberfarb, RM, Hirose, T: Hereditary progressive arthro-ophthalmopathy of Stickler. Am J Ophthal 88:876, 1979.
92. Spallone, A: Stickler's syndrome: a study of 12 families. Br J Ophthal 71:504, 1987.
93. Young, NJA, Hitchings, RA, Sehmi, K, Bird, AC: Stickler's syndrome and neovascular glaucoma. Br J Ophthal 63:826, 1979.
94. Cohen, SM, Brown, FR III, Martyn, L, et al: Ocular histopathologic and biochemical studies of the cerebrohepatorenal syndrome (Zellweger's syndrome) and its relationship to neonatal adrenoleukodystrophy. Am J Ophthal 96:488, 1983.
95. Haddad, R, Font, RL, Friendly, DS: Cerebro-hepato-renal syndrome of Zellweger. Ocular histopathologic findings. Arch Ophthal 94:1927, 1976.
96. Mangitti, E, Lavin, JR: Le Glaucoma Congenital Dans Le Syndrome De Rubinstein-Taybi. Ann Oculist 205:1005, 1972.
97. Weber, U, Bernsmeier, H: Rubinstein-Taybi syndrome and juvenile glaucoma. Klin Monatsbl Augenheilkd 183:47, 1983.
98. Shihab, ZM: Pediatric glaucoma in Rubinstein-Taybi Syndrome. Glaucoma 3:288, 1984.
99. Traboulsi, EI, Parks, MM: Glaucoma in oculo-dento-osseous dysplasia. Am J Ophthal 109:310, 1990.
100. Sugar, HS: Oculodentodigital dysplasia syndrome with angle-closure glaucoma. Am J Ophthal 86:36, 1978.
101. Spellacy, E, Bankes, JLK, Crow, J, et al: Glaucoma in a case of Hurler disease. Br J Ophthal 64:773, 1980.
102. Christiansen, SP, Smith, TJ, Henslee-Downey, PJ: Normal intraocular pressure after a bone marrow transplant in glaucoma associated with mucopolysaccharidosis type I-H. Am J Ophthal 109:230, 1990.
103. Cantor, LB, Disseler, JA, Wilson FM, II: Glaucoma in the Maroteaux-Lamy syndrome. Am J Ophthal 108:426, 1989.
104. Cahane, M, Treister, G, Abraham, FA, Melamed, S: Glaucoma in siblings with Morquio syndrome. Br J Ophthal 74:382, 1990.
105. Wan, WL, Minckler, DS, Rao, NA: Pupillary-block glaucoma associated with childhood cystinosis. Am J Ophthal 101:700, 1986.
106. Hittner, HM, King, RA: Oculocutaneous albinoidism as a manifestation of reduced neural crest derivatives in the Prader-Willi syndrome. Am J Ophthal 94:328, 1982.
107. Futterweit, W, Ritch, R, Teekhasaenee, C, Nelson, ES: Coexistence of Prader-Willi syndrome, congenital ectropion uveae with glaucoma, and factor XI deficiency. JAMA 255:3280, 1986.
108. Enright, KA, Neelon, FA: The eyes have it: Waardenburg's syndrome. N Car Med J 47:592, 1986.
109. Nork, TM, Shihab, ZM, Young, RSL, Price, J: Pigment distribution in Waardenburg's syndrome: a new hypothesis. Graefe's Arch Ophthal 224:487, 1986.
110. Levin, PS, Green, WR, Victor, DI, MacLean, AL: Histopathology of the eye in Cockayne's syndrome. Arch Ophthal 101:1093, 1983.
111. Miller, MT, Gammon, JA, Epstein, RJ, et al: Anterior segment anomalies associated with the fetal alcohol syndrome. J Ped Ophthal Strab 21:8, 1984.
112. Cook, CS, Nowotny, AZ, Sulik, KK: Fetal alcohol syndrome. Eye malformations in a mouse model. Arch Ophthal 105:1576, 1987.

Chapter 13

GLAUCOMAS ASSOCIATED WITH DISORDERS OF THE CORNEAL ENDOTHELIUM

Glaucoma and Corneal Disorders

Glaucoma and disorders of the cornea may be associated in one of three ways[1]. In one set of conditions, the concomitant findings may be due to a *common anterior segment abnormality*. These situations include developmental disorders, such as Peters' anomaly, sclerocornea, aniridia, and the Axenfeld-Rieger syndrome, as well as acquired conditions, such as anterior uveitis and trauma. In a second set of conditions, corneal abnormalities may be *secondary to the glaucoma*. These include pressure-induced changes, such as epithelial and stromal edema with acute or especially high elevations of intraocular pressure (IOP), endothelial changes with chronic pressure elevation, and Haab's striae in childhood glaucomas. Corneal changes may also be secondary to the use of topical antiglaucoma medications.

In the third set of conditions, a *primary corneal disorder* may be associated with secondary IOP elevation. These situations include corneal inflammation with secondary glaucoma resulting from either the inflammation or treatment of the keratopathy (i.e., steroid-induced glaucoma, and glaucomas following penetrating keratoplasty). In addition, certain primary disorders of the corneal endothelium may have an associated secondary glaucoma. Two of these situations, the iridocorneal endothelial syndrome and posterior polymorphous dystrophy, represent spectra of clinical and histopathologic abnormalities, with strong evidence for an association between the glaucoma and the corneal disease. In a third

Table 13.1.
Glaucoma and Corneal Disorders[a]

I. Common anterior segment abnormalities	
A. Developmental disorders	Chapter 12
1. Peters' anomaly	
2. Sclerocornea	
3. Aniridia	
4. Axenfeld-Rieger syndrome	
B. Acquired conditions	
1. Anterior uveitis	Chapter 19
2. Trauma	Chapter 21
II. Glaucoma with secondary corneal abnormalities	
A. Pressure-induced corneal changes	
1. Epithelial and stromal edema (Acute or marked IOP elevation)	Chapter 10
2. Endothelial changes (Chronic IOP elevation)	Present chapter
3. Haab's striae (Childhood glaucomas)	Chapter 11
B. Drug-induced ocular surface changes	
1. Miotics	Chapter 25
2. Epinephrine compounds	Chapter 26
3. Beta blockers	Chapter 27
III. Corneal disorders with secondary glaucoma	
A. Keratitis	
1. Glaucoma secondary to inflammation	Chapter 19
2. Steroid-induced glaucoma	Chapter 20
B. Glaucoma following penetrating keratoplasty	Chapter 23
C. Glaucomas associated with primary disorders of the corneal endothelium	Present chapter
1. Iridocorneal endothelial syndrome	
2. Posterior polymorphous dystrophy	
3. Fuchs' endothelial dystrophy	

[a] Modified from Miller, et al.[1]

condition, Fuchs' endothelial dystrophy, an association with glaucoma has also been suggested. This group of primary corneal endothelial disorders is the subject of the present chapter, while the other conditions noted above are considered in other chapters (Table 13.1).

IRIDOCORNEAL ENDOTHELIAL SYNDROME

Terminology

The term *iridocorneal endothelial (ICE) syndrome* was suggested by Eagle and Yanoff[2–4] to denote a spectrum of disease that is characterized by a primary corneal endothelial abnormality. The endothelial disease is variably associated with corneal edema, anterior chamber angle changes, alterations in the iris, and secondary glaucoma. The following three clinical variations within the ICE syndrome have been distinguished, primarily on the basis of changes in the iris (Table 13.2).

Progressive Iris Atrophy

Harms,[5] in 1903, described a condition that is characterized by extreme atrophy of the iris with hole formation. This variation has been called "essential iris atrophy" or "progressive essential iris atrophy." However, subsequent observations, which are discussed later in this chapter, indicate that iris atrophy is not the "essential" or primary feature in this disease.

Chandler's Syndrome

This variation was described by Chandler[6] in 1956 and differs from progressive

Table 13.2.
Iridocorneal Endothelial (ICE) Syndrome

Major Clinical Variations	Characteristic Features
1. Progressive iris atrophy	Iris features predominate, with marked corectopia, atrophy, and hole formation.
2. Chandler's syndrome	Changes in the iris are mild to absent, while corneal edema, often at normal intraocular pressures, is typical.
3. Cogan-Reese syndrome	Nodular, pigmented lesions of the iris are the hallmark and may be seen with the entire spectrum of corneal and other iris defects.

iris atrophy in that changes in the iris are limited to slight corectopia and mild stromal atrophy or may be absent altogether. In one study of 37 consecutive cases of the ICE syndrome, Chandler's syndrome was the most common clinical variation, accounting for 21 cases (56%), and was characterized by more severe corneal edema despite less severe secondary glaucoma than the rest of the group.[7] Intermediate variations between progressive iris atrophy and Chandler's syndrome are also seen, in which changes in the iris are more extensive than in the latter condition but the hole formation of the former variation is not present.

Cogan-Reese Syndrome

In 1969, Cogan and Reese[8] reported two cases with pigmented nodules of the iris, associated with some features of the ICE syndrome. Subsequent studies have revealed that these nodules may occur on the surface of the iris throughout the complete spectrum of this syndrome.[9,10] Similar cases have been described with diffuse nevi, rather than nodules, on the surface of iris, and this has been called *iris nevus syndrome*.[9] There has been a tendency to lump the Cogan-Reese and iris nevus syndromes together as variants of the ICE syndrome. However, the iris lesions of the two conditions are clinically and histologically different, and there is insufficient evidence at this time to include the iris nevus syndrome as a clinical variation of the ICE syndrome.

General Features[7,11,12]

The ICE syndrome is nearly always clinically unilateral, although subclinical abnormalities of the corneal endothelium in the fellow eye are common. The condition is usually recognized in early to middle adulthood, with a predilection for women. Familial cases are rare, and there is no consistent association with systemic diseases. The most common presenting manifestations are abnormalities of the iris, reduced visual acuity, or pain. The latter two symptoms are usually due to corneal edema but also may result from secondary glaucoma.

Clinicopathologic Features

Corneal Alterations

A common feature throughout the ICE syndrome is a corneal endothelial abnormality, which may be seen by slit-lamp biomicroscopy as a fine hammered silver appearance of the posterior cornea, similar to that of Fuchs' dystrophy (Fig. 13.1). This defect may occur by itself without symptoms or may cause corneal edema with variable degrees of reduced vision and pain.[13] In some cases, the corneal edema may occur at IOP levels that are normal or only slightly elevated. Specular microscopy reveals a characteristic, diffuse abnormality of the corneal endothelial cells, with variable degrees of pleomorphism in size and shape, dark areas within the cells, and loss of the clear hexagonal margins (Fig. 13.2).[14–18] The similarity of these findings among the three main clinical variations of the ICE syndrome is further evidence that they represent a spectrum of disease. Some studies have revealed focal areas of normal and abnormal cells separated by a distinct border,[16,17] with gradual disappearance of the normal areas over time.[17] Decreased endothelial cell counts and cellular pleomorphism have also been observed in fellow,

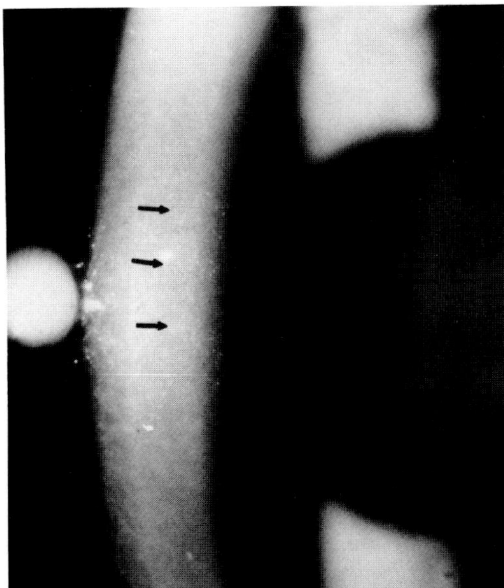

Figure 13.1. Slit-lamp view showing fine hammered silver appearance of corneal endothelial abnormality (*arrows*) in the ICE syndrome. (Reprinted from Am J Ophthal 85:749, 1978, with permission.)

asymptomatic eyes of patients with the ICE syndrome.[19] Endothelial permeability, studied by fluorophotometry, was markedly decreased in the eye with the clinically apparent disorder but normal in the fellow eye.[20]

Electron microscopic studies of the posterior cornea in advanced cases have revealed varied and complex alterations of cells, lining multilayered collagenous tissue posterior to Descemet's membrane (Fig. 13.3).[13,21–28] Most studies agree with regard to the collagenous structures, which consist of the normal prenatal and postnatal layers of Descemet's membrane, lined posteriorly by abnormal collagen zones of variable thickness. However, descriptions of the cellular layer differ among reports, which may relate to the varied response of the corneal endothelium in this syndrome, even within different areas of the same eye. Some cells have evidence of metabolic activity or have undergone division. Filopodial processes and cytoplasmic actin filaments suggest that they are migrating cells.[24,26,28] Groups of blebs are found in some cells, which may explain the dark spots seen by specular microscopy.[24] Other cells are disrupted and necrotic. One clinicopathologic study of a young adult with unilateral corneal endotheliopathy revealed focal necrosis of the

Figure 13.2. Specular microscopic appearance of corneal endothelial cells in the ICE syndrome showing pleomorphism in size and shape, dark areas within the cells, and loss of clear hexagonal margins.

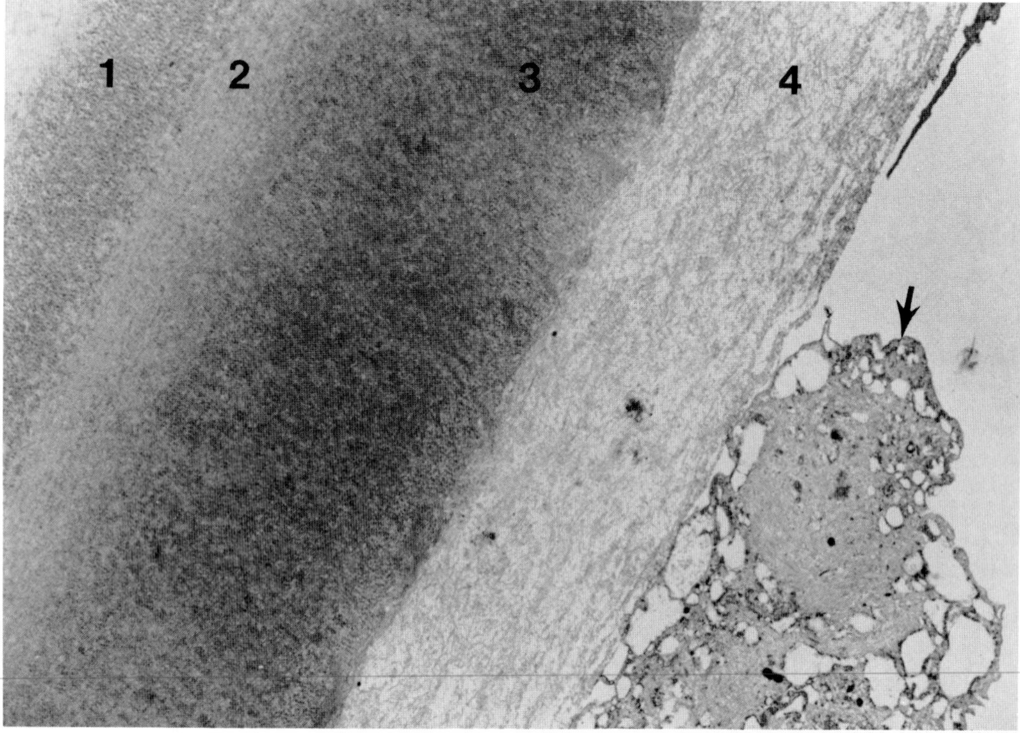

Figure 13.3. Transmission electron microscopic view of inner corneal surface in ICE syndrome showing part of an abnormal cell (*arrow*) on a four-layered membrane, composed of the anterior nonbanded (*1*) and posterior banded (*2*) portions of Descemet's membrane with abnormal compact collagenous (*3*) and loose collagenous (*4*) layers. (Original magnification, ×6875) (Reprinted from Ophthalmology 86:1533, 1979, with permission.)

corneal endothelium, which was thought possibly to represent a forme fruste of the ICE syndrome.[29] Studies differ as to whether the endothelial cells in this syndrome have characteristics of epithelium.[23,24,26–28,30] Cell density varies, with some specimens revealing multiple endothelial layers, suggesting loss of contact inhibition.[24] The typical finding, however, is a monolayer of reduced cell density with occasional acellular zones. Chronic inflammatory cells have also been observed in some cases.[24,26,28]

Anterior Chamber Angle Alterations

Peripheral anterior synechia, usually extending to or beyond Schwalbe's line, is another clinical feature common to all variations of the ICE syndrome (Fig. 13.4). Histologic studies reveal a cellular membrane, consisting of a single layer of endothelial cells and a Descemet's-like membrane, extending down from the peripheral cornea. The membrane may cover an open anterior chamber angle in some areas and may be associated with synechial closure of the angle elsewhere in the same eye.[2,27,31–33]

Secondary glaucoma usually develops as the synechiae progressively close the anterior chamber angle. However, the glaucoma does not correlate precisely with the degree of synechial closure,[11] and it has been reported to occur when the entire angle was open but apparently covered by the cellular membrane.[34,35] Presumably, obstruction to aqueous outflow may result from either the membranes covering the trabecular mesh-

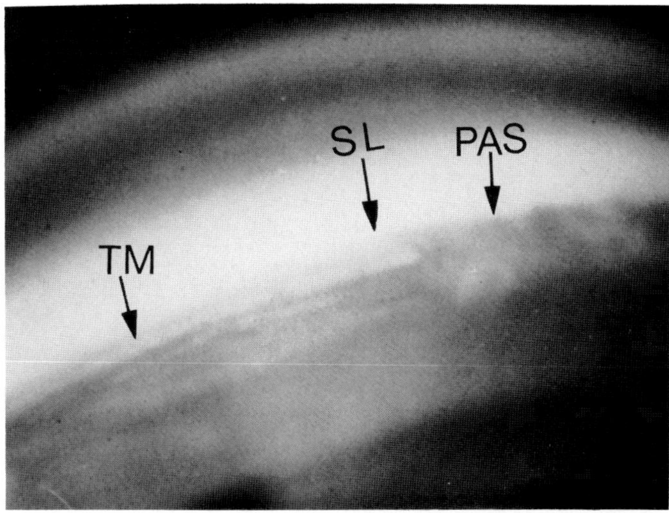

Figure 13.4. Gonioscopic view of patient with the ICE syndrome showing peripheral anterior synechia (*PAS*) extending beyond trabecular meshwork (*TM*) to Schwalbe's line (*SL*). (Reprinted from Am J Ophthal 85:749, 1978, with permission.)

work or synechial closure of the anterior chamber angle.

Alterations of the Iris

The abnormalities of the iris constitute the primary basis for distinguishing clinical variations within the ICE syndrome.

Progressive Iris Atrophy. This variation is characterized by marked atrophy of the iris, associated with variable degrees of corectopia and ectropion uvea. The latter two features are usually directed toward the quadrant with the most prominent area of peripheral anterior synechia.[11,31] The hallmark of progressive iris atrophy is hole formation of the iris, which occurs in two forms.[11] With *stretch holes,* the iris is markedly thinned in the quadrant away from the direction of pupillary distortion, and the holes develop within the area that is being stretched (Fig. 13.5). In other eyes, *melting holes* develop without associated corectopia or thinning of the iris. Fluorescein angiographic studies suggest that this is associated with ischemia of the iris.[10]

Histopathology of the iris in this and all variations of the ICE syndrome includes a cellular membrane on portions of the anterior surface of the iris (Fig. 13.6), which is similar to and continuous with that seen over the anterior chamber angle.[2,31] The membrane is most often found in the quadrant toward which the pupil is distorted.[31]

Chandler's Syndrome. In this clinical form, there is minimal corectopia and mild atrophy of the stroma of the iris (Fig. 13.7).[6] In some cases, there may be no detectable change in the iris.

Cogan-Reese Syndrome. The eyes in this variation of the ICE syndrome may have any degree of iris atrophy but are distinguished by the presence of pigmented, pedunculated nodules on the surface of the iris (Fig. 13.8).[8–10] In some cases, other features of the ICE syndrome may be present for many years before the nodules appear.[10,36] The nodular lesions have an ultrastructure similar to that of the underlying stroma of the iris and are always surrounded by the previously described cellular membrane (Fig. 13.9).[2,31,36–38]

Theories of Mechanism

The membrane theory of Campbell[31] holds that the abnormality of the corneal endothelium is the primary defect in the ICE syndrome (Fig. 13.10). The endothelial defect causes the corneal edema and also leads to the proliferation of the cellular membrane across the anterior chamber angle and onto

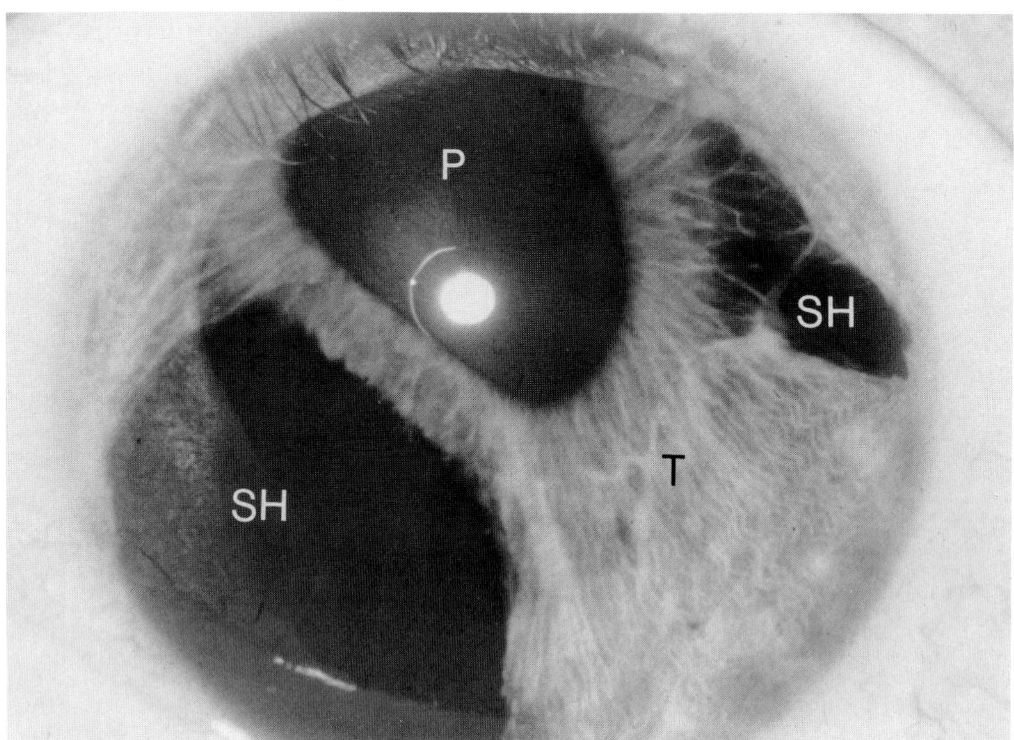

Figure 13.5. Progressive iris atrophy, a variation of the ICE syndrome, with pupillary distortion (*P*), thinning of the iris (*T*), and stretch holes (*SH*). (Reprinted from Am J Ophthal 85:749, 1978, with permission.)

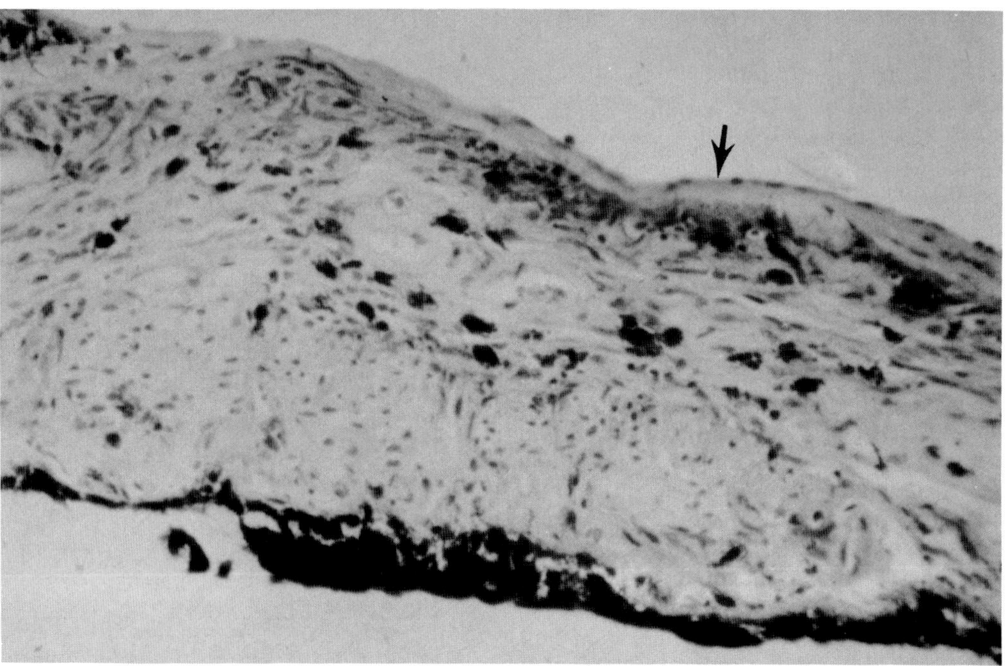

Figure 13.6. Light microscopic view of iris specimen from eye with the ICE syndrome showing Descemet-like membrane and scant monolayer of cells (*arrow*) extending across the stroma. (Hematoxylin-eosin; original magnification, ×250) (Reprinted from Ophthalmology 86:1533, 1979, with permission.)

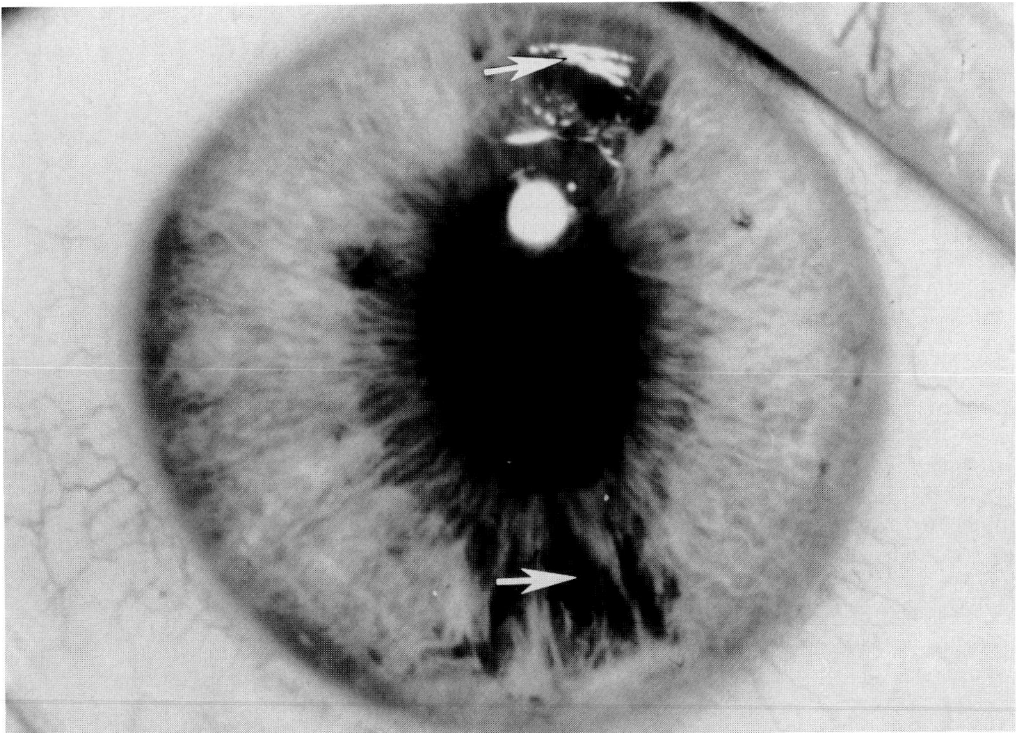

Figure 13.7. Chandler's syndrome, a variation of the ICE syndrome, with slight pupillary distortion and thinning of iris stroma at the vertical poles (*arrows*). (Reprinted from Am J Ophthal 85:749, 1978, with permission.)

the surface of the iris. The observation of filopodial processes, cytoplasmic actin filaments, and apparent loss of contact inhibition are consistent with the concept of migrating cells.[24,26–28] Contracture of the cellular membrane causes the formation of peripheral anterior synechiae, the corectopia, and the ectropion uvea. Stretching of the iris in the direction away from the corectopia, especially when the iris is anchored by peripheral anterior synechiae on both sides, undoubtedly contributes to the atrophy and hole formation, although additional factors, such as ischemia, may also be involved.[12] The cellular membrane is also believed to be responsible for the development of the nodular lesions of the iris in the Cogan-Reese syndrome, possibly by encircling and pinching off portions of the iris stroma to form the nodules.[31,37] As previously noted, the associated glaucoma may be due to obstruction of the trabecular meshwork by either the cellular membrane or, more commonly, the peripheral anterior synechiae.

Each clinical variation is believed to have the same basic mechanism described above. In some cases, the difference in clinical features may simply be due to the time at which the patient is seen. For example, a patient with the initial findings of Chandler's syndrome may later develop iris hole formation and/or nodules, changing the diagnosis to progressive iris atrophy or the Cogan-Reese syndrome, respectively. In other cases, however, patients do not progress and, as previously noted, Chandler's syndrome appears to be the most common variant of the ICE syndrome.[7] It may be that the endothelial cells in these patients are more disrupted and/or less able to migrate, which could explain the more severe corneal edema, as well as the less severe glaucoma and iris changes, as compared with the other variants in this spectrum of disease.[7,24]

The underlying condition that leads to the

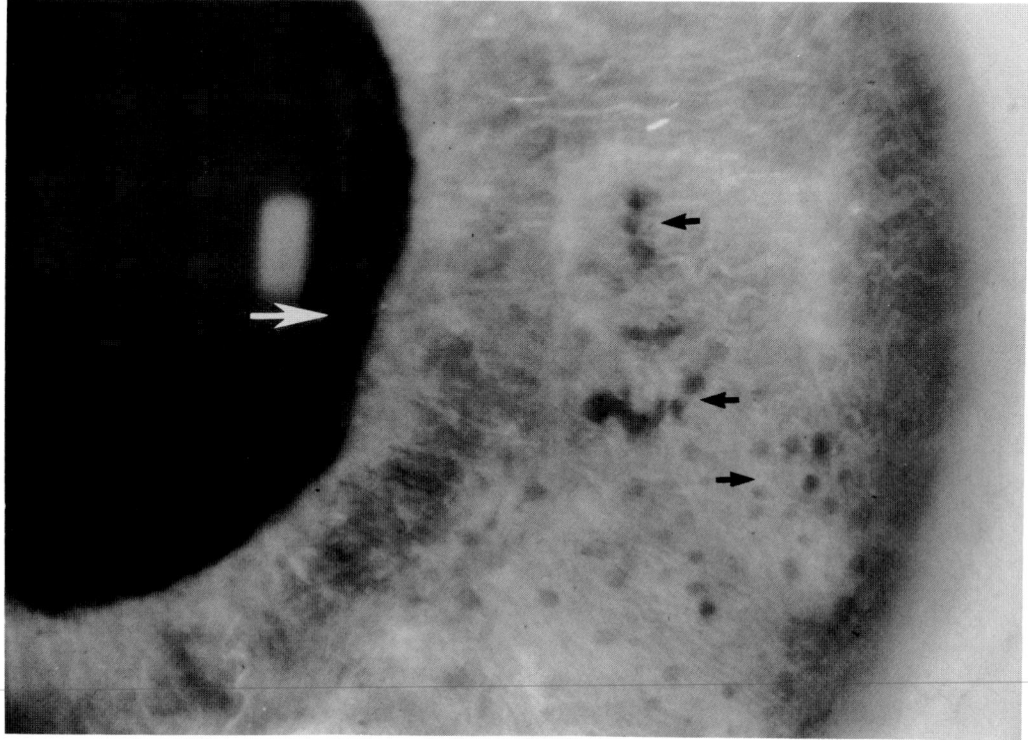

Figure 13.8. Cogan-Reese syndrome, a variation of the ICE syndrome, showing ectropion uvea (*white arrow*) and numerous dark nodules (*black arrows*) on area of flattened iris stroma. (Reprinted from Arch Ophthal 94:406, 1976, with permission.)

corneal endothelial changes is unknown. The absence of a positive family history and the presence of the postnatal layer of Descemet's membrane suggest an acquired disorder. The observation of chronic inflammatory cells has raised the possibility of a viral etiology,[24] although these cells have also been seen in the endothelium of corneas with inherited disease.[26] It has also been suggested that the cellular proliferation in this syndrome could represent a progressive corneal endothelioma.[27]

Differential Diagnosis

Several disorders of the cornea or iris could be confused with the various forms of the ICE syndrome, many of which have associated glaucoma. It is helpful to think of these in the following three categories.[11,12]

Corneal Endothelial Disorders

Posterior polymorphous dystrophy may have associated glaucoma as well as changes of the anterior chamber angle and iris that resemble the ICE syndrome. However, the corneal abnormalities as well as other clinical features clearly distinguish these two spectra of disease. *Fuchs' endothelial dystrophy* has corneal changes that are clinically very similar to those of the ICE syndrome, but none of the chamber angle or iris features of the latter condition. Both conditions are considered later in this chapter.

Dissolution of the Iris

The *Axenfeld-Rieger syndrome* has striking clinical and histopathologic similarities to the ICE syndrome, but the congenital nature and bilaterality as well as the other features described in Chapter 12 help to separate the two conditions. Some advanced cases of progressive iris atrophy might resemble *aniridia,* but the bilaterality of the latter disorder is again a helpful differential feature (Chapter 12). *Iridoschisis* is charac-

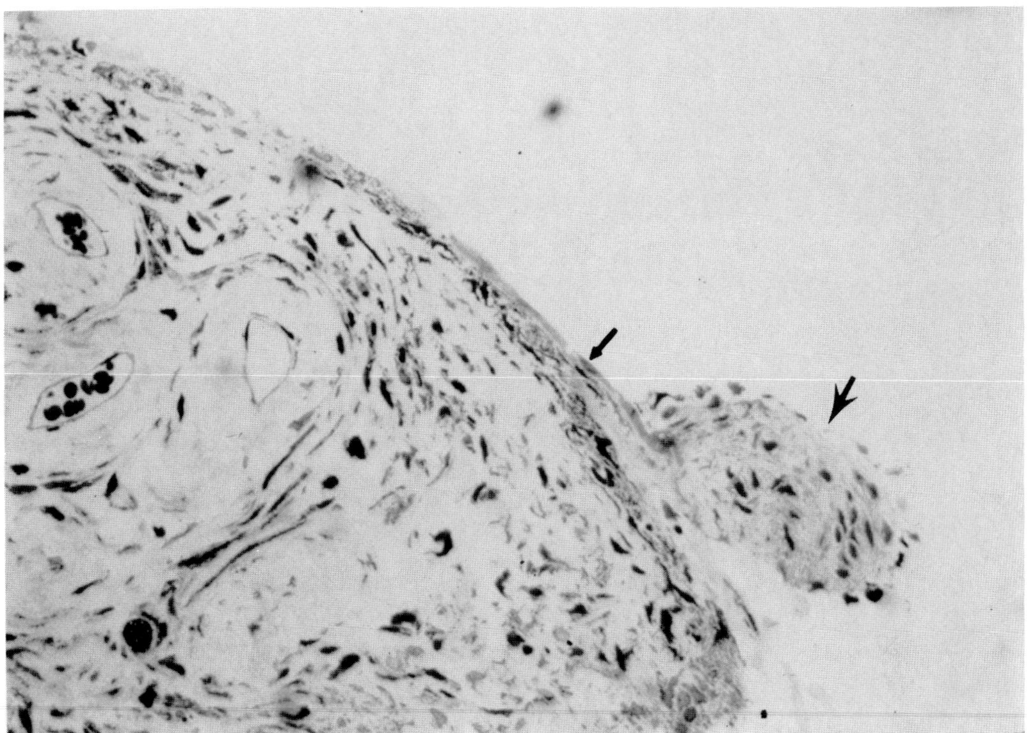

Figure 13.9. Light microscopic view of iridectomy specimen from eye with Cogan-Reese syndrome showing nodule composed of cells resembling the iris stroma (*large arrow*) and portion of a monolayer of spindle-shaped cells (*small arrow*). (Toluidine blue and basic fucsin; original magnification, ×200) (Reprinted from Arch Ophthal 94:406, 1976, with permission.)

terized by separation of superficial layers of iris stroma and may be associated with glaucoma. However, it is typically a disease of the elderly (Chapter 14).

Nodular Lesions of the Iris

Patients with the Cogan-Reese syndrome have had enucleation for presumed *melanomas* of the iris.[8] Patients with *iris melanosis* may also have pedunculated nodules strikingly similar to those of the Cogan-Reese syndrome, but this condition is typically bilateral and may be familial.[39,40] In addition, differentiation must be made from the nodular lesions of *neurofibromatosis,* as well as nodular *inflammatory disorders,* such as sarcoidosis.

Management

Patients with the ICE syndrome may require treatment for corneal edema, secondary glaucoma, or both. The glaucoma can often be controlled medically in the early stages, especially with drugs that reduce aqueous production. Lowering the IOP may also control the corneal edema, although the additional use of hypertonic saline solutions and soft contact lenses may be required. When the IOP can no longer be controlled medically, surgical intervention is indicated. Laser trabeculoplasty is usually not effective in these cases. Filtering surgery is reasonably successful,[11,41] although late failures have occurred as a result of endothelialization of the filtering bleb.[36,41] In some cases, surgical reduction of the IOP is used to relieve the corneal edema. However, even an extremely low pressure may not reverse advanced corneal edema, and penetrating keratoplasty is usually indicated for this situation after the glaucoma has been controlled.[13,42]

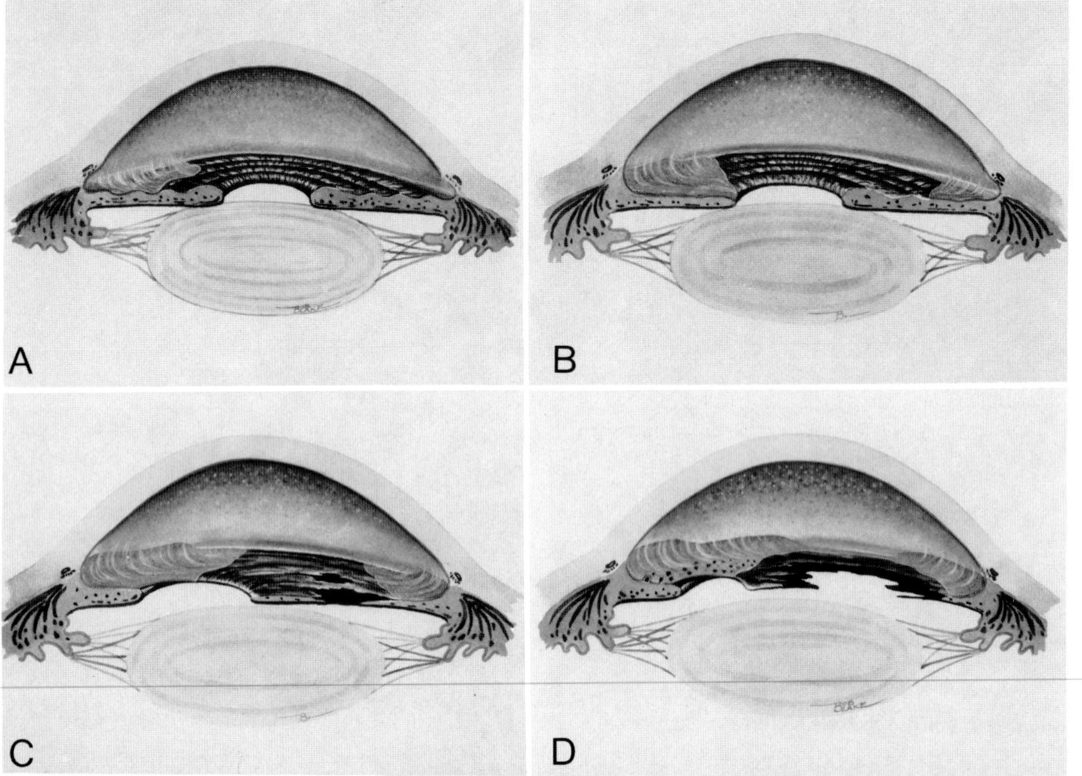

Figure 13.10. Membrane theory of Campbell for pathogenesis of the ICE syndrome: *A,* Extension of membrane from corneal endothelium over anterior chamber angle and onto iris; *B,* Contraction of membrane, creating peripheral anterior synechiae and corectopia; *C,* Thinning and atrophy of iris in quadrants away from corectopia; *D,* Hole formation in area of atrophy (in progressive iris atrophy), ectropion uvea in direction of corectopia, and nodules in area of membrane (in Cogan-Reese syndrome). (Reprinted from Surv Ophthal 24:3, 1979, with permission.)

POSTERIOR POLYMORPHOUS DYSTROPHY

General Features

Posterior polymorphous dystrophy is a bilateral, familial disorder of the corneal endothelium. Inheritance is usually autosomal dominant, and there is no race or sex predilection. Although it is probably congenital, it typically remains asymptomatic until adulthood. As with the ICE syndrome, posterior polymorphous dystrophy represents a spectrum of disorders.[43–45] In one form, the characteristic corneal changes are associated with peripheral iridocorneal adhesions, iris atrophy, and corectopia.[43,45] Glaucoma occurs in approximately 15% of patients with posterior polymorphous dystrophy, both with and without the iridocorneal adhesions.

Clinicopathologic Features

Corneal Alterations

By slit-lamp biomicroscopy, the posterior cornea has the appearance of blisters or vesicles at the level of Descemet's membrane (Fig. 13.11). The vesicles may be linear or in groups and surrounded by an aureole of gray haze.[44,45] Band-like thickenings may also be seen at the level of Descemet's membrane.[46] Two patterns of endothelial abnormality have been identified by slit-lamp biomicroscopy and specular microscopy.[47,48] One is characterized by localized vesicular and band patterns resembling cra-

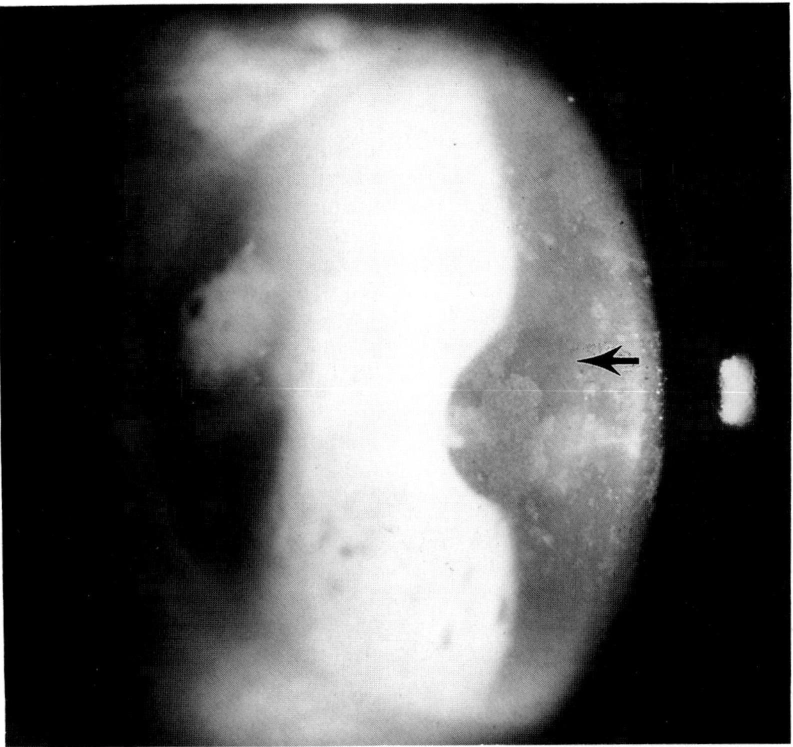

Figure 13.11. Slit-lamp view of patient with posterior polymorphous dystrophy showing typical, irregular lesions (*arrow*) of the posterior corneal surface. (Reprinted with permission from Bourgeois J, Shields MB, Thresher R: Ophthalmology 91:420, 1984.)

ters or doughnut-like lesions and snail tracks, with retention of corneal clarity. The second type has a geographic pattern with associated haze of Descemet's membrane and deep corneal stroma. The latter variety may be associated with iridocorneal adhesions and glaucoma.

Ultrastructural studies reveal an unusually thin Descemet's membrane covered by multiple layers of collagen[49–52] and lined by cells that have been variably described as having features of abnormal endothelium,[53] fibroblasts,[50,52] or epithelium.[49,51,52,54,55] These differences in cellular morphology may represent an evolving process of metaplasia.[50] The incompletely developed Descemet's membrane suggests that the corneal endothelium began to change in late fetal or early adolescent life and subsequently deposited the additional collagen layers.

Clinically, the cornea may remain clear and produce no symptoms, although corneal edema may develop in some cases.

Anterior Chamber Angle and Iris Alterations

A small number of patients may have broad peripheral anterior synechiae extending to or beyond Schwalbe's line, which may be associated with corectopia, ectropion uvea, and atrophy of the iris.[43–45,56] The histopathologic study of such a case revealed a membrane composed of epithelial-like cells and a Descemet's-like membrane extending over the anterior chamber angle and onto the iris (Fig. 13.12).[33,45]

Secondary glaucoma may be present in some of the cases with anterior chamber angle and iris abnormalities, and it has also been observed in eyes with open, normal-appearing angles.[44,45,56,57] In the latter situation, gonioscopy may reveal a high insertion of the iris into the posterior aspect of the trabecular meshwork.[57] An ultrastructural evaluation of such an eye confirmed the high insertion of anterior uvea into the

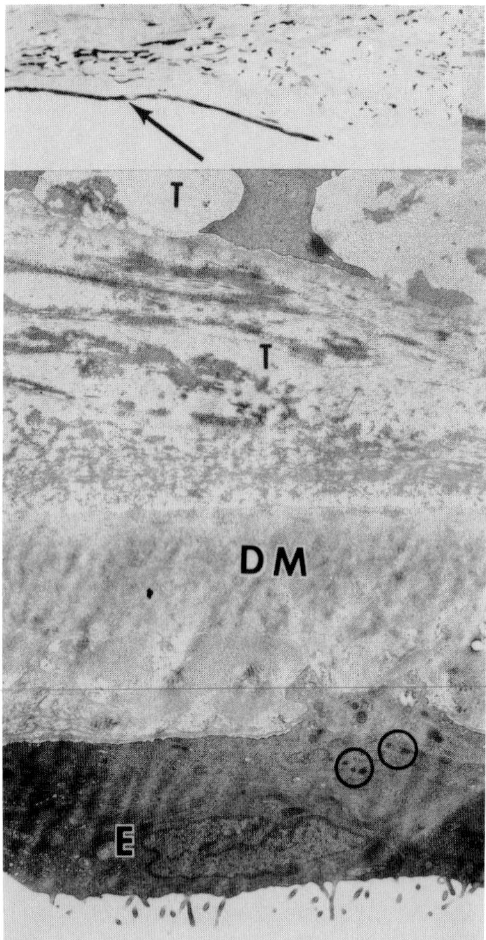

Figure 13.12. Transmission electron microscopic view of trabeculectomy specimen from eye with posterior polymorphous dystrophy showing trabecular beams (*T*) covered by Descemet-like membrane (*DM*) and transformed endothelial cells (*E*) with numerous microvillous projections and desmosomal attachments (*circles*). (Original magnification, ×8200) Inset shows light microscopic appearance of membrane on trabecular meshwork (*arrow*). (Toluidine blue; original magnification, ×130) (Reprinted with permission from Rodrigues MM, Phelps CD, Krachmer JH, et al: Arch Ophthal 98:688, 1980.)

meshwork with collapse of the trabecular beams (Fig. 13.13).[57]

Theories of Mechanism

A membrane theory, similar to that for the ICE syndrome, has been proposed for those cases of posterior polymorphous dystrophy with iridocorneal adhesions. It is postulated that a dystrophic endothelium (or epithelium), producing a basement membrane-like material, extends across the anterior chamber angle and onto the iris, and subsequently causes the synechia formation and changes in the iris.[44,45] The glaucoma may be due to the iridocorneal adhesions in these cases. In the eyes with open angles, the high insertion of the anterior uvea may represent a developmental anomaly of the anterior chamber angle, similar to that seen in several of the developmental glaucomas, and may be responsible for the subsequent collapse of the trabecular meshwork and the secondary glaucoma.[57]

Differential Diagnosis

Conditions that may be confused with posterior polymorphous dystrophy include other forms of posterior corneal dystrophy, such as Fuchs' endothelial dystrophy, congenital hereditary corneal dystrophy, and posterior amorphous corneal dystrophy. The latter is characterized by diffuse gray-white, sheet-like opacities of the posterior stroma, with occasional fine iris processes extending to Schwalbe's line for 360° and various abnormalities of the iris, but no glaucoma.[58] When iridocorneal adhesions are present, the Axenfeld-Rieger syndrome and the ICE syndrome should also be considered. The band-like thickenings of posterior polymorphous dystrophy may be confused with the Haab's striae of congenital glaucoma, although the latter are seen as thinned areas with thickened edges.[46]

Management

Most cases of posterior polymorphous dystrophy are asymptomatic and do not require treatment. However, corneal edema may require conservative management or penetrating keratoplasty. In one series of 21 keratoplasties for posterior polymorphous dystrophy, nine grafts failed, six of which had iridocorneal adhesions and glaucoma, and it has been suggested that keratoplasty should be avoided in these patients until absolutely necessary.[45] Recurrence of posterior polymorphous dystrophy has been reported following penetrating keratoplasty.[59]

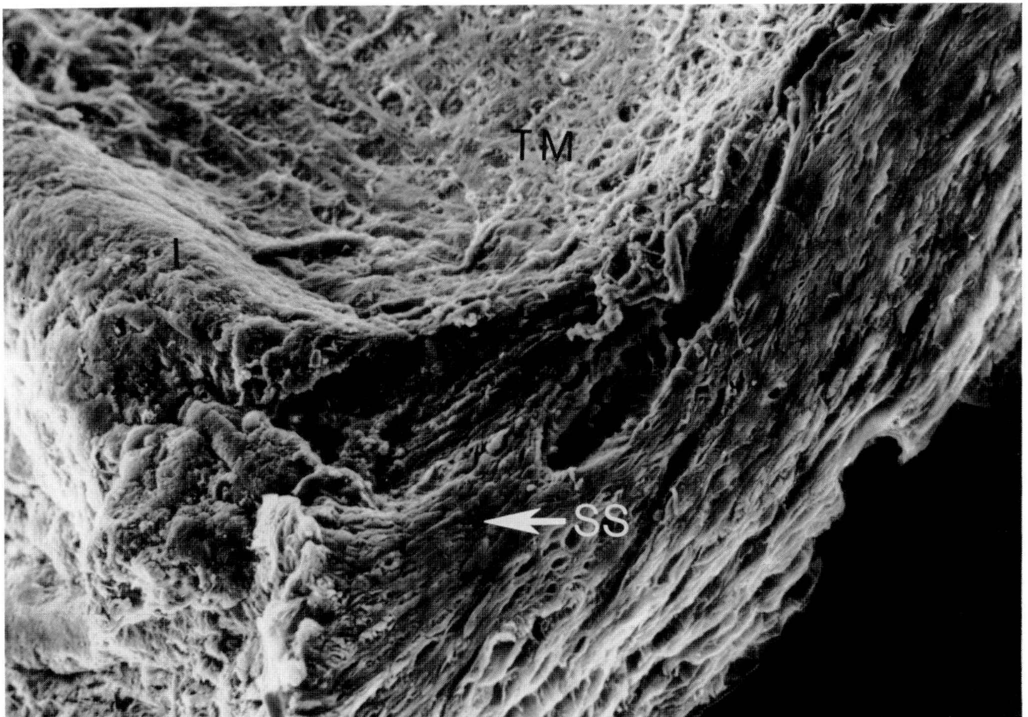

Figure 13.13. Scanning electron microscopic view of trabeculectomy specimen from eye with posterior polymorphous dystrophy showing high insertion of iris (*I*) into posterior aspect of trabecular meshwork (*TM*) well anterior to scleral spur (*SS*). (Original magnification, ×230) (Reprinted with permission from Bourgeois J, Shields MB, Thresher R: Ophthalmology 91:420, 1984.)

The glaucoma, when present, may respond to drugs that lower aqueous production. Laser trabeculoplasty is not likely to be successful in these cases, and filtering surgery generally is indicated when medical therapy is no longer adequate.

FUCHS' ENDOTHELIAL DYSTROPHY

Terminology and Clinicopathologic Features

Cornea Guttata

Cornea guttata is a common condition, the incidence of which increases significantly with age.[60] Slit-lamp biomicroscopy reveals a hammered silver appearance of the central posterior cornea, similar to that seen in the ICE syndrome. However, by specular microscopic study a more characteristic pattern is seen, consisting of enlarged endothelial cells with dark areas that overlap the cell borders.[61] The primary pathology is an alteration in the corneal endothelium that leads to a deposition of collagen on the posterior surface of Descemet's membrane. Histologically, this may appear as warts or excrescences in the pure form of cornea guttata. In other cases, focal accumulations may be covered by additional basement membrane or there may be a uniform thickening of the posterior collagen layers.[62,63]

Fuchs' Endothelial Dystrophy

The vast majority of individuals with cornea guttata have otherwise normal corneas with no visual impairment. However, a small number of patients with the same posterior corneal changes as described above will develop edema of the corneal stroma and epithelium. The clinical entity was described by Fuchs[64] in 1910, and the association with a dystrophy of the corneal endothelium was subsequently recognized. The disorder is bilateral with a predilection for women and an onset usually between the ages of 40 and 70 years. There is a strong familial tendency, and an autosomal dominant inheritance has been described.[62] Viral particles have been found in the corneal endothelium of one eye, suggesting the possibility of an acquired etiology in some cases.[65] Aqueous humor composition is normal, consistent with the theory that Fuchs' dystrophy is a primary disorder of the corneal endothelium.[66] The condition may lead to severe visual reduction, often requiring penetrating keratoplasty.

Association with Glaucoma

Influence of IOP on Corneal Endothelium

Reports are conflicting regarding the association of glaucoma with cornea guttata and Fuchs' endothelial dystrophy. This may be due, at least in part, to the fact that elevated IOP often induces secondary changes in the corneal endothelium. Reduced cell densities have been reported in association with open-angle glaucoma,[67] angle-closure glaucoma,[68–70] and some secondary glaucomas.[70–72] However, the degree of endothelial alteration does not always correlate with the height of IOP elevation, suggesting that other factors may also influence the association between glaucoma and corneal endothelial changes.[67] It has been shown, for example, that the morphology of corneal endothelium is altered by increasing age[73] and anterior uveitis, including glaucomatocyclitic crises.[70,72,74] These observations must be taken into consideration with any reported association between glaucoma and an alteration of the corneal endothelium.

Cornea Guttata and Aqueous Outflow

It has been reported that patients with cornea guttata have a high incidence of abnormal tonographic facilities of outflow.[75] However, in a subsequent study using widefield specular microscopy, the mean value for facility of outflow in patients with cornea guttata was not statistically different from that of the normal population, and there was no correlation between the extent of guttata and facility of outflow.[76] Another study of patients with cornea guttata showed a lower mean IOP in this group as compared with a matched population without guttata.[77]

Fuchs' Endothelial Dystrophy and Glaucoma

Patients with shallow anterior chambers and Fuchs' dystrophy may develop *angle-closure glaucoma,* apparently resulting from a gradual thickening of the cornea with eventual closure of the anterior chamber angle.[78]

It was once estimated that 10–15% of patients with Fuchs' endothelial dystrophy have open-angle glaucoma.[79] However, a study of 64 families with the former condition revealed only one case of open-angle glaucoma.[80] In another study, no genetic overlap between Fuchs' endothelial dystrophy and primary open-angle glaucoma was found on the basis of in vitro lymphocyte responsiveness to corticosteroids.[81]

Management

Although glaucoma is usually not present in eyes with Fuchs' endothelial dystrophy, medical efforts to further reduce the normal IOP may sometimes help to minimize the corneal edema. When glaucoma is present, the open-angle form is managed the same as primary open-angle glaucoma, while the angle-closure form requires an iridectomy or filtering procedure. Prophylactic miotic therapy has not been effective in cases with impending angle closure.[78]

SUMMARY

The iridocorneal endothelial (ICE) syndrome is a primary disorder of the corneal endothelium, which presents in young adulthood as a unilateral abnormality of the cornea, anterior chamber angle, and iris. It appears to be an acquired condition. The abnormal endothelium often causes corneal edema and proliferates over the angle and iris with subsequent contraction, leading to glaucoma and variable degrees of iris distortion. The latter changes are the basis for clinical variations including Chandler's syndrome, progressive iris atrophy, and the Cogan-Reese syndrome. Posterior polymorphous dystrophy is another spectrum of disease in which an endothelial abnormality is the fundamental disorder. Glaucoma is present in a small percentage of these cases, and, in some patients, a proliferation of the abnormal endothelium causes changes of the anterior chamber angle and iris resembling those in the ICE syndrome. The condition differs from the latter syndrome, however, in that it is inherited and bilateral and has a different clinical appearance of the posterior cornea. A third primary disorder of the corneal endothelium, Fuchs' endothelial dystrophy, occasionally has associated glaucoma, usually with an angle-closure mechanism.

References

1. Miller, KN, Carlson, AN, Foulks, GN, Shields, MB: Associated glaucoma and corneal disorders. Focal Points, Am Acad Ophthal, Vol. 7, Module 4, 1989.
2. Eagle, RC Jr, Font, RL, Yanoff, M, Fine, BS: Proliferative endotheliopathy with iris abnormalities. The iridocorneal endothelial syndrome. Arch Ophthal 97:2104, 1979.
3. Yanoff, M: In discussion of Shields, MB, McCracken, JS, Klintworth, GK, Campbell, DG: Corneal edema in essential iris atrophy. Ophthalmology 86:1549, 1979.
4. Yanoff, M: Iridocorneal endothelial syndrome. Unification of a disease spectrum. Surv Ophthal 24:1, 1979.
5. Harms, C: Einseitige spontane Luckenbildung der Iris durch Atrophie ohne mechanische Zerrung. Klin Monatsbl Augenheilkd 41:522, 1903.
6. Chandler, PA: Atrophy of the stroma of the iris. Endothelial dystrophy, corneal edema, and glaucoma. Am J Ophthal 41:607, 1956.
7. Wilson, MC, Shields, MB: A comparison of the clinical variations of the iridocorneal endothelial syndrome. Arch Ophthal 107:1465, 1989.
8. Cogan, DG, Reese, AB: A syndrome of iris nodules, ectopic Descemet's membrane, and unilateral glaucoma. Doc Ophthal 26:424, 1969.
9. Scheie, HG, Yanoff, M: Iris nevus (Cogan-Reese) syndrome. A cause of unilateral glaucoma. Arch Ophthal 93:963, 1975.
10. Shields, MB, Campbell, DG, Simmons, RJ, Hutchinson, BT: Iris nodules in essential iris atrophy. Arch Ophthal 94:406, 1976.
11. Shields, MB, Campbell, DG, Simmons, RJ: The essential iris atrophies. Am J Ophthal 85:749, 1978.
12. Shields, MB: Progressive essential iris atrophy, Chandler's syndrome, and the iris nevus (Cogan-Reese) syndrome: a spectrum of disease. Surv Ophthal 24:3, 1979.
13. Shields, MB, McCracken, JS, Klintworth, GK, Campbell, DG: Corneal edema in essential iris atrophy. Ophthalmology 86:1533, 1979.
14. Setala, K, Vannas, A: Corneal endothelial cells in essential iris atrophy. A specular microscopic study. Acta Ophthal 57:1020, 1979.
15. Hirst, LW, Quigley, HA, Stark, WJ, Shields, MB: Specular microscopy of iridocorneal endothelial syndrome. Am J Ophthal 89:11, 1980.
16. Neubauer, L, Lund, O-E, Leibowitz, HM: Specular microscopic appearance of the corneal endothelium in iridocorneal endothelial syndrome. Arch Ophthal 101:916, 1983.
17. Bourne, WM: Partial corneal involvement in the iridocorneal endothelial syndrome. Am J Ophthal 94:774, 1982.
18. Wang, Y: Specular microscopic studies of the corneal endothelium in iridocorneal endothelial (ICE) syndrome. Eye Science 1:53, 1985.
19. Kupfer, C, Kaiser-Kupfer, MI, Datiles, M, McCain, L: The contralateral eye in the iridocorneal endothelial (ICE) syndrome. Ophthalmology 90:1343, 1983.
20. Bourne, WM, Brubaker, RF: Decreased endothelial permeability in the iridocorneal endothelial syndrome. Ophthalmology 89:591, 1982.
21. Quigley, HA, Forster, RF: Histopathology of cornea and iris in Chandler's syndrome. Arch Ophthal 96:1878, 1978.
22. Richardson, RM: Corneal decompensation in Chandler's syndrome. A scanning and transmission electron microscopic study. Arch Ophthal 97:2112, 1979.
23. Portis, JM, Stamper, RL, Spencer, WH, Webster, RG Jr: The corneal endothelium and Descemet's membrane in the iridocorneal endothelial syndrome. Trans Am Ophthal Soc 83:316, 1985.
24. Alvarado, JA, Murphy, CG, Maglio, M, Hetherington, J: Pathogenesis of Chandler's syndrome, essential iris atrophy and the Cogan-Reese syndrome. I. Alterations of the corneal endothelium. Invest Ophthal Vis Sci 27:853, 1986.
25. Alvarado, JA, Murphy, CG, Juster, RP, Hetherington, J: Pathogenesis of Chandler's syndrome, essential iris atrophy and the Cogan-Reese syndrome. II. Estimated age at disease onset. Invest Ophthal Vis Sci 27:873, 1986.
26. Rodrigues, MM, Stulting, RD, Waring, GO, III: Clinical, electron microscopic, and immunohistochemical study of the corneal endothelium and Descemet's membrane in the iridocorneal endothelial syndrome. Am J Ophthal 101:16, 1986.
27. Eagle, RC Jr, Shields, JA: Iridocorneal endothelial syndrome with contralateral guttate endothelial dystrophy. A light and electron microscopic study. Ophthalmology 94:862, 1987.
28. Rodrigues, MM, Jester, JV, Richards, R, et al: Es-

sential iris atrophy. A clinical, immunohistologic, and electron microscopic study in an enucleated eye. Ophthalmology 95:69, 1988.
29. Stock, EL, Roth, SI, Morimoto, D: Desquamating endotheliopathy. An incipient iridocorneal endothelial syndrome? Arch Ophthal 105:1378, 1987.
30. Hirst, LW, Green, WR, Luckenbvach, M, et al: Epithelial characteristics of the endothelium in Chandler's syndrome. Invest Ophthal Vis Sci 24:603, 1983.
31. Campbell, DG, Shields, MB, Smith, TR: The corneal endothelium and the spectrum of essential iris atrophy. Am J Ophthal 86:317, 1978.
32. Rodrigues, MM, Streeten, BW, Spaeth, GL: Chandler's syndrome as a variant of essential iris atrophy. A clinicopathologic study. Arch Ophthal 96:643, 1978.
33. Rodrigues, MM, Phelps, CD, Krachmer, JH, et al: Glaucoma due to endothelialization of the anterior chamber angle. A comparison of posterior polymorphous dystrophy of the cornea and Chandler's syndrome. Arch Ophthal 98:688, 1980.
34. Benedikt, O, Roll, P: Open-angle glaucoma through endothelialization of the anterior chamber angle. Glaucoma 2:368, 1980.
35. Weber, PA, Gibb, G: Iridocorneal endothelial syndrome: glaucoma without peripheral anterior synechias. Glaucoma 6:128, 1984.
36. Daicker, B, Sturrock, G, Guggenheim, R: Clinicopathological correlation in Cogan-Reese syndrome. Klin Monatsbl Augenheilkd 180:531, 1982.
37. Eagle, RC Jr, Font, RL, Yanoff, M, Fine, BS: The iris naevus (Cogan-Reese) syndrome: light and electron microscopic observations. Br J Ophthal 64:446, 1980.
38. Radius, RL, Herschler, J: Histopathology in the iris-nevus (Cogan-Reese) syndrome. Am J Ophthal 89:780, 1980.
39. Traboulsi, EI, Maumenee, IH: Bilateral melanosis of the iris. Am J Ophthal 103:115, 1987.
40. Joondeph, BC, Goldberg, MF: Familial iris melanosis—a misnomer? Br J Ophthal 73:289, 1989.
41. Kidd, M, Hetherington, J, Magee, S: Surgical results in iridocorneal endothelial syndrome. Arch Ophthal 106:199, 1988.
42. Buxton, JN, Lash, RS: Results of penetrating keratoplasty in the iridocorneal endothelial syndrome. Am J Ophthal 98:297, 1984.
43. Grayson, M: The nature of hereditary deep polymorphous dystrophy of the cornea: its association with iris and anterior chamber dysgenesis. Trans Am Ophthal Soc 72:516, 1974.
44. Cibis, GW, Krachmer, JA, Phelps, CD, Weingeist, TA: The clinical spectrum of posterior polymorphous dystrophy. Arch Ophthal 95:1529, 1977.
45. Krachmer, JH: Posterior polymorphous corneal dystrophy: a disease characterized by epithelial-like endothelial cells which influence management and prognosis. Trans Am Ophthal Soc 83:413, 1985.
46. Cibis, GW, Tripathi, RC: The differential diagnosis of Descemet's Tears (Haab's Striae) and posterior polymorphous dystrophy bands. A clinicopathologic study. Ophthalmology 89:614, 1982.
47. Hirst, LW, Waring, GO III: Clinical specular microscopy of posterior polymorphous endothelial dystrophy. Am J Ophthal 95:143, 1983.
48. Brooks, AMV, Grant, G, Gillies, WE: Differentiation of posterior polymorphous dystrophy from other posterior corneal opacities by specular microscopy. Ophthalmology 96:1639, 1989.
49. Boruchoff, SA, Kuwabara, T: Electron microscopy of posterior polymorphous degeneration. Am J Ophthal 72:879, 1971.
50. Johnson, BL, Brown, SI: Posterior polymorphous dystrophy: a light and electron microscopic study. Br J Ophthal 62:89, 1978.
51. Rodrigues, MM, Sun, T-T, Krachmer, J, Newsome, D: Epithelialization of the corneal endothelium in posterior polymorphous dystrophy. Invest Ophthal Vis Sci 19:832, 1980.
52. Henriquez, AS, Kenyon, KR, Dohlman, CH, et al: Morphologic characteristics of posterior polymorphous dystrophy. A study of nine corneas and review of the literature. Surv Ophthal 29:139, 1984.
53. Polack, FM, Bourne, WM, Forstot, SL, Yamaguchi, T: Scanning electron microscopy of posterior polymorphous corneal dystrophy. Am J Ophthal 89:575, 1980.
54. Richardson, WP, Hettinger, ME: Endothelial and epithelial-like cell formations in a case of posterior polymorphous dystrophy. Arch Ophthal 103:1520, 1985.
55. de Felice, GP, Braidotti, P, Viale, G, et al: Posterior polymorphous dystrophy of the cornea. An ultrastructural study. Graefe's Arch Ophthal 223:265, 1985.
56. Cibis, GW, Krachmer, JH, Phelps, CD, Weingeist, TA: Iridocorneal adhesions in posterior polymorphous dystrophy. Trans Am Acad Ophthal Otol 81:770, 1976.
57. Bourgeois, J, Shields, MB, Thresher, R: Open-angle glaucoma associated with posterior polymorphous dystrophy. A clinicopathologic study. Ophthalmology 91:420, 1984.
58. Dunn, SP, Krachmer, JH, Ching, SST: New findings in posterior amorphous corneal dystrophy. Arch Ophthal 102:236, 1984.
59. Boruchoff, SA, Weiner, MJ, Albert, DM: Recurrence of posterior polymorphous corneal dystrophy after penetrating keratoplasty. Am J Ophthal 109:323, 1990.
60. Lorenzetti, DWC, Uotila, MH, Parikh, N, Kaufman, HE: Central cornea guttata. Incidence in the general population. Am J Ophthal 64:1155, 1967.
61. Laing, RA, Leibowitz, HM, Oak, SS, et al: Endothelial mosaic in Fuch's dystrophy. A qualitative

evaluation with the specular microscope. Arch Ophthal 99:80, 1981.

62. Magovern, M, Beauchamp, GR, McTigue, JW, et al: Inheritance of Fuchs' combined dystrophy. Ophthalmology 86:1897, 1979.
63. Rodrigues, MM, Krachmer, JH, Hackett, J, et al: Fuchs' corneal dystrophy. A clinicopathologic study of the variation in corneal edema. Ophthalmology 93:789, 1986.
64. Fuchs, E: Dystrophis epithelialis corneal. Arch Ophthal 76:478, 1910.
65. Roth, SI, Stock, EL, Jutabha, R: Endothelial viral inclusions in Fuchs' corneal dystrophy. Hum Pathol 18:338, 1987.
66. Wilson, SE, Bourne, WM, Maguire, LJ, et al: Aqueous humor composition in Fuchs' dystrophy. Invest Ophthal Vis Sci 30:449, 1989.
67. Hong, C, Kandori, T, Kitazawa, Y, Tanishima, T: Corneal endothelial cells in ocular hypertension. Jap J Ophthal 26:183, 1982.
68. Bigar, F, Witmer, R: Corneal endothelial changes in primary acute angle-closure glaucoma. Ophthalmology 89:596, 1982.
69. Olsen, T: The endothelial cell damage in acute glaucoma. On the corneal thickness response to intraocular pressure. Acta Ophthal 58:257, 1980.
70. Setala, K: Response of human corneal endothelial cells to increased intraocular pressure. A specular microscopic study. Acta Ophthal (suppl) 144:547, 1980.
71. Vannas, A, Setala, K, Ruusuvaara, P: Endothelial cells in capsular glaucoma. Acta Ophthal 55:951, 1977.
72. Setala, K, Vannas, A: Endothelial cells in the glaucomato-cyclitic crisis. Adv Ophthal 36:218, 1978.
73. Kaufman, HE, Capella, JA, Robbins, JE: The human corneal endothelium. Am J Ophthal 61:835, 1966.
74. Olsen, T: Changes in the corneal endothelium after acute anterior uveitis as seen with the specular microscope. Acta Ophthal 58:250, 1980.
75. Buxton, JN, Preston, RW, Riechers, R, Guilbault, N: Tonography in cornea guttata. A preliminary report. Arch Ophthal 77:602, 1967.
76. Roberts, CW, Steinert, RF, Thomas, JV, Boruchoff, SA: Endothelial guttata and facility of aqueous outflow. Cornea 3:5, 1984.
77. Burns, RR, Bourne, WM, Brubaker, RF: Endothelial function in patients with cornea guttata. Invest Ophthal Vis Sci 20:77, 1981.
78. Stocker, FW: The Endothelium of the Cornea and Its Clinical Implications, 2nd ed. Charles C. Thomas, Springfield, Ill., 1971, p. 79.
79. Kolker, AE, Hetherington, J Jr: Becker, Shaffer's Diagnosis and Therapy of the Glaucomas, 4th ed. CV Mosby, St. Louis, 1976, pp. 265, 266.
80. Krachmer, JH, Purcell, JJ Jr, Yound, CW, Bucher, KD: Corneal endothelial dystrophy. A study of 64 families. Arch Ophthal 96:2036, 1978.
81. Waltman, SR, Palmberg, PF, Becker, B: In vitro corticosteroid sensitivity in patients with Fuchs' dystrophy. Doc Ophthal Proc Series 18:321, 1979.

Chapter 14

GLAUCOMAS ASSOCIATED WITH DISORDERS OF THE IRIS

- I. Conditions with iris disorders and associated glaucoma
- II. Pigmentary glaucoma
  - A. Terminology
  - B. General features
  - C. Clinical features
    1. Slit-lamp biomicroscopic findings
    2. Gonioscopic findings
    3. Fundus findings
    4. Clinical course of glaucoma
  - D. Theories of mechanism
    1. Mechanism of pigment dispersion
    2. Mechanism of IOP elevation
  - E. Differential diagnosis
  - F. Management
- III. Iridoschisis
  - A. General features
  - B. Clinicopathologic features
  - C. Mechanisms of glaucoma
  - D. Differential diagnosis
  - E. Management

Conditions with Iris Disorders and Associated Glaucoma

The iris is involved in many of the secondary glaucomas, either as part of the initial pathologic process or secondary to other ocular events. Most of these conditions are considered in other chapters (Table 14.1). In the present chapter, we will consider two additional conditions in which disorders involving the iris may lead to secondary glaucoma: pigmentary glaucoma and iridoschisis.

PIGMENTARY GLAUCOMA

Terminology

As a normal feature of maturation and aging, a variable amount of uveal pigment is chronically released and dispersed into the anterior ocular segment. This is best appreciated by observing the trabecular meshwork, which is nonpigmented in the infant eye but becomes progressively pigmented to variable degrees with the passage of years, as a result of the accumulation of the dispersed pigment in the aqueous outflow system. There is, therefore, a spectrum of ocular pigment dispersion within the general population. As might be anticipated, this spectrum of pigment dispersion is also found among individuals with various forms of glaucoma, although the pigment in most of these cases is not believed to be a major factor in the mechanism of the glaucoma. However, there are several ocular conditions that are associated with an unusually heavy dispersion of pigment, which may be significantly involved in the increased resistance to aqueous outflow. In 1940, Sugar[1] briefly described one such case with marked pigment dispersion and glaucoma. Sugar and Barbour[2] subsequently (1949) reported the details of this entity, which differed from other forms of pigment dispersion by typical clinical and histopathologic features. They referred to the condition as *pigmentary glaucoma*.[2] When the typical findings are encountered without associated glaucoma, the term *pigment dispersion syndrome* has been advocated.[3]

General Features

The typical patient is a young, myopic male. The disorder appears most frequently

Table 14.1.
Conditions with Iris Disorders and Associated Glaucoma

Condition	Chapter
1. Developmental defects	Chapter 12
a. Axenfeld-Rieger syndrome	
b. Peters' anomaly	
c. Aniridia	
2. Iris atrophy with corneal disease	Chapter 13
a. Iridocorneal endothelial syndrome	
b. Posterior polymorphous dystrophy	
3. Pigmentary glaucoma	Present chapter
4. Iridoschisis	Present chapter
5. Exfoliation syndrome	Chapter 15
6. Neovascular glaucoma	Chapter 16
7. Iris tumors	Chapter 18
8. Anterior uveitis	Chapter 19
9. Trauma	Chapter 22
10. Complications of intraocular surgery	Chapter 23

in the third decade, and it tends to decrease in severity or disappear in later life.[4–5] Most studies agree that the pigment dispersion syndrome is more common among men, with a male/female ratio of approximately 2:1. However, studies differ as to the ratio of men and women converting to pigmentary glaucoma,[3–11] which is considered in more detail later in this chapter. The condition is seen predominantly in Caucasians.[3–11] In one report, 20 black patients were believed to have pigmentary glaucoma on the basis of heavy pigment deposition on the corneal endothelium and trabecular meshwork. However, these patients differed from the typical pigmentary glaucoma population in that most were women, the mean age was 73 years, there was a preponderance of hyperopia, and no iris transillumination defects were noted.[12] A hereditary basis has been suggested[3,7] but has not been clearly established.

Clinical Features

Slit-Lamp Biomicroscopic Findings

Pigment dispersion occurs throughout the anterior ocular segment but is seen by slit-lamp examination primarily on the cornea and iris. *Krukenberg's spindle* is an accumulation of pigment on the posterior surface of the central cornea in a vertical spindle-shaped pattern (Fig. 14.1). Dispersed pigment is deposited on the cornea in this pattern as a result of aqueous convection currents and is then phagocytosed by adjacent endothelial cells.[3] This feature is commonly seen in eyes with pigmentary glaucoma but is neither invariable nor pathognomonic of the disorder. In one study of 43 patients with Krukenberg's spindles, only two developed field loss during a follow-up that averaged 5.8 years.[13] Krukenberg's spindle is actually more common in women[13] and

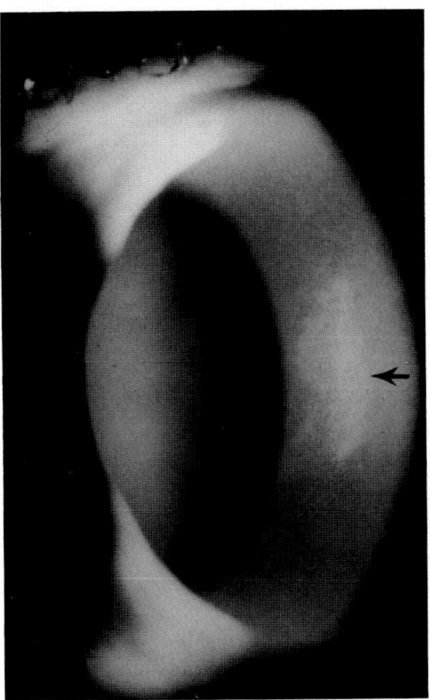

Figure 14.1. Krukenberg's spindle (*arrow*) in patient with pigmentary glaucoma.

may have a hormonal relationship.[14] Despite these corneal findings, patients with the pigment dispersion syndrome appear to have normal corneal endothelial cell counts and central corneal thickness.[15]

Pigment granules are also frequently dispersed on the stroma of the iris, which may give the iris a progressively darker appearance or create heterochromia in asymmetric cases (Fig. 14.2).[9] Other locations where pigment dispersion may be seen by slit-lamp examination include the posterior lens capsule, lens zonules, and the interior of a glaucoma filtering bleb.[9]

Iris transillumination is the most diagnostic clinical feature of pigmentary glaucoma, since it represents the source of the dispersed pigment. The characteristic appearance is a radial spoke-like pattern in the midperiphery of the iris (Fig. 14.3).[16,17] This feature can be seen during slit-lamp biomicroscopy by directing the light beam through the pupil, perpendicular to the plane of the iris, or by using scleral transillumination, and observing the retinal light reflex through the defects in the iris. In some patients, however, a dark, thick iris stroma may prevent transillumination of the defects, so that the absence of this finding does not rule out the diagnosis of pigmentary glaucoma. This could explain the absence of iris transillumination in black patients with pigmentary glaucoma.[12]

Gonioscopic Findings

The principal gonioscopic feature is a dense, homogeneous band of dark brown pigment in the full circumference of the trabecular meshwork (Fig. 14.4). The dispersed pigment may also accumulate along Schwalbe's line, especially inferiorly, creating a thin, dark band. Abundant iris processes inserting anterior to the scleral spur were also observed in one small series of patients with pigmentary glaucoma,[18] but these do not appear to be a consistent finding in this condition.

Fundus Findings

Retinal detachments are more common in this patient population,[19] occurring in 6.4% of one study.[11] Retinal pigment epithelial

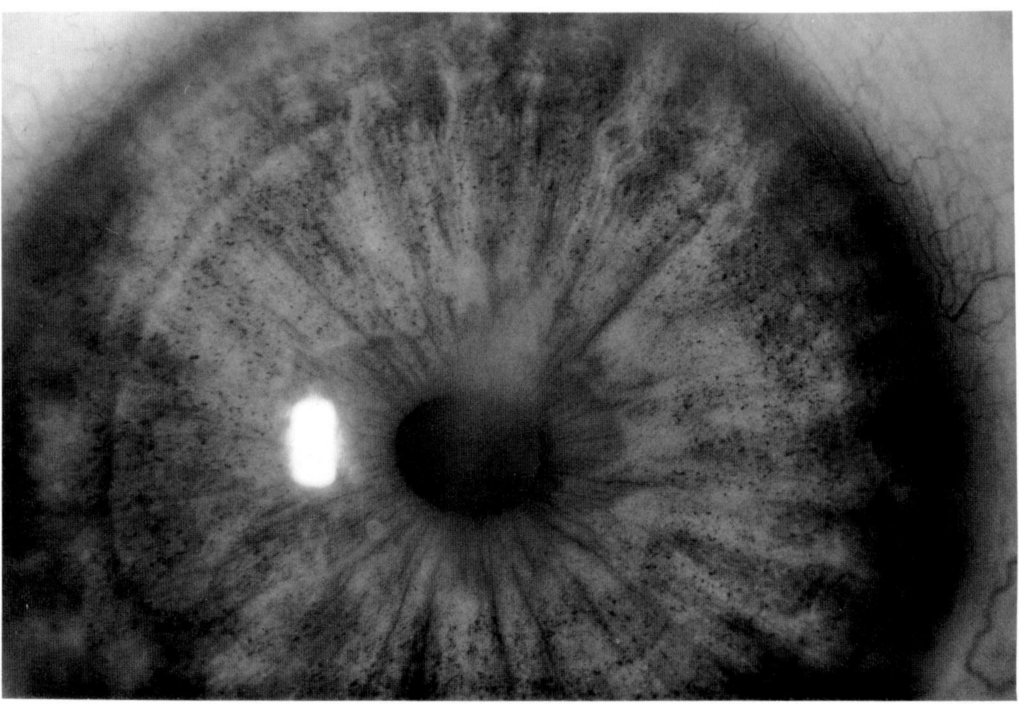

Figure 14.2. Pigment granules on iris stroma in patient with pigmentary glaucoma.

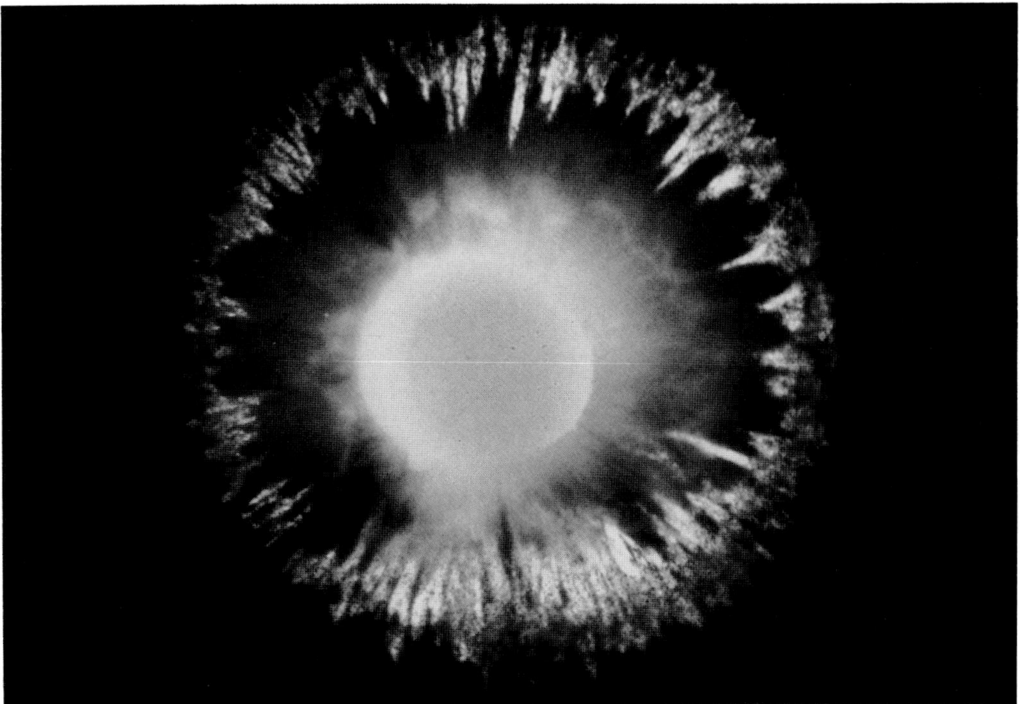

Figure 14.3. Transillumination of the iris in patient with pigmentary glaucoma showing typical peripheral spoke-like defects.

dystrophy has also been reported in two brothers with pigmentary glaucoma.[20]

Clinical Course of the Glaucoma

Patients with the pigment dispersion syndrome may go for years before developing pigmentary glaucoma or may never have a rise in intraocular pressure (IOP). In one study of 97 eyes with pigment dispersion throughout the anterior ocular segment, glaucoma was present in 42,[16] while another study of 407 patients with the dispersion syndrome revealed only one-fourth with glaucoma.[11] In a long-term study that spanned 5–35 years, 13 of 37 patients (35%) with the pigment dispersion syndrome converted to pigmentary glaucoma.[6] The glaucoma usually develops within 15 years of the presentation of the pigment dispersion syndrome, although some may take more than 20 years.[6] In another follow-up study averaging 27 months, progression of the iris transillumination and pigment dispersion could be documented in 31 of 55 patients and correlated with worsening of the glaucoma in most of these.[21] A study of 111 patients with the pigment dispersion syndrome or pigmentary glaucoma indicated that male gender, black race, high myopia, and Krukenberg spindles are risk factors for the development and severity of glaucoma within this population,[10] although another study found that sex did not influence the development or severity of the glaucoma among patients with the pigment dispersion syndrome.[6]

In some cases, the IOP may rise transiently in association with strenuous exercise or spontaneous changes in the pupillary diameter, presumably as a result of increased liberation of pigment,[22] although this does not appear to be clinically significant in most cases.[23] In those cases in which exercise-induced pigment dispersion does cause a significant IOP rise, 0.5% pilocarpine has been effective in inhibiting this phenomenon.[24] Phenylephrine-induced mydriasis will also cause a significant shower of pigment into the anterior chamber in some

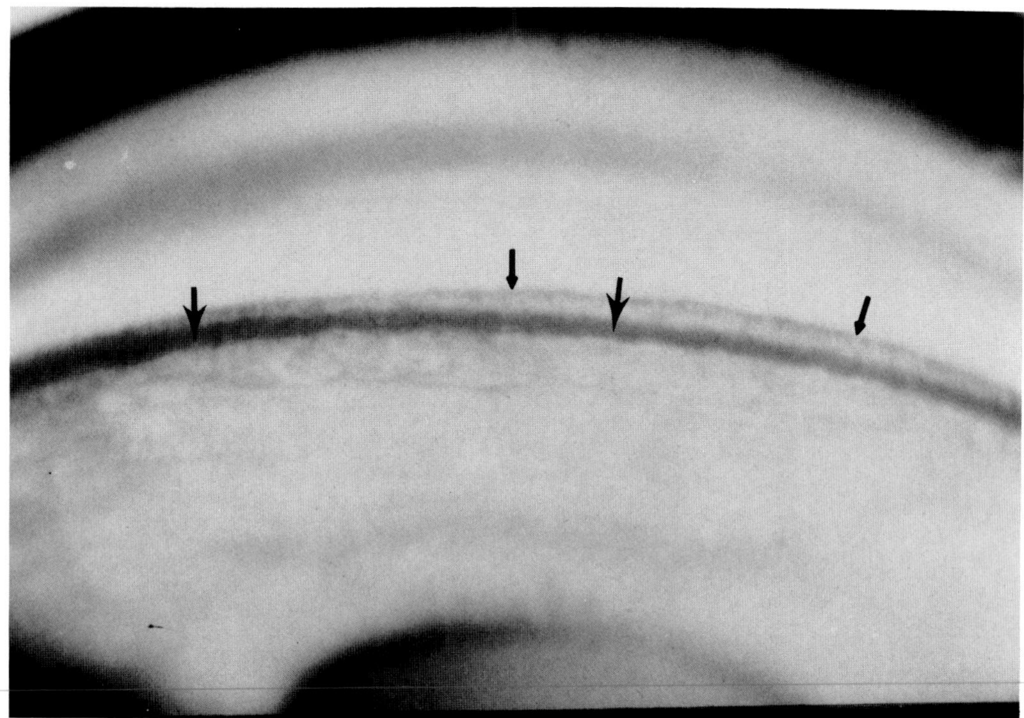

Figure 14.4. Gonioscopic view of patient with pigmentary glaucoma showing typical features of wide-open angle with dense, homogeneous pigmentation of trabecular meshwork (*large arrows*) and heavy pigment accumulation on Schwalbe's line (*small arrows*).

patients with pigmentary glaucoma or the pigment dispersion syndrome, although this transient liberation of pigment is not consistently associated with IOP elevations.[25] Once pigmentary glaucoma becomes established, it may be somewhat more difficult to control than primary open-angle glaucoma, although with increasing age there is a tendency for the condition to become less severe.

Theories of Mechanism

Two fundamental questions must be considered regarding the pathogenesis of the pigment dispersion syndrome and the mechanism of pigmentary glaucoma: (1) What are the factors leading to the pigment dispersion? and (2) How does the dispersed pigment and/or additional features cause the glaucoma?

Mechanism of Pigment Dispersion

Histopathologic observations of the iris in eyes with the pigment dispersion syndrome or pigmentary glaucoma have revealed changes in the iris pigment epithelium, which include focal atrophy and hypopigmentation, an apparent delay in melanogenesis, and a hyperplasia of the dilator muscle.[26–28] In contrast, eyes with primary open-angle glaucoma and varying degrees of pigment dispersion had minimal hypopigmentation of the iris epithelium with normal dilator muscle and melanogenesis.[28] These observations have led some observers to believe that a developmental abnormality of the iris pigment epithelium is the fundamental defect in the pigment dispersion syndrome.[26–28] The additional observation of retinal pigment epithelial dystrophy in two brothers with pigmentary glaucoma raises the possibility of an inherited defect of pigment epithelium in both the anterior and posterior ocular segments.[20] Fluorescein angiography of the iris also suggests that hypovascularity of the iris may play a role in the pigment dispersion syndrome.[29]

Campbell[30] proposed an alternative theory for the mechanism of pigment liberation from the iris. He noted that the peripheral radial defects of the iris correspond in location and number to anterior packets of lens zonules and suggested that mechanical rubbing of these zonules against the peripheral iris leads to the dispersion of pigment. This hypothesis is supported by histologic studies showing a correlation between packets of zonules and deep grooves in the iris pigment epithelium and posterior stroma (Fig. 14.5).[30,31] Sugar[7] has suggested that the radial folds of iris pigment epithelium rubbing against the lens capsule itself may be an additional mechanism of pigment release.

The mechanical theory of Campbell is also supported by biometric[32] and photogrammetric[33] studies of anterior chamber dimensions, which revealed deeper anterior chambers and flatter lenses in the involved eyes of unilateral cases,[32] and a deeper than normal midperipheral chamber depth with corresponding concavity of the iris in eyes with the pigment dispersion syndrome.[33] In addition, the mechanical theory is consistent with clinical observations and helps to explain certain features of the disease. For example, the low incidence of the condition in the nonwhite population may be due to the heavy pigmentation and compactness of the iris stroma in these individuals, which prevents posterior sagging of the midpe-

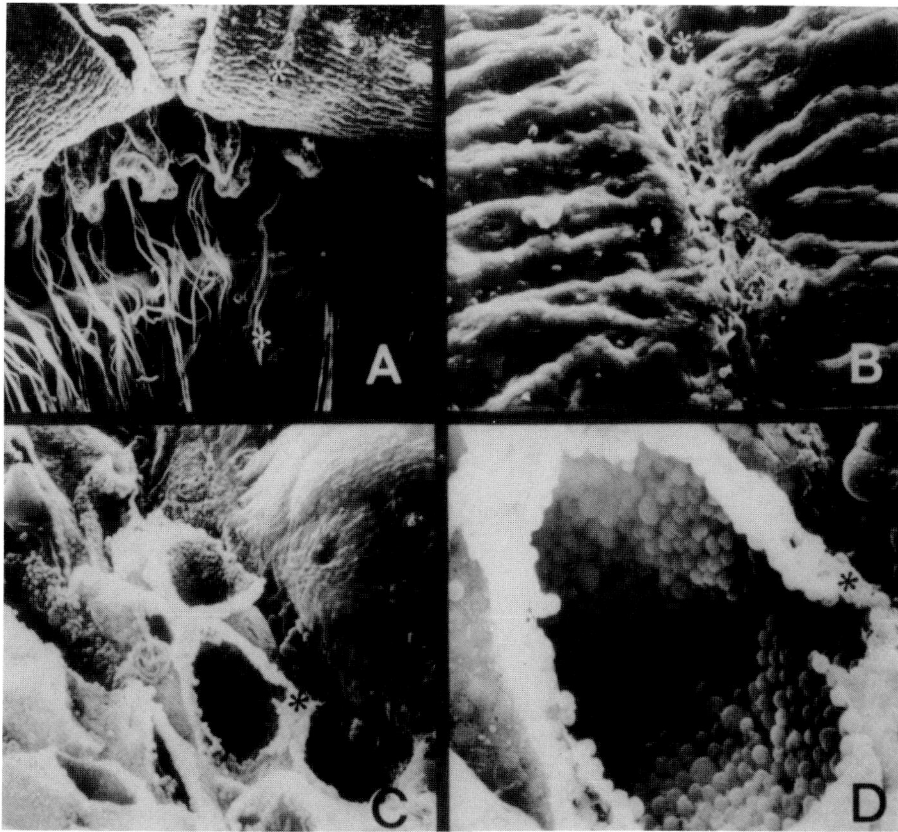

Figure 14.5. Scanning electron microscopic view of peripheral iris from patient with pigment dispersion syndrome showing: *A,* Incomplete radial defect in pigment epithelial layer of iris (*upper asterisk*) and underlying lens zonular packet (*lower asterisk*) (original magnification, ×30); *B,* Radial defect (*asterisk*) with many pigment cells (original magnification, ×260); *C,* Ruptured pigment epithelial cell (*asterisk*) in radial defect (original magnification, ×1300); *D,* Pigment granules lining ruptured cell (*asterisk*) (original magnification, ×4500). (Reprinted with permission from Campbell DG: Arch Ophthal 97:1667, 1979.)

ripheral iris.[34] Furthermore, the tendency for the disease to ameliorate with increasing age may be due to increasing axial length of the lens, which pulls the peripheral iris away from the zonules.[5,30] A case has also been reported in which subluxation of the lens apparently caused remission of pigmentary glaucoma.[35]

The mechanical theory, however, does not fully explain why all eyes with myopia are not subject to the pigment dispersion syndrome, and it may be that additional iris defects, as previously discussed, are necessary for the syndrome to become manifest.

Mechanism of IOP Elevation

In 1963, Grant[36] demonstrated that pigment granules perfused in human autopsy eyes caused a significant obstruction to aqueous outflow. Clinical studies have also shown that pigment release resulting from pharmacologically-induced movement of the iris causes a transient pressure rise in some eyes.[25,37] However, perfusion of living monkey eyes with uveal pigment particles caused only a transient obstruction to aqueous outflow, suggesting that other or additional factors must be involved in the mechanism of pigmentary glaucoma.[38] Histopathologic studies of eyes with pigmentary glaucoma have revealed excessive amounts of pigment granules and cell debris in the trabecular meshwork,[28,39–41] associated with variable degrees of trabecular endothelial cell degeneration (Fig. 14.6).[40,41] Based on these observations, it is generally held that dispersion of pigment into the trabecular meshwork with subsequent alteration of the trabecular beams leads to the elevation of IOP in pigmentary glaucoma.

An alternative theory suggests that a primary developmental anomaly of the ante-

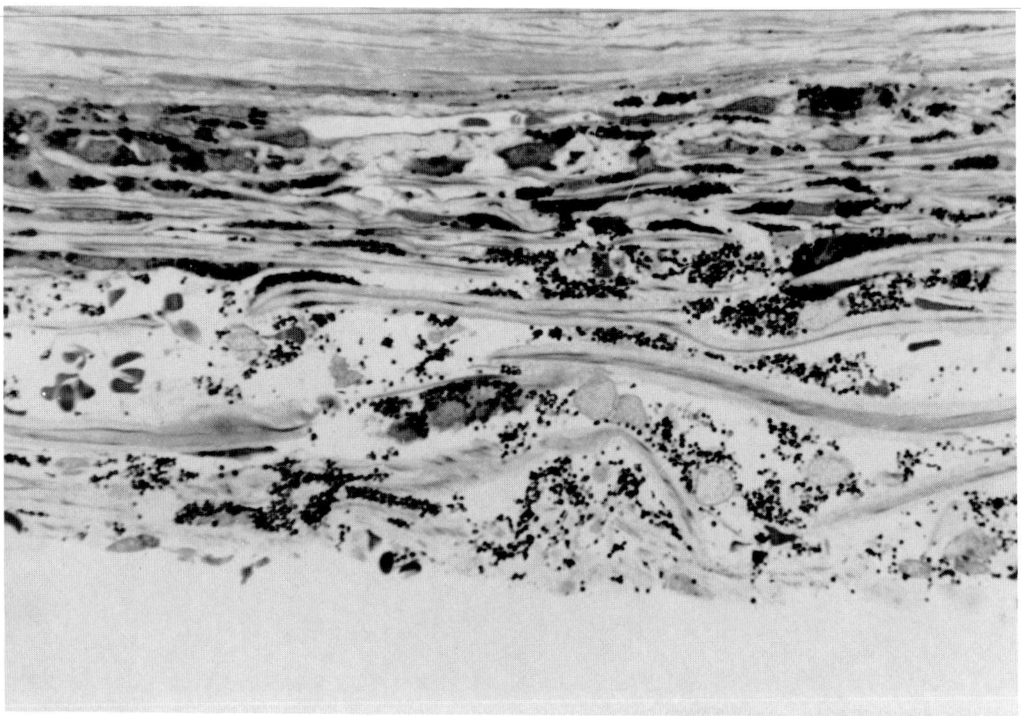

Figure 14.6. Light microscopic view of trabecular meshwork from patient with pigmentary glaucoma showing free pigment granules primarily in the uveal meshwork and in the inner portion of the corneoscleral meshwork, with intracellular pigment in the deeper portions of the meshwork. (Reprinted with permission from Richardson TM: Pigmentary Glaucoma, in The Secondary Glaucomas, ed. Ritch R, Shields, MB, St. Louis, The CV Mosby Co., 1982.)

rior chamber angle may lead to aqueous outflow obstruction.[9] This is based on the previously described abundant iris processes that have been seen in some cases.[18,28] However, this is not a consistent finding and probably plays little, if any, role in the mechanism of pigmentary glaucoma.

A third hypothesis has been that pigmentary glaucoma may be a variation of primary open-angle glaucoma. This theory was derived from observations that both primary open-angle glaucoma and pigmentary glaucoma may be seen in the same family.[18,42] In one study, individuals with Krukenberg's spindles had topical corticosteroid responses that were similar to those seen among close relatives of patients with primary open-angle glaucoma.[42] However, patients with pigmentary glaucoma were not found to have the same corticosteroid sensitivity to in vitro inhibition of lymphocyte transformation as do primary open-angle glaucoma patients.[43] HLA antigen testing reportedly revealed differences between the pigment dispersion syndrome, pigmentary glaucoma, and primary open-angle glaucoma,[44] but another study showed no significant difference among patients with pigmentary glaucoma, the pigment dispersion syndrome, and normal controls.[45] The bulk of the current evidence suggests that pigmentary glaucoma and primary open-angle glaucoma are separate entities.

Differential Diagnosis

As noted at the outset of this chapter, there are several disorders in which an excessive dispersion of pigment may be associated with glaucoma, either with or without a cause-and-effect relationship. These conditions constitute the differential diagnosis for pigmentary glaucoma. One such condition is the exfoliation syndrome (Chapter 15), in which rubbing between the midperipheral lens and peripupillary iris leads to the pigment dispersion. This condition is usually distinguished from pigmentary glaucoma by the typical lens appearance and older age of the patients, although the two conditions have been reported to occur together.[46] Other conditions associated with increased anterior segment pigmentation and glaucoma include some forms of uveitis (Chapter 19), trauma (Chapter 22), ocular melanosis and melanoma (Chapter 18), complications of intraocular surgery (Chapter 23) and primary open-angle glaucoma with excessive pigment dispersion (Chapter 9).

Management

The mechanical theory of Campbell[30] suggests that measures to eliminate contact between the iris and lens zonules would be the most appropriate management for pigmentary glaucoma. Pilocarpine may accomplish this but is usually not tolerated by the young myope because of further induced myopia. The alpha-adrenergic blocker *thymoxamine* may be useful, since it produces miosis without cyclotonia,[30] but it is not available at present in the United States. Pilocarpine in an ocular insert delivery system or gel may provide the desired miosis and improved facility of outflow without excessive induced myopia in these patients. Risk factors for the development and severity of pigmentary glaucoma within populations of patients with the pigment dispersion syndrome, as previously discussed,[10] may help to identify which patients with the syndrome require closer follow-up or the possible initiation of prophylactic miotic therapy. When using miotics in patients with pigmentary glaucoma, special attention must be given to the risk of retinal detachment, which is more common in this population.[19]

Alternative medications to miotic therapy include beta-adrenergic blockers, epinephrine compounds, and carbonic anhydrase inhibitors. When the glaucoma can no longer be controlled medically, laser trabeculoplasty is usually indicated. Patients with pigmentary glaucoma respond well initially to the laser treatment, although the long-term results appear to be poor in patients who are older (e.g., 50s as compared with 30s) or who have had the glaucoma for a longer period of time (10 years as compared with 2–3 years).[47]

When both medical therapy and laser surgery have failed, glaucoma filtering surgery is usually indicated. A higher percentage of patients with pigmentary glaucoma require surgery, as compared with those with primary open-angle glaucoma, and men appear to require it at a much earlier age than women.[10,11]

IRIDOSCHISIS

General Features

Iridoschisis is an uncommon condition and, in contrast to the young age of onset in pigmentary glaucoma, usually appears in the sixth or seventh decade of life, although a case has been reported in a child with associated microphthalmos.[48] The hallmark is a bilateral separation of the layers of iris stroma, typically in the inferior quadrants. The disorder is complicated by glaucoma in approximately half the cases. Corneal edema is also an occasional sequela. Most cases are not associated with other ocular disorders, although concomitant conditions may be seen, such as an elderly patient with coexisting syphilitic interstitial keratitis.[49]

Clinicopathologic Features

Slit-lamp biomicroscopic examination typically reveals sheets or strands of iris stroma that have partly separated from the rest of the iris, especially in the inferior quadrants (Fig. 14.7). In some cases, the loose tissue may touch the corneal endothelium with edema of the cornea. By gonioscopy, the strands of iris tissue may obscure visualization of the anterior chamber angle.

Histopathologic studies of involved iris revealed marked atrophy of the iris stroma with scant or absent collagen fibrils in the area of separation, although there was no evidence of vascular or neural alterations.[50] Specular microscopy of the corneal endothelium has revealed a marked decrease in cell density and a high degree of polymegathism (abnormality in size and shape of cells) in the area directly over the iridoschisis.[51] Histopathology of a corneal button, removed as a result of bullous keratopathy, showed degeneration and focal loss of endothelial cells, patchy posterior banding (110 nm) of Descemet's membrane with irregular connective tissue, and stromal and epithelial edema.[50]

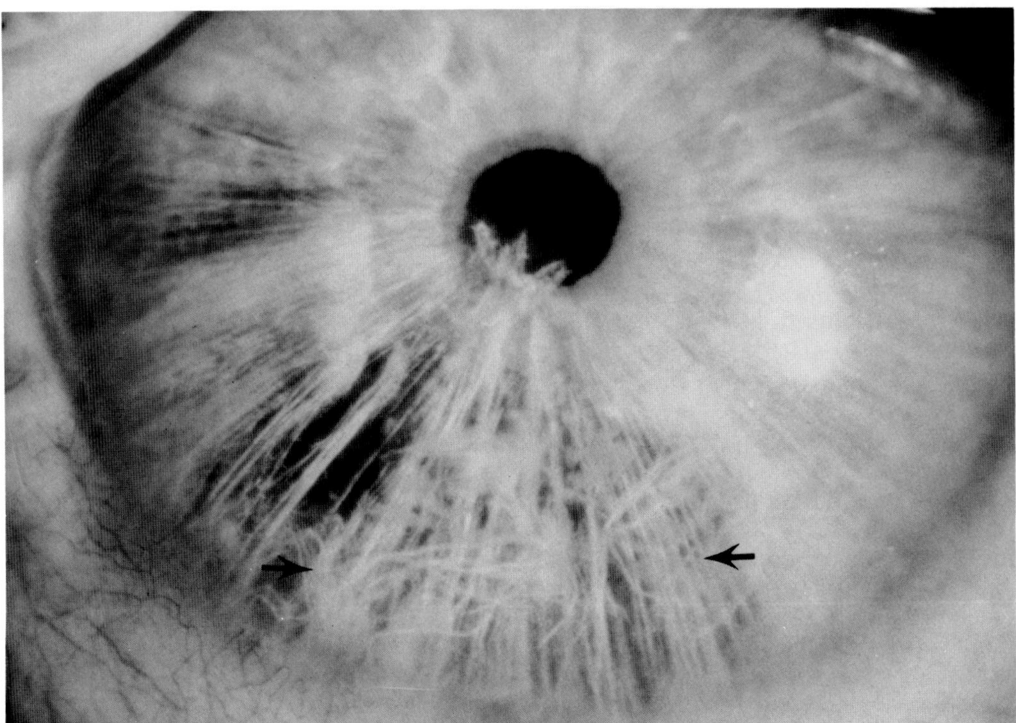

Figure 14.7. Slit-lamp view of patient with iridoschisis showing characteristic strands of iris stroma (*arrows*) that have partly separated from the rest of the iris in the inferior quadrant.

Mechanisms of Glaucoma

Some patients with iridoschisis and glaucoma have angle closure, and it is presumed that a pupillary block mechanism is present, since an iridectomy results in deepening of the anterior chamber.[50] In other patients, the angle is open, in which case the meshwork is apparently obstructed either by release of pigment from the iris or by the shredded iris stroma.[50]

Differential Diagnosis

The main conditions that must be distinguished from iridoschisis are other causes of iris stromal dissolution, such as the iridocorneal endothelial syndrome and Axenfeld-Rieger syndrome, both of which differ from iridoschisis by a much earlier age of onset. It should also be noted that trauma can lead to disruption of the iris, creating clinical findings that resemble iridoschisis. In one patient with iridoschisis, strands of iris floating in the anterior chamber after a trabeculectomy were mistaken for a fungal infection.[52]

Management

Cases with an angle-closure mechanism of glaucoma should be treated with a laser iridotomy, or with conventional surgical iridectomy if corneal edema prevents laser surgery. The open-angle form of glaucoma can be controlled medically in some cases, using an approach similar to that for primary open-angle glaucoma, while other patients require glaucoma filtering surgery.

SUMMARY

Pigmentary glaucoma is typically seen in young adult myopes, with a slight predilection for males. The ocular configuration in these individuals apparently leads to rubbing between the iris and lens zonules that causes liberation of pigment granules. This can be seen clinically as transillumination defects in the peripheral iris and as deposition of the dispersed pigment on the corneal endothelium, iris stroma, and other anterior ocular structures. However, it is in the trabecular meshwork where the accumulation of pigment and subsequent alteration of the trabecular beams leads to a severe form of secondary glaucoma. Another condition, iridoschisis, is an uncommon affliction of the elderly, characterized by a separation of layers of iris stroma with occasional associated glaucoma.

References

1. Sugar, HS: Concerning the chamber angle. I. Gonioscopy. Am J Ophthal 23:853, 1940.
2. Sugar, HS, Barbour, FA: Pigmentary glaucoma. A rare clinical entity. Am J Ophthal 32:90, 1949.
3. Sugar, HS: Pigmentary glaucoma. A 25-year review. Am J Ophthal 62:499, 1966.
4. Speakman, JS: Pigmentary dispersion. Br J Ophthal 65:249, 1981.
5. Ritch, R: Nonprogressive low-tension glaucoma with pigmentary dispersion. Am J Ophthal 94:190, 1982.
6. Migliazzo, CV, Shaffer, RN, Nykin, R, Magee, S: Long-term analysis of pigmentary dispersion syndrome and pigmentary glaucoma. Ophthalmology 93:1528, 1986.
7. Sugar, S: Pigmentary glaucoma and the glaucoma associated with the exfoliation-pseudoexfoliation syndrome: update. Ophthalmology 91:307, 1984.
8. Lichter, PR, Shaffer, RN: Diagnostic and prognostic signs in pigmentary glaucoma. Trans Am Acad Ophthal Otolar 74:984, 1970.
9. Lichter, PR: Pigmentary glaucoma—current concepts. Trans Am Acad Ophthal Otol 78:309, 1974.
10. Farrar, SM, Shields, MB, Miller, KN, Stoup, CM: Risk factors for the development and severity of glaucoma in the pigment dispersion syndrome. Am J Ophthal 108:223, 1989.
11. Scheie, HG, Cameron, JD: Pigment dispersion syndrome: a clinical study. Br J Ophthal 65:264, 1981.
12. Semple, HC, Ball, SF: Pigmentary glaucoma in the black population. Am J Ophthal 109:518, 1990.
13. Wilensky, JT, Buerk, KM, Podos, SM: Krukenberg's spindles. Am J Ophthal 79:220, 1975.
14. Duncan, TE: Krukenberg spindles in pregnancy. Arch Ophthal 91:355, 1974.
15. Murrell, WJ, Shihab, Z, Lamberts, DW, Avera, B: The corneal endothelium and central corneal thickness in pigmentary dispersion syndrome. Arch Ophthal 104:845, 1986.
16. Scheie, HG, Fleischhauer, HW: Idiopathic atrophy of the epithelial layers of the iris and ciliary body. A clinical study. Arch Ophthal 59:216, 1958.
17. Donaldson, DD: Transillumination of the iris. Trans Am Ophthal Soc LXXII:89, 1974.
18. Lichter, PR, Shaffer, RN: Iris processes and glaucoma. Am J Ophthal 70:905, 1970.
19. Delaney, WV Jr: Equatorial lens pigmentation,

myopia, and retinal detachment. Am J Ophthal 79:194, 1975.

20. Piccolino, FC, Calabria, G. Polizzi, A. Fioretto, M: Pigmentary retinal dystrophy associated with pigmentary glaucoma. Graefe's Arch Ophthal 227:335, 1989.
21. Richter, CU, Richardson, TM, Grant, WM: Pigmentary dispersion syndrome and pigmentary glaucoma. A prospective study of the natural history. Arch Ophthal 104:211, 1986.
22. Schenker, HI, Luntz, MH, Kels, B, Podos, SM: Exercise-induced increase of intraocular pressure in the pigmentary dispersion syndrome. Am J Ophthal 89:598, 1980.
23. Smith, DL, Kao, SF, Rabbani, R, Musch, DC: The effects of exercise on intraocular pressure in pigmentary glaucoma patients. Ophthalmic Surg 20:561, 1989.
24. Haynes, WL, Johnson, AT, Alward, WLM: Inhibition of exercise-induced pigment dispersion in a patient with the pigmentary dispersion syndrome. Am J Ophthal 109:601, 1990.
25. Epstein, DL, Boger, WP III, Grant, WM: Phenylephrine provocative testing in the pigmentary dispersion syndrome. Am J Ophthal 85:43, 1978.
26. Fine, BS, Yanoff, M, Scheie, HG: Pigmentary "glaucoma." A histologic study. Trans Am Acad Ophthal Otol 78:314, 1974.
27. Kupfer, C, Kuwabara, T, Kaiser-Kupfer, M: The histopathology of pigmentary dispersion syndrome with glaucoma. Am J Ophthal 80:857, 1975.
28. Rodrigues, MM, Spaeth, GL, Weinreb, S, Sivalingam, E: Spectrum of trabecular pigmentation in open-angle glaucoma: a clinicopathologic study. Trans Am Acad Ophthal Otol 81:258, 1976.
29. Gillies, WE, Tangas, C: Fluorescein angiography of the iris in anterior segment pigment dispersal syndrome. Br J Ophthal 70:284, 1986.
30. Campbell, DG: Pigmentary dispersion and glaucoma. A new theory. Arch Ophthal 97:1667, 1979.
31. Kampik, A, Green, WR, Quigley, HA, Pierce, LH: Scanning and transmission electron microscopic studies of two cases of pigment dispersion syndrome. Am J Ophthal 91:573, 1981.
32. Strasser, G, Hauff, W: Pigmentary dispersion syndrome. A biometric study. Acta Ophthal 63:721, 1985.
33. Davidson, JA, Brubaker, RF, Ilstrup, DM: Dimensions of the anterior chamber in pigment dispersion syndrome. Arch Ophthal 101:81, 1983.
34. Richardson, TM: Pigmentary glaucoma. In: The Secondary Glaucomas, Ritch, R, Shields, MB, eds. CV Mosby, St. Louis, 1982.
35. Ritch, R, Manusow, D, Podos, SM: Remission of pigmentary glaucoma in a patient with subluxed lenses. Am J Ophthal 94:812, 1982.
36. Grant, WM: Experimental aqueous perfusion in enucleated human eyes. Arch Ophthal 69:783, 1963.
37. Mapstone, R: Pigment release. Br J Ophthal 65:258, 1981.
38. Epstein, DL, Freddo, TF, Anderson, PJ, et al: Experimental obstruction to aqueous outflow by pigment particles in living monkeys. Invest Ophthal Vis Sci 27:387, 1986.
39. Rodrigues, MM, Spaeth, GL, Sivalingam, E, Weinreb, S: Value of trabeculectomy specimens in glaucoma. Ophthal Surg 9:29, 1978.
40. Richardson, TM, Hutchinson, BT, Grant, WM: The outflow tract in pigmentary glaucoma. A light and electron microscopic study. Arch Ophthal 95:1015, 1977.
41. Shimizu, T, Hara, K, Futa, R: Fine structure of trabecular meshwork and iris in pigmentary glaucoma. Graefe's Arch Ophthal 215:171, 1981.
42. Becker, B, Podos, SM: Krukenberg's spindles and primary open-angle glaucoma. Arch Ophthal 76:635, 1966.
43. Zink, HA, Palmberg, PF, Sugar, A, et al: Comparison of in vitro corticosteroid response in pigmentary glaucoma and primary open-angle glaucoma. Am J Ophthal 80:478, 1975.
44. Becker, B, Shin, DH, Cooper, DG, Kass, MA: The pigment dispersion syndrome. Am J Ophthal 83:161, 1977.
45. Kaiser-Kupfer, MI, Mittal, KK: The HLA and ABO antigens in pigment dispersion syndrome. Am J Ophthal 85:368, 1978.
46. Layden, WE, Ritch, R, King, DG, Teekhasaenee, C: Combined exfoliation and pigment dispersion syndrome. Am J Ophthal 109:530, 1990.
47. Lunde, MW: Argon laser trabeculoplasty in pigmentary dispersion syndrome with glaucoma. Am J Ophthal 96:721, 1983.
48. Summers, CG, Doughman, DJ, Letson, RD, Lufkin, M: Juvenile iridoschisis and microphthalmos. Am J Ophthal 100:437, 1985.
49. Pearson, PA, Amrien, JM, Baldwin, LB, Smith, TJ: Iridoschisis associated with syphilitic interstitial keratitis. Am J Ophthal 107:88, 1989.
50. Rodrigues, MM, Spaeth, GL, Krachmer, JH, Laibson, PR: Iridoschisis associated with glaucoma and bullous keratopathy. Am J Ophthal 95:73, 1983.
51. Weseley, AC, Freeman, WR: Iridoschisis and the corneal endothelium. Ann Ophthal 15:955, 1983.
52. Zimmerman, TJ, Dabezies, OH Jr, Kaufman, HE: Iridoschisis: a case report. Ann Ophthal 13:297, 1981.

Chapter 15

GLAUCOMAS ASSOCIATED WITH DISORDERS OF THE LENS

Several disorders of the crystalline lens are associated with various forms of glaucoma. In some cases, such as the exfoliation syndrome, a cause-and-effect relationship between the lenticular abnormality and the glaucoma is uncertain. In other situations, including some forms of dislocated lenses and cataracts, the glaucoma clearly results from the alteration of the lens.

THE EXFOLIATION SYNDROME

Terminology

In 1917, Lindberg[1] described cases of chronic glaucoma in which flakes of whitish material adhered to the pupillary border of the iris. Subsequent study revealed that this material is derived, at least in part, from exfoliation of the anterior lens capsule. Two types of exfoliation have now been distinguished, which has led to confusion with the nomenclature.

Capsular Delamination

In this condition, superficial layers of lens capsule separate from the deeper capsular layers to form scroll-like margins and occasionally to float in the anterior chamber as thin, clear membranes (Fig. 15.1). Elschnig[2] first described this condition in glassblowers, leading to the term "glassblower's cataracts", and it was subsequently found that extended exposure to infrared radiation in a variety of occupations was the responsible element. The condition is uncommon since the widespread use of protective goggles by exposed workers, although clinically similar cases may be seen in association with trauma[3] and intraocular inflammation,[4] and idiopathically, usually with advanced

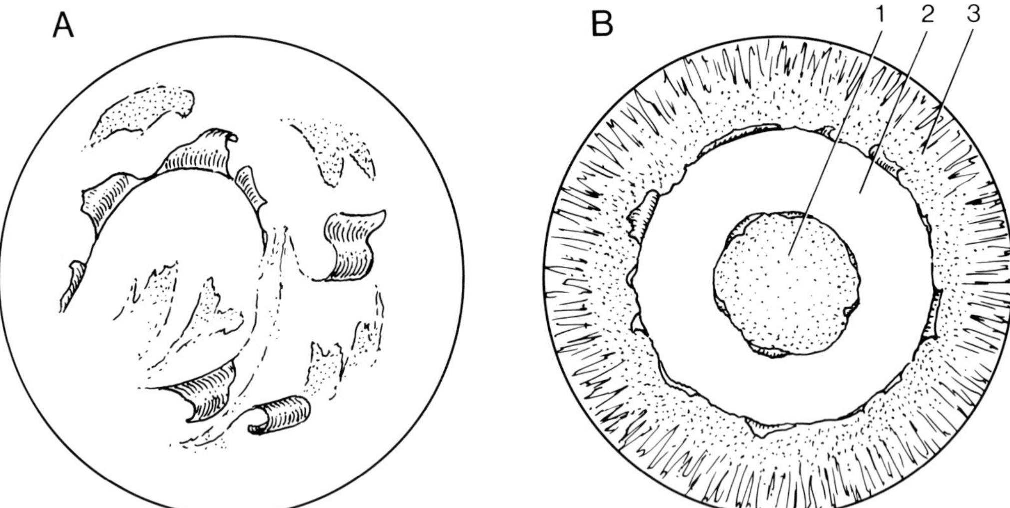

Figure 15.1. Two types of exfoliation of the anterior lens capsule. **A,** Capsular delamination, characterized by thin, clear membranes separating from the anterior lens capsule and often curling at the margins. **B,** The exfoliation syndrome, with three distinct zones: (*1*) central, translucent disc; (*2*) clear zone; and (*3*) peripheral granular zone, often with radial striations.

age.[5–7] Glaucoma is not a common feature of this disorder. The condition has been called *capsular delamination* or *exfoliation of the lens capsule,* and Dvorak-Theobald[8] suggested the term *true exfoliation of the lens capsule* to distinguish it from the condition to be discussed next.

The Exfoliation Syndrome

Vogt,[9] in 1925, described what he believed to be a senile form of capsular delamination, which he called "senile exfoliation." In addition to occurring in an older patient population, this condition differs from the other forms of exfoliation of the lens capsule in clinical appearance (Fig. 15.1) as well as in a frequent association with glaucoma.[9,10] Dvorak-Theobald[8] believed that this disorder is not a true exfoliation of the lens capsule but rather represents precipitates of an unknown substance that are deposited on the anterior lens capsule and other structures in the anterior ocular segment. She recommended the term "pseudo-exfoliation of the lens capsule" to distinguish the condition from capsular delamination, or "true" exfoliation, and the term *pseudoexfoliation syndrome* is commonly used in modern literature. However, more recent ultrastructural studies have suggested that the exfoliative material on the lens capsule is derived, at least in part, from the lens, and it has been proposed that this entity be called *the exfoliation syndrome.*[11–13] Both terms, pseudoexfoliation syndrome and exfoliation syndrome, are still commonly used in current literature. Glaucoma is not always present in eyes with this disorder, but when it does occur in association with the exfoliation syndrome, the condition has been called *capsular glaucoma.*

Epidemiology

Reports vary considerably regarding the prevalence of the exfoliation syndrome, apparently because of differences within the populations that have been studied. Geographic and ethnic differences appear to be important factors, with high prevalences in Scandinavian countries[14–17] and among people of Mediterranean origin.[18] However, considerable geographic variation exists even within countries; for example, three municipalities in middle-Norway had prevalences ranging from 10–21% among persons more than 64 years old.[17] In the United States, the exfoliation syndrome is less common, with one study revealing a prevalence of 1.6% for a population more than 30 years of age and 3.2% for those beyond 60 years,[19] and another showing 0.67% for ages 52–64, 2.6% for 65–74, and 5.0% for 75–85 years.[20]

The reported prevalence of exfoliation syndrome among patients with open-angle glaucoma also shows considerable geographic variation, with 26% in Denmark,[14] 75% in Sweden,[15] and 60% in Norway,[21], compared with reports of 1%,[22] 3%,[12], 6%,[19] and 12%[23] in the United States.

General Features

As noted above, the exfoliation syndrome is more common in older age groups, with most cases occurring in the late 60s and early 70s. The influence of race differs among geographic populations. In South Africa, the exfoliation syndrome was found in 20% of black patients with open-angle glaucoma, compared with 1.4% of the whites in that country,[24] whereas a study in southern Louisiana revealed a prevalance of 0.3% in blacks and 2.0% in whites.[22] The reported influence of sex is also conflicting, with one study showing a preponderance of women[25] and two others of men,[26,27] while most suggest no sex predilection. One study suggested that men may have higher intraocular pressures (IOP) than women with capsular glaucoma.[28] No hereditary pattern has been clearly established for the exfoliation syndrome, and two studies gave conflicting results with regard to a positive correlation with HLA typing.[29,30] A study of married couples showed a higher than expected prevalence among both spouses, suggesting a possible environmental influence.[31] The condition may be unilateral or bilateral, and some unilateral cases will become bilateral with time.[23,25,32]

Clinical Features

Lens Changes

The characteristic appearance of exfoliation material on the anterior lens capsule has three distinct zones (Fig. 15.2): (1) a translucent, central disc with occasional curled up edges; (2) a clear zone, possibly corresponding to contact with the moving iris; and (3) a peripheral granular zone, which may have radial striations.[12] The central zone is not always present, but the peripheral defect is a consistent finding, and the pupil must be dilated before the lens changes can be seen in some cases. Cataracts occur frequently in eyes with the exfoliation syndrome.[20,23,26,28] While this may be, at least in part, a function of the age of the patient population, cataracts in eyes with the exfoliation syndrome have been observed to differ from those without associated diseases by a higher percentage of nuclear cataracts and fewer cortical and supranuclear cataracts in the former group.[33] Phakodonesis and subluxation of the lens may also be seen in some patients, which is apparently due to degenerative changes in the zonular fibers of these individuals.[34]

Iris Changes

Exfoliation material may also be seen as white flecks on the pupillary margin of the iris, with loss of pigment at the pupillary ruff.[35] Iris transillumination typically reveals a "moth-eaten" pattern near the pupillary sphincter,[12,35] and a significant percentage of patients also have diffuse midperipheral transillumination defects[36] (Fig. 15.3). Additional iris changes that may be seen on routine slit-lamp examination include a whorl-like pattern of pigment particles on the iris sphincter and pigment deposition on the peripheral iris.[35] Fluorescein angiographic studies of the iris have revealed hypoperfusion, peripupillary leakage, and neovascularization.[37,38] These findings are more pronounced with increasing age of the patient and duration of the disease and the presence of glaucoma, and they probably represent a secondary feature of the disease.[38] An ultrastructural study suggests that the changes may be due to obstruction of iris vessels causing tissue hypoxia.[39]

Other Slit-Lamp Findings

Exfoliation material may also be seen on lens zonules and on the anterior hyaloid in aphakic eyes.[40] Specular microscopy of the corneal endothelium has revealed a significantly lower than normal cell density in eyes with the exfoliation syndrome.[41] In addi-

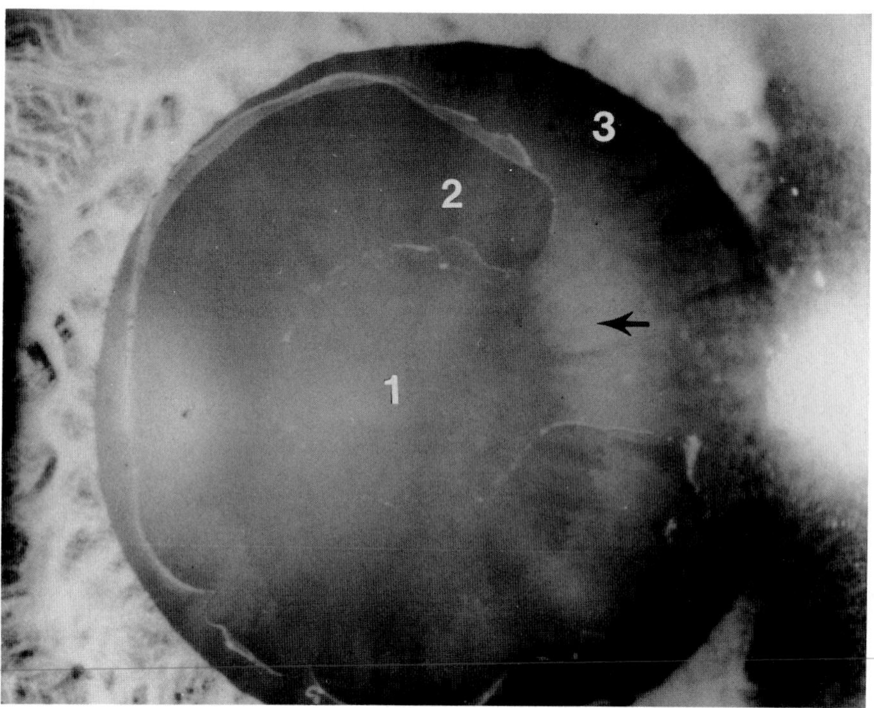

Figure 15.2. Slit-lamp view of lens in patient with the exfoliation syndrome showing three zones on the anterior lens capsule: (*1*) central, translucent disc; (*2*) middle clear zone except for bridge between central and peripheral zones (*arrow*); (*3*) peripheral granular zone with radial striations. (Reprinted with permission from Layden WE: Exfoliation syndrome. In: The Secondary Glaucomas, ed. Ritch R, Shields MB, St. Louis, The CV Mosby Co., 1982.)

tion, significant morphologic changes in cell size and shape have been observed in both the affected and unaffected eye of unilateral cases, and the authors suggested that these corneal endothelial changes might serve as an early sign of the disorder.[41]

Gonioscopic Findings

The exfoliation syndrome is associated with excessive pigment dispersion, which leads to increased trabecular meshwork pigmentation. The pigmentation of the meshwork has a more uneven distribution than that seen in pigmentary glaucoma and may be associated with flecks of exfoliation material (Fig. 15.4). An accumulation of pigment may also be seen along Schwalbe's line (*Sampaolesi's line*). In eyes with marked asymmetry of meshwork pigmentation, glaucoma is more common in the more pigmented eye.[42] However, increased pigmentation of the trabecular meshwork has also been observed in the fellow eye without exfoliation, and it has been suggested that this may be the earliest detectable sign of the exfoliation syndrome.[42] Although the anterior chamber depth is typically normal in eyes with the exfoliation syndrome,[43] the anterior chamber angle is narrow in a high percentage of cases. In one study of 76 patients with the exfoliation syndrome, 18% had angles that were considered to be occludable, and 14% had evidence of angle closure on the basis of peripheral anterior synechiae.[42] When the ciliary processes can be visualized by a special gonioscopic technique (cycloscopy), the exfoliation material may be seen on these structures.[44]

Course of the Glaucoma

As previously noted, not all patients with the exfoliation syndrome develop glau-

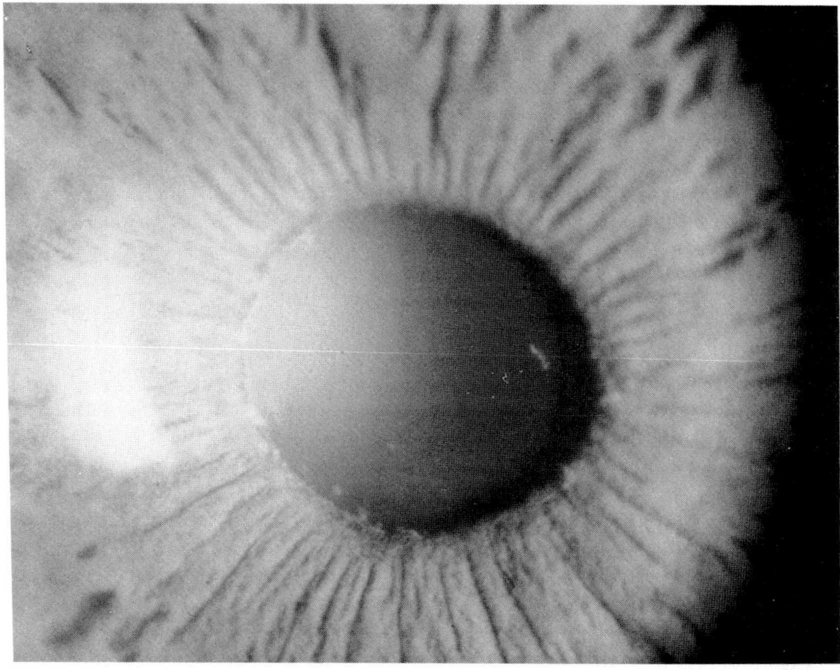

Figure 15.3. Slit-lamp view of iris in patient with the exfoliation syndrome showing white flecks of exfoliative material on the pupillary margin and loss of pigment at the pupillary ruff.

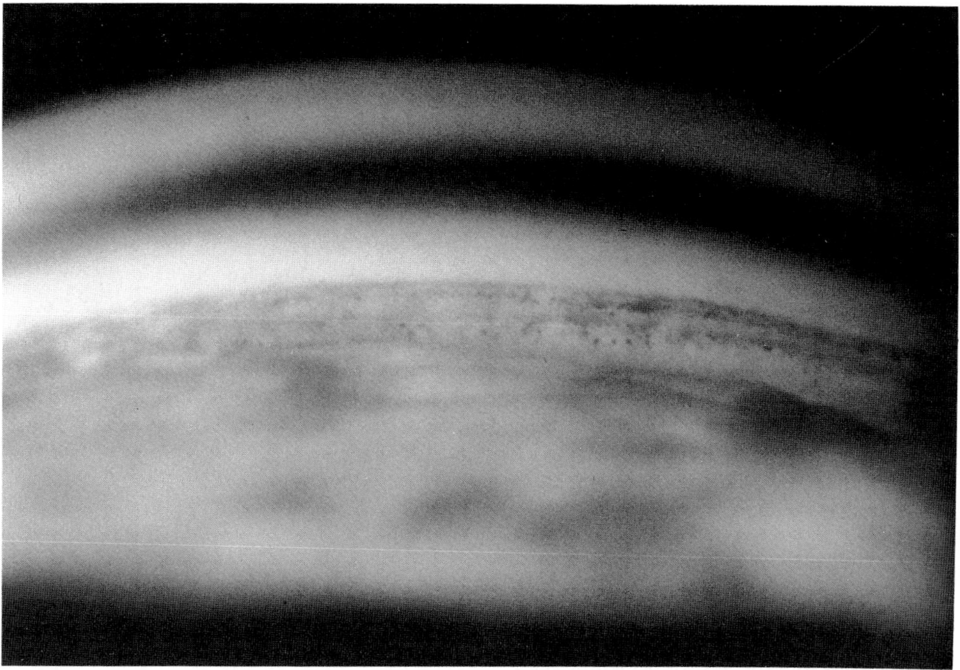

Figure 15.4. Gonioscopic view of eye with exfoliation syndrome showing irregular pigmentation of trabecular meshwork and white flecks of exfoliative material.

coma, and reports vary considerably regarding the frequency of glaucoma in eyes with this condition. Sugar[45] found elevated IOP in 55% of 643 cases in the literature and in 81.8% of his own series. A study of 100 consecutive patients with the exfoliation syndrome revealed 22% with pressure elevations, only one-third of whom had glaucomatous damage,[25] while another series of 518 patients had more than half with glaucoma.[46] In one study of patients with the exfoliation syndrome but without glaucoma on the initial examination, one-third developed glaucoma during a 1.5 year follow-up.[47] Some patients with bilateral exfoliation syndrome will have glaucoma in both eyes, while others will have a pressure rise in only one of the eyes with exfoliation. Less commonly, a patient with unilateral exfoliation may have open-angle glaucoma in both eyes.[15]

Most eyes with capsular glaucoma have an open-angle mechanism, although acute angle closure glaucoma also occurs in a small number of cases.[12,23,46,48] It is not uncommon for a patient to present with an acute onset of high IOP, although the majority of these will have open angles. In one series of 139 exfoliation syndrome patients presenting with acute glaucoma, 86 had open angles, 18 had angle closure, 21 had neovascular glaucoma, and 14 had absolute glaucoma.[48] Once open-angle glaucoma has developed in an eye with exfoliation, the IOP tends to run higher[49] and may be more difficult to control than in cases of primary open-angle glaucoma.[50]

Histopathologic Features and Theories of Mechanism

Questions that must be considered regarding the pathogenesis of the exfoliation syndrome include: (1) the nature and source of the exfoliation material; (2) the mechanism of the associated pigment dispersion; and (3) how these factors contribute to elevation of the IOP.

The Exfoliation Material

Nature. The ultrastructural appearance of the exfoliation material is that of a fibrillar protein,[51] arranged in an irregular meshwork and occasionally coiled as spirals.[52] The material has staining characteristics of oxytalan, a microtubular component of connective and elastic tissues,[53–55] and immunoelectron microscopy has revealed elastin and tropoelastin.[56] These observations have led to the theory that the exfoliation syndrome is a type of elastosis, with elastic microfibrils being abnormally secreted by local ocular cells.[55,56] Other studies indicate that the exfoliation material may be a basement membrane proteoglycan.[57–59] Laminin, a noncollagenous component of basement membrane, has been identified in the fibrillar component of the exfoliation material. These observations suggest that the disease may be caused by a disturbance in the biosynthesis of basement membrane. The presence of glycosaminoglycans in anterior ocular structures and the aqueous humor has also been demonstrated in eyes with the exfoliation syndrome,[52,61,62] and the possibility has been raised that this disease may involve abnormal metabolism of glycosaminoglycans in the iris.[62] Still other studies have suggested that the protein of the exfoliation material may be of the amyloid group,[51,63] and there are clinical similarities between the exfoliation syndrome and primary amyloidosis.[64,65] However, immunohistochemical staining demonstrated amyloid P protein, a minor serum component, on the periphery of the exfoliation fibers, suggesting that it is not an intrinsic fiber component but binds to sites similar to those on normal elastic fibers.[66]

Source. The exfoliation material occurs on and in the *lens* capsule, and adjacent to the lens epithelium.[67–69] The source of the material on the outer surface of the lens capsule has been controversial. Some investigators thought it unlikely that this material could be derived from the lens epithelium, since early ultrastructural studies showed no continuity between the capsular and epithelial exfoliation material,[67] and studies with horseradish peroxidase suggested that this material could not pass through the capsule.[61] These observations led to the theory that the exfoliation material on the lens capsule must have been deposited there from other ocular structures. However, small amounts of fibrillar protein have been seen in the otherwise normal aging lens capsule,[70] and discoid plaques of exfoliation material near the epithelium correspond in location and appearance to material on the capsular surface, with connections between the material at the two levels, suggesting that the lens epithelium does contribute, at least in part, to the exfoliation material on the anterior lens capsule.[68,69,71]

The exfoliation material is also found in the *iris* in the anterior limiting layer, on the posterior aspect of the pigment epithelium, and in the vessel walls.[72] The material is attached in irregular areas to the iris vessels[73] and is located in indentations of the cell membrane of the pigment epithelium, but not in the cytoplasm of those cells.[74] It has been suggested that the iris may be a source of the exfoliation material on the lens capsule,[40,45] which may explain the presence of the material on the anterior hyaloid in aphakic eyes.[75,76]

Exfoliation material has also been found in the *conjunctiva*,[55,77–79] which appears to be another independent source of the material.[80] This has been demonstrated in conjunctival biopsies of eyes that did not have the typical clinical appearance of exfoliation material on the anterior lens capsule but were suspected on the basis of other signs, such as pigment dispersion and iris transillumination defects.[79] The material has also been demonstrated in the ciliary epithelium[81] and on lens zonules, although it is not clear whether these represent additional primary sources or secondary deposition.

Mechanism of Pigment Dispersion

Although the production of exfoliation material appears to be the fundamental feature of the exfoliation syndrome, the associated pigment dispersion in the anterior ocular segment may have an important role in the development of the secondary glaucoma. The precise mechanism of the pigment dispersion is not fully understood. It may be that the pigment is liberated from the epithelium of the iris as a result of rubbing against the rough lens capsule. Sugar,[45] however, believes the pigment dispersion may result from a fundamental defect of the iris.

Mechanism of the Glaucoma

Whatever the principal sources of the exfoliation material and dispersed pigment may be, it is generally thought that these elements are involved in the development of the secondary glaucoma. Studies of aqueous humor dynamics in eyes with unilateral capsular glaucoma revealed higher resistance to aqueous outflow and a lower rate of aqueous flow through the anterior chamber as compared with the normal fellow eye.[82] Ultrastructural studies of eyes with the exfoliation syndrome have revealed both fibrillar material and pigment granules in the trabecular meshwork,[83–85] which may lead to the obstruction of aqueous outflow. However, not all of these eyes had glaucoma,[85] suggesting that additional factors may be involved.

In some cases, the additional factor leading to glaucoma may be a primary disturbance in the facility of aqueous outflow.[86] In support of this theory are the observations that glaucoma does not develop in all eyes with exfoliation, and yet may develop in both eyes of a patient with unilateral exfoliation.[12,23,83,87] However, the increased incidence of glaucoma in eyes with the exfoliation syndrome is thought to indicate a causal relationship between the abnormal material and the elevated IOP.[88] Furthermore, patients with the exfoliation syndrome do not have the same response to topical corticosteroids as do primary open-angle glaucoma patients.[89,90] It appears, therefore, that the condition represents a true secondary glaucoma but may be superimposed on primary open-angle glaucoma in some patients.

Another less common mechanism of glaucoma in patients with the exfoliation syndrome is angle-closure glaucoma.[12,23,42,46,48]

Differential Diagnosis

The exfoliation syndrome must be distinguished from other forms of lens exfoliation as well as other causes of pigment dispersion.

Capsular Delamination

As noted earlier in this chapter, there is another group of disorders that involve exfoliation of the anterior lens capsule and have been referred to as "true" exfoliation of the lens capsule,[5,7,8] or capsular delamination.[6] These cases differ from the exfoliation syndrome in that an underlying precipitating factor, such as trauma,[3,4] exposure to intense heat,[2] or severe uveitis,[4] is often, but not always,[5–7] present. The nature of the lens exfoliation also differs, with thin, clear membrane-like material separating from the anterior lens capsule and often curling at the margins.[5–7] Glaucoma is infrequent with capsular delamination.

Primary Amyloidosis

This generalized, systemic disease, which may be familial[64] or nonfamilial,[65] has numerous ocular manifestations, including glaucoma. The amyloid may be deposited as a white, flaky substance throughout the eye, including the pupillary margin of the iris, the anterior lens capsule, and the anterior chamber angle, creating a clinical picture that resembles the exfoliation syndrome.[64,65]

Pigment Dispersion

A variety of conditions, in addition to the exfoliation syndrome, are characterized by increased pigmentation of the trabecular meshwork. These include the pigment dispersion syndrome and pigmentary glaucoma (Chapter 14), some forms of anterior uveitis (Chapter 19), melanosis and melanomas (Chapter 18), and primary open-angle glaucoma or otherwise normal eyes with unusually heavy pigment dispersion. These conditions usually can be distinguished from the exfoliation syndrome by observing the characteristic appearance of the anterior lens capsule in the latter disorder. As noted in the previous chapter, the exfoliation syndrome has been observed to develop in patients with the pigment dispersion syndrome.[91]

Management

Glaucoma

The glaucoma associated with the exfoliation syndrome is treated basically the same as primary open-angle glaucoma, although it has been emphasized that the former glaucoma is typically more difficult to control.[50] When medical therapy is no longer adequate, laser trabeculoplasty is usually indicated and has a high success rate with this form of secondary glaucoma. When conventional surgical intervention becomes necessary, filtering surgery is generally advocated. The influence of lens removal on the course of the glaucoma is unclear. It has been reported that the exfoliation material diminishes and regresses after intracapsular cataract extraction,[92] although others have observed the development of the exfoliation syndrome years after intracapsular lens removal.[40,75,76]

Cataract

Although lens extraction is not advocated for the management of glaucoma in the exfoliation syndrome, cataract extraction for improvement of visual acuity is frequently indicated and requires special consideration in these patients. With extracapsular cataract surgery, patients with the exfoliation syndrome have a higher than average risk of zonular and capsular breaks.[93–95] This is most likely a result of degeneration of the zonular fibrils[34,96] but may also be associated with a thin posterior lens capsule.[97] Other factors that may complicate cataract surgery in these patients are poor pupillary dilation[94,98] and occasional synechiae between the iris pigment epithelium and the peripheral anterior lens capsule.[99] Preoperatively, the surgeon should look for evidence of zonular dialysis, such as phakodonesis and asymmetric anterior chamber depth,[34,92] and care must be taken during surgery to avoid excessive stress on the zonules or posterior capsule.[93–97] When a successful extracapsular cataract extraction has been performed, the implantation of a posterior chamber intraocular lens appears to be well tolerated in patients with the exfoliation syndrome.[94]

GLAUCOMAS ASSOCIATED WITH DISLOCATION OF THE LENS

Terminology

Several terms have been applied to the clinical situation in which the crystalline lens is displaced from its normal, central position behind the iris. *Subluxation* of the lens implies an incomplete dislocation, in which the lens is still at least partly behind the iris but is tilted or displaced slightly in either an anterior or posterior direction or perpendicular to the optical axis. With *complete dislocation,* the entire lens may be in the anterior chamber or may have fallen posteriorly into the vitreous cavity. The term ectopia of the lens, or *ectopia lentis,* is also applied to cases of lens dislocation but is nonspecific with regard to the degree of lens displacement.

Subluxation or complete dislocation of the lens may be associated with a number of clinical conditions, all of which can lead to secondary glaucoma by a variety of mechanisms. We will first review the more common clinical forms of ectopia lentis and then consider the mechanisms by which these conditions may lead to IOP elevation and how these secondary glaucomas are managed.

Clinical Forms of Ectopia Lentis

Traumatic Dislocation

Trauma is the most common cause of a displaced lens.[100,101] In one series of 166 cases, injury was reported to account for 53% of the total group.[101] The patient population with traumatic dislocation of the lens has a higher than normal incidence of serologic evidence for syphilis,[101] although a direct cause-and-effect relationship between this disease and ectopia lentis has not been established. It may simply be that the patient who is likely to acquire syphilis is also more prone to get into situations that lead to trauma.[101]

Simple Ectopia Lentis

Dislocation of the lens may occur without associated ocular or systemic abnormalities either as a congenital anomaly or as a spontaneous disorder later in life.[102,103] Both forms are typically inherited by an autosomal dominant mode.[103] The condition is usually bilateral and symmetrical, with lens dislocation generally upward and outward. Associated problems include dislocation of the lens into the anterior chamber, secondary glaucoma, and retinal detachment.

Ectopia Lentis et Pupillae

This is a rare, autosomal recessive condition characterized by small, subluxed lenses, and oval or slit-shaped pupils that are displaced, usually in the opposite direction from that of the lens (Fig. 15.5).[102–105] The condition is associated with a wide variety of other ocular abnormalities, including severe axial myopia with related fundus changes, enlarged corneal diameters, iris transillumination defects, poor pupillary di-

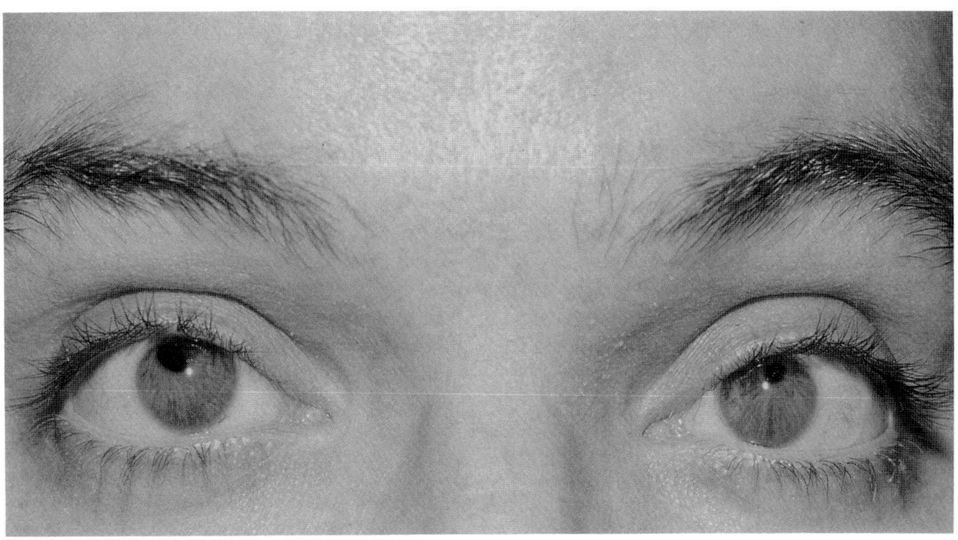

Figure 15.5. Patient with ectopia lentis et pupillae showing typical displacement of pupils.

lation, persistent pupillary membranes, iridohyaloid adhesions, prominent iris processes, cataracts, retinal detachment, and secondary glaucoma.[105] The condition is usually bilateral, although marked variation may be seen between eyes of the same patient.[105]

It has been suggested that simple ectopia lentis may be an incomplete expression of ectopia lentis et pupillae, since both may occur in the same family and have peripheral iris transillumination.[102] In addition, some patients with ectopia lentis et pupillae may have mild systemic changes suggestive of Marfan's syndrome.[102]

Marfan's Syndrome

This autosomal dominant disorder is characteristically seen in a tall, slender individual with long distal limbs (arachnodactyly) and frequent cardiovascular disease.[103,106] In a review of 160 consecutive patients, the most striking ocular abnormality was enlargement of the globe, presumably as a result of scleral stretching.[107] The lens was dislocated in 193 of the eyes, and this correlated with increased ocular axial length, suggesting that stretching and rupture of the zonular fibers leads to the dislocation.[107] The ectopia lentis typically appears in the fourth to fifth decade of life and is rarely complete, but is usually seen as an upward subluxation. Glaucoma may result from the lens dislocation but also occurs in association with surgical aphakia, or as an anomaly of the anterior chamber angle. Retinal detachment is also a common finding in either the phakic or aphakic eye of a patient with Marfan's syndrome.

Homocystinuria

These patients may resemble those with Marfan's syndrome in habitus and ocular problems but differ by an autosomal recessive mode of inheritance and frequent mental retardation.[103,106] Homocystinuria may result from one of several enzyme deficiencies in homocysteine metabolism, and the diagnosis can be confirmed by the demonstration of homocysteine in the urine. The differentiation between Marfan's syndrome and homocystinuria is important since the homocystinuric patient is subject to thromboembolic episodes that can lead to death in early adulthood and create a significant surgical risk. In addition, if the condition is diagnosed in the newborn, appropriate dietary treatment and vitamin supplementation can substantially reduce the risk of ocular complications.[108] The lens dislocation occurs earlier in life than in Marfan's syndrome and is more often in a downward direction, and frequently there is complete dislocation into the vitreous or anterior chamber. Glaucoma is more commonly related to the lens dislocation than in Marfan's syndrome. Retinal detachment is also a frequent problem.

Weill-Marchesani Syndrome

This is the antithesis of the aforementioned conditions with respect to habitus, in that the patients are short and stocky. The principal features of the syndrome are short fingers (brachydactyly) and small, round lenses (microspherophakia). Lens dislocation occurs with equal frequency as compared with Marfan's syndrome and homocystinuria, and glaucoma is more common than in either of the latter two conditions.[109] The small, round lens in this condition also has loose zonules, and the glaucoma may be related to either lens dislocation[109] or a forward shift of the lens, causing pupillary-block glaucoma,[110,111] which can be precipitated or aggravated by miotic therapy. Bilateral angle-closure glaucoma has also been reported following mid-dilation with cyclopentolate in a child with the Weill-Marchesani syndrome but without lens subluxation.[112]

Spontaneous Dislocation

In some middle-aged or older individuals, dislocation of the lens may occur spontaneously, usually in association with cataract formation.[100] Spontaneous dislocation has also been reported in eyes with high myopia, uveitis, buphthalmos, or megalocornea.[100]

Other Conditions with Associated Ectopia Lentis

Other rare congenital disorders associated with lens dislocation include Ehlers-

Table 15.1.
Conditions Associated with Ectopia Lentis[a]

Trauma	Alport's syndrome
Simple ectopia lentis	Mandibulofacial dysostosis
Ectopia lentis et pupillae	Klinefelter's syndrome
Marfan's syndrome	Retinitis pigmentosa
Homocystinuria	Persistent pupillary membrane
Weill-Marchesani syndrome	Axenfeld-Rieger syndrome
High myopia	Dominantly inherited blepharoptosis and high myopia
Uveitis	Marfan-like syndrome with hyaloretinal degeneration
Buphthalmos	Sturge-Weber syndrome
Megalocornea	Syphilis
Ehlers-Danlos syndrome	Crouzon's disease
Hyperlysemia	Refsum's syndrome
Sulfite oxidase deficiency	
Aniridia	
Scleroderma	

[a] Modified from Nelson and Maumenee[103] and Ritch and Wand.[111]

Danlos syndrome, hyperlysemia,[113] sulfite oxidase deficiency,[114] and aniridia.[115] Additional conditions associated with ectopia lentis are included in Table 15.1.

Mechanisms of Associated Glaucoma

Subluxation or complete dislocation of the lens in any of the aforementioned clinical conditions may lead to secondary glaucoma by a variety of mechanisms. In general, these mechanisms of glaucoma apply to all forms of ectopia lentis.

Pupillary Block

The lens may block aqueous flow through the pupil if it is dislocated into the pupil or anterior chamber, or if it is subluxed or tilted forward against the iris without entering the anterior chamber.[100,111,116] This mechanism is particularly common with microspherophakia, as in the Weill-Marchesani syndrome, due to loose zonules of the lens. Pupillary block in the latter condition is often made worse by miotic therapy, which allows further relaxation of zonular support (inverse glaucoma), while cycloplegics may help by pulling the lens posteriorly.[111] Pupillary block may also occur in association with a dislocated lens as a result of herniation of vitreous into the pupil. Peripheral anterior synechiae may develop from a long-standing pupillary block and produce chronic IOP elevation.

Phacolytic Glaucoma

In other cases, the lens may dislocate completely into the vitreous cavity and later undergo degenerative changes with release of material that obstructs aqueous outflow.[117] In one reported case, this condition was associated with retinal perivasculitis, which cleared along with the glaucoma after removal of the lens.[118] Phacolytic glaucoma without dislocation is discussed later in this chapter.

Concomitant Trauma

In cases of traumatic dislocation of the lens, concomitant trauma to the anterior chamber angle from the initial injury may be the cause of the secondary glaucoma.[100,103] In addition, a transient pressure elevation of uncertain etiology may persist for days or weeks after traumatic dislocation of the lens. The mechanisms of glaucoma secondary to trauma are considered in more detail in Chapter 22.

Management

Pupillary Block

If the lens is displaced anteriorly, either in the anterior chamber or partly through the pupil, it may be possible to relieve the condition by dilating the pupil and allowing the lens to reposit back into the posterior chamber.[119] A miotic may then be used to keep the lens behind the iris. As previously noted, however, miotic therapy should be avoided when the pupillary block is a result of loose zonules, since contraction of the ciliary muscle further relaxes the zonular support, making the pupillary block worse.[111] Cycloplegics may help to break the attack by pulling the lens posteriorly. Hyperosmotic agents, carbonic anhydrase inhibitors, or topical beta-blocker may also be useful in breaking the attack. The definitive treatment, however, is a laser iridotomy (or incisional iridectomy if necessary). The iridotomy should be placed peripherally to avoid subsequent obstruction by the lens. Prophylactic iridotomy in cases of microspherophakia, to avoid pupillary block glaucoma, has also been advocated.[111,120] The extraction of a subluxed lens is associated with increased surgical risk and usually should be avoided unless the lens cannot be reposited from the anterior chamber or cataract extraction is needed to improve vision.

Phacolytic Glaucoma

This is the only situation in cases of lens dislocation in which cataract extraction is the procedure of choice.[121] It has been shown that subluxed lenses can be successfully removed through a pars plana approach with vitreous instruments.[118,122]

Chronic Glaucomas

Chronic glaucomas secondary to peripheral anterior synechiae or concomitant trauma in eyes with dislocated lenses are generally managed by standard medical measures. Laser trabeculoplasty has a low success rate in eyes with open-angle glaucoma secondary to trauma, although it is usually reasonable to try this approach when medical therapy is no longer adequate before recommending incisional surgical intervention.

GLAUCOMAS ASSOCIATED WITH CATARACT FORMATION

It has long been recognized clinically that several forms of glaucoma may occur secondary to the formation of cataracts. However, an incomplete understanding of the various mechanisms for these glaucomas has led to a plethora of terms, accompanied by considerable controversy and confusion. More recent observations have provided new explanations and terminology for several of the glaucomas that are associated with cataract formation.

Phacolytic (Lens Protein) Glaucoma

Terminology

In 1900, Gifford[123] described a form of open-angle glaucoma secondary to a hypermature cataract. Among the terms subsequently suggested for this condition were "phacogenetic glaucoma"[124] and "lens-induced uveitis."[125] Flocks and co-workers[126] reported histologic findings that suggested that the glaucoma-inducing mechanism was a macrophagic response to lens material. They proposed that this condition be called *phacolytic glaucoma,* which is the term most often used today. However, Epstein and associates[127,128] have provided evidence that lens protein may be primarily responsible for the obstruction to aqueous outflow in this disorder, and the term *lens protein glaucoma* has been suggested.[129]

Clinical Features

The typical patient presents with the acute onset of monocular pain and redness. There is usually a history of gradual reduction in visual acuity over the preceding months or years, and vision at the time of presentation may be reduced to only inaccurate light perception. The examination reveals a high IOP, conjunctival hyperemia, and diffuse corneal edema. It is important to note that the anterior chamber angle is open and usually grossly normal. A heavy flare is typically seen in the anterior chamber, often associated with iridescent or hyperrefringent particles. The latter have been variably reported to represent calcium oxalate[130] or cholesterol[131] crystals and are a helpful diagnostic sign in phacolytic glaucoma. Chunks of white material may also be seen in the aqueous and on the anterior lens capsule and corneal endothelium. Specular microscopy in five cases revealed regular round cells about three times the size of an erythrocyte that were found by histologic study of aqueous aspirates to represent macrophages.[131] The cataract is typically mature (totally opaque) or hypermature (liquid cortex) but may rarely be immature. A less common variation of phacolytic glaucoma is the previously discussed situation in which the lens has dislocated into the vitreous and undergone phacolysis. The latter cases differ clinically in that the glaucoma tends to be more subacute.

Theories of Mechanism

It is generally accepted that part of the pathogenesis in phacolytic glaucoma is the release of soluble lens protein into the aqueous through microscopic defects in the lens capsule. However, theories vary as to how this protein leads to the elevated IOP.

As previously noted, it has been postulated that macrophages, laden with phagocytosed lens material, block the trabecular meshwork to produce the acute glaucoma.[126] This theory has been supported by the demonstration of macrophages in the aqueous[132] and trabecular meshwork[133] of eyes with phacolytic glaucoma. By electron microscopic study, these macrophages were found to have phagocytized degenerated lens material.[134] Against the macrophage theory, however, is the observation that lens-laden macrophages in the anterior chamber do not invariably lead to elevated IOP. For example, a macrophagic cellular reaction may be found in the anterior chamber aspirate following needling and aspiration of a cataract, but it does not appear to obstruct aqueous outflow.[135] However, the number of macrophages in the aqueous may be greater in phacolytic glaucoma.

An alternative theory is that heavy-molecular-weight (HMW) soluble protein from the lens directly obstructs the outflow of aqueous.[127–129] Such protein has been shown to cause a significant decrease in outflow when perfused in enucleated human eyes.[127] HMW soluble protein is known to increase in the cataractous lens[136] and has been demonstrated in the aqueous of eyes with phacolytic glaucoma in quantities sufficient to obstruct aqueous outflow.[128] HMW protein is rare in childhood lenses,[137,138] which may explain why phacolytic glaucoma rarely, if ever, occurs in children. Electron microscopy has also demonstrated free-floating degenerated lens material in the aqueous and trabecular meshwork of an eye with phacolytic glaucoma.[134]

Differential Diagnosis

Several forms of glaucoma may present with the sudden onset of pain and redness, creating diagnostic confusion with phacolytic glaucoma. *Acute angle-closure glaucoma,* of primary or secondary etiology, must be ruled out on the basis of the gonioscopic examination. *Open-angle glaucoma secondary to uveitis* may be more difficult to distinguish. In some cases, a paracentesis and microscopic examination of the aqueous may be helpful by demonstrating amorphous protein-like fluid and occasional macrophages in eyes with phacolytic glaucoma.[129] A therapeutic trial of topical steroids will produce only temporary remission when phacolysis is the underlying problem, which may help to distinguish it from a primary uveitis. Other conditions, such as neovascular glaucoma and trauma, may also cause a sudden IOP rise but usually can be distinguished on the basis of history and/or clinical findings.

Management

Phacolytic glaucoma should be handled as an emergency, ultimately by removal of the lens.[139,140] It is desirable, however, to first bring the IOP under medical control with hyperosmotics, carbonic anhydrase inhibitors, and topical beta-blockers, and possibly to minimize associated inflammation with topical steroid therapy.[129] When the pressure cannot be lowered medically, it may be necessary to accomplish this at the time of surgery by gradual release of aqueous through a paracentesis incision. Opinions differ regarding the advisability of intracapsular versus extracapsular cataract extraction for this particular condition. If the former is chosen, special care must be taken to avoid rupturing the fragile lens capsule, and it has been suggested that a sector iridectomy with the use of alpha-chymotrypsin enzyme may be helpful.[129] Extracapsular cataract extraction with posterior chamber intraocular lens implantation was performed in five patients with phacolytic glaucoma with uniformly good results, and the authors point out the advantages of better visual rehabilitation and a surgical technique with which more surgeons are currently familiar.[141] If the lens capsule is ruptured intentionally or unintentionally, the anterior chamber should be thoroughly irrigated and all lens material removed to avoid postoperative IOP rise. Following uncomplicated cataract surgery, the glaucoma usually clears and there is often a return of good vision, despite a significant preoperative reduction.

Lens Particle Glaucoma

Terminology

It was once thought that a primary toxicity of cataractous lens material caused an inflammatory reaction called "phacotoxic uveitis," which led to secondary glaucoma in some cases. Subsequent studies, however, have not supported the concept that liberated lens material is toxic.[142] It appears that cases incorrectly given this diagnosis are actually a result of liberation of lens particles and debris following disruption of the lens capsule, and the term *lens particle glaucoma* has been proposed for this entity.[129]

Clinical Features

This condition is typically associated with disruption of the lens capsule either by an extracapsular cataract extraction or a penetrating injury. The onset of IOP elevation usually occurs soon after the primary event and is generally proportional to the amount of "fluffed up" lens cortical material in the anterior chamber. Uncommon clinical variations include an onset of glaucoma many years after capsular disruption or following a spontaneous rupture in the lens capsule. The latter condition may be hard to distinguish from phacolytic glaucoma, although cases of lens particle glaucoma tend to have a greater inflammatory component, often associated with posterior and anterior synechiae and inflammatory pupillary membranes.[129]

Theories of Mechanism

It has been demonstrated by perfusion studies with enucleated human eyes that small amounts of free particulate lens material significantly reduce outflow.[127] This is presumed to be the principal mechanism of trabecular meshwork obstruction in cases of lens particle glaucoma. However, it is possible that the associated inflammation, whether in response to the surgery, trauma, or retained lens material, may also contribute to the glaucoma in this condition.

Differential Diagnosis

In its typical form, the diagnosis of lens particle glaucoma is usually easy to make on the basis of history and physical findings. In atypical forms, such as delayed onset or spontaneous capsule rupture, the diagnosis might be confused with phacoanaphylaxis, phacolytic glaucoma, or other types of secondary open-angle glaucoma. When doubt exists, microscopic examination of aqueous from an anterior chamber tap may help to establish the diagnosis of lens particle glaucoma by demonstrating leukocytes and macrophages along with lens cortical material.[129]

Management

In some cases, it is possible to control the IOP medically with drugs that reduce aqueous production. Because inflammation is also present, the pupil should be dilated and topical steroids should be used, although it may be advisable to use the latter only in moderate amounts, since steroid therapy may delay absorption of the lens material.[129] The IOP will usually return to normal after the lens material has been absorbed. When the pressure cannot be adequately controlled medically, the residual lens material should be surgically removed, either by irrigation if the material is loose or with vitrectomy instruments when it is adherent to ocular structures.

Phacoanaphylaxis

Terminology

In 1922, Verhoeff and Lemoine[143] reported that a small percentage of individuals are hypersensitive to lens protein and that rupture of the lens capsule in these cases leads to an intraocular inflammation, which they called "endophthalmitis phacoanaphylactica." Although such cases are apparently rare, there is evidence that a true *phacoanaphylaxis* does occur in response to lens protein antigen,[144] with secondary inflammation and occasional open-angle glaucoma.

Clinical Features

As in the case of lens particle glaucoma, there is usually preceding disruption of the lens capsule by extracapsular cataract surgery or penetrating injury.[145] The distinguishing feature, however, is a latent period during which time sensitization to lens protein occurs. A particularly likely setting for the development of phacoanaphylaxis is when lens material, especially the nucleus, is retained in the vitreous. The typical physical finding is a chronic, relentless "granulomatous-type" of inflammation, which is centered around lens material either in the primarily involved eye or in the fellow eye after it has undergone extracapsular cataract surgery. Secondary glaucoma is only rarely a feature of phacoanaphylaxis.

Theories of Mechanism

It has been demonstrated in rabbits that autologous lens protein is antigenic,[144] and it is assumed that the lens capsule isolates the lenticular antigens from the immune response, with sensitization occurring only when the capsule is violated. However, this concept was not supported by human studies that failed to demonstrate lens antibodies after injury to the lens and that showed an equal incidence of antibody in cataract patients and controls.[146] The same study did show a higher prevalence of antibodies in a small group with hypermature cataracts and more frequent postoperative uveitis in patients with antibodies in preoperative blood specimens, although the latter observation was not statistically significant. In the rabbit study cited above, there was considerable variation in the response to autologous lens antigen,[144] which may explain the infrequency with which phacoanaphylaxis is seen clinically. The cellular appearance of the immune response is characterized by polymorphonuclear leukocytes and lymphoid, epithelioid, and giant cells, usually around a nidus of lens material. It may be that the occasional glaucoma in phacoanaphylaxis is related to the accumulation of these cells in the trabecular meshwork, although lens protein or particles may also be present and could account for the glaucoma.

Differential Diagnosis

Other chronic forms of uveitis, especially sympathetic ophthalmia, may occur in association with phacoanaphylaxis. Phacolytic and lens particle glaucomas must also be considered. Microscopic examination of the aqueous may be helpful, although variations in cytology have not been fully studied in this condition, and the diagnosis may require histologic examination of the surgically removed lens material.

Management

Steroid therapy should be used to control the uveitis, with antiglaucoma medication as required. When medical measures are inadequate, the retained lens material should be surgically removed.

Intumescent Lens

In some eyes with advanced cataract formation, the lens may become swollen or intumescent, with progressive reduction in the anterior chamber angle, eventually leading to a form of secondary angle-closure glaucoma. This has been referred to as "phacomorphic glaucoma."[147] The angle closure may be secondary to either an enhanced pupillary block mechanism or to forward displacement of the lens-iris diaphragm. In either case, the diagnosis is usually made by observing a mature, intumescent cataract associated with a central anterior chamber depth that is significantly shallower than that of the fellow eye. The treatment is initial medical reduction of the IOP with hyperosmotics, carbonic anhydrase inhibitors, and topical beta-blockers, followed by extraction of the cataract.

SUMMARY

The exfoliation syndrome, a relatively common disorder among older individuals and within certain ethnic populations, is characterized by a protein-like material of the lens, iris, and various other anterior ocular structures. It is recognized clinically by the typical appearance of the exfoliative material on the anterior lens capsule. The condition may be unilateral or bilateral, and some cases have associated glaucoma resulting from the accumulation of exfoliative material and iris pigment granules in the trabecular meshwork.

The lens may also be associated with glaucoma when it is dislocated, which may occur with trauma or certain inherited disorders, such as Marfan's syndrome, homocystinuria, and the Weill-Marchesani syndrome. Mechanisms by which a dislocated lens may be associated with glaucoma include pupillary block, degenerative changes of the lens, and concomitant damage of the anterior chamber angle.

A cataractous lens may also lead to secondary glaucoma by obstruction of the trabecular meshwork with lens protein and macrophages (phacolytic glaucoma), lens particles and debris (lens particle glaucoma), or inflammatory cells as part of an immune response (phacoanaphylaxis). In addition, an intumescent lens may lead to angle-closure glaucoma.

References

1. Lindberg, JG: Clinical investigations on depigmentation of the pupillary border and translucency of the iris. In cases of senile cataract and in normal eyes in elderly persons. Academic Dissertation, Helsinki, 1917. English translation by Tarkkanen, A, Forsius, H, Acta Ophthal Suppl 190, vol. 66, University Press, Helsinki, 1989.
2. Elschnig, A: Ablosung der Zonulalamelle bei Glasblasern. Klin Monatsbl Augenheilkd 69:732, 1922.
3. Kraupa, E: Linsenkapselrisse ohne Wundstar. Zeitschrift fur Augenheilkunde 48:93, 1922.
4. Butler, TH: Capsular glaucoma. Trans Ophthal Soc UK 68:575, 1938.
5. Radda, TM, Klemen, UM: Idiopathic true exfoliation. Klin Monatsbl Augenheilkd 181:276, 1982.
6. Brodrick, JD, Tate, GW Jr: Capsular delamination (true exfoliation) of the lens. Report of a case. Arch Ophthal 97:1693, 1979.
7. Cashwell, LF Jr, Holleman, IL, Weaver, RG, van Rens, GH: Idiopathic true exfoliation of the lens capsule. Ophthalmology 96:348, 1989.
8. Dvorak-Theobald, G: Pseudo-exfoliation of the lens capsule. Relation to "true" exfoliation of the lens capsule as reported in the literature and role in the production of glaucoma capsulocuticulare. Am J Ophthal 37:1, 1954.
9. Vogt, A: Ein neues Spaltlampenbild des Pupillengebietes: Hellblauer Pupillensaumfilz mit Hautchenbildung auf der Linsenvorderkapsel. Klin Monatsbl Augenheilkd 75:1, 1925.
10. Vogt, A: Vergleichende Uebersicht uber Klinik und Histologie der Alters—und Feuerlamelle der Linsenvorderkapsel. Klin Monatsbl Augenheilkd 89:587, 1932.
11. Sunde, OA: Senile exfoliation of the anterior lens capsule. Acta Ophthal Suppl 45:27, 1956.
12. Layden, WE, Shaffer, RN: Exfoliation syndrome. Am J Ophthal 78:835, 1974.
13. Tarkkanen, A, Forsius, H (eds): Exfoliation Syndrome. Acta Ophthal Suppl 184, vol. 66, Scriptor, Copenhagen, 1988.
14. Ohrt, V, Nehen, JH: The incidence of glaucoma capsulare based on a Danish hospital material. Acta Ophthal 59:888, 1981.
15. Lindblom, B, Thorburn, W: Observed incidence of glaucoma in Halsingland, Sweden. Acta Ophthal 62:217, 1984.
16. Lindblom, B, Thorburn, W: Prevalence of visual field defects due to capsular and simple glaucoma in Halsingland, Sweden. Acta Ophthal 60:353, 1982.
17. Ringvold, A, Blika, S, Elsas, T, et al: The prevalence of pseudoexfoliation in three separate municipalities of Middle-Norway. A preliminary report. Acta Ophthal 65/suppl 182:17, 1987.
18. Meyer, E, Haim, T, Zonis, S, et al: Pseudoexfoliation: epidemiology, clinical and scanning electron microscopic study. Ophthalmologica 188:141, 1984.
19. Cashwell, LF, Shields, MB: Exfoliation syndrome. Prevalence in a southeastern United States population. Arch Ophthal 106:335, 1988.
20. Hiller, R, Sperduto, RD, Krueger, DE: Pseudoexfoliation, intraocular pressure, and senile lens changes in a population-based survey. Arch Ophthal 100:1080, 1982.
21. Blika, S, Ringvold, A: The occurrence of simple and capsular glaucoma in Middle-Norway. Acta Ophthal 65/Suppl 182:11, 1987.
22. Ball, SF, Graham, S, Thompson, H: The racial prevalence and biomicroscopic signs of exfoliation syndrome in the glaucoma population of southern Louisiana. Glaucoma 11:169, 1989.
23. Roth, M, Epstein, DL: Exfoliation syndrome. Am J Ophthal 89:477, 1980.
24. Luntz, MH: Prevalence of pseudo-exfoliation syndrome in an urban South African clinic population. Am J Ophthal 74:581, 1972.
25. Kozart, DM, Yanoff, M: Intraocular pressure status in 100 consecutive patients with exfoliation syndrome. Ophthalmology 89:214, 1982.
26. Taylor, HR: The environment and the lens. Br J Ophthal 64:303, 1980.
27. Khanzada, AM: Exfoliation syndrome in Pakistan. Pak J Ophthal 2:7, 1986.
28. Madden, JG, Crowley, MJ: Factors in the exfoliation syndrome. Br J Ophthal 66:432, 1982.
29. Olivius, E, Polland, WP: Histocompatibility (HLA) antigens in capsular glaucoma and simplex glaucoma. Acta Ophthal 58:406, 1980.
30. Slagsvold, JE, Nordhagen, R: The HLA system in primary open angle glaucoma and in patients with pseudoexfoliation of the lens capsule (exfoliation or fibrillopathia epitheliocapsularis). Acta Ophthal 58:188, 1980.
31. Ringvold, A, Blika, S, Elsas, T, et al: The Middle-Norway eye-screening study. I. Epidemiology of

the pseudo-exfoliation syndrome. Acta Ophthal 66:652, 1988.

32. Crittendon, JJ, Shields, MB: Exfoliation syndrome in the southeastern United States. II. Characteristics of patient population and clinical courses. Acta Ophthal 66/suppl 184:103, 1988.
33. Seland, JH, Chylack, LT Jr.: Cataracts in the exfoliation syndrome (fibrillopathia epitheliocapsularis). Trans Ophthal Soc UK 102:375, 1982.
34. Futa, R, Furoyoshi, N: Phakodonesis in capsular glaucoma: a clinical and electron microscopic study. Jap J Ophthal 33:311, 1989.
35. Prince, AM, Ritch, R: Clinical signs of the pseudoexfoliation syndrome. Ophthalmology 93:803, 1986.
36. Repo, LP, Teräsvirta, ME, Tuovinen, EJ: Generalized peripheral iris transluminance in the pseudoexfoliation syndrome. Ophthalmology 97:1027, 1990.
37. Sakai, K, Kojima, K: Fluorescein angiography and electron microscopic study of the iris with exfoliation syndrome. Folia Ophthal Jap 33:72, 1982.
38. Brooks, AMV, Gillies, WE: The development of microneovascular changes in the iris in pseudoexfoliation of the lens capsule. Ophthalmology 94:1090, 1987.
39. Ringvold, A, Davanger, M: Iris neovascularisation in eyes with pseudoexfoliation syndrome. Br J Ophthal 65:138, 1981.
40. Sugar, HS: Onset of the exfoliation syndrome after intracapsular lens extraction. Am J Ophthal 89:601, 1980.
41. Miyake, K, Matsuda, M, Inaba, M: Corneal endothelial changes in pseudoexfoliation syndrome. Am J Ophthal 108:49, 1989.
42. Wishart, PK, Spaeth, GL, Poryzees, EM: Anterior chamber angle in the exfoliation syndrome. Br J Ophthal 69:103, 1985.
43. Bartholomew, RS: Anterior chamber depth in eyes with pseudoexfoliation. Br J Ophthal 64:322, 1980.
44. Mizuno, K, Muroi, S: Cycloscopy of pseudoexfoliation. Am J Ophthal 87:513, 1979.
45. Sugar, S: Pigmentary glaucoma and the glaucoma associated with the exfoliation-pseudoexfoliation syndrome: update. Ophthalmology 91:307, 1984.
46. Brooks, AMV, Gillies, WE: The presentation and prognosis of glaucoma in pseudoexfoliation of the lens capsule. Ophthalmology 95:271, 1988.
47. Slagsvold, JE: The follow-up in patients with pseudoexfoliation of the lens capsule with and without glaucoma. 2. The development of glaucoma in persons with pseudoexfoliation. Acta Ophthal 64:241, 1986.
48. Gillies, WE, Brooks, AMV: The presentation of acute glaucoma in pseudoexfoliation of the lens capsule. Aust New Zeal J Ophthal 16:101, 1988.
49. Lindblom, B, Thorburn, W: Functional damage at diagnosis of primary open-angle glaucoma. Acta Ophthal 62:223, 1984.
50. Olivius, E, Thorburn, W: Prognosis of glaucoma simplex and glaucoma capsulare. A comparative study. Acta Ophthal 56:921, 1978.
51. Dark, AJ, Streeten, BW, Cornwall, CC: Pseudoexfoliative disease of the lens: a study in electron microscopy and histochemistry. Br J Ophthal 61:462, 1977.
52. Davanger, M: The pseudo-exfoliation syndrome. A scanning electron microscopic study. I. The anterior lens surface. Acta Ophthal 53:809, 1975.
53. Garner, A, Alexander, RA: Pseudoexfoliative disease: histochemical evidence of an affinity with zonular fibres. Br J Ophthal 68:574, 1984.
54. Streeten, BW, Dark, AJ, Barnes, CW: Pseudoexfoliative material and oxytalan fibers. Exp Eye Res 38:523, 1984.
55. Streeten, BW, Bookman, L, Ritch, R, et al: Pseudoexfoliative fibrillopathy in the conjunctiva. A relation to elastic fibers and elastosis. Ophthalmology 94:1439, 1987.
56. Li, Z-Y, Streeten, BW, Wallace, RN: Association of elastin with pseudoexfoliative material: an immunoelectron microscopic study. Curr Eye Res 7:1163, 1988.
57. Eagle, RC Jr, Font, RL, Fine, BS: The basement membrane exfoliation syndrome. Arch Ophthal 97:510, 1979.
58. Bertelsen, TI, Drablos, PA, Flood, PR: The so-called senile exfoliation (pseudoexfoliation) of the anterior lens capsule. A product of the lens epithelium. Fibrillopathia epitheliocapsularis. A microscopic, histochemical and electron microscopic investigation. Acta Ophthal 42:1096, 1964.
59. Harnisch, JP, Barrach, HJ, Hassell, JR, Sinha, PK: Identification of a basement membrane proteoglycan in exfoliation material. Graefe's Arch Ophthal 215:273, 1981.
60. Konstas, AG, Marshall, GE, Lee, WR: Immunogold localisation of laminin in normal and exfoliative iris. Br J Ophthal 74:450, 1990.
61. Davanger, M, Pedersen, OO: Pseudo-exfoliation material on the anterior lens surface. Demonstration and examination of an interfibrillar ground substance. Acta Ophthal 53:3, 1975.
62. Baba, H: Histochemical and polarization optical investigation for glycosaminoglycans in exfoliation syndrome. Graefe's Arch Ophthal 221:106, 1983.
63. Ringvold, A, Husby, G: Pseudo-exfoliation material—an amyloid-like substance. Exp Eye Res 17:289, 1973.
64. Tsukahara, S, Matsuo, T: Secondary glaucoma accompanied with primary familial amyloidosis. Ophthalmologica 175:250, 1977.
65. Schwartz, MF, Green, RW, Michels, RG, et al: An unusual case of ocular involvement in primary

systemic nonfamilial amyloidosis. Ophthalmology 89:394, 1982.
66. Li, Z-Y, Streeten, BW, Yohai, N: Amyloid P protein in pseudoexfoliative fibrillopathy. Curr Eye Res 8:217, 1989.
67. Benedikt, O, Aubock, L, Gottinger, W, Waltinger, H: Comparative transmission and scanning electronmicroscopical studies on lenses in so-called exfoliation syndrome. Graefe's Arch Ophthal 187:249, 1973.
68. Seland, JH: The ultrastructure of the deep layer of the lens capsule in fibrillopathia epitheliocapsularis (FEC), so-called senile exfoliation or pseudoexfoliation. A scanning electron microscopic study. Acta Ophthal 56:335, 1978.
69. Seland, JH: Histopathology of the lens capsule in fibrillopathia epitheliocapsularis (FEC) or so-called senile exfoliation or pseudoexfoliation. An electron microscopic study. Acta Ophthal 57:477, 1979.
70. Dark, AJ, Streeten, BW, Jones, D: Accumulation of fibrillar protein in the aging human lens capsule. With special reference to the pathogenesis of pseudoexfoliative disease of the lens. Arch Ophthal 82:815, 1969.
71. Bergmanson, JPG, Jones, WL, Chu, LW-F: Ultrastructural observations on (pseudo-) exfoliation of the lens capsule: a re-examination of the involvement of the lens epithelium. Br J Ophthal 68:118, 1984.
72. Ghosh, M, Speakman, JS: The iris in senile exfoliation of the lens. Can J Ophthal 9:289, 1974.
73. Shimizu, T: Changes of iris vessels in capsular glaucoma: three-dimensional and electron microscopic studies. Jap J Ophthal 29:434, 1985.
74. Shimizu, T, Futa, R: The fine structure of pigment epithelium of the iris in capsular glaucoma. Graefe's Arch Ophthal 223:77, 1985.
75. Radian, AB, Radian, AL: Senile pseudoexfoliation in aphakic eyes. Br J Ophthal 59:577, 1975.
76. Caccamise, WC: The exfoliation syndrome in the aphakic eye. Am J Ophthal 91:111, 1981.
77. Speakman, JS, Ghosh, M: The conjunctiva in senile lens exfoliation. Arch Ophthal 94:1757, 1976.
78. Roh, YB, Ishibashi, T, Ito, N, Inomata, H: Alteration of microfibrils in the conjunctiva of patients with exfoliation syndrome. Arch Ophthal 105:978, 1987.
79. Prince, AM, Streeten, BW, Ritch, R, et al: Preclinical diagnosis of pseudoexfoliation syndrome. Arch Ophthal 105:1076, 1987.
80. Ringvold, A, Davanger, M: Notes on the distribution of pseudo-exfoliation material with particular reference to the uveoscleral route of aqueous humour. Acta Ophthal 55:807, 1977.
81. Ghosh, M, Speakman, JS: The ciliary body in senile exfoliation of the lens. Can J Ophthal 8:394, 1973.
82. Johnson, DH, Brubaker, RF: Dynamics of aqueous humor in the syndrome of exfoliation with glaucoma. Am J Ophthal 93:629, 1982.
83. Sampaolesi, R, Argento, C: Scanning electron microscopy of the trabecular meshwork in normal and glaucomatous eyes. Invest Ophthal Vis Sci 16:302, 1977.
84. Rodrigues, MM, Spaeth, GL, Sivalingam, E, Weinreb, S: Value of trabeculectomy specimens in glaucoma. Ophthal Surg 9:29, 1978.
85. Benedikt, O, Roll, P: The trabecular meshwork of a non-glaucomatous eye with the exfoliation syndrome. Electronmicroscopic study. Virchows Arch A Path Anat and Histol 384:347, 1979.
86. Pohjanpelto, PEJ: The fellow eye in unilateral hypertensive pseudoexfoliation. Am J Ophthal 75:216, 1973.
87. Cebon, L, Smith, RJH: Pseudoexfoliation of lens capsule and glaucoma. Case report. Br J Ophthal 60:279, 1976.
88. Aasved, H: Intraocular pressure in eyes with and without fibrillopathia epitheliocapsularis (so-called senile exfoliation or pseudoexfoliation). Acta Ophthal 49:601, 1971.
89. Pohjola, S, Horsmanheimo, A: Topically applied corticosteroids in glaucoma capsulare. Arch Ophthal 85:150, 1971.
90. Gillies, WE: Corticosteroid-induced ocular hypertension in pseudo-exfoliation of lens capsule. Am J Ophthal 70:90, 1970.
91. Layden, WE, Ritch, R, King, DG, Teekhasaenee, C: Combined exfoliation and pigment dispersion syndrome. Am J Ophthal 109:530, 1990.
92. Gillies, WE: Effect of lens extraction in pseudoexfoliation of the lens capsule. Br J Ophthal 57:46, 1973.
93. Skuta, GL, Parrish, RK II, Hodapp, E, et al: Zonular dialysis during extracapsular cataract extraction in pseudoexfoliation syndrome. Arch Ophthal 105:632, 1987.
94. Raitta, C, Tarkkanen, A: Posterior chamber lens implantation in capsular glaucoma. Acta Ophthal 65/suppl 182:24, 1987.
95. Hovding, G: The association between fibrillopathy and posterior capsular/zonular breaks during extracapsular cataract extraction and posterior chamber IOL implantation. Acta Ophthal 66:662, 1988.
96. Chijiiwa, T, Araki, H, Ishibashi, T, Inomata, H: Degeneration of zonular fibrils in a case of exfoliation glaucoma. Ophthalmologica 199:16, 1989.
97. Ruotsalainen, J, Tarkkanen, A: Capsule thickness of cataractous lenses with and without exfoliation syndrome. Acta Ophthal 65:444, 1987.
98. Carpel, EF: Pupillary dilation in eyes with pseudoexfoliation syndrome. Am J Ophthal 105:692, 1988.
99. Dark, AJ: Cataract extraction complicated by capsular glaucoma. Br J Ophthal 63:465, 1979.

100. Chandler, PA: Choice of treatment in dislocation of the lens. Arch Ophthal 71:765, 1964.
101. Jarrett, WH: Dislocation of the lens. A study of 166 hospitalized cases. Arch Ophthal 78:289, 1967.
102. Luebbers, JA, Goldberg, MF, Herbst, R, et al: Iris transillumination and variable expression in ectopia lentis et pupillae. Am J Ophthal 83:647, 1977.
103. Nelson, LB, Maumenee, IH: Ectopia lentis. Surv Ophthal 27:143, 1982.
104. Townes, PL: Ectopia lentis et pupillae. Arch Ophthal 94:1126, 1976.
105. Goldberg, MF: Clinical manifestations of ectopia lentis et pupillae in 16 patients. Ophthalmology 95:1080, 1988.
106. Cross, HE, Jensen, AD: Ocular manifestations in the Marfan syndrome and homocystinuria. Am J Ophthal 75:405, 1973.
107. Maumenee, IH: The eye in the Marfan syndrome. Trans Am Ophthal Soc 79:684, 1981.
108. Burke, JP, O'Keefe, M, Bowell, R, Naughten, ER: Ocular complications in homocystinuria—early and late treated. Br J Ophthal 73:427, 1989.
109. Jensen, AD, Cross, HE, Patton, D: Ocular complications in the Weill-Marchesani syndrome. Am J Ophthal 77:261, 1974.
110. Willi, M, Kut, L, Cotlier, E: Pupillary-block glaucoma in the Marchesani syndrome. Arch Ophthal 90:504, 1973.
111. Ritch, R, Wand, M: Treatment of the Weill-Marchesani Syndrome. Ann Ophthal 13:665, 1981.
112. Wright, KW, Chrousos, GA: Weill-Marchesani syndrome with bilateral angle-closure glaucoma. J Ped Ophthal Strab 22:129, 1985.
113. Smith, TH, Holland, MG, Woody, NC: Ocular manifestations of familial hyperlysinemia. Trans Am Acad Ophthal Otol 75:355, 1971.
114. Shih, VE, Abroms, IF, Johnson, JL, et al: Sulfite oxidase deficiency. Biochemical and clinical investigations of a hereditary metabolic disorder in sulfur metabolism. N Engl J Med 297:1022, 1977.
115. David, R, MacBeath, L, Jenkins, T: Aniridia associated with microcornea and subluxated lenses. Br J Ophthal 62:118, 1978.
116. Hein, HF, Maltzman, B: Long-standing anterior dislocation of the crystalline lens. Ann Ophthal 7:66, 1975.
117. Pollard, ZF: Phacolytic glaucoma secondary to ectopia lentis. Ann Ophthal 7:999, 1975.
118. Friberg, TR: Retinal perivasculitis in phacolytic glaucoma. Am J Ophthal 91:761, 1981.
119. Jay, B: Glaucoma associated with spontaneous displacement of the lens. Br J Ophthal 56:258, 1972.
120. Johnson, GJ, Bosanquet, RC: Spherophakia in a Newfoundland family: 8 years' experience. Can J Ophthal 18:159, 1983.
121. Chandler, PA: Completely dislocated hypermature cataract and glaucoma. Trans Am Ophthal Soc 57:242, 1959.
122. Treister, G, Machemer, R: Pars plana surgical approach for various anterior segment problems. Arch Ophthal 97:909, 1979.
123. Gifford, H: Danger of the spontaneous cure of senile cataracts. Am J Ophthal 17:289, 1900.
124. Zeeman, WPC: Zwei Falle von Glaucoma phacogeneticum mit anatomischem Befund. Ophthalmologica 106:136, 1943.
125. Irvine, SR, Irvine, AR Jr: Lens-induced uveitis and glaucoma. Part III. "Phacogenetic glaucoma": lens-induced glaucoma; mature or hypermature cataract; open iridocorneal angle. Am J Ophthal 35:489, 1952.
126. Flocks, M, Littwin, CS, Zimmerman, LE: Phacolytic glaucoma. A clinicopathologic study of one hundred thirty-eight cases of glaucoma associated with hypermature cataract. Arch Ophthal 54:37, 1955.
127. Epstein, DL, Jedziniak, JA, Grant, WM: Obstruction of aqueous outflow by lens particles and by heavy-molecular-weight soluble lens proteins. Invest Ophthal Vis Sci 17:272, 1978.
128. Epstein, DL, Jedziniak, JA, Grant, WM: Identification of heavy-molecular-weight soluble protein in aqueous humor in human phacolytic glaucoma. Invest Ophthal Vis Sci 17:398, 1978.
129. Epstein, DL: Diagnosis and management of lens-induced glaucoma. Ophthalmology 89:227, 1982.
130. Bartholomew, RS, Rebello, PF: Calcium oxalate crystals in the aqueous. Am J Ophthal 88:1026, 1979.
131. Brooks, AMV, Grant, G, Gillies, WE: Comparison of specular microscopy and examination of aspirate in phacolytic glaucoma. Ophthalmology 97:85, 1990.
132. Goldberg, MF: Cytological diagnosis of phacolytic glaucoma utilizing Millipore filtration of the aqueous. Br J Ophthal 51:847, 1967.
133. Tomita, G, Watanabe, K, Funahashi, M, et al: Lens induced glaucoma—histopathological study of the filtrating angle. Folia Ophthal Jap 35:1345, 1984.
134. Ueno, H, Tamai, A, Iyota, K, Moriki, T: Electron microscopic observation of the cells floating in the anterior chamber in a case of phacolytic glaucoma. Jap J Ophthal 33:103, 1989.
135. Yanoff, M, Scheie, HG: Cytology of human lens aspirate. Its relationship to phacolytic glaucoma and phacoanaphylactic endophthalmitis. Arch Ophthal 80:166, 1968.
136. Jedziniak, JA, Kinoshita, JH, Yates, EM, et al: On the presence and mechanism of formation of heavy molecular weight aggregates in human normal and cataractous lenses. Exp Eye Res 15:185, 1973.
137. Spector, A, Li, S, Sigelman, J: Age-dependent

changes in the molecular size of human lens proteins and their relationship to light scatter. Invest Ophthal 13:795, 1974.
138. Jedziniak, JA, Nicoli, DF, Baram, H, Benedek, GB: Quantitative verification of the existence of high molecular weight protein aggregates in the intact normal human lens by light-scattering spectroscopy. Invest Ophthal Vis Sci 17:51, 1978.
139. Chandler, PA: Problems in the diagnosis and treatment of lens-induced uveitis and glaucoma. Arch Ophthal 60:828, 1958.
140. Volcker, HE, Naumann, G: Clinical findings in phakolytic glaucoma. Klin Monatsbl Augenheilkd 166:613, 1975.
141. Lane, SS, Kopietz, LA, Lindquist, TD, Leavenworth, N: Treatment of phacolytic glaucoma with extracapsular cataract extraction. Ophthalmology 95:749, 1988.
142. Muller, H: Phacolytic glaucoma and phacogenic ophthalmia. (Lens induced uveitis). Trans Ophthal Soc UK 83:689, 1963.
143. Verhoeff, FH, Lemoine, AN: Endophthalmitis phacoanaphylactica. In: Trans Int Cong Ophthal, Washington, DC, Philadelphia, William F. Fell Co., 1922, p. 234.
144. Rahi, AHS, Misra, RN, Morgan, G: Immunopathology of the lens. III. Humoral and cellular immune responses to autologous lens antigens and their roles in ocular inflammation. Br J Ophthal 61:371, 1977.
145. Perlman, EM, Albert, DM: Clinically unsuspected phacoanaphylaxis after ocular trauma. Arch Ophthal 95:244, 1977.
146. Nissen, SH, Andersen, P, Andersen, HMK: Antibodies to lens antigens in cataract and after cataract surgery. Br J Ophthal 65:63, 1981.
147. Duke-Elder, S: System of Ophthalmology. Vol II. Henry Kimpton Publishers, London, 1969, p. 662.

Chapter 16

GLAUCOMAS ASSOCIATED WITH DISORDERS OF THE RETINA, VITREOUS, AND CHOROID

Several types of glaucoma are associated with diseases of the retina. The most common of these is neovascular glaucoma, which is usually secondary to one of several retinal disorders, although some cases are associated with other ocular or extraocular conditions. In addition, retinal detachments and a variety of less common disorders of the retina, vitreous, or choroid may cause or occur in association with various forms of glaucoma.

NEOVASCULAR GLAUCOMA

Terminology

In 1906, Coats[1] described new vessel formation on the iris in eyes with central retinal vein occlusion. This neovascularization of the iris has become commonly known as *rubeosis iridis* and is now recognized as a complication of many diseases of the retina and other ocular and extraocular disorders. Rubeosis iridis is frequently associated with a severe form of secondary glaucoma, which has been given several different names on the basis of various clinical features: "hemorrhagic glaucoma," referring to the hyphema that is present in some cases; "congestive glaucoma," describing the frequently acute nature of the condition; and "thrombotic glaucoma," implying an underlying vascular thrombotic etiology. However, none of these terms accurately describes the glaucoma in all cases, and more nonspecific names are preferable, such as *rubeotic glaucoma*[2] or *neovascular glaucoma,* the latter of which was proposed by Weiss and co-workers[3] and is found most often in current literature.

Factors Predisposing to Rubeosis Iridis

Most cases of rubeosis iridis are preceded by a hypoxic disease of the retina. Diabetic retinopathy and occlusion of major retinal vessels account for more than half of these with the former possibly being slightly more common.[4,5] However, many additional retinal diseases, as well as certain other ocular or extraocular disorders, have now been recognized, resulting in a long list of conditions that may predispose to the development of rubeosis iridis (Table 16.1).

Table 16.1.
Factors Predisposing to Rubeosis Iridis and Neovascular Glaucoma[a]

Diabetic retinopathy
Retinal vascular occlusive disorders
- Central retinal vein occlusion
- Central retinal artery occlusion[26,27]
- Branch retinal vein occlusion[29]
- Branch retinal artery occlusion[26,30]

Other retinal disorders
- Retinal detachment
- Choroidal melanoma
- Retinoblastoma[32]
- Hemorrhagic retinal disorders
- Coat's exudative retinopathy
- Retinopathy of prematurity
- Sickle cell retinopathy[33]
- Syphilitic retinal vasculitis[34]
- Retinoschisis[35]
- Stickler's syndrome (inherited vitreoretinal degeneration)[36]
- Optic nerve glioma with subsequent venous stasis retinopathy[37]
- Photoradiation[38] and helium ion irradiation[39] for uveal melanoma

Other ocular disorders
- Uveitis
- Intraocular lens implantation[40]
- Iris melanoma[41]

Extraocular vascular disorders
- Carotid artery obstructive disease[42]
- Carotid-cavernous fistula[43,44]
- Internal carotid artery occlusion[45]

[a] Modified from Hoskins[4] and Brown, et al.[5]

Diabetic Retinopathy

Approximately one-third of the patients with rubeosis iridis have diabetic retinopathy.[4,5] The frequency with which this condition occurs in association with diabetic retinopathy is greatly influenced by surgical interventions. Following pars plana vitrectomy for diabetic retinopathy, the reported incidence of rubeosis iridis ranges from 25 to 42%, while neovascular glaucoma ranges from 10 to 23%.[6–10] In these cases, the occurrence of rubeosis iridis and neovascular glaucoma are much higher in aphakic eyes.[9–15] In one series, vitreous cavity lavage of hemorrhage following pars plana vitrectomy for diabetic retinopathy was associated with rubeosis iridis in 76% of aphakic eyes and 14% of phakic eyes.[15] Postoperative neovascular glaucoma is also more common when rubeosis iridis is present before the vitrectomy.[16] In contrast, successful surgical reattachment of the retina during vitrectomy for diabetic retinopathy often leads to regression of preoperative rubeosis iridis, especially when the lens is retained.[17] A completely attached retina and aggressive panretinal photocoagulation have been shown to be the most important factors in preventing neovascular glaucoma after vitrectomy for proliferative diabetic retinopathy.[18] Intraocular silicone oil also reduces the incidence of anterior segment neovascularization, apparently by acting as a diffusion/convection barrier to the posterior movement of oxygen in the anterior chamber.[19] Long-term diabetic vitrectomy results indicate that rubeosis iridis and neovascular glaucoma develop most often during the first 6 months after surgery.[20]

Intracapsular cataract surgery alone in eyes with diabetic retinopathy is also associated with an increased incidence of postoperative rubeosis iridis and neovascular glaucoma.[21] The incidence is similar with extracapsular extraction and a primary capsulotomy.[22] Leaving the posterior capsule intact appears to prevent this complication,[22] although a subsequent laser capsulotomy in diabetic patients may lead to neovascular glaucoma.[23]

Retinal Vascular Occlusive Disorders

Central retinal vein occlusion accounted for 28% of all rubeosis iridis in one series.[4] Conversely, elevated intraocular pressure (IOP), with or without glaucomatous damage, is believed to be a predisposing factor for the development of retinal vein occlusion,[24] although others believe that systemic hypertension and other medical disorders may be more important in the development of retinal vein occlusion.[25] Much less often, rubeosis iridis and neovascular glaucoma may be associated with *central retinal artery occlusion*.[26] In a series of 168 patients with central retinal artery occlusion, the incidence of rubeosis iridis was 16.67%.[27] Patients who develop neovascular glaucoma in association with central retinal artery occlusion are usually elderly with severe carotid artery disease and atherosclerosis, which may be predisposing factors for development of the retinal artery occlusion[28] as well as the ocular neovascularization.[26] *Branch retinal vein occlusion* may rarely cause rubeosis iridis[4] and neovascular glaucoma.[29] *Branch retinal artery occlusion* has also been reported as a rare cause of rubeosis iridis,[26,30] although the association with neovascular glaucoma is uncertain.

Other Retinal Disorders

Rubeosis iridis may be associated with a *retinal detachment,* which is usually chronic and often overlies a *choroidal melanoma*. A rhegmatogenous retinal detachment along with a vitrectomy and lensectomy has been used to create a model of rubeosis iridis in cats.[31] Many other retinal disorders have also been reported in association with rubeosis iridis and neovascular glaucoma (Table 16.1).

Other Ocular Disorders

Uveitis was present in 11% of rubeotic eyes in one series[4] and in 1.5% in another study.[5] One case has been reported in which neovascular glaucoma followed implantation of a posterior chamber intraocular lens.[40] An iris melanoma has also been associated with neovascular glaucoma, which resolved after the tumor was excised.[41] End stage glaucoma (open-angle or angle-closure) has been said to give rise to rubeosis iridis,[4] which may be related to associated central retinal vein occlusion.

Extraocular Vascular Disorders

Carotid artery obstructive disease is probably the third most common cause of neovascular glaucoma, accounting for 13% of all cases in one series.[5] These eyes may initially be normotensive or even hypotensive as a result of decreased perfusion of the ciliary body with reduced aqueous production, and fluorescein angiography may reveal an increased arm-to-retina time and leakage from the major retinal arterioles.[42] A *carotid-cavernous fistula* may also cause rubeosis iridis and neovascular glaucoma as a result of decreased arterial flow and subsequent reduction in the ocular perfusion pressure, which may occur either before or after treatment of the fistula.[3,43,44] It has also been reported that internal carotid artery occlusion may create an "ophthalmic artery steal phenomenon" with associated rubeosis iridis.[45]

Theories of Neovasculogenesis

The mechanism(s) by which the aforementioned clinical situations lead to the development of rubeosis iridis is not fully understood, although the following theories have been proposed.

Retinal Hypoxia

Since most, but not all, of the conditions associated with rubeosis iridis involve diminished perfusion of the retina, it may be that retinal hypoxia is at least one factor in the formation of new vessels on the iris and anterior chamber angle, as well as on the retina and optic nerve head.[46] This concept is supported by the clinical observation that rubeosis iridis in association with either proliferative diabetic retinopathy[47] or central retinal vein occlusion[48] is more likely to occur when significant capillary nonperfusion is present. However, retinal capillary obliteration may represent an epiphenomenon of retinal ischemia, since the hypotony and neovascularization following experimental occlusion of the major temporal retinal vein in monkeys did not correlate with capillary loss but did correlate with retinal vascular leakage.[49] Another study with monkeys showed no significant difference in vitreous oxygen tension over nonperfused retina with intraretinal neovascularization as compared with normal retinal areas,[50] although vitreous body measurements may not accurately reflect retinal oxygen levels.

Angiogenesis Factors

It has been demonstrated that tumors possess a diffusible factor, "tumor angiogenesis factor," that is capable of eliciting new vessel growth toward the tumor.[51] Subsequent studies have suggested that human and animal retinas, as well as other vascular ocular tissues, have similar angiogenic activity, which may explain why ocular neovascularization can occur in areas remote from the site of retinal capillary nonperfusion.[52–54] Tissue culture studies have revealed vasoproliferative activity in the aqueous and vitreous of human eyes with neovascular glaucoma or proliferative diabetic retinopathy, as well as in animal models of neovascularization, but not in fluids from normal eyes.[55] The exact nature of this angiogenic factor is unknown. It was characterized in one study as diffusible, heat labile, and noninflammatory,[53] and possibilities that have been considered regarding the identity of this substance include lactic acid,[56] biogenic amines,[57] and prostaglandins.[58]

Chronic Dilation of Ocular Vessels

It has also been proposed that dilation of vessels is the stimulus that leads to new vessel growth in response to hypoxia, or any other factor that causes a vessel to dilate.[59,60] According to this theory, rubeosis iridis results from local hypoxia of the iris, which causes dilation of iris vessels and subsequent new vessel formation.

Vasoinhibitory Factors

It has also been postulated that ocular tissues may produce substances that inhibit neovascularization. The vitreous[61] and lens[62] have been suggested as possible sources of these vasoinhibitory factors, which could explain why vitrectomy or lensectomy increases the risk of rubeosis iridis in eyes with diabetic retinopathy. More recently, retinal pigment epithelial cells have been shown to release an inhibitor of neovascularization.[63]

Clinicopathologic Course

The clinical and histologic events that lead from a predisposing factor, through rubeosis iridis, to advanced neovascular glaucoma may be thought of in the following four stages (Fig. 16.1).

Pre-rubeosis Stage

In patients with a predisposing factor, such as diabetic retinopathy or central retinal vein occlusion, it is helpful to understand what the likelihood is for developing rubeosis iridis and what the chances are that this may progress to neovascular glaucoma. There are additional circumstances, especially with the two predisposing factors noted above, that may increase the risk of neovascular glaucoma to the extent that treatment is indicated even before rubeosis is detected.

Diabetic Retinopathy. The prevalence of rubeosis iridis among patients with diabetes mellitus ranges from 0.25 to 20% according to various reports.[64] The diabetes will generally have been present for many years before rubeosis develops, and concomitant proliferative diabetic retinopathy is usually found. In patient populations with proliferative diabetic retinopathy, rubeosis iridis is reported to occur in approximately half of the cases.[64,65] Rubeosis iridis may also rarely occur in an eye with nonproliferative retinopathy,[64] although other predisposing factors, such as carotid artery disease, should be considered in these cases.

As previously discussed, the risk of rubeosis iridis and neovascular glaucoma in patients with diabetic retinopathy is greatly increased when arteriolar or capillary nonperfusion is present[47] or following vitrectomy or lensectomy.[6–15] There is also a highly significant correlation between rubeosis iridis and optic disc neovasculari-

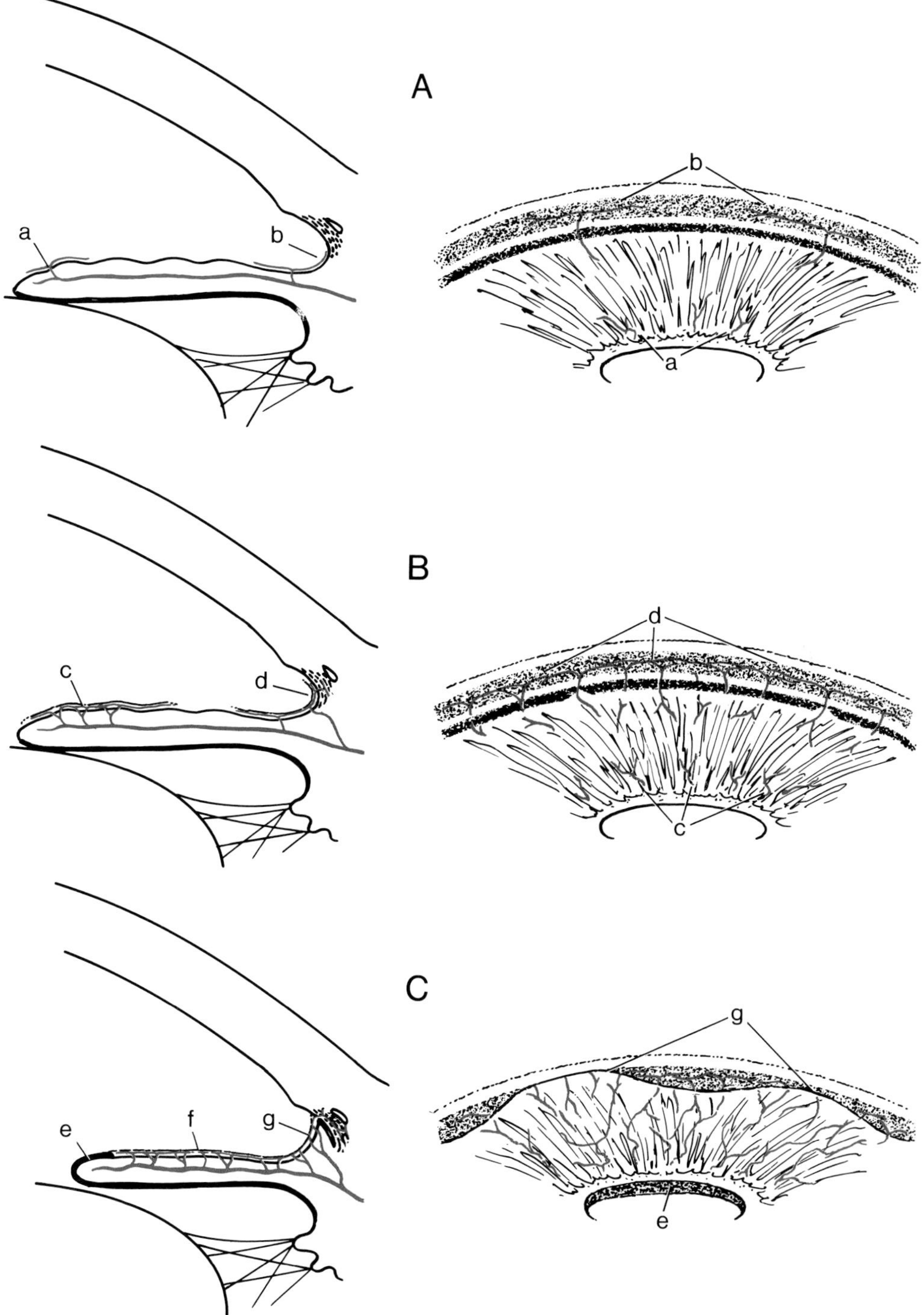

Figure 16.1. Clinicopathologic stages of neovascular glaucoma (Pre-rubeosis stage not depicted, since no anterior segment abnormalities are present at this stage): **A,** Preglaucoma stage (rubeosis iridis), characterized by new vessels on the surface of the iris (*a*) and in the anterior chamber angle (*b*); **B,** Open-angle glaucoma stage, characterized by an increase in neovascularization and a fibrovascular membrane on the iris (*c*) and in the anterior chamber angle (*d*); **C,** Angle-closure glaucoma stage, characterized by contracture of the fibrovascular membrane, causing corectopia, ectropion uvea (*e*), flattening of the iris (*f*), and peripheral anterior synechiae (*g*).

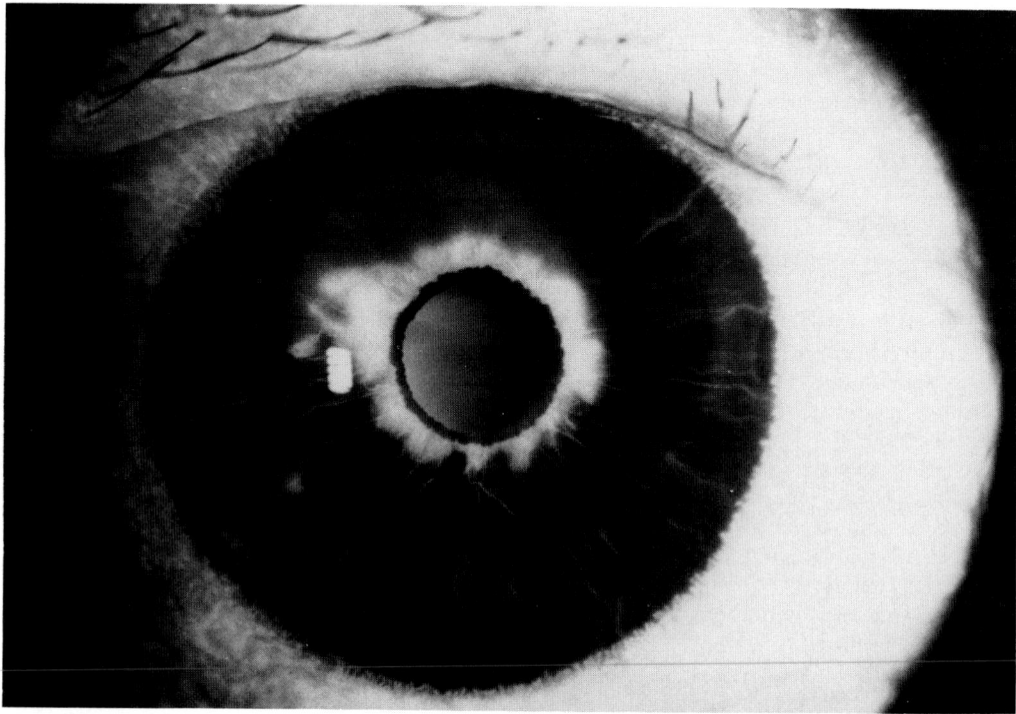

Figure 16.2. Fluorescein angiographic view of the iris in patient with proliferative diabetic retinopathy showing peripupillary microvascular leakage despite absence of clinically apparent rubeosis. (Reprinted with permission from Ehrenberg M, McCuen BW, Schindler RH, Machemer R: Ophthalmology 91:321, 1980.)

zation,[66] as well as a rhegmatogenous retinal detachment.[17,18] Peripupillary leakage with iris fluorescein angiography correlates with the risk of developing rubeosis iridis following vitrectomy for diabetic retinopathy (Fig. 16.2).[67–69]

Central Retinal Vein Occlusion. During the early months after a central retinal vein occlusion, hypotony may develop.[70,71] The explanation for this is unclear, although the possible influences of anterior segment ischemia or an angiogenic factor have been considered.[70,71]

As in diabetic retinopathy, the incidence of rubeosis iridis and neovascular glaucoma in eyes with central retinal vein occlusion is significantly correlated with the extent of retinal capillary nonperfusion.[48,72–75] In one study, the incidence of rubeosis iridis following central retinal vein occlusion was 60% when retinal ischemia was demonstrated by fluorescein angiography, compared with 1% in those eyes with good capillary perfusion.[73] While fluorescein angiography may be the most direct method of evaluating capillary nonperfusion, it is not always feasible, because of obstruction of visualization by the blood or other media opacities, and alternative evidence of poor perfusion must be considered. The ophthalmoscopic findings may be helpful in this regard. Neovascular glaucoma has been reported in 14[76]–27%[77] of eyes with hemorrhagic retinopathy (complete venous occlusion) but in none of the cases of venous stasis retinopathy (incomplete occlusion).[76–78] Fluorescein angiography of the iris is another helpful technique, in that virtually all eyes with extensive retinal capillary closure following central retinal vein occlusion have abnormal, leaking vessels of the iris.[79] Other methods of differentiating ischemic from nonischemic central retinal vein occlusion include the demonstration of a relative afferent pupillary defect[80] and electroretinography.[81–83] The most useful findings in the latter test include a b-wave implicit time delay and a reduced b-wave/a-wave amplitude ratio,[81–83] and it has been suggested that these findings are better than retinal fluorescein angiography in predicting neovascular glaucoma after central retinal vein occlusion.[83]

Pre-glaucoma Stage (rubeosis iridis)

Clinical Features. This stage is characterized by a normal IOP, unless preexisting primary open-angle glaucoma is present. Slit-lamp biomicroscopy early in the disease process typically reveals dilated tufts of preexisting capillaries and fine, randomly oriented vessels on the surface of the iris near the pupillary margin[84] (Fig. 16.3). The new vessels are also characterized by leakage of fluorescein.[84,85] Reports differ as to whether true neovascularization is first seen on the peripupillary iris[84] or in the anterior chamber angle.[86] In most cases, however, it appears to progress from the pupillary margin toward the root of the iris. Gonioscopy may reveal a normal anterior chamber angle or may show a variable amount of angle neovascularization. The latter is characterized by single vascular trunks crossing the ciliary body band and scleral spur and arborizing on the trabecular meshwork.

Histopathologic Features. The rubeosis iridis begins intrastromally and then develops on the surface of the iris.[61,87] Experimental retinal vein occlusion in monkey eyes indicates that the rubeosis iridis begins with dilation of normal iris vessels and marked increase in metabolism of vascular endothelial cells followed by new vessel formation.[88] Silicone injection studies indicate that the new vessels on the iris arise from normal iris arteries and drain primarily into iris and ciliary body veins, while new vessels in the angle arise from arteries of the iris and ciliary body and connect with the peripheral neovascular network on the iris.[89] Although the clinical appearance of rubeosis iridis is said to be the same in cases

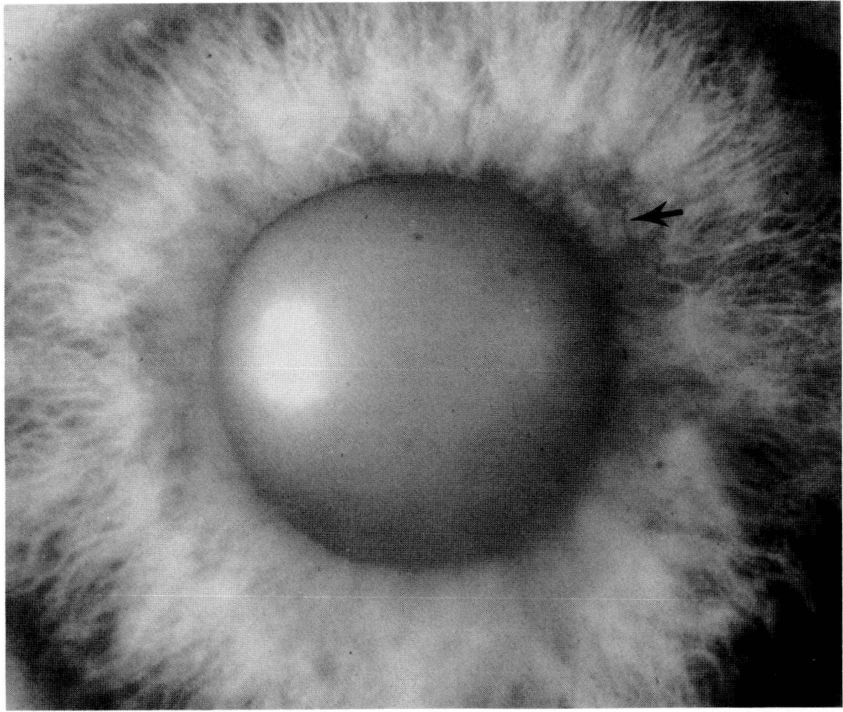

Figure 16.3. Slit-lamp view of iris in patient with rubeosis iridis showing fine, tortuous vessels on surface of peripupillary iris (*arrow*).

of diabetes and central retinal vein occlusion,[85] the silicone injections show tighter and more evenly distributed neovascularization in the diabetic eye.[89] The silicone injection studies also show that new vessels in the angle run circumferentially in the trabecular meshwork, with branches coursing into the fibrosed Schlemm's canal and occasionally into collector channels.[89] The new vessels are characterized histologically as having thin fenestrated walls[87,90,91] and are arranged in irregular patterns.[87] The ultrastructure of iris neovascularization associated with sickle cell retinopathy is said to be similar to that in diabetes and retinal occlusive disease with open interendothelial cell junctions, attenuated intraendothelial cytoplasm, and pericyte formation.[92]

Open-Angle Glaucoma Stage

Clinical Features. Neovascular glaucoma does not invariably follow the development of rubeosis iridis,[64,65,70,84] and the latter condition may rarely resolve spontaneously, especially that associated with diabetic retinopathy.[64] The reported incidence of neovascular glaucoma in diabetic patients with rubeosis iridis ranges from 13 to 22%,[64,65,84] while that associated with central retinal vein occlusion is probably significantly higher. The latter condition typically occurs 8–15 weeks after the vascular occlusive event[70] and has been called "90 day glaucoma", because the average time interval was thought to be 3 months. However, it is important to note that the glaucoma can develop during the first month or any time after a central retinal vein occlusion.

The rubeosis iridis is typically more florid in this stage, and biomicroscopic examination of the aqueous often reveals an inflammatory reaction (Fig. 16.4). As shown by gonioscopy, the anterior chamber angle is still open, but the neovascularization is intense (Fig. 16.5). The IOP is now elevated and may rise suddenly, causing the patient to present with acute onset glaucoma. Hyphema may also be present in this stage.

Histopathologic Features. The hallmark of this stage is a fibrovascular membrane that covers the anterior chamber angle and anterior surface of the iris[87,90] and may even extend onto the posterior iris.[90] Chronic in-

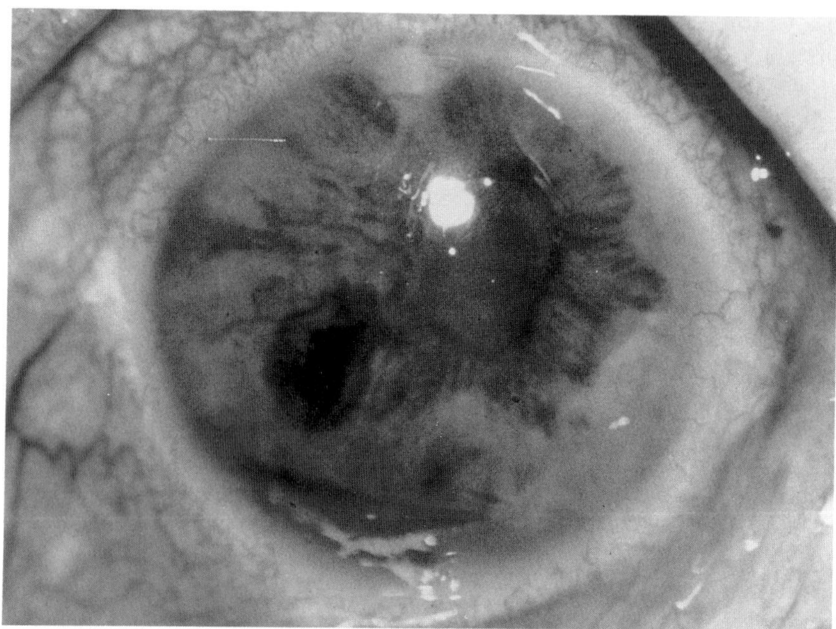

Figure 16.4. Slit-lamp appearance of iris in patient with neovascular glaucoma showing marked rubeosis and hyphema.

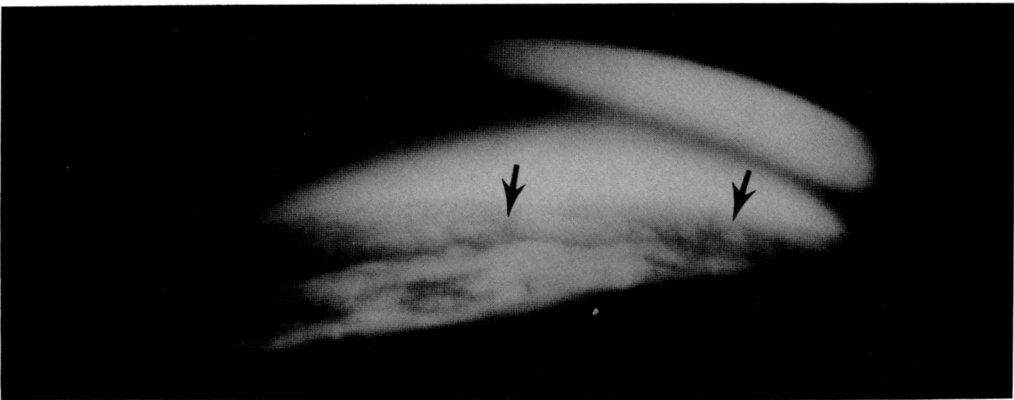

Figure 16.5. Gonioscopic view of patient with open-angle stage of neovascular glaucoma showing intense neovascularization (*arrows*) in an open anterior chamber angle. (Courtesy of Brooks W. McCuen, II, M.D.)

flammatory changes are also typically seen on histologic examination.[87,90] The glaucoma in this stage probably results from obstruction of the trabecular meshwork by the fibrovascular membrane, with variable contribution from the inflammation and hemorrhage.

Angle-Closure Glaucoma Stage

Clinical Features. In this stage, the stroma of the iris has become flattened, with a smooth, glistening appearance. Ectropion uvea is frequently present, and the iris is often dilated and pulled anteriorly from the lens (Fig. 16.6). In the anterior chamber angle, the contracture leads to peripheral anterior synechia formation, with eventual total synechial closure of the angle. The glaucoma in this stage is typically severe and usually requires surgical intervention.

Histopathologic Features. The clinically observed alterations of the iris and anterior chamber angle in this stage result from contracture of tissue overlying these structures. Histopathologic studies reveal peripheral anterior synechiae and flattening of the anterior iris surface by a confluent fibrovascular membrane.[93,94] Overlying the new vessels is a clinically inapparent, superficial layer of myofibroblasts (fibroblastic cells with smooth muscle differentiation), which may be responsible for the tissue contraction.[93] A layer of endothelium, continuous with the corneal endothelium at the pseudoangle, is also seen in some cases[94–96] and has been observed to possess features of myoblastic differentiation,[96] which may explain the origin of these cells.

Differential Diagnosis

In the open-angle glaucoma stages, neovascular glaucoma must be distinguished from other glaucomas with acute onset, such as angle-closure glaucoma and glaucoma associated with anterior uveitis. This differentiation can usually be made on the basis of new vessels on the iris and in the anterior chamber angle with neovascular glaucoma, although eyes with uveitis often have dilation of normal iris vessels that may be confused with neovascularization, especially with blue irides. Patients with Fuchs' heterochromic iridocyclitis also typically have new vessels in the anterior chamber angle (Chapter 19). In the angle-closure stage of neovascular glaucoma, the new vessels may be less apparent, and the differential diagnosis must include other causes of iris distortion and peripheral anterior synechiae, such as the iridocorneal endothelial syndrome (Chapter 13) and old trauma (Chapter 22).

Management

Panretinal Photocoagulation

Ablation of peripheral retina with laser (usually argon) or xenon arc photocoagula-

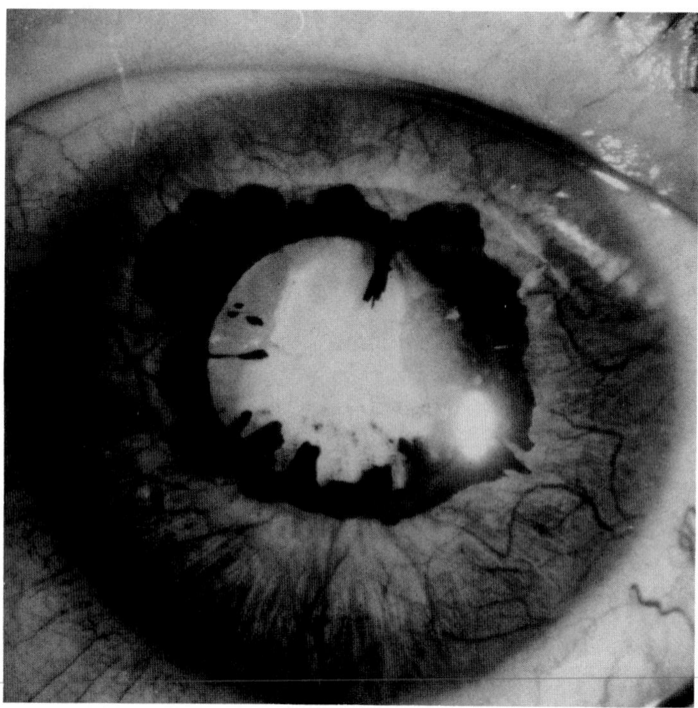

Figure 16.6. Slit-lamp view of patient with angle-closure stage of neovascular glaucoma showing numerous new vessels on iris, with pupillary dilation and ectropion uvea resulting from contracture of the fibrovascular membrane.

tion is the first line of therapy for most cases of neovascular glaucoma. This procedure has been shown to significantly reduce or eliminate anterior segment neovascularization in many cases[97–102] and to reduce the chances of developing rubeosis iridis in eyes with diabetic retinopathy or central retinal vein occlusion.[73,84,103–107] The mechanism by which panretinal photocoagulation influences neovascularization is uncertain, although it may be related to decreasing the retinal oxygen demand, which is consistent with the reported observation that the photoreceptor-retinal pigment epithelial complex accounts for two-thirds of the total retinal oxygen consumption.[108] This, in turn, may reduce the stimulus for release of an angiogenesis factor and/or may reduce the hypoxia in the anterior ocular segment.

Prophylactic Therapy. Panretinal photocoagulation is most effective as prophylaxis against the development of rubeosis iridis and neovascular glaucoma. It should be considered, therefore, during the *prerubeosis stage,* if the risk of developing rubeosis iridis is sufficiently high. The prime example of this is central retinal vein occlusion in which there is evidence of significant retinal capillary nonperfusion, as discussed earlier in this chapter. The risk of rubeosis iridis in eyes with diabetic retinopathy is more difficult to predict, but vitrectomy or lensectomy, especially in association with peripupillary fluorescein leakage, may be indications for prophylactic therapy. The latter is often performed as endophotocoagulation in conjunction with pars plana vitrectomy for diabetic retinopathy. By the time rubeosis iridis appears (*preglaucoma stage*), panretinal photocoagulation is indicated in all cases, including those resulting from central retinal artery occlusion[109] and carotid artery insufficiency. Even though neovascular glaucoma does not invariably follow rubeosis iridis, it does so with sufficient frequency that prophylactic laser therapy is justified in nearly all cases.

Treatment of Glaucoma. It is reported that panretinal photocoagulation may reverse IOP elevation in the open-angle glaucoma stage[97,98,110] and in some cases of early angle-closure neovascular glaucoma, provided the synechial closure has not exceeded 270°.[100] Even in the latter situation, panretinal photocoagulation may be useful in reducing anterior segment neovascularization prior to intraocular surgery.[111] However, one study showed that panretinal photocoagulation prior to vitrectomy for diabetic retinopathy did not prevent postoperative rubeosis iridis.[112] In these cases, intraocular panretinal photocoagulation at the time of vitrectomy may be the procedure of choice.[113]

Panretinal Cryotherapy

When cloudy media precludes panretinal photocoagulation, it has been reported that transscleral panretinal cryotherapy, often combined with cyclocryotherapy, in eyes with neovascular glaucoma will control the IOP and reduce or abolish the neovascularization.[114,115]

Goniophotocoagulation

This technique involves the direct application of argon laser therapy to new vessels in the anterior chamber angle.[116] It is most effective when used in the early stages of the disease to prevent the progressive angle changes and eventual intractable neovascular glaucoma.[117] Although no longer commonly used, it may be beneficial in patients with a high risk of developing neovascular glaucoma, when panretinal photocoagulation has not been successful or is not possible or advisable, and prior to intraocular surgery.[117]

Medical Management

Once the IOP begins to rise, medical therapy is usually required and is frequently sufficient to control the pressure during the *open-angle glaucoma stage*. The mainstay of the therapy at this stage is drugs that reduce aqueous production, such as carbonic anhydrase inhibitors and topical beta-blockers. Miotics rarely are helpful and usually should be avoided because of the complications with inflammation. Topical corticosteroids may be useful in minimizing the inflammation and pain.[118] In addition, intravitreal triamcinolone has been shown to reduce retinal neovascularization in rabbit eyes,[119] raising the question of a possible direct benefit of topical steroids on rubeotic vessels. In far advanced or blind eyes, atropine is helpful for relief of pain. Hyperosmotic agents may also be required for temporary control of cases with marked IOP elevation.

Cyclodestructive Procedures

If the disease follows its natural course to the *angle-closure glaucoma stage,* medical therapy nearly always becomes ineffective and surgical intervention is required. Even at this stage, panretinal photocoagulation may be beneficial by reducing the anterior segment neovascularization to allow filtration surgery. With active rubeosis, however, standard filtering surgery has a low chance of success, and a cyclodestructive procedure may be preferable.

While good results have been reported by some surgeons with the use of *cyclocryotherapy* for neovascular glaucoma,[120,121] other reports have been less encouraging.[122–124] In one 2-year follow-up of 50 eyes, one-third were uncontrolled and one-third developed phthisis.[122] An alternative cyclodestructive procedure is *transscleral Nd:YAG cyclophotocoagulation,* and preliminary experience suggests that this may become the surgical procedure of choice for neovascular glaucoma, when filtering surgery is not believed to be indicated.[125]

Filtering Surgery

It has been a general belief that standard filtering procedures in eyes with neovascular glaucoma are rarely successful, primarily because of the high risk of intraoperative bleeding and postoperative progression of the fibrovascular membrane. As noted above, however, a successful panretinal photocoagulation, possibly combined with goniophotocoagulation, will often reduce the neovascularization sufficiently to make it possible to perform a standard filtering operation, such as trabeculectomy or a full-thickness filtering procedure.[126] In addition, newer techniques of filtering surgery for neovascular glaucoma have been described, which include a modified trabeculectomy with intraocular bipolar cautery of peripheral iris and ciliary processes,[127,128] and creation of a limbal fistula with a carbon dioxide laser.[129] Encouraging preliminary experience has also been reported with the implantation of tubes[130–133] or valves[134] into the anterior chamber in eyes with neovascular glaucoma. Details regarding the techniques and reported results of these procedures are considered in Section Three.

Other Surgical Procedures

Several new techniques have been evaluated for the treatment of neovascular glaucoma. Silicone oil injection during revision of vitrectomy after unsuccessful diabetic vitreous surgery achieved stabilization or regression of anterior ocular neovascular changes in 83% of eyes in one study.[135] Vascular occlusion has been created in experimental models following photosensitization of vessels with intravenous hematoporphyrin and exposure to red light[136] or intravenous injection of rose bengal and exposure to filtered light with a wavelength of 550 nm (the absorption maximum of rose bengal).[137] Exposure to 100% oxygen under hyperbaric conditions has been shown to significantly increase the partial pressure of oxygen in the aqueous humor of animal eyes, which may have an application in treating hypoxic diseases of the anterior segment, including rubeosis iridis.[138]

Hypophysectomy is mentioned only for historical interest. Its efficacy was never established with regard to rubeosis iridis and neovascular glaucoma. In one study, 62 patients were treated and compared with 73 untreated cases. Rubeosis iridis developed in 29% of the former group and 33% of the latter, while the incidence of neovascular glaucoma in eyes with rubeosis iridis was 27% and 33%, respectively.[65]

ALTERATIONS OF INTRAOCULAR PRESSURE ASSOCIATED WITH RETINAL DETACHMENT

Reduced IOP and Retinal Detachment

An eye with a rhegmatogenous retinal detachment typically has a reduced IOP. Experimental studies with retinal detachments in monkeys suggest that an early, transient pressure drop may result from inflammation and reduced aqueous production,[139] while a more prolonged hypotony may be due to posterior flow of aqueous through the retinal hole.[140] A study with kinetic vitreous fluorophotometry indicated a posterior flow, presumably through a break in the retinal pigment epithelium, in patients with vitreous and rhegmatogenous retinal detachments.[141] Campbell[142] has described a condition, the *iris retraction syndrome,* in which a patient presents with a rhegmatogenous retinal detachment, a secluded pupil, and angle closure secondary to iris bombé. Pharmacologic suppression of aqueous production in these individuals leads to hypotony and a posterior retraction of the iris, presumably because of a shift in the predominant direction of aqueous flow toward the subretinal space.

Glaucomas Associated with Retinal Detachment

The coexistence of glaucoma and a retinal detachment in the same eye occurs under three circumstances: (1) glaucomas associated with retinal detachment, in which a cause-and-effect relationship is uncertain; (2) glaucoma secondary to retinal detachment; and (3) glaucomas secondary to treatment for retinal detachment. The first two situations are discussed in this chapter, and the third is considered in Chapter 23.

Primary Open-Angle Glaucoma and Retinal Detachment

Epidemiology. Primary open-angle glaucoma is more common in eyes with a rhegmatogenous retinal detachment than in the general population. In one study of 817 cases of retinal detachment, primary open-angle glaucoma was present in 4%, and an additional 6.5% had elevated IOP without glaucomatous damage.[143]

Theories of Mechanism. It is not known why primary open-angle glaucoma and rhegmatogenous retinal detachment occur in the same eye more frequently than would be anticipated on the basis of chance occurrence. Neither myopia nor the use of miotics has been found to be the common denominator.[143] In 30 cases of spontaneous rhegmatogenous retinal detachment, 53% had a cup/disc ratio greater than 0.3 and 20% were high topical steroid responders.[144] These values are significantly higher than these in the general population and resemble the findings in groups of patients with primary open-angle glaucoma, which led the authors to suggest that the two diseases may be related genetically by multifactorial inheritance.

Management. When primary open-angle glaucoma and retinal detachment coexist, one disorder may mask the presence of the other, necessitating careful attention to certain details during the management of either condition. When following a patient with primary open-angle glaucoma, the physician should examine the peripheral retina before initiating therapy and at least annually or whenever warning signs appear, such as floaters, flashing lights, loss of peripheral vision, or a sudden decrease in the IOP. Although the role of miotics in the pathogenesis of rhegmatogenous retinal detachment has not been clearly established, circumstantial evidence indicates that particular caution is warranted when these drugs are used.[145,146]

In an eye with a rhegmatogenous retinal detachment, the reduced IOP may mask a preexisting glaucoma. In addition, retinal detachment surgery lowers ocular rigidity, which will cause a Schiøtz tonometer to read falsely low.[147,148] In one study of 115 eyes, the mean disparity between applanation and Schiøtz pressure measurements averaged 8.6 mm Hg 1 month after retinal detachment surgery and 5.8 mm Hg 6 months postoperatively.[147] Therefore, an applanation tonometer should be used following retinal detachment surgery, and the optic nerve head should be inspected carefully during the fundus examination to avoid missing coexisting glaucoma.

The success of retinal detachment surgery is not adversely affected by the presence of glaucoma,[143] although the visual outcome may be worse because of the concomitant glaucomatous optic atrophy.[143,149] Following retinal detachment surgery, special caution should be given to the use of topical steroids, because of the increased incidence of high topical steroid responders,[144] and miotics should be used with caution in either eye.

Pigmentary Glaucoma and Retinal Detachment

Patients with the pigment dispersion syndrome, with or without glaucoma, may have an increased incidence of retinal detachment. In addition, patients with retinal detachment are reported to have varying degrees of pigment dispersion in the anterior chamber angle in a significant number of cases.[150] As in the case of primary open-angle glaucoma, no definite cause-and-effect relationship has been established, but the same considerations as mentioned above must be employed in the management of coexisting pigmentary glaucoma and retinal detachment.

Glaucoma Secondary to Rhegmatogenous Retinal Detachment (Schwartz Syndrome)

As previously noted, a rhegmatogenous retinal detachment is typically associated with a slight reduction in the IOP. However, Schwartz described a rare condition in which the patient presents with unilateral pressure elevation, a retinal detachment, and an open anterior chamber angle with aqueous cells and flare.[151] The condition has become known as the *Schwartz syndrome*.

Theories of Mechanism. The mechanism of the glaucoma is unclear, although many patients have a history of ocular trauma,[143,151] and concomitant damage to the trabecular meshwork may cause reduced aqueous outflow in some cases. Other suggested mechanisms include anterior uveitis secondary to the retinal detachment[151] and obstruction of the trabecular meshwork by pigment from the retinal pigment epithelium[152] or glycosaminoglycans from the visual cells.[153] More recently, photoreceptor outer segments with few inflammatory cells have been demonstrated in the aqueous of patients with the Schwartz syndrome,[154] and the injection of rod outer segments into human autopsy and living cat eyes has been shown to significantly reduce outflow facility by obstructing the trabecular meshwork.[155]

Management. The treatment of both the rhegmatogenous retinal detachment and the secondary glaucoma is repair of the detachment, which typically results in resolution of the glaucoma within a few days.[151] In the differential diagnosis, it is important to remember that an eye with a retinal detachment and glaucoma may harbor a malignant melanoma.[156]

Glaucoma Secondary to Other Forms of Retinal Detachment

In addition to rhegmatogenous retinal detachment, several other forms of retinal detachment may be associated with a secondary glaucoma. These include traction detachments, as with proliferative diabetic retinopathy and retinopathy of prematurity (discussed in this chapter), exudative retinal detachments (Chapter 19), and detachments associated with neoplasia, such as melanomas and retinoblastoma (Chapter 18). Each of these conditions may lead to either a neovascular or angle-closure mechanism of glaucoma.

ANGLE-CLOSURE GLAUCOMAS ASSOCIATED WITH DISORDERS OF THE RETINA, VITREOUS, AND CHOROID

Central Retinal Vein Occlusion

The neovascular glaucoma following retinal vascular occlusive disease was discussed earlier in this chapter. In addition, a small number of cases have been described in which shallowing of the anterior chamber after a central retinal vein occlusion led to transient angle-closure glaucoma.[157–160]

Examination typically reveals a forward shift of the lens-iris diaphragm in the involved eye and a normal anterior chamber depth in the fellow eye. The mechanism of the angle-closure is uncertain, although it has been postulated that transudation of fluid from the retinal vessels into the vitreous leads to forward displacement of the lens with a subsequent pupillary block.[157] The differential diagnosis should include primary angle-closure glaucoma, which may secondarily cause occlusion of the central retinal vein, and neovascular glaucoma, which can lead to synechial closure of the anterior chamber angle. The former situation might be recognized by a potentially occludable angle in the fellow eye, while the latter usually can be identified by the presence of rubeosis iridis.

Treatment usually should be medical, since the angle returns to normal depth over a period of several weeks. Carbonic anhydrase inhibitors and topical beta-blockers may be helpful, and success has been reported with both pilocarpine[157,158] and cycloplegics.[159]

Hemorrhagic Retinal or Choroidal Detachment

Acute angle-closure glaucoma may occur secondary to a spontaneous massive hemorrhagic retinal or choroidal detachment.[161] The hemorrhagic detachment is typically the result of a disciform macular lesion, and associated conditions include systemic hypertension, primary clotting disorders, and the systemic use of anticoagulants and thrombolytic agents.[161,162] The mechanism of the angle closure is believed to be the abrupt forward displacement of the lens-iris diaphragm by the massively detached retina and choroid.[161] Visual prognosis is poor in these eyes, and the management is directed primarily at relief of pain through IOP control with antiglaucoma medications or cyclodestructive surgery. Retrobulbar alcohol injection or enucleation occasionally may be necessary.

Ciliochoroidal Effusion

In the following conditions, uveal effusion with ciliochoroidal detachment may lead to a forward rotation of the lens-iris diaphragm and angle-closure glaucoma.

Nanophthalmos

This rare ocular anomaly is characterized by a small eye, with a small cornea, shallow anterior chamber, narrow angle, and high lens/eye volume ratio.[163–165] The eyes are highly hyperopic because of the short axial length (<20 mm by most definitions) and frequently develop angle-closure glaucoma in the fourth to sixth decades of life. Additional reported retinal disorders include pigmentary retinal dystrophy[166] and pigmentary retinal degeneration and cystic macular degeneration in a family with an autosomal-recessive syndrome.[167] Uveal effusion and nonrhegmatogenous retinal detachment have been found following intraocular surgery in these cases.[163–165,168] There is evidence that the uveal effusion and retinal detachment, in some patients, may precede the surgery and actually cause the angle-closure glaucoma by producing a forward shift of the lens-iris diaphragm, leading to a pupillary block mechanism.[169]

Histopathologic studies reveal an unusually thick sclera with irregular interlacing collagen bundles,[170,171] reduced glycosaminoglycans,[171] and elevated fibronectin.[172] Altered metabolism of glycosaminoglycans and fibronectin may be related to the development of abnormal sclera in nanophthalmos.[170–172] It has been proposed that the uveal effusion may result from reduced scleral permeability to proteins by the thickened sclera,[173] or compression of venous drainage channels by the dense collagen around the vortex veins.[174]

This form of secondary glaucoma responds poorly to conventional surgical therapy, with a high complication rate, associated primarily with the uveal effusion.[164,168] Medical therapy may be effective, although miotics may increase the pupillary block.[164] Laser iridotomy and laser gonioplasty (retraction of the peripheral iris) appear to have the highest success rate and are the procedures of choice.[164,169] A suggested approach to managing the uveal effusion is vortex vein decompression and, in some cases, drainage of choroidal and/or subretinal fluid with air injection into the vitreous cavity.[174]

Uveal Effusion Syndrome

This condition has similarities to nanophthalmos, with the main exception being an eye of normal size. It occurs more frequently in males and is characterized by dilated episcleral vessels, thickened or detached choroid and ciliary body, and nonrhegmatogenous retinal detachment.[173] As with nanophthalmos, the sclera may be thickened and impermeable, although one ultrastructural study revealed increased glycosaminoglycan-like deposits between the scleral fibers as well as dilated rough endoplasmic reticulum and large intracellular glycogen-like granules in scleral cells.[175] The IOP may be normal, unless secondary angle-closure glaucoma is present, which reportedly responds to cycloplegics, aqueous suppressants, and corticosteroids.[176]

Other Causes of Ciliochoroidal Effusion

Several additional causes of ciliochoroidal effusion are considered in subsequent chapters: inflammatory conditions (Chapter 19), arteriovenous malformation (Chapter 17), tumors (Chapter 18), trauma (Chapter 22), and surgery (Chapter 23).

Retinopathy of Prematurity (Retrolental Fibroplasia)

Contracture of the retrolental mass in retinopathy of prematurity can cause progressive shallowing of the anterior chamber with eventual angle-closure glaucoma. This complication coincides with the cicatricial phase of the disease, which usually has its onset at 3–6 months of age. However, the angle-closure glaucoma may occur later in childhood, and there is a need for continued observation. In one series of five patients with secondary angle-closure glaucoma, the glaucoma in each case occurred after age 2 years,[177] while another series described the onset of angle-closure glaucoma secondary to retinopathy of prematurity in three adults in their 20s.[178] Although the typical mechanism of glaucoma is angle closure resulting from the retrolental mass, anterior chamber angle abnormalities, including hypopigmentation of the iris root, a translucent material in the angle, and a prominent Schwalbe's line, suggest a developmental origin in some cases.[179]

The glaucoma usually does not respond well to medical therapy, although some success has been reported with the use of cycloplegics[180] and topical corticosteroids.[181] Lens aspiration, with anterior vitrectomy in some cases, has been used successfully to control the IOP, although the procedure usually is used only to relieve pain and avoid enucleation since useful vision is typically lost by this stage.[177,182,183]

However, vitrectomy techniques to reattach the retina are resulting in improved vision in some cases.[184,185]

Persistent Hyperplastic Primary Vitreous

Retention and hyperplasia of the primary vitreous is usually unilateral and often associated with microphthalmia and elongated ciliary processes.[186] Shallowing of the anterior chamber with subsequent angle-closure glaucoma may result from contracture of the fibrous retrolenticular mass and swelling of a cataractous lens. Small pupillary notches, resulting from anastomotic vessels between the anterior and posterior tunica vasculosa lentis, may be a helpful sign of persistent hyperplastic primary vitreous, especially when the diagnosis is obscured by an opaque lens.[187] The appearance of persistent hyperplastic primary vitreous by computed tomography is sufficiently characteristic to also make this a useful diagnostic modality.[188]

If left untreated, the vast majority of these eyes will show progressive deterioration.[189] The recommended treatment is aspiration of the lens and removal of the fibrovascular mass with scissors[190] or vitrectomy instruments.[189,190–194] Since the retina in these cases often extends as far anteriorly as the pars plicata, a pars plana incision is believed to be contraindicated,[194] and success with a limbal incision has been reported.[189] This treatment may prevent or eliminate the angle-closure glaucoma, although postoperative visual rehabilitation is difficult and treatment to avoid amblyopia is usually required.[190,191]

Attention should also be given to the fellow eye in these cases, since two adult patients with uncomplicated unilateral persistent hyperplastic primary vitreous were found to have open-angle glaucoma in the contralateral eye, associated with anomalous blood vessels in the entire circumference of the anterior chamber angle, band keratopathy, and heterochromia iridis.[195]

Retinal Dysplasia

This condition is usually bilateral and associated with multiple congenital anomalies, especially in trisomy 13–15.[196] The dysplastic retina may be pulled up behind the lens, and glaucoma may result from angle closure or an associated dysgenesis of the anterior chamber angle.

RETINITIS PIGMENTOSA

Retinitis pigmentosa has been described in association with primary glaucoma, which most often appears to be of the open-angle type.[197] However, the association is infrequent, and a true cause-and-effect relationship has not been established.

SUMMARY

Neovascular glaucoma is a relatively common and serious complication of several retinal disorders, especially diabetic retinopathy and central retinal vein occlusion, as well as several other ocular and extraocular conditions. By mechanisms that are not fully understood, a fibrovascular membrane develops on the iris and in the anterior chamber angle, which initially obstructs aqueous outflow in an open angle and then contracts to produce an angle-closure form of glaucoma. The most effective treatment is panretinal photocoagulation in the early stages of the disease to reduce the stimulus for anterior segment neovascularization.

Retinal detachments are usually associated with a reduction in IOP, although some patients may have concomitant retinal detachment and glaucoma, which may or may not have a cause-and-effect relationship. There is also a group of conditions in which angle-closure glaucoma may be associated with a retinal, choroidal, or vitreous disorder, including central retinal vein occlusion, nanophthalmos, retinopathy of prematurity, persistent hyperplastic primary vitreous, and retinal dysplasia.

References

1. Coats, G: Further cases of thrombosis of the central vein. Royal Lond Ophthal Hosp Rep 16:516, 1906.
2. Smith, RJH: Rubeotic glaucoma. Br J Ophthal 65:606, 1981.
3. Weiss, DI, Shaffer, RN, Nehrenberg, TR: Neo-

vascular glaucoma complicating carotid-cavernous fistula. Arch Ophthal 69:304, 1963.

4. Hoskins, HD Jr: Neovascular glaucoma: current concepts. Trans Am Acad Ophthal Otol 78:330, 1974.
5. Brown, GC, Magargal, LE, Schachat, A, Shah, H: Neovascular glaucoma: etiologic considerations. Ophthalmology 91:315, 1984.
6. Mandelcorn, MS, Blankenship, G, Machemer, R: Pars plana vitrectomy for the management of severe diabetic retinopathy. Am J Ophthal 81:561, 1976.
7. Aaberg, TM, Van Horn, DL: Late complications of pars plana vitreous surgery. Ophthalmology 85:126, 1978.
8. Michels, RG: Vitrectomy for complications of diabetic retinopathy. Arch Ophthal 96:237, 1978.
9. Blankenship, G, Cortez, R, Machemer, R: The lens and pars plana vitrectomy for diabetic retinopathy complications. Arch Ophthal 97:1263, 1979.
10. Machemer, R, Blankenship, G: Vitrectomy for proliferative diabetic retinopathy associated with vitreous hemorrhage. Ophthalmology 88:643, 1981.
11. Schachat, AP, Oyakawa, RT, Michels, RG, Rice, TA: Complications of vitreous surgery for diabetic retinopathy. II. Postoperative complications. Ophthalmology 90:522, 1983.
12. Blankenship, GW: The lens influence on diabetic vitrectomy results. Report of a prospective randomized study. Arch Ophthal 98:2196, 1980.
13. Aaberg, TM: Pars plana vitrectomy for diabetic traction retinal detachment. Ophthalmology 88:639, 1981.
14. Rice, TA, Michels, RG, Maguire, MG, Rice, EF: The effect of lensectomy on the incidence of iris neovascularization and neovascular glaucoma after vitrectomy for diabetic retinopathy. Am J Ophthal 95:1, 1983.
15. Blankenship, GW: Management of vitreous cavity hemorrhage following pars plana vitrectomy for diabetic retinopathy. Ophthalmology 93:39, 1986.
16. Blankenship, GW: Preoperative iris rubeosis and diabetic vitrectomy results. Ophthalmology 87:176, 1980.
17. Scuderi, JJ, Blumenkranz, MS, Blankenship, GW: Regression of diabetic rubeosis iridis following successful surgical reattachment of the retina by vitrectomy. Retina 2:193, 1982.
18. Wand, M, Madigan, JC, Gaudio, AR, Sorokanich, S: Neovascular glaucoma following pars plana vitrectomy for complications of diabetic retinopathy. Ophthal Surg 21:113, 1990.
19. de Juan, E Jr, Hardy, M, Hatchell, DL, Hatchell, MC: The effect of intraocular silicone oil on anterior chamber oxygen pressure in cats. Arch Ophthal 104:1063, 1986.
20. Blankenship, GW, Machemer, R: Long-term diabetic vitrectomy results. Report of 10 year follow-up. Ophthalmology 92:503, 1985.
21. Aiello, LM, Wand, M, Liang, G: Neovascular glaucoma and vitreous hemorrhage following cataract surgery in patients with diabetes mellitus. Ophthalmology 90:814, 1983.
22. Poliner, LS, Christianson, DJ, Escoffery, RF, et al: Neovascular glaucoma after intracapsular and extracapsular cataract extraction in diabetic patients. Am J Ophthal 100:637, 1985.
23. Weinreb, RN, Wasserstrom, JP, Parker, W: Neovascular glaucoma following Neodymium-YAG laser posterior capsulotomy. Arch Ophthal 104:730, 1986.
24. David, R, Zangwill, L, Badarna, M, Yassur, Y: Epidemiology of retinal vein occlusion and its association with glaucoma and increased intraocular pressure. Ophthalmologica 197:69, 1988.
25. Cole, MD, Dodson, PM, Hendeles, S: Medical conditions underlying retinal vein occlusion in patients with glaucoma or ocular hypertension. Br J Ophthal 73:693, 1989.
26. Hayreh, SS, Podhajsky, P: Ocular neovascularization with retinal vascular occlusion. II. Occurrence in central and branch retinal artery occlusion. Arch Ophthal 100:1585, 1982.
27. Duker, JS, Brown, GC: Iris neovascularization associated with obstruction of the central retinal artery. Ophthalmology 95:1244, 1988.
28. Peternel, P, Keber, D, Videcnik, V: Carotid arteries in central retinal vessel occlusion as assessed by Doppler ultrasound. Br J Ophthal 73:880, 1989.
29. Magargal, LE, Brown, GC, Augsburger, JJ, Parrish, RK: Neovascular glaucoma following branch retinal vein obstruction. Glaucoma 3:333, 1981.
30. Bresnick, GH, Gay, AJ: Rubeosis iridis associated with branch retinal arteriolar occlusions. Arch Ophthal 77:176, 1967.
31. Stefansson, E, Landers, MB III, Wolbarsht, ML, Klintworth, GK: Neovascularization of the iris: an experimental model in cats. Invest Ophthal Vis Sci 25:361, 1984.
32. Walton, DS, Grant, WM: Retinoblastoma and iris neovascularization. Am J Ophthal 65:598, 1968.
33. Goldberg, MF, Tso, MOM: Rubeosis iridis and glaucoma associated with sickle cell retinopathy: a light and electron microscopic study. Ophthalmology 85:1028, 1978.
34. Savir, H, Kurz, O: Fluorescein angiography in syphilitic retinal vasculitis. Ann Ophthal 8:713, 1976.
35. Hung, JY, Hilton, GF: Neovascular glaucoma in a patient with X-linked juvenile retinoschisis. Ann Ophthal 12:1054, 1980.
36. Young, NJA, Hitchings, RA, Sehmi, K, Bird,

AC: Stickler's syndrome and neovascular glaucoma. Br J Ophthal 63:826, 1979.
37. Buchanan, TAS, Hoyt, WF: Optic nerve glioma and neovascular glaucoma: report of a case. Br J Ophthal 66:96, 1982.
38. Lewis, RA, Tse, DT, Phelps, CD, Weingeist, TA: Neovascular glaucoma after photoradiation therapy for uveal melanoma. Arch Ophthal 102:839, 1984.
39. Kim, MK, Char, DH, Castro, JL, et al: Neovascular glaucoma after helium ion irradiation for uveal melanoma. Ophthalmology 93:189, 1986.
40. Apple, DJ, Craythorn, JM, Olson, RJ, et al: Anterior segment complications and neovascular glaucoma following implantation of a posterior chamber intraocular lens. Ophthalmology 91:403, 1984.
41. Shields, MB, Proia, AD: Neovascular glaucoma associated with an iris melanoma. A clinicopathologic report. Arch Ophthal 105:672, 1987.
42. Coppeto, JR, Wand, M, Bear, L, Sciarra, R: Neovascular glaucoma and carotid artery obstructive disease. Am J Ophthal 99:567, 1985.
43. Sugar, HS: Neovascular glaucoma after carotid-cavernous fistula formation. Ann Ophthal 11:667, 1979.
44. Harris, GJ, Rice, PR: Angle closure in carotid-cavernous fistula. Ophthalmology 86:1521, 1979.
45. Huckman, MS, Haas, J: Reversed flow through the ophthalmic artery as a cause of rubeosis iridis. Am J Ophthal 74:1094, 1972.
46. Wise, GN: Retinal neovascularization. Trans Am Ophthal Soc 54:729, 1956.
47. Bresnick, GH, De Venecia, G, Myers, FL, et al: Retinal ischemia in diabetic retinopathy. Arch Ophthal 93:1300, 1975.
48. Laatikainen, L, Kohner, EM: Fluorescein angiography and its prognostic significance in central retinal vein occlusion. Br J Ophthal 60:411, 1976.
49. Virdi, PS, Hayreh, SS: Ocular neovascularization with retinal vascular occlusion. I. Association with experimental retinal vein occlusion. Arch Ophthal 100:331, 1982.
50. Ernest, JT, Archer, DB: Vitreous body oxygen tension following experimental branch retinal vein obstruction. Invest Ophthal Vis Sci 18:1025, 1979.
51. Folkman, J, Merler, E, Abernathy, C, Williams, G: Isolation of a tumor factor responsible for angiogenesis. J Exp Med 133:275, 1971.
52. Glaser, BM, D'Amore, PA, Michels, RG, et al: The demonstration of angiogenic activity from ocular tissues. Preliminary report. Ophthalmology 87:440, 1980.
53. Federman, JL, Brown, GC, Felberg, NT, Felton, SM: Experimental ocular angiogenesis. Am J Ophthal 89:231, 1980.
54. Patz, A: Studies on retinal neovascularization. Invest Ophthal Vis Sci 19:1133, 1980.
55. Gu, XQ, Fry, GL, Lata, GF, et al: Ocular neovascularization. Tissue culture studies. Arch Ophthal 103:111, 1985.
56. Imre, G: Studies on the mechanism of retinal neovascularization. Role of lactic acid. Br J Ophthal 48:75, 1964.
57. Zauberman, H, Michaelson, IC, Bergmann, F, Maurice, DM: Stimulation of neovascularization of the cornea by biogenic amines. Exp Eye Res 8:77, 1969.
58. Ben Ezra, D: Neovasculogenesis. Triggering factors and possible mechanisms. Surv Ophthal 24:167, 1979.
59. Wolbarsht, ML, Landers, MB III, Stefansson, E: Vasodilation and the etiology of diabetic retinopathy: a new model. Ophthal Surg 12:104, 1981.
60. Stefansson, E, Landers, MB III, Wolbarsht, ML: Oxygenation and vasodilatation in relation to diabetic and other proliferative retinopathies. Ophthal Surg 14:209, 1983.
61. Henkind, P: Ocular neovascularization. Am J Ophthal 85:287, 1978.
62. Williams, GA, Eisenstein, R, Schumacher, B, et al: Inhibitor of vascular endothelial cell growth in the lens. Am J Ophthal 97:366, 1984.
63. Glaser, BM, Campochiaro, PA, Davis, JL Jr, Jerdan, JA: Retinal pigment epithelial cells release inhibitors of neovascularization. Ophthalmology 94:780, 1987.
64. Ohrt, V: The frequency of rubeosis iridis in diabetic patients. Acta Ophthal 49:301, 1971.
65. Madsen, PH: Rubeosis of the iris and haemorrhagic glaucoma in patients with proliferative diabetic retinopathy. Br J Ophthal 55:368, 1971.
66. Bonnet, M, Jourdain, M, Francoz-Taillanter, N: Clinical correlation between rubeosis iridis and optic disc neovascularization. J Fr Ophthal 4:405, 1981.
67. Kluxen, G, Friedburg, D, Ruppert, A: Circular neovascularization of the circulus arteriosus iridis minor. Klin Monatsbl Augenheilkd 176:160, 1980.
68. Laqua, H: Rubeosis iridis following pars plana vitrectomy. Klin Monatsbl Augenheilkd 177:24, 1980.
69. Ehrenberg, M, McCuen, BW II, Schindler, RH, Machemer, R: Rubeosis iridis: preoperative iris fluorescein angiography and periocular steroids. Ophthalmology 91:321, 1984.
70. Cappin, JM, Whitelocke, R: The iris in central retinal vein thrombosis. Proc Royal Soc Med 67:1048, 1974.
71. Hayreh, S, March, W, Phelps, CD: Ocular hypotony following retinal vein occlusion. Arch Ophthal 96:827, 1978.
72. Sinclair, SH, Gragoudas, ES: Prognosis for rubeosis iridis following central retinal vein occlusion. Br J Ophthal 63:735, 1979.
73. Tasman, W, Magargal, LE, Augsburger, JJ: Effects of argon laser photocoagulation on rubeosis

iridis and angle neovascularization. Ophthalmology 87:400, 1980.

74. Magargal, LE, Donoso, LA, Sanborn, GE: Retinal ischemia and risk of neovascularization following central retinal vein obstruction. Ophthalmology 89:1241, 1982.
75. Hayreh, SS, Rojas, P, Podhajsky, P, et al: Ocular neovascularization with retinal vascular occlusion. III. Incidence of ocular neovascularization with retinal vein occlusion. Ophthalmology 90:488, 1983.
76. Priluck, IA, Robertson, DM, Hollenhorst, RW: Long-term follow-up of occlusion of the central retinal vein in young adults. Am J Ophthal 90:190, 1980.
77. Zegarra, H, Gutman, FA, Conforto, J: The natural course of central retinal vein occlusion. Ophthalmology 86:1931, 1979.
78. Zegarra, H, Gutman, FA, Zakov, N, Carim, M: Partial occlusion of the central retinal vein. Am J Ophthal 96:330, 1983.
79. Laatikainen, L, Blach, RK: Behavior of the iris vasculature in central retinal vein occlusion: a fluorescein angiographic study of the vascular response of the retina and the iris. Br J Ophthal 61:272, 1977.
80. Servais, GE, Thompson, HS, Hayreh, SS: Relative afferent pupillary defect in central retinal vein occlusion. Ophthalmology 93:301, 1986.
81. Sabates, R, Hirose, T, McMeel, JW: Electroretinography in the prognosis and classification of central retinal vein occlusion. Arch Ophthal 101:232, 1983.
82. Kaye, SB, Harding, SP: Early electroretinography in unilateral central retinal vein occlusion as a predictor of rubeosis iridis. Arch Ophthal 106:353, 1988.
83. Johnson, MA, Marcus, S, Elman, MJ, McPhee, TJ: Neovascularization in central retinal vein occlusion: electroretinographic findings. Arch Ophthal 106:348, 1988.
84. Wand, M, Dueker, DK, Aiello, LM, Grant, WM: Effects of panretinal photocoagulation on rubeosis iridis, angle neovascularization, and neovascular glaucoma. Am J Ophthal 86:332, 1978.
85. Madsen, PH: Haemorrhagic glaucoma. Comparative study in diabetic and nondiabetic patients. Br J Ophthal 55:444, 1971.
86. Laatikainen, L: Development and classification of rubeosis iridis in diabetic eye disease. Br J Ophthal 63:150, 1979.
87. Schulze, RR: Rubeosis iridis. Am J Ophthal 63:487, 1967.
88. Nork, TM, Tso, MOM, Duvall, J, Hayreh, SS: Cellular mechanisms of iris neovascularization secondary to retinal vein occlusion. Arch Ophthal 107:581, 1989.
89. Jocson, VL: Microvascular injection studies in rubeosis iridis and neovascular glaucoma. Am J Ophthal 83:508, 1977.
90. Anderson, DM, Morin, JD, Hunter, WS: Rubeosis iridis. Can J Ophthal 6:183, 1971.
91. Peyman, GA, Raichand, M, Juarez, CP, et al: Hypotony and experimental rubeosis iridis in primate eyes. A clinicopathologic study. Graefe's Arch Ophthal 224:435, 1986.
92. Goldberg, MF, Tso, MOM: Rubeosis iridis and glaucoma associated with sickle cell retinopathy: a light and electron microscopic study. Ophthalmology 85:1028, 1978.
93. John, T, Sassani, JW, Eagle, RC Jr: The myofibroblastic component of rubeosis iridis. Ophthalmology 90:721, 1983.
94. Nomura, T: Pathology of anterior chamber angle in diabetic neovascular glaucoma: extension of corneal endothelium onto iris surface. Jap J Ophthal 27:193, 1983.
95. Gartner, S, Taffet, S, Friedman, AH: The association of rubeosis iridis with endothelialisation of the anterior chamber: report of a clinical case with histopathological review of 16 additional cases. Br J Ophthal 61:267, 1977.
96. Harris, M, Tso, AY, Kaba, FW, et al: Corneal endothelial overgrowth of angle and iris. Evidence of myoblastic differentiation in three cases. Ophthalmology 91:1154, 1984.
97. Little, HL, Rosenthal, AR, Dellaporta, A, Jacobson, DR: The effect of pan-retinal photocoagulation on rubeosis iridis. Am J Ophthal 81:804, 1976.
98. Laatikainen, L: Preliminary report on effect of retinal panphotocoagulation on rubeosis iridis and neovascular glaucoma. Br J Ophthal 61:278, 1977.
99. Laatikainen, L, Kohner, EM, Khoury, D, Blach, RK: Panretinal photocoagulation in central retinal vein occlusion: a randomised controlled clinical study. Br J Ophthal 61:741, 1977.
100. Jacobson, DR, Murphy, RP, Rosenthal, AR: The treatment of angle neovascularization with panretinal photocoagulation. Ophthalmology 86:1270, 1979.
101. Murphy, RP, Egbert, PR: Regression of iris neovascularization following panretinal photocoagulation. Arch Ophthal 97:700, 1979.
102. Pavan, PR, Folk, JC, Weingeist, TA, et al: Diabetic rubeosis and panretinal photocoagulation. A prospective, controlled, masked trial using iris fluorescein angiography. Arch Ophthal 101:882, 1983.
103. May, DR, Klein, ML, Peyman, GA: A prospective study of xenon arc photocoagulation for central retinal vein occlusion. Br J Ophthal 60:816, 1976.
104. Magargal, LE, Brown, GC, Augsburger, JJ, Parrish, RK II: Neovascular glaucoma following cen-

tral retinal vein obstruction. Ophthalmology 88:1095, 1981.
105. Magargal, LE, Brown, GC, Augsburger, JJ, Donoso, LA: Efficacy of panretinal photocoagulation in preventing neovascular glaucoma following ischemic central retinal vein obstruction. Ophthalmology 89:780, 1982.
106. Laatikainen, L: A prospective follow-up study of panretinal photocoagulation in preventing neovascular glaucoma following ischaemic central retinal vein occlusion. Graefe's Arch Ophthal 220:236, 1983.
107. Kaufman, SC, Ferris, FL, III, Swartz, M, et al: Intraocular pressure following panretinal photocoagulation for diabetic retinopathy. Diabetic Retinopathy Report No. 11. Arch Ophthal 105:807, 1987.
108. Weiter, JJ, Zuckerman, R: The influence of the photoreceptor-RPE complex on the inner retina. An explanation of the beneficial effects of photocoagulation. Ophthalmology 87:1133, 1980.
109. Duker, JS, Brown, GC: The efficacy of panretinal photocoagulation for neovascularization of the iris after central retinal artery obstruction. Ophthalmology 96:92, 1989.
110. Teich, SA, Walsh, JB: A grading system for iris neovascularization. Prognostic implications for treatment. Ophthalmology 88:1102, 1981.
111. Flanagan, DW, Blach, RK: Place of panretinal photocoagulation and trabeculectomy in the management of neovascular glaucoma. Br J Ophthal 67:526, 1983.
112. Goodart, R, Blankenship, G: Panretinal photocoagulation influence on vitrectomy results for complications of diabetic retinopathy. Ophthalmology 87:183, 1980.
113. Miller, JB, Smith, MR, Boyer, DS: Intraocular carbon dioxide laser photocautery. Indications and contraindications at vitrectomy. Ophthalmology 87:1112, 1980.
114. May, DR, Bergstrom, TJ, Parmet, AJ, Schwartz, JG: Treatment of neovascular glaucoma with transscleral panretinal cryotherapy. Ophthalmology 87:1106, 1980.
115. Vernon, SA, Cheng, H: Panretinal cryotherapy in neovascular disease. Br J Ophthal 72:401, 1988.
116. Simmons, RJ, Dueker, DK, Kimbrough, RL, Aiello, LM: Goniophotocoagulation for neovascular glaucoma. Trans Am Acad Ophthal Otol 83:80, 1977.
117. Simmons, RJ, Deppermann, SR, Dueker, DK: The role of gonio-photocoagulation in neovascularization of the anterior chamber angle. Ophthalmology 87:79, 1980.
118. Drews, RC: Corticosteroid management of hemorrhagic glaucoma. Trans Am Acad Ophthal Otol 78:334, 1974.
119. Tano, Y, Chandler, D, Machemer, R: Treatment of intraocular proliferation with intravitreal injection of triamcinolone acetonide. Am J Ophthal 90:810, 1980.
120. Feibel, RM, Bigger, JF: Rubeosis iridis and neovascular glaucoma. Evaluation of cyclocryotherapy. Am J Ophthal 74:862, 1972.
121. Boniuk, M: Cryotherapy in neovascular glaucoma. Trans Am Acad Ophthal Otol 78:337, 1974.
122. Krupin, T, Mitchell, KB, Becker, B: Cyclocryotherapy in neovascular glaucoma. Am J Ophthal 86:24, 1978.
123. Faulborn, J, Birnbaum, F: Cyclocryotherapy of haemorrhagic glaucoma: Clinical long time and histopathologic results. Klin Monatsbl Augenheilkd 170:651, 1977.
124. Faulborn, J, Hoster, K: Results of cyclocryotherapy in case of hemorrhagic glaucoma. Klin Monatsbl Augenheilkd 162:513, 1973.
125. Hampton, C, Shields, MB, Miller, KN, Blasini, M: Evaluation of a protocol for transscleral Neodymium:YAG cyclophotocoagulation in one hundred patients. Ophthalmology 97:910, 1990.
126. Allen, RC, Bellows, AR, Hutchinson, BT, Murphy, SD: Filtration surgery in the treatment of neovascular glaucoma. Ophthalmology 89:1181, 1982.
127. Herschler, J, Agness, D: A modified filtering operation for neovascular glaucoma. Arch Ophthal 97:2339, 1979.
128. Parrish, R, Herschler, J: Eyes with end-stage neovascular glaucoma. Natural history following successful modified filtering operation. Arch Ophthal 101:745, 1983.
129. L'Esperance, FA Jr, Mittl, RN, James, WA Jr: Carbon dioxide laser trabeculostomy for the treatment of neovascular glaucoma. Ophthalmology 90:821, 1983.
130. Molteno, ACB, Van Rooyen, MMB, Bartholomew, RS: Implants for draining neovascular glaucoma. Br J Ophthal 61:120, 1977.
131. Egerer, I: Clinical experience in glaucoma surgery utilizing silicon catheters. Klin Monatsbl Augenheilkd 174:434, 1979.
132. Ancker, E, Molteno, ACB: Molteno drainage implant for neovascular glaucoma. Trans Ophthal Soc UK 102:122, 1982.
133. Honrubia, RM, Gómez, ML, Hernández, A, Grijalbo, MP: Long-term results of silicone tube in filtering surgery for eyes with neovascular glaucoma. Am J Ophthal 97:501, 1984.
134. Krupin, R, Kaufman, P, Mandell, A, et al: Filtering valve implant surgery for eyes with neovascular glaucoma. Am J Ophthal 89:338, 1980.
135. McCuen, BW II, Rinkoff, JS: Silicone oil for progressive anterior ocular neovascularization after failed diabetic vitrectomy. Arch Ophthal 107:677, 1989.
136. Packer, AJ, Tse, DT, Gu, X-Q, Hayreh, SS: Hematoporphyrin photoradiation therapy for iris

neovascularization. A preliminary report. Arch Ophthal 102:1193, 1984.
137. Nanda, SK, Hatchell, DL, Tiedeman, JS, et al: A new method for vascular occlusion. Photochemical initiation of thrombosis. Arch Ophthal 105:1121, 1987.
138. Jampol, LM, Orlin, C, Cohen, SB, et al: Hyperbaric and transcorneal delivery of oxygen to the rabbit and monkey anterior segment. Arch Ophthal 106:825, 1988.
139. Pederson, JE, MacLellan, HM: Experimental retinal detachment. I. Effect of subretinal fluid composition on reabsorption rate and intraocular pressure. Arch Ophthal 100:1150, 1982.
140. Cantrill, HL, Pederson, JE: Experimental retinal detachment. III. Vitreous fluorophotometry. Arch Ophthal 100:1810, 1982.
141. Tsuboi, S, Taki-Noie, J, Emi, K, Manabe, R: Fluid dynamics in eyes with rhegmatogenous retinal detachments. Am J Ophthal 99:673, 1985.
142. Campbell, DG: Iris retraction associated with rhegmatogenous retinal detachment syndrome and hypotony. A new explanation. Arch Ophthal 102:1457, 1984.
143. Phelps, CD, Burton, TC: Glaucoma and retinal detachment. Arch Ophthal 95:418, 1977.
144. Shammas, HF, Halasa, AH, Faris, BM: Intraocular pressure, cup-disc ratio, and steroid responsiveness in retinal detachment. Arch Ophthal 94:1108, 1976.
145. Pape, LG, Forbes, M: Retinal detachment and miotic therapy. Am J Ophthal 85:558, 1978.
146. Beasley, H, Fraunfelder, FT: Retinal detachments and topical ocular miotics. Ophthalmology 86:95, 1979.
147. Pemberton, JW: Schiøtz-applanation disparity following retinal detachment surgery. Arch Ophthal 81:534, 1969.
148. Syrdalen, P: Intraocular pressure and ocular rigidity in patients with retinal detachment. II. Postoperative study. Acta Ophthal 48:1036, 1970.
149. Burton, TC, Lambert, RW Jr: A predictive model for visual recovery following retinal detachment surgery. Ophthalmology 85:619, 1978.
150. Sebestyen, JG, Schepens, CL, Rosenthal, ML: Retinal detachment and glaucoma. I. Tonometric and gonioscopic study of 160 cases. Arch Ophthal 67:736, 1962.
151. Schwartz, A: Chronic open-angle glaucoma secondary to rhegmatogenous retinal detachment. Am J Ophthal 75:205, 1973.
152. Davidorf, FH: Retinal pigment epithelial glaucoma. Ophthal Digest 38:11, 1976.
153. Baba, H: Probability of the presence of glycosaminoglycans in aqueous humor. Graefe's Arch Ophthal 220:117, 1983.
154. Matsuo, N, Takabatake, M, Ueno, H, et al: Photoreceptor outer segments in the aqueous humor in rhegmatogenous retinal detachment. Am J Ophthal 101:673, 1986.
155. Lambrou, FH, Vela, MA, Woods, W: Obstruction of the trabecular meshwork by retinal rod outer segments. Arch Ophthal 107:742, 1989.
156. Yanoff, M: Glaucoma mechanisms in ocular malignant melanoma. Am J Ophthal 70:898, 1970.
157. Hyams, SW, Neumann, E: Transient angle-closure glaucoma after retinal vein occlusion. Report of two cases. Br J Ophthal 56:353, 1972.
158. Grant, WM: Shallowing of the anterior chamber following occlusion of the central retinal vein. Am J Ophthal 75:384, 1973.
159. Bloome, MA: Transient angle-closure glaucoma in central retinal vein occlusion. Ann Ophthal 9:44, 1977.
160. Mendelsohn, AD, Jampol, LM, Shoch, D: Secondary angle-closure glaucoma after central retinal vein occlusion. Am J Ophthal 100:581, 1985.
161. Pesin, SR, Katz, LJ, Augsburger, JJ, et al: Acute angle-closure glaucoma from spontaneous massive hemorrhagic retinal or choroidal detachment. An updated diagnostic and therapeutic approach. Ophthalmology 97:76, 1990.
162. Steinemann, T, Goins, K, Smith, T, et al: Acute closed-angle glaucoma complicating hemorrhagic choroidal detachment associated with parenteral thrombolytic agents. Am J Ophthal 106:752, 1988.
163. Brockhurst, RJ: Nanophthalmos with uveal effusion. A new clinical entity. Arch Ophthal 93:1289, 1975.
164. Singh, OS, Simmons, RJ, Brockhurst, RJ, Trempe, CL: Nanophthalmos: a perspective on identification and therapy. Ophthalmology 89:1006, 1982.
165. Ryan, EA, Zwann, J, Chylack, LT Jr: Nanophthalmos with uveal effusion. Clinical and embryologic considerations. Ophthalmology 89:1013, 1982.
166. Ghose, S, Sachdev, MS, Kumar, H: Bilateral nanophthalmos, pigmentary retinal dystrophy, and angle closure glaucoma—a new syndrome? Br J Ophthal 69:624, 1985.
167. MacKay, CJ, Shek, MS, Carr, RE, et al: Retinal degeneration with nanophthalmos, cystic macular degeneration, and angle closure glaucoma. A new recessive syndrome. Arch Ophthal 105:366, 1987.
168. Calhoun, FP Jr: The management of glaucoma in nanophthalmos. Trans Am Ophthal Soc 73:97, 1975.
169. Kimbrough, RL, Trempe, CS, Brockhurst, RJ, Simmons, RF: Angle-closure glaucoma in nanophthalmos. Am J Ophthal 88:572, 1979.
170. Trelstad, RL, Silbermann, NN, Brockhurst, RJ: Nanophthalmic sclera: ultrastructural, histochemical, and biochemical observations. Arch Ophthal 100:1935, 1982.
171. Yue, BYJT, Duvall, J, Goldberg, MF, et al: Na-

nophthalmic sclera. Morphologic and tissue culture studies. Ophthalmology 93:534, 1986.
172. Yue, BYJT, Kurosawa, A, Duvall, J, et al: Nanophthalmic sclera. Fibronectin studies. Ophthalmology 95:56, 1988.
173. Gass, JDM: Uveal effusion syndrome. A new hypothesis concerning pathogenesis and technique of surgical treatment. Retina 3:159, 1983.
174. Brockhurst, RJ: Vortex vein decompression for nanophthalmic uveal effusion. Arch Ophthal 98:1987, 1980.
175. Ward, RC, Gragoudas, ES, Pon, DM, Albert, DM: Abnormal scleral findings in uveal effusion syndrome. Am J Ophthal 106:139, 1988.
176. Fourman, S: Angle-closure glaucoma complicating ciliochoroidal detachment. Ophthalmology 96:646, 1989.
177. Pollard, ZF: Secondary angle-closure glaucoma in cicatricial retrolental fibroplasia. Am J Ophthal 89:651, 1980.
178. Smith, J, Shivitz, I: Angle-closure glaucoma in adults with cicatricial retinopathy of prematurity. Arch Ophthal 102:371, 1984.
179. Hartnett, ME, Gilbert, MM, Richardson, TM, et al: Anterior segment evaluation of infants with retinopathy of prematurity. Ophthalmology 97:122, 1990.
180. Kushner, BJ: Ciliary block glaucoma in retinopathy of prematurity. Arch Ophthal 100:1078, 1982.
181. Kushner, BJ, Sondheimer, S: Medical treatment of glaucoma associated with cicatricial retinopathy of prematurity. Am J Ophthal 94:313, 1982.
182. Hittner, HM, Rhodes, LM, McPherson, AR: Anterior segment abnormalities in cicatricial retinopathy of prematurity. Ophthalmology 86:803, 1979.
183. Pollard, ZF: Lensectomy for secondary angle-closure glaucoma in advanced cicatricial retrolental fibroplasia. Ophthalmology 91:395, 1984.
184. Machemer, R: Closed vitrectomy for severe retrolental fibroplasia in the infant. Ophthalmology 90:436, 1983.
185. Trese, MT: Surgical results of Stage V retrolental fibroplasia and timing of surgical repair. Ophthalmology 91:461, 1984.
186. Reese, AB: Persistent hyperplastic primary vitreous. Am J Ophthal 40:317, 1955.
187. Meisels, HI, Goldberg, MF: Vascular anastomoses between the iris and persistent hyperplastic primary vitreous. Am J Ophthal 88:179, 1979.
188. Goldberg, MF, Mafee, M: Computed tomography for diagnosis of persistent hyperplastic primary vitreous (PHPV) Ophthalmology 90:442, 1983.
189. Stark, WJ, Lindsey, PS, Fagadau, WR, Michels, RG: Persistent hyperplastic primary vitreous. Surgical treatment. Ophthalmology 90:452, 1983.
190. Smith, RE, Maumenee, AE: Persistent hyperplastic primary vitreous: results of surgery. Trans Am Acad Ophthal Otol 78:911, 1974.
191. Nankin, SJ, Scott, WE: Persistent hyperplastic primary vitreous. Roto-extraction and other surgical experience. Arch Ophthal 95:240, 1977.
192. Laatikainen, L, Tarkkanen, A: Microsurgery of persistent hyperplastic primary vitreous. Ophthalmologica 185:193, 1982.
193. Federman, JL, Shields, JA, Altman, B, Koller, H: The surgical and nonsurgical management of persistent hyperplastic primary vitreous. Ophthalmology 89:20, 1982.
194. Volcker, HE, Lang, GK, Naumann, GOH: Surgery for posterior polar cataract in cases of persistent hyperplastic primary vitreous. Klin Monatsbl Augenheilkd 183:79, 1983.
195. Awan, KJ, Humayun, M: Changes in the contralateral eye in uncomplicated persistent hyperplastic primary vitreous in adults. Am J Ophthal 99:122, 1985.
196. Hoepner, J, Yanoff, M: Ocular anomalies in trisomy 13-15: an analysis of 13 eyes with two new findings. Am J Ophthal 74:729, 1972.
197. Kogbe, OI, Follmann, P: Investigations into the aqueous humour dynamics in primary pigmentary degeneration of the retina. Ophthalmologica 171:165, 1975.

Chapter 17

GLAUCOMAS ASSOCIATED WITH ELEVATED EPISCLERAL VENOUS PRESSURE

Episcleral Venous Pressure

The episcleral venous pressure, as discussed in Chapter 2, is one factor that contributes to the intraocular pressure (IOP). The normal episcleral venous pressure is approximately 8–10 mm Hg,[1–5] although values vary according to the measurement technique. The several instruments that have been devised for measuring episcleral venous pressure were described in Chapter 3.[1,2,4,5]

It is commonly believed that the IOP rises mm Hg for mm Hg with an increase in the episcleral venous pressure, although it has been suggested that the magnitude of IOP rise may be greater than the rise in venous pressure.[6] Studies of primary open-angle glaucoma have shown no abnormality of episcleral venous pressure.[2,5,7] In fact, there appears to be a negative correlation between episcleral venous pressure and IOP in most situations, with ocular hypertensives having significantly lower episcleral venous pressures.[5] However, a variety of conditions can cause an elevation of episcleral venous pressure and produce characteristic forms of secondary glaucoma.

General Features of Elevated Episcleral Venous Pressure

The following findings are common to most cases of elevated episcleral venous pressure.

External Examination

The most consistent feature is variable degrees of dilation and tortuosity of the episcleral and bulbar conjunctival vessels (Fig. 17.1). Additional findings may include chemosis, proptosis, and a bruit and pulsations over the orbit, although these are inconsistent findings that depend upon the underlying cause of the elevated episcleral venous pressure.

Intraocular Pressure

As noted above, the rise in IOP is approximately equal to the rise in episcleral venous

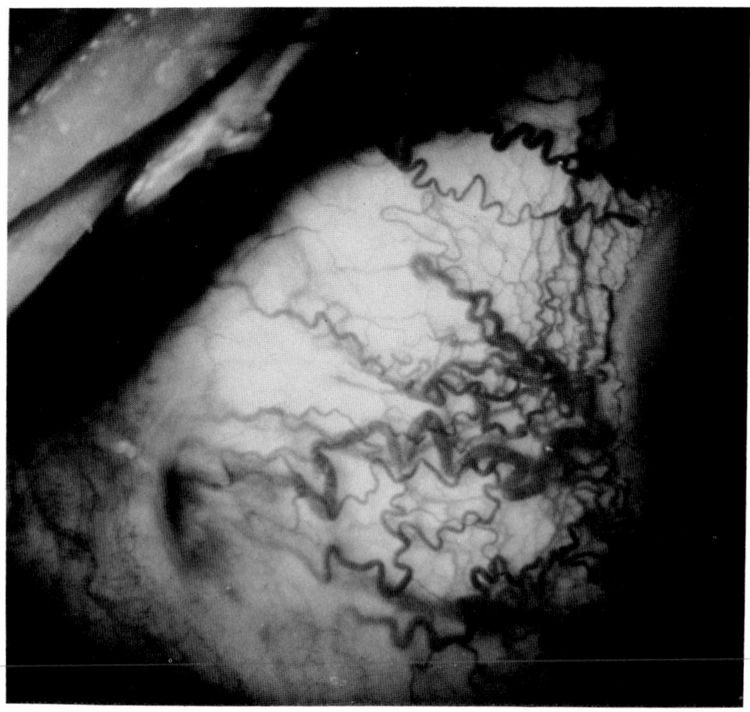

Figure 17.1. External view of patient with elevated episcleral venous pressure showing characteristic dilation and tortuosity of the episcleral and bulbar conjunctival vessels.

pressure. The resultant tension is typically in the mid-20s to mid-30s, and an increased ocular pulse is often present.[8]

Gonioscopy

The anterior chamber angle is typically open, and the only abnormality may be blood reflux into Schlemm's canal. However, the latter feature has limited diagnostic value, since it is an inconsistent finding in cases of elevated episcleral venous pressure and may be seen in normal eyes.

Tonography

The facility of aqueous outflow is characteristically normal. In fact, a study with monkeys revealed that elevated venous pressure was associated with increased outflow,[9] which may result, at least in part, from a widening of Schlemm's canal. However, prolonged elevation of episcleral venous pressure often leads to a reduction in outflow facility, which may persist after normalization of the venous pressure.[8]

CLINICAL FORMS OF ELEVATED EPISCLERAL VENOUS PRESSURE

The various causes of elevated episcleral venous pressure may be considered in three categories: (1) obstruction to venous flow; (2) arteriovenous fistulas; and (3) idiopathic episcleral venous pressure elevation.[5] The mechanisms by which these conditions lead to glaucoma and their management are considered in separate sections at the end of this chapter.

Venous Obstruction

Thyrotropic Ophthalmopathy

This disorder is also referred to as endocrine exophthalmos or Graves' disease. The precise hormonal basis of the condition is uncertain, although the ocular pathology consists of orbital infiltration with lymphocytes, mast cells, and plasma cells. This is the most common cause of unilateral, as well as bilateral, proptosis and may lead to glaucoma by several mechanisms.

Elevated episcleral venous pressure may occur in severe cases with marked proptosis and orbital congestion (Fig. 17.2). The contracture of extraocular muscles, which occurs in the later phases of this infiltrative ophthalmopathy, may influence the IOP in different fields of gaze. Typically, fibrosis of the inferior rectus muscle causes resistance to upgaze, which is associated with a rise in the IOP when the patient looks up. In some cases, an artificial pressure elevation may be recorded with gaze in the usual straight-ahead position, and the patient must be allowed to change the direction of gaze to his or her "resting" position.[10] Ideally, the IOP should be measured in several fields of gaze to avoid this potential testing artifact.

It must be kept in mind, as discussed in Chapter 4, that thyroid dysfunction may be associated with abnormal scleral rigidity, and the IOP in these individuals should be measured by applanation tonometry. In addition to glaucoma, other serious complications of thyrotropic ophthalmopathy include corneal exposure resulting from proptosis and lid retraction, and optic nerve compression from the orbital mass. The corneal exposure can lead to a corneal ulcer and anterior chamber inflammation, which can be another mechanism of glaucoma.

Superior Vena Cava Syndrome

Lesions of the upper thorax may obstruct venous return from the head, causing elevated episcleral venous pressure in association with exophthalmos, edema and cyanosis of the face and neck, and dilated veins of the head, neck, chest, and upper extremities.[11]

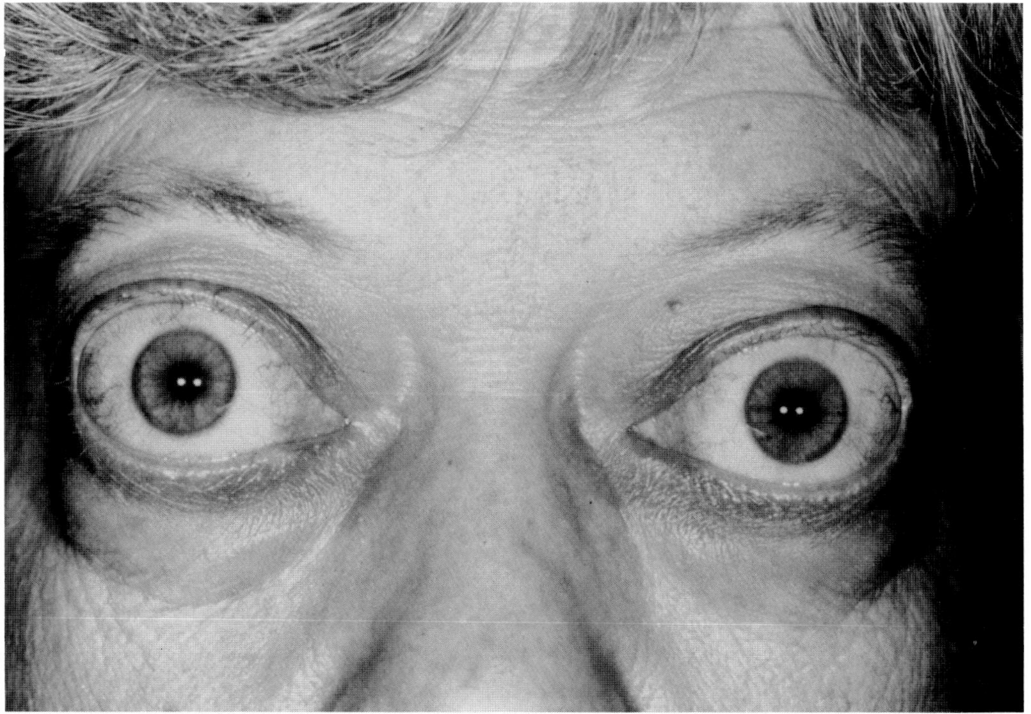

Figure 17.2. Patient with thyrotropic ophthalmopathy showing typical exophthalmos. Such patients may develop elevated episcleral venous pressure and secondary glaucoma. (Courtesy of Jonathan Dutton, M.D.)

Other conditions that may occasionally obstruct orbital venous drainage include *retrobulbar tumors* and *cavernous sinus thrombosis*.

Arteriovenous Fistulas

Carotid Cavernous Sinus Fistulas

Carotid cavernous sinus fistulas can be subdivided into two categories. The majority (about three-fourths) are secondary to trauma and are characterized by a direct vascular communication and high blood flow, while the remainder have a spontaneous etiology and typically have an indirect or dural communication with low flow.[12]

Traumatic. The typical trauma is severe head injury, which results in a large fistula between the internal carotid artery and the surrounding cavernous sinus venous plexus. This condition is characterized by pulsating exophthalmos, a bruit over the globe, conjunctival chemosis, engorgement of epibulbar veins, restriction of motility, and evidence of ocular ischemia.[12–15] The shunting of the internal carotid cavernous sinus fistula causes high flow and high pressure.[12,16]

Spontaneous. This form of carotid cavernous sinus fistula occurs most often in middle-aged to elderly women with no history of trauma. A small fistula in these cases is fed by a meningeal branch of the intracavernous internal carotid artery or external carotid artery, which empties directly into the cavernous sinus or an adjacent dural vein that connects with the cavernous sinus.[16,17] The mixing of arterial and venous blood leads to both a reduction in arterial pressure and an increase in orbital venous pressure, which increases the episcleral venous pressure. These patients have prominent episcleral and conjunctival veins, which is often the presenting complaint, but minimal proptosis and no pulsations or bruit. The small fistula results in low-flow, low-pressure shunting.[16] The condition has been called "red-eyed shunt syndrome"[16] or "dural shunt syndrome."[17]

Orbital Varices

This condition is characterized by intermittent exophthalmos and elevated episcleral venous pressure, usually associated with stooping over or the Valsalva maneuver.[6,18] Since venous pressure is typically normal between episodes, secondary glaucoma is not common. However, glaucomatous damage has been reported to occur, and it has been suggested that management with antiglaucoma medications may be effective and should be tried before considering surgical intervention.[6]

Sturge-Weber Syndrome

One mechanism of IOP elevation in this condition is believed to be elevated episcleral venous pressure resulting from the episcleral hemangiomas with arteriovenous fistulas.[19,20] The Sturge-Weber syndrome is discussed in more detail in the next chapter.

Idiopathic Episcleral Venous Pressure Elevation

Several cases have been reported of dilated episcleral veins and open-angle glaucoma without exophthalmos or any explanation for the venous congestion.[21–27] The typical patient is elderly with no family history of the condition, although it may be seen in young adults and has been described in a mother and daughter.[21] Most cases are unilateral, and those in which episcleral venous pressure has been measured have all had elevated venous pressures.[21,24,27] The cause of the elevated episcleral venous pressure is unknown. In one series of five patients with unilateral elevation of episcleral venous pressure and open-angle glaucoma, venous outflow was shown to be normal by orbital venography, and the authors presumed the mechanism to be a localized venous obstruction in the region of the extraocular muscles.[27] The associated glaucoma may be severe, with advanced glaucomatous damage.

MECHANISMS OF SECONDARY GLAUCOMA

There are several mechanisms by which elevated episcleral venous pressure may lead to secondary glaucoma. Some are common to all forms of episcleral venous pressure elevation, while others are associated with specific conditions.

Direct Effect

As noted at the outset of this chapter, episcleral venous pressure is a component of the normal IOP, and a rise in episcleral venous pressure is associated with approximately the same amount of increase in IOP. These eyes typically have a wide-open anterior chamber angle, often with blood in Schlemm's canal. This is the most common mechanism of glaucoma associated with episcleral venous pressure elevation. However, IOP elevation is not present in all patients with elevated venous pressure. For example, in patients with carotid cavernous sinus fistula, elevated IOP is more common in the atypical dural shunt syndrome, occurring in nearly all of these cases.[16,17]

Outflow Resistance

While facility of outflow is typically normal, if not improved,[9] during elevated episcleral venous pressure, prolonged venous pressure elevation may lead to reduced outflow even after venous pressure is normalized.[8] A trabeculectomy specimen from one idiopathic case revealed compression of the trabecular meshwork near Schlemm's canal, with extracellular deposits and hyalinization of the trabecular beams,[26] although it is not clear whether this represented a primary or secondary alteration.

Acute Angle Closure

Angle-closure glaucoma has been associated with arteriovenous fistulas.[28–30] The mechanism appears to be venous stasis within the vortex veins leading to either a serous choroidal detachment[28,29,31] or a suprachoroidal hemorrhage[30] and subsequent forward displacement of the lens-iris diaphragm. These have been reported in association with the dural shunt syndrome[28–30] and an orbital arteriovenous fistula.[29]

Neovascular Glaucoma

The reduced arterial flow, especially associated with the dural shunt syndrome, may also lead to ocular ischemia with rubeosis iridis and neovascular glaucoma.[14,32,33]

It has also been proposed, based on model experiments and mathematical analysis, that the visual field loss in glaucoma secondary to elevated venous pressure is associated with intraocular vein collapse and retardation of intraocular blood flow.[34]

MANAGEMENT

In many cases, the initial therapy should be directed toward eliminating the cause of the elevated episcleral venous pressure. This is particularly true in patients with thyrotropic ophthalmopathy, superior vena cava syndrome, retrobulbar tumors, or cavernous sinus thrombosis. However, in cases of carotid cavernous sinus fistula and orbital varices, the risk of surgical intervention may be such that other measures of glaucoma control should be considered first.[6,14,15] Surgical intervention in these cases usually consists of intraarterial balloon occlusion or embolization.[12,35] While reported success rates vary from 58 to 100%,[12] complications do occur, including anterior segment ischemia, ischemia of the optic nerve, and cerebral ischemia.[14,15] More recently, a transvenous approach via the ipsilateral superior ophthalmic vein has been described as a safer way to pass a detachable balloon into the cavernous sinus.[36] However, since many fistulas close spontaneously, especially with the dural shunt syndrome, conservative management is advisable in mild cases, with embolization for those with visual disability or progressive signs.[35]

When treatment of the glaucoma is required, drugs that reduce aqueous production (such as beta-blockers and carbonic anhydrase inhibitors) should be used, since those that improve outflow are rarely effective. Cases with acute angle closure associated with the dural shunt syndrome and uveal effusion may also respond to these medications,[29] while those with a suprachoroidal hemorrhage may require drainage of the blood.[30] If surgical intervention becomes necessary, in most cases a filtering procedure should be employed. However, there is an increased risk of uveal effusion and expulsive hemorrhage when filtering eyes with elevated episcleral venous pressure, especially in the Sturge-Weber syndrome, and it has been recommended that drainage of the suprachoroid be routinely performed at the time of surgery.[37]

SUMMARY

The episcleral venous pressure normally contributes 8–10 mm Hg to the IOP. An elevated episcleral venous pressure may be associated with several forms of secondary glaucoma. Conditions that may cause elevated episcleral venous pressure include: (1) obstruction to venous flow, as with thyrotropic ophthalmopathy, superior vena cava syndrome, retrobulbar tumors, and cavernous sinus thrombosis; (2) arteriovenous fistulas, which include carotid cavernous sinus fistula, orbital varices, and the Sturge-Weber syndrome; and (3) idiopathic cases. Mechanisms of associated secondary glaucoma include: (1) the direct effect of elevated episcleral venous pressure on IOP; (2) chronic outflow obstruction; (3) acute angle closure; and (4) neovascular glaucoma. Management is usually directed first at the cause of the venous pressure elevation, with medical and surgical glaucoma therapy as required.

References

1. Brubaker, RF: Determination of episcleral venous pressure in the eye. A comparison of three methods. Arch Ophthal 77:110, 1967.
2. Podos, SM, Minas, TF, Macri, FJ: A new instrument to measure episcleral venous pressure. Comparison of normal eyes and eyes with primary open-angle glaucoma. Arch Ophthal 80:209, 1968.
3. Krakau, CET, Widakowich, J, Wilke, K: Measurements of the episcleral venous pressure by means of an air jet. Acta Ophthal 51:185, 1973.
4. Phelps, CD, Armaly, MF: Measurement of episcleral venous pressure. Am J Ophthal 85:35, 1978.
5. Talusan, ED, Schwartz, B: Episcleral venous pressure. Differences between normal, ocular hypertensive, and primary open-angle glaucomas. Arch Ophthal 99:824, 1981.
6. Kollarits, CR, Gaasterland, D, Di Chiro, G, et al: Management of a patient with orbital varices, visual loss, and ipsilateral glaucoma. Ophthal Surg 8:54, 1977.
7. Linner, E: The outflow pressure in normal and glaucomatous eyes. Acta Ophthal 33:101, 1955.
8. Chandler, PA, Grant, WM: Glaucoma, 2nd ed. Lea and Febiger, Philadelphia, 1979, p. 267.
9. Barany, EH: The influence of extraocular venous pressure on outflow facility in *Cercopithecus ethiops* and *Macaca fascicularis*. Invest Ophthal Vis Sci 17:711, 1978.
10. Buschmann, W: Glaucoma and Graves' disease. Klin Monatsbl Augenheilkd 188:138, 1986.
11. Alfano, JE, Alfano, PA: Glaucoma and the superior vena caval obstruction syndrome. Am J Ophthal 42:685, 1956.
12. Keltner, JL, Satterfield, D, Dublin, AB, Lee, BCP: Dural and carotid cavernous sinus fistulas. Diagnosis, management, and complications. Ophthalmology 94:1585, 1987.
13. Henderson, JW, Schneider, RC: The ocular findings in carotid cavernous fistula in a series of 17 cases. Am J Ophthal 48:585, 1959.
14. Sanders, MD, Hoyt, WF: Hypoxic ocular sequelae of carotid-cavernous fistulae. Study of the causes of visual failure before and after neurosurgical treatment in a series of 25 cases. Br J Ophthal 53:82, 1969.
15. Palestine, AG, Younge, BR, Piepgras, DG: Visual prognosis in carotid-cavernous fistula. Arch Ophthal 99:1600, 1981.
16. Phelps, CD, Thompson, HS, Ossoinig, KC: The diagnosis and prognosis of atypical carotid-cavernous fistula (red-eyed shunt syndrome). Am J Ophthal 93:423, 1982.
17. Grove, AS Jr: The dural shunt syndrome. Pathophysiology and clinical course. Ophthalmology 90:31, 1983.
18. Wright, JE: Orbital vascular anomalies. Trans Am Acad Ophthal Otol 78:606, 1974.
19. Weiss, DI: Dual origin of glaucoma in encephalotrigeminal hemangiomatosis. Trans Ophthal Soc UK 93:477, 1971.
20. Phelps, CD: The pathogenesis of glaucoma in Sturge-Weber syndrome. Ophthalmology 85:276, 1978.
21. Minas, TF, Podos, SM: Familial glaucoma associated with elevated episcleral venous pressure. Arch Ophthal 80:202, 1968.
22. Radius, RL, Maumenee, AE: Dilated episcleral vessels and open-angle glaucoma. Am J Ophthal 86:31, 1978.
23. Benedikt, O, Roll, P: Dilatation and tortuosity of episcleral vessels in open-angle glaucoma. I: Clinical picture. Klin Monatsbl Augenheilkd 176:292, 1980.
24. Talusan, ED, Fishbein, SL, Schwartz, B: Increased pressure of dilated episcleral veins with open-angle glaucoma without exophthalmos. Ophthalmology 90:257, 1983.
25. Ruprecht, KW, Naumann, GOH: Unilateral secondary open-angle glaucoma associated with idiopathically dilated episcleral vessels. Klin Monatsbl Augenheilkd 184:23, 1984.
26. Roll, P, Benedikt, O: Dilatation and tortuosity of episcleral vessels in open-angle glaucoma. II:

Electron-microscopic findings in the trabecular lamellae. Klin Monatsbl Augenheilkd 176:297, 1980.

27. Jorgensen, JS, Guthoff, R: Pathogenesis of glaucoma in patients with idiopathically dilated episcleral vessels. Klin Monatsbl Augenheilkd 190:428, 1987.
28. Harris, GJ, Rice, PR: Angle closure in carotid-cavernous fistula. Ophthalmology 86:1521, 1979.
29. Fourman, S: Acute closed-angle glaucoma after arteriovenous fistulas. Am J Ophthal 107:156, 1989.
30. Buus, DR, Tse, DT, Parrish, RK II: Spontaneous carotid cavernous fistula presenting with acute angle closure glaucoma. Arch Ophthal 107:596, 1989.
31. Jorgensen, JS, Payer, H: Elevated episcleral venous pressure and uveal effusion. Klin Monatsbl Augenheilkd 195:14, 1989.
32. Spencer, WH, Thompson, HS, Hoyt, WF: Ischaemic ocular necrosis from carotid-cavernous fistula. Pathology of stagnant anoxic "inflammation" in orbital and ocular tissues. Br J Ophthal 57:145, 1973.
33. Weiss, DI, Shaffer, RN, Nehrenberg, TR: Neovascular glaucoma complicating carotid-cavernous fistula. Arch Ophthal 69:304, 1963.
34. Moses, RA, Grodzki, WJ Jr: Mechanism of glaucoma secondary to increased venous pressure. Arch Ophthal 103:1701, 1985.
35. Kupersmith, MJ, Berenstein, A, Choi, IS, et al: Management of nontraumatic vascular shunts involving the cavernous sinus. Ophthalmology 95:121, 1988.
36. Hanneken, AM, Miller, NR, Debrun, GM, Nauta, HJW: Treatment of carotid-cavernous sinus fistulas using a detachable balloon catheter through the superior ophthalmic vein. Arch Ophthal 107:87, 1989.
37. Bellows, RA, Chylack, LT, Epstein, DL, Hutchinson, BT: Choroidal effusion during glaucoma surgery in patients with prominent episcleral vessels. Arch Ophthal 97:493, 1979.

Chapter 18

GLAUCOMAS ASSOCIATED WITH INTRAOCULAR TUMORS

A variety of intraocular tumors can give rise to secondary glaucoma. In one survey of 2597 patients with intraocular tumors, 5% of the tumor-containing eyes had tumor-induced elevated intraocular pressure (IOP) at the time of diagnosis of the tumor.[1] In some cases, the mass lesions represent life-threatening malignancies, while other tumors are benign, creating significant problems in diagnosis and management. For patients with an intraocular malignancy, the emphasis shifts from the prevention of blindness to the preservation of life, while care must be taken in eyes with benign lesions to avoid loss of vision from unnecessary treatment. In this chapter, we will consider the differential diagnosis and management of glaucomas associated with intraocular tumors.

PRIMARY UVEAL MELANOMAS

Melanomas of the uveal tract, the most common primary intraocular malignancy, are frequently associated with glaucoma by several mechanisms and with a variety of clinical presentations. In one large histopathologic study of eyes with malignant melanomas involving one or more portions of the uveal tract, the overall prevalence of glaucoma was 20%.[2] Anterior uveal melanomas lead to IOP elevation more frequently than posterior melanomas, with reports of 41%[2] and 45%[3] in two series, while choroidal melanomas were found to have associated glaucoma in only 14% of one study.[2] These figures are undoubtedly skewed, however, since one series represents histopathologic material,[2] while the other represents patients primarily referred to a glaucoma service.[3] A clinical series from an oncology service may provide more meaningful statistics, in which 3% of 2111 eyes with uveal melanomas had secondary IOP elevation, including 7% with iris melanomas, 17% with ciliary body melanomas, and 2% with choroidal melanomas.[1] Metastatic melanomas are rarely found in the eye but can cause glaucoma, and these are discussed later in this chapter under "Systemic Malignancies."

Anterior Uveal Melanomas

Clinical Presentations and Mechanisms of Glaucoma

Melanomas of the anterior uveal tract most often arise from the ciliary body. These may be difficult to visualize directly, often presenting as a smooth-domed elevation of the overlying iris. However, wide dilation may allow gonioscopic visualization of the lesion, which is typically seen as a chocolate-brown mass between the iris and lens. In other cases, a primary melanoma of the ciliary body may extend through the peripheral iris and become visible as a nodular mass on the iris stroma and in the anterior chamber angle (Fig. 18.1). Primary melanomas of the iris are usually easily seen by slit-lamp biomicroscopy and gonioscopy, typically as slightly elevated, brown masses on the stroma (Fig. 18.2). However, some melanomas of the iris may be amelanotic, often with an associated secondary vasculature (Fig. 18.3).

Melanomas of the anterior uvea may lead to glaucoma by either open-angle or angle-closure mechanisms, with the former being more common. Aqueous humor outflow in the open anterior chamber angle can be obstructed by direct extension of the tumor or by seeding of tumor cells or melanin granules (Fig. 18.4).[2–4] In some eyes, the melanoma may arise from either iris, ciliary body, or the iridociliary junction and spread circumferentially, creating a *ring melanoma*. It may extend posteriorly, causing a retinal detachment and the impression of a choroidal tumor. Others may extend into the anterior chamber, causing elevated IOP

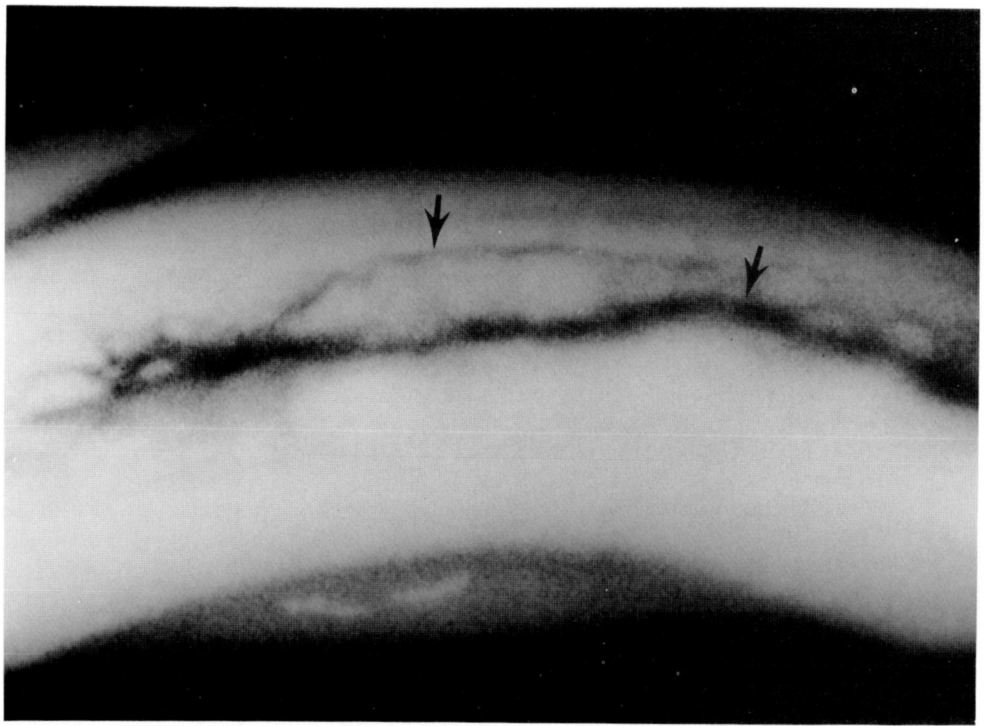

Figure 18.1. Gonioscopic view of malignant melanoma of the ciliary body presenting as multiple, pale tumors (*arrows*) on the peripheral iris and in the anterior chamber angle. (Reprinted from The Secondary Glaucomas, ed. Ritch R, Shields MB, St. Louis, The CV Mosby Co., 1982, with permission.)

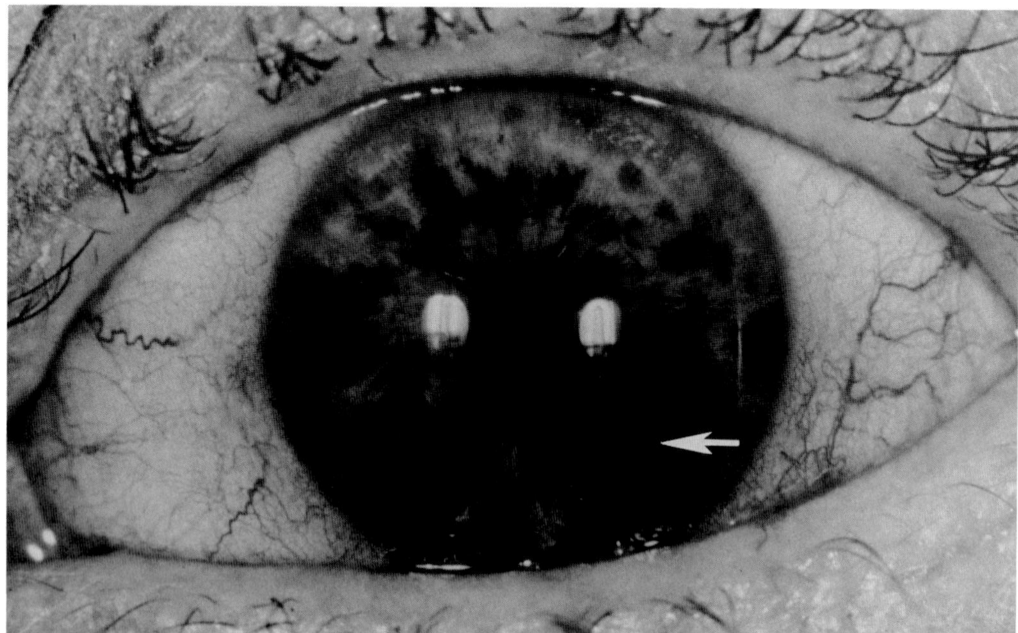

Figure 18.2. Slit-lamp view of malignant melanoma of the iris (*arrow*). (Reprinted with permission from Shields MB, Klintworth GK: Ophthalmology 87:503, 1980.)

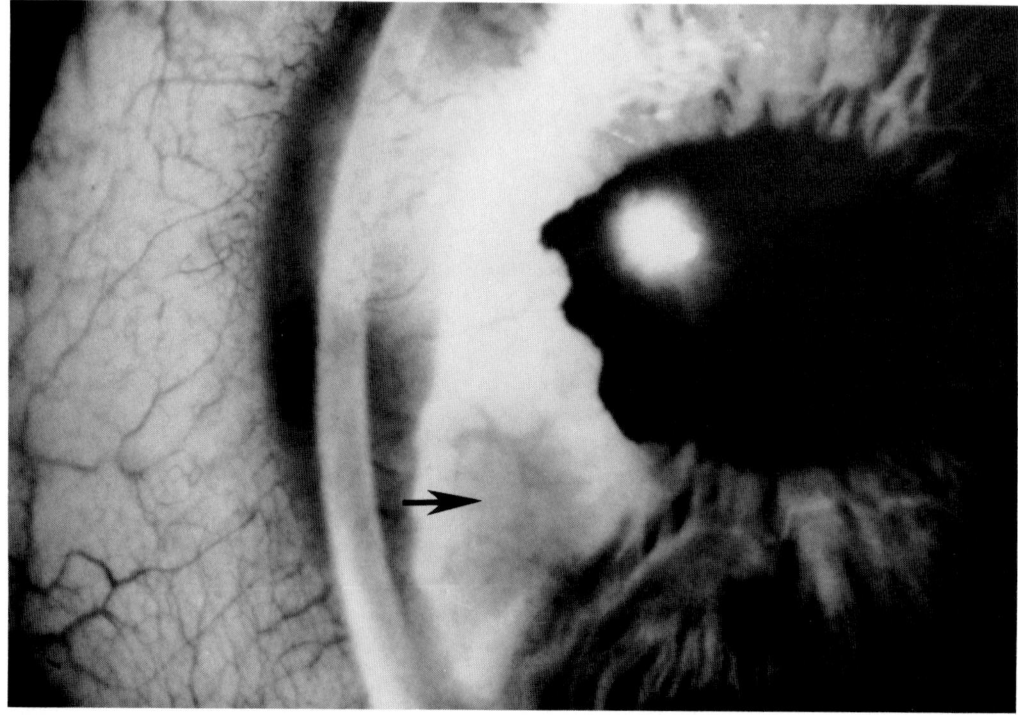

Figure 18.3. Slit-lamp view of amelanotic malignant melanoma of the iris (*arrow*). (Courtesy of David G. Campbell, M.D.)

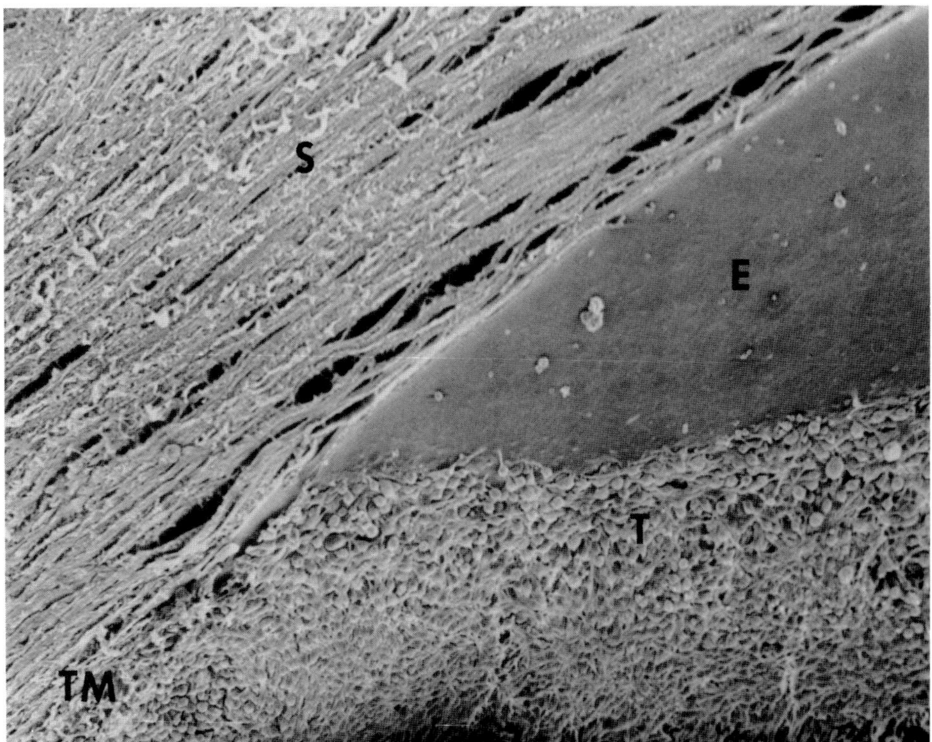

Figure 18.4. Scanning electron microscopic view of eye with malignant melanoma of the ciliary body showing tumor cells (*T*) in anterior chamber angle and on cornea; corneal endothelium (*E*); corneal stroma (*S*); and trabecular meshwork (*TM*). (Original magnification, ×120) (Reprinted with permission from Shields MB, Klintworth GK: Ophthalmology 87:503, 1980.)

as a result of infiltration of the angle with occasional iris nodularity and heterochromia.[5]

In another condition, referred to as *melanomalytic glaucoma,* macrophages containing melanin from a necrotic melanoma obstruct the trabecular meshwork.[2,6] Ultrastructural studies reveal not only infiltration of the angle with melanin-laden macrophages but also phagocytosis of melanin by trabecular-endothelial cells, as well as tumor cells on the iris and in the meshwork.[7,8]

Yet another variation of anterior uveal melanoma and glaucoma occurs with a *tapioca melanoma*. This rare melanoma of the iris creates a nodular appearance resembling tapioca pudding[9] and typically consists of low-grade spindle-type cells, although a case with epithelioid-type cells and metastases has been reported.[10] Glaucoma is reported to occur in one-third of the cases with tapioca melanoma.[9] Another reported mechanism of IOP elevation with an iris melanoma is neovascular glaucoma, which resolved after excision of the tumor.[11]

Ciliary body melanomas may also cause an angle-closure form of secondary glaucoma as a result of compression of the root of the iris into the anterior chamber angle[4] or forward displacement of the lens-iris diaphragm (Fig. 18.5). It should also be noted that some eyes with a melanoma confined to the ciliary body may have a slightly lower IOP than the fellow eye.[12] Any alteration in tension, therefore, can be an indication of an anterior uveal melanoma.

Differential Diagnosis

A number of conditions can be confused with glaucoma and an anterior uveal mela-

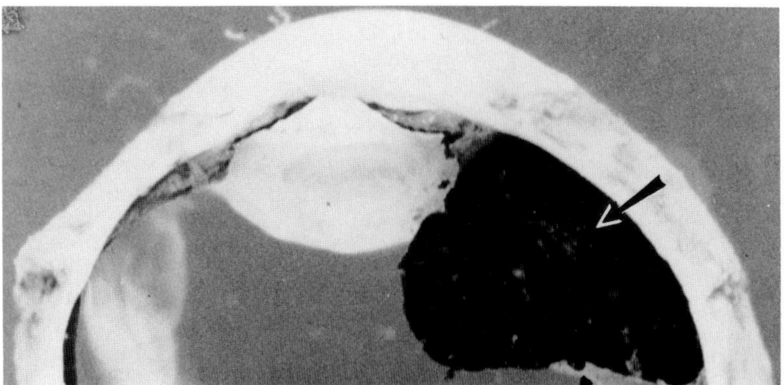

Figure 18.5. Gross appearance of sectioned eye showing malignant melanoma of the ciliary body (*arrow*) adjacent to the lens, creating closure of the anterior chamber angle. (Reprinted with permission from Shields MB, Klintworth GK: Ophthalmology 87:503, 1980.)

noma. Associated changes may mask an underlying melanoma, while other mass lesions may simulate an anterior uveal melanoma. For example, *iritis* may appear to be present in some cases of glaucoma and melanoma, which usually represents tumor cells in the anterior chamber,[3] while other eyes may have primary iritis with inflammatory nodules that might be confused with a malignancy.[13] In one large series, a primary *cyst of the iris* was the most common lesion to be confused with a melanoma of the iris.[14] However, it is important to note that anterior uveal melanomas can masquerade as cysts of the iris or ciliary body due to separation of the two epithelial layers by an eosinophilic exudate (Fig. 18.6).[3,4] Other mass lesions that may be confused with melanomas of the anterior uvea include metastatic malignancies and benign tumors,[14] which are discussed later in this chapter.

Choroidal Melanomas

Occasionally, a patient with a melanoma of the choroid may present with acute angle-closure glaucoma.[2,15] This is usually a result of the forward displacement of the lens-iris diaphragm by a large posterior tumor, which is commonly associated with a total retinal detachment.[2] Therefore, the finding of a retinal detachment and glaucoma in the same eye should alert the clinician to the possibility of an underlying malignant melanoma. Other reported mechanisms of IOP elevation in association with choroidal melanomas include neovascular glaucoma[2] and pigment dispersion in the vitreous with melanomalytic glaucoma.[16] In addition to retinal detachment, other conditions that may mask the presence of a choroidal melanoma include intraocular inflammation and hemorrhage,[17] while a dislocated lens nucleus may mimic a choroidal melanoma, especially when inflammatory glaucoma is also present.[18]

Diagnostic Adjuncts

The difficulty in detecting a uveal melanoma and distinguishing it from other intraocular tumors occasionally necessitates the use of special diagnostic measures.

Ultrasonography

Ultrasonography may be useful in demonstrating the presence of a ciliary body melanoma (Fig. 18.7) or a choroidal melanoma when the latter is masked by a retinal detachment, vitreous hemorrhage, or other opacity in the ocular media. However, this technique does not, with absolute certainty, distinguish a neoplasm from other masses of the posterior ocular segment.[19]

Radioactive Phosphorous Uptake

The 32P test is said to be helpful in differentiating benign from malignant lesions of the choroid.[20,21] However, the study is not

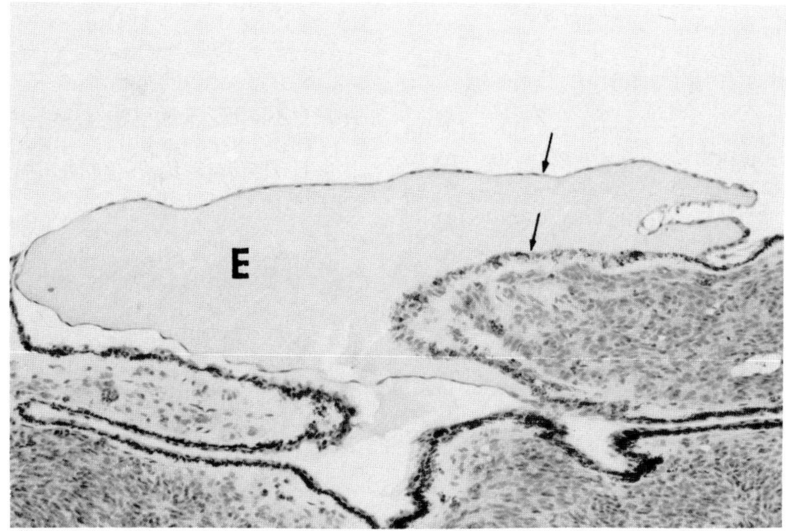

Figure 18.6. Light microscopic view of epithelial layers (*arrows*) of ciliary body separated by prominent eosinophilic exudate (*E*). Stroma of ciliary body contains malignant melanoma. (Hematoxylin-eosin; original magnification, ×100) (Reprinted with permission from Shields MB, Klintworth GK: Ophthalmology 87:503, 1980.)

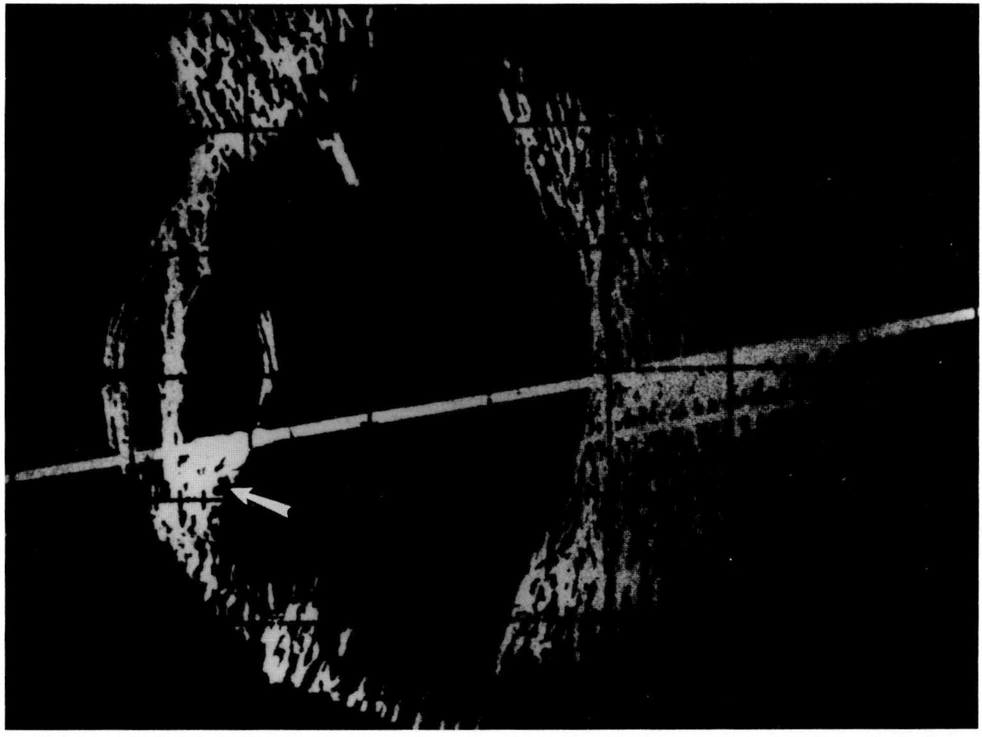

Figure 18.7. B-scan ultrasonographic view of ciliary body mass (*arrow*) in eye with malignant melanoma of ciliary body. (Reprinted from The Secondary Glaucomas, ed. Ritch R, Shields MB, St. Louis, The CV Mosby Co., 1982, with permission.)

as useful in diagnosing the smaller tumors of the iris[20] and ciliary body.[21]

Fluorescein Angiography of the Iris

This test is reported to be useful in distinguishing melanomas from benign lesions of the iris, such as leiomyomas[22,23] and benign melanocytic tumors.[24] The angiographic characteristic of a melanoma of the iris is diffuse and eventually confluent fluorescence emanating from ill-defined vascular foci.[24]

Cytopathologic Studies

An *aqueous or vitreous aspirate* may provide sufficient material for a histopathologic diagnosis of either a primary or metastatic malignancy.[25,26] This may be especially useful for suspected melanomas of the anterior uvea when cells can be seen in the aqueous by slit-lamp biomicroscopy (Fig. 18.8). The technique involves aspiration of aqueous with a small-gauge needle through the limbus. For neoplastic cells, cytologic preservation is best with a Millipore filter.[26]

A *fine needle aspiration biopsy* may also be used to obtain material for cytopathologic study from a suspected anterior uveal or choroidal melanoma.[27] In one case, this allowed differentiation of a diffuse iris melanoma from a focal tumor.[28]

Frozen Section Diagnoses

A frozen section may be helpful in identifying a tumor of the iris and in determining the surgical resection margins of the lesion.[29] In sending the iridectomy specimen to the pathologist, care must be taken to identify the orientation of the tissue and to avoid curling of the edges.[29]

Prognosis

When a uveal melanoma is associated with glaucoma, the prognosis appears to be

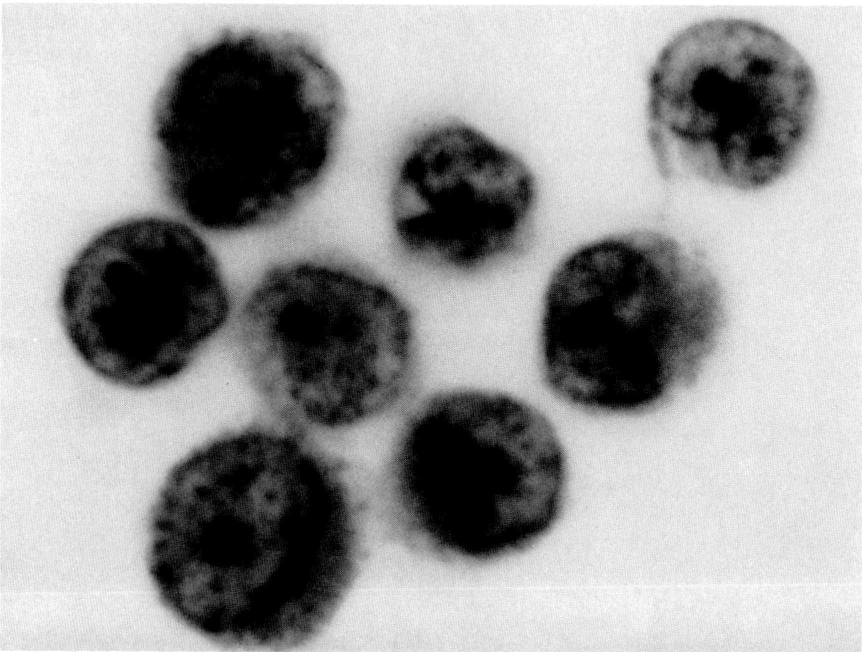

Figure 18.8. Light microscopic view of melanoma cells aspirated from aqueous of eye with anterior uveal melanoma. (Papanicolaou; original magnification, ×400) (Reprinted from The Secondary Glaucomas, ed. Ritch R, Shields MB, St. Louis, The CV Mosby Co., 1982, with permission.)

worse for metastasis and death as opposed to a melanoma without glaucoma. In one study, three of four patients with a primary melanoma of the ciliary body and glaucoma died of metastatic disease within 2½ years after enucleation,[3] while another investigation of uveal melanomas in children and adolescents identified glaucoma as a predominant factor relating to a fatal outcome.[30] Histopathologic studies of eyes with a ciliary body melanoma and glaucoma often reveal tumor cells in the aqueous outflow system, which is a potential route of extraocular metastasis.[3] Patients with choroidal melanomas and glaucoma also have a more guarded prognosis, because the tumor is usually large by the time the glaucoma has developed.

Melanomas of the iris, in general, have a better prognosis than that of other uveal melanomas.[31,32] However, metastases have been reported,[10,31,33–38] and the better prognosis may be due to the earlier detection allowed by the more obvious location, rather than a more benign nature of iris melanomas than other uveal melanomas.[34] In one series of 1043 reported iris melanomas, 31 (3%) metastasized, with cell type influencing the rate of metastasis (none with spindle A, 2.6% with spindle B, 6.9% with epithelioid, and 10.5% with mixed-cell).[35] Observed growth of iris lesions may be the best indicator of malignant potential. However, in one study of 175 patients with melanocytic tumors of the iris, followed for 1–12 years, there was only a 4.6% incidence of tumor growth, and the growth was not always indicative of the presence of malignant cells.[36] The presence of glaucoma with an iris melanoma may also increase the risk of metastasis.

Management

Considering the poor prognosis in cases of ciliary body or choroidal melanoma associated with glaucoma, the recommended management most often is enucleation. By the time glaucoma has developed, the melanoma is usually too large or diffuse for local treatment. However, there are exceptions, especially when the eye with the melanoma is the patient's only eye with useful vision. In such cases, local excision of an anterior uveal melanoma[39,40] or radiotherapy of anterior or posterior tumors[41] is occasionally attempted. In one series of 52 patients undergoing iridocyclectomy for lesions of the iris or ciliary body, half of the excised lesions were benign and nearly one-third of the group eventually required enucleation.[40] Radiotherapy, especially with anterior tumors, may be complicated by hemorrhage and further pressure elevation, as well as failure to eradicate the melanoma.[41]

Care must be taken to avoid artificial elevation of the IOP during both diagnostic and surgical maneuvers for fear that this may accelerate extraocular dissemination of tumor cells.[42–45] Enucleation techniques have been developed to minimize intraoperative pressure elevation, which include manometric pressure regulating systems[43,44] and the use of a wire snare to cut the optic nerve.[45]

Cases of iris melanoma and glaucoma are usually managed more conservatively, since the tumors are typically small when first detected and can be observed for evidence of growth. However, as previously discussed, iris melanomas may metastasize,[31,33–38] and the degree to which associated glaucoma increases this risk is uncertain. In general, iris melanomas should be photographed and followed for evidence of growth. If slight growth is detected, continued close observation is still reasonable, whereas pronounced and progressive growth requires surgical intervention.[37] This usually consists of complete excision by a sector iridectomy. Xenon arc photocoagulation has also been used to eradicate an iris melanoma.[46] However, if the tumor has disseminated or diffusely extended into the anterior segment, as is often the case when glaucoma is also present, enucleation may be indicated.

The management of the associated glaucoma in eyes with a uveal melanoma is best limited to medical therapy. Filtering surgery should probably be avoided, since extraocular dissemination and fatal metastases have been documented in such cases.[36] When surgical intervention for the glaucoma is required, especially in eyes with iris melanomas, a cyclodestructive procedure may be reasonable.

SYSTEMIC MALIGNANCIES

Metastatic Carcinomas

Two large studies have been reported in which at least one eye from autopsy cases with known malignancies were examined for ocular metastases.[47,48] The most common primary sites for metastasis to the eye were the lung and breast. The two studies agreed regarding the incidence of ocular metastases from the lung (6%[47] and 6.7%[48]), although the results differed for metastases from the breast (37%[47] and 9.7%[48]) as well as for the overall incidence from all primary carcinomas (12%[47] and 4%[48]). In any event, metastatic carcinoma of the eye is not uncommon and is said by some to be the most common form of intraocular malignancy.[49]

The most common site of ocular metastasis is the posterior uvea,[47,48,50] although glaucoma is more often associated with metastases to the anterior segment.[51] In one study of 227 cases of carcinoma metastatic to the eye and orbit, glaucoma was detected in 7.5% of the total group[50] and in 56% of the 26 with anterior ocular metastasis.[51] In another series of 256 eyes with uveal metastases, secondary IOP elevation was present in 5% of the total group but in 64% and 67% of eyes with iris and ciliary body metastases, respectively.[1] The clinical appearance of metastatic carcinomas of the anterior uvea is that of a gelatinous or translucent mass, which may be a single lesion or multiple nodules on the iris, often associated with rubeosis iridis, iridocyclitis, or hyphema (Fig. 18.9).[51–55]

Mechanisms of glaucoma in eyes with anterior uveal metastatic carcinoma include open-angle forms in which the trabecular meshwork may be covered by sheets of tumor cells or may be infiltrated with neoplastic tissue.[1,51] Other patients have angle-closure glaucoma resulting from compres-

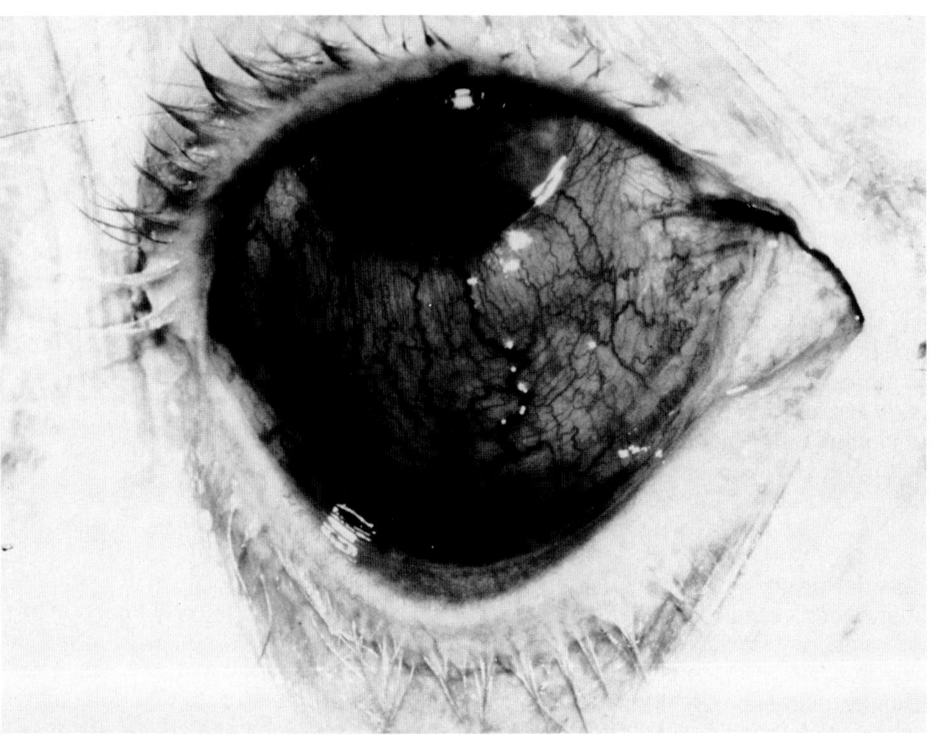

Figure 18.9. External view of patient with metastatic carcinoma showing inferior subconjunctival mass and layered hyphema and hypopyon, obscuring a mass of the ciliary body and iris. (Reprinted from The Secondary Glaucomas, ed. Ritch R, Shields MB, St. Louis, The CV Mosby Co., 1982, with permission.)

sion of the iris by the tumor or resulting from peripheral anterior synechiae.[1,51] An unusual case has also been described in which a nasal carcinoma caused bilateral glaucoma by infiltrating Schlemm's canal and intrascleral and episcleral collector channels.[56]

In the management of metastatic carcinoma to the anterior uvea, an aqueous paracentesis for cytopathologic examination is often helpful in establishing the diagnosis.[49,54] When the cytology is nondiagnostic, a serologic tumor marker in the aqueous has been used to make the diagnosis.[57] Treatment of the metastatic carcinoma usually includes radiation therapy and occasional chemotherapy.[49,53,54] Enucleation is usually reserved for blind, painful eyes. If the associated glaucoma persists, it should be controlled medically whenever possible.

Metastatic Melanomas

Although ocular melanomas are nearly always primary malignancies, metastatic melanomas of the eye have been reported and may occasionally cause secondary glaucoma.[25] A unique form has been called *black hypopyon,* in which a disseminated cutaneous malignant melanoma metastasized to the eye, where it became necrotic, possibly in response to immunotherapy or irradiation, resulting in a hypopyon of tumor cells and pigment-laden macrophages with secondary glaucoma.[58]

Leukemias

In an autopsy survey of 117 eyes of individuals who died of acute or chronic leukemia, the incidence of leukemic infiltrates in the ocular tissues was 28%.[48] In a slit-lamp study of 39 children with acute leukemia, the same percentage of cases was found to have flare or cells in the anterior chamber.[59] A leukemic infiltration of the anterior ocular segment leads to secondary glaucoma in some cases, which may present in association with hyphema and hypopyon.[60–62] These patients more often have acute lymphocytic leukemia. Apparent uveitis in children with acute leukemia should be regarded as evidence of relapse, and anterior chamber aspiration and iris biopsy are said to be essential procedures in establishing this diagnosis.[63] In a series of 135 patients who had fatal leukemia, ocular leukemic infiltration was found in one-third of the cases, most often in the choroid.[64] Chronic leukemias in adults may also have ocular involvement, with one case presenting as recurring bilateral hypopyon,[65] and another as a massive subretinal hemorrhage with acute angle-closure glaucoma.[66] In most cases, after the diagnosis has been established by cytologic examination of an aqueous aspirate, treatment usually includes irradiation and chemotherapy.

Other Neoplasias

Lymphomas

An autopsy review of 60 eyes from patients with lymphomas revealed ocular involvement in four (6.7%).[48] The anterior ocular segment may be involved, presenting as iridocyclitis, with occasional IOP elevation.[67] A case of open-angle glaucoma has also been reported in association with a subconjunctival malignant lymphoma.[68]

Histiocytosis X

This uncommon multisystem disorder, characterized by accumulation of histiocytes in various tissues, includes three clinical subsets: eosinophilic granuloma (lesions confined to bone), Hand-Schüller-Christian disease (bone and soft tissue involvement), and Letterer-Siwe disease (predominantly soft tissue involvement in infants). Histiocytosis X has been reported to involve the anterior chamber with associated secondary glaucoma.[69] However, this is apparently extremely rare, since a study of 76 children with histiocytosis X revealed 18 with orbital but none with intraocular involvement.[70]

Multiple Myeloma

Apparent nongranulomatous anterior uveitis with secondary glaucoma in a patient with multiple myeloma was found by cytologic examination to represent an infiltrate of neoplastic plasma cells.[71]

OCULAR TUMORS OF CHILDHOOD

Retinoblastoma

Incidence of Glaucoma

Although secondary glaucoma is not commonly recognized clinically in children with retinoblastoma, histopathologic studies suggest that it is a frequent complication of this disease. In one study of 149 eyes, there was histologic evidence of a glaucoma-inducing mechanism in 50% of the cases, although an elevated IOP had been clinically recorded in only 23%.[72] In another series of 303 eyes with retinoblastoma, 17% had documented pressure elevation.[1] Glaucoma was found in one study to be the presenting sign in 7% of eyes with retinoblastoma, with leukocoria (white pupillary reflex) and strabismus being the most common presentations, at 60% and 20%, respectively.[73]

Mechanisms of Glaucoma

Neovascularization of the iris is a frequent histopathologic finding in eyes with retinoblastoma and is the most common cause of the associated glaucoma.[1,72,74,75] Both the rubeosis iridis and neovascular glaucoma are frequently overlooked clinically and should be considered in all cases of retinoblastoma. Two additional causes of glaucoma are pupillary block with secondary angle-closure resulting from massive exudative retinal detachment[1] and obstruction of the anterior chamber angle by inflammatory cells or necrotic tumor tissue.[72] In a review of 1500 patients with retinoblastoma, anterior chamber involvement was seen in 30 cases and was found to indicate a poor prognosis.[76] Specular microscopy has been shown to demonstrate clusters of retinoblastoma cells on the corneal endothelium as a bright, lacy network of reflections within a dark area.[77]

Differential Diagnosis

Conditions that simulate retinoblastoma have been called "pseudogliomas" and include retrolental fibroplasia, persistent hyperplastic primary vitreous, retinal dysplasia, Coats' disease, toxocariasis, and infantile retinal detachment.[78,79] Each of these conditions also has a high incidence of rubeosis iridis, so that this factor is not helpful in distinguishing retinoblastoma from the pseudogliomas.[75,78]

Management

The presence of rubeosis iridis, with or without glaucoma,[75] as well as the presence of glaucoma without iris neovascularization, which usually indicates a large tumor with angle closure or dissemination of tumor cells into the anterior chamber,[76] all indicate a more grave prognosis in patients with retinoblastoma. In most of these cases, enucleation is indicated.

Juvenile Xanthogranuloma

This is a benign, self-limiting disease of infants and young children, with rare cases in young adults.[80] It is characterized by discrete, yellow, papular cutaneous lesions, primarily of the head and neck, as well as salmon-colored to lightly pigmented lesions of the iris.[81,82] The latter feature is usually unilateral and may cause spontaneous hyphema. Secondary glaucoma may occur from invasion of the anterior chamber angle with histiocytes or in association with the hyphema or a secondary uveitis. Treatment for eyes with juvenile xanthogranuloma and secondary glaucoma includes topical corticosteroids and occasionally external beam irradiation.[83–87]

Medulloepithelioma

A medulloepithelioma, or diktyoma, is a primary tumor of childhood, which arises most often from nonpigmented ciliary epithelium. The clinical appearance is that of a whitish-gray mass or cyst of the iris or ciliary body. In a study of 56 cases, glaucoma was observed clinically in 26 eyes.[88] Histopathologic evidence of secondary glaucoma was seen in 18 cases, 11 of which had rubeosis iridis. Peripheral anterior synechiae and shallow anterior chambers were also commonly observed. In one report, glaucoma was associated with two white flocculi floating in the anterior chamber, delicate iris neovascularization, and a globular ciliary body mass.[89] Some medulloepitheliomas are malignant, although the mortality rate is low. While enucleation is the most common treatment, success has been reported with iridocyclectomy, and local excision has been recommended when the tumor is small and well circumscribed.[88]

BENIGN TUMORS OF THE ANTERIOR UVEA

In the differential diagnosis of anterior uveal tumors, several benign lesions must be considered. These include nevi, cysts, melanocytoses, melanocytomas, adenomas, and leiomyomas. Secondary glaucoma may be associated with several of these conditions, further compounding the diagnostic problem.

Nevi of the Iris

One or more nevi on the stromal surface of the iris is not an uncommon clinical finding. They are usually recognized as small, discrete, flat or slightly elevated lesions of variable pigmentation. However, some may be confused with melanomas, which has led to unnecessary surgical intervention. In a retrospective clinicopathologic study of 189 lesions of the anterior uvea that were originally diagnosed as melanomas, 80% were reclassified as nevi of several cell types.[90] These authors found no clinical features to distinguish benign from malignant tumors, including diffuse spread or the presence of glaucoma. Diffuse, pigmented and nonpigmented nevi of the iris can cause glaucoma by direct extension across the trabecular meshwork.[90,91] As previously noted in this chapter, fluorescein angiography of the iris, aqueous aspiration for cytologic examination, or a biopsy may aid in the important differentiation between melanomas and benign lesions of the iris.

A specific form of iris nevus with associated glaucoma is the *iris nevus syndrome.* In these cases, diffuse nevi of the iris are associated with progressive synechial closure of the angle and secondary IOP elevation.[92] A subset of the iridocorneal endothelial syndrome, the *Cogan-Reese syndrome,* has a similar clinical appearance, but the pedunculated nodules on the surface of the iris are composed of tissue resembling iris stroma.[93] The benign lesions of the iris in both of these conditions have been mistaken for malignant melanomas, which has led to enucleation in some patients. These conditions are discussed further in Chapter 13.

Cysts

Cysts of the iris have been classified as primary and secondary, with the former arising from the epithelial layers of the iris and ciliary body or, less often, from the iris stroma.[94] The majority of the primary cysts are stationary lesions, rarely progressing or causing visual complications. However, families have been described in which multiple cysts of the iris and ciliary body, presumably of autosomal dominant inheritance, caused angle-closure glaucoma.[95] These have been successfully treated by laser cystotomy.[95,96] Secondary cysts of the iris, which may result from trauma or neoplasia, are more likely than primary cysts to lead to inflammation and glaucoma.[94]

Melanocytomas

These tumors are classified as benign nevi and are seen clinically as darkly pigmented lesions, usually on the optic nerve head and less often in the choroid, ciliary body, or iris. Those in the latter location have been reported to cause glaucoma, either by direct spread into the anterior chamber angle[97] or dispersion of pigment into the angle from a necrotic melanocytoma.[98]

Melanoses

Melanosis iridis is characterized by verrucous-like elevations on the surface of a darkly pigmented, velvety iris. It is usually unilateral and sometimes sectorial, although bilateral involvement has been reported.[99] *Melanosis oculi* has additional hyperpigmentation of the episclera, choroid, or both and has been reported in association with open-angle glaucoma, in which the mechanism appears to be heavy pigmentation of the trabecular meshwork.[100] A similar condition has been observed in oculodermal melanocytosis (nevus of Ota), which is considered further in the next section of this chapter.

Adenomas

Benign adenomas may arise from the epithelium of the anterior uvea, especially the ciliary body (Fuchs' adenoma). They occur predominantly in adults, although one has been observed in a child with associated hyperplastic primary vitreous.[101] While common among the elderly, they are rarely noted clinically.[102] Some, however, can involve the iris, primarily or secondarily,[103] and have been reported to cause glaucoma from pigment dispersion.[104] Adenomas must be distinguished from anterior uveal cysts and melanomas.[103] Adenocarcinomas may also arise from the ciliary body epithelium and have been reported to cause glaucoma.[105]

Leiomyomas

These rare tumors may appear as a slow-growing grayish-white, vascularized nodule on the surface of the iris. Glaucoma is not a typical complication.

PHAKOMATOSES

In 1932, Van der Hoeve[106] coined the term *phakomatosis,* meaning "mother-spot" or "birthmark," to denote a group of disorders that are characterized by hamartomas, which are congenital tumors arising from tissue that is normally found in the involved area. The hamartomas primarily involve the eye, skin, and nervous system, although other systems may be involved to a lesser degree, including pulmonary, cardiovascular, gastrointestinal, renal, and skeletal. In some cases, the anomalies are present at birth, while others become manifest later in life. The four conditions that traditionally comprise the phakomatoses are: (1) von Hippel-Lindau syndrome; (2) von Recklinghausen's neurofibromatosis; (3) tuberous sclerosis or Bourneville's disease; and (4) Sturge-Weber syndrome. Several other disorders have subsequently been included by various authors. The following discussion is limited to those phakomatoses that may frequently or occasionally have associated glaucoma.

Sturge-Weber Syndrome (encephalotrigeminal angiomatosis)

General Features

The hamartoma in this condition arises from vascular tissue and produces a characteristic port wine hemangioma of the skin along the trigeminal distribution (Fig. 18.10) and an ipsilateral leptomeningeal angioma. The angiomata are present at birth and are usually unilateral, although bilateral cases also occur. The nervous system involvement frequently causes seizure disorders, hemispheric motor or sensory defects, and intellectual deficiency. A characteristic radiographic finding is cortical calcifications that develop after several years and appear as double densities or "railroad tracks." There is no race or sex predilection, and no hereditary pattern has been established.

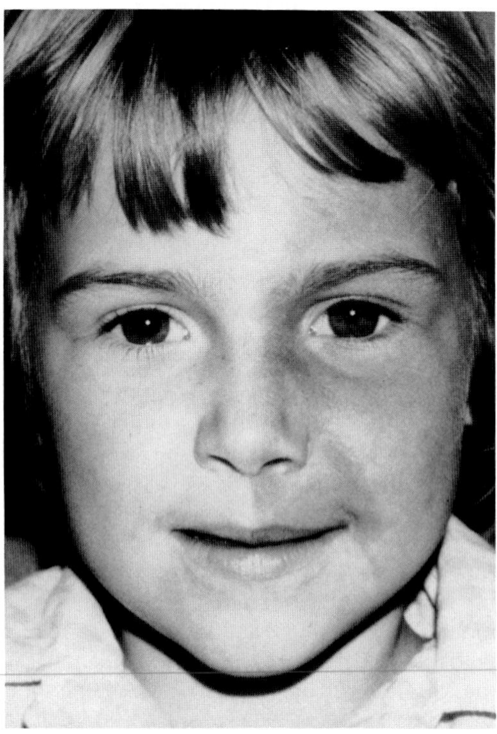

Figure 18.10. Child with Sturge-Weber syndrome and unilateral secondary glaucoma showing typical port wine hemangioma of the skin along the distribution of the left trigeminal nerve.

Ocular Features

In approximately half of the cases in which the port wine stain involves both the ophthalmic and maxillary divisions of the trigeminal nerve, glaucoma will be present. Slit-lamp examination typically reveals a dense episcleral vascular plexus and occasional ampulliform dilations of conjunctival vessels. These findings are always on the side of the cutaneous lesion. Some patients also have a choroidal hemangioma.

Theories of Glaucoma Mechanism

The cause of glaucoma in the Sturge-Weber syndrome is a controversial issue. Weiss[107] described two mechanisms, the more common of which occurs in infants, with a developmental anomaly of the anterior chamber angle similar to that of primary congenital glaucoma. One histopathologic report described hemangiomas of the choroid and episclera, as well as a partial developmental anomaly of the anterior chamber angle.[108] The other mechanism of glaucoma appears later in life and is associated with an open anterior chamber angle and small arteriovenous fistulas in the episcleral vessels. Phelps,[109] however, observed episcleral hemangiomas in all cases and elevated episcleral venous pressure whenever this parameter could be studied, but he saw no abnormalities of the anterior chamber angle. He believed that elevated episcleral venous pressure was the most common glaucoma mechanism in all ages of patients with the Sturge-Weber syndrome. Cibis and associates[110] found aging changes, similar to those seen in primary open-angle glaucoma, in the trabecular meshwork of three eyes with Sturge-Weber syndrome. They postulated that this alteration, and not elevated episcleral venous pressure, is the mechanism of the later onset cases.

Management

Medical therapy may suffice to control the glaucoma that occurs in later life, while the infantile form usually requires surgical intervention.[107] Success has been reported with a trabeculectomy in children and adults.[111,112] However, filtering surgery in these patients is commonly associated with intraoperative choroidal effusion[112–114] and occasionally with expulsive hemorrhage.[108,113–115] In one study of 30 patients, goniotomy was not associated with these complications and was the author's first choice in most cases.[112] Since it may not be certain whether the glaucoma results from an anterior chamber angle anomaly or elevated episcleral venous pressure, a combined trabeculotomy-trabeculectomy may improve the chances of success, by treating both possible sources of elevated IOP,[113] although it does not reduce the potential for serious complications. Another alternative to reduce the risk of massive choroidal effusion and expulsive hemorrhage is a cyclodestructive procedure.

von Recklinghausen's Neurofibromatosis

General Features

The principal systemic lesions in this condition involve the skin and include café au lait spots, which are flat, hyperpigmented lesions with well-circumscribed borders, and neurofibromas, which appear as soft, flesh-colored, pedunculated masses. The latter lesions arise from Schwann cells. Central nervous system involvement is uncommon, although neurofibromas may develop from cranial nerves, especially the acoustic nerve. Two subsets of neurofibromatosis have been distinguished: *peripheral* (von Recklinghausen's), characterized by the skin lesions; and *central,* characterized by bilateral acoustic schwannomas.[116] Both are inherited by an autosomal dominant mode with variable expressivity. Genetic analysis of a kindred with von Recklinghausen's neurofibromatosis indicated that the responsible gene is located near the centromere on chromosome 17.[117]

Ocular Features

In the peripheral form, the eyelids, conjuctiva, iris, ciliary body, and choroid may be involved with the neurofibromas. The hamartomatous lesions of the iris are called *Lisch nodules*. They are usually bilateral and characterized by well-defined, clear to yellow or brown dome-shaped gelatinous elevations on the iris stroma (Fig. 18.11). An ultrastructural study indicates that they are of melanocytic origin.[118] Lisch nodules are a nearly constant feature of von Recklinghausen's neurofibromatosis, occurring in 92% of one series of 77 patients.[119] In another study of 64 patients, the nodules were seen in 95% and in all patients aged 16 years or older.[120] In addition, chorioretinal hamartomas and gliomas of the optic nerve are occasionally present. A fluorescein angiographic study of the choroidal lesions revealed avascular patches of hypofluorescence similar to multiple small choroidal

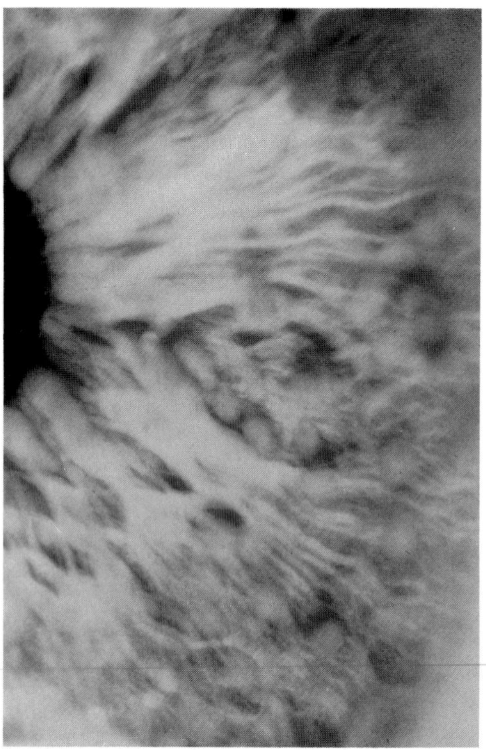

Figure 18.11. Slit-lamp view of Lisch nodules on the iris of a patient with von Recklinghausen's neurofibromatosis. (Courtesy of George Rosenwasser, M.D.).

nevi.[120] The central form of neurofibromatosis does not typically have ocular findings, other than presenile posterior subcapsular or nuclear cataracts.[116]

Intraocular pressure elevation is more likely to occur in neurofibromatosis when the lids are involved with neurofibromas. The several possible mechanisms of glaucoma include: (1) infiltration of the angle with neurofibromatous tissue; (2) closure of the anterior chamber angle as a result of nodular thickening of the ciliary body and choroid; (3) fibrovascular membrane resembling neovascular glaucoma; and (4) failure of normal anterior chamber angle development.[121,122]

Management

In treating the glaucoma, medical measures should be attempted first, since surgical approaches are often not satisfactory. An infant with unilateral glaucoma underwent five unsuccessful operations before ocular neurofibromatosis was discovered 2 years later.[123]

von Hippel-Lindau Disease

This phakomatosis is characterized by angiomatosis of the retina and, in a small percentage of cases, the cerebellum. Most cases are not familial. Glaucoma may occur as a late sequelae as a result of rubeosis iridis or iridocyclitis.

Nevus of Ota (oculodermal melanocytosis)

This condition is not included in all reported classifications of the phakomatoses but does fit the broader definition of the disease group.

General Features

The hamartoma in this condition represents an abnormally large accumulation of melanocytes in ocular tissues, especially the episclera (Fig. 18.12), as well as the skin in the distribution of the trigeminal nerve and occasionally the nasal or buccal mucosa. In a study of 194 patients, 67 had only dermal involvement, 12 had only ocular involvement, and 115 had both.[124] It is nearly always unilateral, with a preponderance of females and a tendency toward dark races.[125] Degeneration to malignant melanomas may occur in Caucasian patients but rarely in non-Caucasians.[126–129]

Glaucoma

Evidence of chronic glaucoma has been observed in patients with the nevus of Ota.[130–133] Elevated IOP, with or without glaucomatous damage, was seen in 10% of one series.[124] The involved eye typically has unusually heavy pigmentation of the trabecular meshwork, and histopathologic studies have revealed melanocytes in the meshwork.[132,133]

Management

Medical management, as with other forms of open-angle glaucoma, should be tried first. When this fails, laser trabecu-

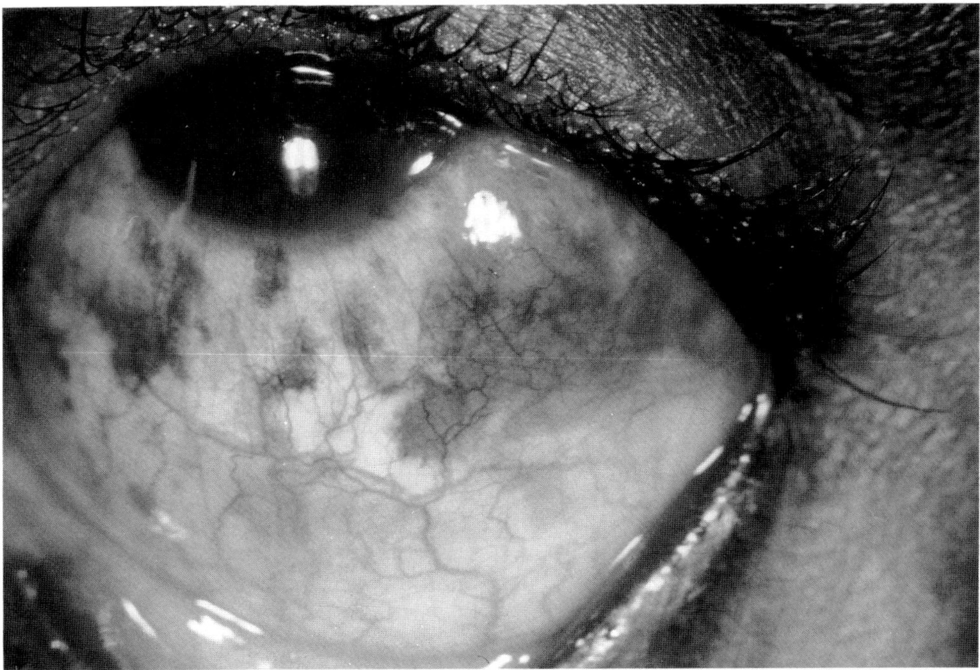

Figure 18.12. Abnormal pigmentation of the episclera in a patient with oculodermal melanocytosis (nevus of Ota).

loplasty may be effective.[100] Otherwise, filtering surgery is indicated.

SUMMARY

Primary malignant melanomas of the uvea may cause secondary open-angle glaucoma by either direct extension or seeding of tumor cells, pigment granules, or macrophages into the anterior chamber angle. Less often, these tumors may cause angle-closure glaucoma by a mass effect behind the iris or lens. Ultrasonography and cytology of aqueous aspirates are useful diagnostic adjuncts, and most confirmed cases are managed by enucleation. Systemic malignancies, including metastatic carcinomas and melanomas, leukemias, and lymphomas, may occasionally cause secondary glaucomas, usually by invasion of the anterior chamber angle. Ocular tumors of childhood that may cause glaucoma include retinoblastoma, juvenile xanthogranuloma, and medulloepithelioma. Other benign tumors of the anterior uvea that may be associated with glaucoma are nevi, cysts, melanocytomas, melanosis, adenomas, and leiomyomas. Some of the phakomatoses, most notably the Sturge-Weber syndrome, von Recklinghausen's neurofibromatosis, and the nevus of Ota, may also have associated glaucoma.

References

1. Shields, CL, Shields, JA, Shields, MB, Augsburger, JJ: Prevalence and mechanisms of secondary intraocular pressure elevation in eyes with intraocular tumors. Ophthalmology 94:839, 1987.
2. Yanoff, M: Glaucoma mechanisms in ocular malignant melanomas. Am J Ophthal 70:898, 1970.
3. Shields, MB, Klintworth, GK: Anterior uveal melanomas and intraocular pressure. Ophthalmology 87:503, 1980.
4. Hopkins, RE, Carriker, FR: Malignant melanoma of the ciliary body. Am J Ophthal 45:835, 1958.
5. Omulecki, W, Pruszczynski, M, Borowski, J: Ring melanoma of the iris and ciliary body. Br J Ophthal 69:514, 1985.
6. Yanoff, M, Scheie, HG: Melanomalytic glaucoma. Report of a case. Arch Ophthal 84:471, 1970.
7. Van Buskirk, EM, Leure-duPree, AE: Patho-

physiology and electron microscopy of melanomalytic glaucoma. Am J Ophthal 85:160, 1978.
8. McMenamin, PG, Lee, WR: Ultrastructural pathology of melanomalytic glaucoma. Br J Ophthal 70:895, 1986.
9. Reese, AB, Mund, ML, Iwamoto, T: Tapioca melanoma of the iris. Part 1. Clinical and light microscopy studies. Am J Ophthal 74:840, 1972.
10. Zakka, KA, Foos, RY, Sulit, H: Metastatic tapioca iris melanoma. Br J Ophthal 63:744, 1979.
11. Shields, MB, Proia, AD: Neovascular glaucoma associated with an iris melanoma. A clinicopathologic report. Arch Ophthal 105:672, 1987.
12. Foos, RY, Hull, SN, Straatsma, BR: Early diagnosis of ciliary body melanomas. Arch Ophthal 81:336, 1969.
13. Gupta, K, Hoepner, JA, Streeten, BW: Pseudomelanoma of the iris in herpes simplex keratoiritis. Ophthalmology 93:1524, 1986.
14. Shields, JA, Sanborn, GE, Augsburger, JJ: The differential diagnosis of malignant melanoma of the iris. A clinical study of 200 patients. Ophthalmology 90:716, 1983.
15. Singer, PR, Krupin, T, Smith, ME, Becker, B: Recurrent orbital and metastatic melanoma in a patient undergoing previous glaucoma surgery. Am J Ophthal 87:766, 1979.
16. El Baba, F, Hagler, WS, De La Cruz, A, Green, WR: Choroidal melanoma with pigment dispersion in vitreous and melanomalytic glaucoma. Ophthalmology 95:370, 1988.
17. Fraser, DJ, Font, RL: Ocular inflammation and hemorrhage as initial manifestations of uveal malignant melanoma. Incidence and prognosis. Arch Ophthal 97:1311, 1979.
18. Alward, WLM, Frazier Byrne, S, Hughes, JR, Hodapp, EA: Dislocated lens nuclei simulating choroidal melanomas. Arch Ophthal 107:1463, 1989.
19. Gitter, KA, Meyer, D, Sarin, LK: Ultrasound to evaluate eyes with opaque media. Am J Ophthal 64:100, 1967.
20. Shields, JA: Accuracy and limitations of the 32P test in the diagnosis of ocular tumors: an analysis of 500 cases. Ophthalmology 85:950, 1978.
21. Goldberg, B, Kara, GB, Previte, LR: The use of radioactive phosphorus (32P) in the diagnosis of ocular tumors. Am J Ophthal 90:817, 1980.
22. Christiansen, JM, Wetzig, PC, Thatcher, DB, Green, WR: Diagnosis and management of anterior uveal tumors. Ophthal Surg 10:81, 1979.
23. Brovkina, AF, Chichua, AG: Value of fluorescein iridography in diagnosis of tumours of the iridociliary zone. Br J Ophthal 63:157, 1979.
24. Jakobiec, FA, Depot, MJ, Henkind, P, Spencer, WH: Fluorescein angiographic patterns of iris melanocytic tumors. Arch Ophthal 100:1288, 1982.
25. Char, DH, Schwartz, A, Miller, TR, Abele, JS: Ocular metastases from systemic melanoma. Am J Ophthal 90:702, 1980.
26. Green, WR: Diagnostic cytopathology of ocular fluid specimens. Ophthalmology 91:726, 1984.
27. Midena, E, Segato, T, Piermarocchi, S, Boccato, P: Fine needle aspiration biopsy in ophthalmology. Surv Ophthal 29:410, 1985.
28. Char, DH, Crawford, JB, Gonzales, J, Miller, T: Iris melanoma with increased intraocular pressure. Differentiation of focal solitary tumors from diffuse or multiple tumors. Arch Ophthal 107:548, 1989.
29. Karcioglu, ZA, Caldwell, DR: Frozen section diagnosis in ophthalmic surgery. Surv Ophthal 28:323, 1984.
30. Barr, CC, McLean, IW, Zimmerman, LE: Uveal melanoma in children and adolescents. Arch Ophthal 99:2133, 1981.
31. Rones, B, Zimmerman, LE: The prognosis of primary tumors of the iris treated by iridectomy. Arch Ophthal 60:193, 1958.
32. Dunphy, EB, Dryja, TP, Albert, DM, Smith, TR: Melanocytic tumor of the anterior uvea. Am J Ophthal 86:680, 1978.
33. Sunba, MSN, Rahi, AHS, Morgan, G: Tumors of the anterior uvea. I. Metastasizing malignant melanoma of the iris. Arch Ophthal 98:82, 1980.
34. Kersten, RC, Tse, DT, Anderson, R: Iris melanoma. Nevus or malignancy? Surv Ophthal 29:423, 1985.
35. Geisse, LJ, Robertson, DM: Iris melanomas. Am J Ophthal 99:638, 1985.
36. Territo, C, Shields, CL, Shields, JA, et al: Natural course of melanocytic tumors of the iris. Ophthalmology 95:1251, 1988.
37. McGalliard, JN, Johnston, PB: A study of iris melanoma in Northern Ireland. Br J Ophthal 73:591, 1989.
38. Shields, JA, Shields, CL: Hepatic metastases of diffuse iris melanoma 17 years after enucleation. Am J Ophthal 106:749, 1989.
39. Sugar, HS: Removal of some intraocular tumors: report of twelve cases. Ann Ophthal 13:633, 1981.
40. Memmen, JE, McLean, IW: The long-term outcome of patients undergoing iridocyclectomy. Ophthalmology 97:429, 1990.
41. Foulds, WS, Lee, WR: The significance of glaucoma in the management of melanomas of the anterior segment. Trans Ophthal Soc UK 103:59, 1983.
42. Zimmerman, LE, McLean, IW, Foster, WD: Statistical analysis of follow-up data concerning uveal melanomas, and the influence of enucleation. Ophthalmology 87:557, 1980.
43. Kramer, KK, LaPiana, FG, Whitmore, PV: Enucleation with stabilization of intraocular pressure in the treatment of uveal melanomas. Ophthal Surg 11:39, 1980.
44. Blair, CJ, Guerry, RK, Stratford, TP: Normal in-

traocular pressure during enucleation for choroidal melanoma. Arch Ophthal 101:1900, 1983.
45. Migdal, C: Effect of the method of enucleation on the prognosis of choroidal melanoma. Br J Ophthal 67:385, 1983.
46. Cleasby, GW, Van Westenbrugge, JA: Treatment of iris melanoma by photocoagulation: a case report. Ophthal Surg 18:42, 1987.
47. Bloch, RS, Gartner, S: The incidence of ocular metastatic carcinoma. Arch Ophthal 85:673, 1971.
48. Nelson, CC, Hertzberg, BS, Klintworth, GK: A histopathologic study of 716 unselected eyes in patients with cancer at the time of death. Am J Ophthal 95:788, 1983.
49. Scholz, R, Green, WR, Baranano, EC, et al: Metastatic carcinoma to the iris. Diagnosis by aqueous paracentesis and response to irradiation and chemotherapy. Ophthalmology 90:1524, 1983.
50. Ferry, AP, Font, RL: Carcinoma metastatic to the eye and orbit. I. A clinicopathologic study of 227 cases. Arch Ophthal 92:276, 1974.
51. Ferry, AP, Font, RL: Carcinoma metastatic to the eye and orbit. II. A clinicopathological study of 26 patients with carcinoma metastatic to the anterior segment of the eye. Arch Ophthal 93:472, 1975.
52. Freeman, TR, Friedman, AH: Metastatic carcinoma of the iris. Am J Ophthal 80:947, 1975.
53. Frank, KW, Sugar, HS, Sherman, AI, et al: Anterior segment metastases from an ovarian choriocarcinoma. Am J Ophthal 87:778, 1979.
54. Woog, JJ, Chess, J, Albert, DM, et al: Metastatic carcinoma of the iris simulating iridocyclitis. Br J Ophthal 68:167, 1984.
55. Kurosawa, A, Sawaguchi, S: Iris metastasis from squamous cell carcinoma of the uterine cervix. Arch Ophthal 105:618, 1987.
56. Johnson, BL: Bilateral glaucoma caused by nasal carcinoma obstructing Schlemm's canal. Am J Ophthal 96:550, 1983.
57. Rotkis, WM, Kulander, BG, Chandler, JW, Kaiser, FS: Diagnosis of anterior chamber metastasis by serologic marker found during anterior chamber paracentesis. Am J Ophthal 102:179, 1986.
58. Wormald, RPL, Harper, JI: Bilateral black hypopyon in a patient with self-healing cutaneous malignant melanoma. Br J Ophthal 67:231, 1983.
59. Abramson, A: Anterior chamber activity in children with acute leukemia. Ann Ophthal 12:553, 1980.
60. Zakka, KA, Yee, RD, Shorr, N, et al: Leukemic iris infiltration. Am J Ophthal 89:204, 1980.
61. Kincaid, MC, Green, WR: Ocular and orbital involvement in leukemia. Surv Ophthal 27:211, 1983.
62. Rosenthal, AR: Ocular manifestations of leukemia. A review. Ophthalmology 90:899, 1983.
63. Novakovic, P, Kellie, SJ, Taylor, D: Childhood leukaemia: relapse in the anterior segment of the eye. Br J Ophthal 73:354, 1989.
64. Leonardy, NJ, Rupani, M, Dent, G, Klintworth, GK: Analysis of 135 autopsy eyes for ocular involvement in leukemia. Am J Ophthal 109:436, 1990.
65. Santoni, G, Fiore, C, Lupidi, G, Bibbiani, U: Recurring bilateral hypopyon in chronic myeloid leukemia in blastic transformation. A case report. Graefe's Arch Ophthal 223:211, 1985.
66. Kozlowski, IMD, Hirose, T, Jalkh, AE: Massive subretinal hemorrhage with acute angle-closure glaucoma in chronic myelocytic leukemia. Am J Ophthal 103:837, 1987.
67. Saga, T, Ohno, S, Matsuda, H, et al: Ocular involvement by a peripheral T-cell lymphoma. Arch Ophthal 102:399, 1984.
68. Sato, M, Futa, R: A case of secondary open-angle glaucoma associated with subconjunctival malignant melanoma. Jap J Clin Ophthal 40:57, 1986.
69. Epstein, DL, Grant, WM: Secondary open-angle glaucoma in histiocytosis X. Am J Ophthal 84:332, 1977.
70. Moore, AT, Pritchard, J, Taylor, DSI: Histiocytosis X: an ophthalmological review. Br J Ophthal 69:7, 1985.
71. Shakin, EP, Augsburger, JJ, Eagle, RC Jr, et al: Multiple myeloma involving the iris. Arch Ophthal 106:524, 1988.
72. Yoshizumi, MO, Thomas, JV, Smith, TR: Glaucoma-inducing mechanisms in eyes with retinoblastoma. Arch Ophthal 96:105, 1978.
73. Ellsworth, RM: The practical management of retinoblastoma. Trans Am Ophthal Soc 67:462, 1969.
74. Walton, DS, Grant, WM: Retinoblastoma and iris neovascularization. Am J Ophthal 65:598, 1968.
75. Spaulding, AG: Rubeosis iridis in retinoblastoma and pseudoglioma. Trans Am Ophthal Soc LXXVI:584, 1978.
76. Haik, BG, Dunleavy, SA, Cooke, C, et al: Retinoblastoma with anterior chamber extension. Ophthalmology 94:367, 1987.
77. Roberts, CW, Iwamoto, M, Haik, BC: Ultrastructural correlation of specular microscopy in retinoblastoma. Am J Ophthal 102:182, 1986.
78. Moazed, K, Albert, D, Smith, TR: Rubeosis iridis in "pseudogliomas." Surv Ophthal 25:85, 1980.
79. Shields, JA: Ocular toxocariasis. A review. Surv Ophthal 28:361, 1984.
80. Bruner, WE, Stark, WJ, Green, WR: Presumed juvenile xanthogranuloma of the iris and ciliary body in an adult. Arch Ophthal 100:457, 1982.
81. Zimmerman, L: Ocular lesions of juvenile xanthogranuloma (nevoxanthoendothelioma). Trans Am Acad Ophthal Otol 69:412, 1965.
82. Schwartz, LW, Rodrigues, MM, Hallett, JW: Ju-

venile xanthogranuloma diagnosed by paracentesis. Am J Ophthal 77:243, 1974.
83. Gass, JDM: Management of juvenile xanthogranuloma of the iris. Arch Ophthal 71:344, 1964.
84. Hadden, OB: Bilateral juvenile xanthogranuloma of the iris. Br J Ophthal 59:699, 1975.
85. Witmer, R, Landolt, E: Juvenile xanthogranuloma of the iris. Klin Monatsbl Augenheilkd 176:658, 1980.
86. Thieme, R, Lukassek, B, Keinert, K: Problems in juvenile xanthogranuloma of the anterior uvea. Klin Monatsbl Augenheilkd 176:893, 1980.
87. Cadera, W, Silver, MM, Burt, L: Juvenile xanthogranuloma. Can J Ophthal 18:169, 1983.
88. Broughton, WL, Zimmerman, LE: A clinicopathologic study of 56 cases of intraocular medulloepitheliomas. Am J Ophthal 85:407, 1978.
89. Jakobiec, FA, Howard, GM, Ellsworth, RM, Rosen, M: Electron microscopic diagnosis of medulloepithelioma. Am J Ophthal 79:321, 1975.
90. Jakobiec, FA, Silbert, G: Are most iris 'melanomas' really nevi? A clinicopathologic study of 189 lesions. Arch Ophthal 99:2117, 1981.
91. Nik, NA, Hidayat, A, Zimmerman, LE, Fine, BS: Diffuse iris nevus manifested by unilateral open angle glaucoma. Arch Ophthal 99:125, 1981.
92. Scheie, HG, Yanoff, M: Iris nevus (Cogan-Reese) syndrome. A cause of unilateral glaucoma. Arch Ophthal 93:963, 1975.
93. Cogan, DG, Reese, AB: A syndrome of iris nodules, ectopic Descemet's membrane, and unilateral glaucoma. Doc Ophthal 26:424, 1969.
94. Shields, JA, Kline, WM, Augsburger, JJ: Primary iris cysts: a review of the literature and report of 62 cases. Br J Ophthal 68:152, 1984.
95. Vela, A, Rieser, JC, Campbell, DG: The heredity and treatment of angle-closure glaucoma secondary to iris and ciliary body cysts. Ophthalmology 91:332, 1983.
96. Bron, AJ, Wilson, CB, Hill, AR: Laser treatment of primary ring-shaped epithelial iris cyst. Br J Ophthal 68:859, 1984.
97. Nakazawa, M, Tamai, M: Iris melanocytoma with secondary glaucoma. Am J Ophthal 97:797, 1984.
98. Shields, JA, Annesley, WH Jr, Spaeth, GL: Necrotic melanocytoma of iris with secondary glaucoma. Am J Ophthal 84:826, 1977.
99. Traboulsi, EI, Maumenee, IH: Bilateral melanosis of the iris. Am J Ophthal 103:115, 1987.
100. Goncalves, V, Sandler, T, O'Donnell, FE Jr: Open angle glaucoma in melanosis oculi: response to laser trabeculoplasty. Ann Ophthal 17:33, 1985.
101. Doro, S, Werblin, TP, Haas, B, et al: Fetal adenoma of the pigmented ciliary epithelium associated with persistent hyperplastic primary vitreous. Ophthalmology 93:1343, 1986.
102. Zaidman, GW, Johnson, BL, Salamon, SM, Mondino, BJ: Fuchs' adenoma affecting the peripheral iris. Arch Ophthal 101:771, 1983.
103. Shields, CL, Shields, JA, Cook, GR, et al: Differentiation of adenoma of the iris pigment epithelium from iris cyst and melanoma. Am J Ophthal 100:678, 1985.
104. Shields, JA, Augsburger, JJ, Sanborn, GE, Klein, RM: Adenoma of the iris-pigment epithelium. Ophthalmology 90:735, 1983.
105. Papale, JJ, Akiwama, K, Hirose, T, et al: Adenocarcinoma of the ciliary body pigment epithelium in a child. Arch Ophthal 102:100, 1984.
106. Van der Hoeve, J: Eye symptoms in phakomatoses. Trans Ophthal Soc UK 52:380, 1932.
107. Weiss, DI: Dual origin of glaucoma in encephalotrigeminal haemangiomatosis. Trans Ophthal Soc UK 93:477, 1973.
108. Christensen, GR, Records, RE: Glaucoma and expulsive hemorrhage mechanisms in the Sturge-Weber syndrome. Ophthalmology 86:1360, 1979.
109. Phelps, CD: The pathogenesis of glaucoma in Sturge-Weber syndrome. Ophthalmology 85:276, 1978.
110. Cibis, GW, Tripathi, RC, Tripathi, BJ: Glaucoma in Sturge-Weber syndrome. Ophthalmology 91:1061, 1984.
111. Ali, MA, Fahmy, IA, Spaeth, GL: Trabeculectomy for glaucoma associated with Sturge-Weber syndrome. Ophthal Surg 21:352, 1990.
112. Iwach, AG, Hoskins, HD Jr, Hetherington, J Jr, Shaffer, RN: Analysis of surgical and medical management of glaucoma in Sturge-Weber syndrome. Ophthalmology 97:904, 1990.
113. Board, RJ, Shields, MB: Combined trabeculotomy-trabeculectomy for the management of glaucoma associated with Sturge-Weber syndrome. Ophthal Surg 12:813, 1981.
114. Bellows, AR, Chylack, LT Jr, Epstein, DL, Hutchinson, BT: Choroidal effusion during glaucoma surgery in patients with prominent episcleral vessels. Arch Ophthal 97:493, 1979.
115. Theodossiadis, G, Damanakis, A, Koutsandrea, C: Expulsive choroidal effusion during glaucoma surgery in a child with Sturge-Weber syndrome. Klin Monatsbl Augenheilkd 186:300, 1985.
116. Pearson-Webb, MA, Kaiser-Kupfer, MI, Eldridge, R: Eye findings in bilateral acoustic (central) neurofibromatosis: association with presenile lens opacities and cataracts but absence of Lisch nodules. N Engl J Med 315:1553, 1986.
117. Barker, D, Wright, E, Nguyen, K, et al: Gene for von Recklinghausen neurofibromatosis is in the pericentromeric region of chromosome 17. Science 236:1100, 1987.
118. Perry, HD, Font, RL: Iris nodules in von Recklinghausen's neurofibromatosis. Electon microscopic confirmation of their melanocytic origin. Arch Ophthal 100:1635, 1982.
119. Lewis, RA, Riccardi, VM: von Recklinghausen

neurofibromatosis. Incidence of iris hamartomata. Ophthalmology 88:348, 1981.

120. Huson, S, Jones, D, Beck, L: Ophthalmic manifestations of neurofibromatosis. Br J Ophthal 71:235, 1987.

121. Grant, WM, Walton, DS: Distinctive gonioscopic findings in glaucoma due to neurofibromatosis. Arch Ophthal 79:127, 1968.

122. Wolter, JR, Butler, RG: Pigment spots of the iris and ectropion uveae. With glaucoma in neurofibromatosis. Am J Ophthal 56:964, 1963.

123. Brownstein, S, Little, JM: Ocular neurofibromatosis. Ophthalmology 90:1595, 1983.

124. Teekhasaenee, C, Ritch, R, Rutnin, U, Leelawongs, N: Ocular findings in oculodermal melanocytosis. Arch Ophthal 108:1114, 1990.

125. Mishima, Y, Mevorah, B: Nevus Ota and nevus Ito in American Negroes. J Invest Dermatol 36:133, 1961.

126. Albert, DM, Scheie, HG: Nevus of Ota with malignant melanoma of the choroid. Report of a case. Arch Ophthal 69:774, 1963.

127. Font, RL, Reynolds, AM, Zimmerman, LE: Diffuse malignant melanoma of the iris in the nevus of Ota. Arch Ophthal 77:513, 1967.

128. Sabates, FN, Yamashita, T: Congenital melanosis oculi. Complicated by two independent malignant melanomas of the choroid. Arch Ophthal 77:801, 1967.

129. Velazquez, N, Jones, IS: Ocular and oculodermal melanocytosis associated with uveal melanoma. Ophthalmology 90:1472, 1983.

130. Fishman, GRA, Anderson, R: Nevus of Ota. Report of two cases, one with open-angle glaucoma. Am J Ophthal 54:453, 1962.

131. Foulks, GN, Shields, MB: Glaucoma in oculodermal melanocytosis. Ann Ophthal 9:1299, 1977.

132. Sugar, HS: Glaucoma with trabecular melanocytosis. Ann Ophthal 14:374, 1982.

133. Futa, R, Shimizu, T, Okura, F, Yasutake, T: A case of open-angle glaucoma associated with nevus Ota—electron microscopic study of the anterior chamber angle and iris. Folia Ophthal Jap 35:501, 1984.

Chapter 19

GLAUCOMAS ASSOCIATED WITH OCULAR INFLAMMATION

- I. Iridocyclitis
  - A. Terminology
  - B. Clinical forms of iridocyclitis and glaucoma
    - 1. Acute anterior iridocyclitis
    - 2. Sarcoidosis
    - 3. Juvenile rheumatoid arthritis
    - 4. Ankylosing spondylitis
    - 5. Pars planitis
    - 6. Glaucomatocyclitic crisis
    - 7. Fuchs' heterochromic cyclitis
    - 8. Behçet's disease
    - 9. Reiter's syndrome
    - 10. Glaucoma with precipitates on trabecular meshwork
    - 11. Epidemic dropsy
    - 12. Infectious diseases
      - a. Congenital rubella
      - b. Syphilis
      - c. Hansen's disease
      - d. Disseminated meningococcemia
      - e. Hemorrhagic fever with renal syndrome
      - f. Acquired immune deficiency syndrome
  - C. Theories of mechanisms for associated glaucomas
    - 1. Aqueous production
    - 2. Aqueous outflow
      - a. Acute mechanisms of obstruction
      - b. Chronic mechanisms of obstruction
  - D. Management
    - 1. Management of the inflammation
    - 2. Management of the glaucoma
- II. Other forms of ocular inflammation
  - A. Choroiditis and retinitis
    - 1. Vogt-Koyanagi-Harada syndrome
    - 2. Sympathetic ophthalmia
    - 3. Cytomegalic inclusion retinitis
    - 4. Toxocariasis
  - B. Keratitis
    - 1. Interstitial keratitis
    - 2. Herpes simplex keratouveitis
    - 3. Herpes zoster keratouveitis
  - C. Scleritis
  - D. Episcleritis

The form of ocular inflammation that most frequently produces intraocular pressure (IOP) elevation is primary iridocyclitis. In addition, when glaucoma is associated with other types of ocular inflammation, usually there is secondary involvement of the anterior uveal tract. Therefore, we will consider first the clinical forms of iridocyclitis and the mechanisms and management of the associated glaucomas, and then review the other forms of ocular inflammation that may lead to secondary glaucoma.

IRIDOCYCLITIS

Terminology

The general forms of iridocyclitis are classified primarily according to the clinical presentation and duration of active disease. However, a specific case of iridocyclitis may manifest one or all of these clinical forms at different times during the course of the disease.

Acute Iridocyclitis

The characteristic history for this type of iridocyclitis is the sudden onset of mild to moderate ocular pain, photophobia, and blurred vision. Physical examination typically reveals ciliary flush and a slight constriction of the pupil (Fig. 19.1). Slit-lamp biomicroscopy shows variable degrees of aqueous flare and cells, and fine inflammatory precipitates may be seen on the corneal endothelium (keratic precipitates). The IOP

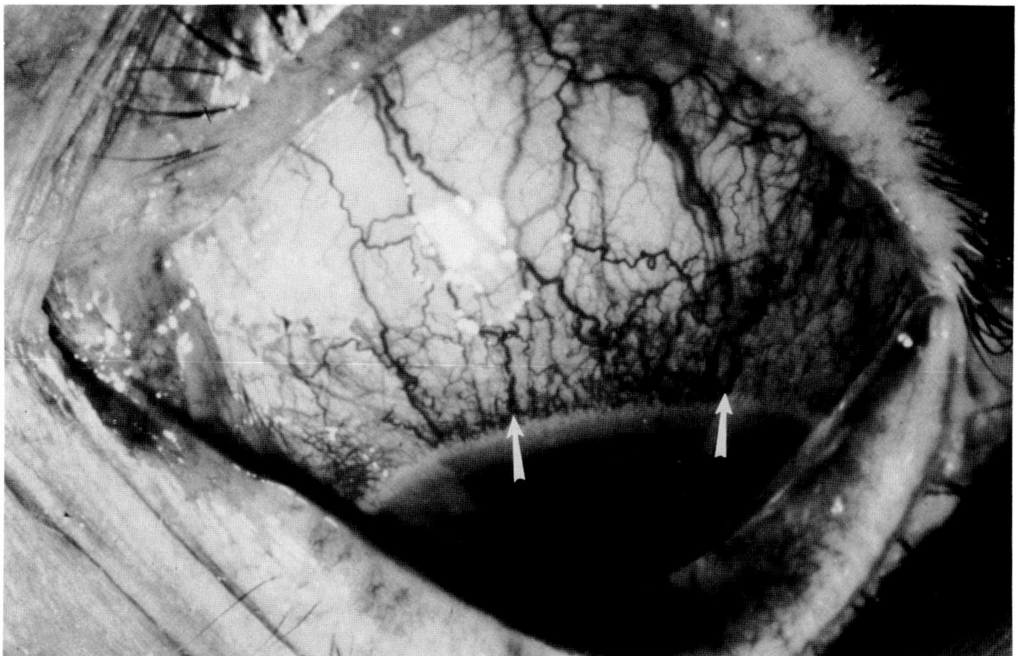

Figure 19.1. Slit-lamp view of eye with acute iritis showing typical ciliary flush (*arrows*). (Courtesy of Gary N. Foulks, M.D.)

is often lower than in the fellow eye, although some patients will present with a marked elevation of the pressure, which may be associated with severe pain and corneal edema.

Subacute Iridocyclitis

Some cases of ocular inflammation produce minimal or no symptoms. The diagnosis may be made during a routine eye examination or as part of a work-up for a related systemic disease. This form of iridocyclitis can have serious consequences because complications, such as secondary glaucoma, may go undetected until advanced damage has occurred.

Chronic Iridocyclitis

The clinical presentation in this form of iridocyclitis ranges from acute to subacute but is characterized by a protracted course of months to years, often with remissions and exacerbations. Complicating sequelae include the formation of posterior and peripheral anterior synechiae, cataracts, and band keratopathy (Fig. 19.2). It is this form of iridocyclitis that is particularly prone to cause secondary glaucoma. In a study of 100 patients with uveitis, all of whom had anterior uveal involvement, secondary glaucoma was present in 23 cases, of which 20 represented chronic uveitis and 3 acute uveitis.[1]

Clinical Forms of Iridocyclitis and Glaucoma

Acute Anterior Uveitis

This is the most common form of ocular inflammation, although it probably represents a group of conditions characterized by short-term acute iridocyclitis. Approximately half of the white patients are HLA-B27 positive,[2] which appears to represent a distinct clinical entity. As compared with HLA-B27 negative acute anterior uveitis, the former has an earlier age of onset; frequent unilateral, alternating eye involvement; severe ocular findings, such as fibrin in the anterior chamber, but no mutton fat keratic precipitates; and a frequent association with sero-negative spondyloarthropa-

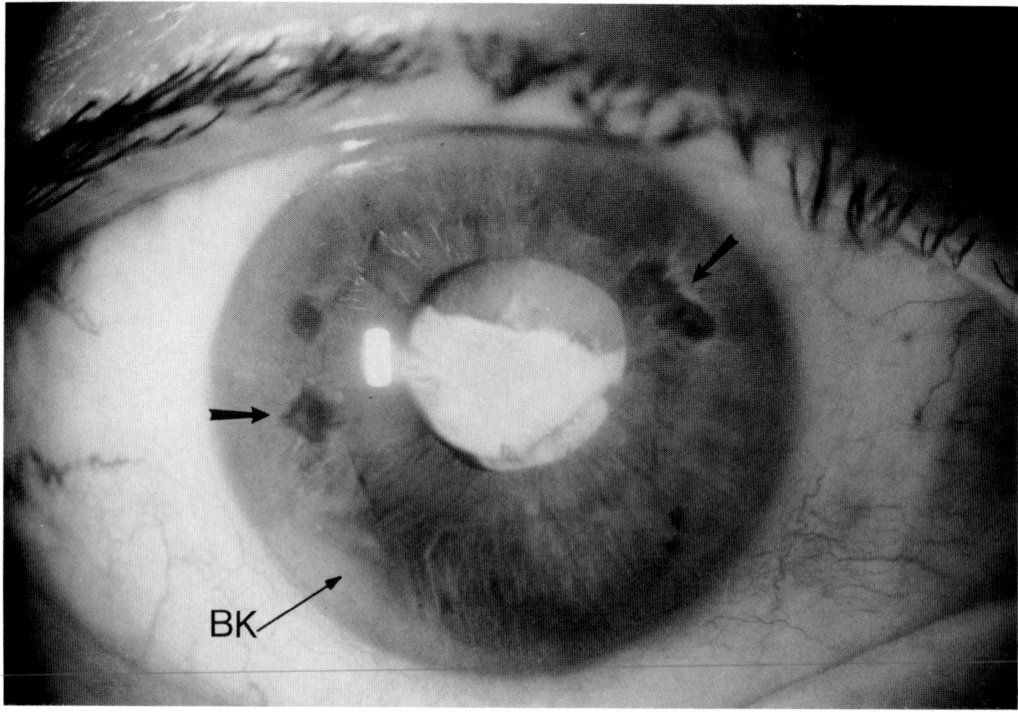

Figure 19.2. Slit-lamp view of eye with chronic iritis showing anterior synechiae (*arrows*), dense cataract, and band keratopathy (*BK*).

thies.[3] Although it has a higher incidence of ocular complications than HLA-B27 negative cases, the long-term visual outcome is not significantly worse.[3] Anterior segment fluorophotometry suggests that the HLA-B27 positive patients have more severe inflammation on the basis of blood-aqueous barrier disruption.[4] These patients also have a higher than normal prevalence of first-degree relatives with HLA-B27 positive acute anterior uveitis (13%) and ankylosing spondylitis (11%).[5] These cases usually respond to nonspecific antiinflammatory therapy, as discussed later in this chapter, although it is important to rule out related ocular or systemic disease.

Sarcoidosis

This is a multisystem inflammatory disorder of uncertain etiology, which has a predilection for young adults and black individuals. The typical histopathologic finding is noncaseating granulomas, and systemic involvement commonly includes pulmonary hilar lymphadenopathy, peripheral lymphadenopathy, and cutaneous lesions. In a review of 532 cases of sarcoidosis, 202 (38%) had ocular involvement, which included chorioretinitis, retinal periphlebitis, and occasional involvement of the optic nerve, orbit, or lacrimal glands.[6] However, by far the most common ocular abnormality was anterior uveitis.

Iridocyclitis. Acute iridocyclitis, with the previously described features of ciliary flush, aqueous flare and cells, and occasional fine or large (mutton fat) keratic precipitates, was noted in 30 (14.9%) of the 202 patients with ocular sarcoid.[6] In the acute phase, the inflammation was usually unilateral. A more frequent finding, indeed the most common ocular manifestation of sarcoidosis, was a "chronic granulomatous uveitis," which was reported in 106 (52.5%) of the 202 cases. This is more often bilateral, has a protracted course, and is typified by mutton fat keratic precipitates, synechiae, and iris nodules (Fig. 19.3). The nodules, which were seen in 23 (11.4%) of the 202

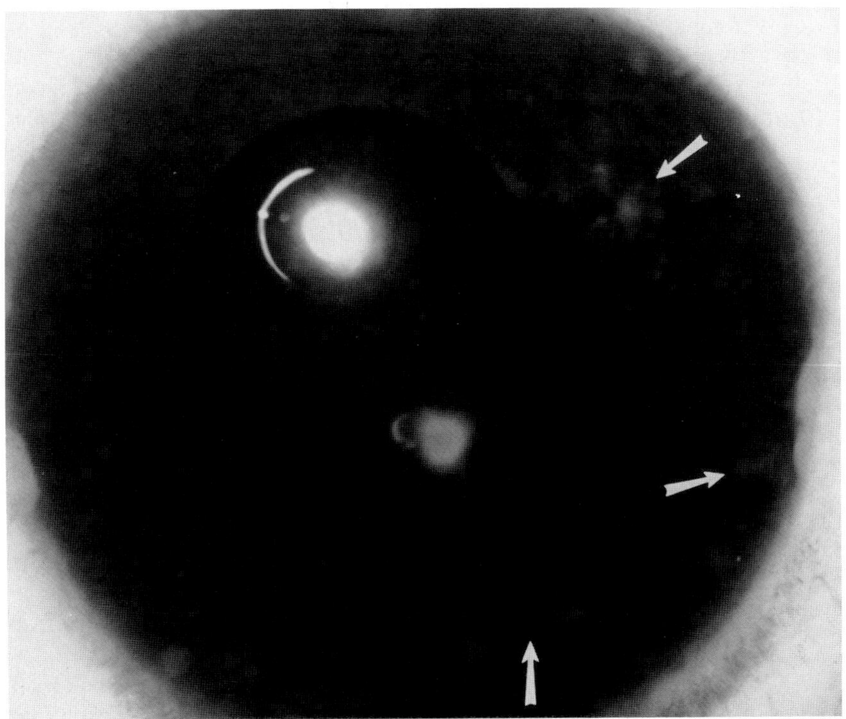

Figure 19.3. Slit-lamp view of eye with sarcoid uveitis showing typical iridic nodules (*arrows*). (Courtesy of John W. Reed, M.D.)

cases of ocular sarcoidosis, may involve the pupillary border (Koeppe nodules) and stroma of the iris (Busacca nodules), as well as the anterior chamber angle and the ciliary body. In one series of 102 eyes of 52 patients with ocular sarcoidosis, 35% of eyes had iris nodules, 49% had nodules in the angle, and 42% had ciliary nodules.[7] Gonioscopy may also reveal inflammatory precipitates on the trabecular meshwork[8] and whitish spots on the ciliary body band, which hyperfluoresce during fluorescein gonioangiography and may represent granulomas of the ciliary body.[9]

Chronic ocular sarcoidosis is associated with a worse visual prognosis. In a series of 21 patients with sarcoid uveitis, eight had a monophasic course and a favorable visual outcome, while 13 had a relapsing course with severe visual loss in five eyes.[10] The course of the ocular disease does not always parallel that of the systemic manifestations. In one series of 33 patients with chronic sarcoidosis, defined as a minimum duration of 5 years, and anterior uveitis, the uveitis was chronic in only 18 patients.[11] In another series of 33 patients with chronic ocular sarcoidosis, 15 had no systemic manifestations, although the serum angiotensin converting enzyme level was increased in a significantly greater proportion of those 15 patients than in those who had totally recovered from sarcoidosis.[10]

Glaucoma. This complication of the iridocyclitis occurred in 22 (10.9%) of the 202 patients with ocular sarcoid.[6] Chronic uveitis and secondary glaucoma are poor prognostic signs, with eight of 11 such patients suffering severe visual loss in one study.[11] The most common mechanism of secondary glaucoma associated with the iridocyclitis of sarcoidosis is obstruction of the trabecular meshwork by inflammatory debris or the nodules.[12] A more chronic form of glaucoma may also occur in association with iris bombé or goniosynechiae,[12] and a subacute form has been described with the precipitates on the trabecular meshwork.[8] Neovascularization of the iris and angle has also been reported as a mechanism of glaucoma in association with sarcoidosis.[13]

Juvenile Rheumatoid Arthritis

Juvenile rheumatoid arthritis (JRA) is a spectrum of arthritic disorders in children. One form is characterized by monoarticular or pauciarticular (involvement of four joints or less) onset, a predilection for girls, and minimal additional systemic manifestations. Other types of JRA have polyarticular onset or additional acute systemic involvement.

Iridocyclitis. The reported prevalence of iridocyclitis in patients with the monoarticular or pauciarticular form of JRA ranges from 19%[14] to 29%,[15] while the other types of JRA are rarely associated with this ocular finding.[14–18] In addition, JRA is by far the most common systemic finding in children who have anterior uveitis associated with a specific systemic disease, accounting for 81% of one large series.[19] The ocular inflammation may have an acute onset, with the typical features of acute iridocyclitis. However, many cases are asymptomatic, emphasizing the need for periodic ocular examinations of children with JRA.[14,15] The onset of the arthritis typically precedes that of the uveitis, although iridocyclitis may persist in adult life whereas the arthritis usually disappears.[16] Children with iridocyclitis rarely have a positive serology for rheumatoid factor, but they frequently have antinuclear antibody[16,18] and HLA-B27 antigen,[18] and some eventually are found to have typical ankylosing spondylitis.[18]

Complications associated with significant visual loss in children with iridocyclitis and JRA include cataracts, band keratopathy, and glaucoma. These are more common when the uveitis is the initial manifestation. In one series, 67% of such patients had a poor visual outcome, compared with only 6% of those in whom the arthritis preceded the uveitis.[20] The prevalence and severity of the complications and visual loss also correlates with the degree and duration of the ocular inflammation.

Glaucoma. The reported prevalence of glaucoma in children with JRA and iridocyclitis ranges from 14 to 27%.[16–18,20] Glaucoma is a particularly serious complication, with half of the eyes in one study having a vision of 20/200 or less.[18] The glaucoma mechanism is usually a pupillary block, although it may be related to alterations in the trabecular meshwork early in the course of the disease. Histopathologic studies of advanced cases revealed peripheral anterior synechiae and occlusion of the pupil in one case,[21] and a dense inflammatory infiltrate composed primarily of plasma cells in the iris and ciliary body with angle closure in another patient.[22] Treatment is typically difficult, with many eyes responding only partly to corticosteroids. The addition of nonsteroidal antiinflammatory agents may be helpful in these cases.[17,18] Antiglaucoma drugs may be required to control IOP elevation, and glaucoma surgery is occasionally needed, although reported results in these cases are poor.[16]

Ankylosing Spondylitis (Marie-Strümpell Disease)

This form of arthritis typically involves the cervical or lumbosacral spine and is associated with an intermittent acute iridocyclitis in 3.5–12.5% of reported cases.[23] A high percentage of these patients have the HLA-B27 antigen.[24] Recurrent uveitis may precede the arthritic symptoms, and there is evidence, based on HLA typing and sensitive bone scans, that the ocular inflammation may occur in the absence of overt symptoms or radiologic evidence of the spondylitis.[23] As previously noted, there is an apparent overlap between this condition and HLA-B27 positive acute anterior uveitis[3,5] and the iridocyclitis with JRA.[18] Glaucoma may result from trabecular damage or synechiae formation.

Pars Planitis (Chronic Cyclitis)

This protracted ocular inflammatory disorder, which represents one subtype of peripheral uveitis, primarily involves the ciliary body. Typical findings include a "snowbank" appearance of the vitreous base overlying the pars plana inferiorly, retinal phlebitis, and a cystoid maculopathy.[25] In a series of 100 cases with a 4–20 year follow-up, the incidence of glaucoma was 8%,[26] while another group of 58 eyes had glaucoma in 7%.[25] A clinicopathologic study of seven cases of pars planitis revealed glaucoma in five, and possible mechanisms of pressure elevation included peripheral anterior synechiae, iris bombé, and rubeosis iridis.[27] Topical corticosteroid and antiglaucoma therapy may be effective in some cases. Decreased visual acuity, which is usually due to cystoid maculopathy, may require the chronic use of oral and/or periocular steroids, cryotherapy in the area of the "snowbank", and systemic antimetabolites as the final step.[25]

Glaucomatocyclitic Crisis (Posner-Schlossman Syndrome)

In 1948, Posner and Schlossman[28] described a uniocular disease in young to middle-aged adults, which was characterized by recurrent attacks of mild anterior uveitis with marked elevations of IOP. Many patients have associated systemic disorders, including various allergic conditions and gastrointestinal diseases, most notably peptic ulcers.[29] In one series of 22 patients, HLA-Bw54 was present in 41%, suggesting that immunogenetic factors play an important role in the pathogenesis of glaucomatocyclitic crisis.[30]

Iridocyclitis. The typical symptoms are slight ocular discomfort, blurred vision, and halos, which last from several hours up to a few weeks or rarely more, and tend to recur on a monthly or yearly basis.[28] Physical findings are minimal, with occasional mild ciliary flush, slight pupillary constriction, and corneal epithelial edema. Hypochromia of the iris is not a consistent finding, but has been reported in up to 40% of various series.[31] Early segmental iris ischemia with late congestion and leakage on fluorescein angiography has also been described.[32] Slit-lamp biomicroscopy reveals occasional faint flare and a few fine, nonpigmented keratic precipitates, while gonioscopy shows a normal, open angle with occasional debris and the characteristic absence of synechiae.[28,31]

Glaucoma. The IOP is typically elevated in the range of 40–60 mm Hg and coincides with the duration of the uveitis. Intraocular pressure and facility of aqueous outflow usually return to normal between attacks, although severe cases with optic nerve head and visual field damage have been reported.[33,34] The glaucoma may be related to inflammatory changes in the trabecular meshwork. Histologic evaluation of a trabeculectomy specimen obtained during an acute attack revealed numerous mononuclear cells in the meshwork.[35] Other theories of mechanism include increased aqueous production, possibly resulting from elevated levels of aqueous prostaglandins,[36] and an association with primary open-angle glaucoma.[32,33] Most cases can be controlled during attacks with corticosteroids and antiglaucoma agents that reduce aqueous production,[31,37] although rare, severe cases may require filtering surgery.[34,35]

Fuchs' Heterochromic Cyclitis

In 1906, Fuchs[38] described a condition characterized by mild anterior uveitis, heterochromia, cataracts, and occasional glaucoma. The similarities and differences between this disease and glaucomatocyclitic crisis should be noted to avoid confusing the two. Fuchs' heterochromic cyclitis is usually unilateral, although bilateral involvement has been reported in up to 13% of the cases.[39] The typical age of onset is in the third or fourth decade,[40] and there is an equal incidence among men and women.[39] It is said to be the most commonly misdiagnosed form of uveitis,[41] especially in black patients, in whom the heterochromia may be less obvious.[42] Several theories of etiology have been considered, with the most likely being a true inflammation of immunologic origin, possibly related to depression of suppressor T-cell activity.[41] Cellular immunity to corneal antigens has been found in the majority of patients,[43] with autoantibodies against corneal epithelium in almost 90% of cases.[44] The search for HLA-linked genetic factors is inconclusive, although preliminary evidence suggests a decrease in the frequency of HLA-CW3.[45] A few patients have associated congenital Horner's syndrome, suggesting the possibility of a neurogenic mechanism in these cases.[46]

Iridocyclitis. The uveitis in this disease is mild and tends to run a single, very protracted course, although it may be intermittent initially. The patient is usually unaware of any difficulty until visual disturbance, primarily from cataract formation, becomes apparent. While hypochromia of the iris is more common than in glaucomatocyclitic crisis, it is not a constant feature and tends to develop gradually during the course of the disease.[39,40] In one series it was seen in 92% of 54 white patients and 76% of 13 black individuals.[42]

Gross signs of ocular inflammation are typically absent, although slit-lamp biomicroscopy may reveal minimal aqueous flare and cells. Characteristic fine stellate keratic precipitates are usually seen on the lower half of the cornea but may involve the upper half also.[47] The iris frequently has extensive stromal atrophy, and transillumination of the iris is reported to demonstrate a characteristic light, even translucence.[48] Electron microscopic studies of the iris have revealed a scant number of deep stromal melanocytes with immature melanin granules, abundant plasma cells, an increase in mast cells, and a membranous degeneration of nerve fibers.[49,50]

Patients may also have neovascularization of both the anterior chamber angle and iris, as well as nodules on the iris.[45] The nodules typically occur along the pupillary border, similar to the Koeppe nodules of sarcoidosis. They are generally believed to be uncommon, often leading to a misdiagnosis,[41] although in one series they were seen in 20% of whites and 30% of blacks.[42] Anterior segment fluorescein angiography has shown delayed filling, sector ischemia, leakage, and neovascularization,[51,52] and fluorophotometry has revealed an abnormal permeability of the blood-aqueous barrier.[53] A high percentage of patients may also have chorioretinal scars,[38] which are commonly associated with toxoplasmosis.[54,55]

Glaucoma. Secondary IOP elevation is not as common as with glaucomatocyclitic crisis but may occur as a late, serious complication. The reported incidence varies from 13 to 59%,[47,56,57] with the higher figures seen in series with long-term follow-up.[47] The glaucoma typically persists after the uveitis has subsided. The anterior chamber angle is open and characteristically free of synechiae, although fine vessels, which may hemorrhage, are often seen extending onto the trabecular meshwork.[56] Histopathologic examination of the anterior chamber angle structures in one case revealed rubeosis, trabeculitis, and an inflammatory membrane over the angle,[58] while another study showed extensive atrophy of Schlemm's canal and the trabecular endothelium.[59] The glaucoma typically does not respond to steroid therapy but requires standard medical or surgical management.[40,47]

Behçet's Disease

This multiple system disease is the result of an occlusive vasculitis and is characterized by uveitis, aphthous lesions of the mouth, and ulcerations of the genitalia.[60,61] Additional systemic findings include erythema nodosum, arthropathy, thrombophlebitis, and a necrotizing vasculitis of the central nervous system, which may be fatal. The most common ocular disorder is iridocyclitis, which may be associated with a sterile hypopyon. In a study of 49 patients, followed over a 10-year period, 17 developed a hypopyon, which typically appears late in the course of the disease but was the initial finding in three patients.[62] Posterior uveitis and necrotizing retinal vasculitis are also commonly found in this disorder.[61,63] In the 10-year study, all patients developed both anterior and posterior involvement within 2 years.[62] The uveitis tends to occur late in the course of the disease and is eventually bilateral. The anterior uveitis may lead to secondary glaucoma. All patients initially respond to steroid treatment, although the uveitis usually requires cytotoxic-immunosuppressive agents, such as chlorambucil, in most cases.[62] Even with this therapy, the prognosis is poor, with loss of useful visual acuity in 74% of eyes in the 10-year study.[62]

Reiter's Syndrome

This multisystem disease is characterized by conjunctivitis, urethritis, arthritis, and mucocutaneous lesions. It typically afflicts young men, with a high frequency of the HLA-B27 genotype.[64] In a review of 113 patients, 98% had rheumatologic manifestations; 74%, genitourinary; 58%, ocular; and 42%, mucocutaneous findings.[64] Conjunctivitis was seen in all patients with ocular manifestations and is characterized by a papillary reaction with a mucopurulent discharge. A nongranulomatous iridocyclitis without hypopyon was the second most common ocular manifestation, occurring in 12% of the total group, although secondary glaucoma was seen in only one of the 113 patients.

Glaucoma Associated with Precipitates on the Trabecular Meshwork (Grant's Syndrome)

Chandler and Grant[65] described an uncommon form of secondary open-angle glaucoma in which the only evidence of ocular inflammation is precipitates on the trabecular meshwork. Since the condition is usually bilateral, it may be mistaken for primary open-angle glaucoma. However, careful gonioscopy reveals gray or slightly yellow precipitates on the meshwork and irregular peripheral anterior synechiae, which often attach to the trabecular precipitates.[8] The cause is unknown, although some patients eventually develop sarcoidosis, rheumatoid arthritis, ankylosing spondylitis, episcleritis, glaucomatocyclitic crisis, or chronic uveitis.[8] The glaucoma, which is presumed to be due to inflammatory changes in the trabecular meshwork, usually clears promptly with topical corticosteroid therapy, although antiglaucoma drugs that reduce aqueous production may be required temporarily for pressure control. The condition often recurs, and the patients must be followed closely. Untreated cases may progress to synechial closure of the angle.

Epidemic Dropsy

This acute toxic disease, which results from the unintentional ingestion of sanguinarine in *Argemone mexicana* oil as an adulterant of cooking oils, is characterized by the explosive onset of leg edema, with tenderness, erythema, and rash over the edematous parts, gastrointestinal symptoms, low-grade fever, and congestive heart failure, which may be fatal.[66,67] Ocular features include glaucoma and retinal vascular dilation, tortuosity, and hemorrhage.[66] The glaucoma is bilateral with open angles, normal outflow facility, and normal trabecular meshwork by histopathologic and histochemical testing.[67] Although there are no signs of anterior segment inflammation, aqueous assays reveal elevated prostaglandin E_2 levels, histamine activity, and total protein levels, suggesting hypersecretion as the mechanism of the elevated IOP.[67]

Infectious Diseases

The following infectious processes may cause an iridocyclitis with the occasional association of glaucoma.

Congenital Rubella. This disorder predominantly affects the heart, auditory apparatus, and eyes,[68] although virtually any organ may be involved. Ocular defects occur in 30–60% of the cases and include cataracts, microphthalmia, retinopathy, and glaucoma.[69] Corneal edema may occur as a result of coexistent glaucoma or in the absence of elevated IOP.[70] The secondary glaucoma is reported to occur in 2–15% of children with congenital rubella.[71] Contrary to earlier reports, the cataracts and glaucoma occur together at a frequency that would be anticipated with each occurring independently.[71] The glaucoma may be associated with hypoplasia of the iris stroma and hypoperfusion by iris angiography.[72] The glaucoma is particularly severe, with blindness occurring in 8 of 15 children in one follow-up study.[73] Mechanisms of the glaucoma include iridocyclitis, angle anomalies, and angle-closure glaucoma resulting from microphthalmia, an intumescent lens, or pupillary block after cataract extraction. Although the ocular abnormalities are most often observed in the neonatal period, the glaucoma may also occur later in childhood, or in young adulthood, usually in association with microphthalmia and cataracts.[74]

Syphilis. Congenital syphilis may cause iridocyclitis with secondary glaucoma in either the early or late stages of the disease. Glaucoma associated with the interstitial keratitis of congenital syphilis is discussed later in this chapter. Acquired syphilis in adults may also cause iridocyclitis and IOP elevation.[75] Mass lesions of the iris and ciliary body have also been associated with this condition.[76]

Hansen's Disease. Uveitis is common in *lepromatous leprosy* and typically involves the iris and ciliary body,[77,78] with four forms having been described: (1) chronic iridocyclitis; (2) acute plastic iridocyclitis; (3) iris pearls or miliary lepromata, which is pathognomonic of the disease; and (4) nodular lepromata, characterized by larger, less discrete masses on the iris.[77] Complications of keratitis and iridocyclitis are the main causes of blindness in this disease. The chronic iridocyclitis may be associated with iris atrophy and small nonreacting pupils, which aggravate the visual impairment.[79,80] In a study of 100 cases, 19 had acute or chronic iridocyclitis and 12 had evidence of glaucoma, which was usually secondary to chronic anterior uveitis.[81] However, patients with chronic plastic iridocyclitis tend to have lower than normal IOP with significant postural influence.[80,82,83] The pupillary and IOP abnormalities suggest ocular autonomic dysfunction, although the lack of correlation between these two findings suggests that there may be another mechanism for the hypotension, such as reduced aqueous production or increased uveoscleral outflow secondary to the inflammation.[80,83] Active iridocyclitis is reported to respond to treatment with dapsone, corticosteroids, and rifampin.[77] There is evidence that effective antimicrobial and antiinflammatory therapy may significantly minimize the ocular complications.[84]

Disseminated Meningococcemia. These patients may have associated iridocyclitis[85] or endophthalmitis[86] with acute glaucoma, which is presumably due to obstruction of the anterior chamber by a blanket of cells.

Hemorrhagic Fever with Renal Syndrome (nephropathia epidemica). This viral disease is characterized by fever, chills, malaise, nausea, vomiting, and headache, which progresses to back and abdominal pain, uremia, hematuria, oliguria, and proteinuria. Three patients have been described with associated transient angle-closure glaucoma, which was believed to be due to swelling of the ciliary body.[87]

Acquired Immune Deficiency Syndrome (AIDS). This viral disorder has severe defects of immunoregulation, leading to life-threatening opportunistic infections, Kaposi's sarcoma, or both. Bilateral acute angle-closure glaucoma has been reported in these patients,[88,89] which appears to be due to choroidal effusion with anterior rotation of the ciliary body.[88] Such cases do not respond to miotics or iridectomy, although peripheral iridoplasty was successful in one case.[89] Cycloplegics and, if necessary, drainage of suprachoroidal fluid may also be effective.[88]

Theories of Mechanisms for Associated Glaucoma

The possible mechanisms by which iridocyclitis may lead to an elevated IOP have already been mentioned with regard to certain specific forms of iridocyclitis and will now be summarized. In general, iridocyclitis affects both aqueous production and resistance to aqueous outflow, with the subsequent change in IOP representing a balance between these two factors.

Aqueous Production

Inflammation of the ciliary body usually leads to reduced aqueous production. If this outweighs a concomitant increased resistance to outflow, the IOP will be reduced, which is often the case with acute iridocyclitis. Experimental iridocyclitis in monkeys suggests that the hypotony may be due to both a reduction in aqueous humor flow and an increase in uveoscleral outflow.[90] However, prostaglandins, which have been demonstrated in the aqueous of eyes with uveitis, are known to cause elevated IOP without a reduction in outflow facility,[91–94] suggesting that increased aqueous production may possibly occur in some cases of uveitis.

Aqueous Outflow

When the aqueous outflow system is involved in an ocular inflammatory disease, increased resistance to outflow may result from a variety of acute and chronic mechanisms.

Acute Mechanisms of Obstruction. During the active phase of iridocyclitis, several mechanisms of obstruction to aqueous outflow may lead to a relatively sudden, but usually reversible, rise in IOP. In the majority of cases, the anterior chamber angle is open, which is an important observation in ruling out primary angle-closure glaucoma. Obstruction of the trabecular meshwork may occur in several ways.

A disruption in the blood-aqueous barrier allows inflammatory cells and fibrin to enter the aqueous and accumulate in the trabecular meshwork. Normal serum components have been shown to reduce outflow when perfused in enucleated human eyes.[95] Prostaglandins were demonstrated to increase aqueous protein content,[93,94,96,97] and it has been suggested that an accumulation of cyclic adenosine monophosphate (cAMP), resulting from prostaglandins or certain nonprostaglandin agents, causes the barrier damage.[98]

In other cases, swelling or dysfunction of the trabecular lamellae or endothelium may lead to aqueous outflow obstruction. Precipitates on the trabecular meshwork, as previously discussed, may also occur in eyes with ocular inflammation and elevated IOP.[8,65] It must also be kept in mind that the use of corticosteroids in treating the inflammation may create yet another mechanism of IOP elevation (steroid-induced glaucoma), which is discussed in the next chapter.

Much less commonly, ocular inflammation may lead to acute closure of the anterior chamber angle by uveal effusion with forward rotation of the ciliary body. In addition, if a significant posterior uveitis is present, angle closure may result from displacement of the lens-iris diaphragm as a result of massive exudative retinal detachment.

Chronic Mechanisms of Obstruction. Several sequelae of inflammation may lead to a chronic elevation of IOP. Obstruction of aqueous outflow may result from scarring and obliteration of outflow channels, or from the overgrowth of an endothelial-cuticular or fibrovascular membrane in the open angle. The membranes may eventually contract, leading to synechial closure of the angle. In addition to the influence of membrane contraction, peripheral anterior synechiae may result from the protein and inflammatory cells in the angle, which pull the iris toward the cornea. Posterior synechiae may also be a sequelae of anterior uveitis and can cause iris bombé, with closure of the anterior chamber angle.

Management

In treating an eye with iridocyclitis and glaucoma, control of the inflammatory component alone frequently leads to normalization of the IOP, and this is usually the first approach in the treatment plan. However, if the magnitude of the pressure elevation poses an immediate threat to vision, or if the IOP does not respond adequately to antiinflammatory therapy, medical and even surgical management of the glaucoma may also be indicated. The following basic principles of management apply to most cases of iridocyclitis as well as other forms of ocular inflammation, with exceptions as noted in the discussions of the specific diseases.

Management of the Inflammation

Corticosteroids. This group of drugs constitutes the first line of defense in most cases of ocular inflammation. Topical administration is preferred for anterior segment disease, and commonly used steroids include prednisolone 1.0% and dexamethasone 0.1%. In a rabbit model of anterior uveitis, frequent topical administration of prednisolone acetate 1.0% caused a significant decrease in protein levels and leukocytes in the anterior chamber.[99] Administration of the steroid every hour may be required initially, with gradual reduction in frequency as the inflammation subsides. In a rabbit model of keratitis, instillation every 15 minutes was even more effective than the hourly regimen, although five doses at 1-minute intervals each hour was equivalent to the effect achieved by administration every 15 minutes.[100] When the response to topical administration is insufficient, periocular injections (e.g., dexamethasone phosphate, prednisolone succinate, triamcinolone acetate, or methylprednisolone acetate) or a systemic corticosteroid (e.g., prednisone) may be required. With any form of administration, the many side effects of corticosteroids must be considered, including steroid-induced glaucoma.

Nonsteroidal Antiinflammatory Agents. When the use of corticosteroids is contraindicated or inadequate, other antiinflammatory drugs may be helpful. *Prostaglandin synthetase inhibitors,* such as aspirin,[101] imidazole,[102] indoxole,[103] indomethacin,[103] and dipyridamole,[104] have been effective in some cases of uveitis. With severe cases, *immunosuppressive agents*, such as methotrexate,[105] azathioprine,[106] or chlorambucil,[106] may be indicated. In a study of 25 patients with severe chronic uveitis who were poorly responsive or unresponsive to corticosteroid therapy, all responded to long-term daily administration of prednisone 10–15 mg combined with azathioprine 2.0–2.5 mg or chlorambucil 6–8 mg.[106] These patients must be monitored closely for hematologic reactions. Short-term plasma exchange is also reported to be of value in treating endogenous uveitis.[107]

In conjunction with antiinflammatory agents, a mydriatic-cycloplegic drug, such as atropine 1%, homatropine 1–5%, or cyclopentolate 0.5–1%, is usually indicated to avoid posterior synechiae and to relieve the discomfort of ciliary muscle spasm.

Management of the Glaucoma

Medical. Since miotics are generally contraindicated in the inflamed eye, a topical beta-blocker or epinephrine compound is usually the first line antiglaucoma drug in the treatment of glaucoma secondary to ocular inflammation. A carbonic anhydrase inhibitor may also be needed, and a hyperosmotic agent is occasionally required as a short-term emergency measure.

Surgical. Intraocular surgery should be avoided whenever possible in eyes with active inflammation. However, when medical therapy is inadequate, surgery may be required. In these cases, it is best to do the least amount of surgery possible. A laser iridotomy may be safer than an incisional iridectomy when an angle-closure mechanism is present, although fibrin may tend to close a small iridotomy in an inflamed eye. Laser trabeculoplasty is usually not effective in eyes with open-angle glaucoma secondary to uveitis and may cause an additional, significant rise in IOP if the inflammation is still active. Filtering surgery with heavy steroid therapy is usually indicated in open-angle cases that are uncontrolled on maximum tolerable medical therapy. Adjuvant use of subconjunctival 5-fluorouracil has been shown to significantly improve the success rate in these cases.[108] A technique called *trabeculodialysis* has been described, in which a goniotomy knife is used to incise above the trabecular meshwork and then peel the meshwork downward.[109] This was successful in a preliminary series of eyes with anterior uveitis and glaucoma,[109] although a subsequent study of 30 eyes in 23 children and young adults achieved success in only 60%, with most of these requiring concomitant antiglaucoma medication.[110] Cyclodestructive surgery, such as transscleral Nd:YAG cyclophotocoagulation, may be another reasonable surgical option, especially in aphakic and pseudophakic eyes.

OTHER FORMS OF OCULAR INFLAMMATION

Choroiditis and Retinitis

In the following conditions, an inflammation that is predominantly posterior may cause secondary glaucoma either by an associated anterior inflammatory component or by angle closure from a posterior mass effect.

Vogt-Koyanagi-Harada Syndrome

The systemic findings in this disorder include alopecia, poliosis, and meningeal signs. Ocular manifestations consist of anterior and posterior uveitis with exudative retinal detachment. In a review of 51 cases, secondary glaucoma was found in 20% of the patients.[111] Within the total group, a mild anterior uveitis was seen in all patients, and posterior synechiae occurred in 36%, keratic precipitates in 30%, and nodules on the iris in 8.4%.[111] These patients may also present with a transient shallow anterior chamber, which is apparently due to swelling of the ciliary body secondary to severe choroiditis, and which may lead to angle-closure glaucoma.[112–114] These findings are usually reversible with corticosteroid therapy.[112]

Sympathetic Ophthalmia

This form of ocular inflammation typically occurs weeks or months after traumatic or surgical penetration of the fellow eye. The severity of the inflammation is related to the degree of ocular pigmentation, and the choroid is predominantly affected, with frequent involvement of the overlying retina.[115,116] The condition bears striking clinical and histopathologic similarities to the Vogt-Koyanagi-Harada syndrome, and the two disorders may share a common immunopathologic inflammatory mechanism.[116] In a study of 17 cases with an average follow-up of 10.6 years, seven (43%) had secondary glaucoma.[115] The mechanism of the glaucoma is unknown, although in a histopathologic study of 105 cases, a high percentage had plasma cell infiltration of the iris and ciliary body,[115] suggesting an immune reaction near the area of aqueous outflow. Whatever the cause, the glaucoma is typically difficult to treat, requiring frequent adjustments of corticosteroids and occasional surgical intervention.[117]

Cytomegalic Inclusion Retinitis

This disorder was described in two adult renal transplant patients, both of whom developed a secondary open-angle glaucoma presumably resulting from an associated anterior uveitis.[118]

Toxocariasis

The common ocular form of this disease, characterized by retinitis and vitritis, may also have anterior uveitis with posterior synechiae, iris bombé, and secondary glaucoma.[119]

Keratitis

Interstitial Keratitis

As a feature of *congenital syphilis,* interstitial keratitis typically appears late in the course of the disease, between the ages of 5 and 16, although it may appear as early as birth or as late as 30 years of age.[120] The presenting symptoms of interstitial keratitis include marked ciliary flush, lacrimation, photophobia, and pain. The mechanisms of glaucoma associated with interstitial keratitis, in addition to the previously discussed concomitant iridocyclitis, include open-angle and angle-closure forms that usually appear later in life.[121,122]

With secondary open-angle glaucoma, the eye may have irregular pigmentation of the anterior chamber angle, with occasional columnar peripheral anterior synechiae, and one histopathologic study revealed endothelium and a glassy membrane over the angle.[121] This condition responds poorly to medical therapy but may be controlled by filtering surgery. Another mechanism of secondary open-angle glaucoma in the adult is the recurrence of iridocyclitis in an eye that had interstitial keratitis in younger life.[121] The residual ghost vessels in the cornea may help in making this diagnosis.

Eyes with interstitial keratitis in infancy often have small anterior segments and narrow angles, which can lead to angle-closure glaucoma later in life. This is usually subacute and responds well to peripheral iridectomy.[121,123] In some cases, multiple cysts of the iris may lead to angle-closure.

Interstitial keratitis may also be associated with vertigo, tinnitus, and deafness, which is referred to as *Cogan's syndrome.* An atypical form may have noncorneal ocular inflammation,[124] which may involve the anterior uvea with secondary glaucoma.

Herpes Simplex Keratouveitis

This viral infection may cause recurrent conjunctivitis, keratitis, and uveitis. In one study of patients with herpes simplex keratouveitis, 28% had IOP elevation and 10% had glaucomatous damage.[125] The keratitis in cases with associated IOP elevation is typically disciform or stromal, rather than that of a superficial ulcer.[125] The pressure usually remains elevated for several weeks, and a rabbit model suggests a biphasic IOP response in which the uveitis during the first few days represents active infection but subsequently is due to immune mechanisms.[126] An analysis of aqueous from 33 herpes patients revealed herpes simplex virus in eight cases, all of which had secondary glaucoma.[127] Histopathology of rabbit eyes with experimental herpetic keratouveitis showed mononuclear cells in the trabecular meshwork and peripheral anterior synechiae.[128]

Management of this condition requires attention to the infection, inflammation, and glaucoma, and one suggested regimen includes topical trifluorothymidine, corticosteroids, and cycloplegics along with antiglaucoma agents that reduce aqueous production.[127] One study indicated that the severity of the uveitis and IOP rise in experimental secondary herpes simplex uveitis was lessened with dexamethasone 0.1% twice daily, but not with aspirin or cyclophosphamide.[129]

Herpes Zoster Keratouveitis

In addition to causing the characteristic cutaneous vesicular eruptions along the trigeminal distribution, this viral disease may produce a keratitis and uveitis. The anterior uveitis not uncommonly leads to a secondary glaucoma. In one series of 86 patients with herpes zoster ophthalmicus, 37 had uveitis, and 10 of these had secondary glaucoma.[130] In another study, five of 14 patients with keratouveitis had transient high IOP.[131] Topical acyclovir has been shown to be superior to topical steroids in the treatment of herpes zoster keratouveitis.[132]

Adenovirus Type 10

This viral agent has been reported to cause keratoconjunctivitis with a transient increased IOP.[133]

Scleritis

This is an extremely painful, potentially disastrous form of ocular inflammation, which may primarily involve either the anterior or posterior segment of the eye.[134] The anterior forms may present as *diffuse* or *nodular anterior scleritis,* characterized by episcleral congestion and scleral edema. These are painful and often recurrent, but relatively benign. *Necrotizing scleritis* is a more severe condition, with extensive granulomatous infiltration of the conjunctiva, episclera, and sclera and degradation of scleral collagen.[135,136] It is typically painful and progressive, although a variation, *scleromalacia perforans,* which is seen primarily in patients with rheumatoid arthritis, has no pain or redness. Anterior segment fluorescein angiography helps to distinguish the more benign forms, with vasodilation and rapid flow, from the necrotizing cases, with gross vascular abnormalities and delayed flow.[137] Posterior scleritis, which is more difficult to diagnose, may present with pars planitis, exudative retinal detachment, optic nerve head edema, or proptosis.

In one study of 301 cases, glaucoma was present in 11.6%,[134] while in another series, the prevalence of elevated IOP was 18.7% with rheumatoid scleritis and 12% with nonrheumatoid scleritis.[138] A histopathologic study of 92 enucleated eyes revealed evidence of increased IOP in 49%.[139] In the vast majority of cases, the glaucoma is associated with anterior scleritis, and mechanisms of pressure elevation in these patients include trabecular meshwork damage by iridocyclitis, overlying corneoscleral inflammation, and peripheral anterior synechiae.[139] Other mechanisms include steroid-induced glaucoma, iris neovascularization,[139] and elevated episcleral venous pressure in an eye with anterior diffuse scleritis in relapsing polychondritis.[140] Glaucoma associated with posterior scleritis is much less common but may result from a forward shift of the lens-iris diaphragm or an anterior rotation of the ciliary body in association with choroidal effusion.[141]

Treatment of the scleritis generally consists of topical and systemic corticosteroids and nonsteroidal antiinflammatory agents. A combination of oral prednisone and indomethacin proved to be more effective than either drug used alone and allowed lower doses of each (10–60 mg and 50–150 mg daily, respectively).[142] Antiglaucoma agents are used as needed, and surgical intervention for the glaucoma should be resorted to only when absolutely necessary.

Episcleritis

In contrast to scleritis, episcleritis produces only mild discomfort and does not typically lead to serious sequelae. The characteristic appearance is congestion of the episcleral vessels, which may be diffuse with chemosis and occasional lid edema (simple episcleritis) or localized with nodules in the episcleral tissue (nodular episcleritis).[134] Secondary glaucoma is uncommon in this condition[134,138] but has been reported.[143] Presumed mechanisms of open-angle glaucoma include inflammation of the angle structures[143] and steroid-induced glaucoma.[134] Angle-closure glaucoma has also been observed in association with episcleritis.[138] In most cases, both the episcleritis and the secondary glaucoma respond to topical corticosteroids.

SUMMARY

The type of ocular inflammation most often associated with IOP elevation is iridocyclitis, either in a primary form or secondary to inflammation elsewhere in the eye. The anterior uveitis may be acute, subacute, or chronic, and may occur as an isolated finding of uncertain etiology (e.g., acute anterior uveitis, pars planitis, glaucomatocyclitic crises, and Fuchs' heterochromic cyclitis) or in association with a systemic inflammatory disorder (e.g., sarcoidosis, some forms of rheumatoid arthritis, Behçet's disease, and many infectious conditions). The mechanisms by which iridocyclitis leads to obstruction of aqueous outflow include acute, usually reversible forms (e.g., accumulation of inflammatory elements in the intertrabecular spaces, edema of the trabecular lamellae, or angle closure resulting from ciliary body swelling) and chronic forms (e.g., scar formation or membrane overgrowth in the anterior chamber angle). There is also a suggestion that uveitis may cause increased aqueous production. Treatment of combined iridocyclitis and glaucoma involves steroidal and nonsteroidal antiinflammatory agents and antiglaucoma drugs, with surgical intervention reserved for medical failures. Other forms of ocular inflammation that may be associated with glaucoma include choroiditis and retinitis, keratitis, scleritis, and episcleritis.

References

1. Panek, WC, Holland, GN, Lee, DA, Christensen, RE: Glaucoma in patients with uveitis. Br J Ophthal 74:223, 1990.
2. Brewerton, DA, Caffrey, M, Nicholls, A, et al: Acute anterior uveitis and HLA 27. Lancet 2:994, 1973.
3. Rothova, A, van Veenendaal, WG, Linssen, A, et al: Clinical features of acute anterior uveitis. Am J Ophthal 103:137, 1987.
4. Fearnley, IR, Spalton, DJ, Smith, SE: Anterior segment fluorophotometry in acute anterior uveitis. Arch Ophthal 105:1550, 1987.
5. Derhaag, PJFM, Linssen, A, Broekema, N, et al: A familial study of the inheritance of HLA-B27-positive acute anterior uveitis. Am J Ophthal 105:603, 1988.
6. Obenauf, CD, Shaw, HE, Sydnor, CF, Klintworth, GK: Sarcoidosis and its ophthalmic manifestations. Am J Ophthal 86:648, 1978.
7. Mizuno, K, Takahashi, J: Sarcoid cyclitis. Ophthalmology 93:511, 1986.
8. Roth, M, Simmons, RJ: Glaucoma associated with precipitates on the trabecular meshwork. Ophthalmology 86:1613, 1979.
9. Kimura, R: Hyperfluorescent dots in the ciliary body band in patients with granulomatous uveitis. Br J Ophthal 66:322, 1982.
10. Karma, A, Huhti, E, Poukkula, A: Course and outcome of ocular sarcoidosis. Am J Ophthal 106:467, 1988.
11. Jabs, DA, Johns, CJ: Ocular involvement in chronic sarcoidosis. Am J Ophthal 102:297, 1986.
12. Iwata, K, Nanba, K, Sobue, K, Abe, H: Ocular sarcoidosis: evaluation of intraocular findings. Ann NY Acad Sci 278:445, 1976.
13. Mayer, J, Brouillette, G, Corriveau, LA: Sarcoidose et rubeosis iridis. Can J Ophthal 18:197, 1983.
14. Calabro, JJ, Parrino, GR, Atchoo, PD, et al: Chronic iridocyclitis in juvenile rheumatoid arthritis. Arthritis Rheumatism 13:406, 1970.
15. Schaller, J, Kupfer, C, Wedgwood, RJ: Iridocyclitis in juvenile rheumatoid arthritis. Pediatrics 44:92, 1969.
16. Key, SN III, Kimura, SJ: Iridocyclitis associated with juvenile rheumatoid arthritis. Am J Ophthal 80:425, 1975.
17. Chylack, LT Jr, Bienfang, DC, Bellows, R, Stillman, JS: Ocular manifestations of juvenile rheumatoid arthritis. Am J Ophthal 79:1026, 1975.
18. Kanski, JJ: Anterior uveitis in juvenile rheumatoid arthritis. Arch Ophthal 95:1794, 1977.
19. Kanski, JJ, Shun-Shin, GA: Systemic uveitis syndromes in childhood: an analysis of 340 cases. Ophthalmology 91:1247, 1984.
20. Wolf, MD, Lichter, PR, Ragsdale, CG: Prognostic factors in the uveitis of juvenile rheumatoid arthritis. Ophthalmology 94:1242, 1987.
21. Sabates, R, Smith, T, Apple, D: Ocular histopathology in juvenile rheumatoid arthritis. Ann Ophthal 11:733, 1979.
22. Merriam, JC, Chylack, LT, Albert, DM: Early-onset pauciarticular juvenile rheumatoid arthritis. A histopathologic study. Arch Ophthal 101:1085, 1983.
23. Russell, AS, Lentle, BC, Percy, JS, Jackson, FI: Scintigraphy of sacroiliac joints in acute anterior uveitis. A study of thirty patients. Ann Intern Med 85:606, 1976.
24. Brewerton, DA, Hart, FD, Nicholls, A, et al: Ankylosing spondylitis and HL-A 27. Lancet 1:904, 1973.

25. Henderly, DE, Genstler, AJ, Rao, NA, Smith, RE: Pars planitis. Trans Ophthal Soc UK 105:227, 1986.
26. Smith, RE, Godfrey, WA, Kimura, SJ: Complications of chronic cyclitis. Am J Ophthal 82:277, 1976.
27. Pederson, JE, Kenyon, KE, Green, WR, Maumenee, AE: Pathology of pars planitis. Am J Ophthal 86:762, 1978.
28. Posner, A, Schlossman, A: Syndrome of unilateral recurrent attacks of glaucoma with cyclitic symptoms. Arch Ophthal 39:517, 1948.
29. Knox, DL: Glaucomatocyclitic crises and systemic disease: peptic ulcer, other gastrointestinal disorders, allergy and stress. Trans Am Ophthal Soc 86:473, 1988.
30. Hirose, S, Ohno, S, Matsuda, H: HLA-Bw54 and glaucomatocyclitic crisis. Arch Ophthal 103:1837, 1985.
31. Hollwich, F: Clinical aspects and therapy of the Posner-Schlossmann-syndrome. Klin Monatsbl Augenheilkd 172:736, 1978.
32. Raitta, C, Vannas, A: Glaucomatocyclitic crisis. Arch Ophthal 95:608, 1977.
33. Kass, MA, Becker, B, Kolker, AE: Glaucomatocyclitic crisis and primary open-angle glaucoma. Am J Ophthal 75:668, 1973.
34. Hung, PT, Chang, JM: Treatment of glaucomatocyclitic crises. Am J Ophthal 77:169, 1974.
35. Harstad, HK, Ringvold, A: Glaucomatocyclitic crises (Posner-Schlossman syndrome). A case report. Acta Ophthal 64:146, 1986.
36. Nagataki, S, Mishima, S: Aqueous humor dynamics in glaucomato-cyclitic crisis. Invest Ophthal 15:365, 1976.
37. de Roetth, A Jr: Glaucomatocyclitic crisis. Am J Ophthal 69:370, 1970.
38. Fuchs, E: Uber Komplikationen der Heterochromie. Ztschr Augenh 15:191, 1906.
39. Franceschetti, A: Heterochromic cyclitis (Fuchs' syndrome). Am J Ophthal 39:50, 1955.
40. Kimura, SJ, Hogan, MJ, Thygeson, P: Fuchs' syndrome of heterochromic cyclitis. Arch Ophthal 54:179, 1955.
41. O'Connor, GR: Heterochromic iridocyclitis. Trans Ophthal Soc UK 104:219, 1985.
42. Tabbut, BR, Tessler, HH, Williams, D: Fuchs' heterochromic iridocyclitis in blacks. Arch Ophthal 106:1688, 1988.
43. van der Gaag, R, Broersma, L, Rothova, A, et al: Immunity to a corneal antigen in Fuchs' heterochromic cyclitis patients. Invest Ophthal Vis Sci 30:443, 1989.
44. La Hey, E, Baarsma, GS, Rothova, A, et al: High incidence of corneal epithelium antibodies in Fuchs' heterochromic cyclitis. Br J Ophthal 72:921, 1988.
45. De Bruyere, M, Dernouchamps, J-P, Sokal, G: HLA antigens in Fuchs' heterochromic iridocyclitis. Am J Ophthal 102:392, 1986.
46. Regenbogen, LS, Naveh-Floman, N: Glaucoma in Fuchs' heterochromic cyclitis associated with congenital Horner's syndrome. Br J Ophthal 71:844, 1987.
47. Liesegang, TJ: Clinical features and prognosis in Fuchs' uveitis syndrome. Arch Ophthal 100:1622, 1982.
48. Saari, M, Vuorre, I, Nieminen, H: Infra-red transillumination stereophotography of the iris in Fuchs's heterochromic cyclitis. Br J Ophthal 62:110, 1978.
49. Melamed, S, Lahav, M, Sandbank, U, et al: Fuch's heterochromic iridocyclitis: an electron microscopic study of the iris. Invest Ophthal Vis Sci 17:1193, 1978.
50. McCartney, ACE, Bull, TB, Spalton, DJ: Fuchs' heterochromic cyclitis: an electron microscopy study. Trans Ophthal Soc UK 105:324, 1986.
51. Saari, M, Vuorre, I, Nieminen, H: Fuchs's heterochromic cyclitis: a simultaneous bilateral fluorescein angiographic study of the iris. Br J Ophthal 62:715, 1978.
52. Berger, BB, Tessler, HH, Kottow, MH: Anterior segment ischemia in Fuchs' heterochromic cyclitis. Arch Ophthal 98:499, 1980.
53. Johnson, D, Liesegang, TJ, Brubaker, RF: Aqueous humor dynamics in Fuchs' uveitis syndrome. Am J Ophthal 95:783, 1983.
54. Arffa, RC, Schlaegel, TF: Chorioretinal scars in Fuchs' heterochromic iridocyclitis. Arch Ophthal 102:1153, 1984.
55. De Abreu, MT, Belfort, R Jr, Hirata, PS: Fuchs' heterochromic cyclitis and ocular toxoplasmosis. Am J Ophthal 93:739, 1982.
56. Huber, A: Das Glaukom bei komplizierter Heterochromic Fuchs. Ophthalmologica 142:66, 1961.
57. Daus, W, Kraus-Mackiw, E: Fuchs' heterochromic cyclitis. Case reports of patients treated at Heidelberg University Eye Hospital since 1978. Klin Monatsbl Augenheilkd 185:410, 1984.
58. Perry, HD, Yanoff, M, Scheie, HG: Rubeosis in Fuchs heterochromic iridocyclitis. Arch Ophthal 93:337, 1975.
59. Benedikt, O, Roll, P, Zirm, M: The glaucoma in heterochromic cyclitis Fuchs. Gonioscopic studies and electron microscopic investigations of the trabecular meshwork. Klin Monatsbl Augenheilkd 173:523, 1978.
60. Colvard, DM, Robertson, DM, O'Duffy, JD: The ocular manifestations of Behçet's disease. Arch Ophthal 95:1813, 1977.
61. Michelson, JB, Chisari, FV: Behçet's disease. Surv Ophthal 26:190, 1982.
62. Benezra, D, Cohen, E: Treatment and visual prognosis in Behçet's disease. Br J Ophthal 70:589, 1986.

63. James, DG, Spiteri, MA: Behçet's disease. Ophthalmology 89:1279, 1982.
64. Lee, DA, Barker, SM, Su, WPD, et al: The clinical diagnosis of Reiter's syndrome. Ophthalmic and nonophthalmic aspects. Ophthalmology 93:350, 1986.
65. Chandler, PA, Grant, WM: Lectures on Glaucoma. Lea and Febiger, Philadelphia, 1954, p. 257.
66. Rathore, MK: Ophthalmological study of epidemic dropsy. Br J Ophthal 66:573, 1982.
67. Sachdev, MS, Sood, NN, Verma, LK, et al: Pathogenesis of epidemic dropsy glaucoma. Arch Ophthal 106:1221, 1988.
68. Cooper, LZ, Ziring, PR, Ockerse, AB, et al: Rubella. Clinical manifestations and management. Am J Dis Child 118:18, 1969.
69. Rudolph, AJ, Desmond, MM: Clinical manifestations of the congenital rubella syndrome. Int Ophthal Clin 12:3, 1972.
70. deLuise, VP, Cobo, LM, Chandler, D: Persistent corneal edema in the congenital rubella syndrome. Ophthalmology 90:835, 1983.
71. Boniuk, M: Glaucoma in the congenital rubella syndrome. Int Ophthal Clin 12:121, 1972.
72. Brooks, AMV, Gillies, WE: Glaucoma associated with congenital hypoplasia of the iris stroma in rubella. Glaucoma 11:36, 1989.
73. Wolff, SMacK: The ocular manifestations of congenital rubella. Trans Am Ophthal Soc 70:577, 1972.
74. Boger, WP III: Late ocular complications in congenital rubella syndrome. Ophthalmology 87:1244, 1980.
75. Schwartz, LK, O'Connor, GR: Secondary syphilis with iris papules. Am J Ophthal 90:380, 1980.
76. Scully, RE, Mark, EJ, McNeely, BU: Mass in the iris and a skin rash in a young man. N Engl J Med 310:972, 1984.
77. Michelson, JB, Roth, AM, Waring, GO III: Lepromatous iridocyclitis diagnosed by anterior chamber paracentesis. Am J Ophthal 88:674, 1979.
78. Malla, OK, Brandt, F, Anten, JGF: Ocular findings in leprosy patients in an institution in Nepal (Khokana). Br J Ophthal 65:226, 1981.
79. Ffytche, TJ: Role of iris changes as a cause of blindness in lepromatous leprosy. Br J Ophthal 65:231, 1981.
80. Lewallen, S, Courtright, P, Lee, H-S: Ocular autonomic dysfunction and intraocular pressure in leprosy. Br J Ophthal 73:946, 1989.
81. Shields, JA, Waring, GO III, Monte, LG: Ocular findings in leprosy. Am J Ophthal 77:880, 1974.
82. Brandt, F, Malla, OK, Anten, JGF: Influence of untreated chronic plastic iridocyclitis on intraocular pressure in leprous patients. Br J Ophthal 65:240, 1981.
83. Hussein, N, Courtright, P, Ostler, HB, et al: Low intraocular pressure and postural changes in intraocular pressure in patients with Hansen's Disease. Am J Ophthal 108:80, 1989.
84. Spaide, R, Nattis, R, Lipka, A, D'Amico, R: Ocular findings in leprosy in the United States. Am J Ophthal 100:411, 1985.
85. deLuise, VP, Stern, JT, Paden, P: Uveitic glaucoma caused by disseminated meningococcemia. Am J Ophthal 95:707, 1983.
86. Jensen, AD, Naidoff, MA: bilateral meningococcal endophthalmitis. Arch Ophthal 90:396, 1973.
87. Saari, KM: Acute glaucoma in hemorrhagic fever with renal syndrome (nephropathia epidemica). Am J Ophthal 81:455, 1976.
88. Ullman, S, Wilson, RP, Schwartz, L: Bilateral angle-closure glaucoma in association with the acquired immune deficiency syndrome. Am J Ophthal 101:419, 1986.
89. Koster, HR, Liebmann, JM, Ritch, R, Hudock, S: Acute angle-closure glaucoma in a patient with acquired immunodeficiency syndrome successfully treated with argon laser peripheral iridoplasty. Ophthal Surg 21:501, 1990.
90. Toris, CB, Pederson, JE: Aqueous humor dynamics in experimental iridocyclitis. Invest Ophthal Vis Sci 28:477, 1987.
91. Chiang, TS, Thomas, RP: Ocular hypertension following intravenous infusion of prostaglandin E_1. Arch Ophthal 88:418, 1972.
92. Chiang, TS, Thomas, RP: Consensual ocular hypertensive response to prostaglandin E_2. Invest Ophthal 11:845, 1972.
93. Kass, MA, Podos, SM, Moses, RA, Becker, B: Prostaglandin E_1 and aqueous humor dynamics. Invest Ophthal 11:1022, 1972.
94. Podos, SM, Becker, B, Kass, MA: Prostaglandin synthesis, inhibition, and intraocular pressure. Invest Ophthal 12:426, 1973.
95. Epstein, DL, Hashimoto, JM, Grant, WM: Serum obstruction of aqueous outflow in enucleated eyes. Am J Ophthal 86:101, 1978.
96. Neufeld, AH, Sears, ML: The site of action of prostaglandin E_2 on the disruption of the blood-aqueous barrier in the rabbit eye. Exp Eye Res 17:445, 1973.
97. Kulkarni, PS, Srinivasan, BD: The effect of intravitreal and topical prostaglandins on intraocular inflammation. Invest Ophthal Vis Sci 23:383, 1982.
98. Bengtsson, E: The effect of theophylline on the breakdown of the blood-aqueous barrier in the rabbit eye. Invest Ophthal Vis Sci 16:636, 1977.
99. Bolliger, GA, Kupferman, A, Leibowitz, HM: Quantitation of anterior chamber inflammation and its response to therapy. Arch Ophthal 98:1110, 1980.
100. Leibowitz, HM, Kupferman, A: Optimal frequency of topical prednisolone administration. Arch Ophthal 97:2154, 1979.

101. Marsetio, M, Siverio, CE, Oh, JO: Effects of aspirin and dexamethasone on intraocular pressure in primary uveitis produced by herpes simplex virus. Am J Ophthal 81:636, 1976.
102. Kass, MA, Palmberg, P, Becker, B: The ocular anti-inflammatory action of imidazole. Invest Ophthal Vis Sci 16:66, 1977.
103. Spinelli, HM, Krohn, DL: Inhibition of prostaglandin-induced iritis. Topical indoxole vs indomethacin therapy. Arch Ophthal 98:1106, 1980.
104. Podos, SM: Effect of dipyridamole on prostaglandin-induced ocular hypertension in rabbits. Invest Ophthal Vis Sci 18:646, 1979.
105. Wong, VG, Hersh, EM: Methotrexate in the therapy of cyclitis. Trans Am Acad Ophthal Otol 69:279, 1965.
106. Andrasch, RH, Pirofsky, B, Burns, RP: Immunosuppressive therapy for severe chronic uveitis. Arch Ophthal 96:247, 1978.
107. Wizemann, AJS, Wizemann, V: Therapeutic effects of short-term plasma exchange in endogenous uveitis. Am J Ophthal 97:565, 1984.
108. Jampel, HD, Jabs, DA, Quigley, HA: Trabeculectomy with 5-fluorouracil for adult inflammatory glaucoma. Am J Ophthal 109:168, 1990.
109. Hoskins, HD Jr, Hetherington, J Jr, Shaffer, RN: Surgical management of the inflammatory glaucomas. Pers Ophthal 1:173, 1977.
110. Kanski, JJ, McAllister, JA: Trabeculodialysis for inflammatory glaucoma in children and young adults. Ophthalmology 92:927, 1985.
111. Ohno, S, Char, DH, Kimura, SJ, O'Connor, GR: Vogt-Koyanagi-Harada syndrome. Am J Ophthal 83:735, 1977.
112. Shirato, S, Hayashi, K, Masuda, K: Acute angle closure glaucoma as an initial sign of Harada's disease: report of two cases. Jap J Ophthal 24:260, 1980.
113. Kimura, R, Sakai, M, Okabe, H: Transient shallow anterior chamber as initial symptom in Harada's syndrome. Arch Ophthal 99:1604, 1981.
114. Kimura, R, Kasai, M, Shoji, K, Kanno, C: Swollen ciliary processes as an initial symptom in Vogt-Koyanagi-Harada syndrome. Am J Ophthal 95:402, 1983.
115. Lubin, JR, Albert, DM, Weinstein, M: Sixty-five years of sympathetic ophthalmia. A clinicopathologic review of 105 cases (1913–1978). Ophthalmology 87:109, 1980.
116. Marak, GE Jr: Recent advances in sympathetic ophthalmia. Surv Ophthal 24:141, 1979.
117. Makley, TA Jr, Azar, A: Sympathetic ophthalmia. A long-term follow-up. Arch Ophthal 96:257, 1978.
118. Merritt, JC, Callender, CO: Adult cytomegalic inclusion retinitis. Ann Ophthal 10:1059, 1978.
119. Shields, JA: Ocular toxocariasis. A review. Surv Ophthal 28:361, 1984.
120. Tavs, LE: Syphilis. Maj Prob Clin Ped 19:222, 1978.
121. Grant, WM: Late glaucoma after interstitial keratitis. Am J Ophthal 79:87, 1975.
122. Tsukahara, S: Secondary glaucoma due to inactive congenital syphilitic interstitial keratitis. Ophthalmologica 174:188, 1977.
123. Sugar, HS: Late glaucoma associated with inactive syphilitic interstitial keratitis. Am J Ophthal 53:602, 1962.
124. Cobo, LM, Haynes, BF: Early corneal findings in Cogan's syndrome. Ophthalmology 91:903, 1984.
125. Falcon, MG, Williams, HP: Herpes simplex kerato-uveitis and glaucoma. Trans Ophthal Soc UK 98:101, 1978.
126. Oh, JO: Effect of cyclophosphamide on primary herpes simplex uveitis in rabbits. Invest Ophthal Vis Sci 17:769, 1978.
127. Sundmacher, R, Neumann-Haefelin, D: Herpes simplex virus isolations from the aqueous of patients suffering from focal iritis, endothelitis, and prolonged disciform keratitis with glaucoma. Klin Monatsbl Augenheilkd 175:488, 1979.
128. Townsend, WM, Kaufman, HE: Pathogenesis of glaucoma and endothelial changes in herpetic kerato-uveitis in rabbits. Am J Ophthal 71:904, 1971.
129. Dennis, RF, Oh, JO: Aspirin, cyclophosphamide, and dexamethasone effects on experimental secondary herpes simplex uveitis. Arch Ophthal 97:2170, 1979.
130. Womack, LW, Liesegang, TJ: Complications of herpes zoster ophthalmicus. Arch Ophthal 101:42, 1983.
131. Reijo, A, Antti, V, Jukka, M: Endothelial cell loss in herpes zoster keratouveitis. Br J Ophthal 67:751, 1983.
132. McGill, J, Chapman, C: A comparison of topical acyclovir with steroids in the treatment of herpes zoster keratouveitis. Br J Ophthal 67:746, 1983.
133. Hara, J, Ishibashi, T, Fujimoto, F, et al: Adenovirus type 10 keratoconjunctivitis with increased intraocular pressure. Am J Ophthal 90:481, 1980.
134. Watson, PG, Hayreh, SS: Scleritis and episcleritis. Br J Ophthal 60:163, 1976.
135. Young, RD, Watson, PG: Microscopical studies of necrotising scleritis. I. Cellular aspects. Br J Ophthal 68:770, 1984.
136. Young, RD, Watson, PG: Microscopical studies of necrotising scleritis. II. Collagen degradation in the scleral stroma. Br J Ophthal 68:781, 1984.
137. Watson, PG, Bovey, E: Anterior segment fluorescein angiography in the diagnosis of scleral inflammation. Ophthalmology 92:1, 1985.
138. McGavin, DDM, Williamson, J, Forrester, JV, et al: Episcleritis and scleritis. A study of their clinical manifestations and association with rheumatoid arthritis. Br J Ophthal 60:192, 1976.
139. Wilhelmus, KR, Grierson, I, Watson, PG: Histo-

pathologic and clinical associations of scleritis and glaucoma. Am J Ophthal 91:697, 1981.

140. Chen, CJ, Harisdangkul, V, Parker, L: Transient glaucoma associated with anterior diffuse scleritis in relapsing polychondritis. Glaucoma 4:109, 1982.

141. Quinlan, MP, Hitchings, RA: Angle-closure glaucoma secondary to posterior scleritis. Br J Ophthal 62:330, 1978.

142. Mondino, BJ, Phinney, RB: Treatment of scleritis with combined oral prednisone and indomethacin therapy. Am J Ophthal 106:473, 1988.

143. Harbin, TS Jr, Pollack, IP: Glaucoma in episcleritis. Arch Ophthal 93:948, 1975.

Chapter 20

STEROID-INDUCED GLAUCOMA

As discussed in Chapter 9, a certain percentage of the general population will respond to repeated instillation of topical corticosteroids with a variable increase in the intraocular pressure (IOP). This occurs more commonly in individuals who have primary open-angle glaucoma or a family history of the disease. There are many unknown facets regarding the pressure response to steroids, such as the precise distribution of steroid responders in the general population, the reproducibility of these responses, and hereditary influences. Nevertheless, the critical fact is that certain people do manifest this response to chronic steroid therapy, and the IOP elevation can lead to glaucomatous optic atrophy and loss of vision. Such a condition is referred to as steroid-induced glaucoma.

Historical Background

In 1950, McLean[1] reported an IOP rise in response to the systemic administration of ACTH for the treatment of uveitis. Francois,[2] in 1954, noted that a similar elevation in tension could occur after local therapy with cortisone. Numerous reports followed these early observations, which confirmed that IOP rise may occur with topical, systemic, or periocular administration of corticosteroids, although more often after local therapy.

Clinical Features

The typical clinical presentation is associated with topical steroid therapy. Intraocular pressure elevation usually develops within a few weeks with potent corticosteroids or in months with the weaker steroids.[3] The clinical picture resembles that of primary open-angle glaucoma with an open, normal-appearing anterior chamber angle and absence of symptoms. Much less often, the condition may have an acute presentation, in which pressure rises have been observed within hours after steroid administration in eyes with open angles.[3,4] This has been seen with intensive systemic steroid therapy or the topical use of potent corticosteroids.

Variations of the above clinical forms depend on the patient's age and the condition of the eyes. Although children are reported to have a lower incidence of positive steroid responders than adults,[5] glaucoma has been precipitated by treating external diseases in infants with corticosteroids.[6] It has also been reported that IOP elevation may occur in the first few weeks after a trabeculectomy despite a good filtering bleb, possibly because of the influence of topical steroid therapy.[7] Another clinical variation of steroid-induced glaucoma is apparent low-tension glaucoma, which may result when the steroid-induced pressure elevation has damaged the optic nerve head and visual field and then returned to normal with cessation of the steroid.[8]

Theories of Mechanism

It is generally agreed that the IOP elevation caused by steroid administration results from reduction in facility of aqueous outflow.[9–11] In the rabbit eye, intravenously administered glucocorticoids are specifically bound in the nuclei of cells in the outflow pathway.[12] When cultured human trabecular cells were incubated with dexamethasone, a high binding affinity for the glucocorticoid was demonstrated, with two-thirds of the binding occurring in the nuclear fraction.[13] The binding affinity of rabbit iris-ciliary body for dexamethasone was found to be virtually identical to that of rabbit liver, although the concentration of glucocorticoid receptors was nearly two-fold higher in the ocular tissue.[14] It has also been shown that topical administration of steroids in rabbits is associated with a translocation of glucocorticoid receptors from the cytoplasm to the nucleus in iris-ciliary body and adjacent corneoscleral tissue.[15] This may be a necessary event in steroid-induced elevation of IOP, since the degree to which a glucocorticoid is able to produce translocation correlates with the in vivo pressure-inducing tendency of that drug.[15] Other studies have shown that dihydrocortisols, which are intermediate glucocorticoid metabolites, accumulate abnormally in trabecular cells from patients with primary open-angle glaucoma and potentiate the effect of topical dexamethasone on IOP elevation in rabbits.[16]

The above studies suggest that trabecular and anterior uveal tissue have a high concentration of glucocorticoid receptors and probably represent the target tissue in the steroid-induced mediation of reduced aqueous outflow facility. The precise mechanism responsible for the obstruction to outflow is unknown, but the following observations and theories have been reported.

Influence on Extracellular Matrix. Hyaluronidase-sensitive glycosaminoglycans (mucopolysaccharides) are normally present in the aqueous outflow system. Francois[17–19] postulated that glycosaminoglycans in the polymerized form become hydrated, producing a "biological edema" that may increase resistance to aqueous outflow. Hyaluronidase within lysosomes depolymerizes hyaluronate, and corticosteroids stabilize the lysosomal membrane, which leads to an accumulation of polymerized glycosaminoglycans in the trabecular meshwork. Francois also suggested that the lysosomes reside primarily in fibroblasts in the meshwork, which he called goniocytes. He believed that clones of goniocytes may have variable sensitivity to corticosteroids, accounting for the differences in individual pressure responses. Lysosomal hyaluronidase activity has been demonstrated in the corneoscleral junction of rabbit and human eyes, although the role of the enzyme in aqueous outflow regulation is unclear.[20] Examinations of trabecular specimens from eyes with steroid-induced glaucoma have also been inconclusive, although there is some evidence, both in human eyes[21] as well as in experimental rabbit studies,[22] that an excess accumulation of glycosaminoglycans in the aqueous outflow system may be an important factor in steroid-induced glaucoma.

Topical dexamethasone-induced IOP elevation in rabbits was associated with an increase in chondroitin sulfate within the aqueous outflow pathway, but a decrease in hyaluronic acid.[23] Dexamethasone has also been shown to decrease the synthesis of collagen in normal human trabecular meshwork explants.[24] Thus, corticosteroids appear to influence both the glycosaminoglycans and collagen of the extracellular matrix in trabecular meshwork tissue, although the precise role in IOP elevation is not fully established.

Influence on Phagocytosis. Endothelial cells lining the trabecular meshwork have phagocytic properties, which may help to clean the aqueous of debris before it reaches the inner wall of Schlemm's canal. Corticosteroids are known to suppress phagocytic activity, and the possibility has been raised that suppressed phagocytosis of the trabecular endothelium may allow debris in the aqueous to accumulate in the meshwork and act as a barrier to outflow.[25] This theory is consistent with ultrastructural studies showing marked depositions of amorphous and fibrous or linear material in the juxtacanalicular meshwork of eyes with steroid-induced glaucoma.[26,27]

Additional Observations. It has also been observed in rabbits that long-term topical steroid administration is associated with a shift toward an alkaline aqueous and reduced ascorbic acid content.[28,29] The authors suggest that these changes may be related to steroid-induced glaucoma, although more study is needed to establish this theory. Additional ocular responses that may occur in some individuals on chronic topical corticosteroid therapy include a slight mydriasis and ptosis, and an increase in corneal thickness. However, none of these changes appears to correlate with the IOP response.[10,30] The influence of corticosteroid therapy on aqueous production is uncertain, with one fluorophotometric study showing an increased rate of aqueous flow associated with the oral administration of hydrocortisone,[31] while another study found no alteration in flow after 1 week of topical dexamethasone therapy.[32]

PREVENTION

To avoid loss of vision from steroid-induced glaucoma, the physician must know how to prevent or minimize the chances of its occurrence. This requires close attention to the patient's history and to the selection and use of steroids.

Patient Selection

As previously noted, individuals with primary open-angle glaucoma or a family history of the disease are more likely to respond to chronic steroid therapy with a significant rise in IOP. In addition, it has been noted that high myopes,[33] diabetics,[34] and patients with connective tissue diseases (especially rheumatoid arthritis),[35] have a similar predisposition. Therefore, these patients are at a somewhat higher risk of developing steroid-induced glaucoma. However, since it is not possible to predict which additional individuals without these predisposing factors will also have a pressure rise, all patients must be treated cautiously. This involves avoiding steroids when a safer drug will suffice, using the least amount of steroid necessary, establishing a baseline IOP before initiating therapy, and monitoring the tension closely for the duration of the corticosteroid therapy.

Drug Selection

When corticosteroid therapy is required for any disorder, the optimum drug is the one that will achieve the desired therapeutic response by the safest route of administration, in the lowest concentration, and with the fewest potential adverse reactions. With regard to the IOP response, the following facts should be considered.

Routes of Administration

Topical corticosteroid therapy is more often associated with an IOP rise than is the case with systemic administration. This may occur not only with drops or ointment applied directly to the eye but also with steroid preparations used in treating the skin of the eyelids.[36–38]

Periocular injection is the most dangerous route of corticosteroid administration from the standpoint of steroid-induced glaucoma. Intraocular pressure elevation may occur in response to subconjunctival, sub-Tenon's, or retrobulbar injections of steroids.[39–43] The patient's response to earlier topical steroid therapy does not always predict how that individual will respond to periocular corticosteroids.[42] Repository steroids are particularly dangerous because of their prolonged duration of action, and it may occasionally be necessary to surgically excise the remaining drug before the pressure can be brought under control.[41–43] Histopathologic study of excised specimens reveals granular or foamy, eosinophilic material in the subepithelial connective tissue.[43] If repository steroids must be used, they should be injected in an inferior quadrant to avoid compromising the superior sites for possible future filtering surgery.

Systemic administration of corticosteroids is least likely to induce glaucoma, although cases have been described.[44–48] In one study of 62 patients receiving systemic steroids following renal transplantation, six developed IOP elevation, and five of these had HLA-B12.[48] It is reported that this response does not correlate with the dosage or duration of treatment but is associated with the degree of pressure response to topical steroids.[46,47] It has been noted that amounts of corticosteroids, sufficient to influence the IOP, can be absorbed from skin application in areas remote from the eyes.[21]

Relative Pressure-Inducing Effects of Topical Steroids

Although topical corticosteroids are more likely to cause an elevation of the IOP than are systemic steroids, the topical route of administration is still generally preferred to avoid the additional dangers associated with systemic corticosteroid therapy. While no topical steroid is totally free of a pressure-inducing effect, the following observations have been reported regarding the relative tendencies of these drugs to induce an elevation of the IOP.

Corticosteroids. In general, the antiinflammatory potency of a topical steroid is proportional to its pressure-inducing effect. *Betamethasone, dexamethasone,* and *prednisolone* are commonly used, potent corticosteroids with a significant tendency to produce steroid-induced glaucoma. However, as might be anticipated, the pressure-inducing potency is related to the dosage of the drug. In a study of high topical steroid responders, betamethasone 0.01% caused significantly less pressure elevation than the 0.1% concentration.[49] In addition, the formulation may cause some dissociation of antiinflammatory and pressure-inducing effects. In a rabbit study, dexamethasone acetate 0.1% had a better antiinflammatory effect than dexamethasone alcohol 0.1% or dexamethasone sodium phosphate 0.1%, while the acetate and sodium phosphate preparations had the same effect on IOP elevation in humans.[50]

Flurandrenolide, a less commonly used corticosteroid, has also been reported to cause steroid-induced glaucoma.[51] A newer corticosteroid with high topical activity, *clobetasone butyrate* 0.1%, was compared with prednisolone phosphate 0.5% and betamethasone phosphate 0.1%.[52–54] While the results varied somewhat among studies, clobetasone butyrate was comparable or slightly weaker in antiinflammatory action but also had less of a tendency to produce IOP elevation.

Nonadrenal Steroids. A group of drugs closely related to progesterone has been shown to have useful antiinflammatory properties with significantly less pressure-inducing effects than most corticosteroids. *Medrysone* is primarily of value in the treatment of extraocular disorders, since it has limited corneal penetration, although one study found it to be effective in treating iritis.[55] Most reports describe little or no associated IOP elevation,[55–57] although a slight pressure response in some patients has been observed.[49,58] The steroid antagonist mifepristone has been shown to reduce the hypertensive effect of medrysone in rabbits.[59] *Fluorometholone* 0.1% is more efficacious than medrysone in treating inflammation of the anterior ocular segment. Although the pressure-inducing effect of fluoromethalone is substantially less than that of the potent corticosteroids,[58,60–62] significant pressure rises have been observed with the use of this drug.[62,63] Fluorometholone 0.25% may have a significantly greater therapeutic effect than the 0.1% but is still less likely to increase IOP in corticosteroid responders than is dexamethasone 0.1%.[64] However, the same precautions must be taken with the nonadrenal steroids as with the corticosteroids.

Nonsteroidal Antiinflammatory Drugs. Preliminary experience with topical *oxyphenbutazone*[65] and *flurbiprofen*[66] indicates that these nonsteroidal antiinflammatory agents do not cause an elevation of IOP. It has also been shown that flurbiprofen does not block corticosteroid-induced pressure elevation.[66]

MANAGEMENT

Discontinuation of the Steroid. Discontinuation is the first line of defense and is often all that is required. The chronic form is said to normalize in 1–4 weeks, while the acute form typically resolves within days of stopping the steroid.[4] In rare cases, the glaucoma may persist despite stopping all steroids. The latter situation occurred in 6 of 210 patients (2.8%) in one series, and all of these patients had a family history of glaucoma.[3] The duration of steroid therapy also appears to influence the reversibility of the IOP elevation. In a study of 22 patients with steroid-induced glaucoma, the pressures normalized in all cases in which the drug was used for less than 2 months, while the tension remained chronically elevated in all patients who used the steroid for more than 4 years.[67] If continued corticosteroid therapy is essential, it may be possible to control the IOP with the additional use of antiglaucoma medications or by changing to a steroid with less pressure-inducing potential.

Glaucoma Therapy. The medical management of these cases is essentially the same as for primary open-angle glaucoma. Surgical intervention is indicated when the glaucoma is uncontrolled on maximum tolerable medication. As previously noted, it may occasionally be necessary to excise a depot of periocular steroid if this appears to be responsible for the persistent pressure elevation.[41–43] In other cases of medically uncontrollable glaucoma, laser trabeculoplasty is usually indicated, followed by filtering surgery if necessary.

SUMMARY

The prolonged use of steroids, especially the topical administration of corticosteroids, will cause an IOP elevation in some patients, with clinical findings that typically resemble primary open-angle glaucoma. The mechanism of the secondary glaucoma is uncertain, although an unusual sensitivity to steroids in the aqueous outflow pathways may lead to increased resistance to outflow, possibly through an influence on glycosaminoglycans or phagocytic activity in the trabecular meshwork. The problem is best managed by attempting to prevent it through the judicious use of antiinflammatory agents. When steroid-induced glaucoma does occur, the steroid should be stopped, if possible, and persisting pressure elevation should be managed with medication or surgery as required.

References

1. McLean, JM: Use of ACTH and cortisone. Discussion of paper of Woods, AC. Trans Am Ophthal Soc 48:293, 1950.
2. Francois, J: Cortisone et tension oculaire. Ann D'Oculist 187:805, 1954.
3. Francois, J: Corticosteroid glaucoma. Ann Ophthal 9:1075, 1977.
4. Weinreb, RN, Polansky, JR, Kramer, SG, Baxter, JD: Acute effects of dexamethasone on intraocular pressure in glaucoma. Invest Ophthal Vis Sci 26:170, 1985.
5. Biedner, B-A, David, R, Grudsky, A, Sachs, U: Intraocular pressure response to corticosteroids in children. Br J Ophthal 64:430, 1980.
6. Gnad, HD, Martenet, AC: Kongenitales Glaukom and Cortison. Klin Monatsbl Augenheilkd 162:86, 1973.
7. Wilensky, JT, Snyder, D, Gieser, D: Steroid-induced ocular hypertension in patients with filtering blebs. Ophthalmology 87:240, 1980.
8. Sugar, HS: Low tension glaucoma: a practical approach. Ann Ophthal 11:1155, 1979.
9. Armaly, MF: Effect of corticosteroids on intraocular pressure and fluid dynamics. II. The effect of dexamethasone in the glaucomatous eye. Arch Ophthal 70:492, 1963.
10. Miller, D, Peczon, JD, Whitworth, CG: Corticosteroids and functions in the anterior segment of the eye. Am J Ophthal 59:31, 1965.
11. Kupfer, C, Ross, K: Studies of aqueous humor dynamics in man. I. Measurements in young normal subjects. Invest Ophthal 10:518, 1971.
12. Tchernitchin, A, Wenk, EJ, Hernandez, MR, et al: Glucocorticoid localization by radioautography in the rabbit eye following systemic administration of ^{3}H-dexamethasone. Invest Ophthal Vis Sci 19:1231, 1980.
13. Weinreb, RN, Bloom, E, Baxter, JD, et al: Detection of glucocorticoid receptors in cultured human trabecular cells. Invest Ophthal Vis Sci 21:403, 1981.
14. McCarty, GR, Schwartz, B: Increased concentration of glucocorticoid receptors in rabbit iris-ciliary body compared to rabbit liver. Invest Ophthal Vis Sci 23:525, 1982.
15. Southren, AL, Dominguez, MO, Gordon, GG, et al: Nuclear translocation of the cytoplasmic glucocorticoid receptor in the iris-ciliary body and adjacent corneoscleral tissue of the rabbit following topical administration of various glucocorticoids. Invest Ophthal Vis Sci 24:147, 1983.
16. Southren, AL, Gordon, GG, l'Hommedieu, D, et al: 5B-Dihydrocortisol: possible mediator of the ocular hypertension in glaucoma. Invest Ophthal Vis Sci 26:393, 1985.
17. Francois, J, Victoria-Troncoso, V: Mucopolysaccharides and pathogenesis of cortisone glaucoma. Klin Monatsbl Augenheilkd 165:5, 1974.
18. Francois, J: The importance of the mucopolysaccharides in intraocular pressure regulation. Invest Ophthal 14:173, 1975.

19. Francois, J: Tissue culture of ocular fibroblasts. Ann Ophthal 11:1551, 1975.
20. Hayasaka, S: Lysosomal enzymes in ocular tissues and diseases. Surv Ophthal 27:245, 1983.
21. Spaeth, GL, Rodrigues, MM, Weinreb, S: Steroid-induced glaucoma: A. Persistent elevation of intraocular pressure. B. Histopathological aspects. Trans Am Ophthal Soc LXXV:353, 1977.
22. Ticho, U, Lahav, M, Berkowitz, S, Yoffe, P: Ocular changes in rabbits with corticosteroid-induced ocular hypertension. Br J Ophthal 63:646, 1979.
23. Knepper, PA, Collins, JA, Frederick, R: Effect of dexamethasone, progesterone, and testosterone on IOP and GAGs in the rabbit eye. Invest Ophthal Vis Sci 26:1093, 1985.
24. Hernandez, MR, Weinstein, BI, Dunn, MW, et al: The effect of dexamethasone on the synthesis of collagen in normal human trabecular meshwork explants. Invest Ophthal Vis Sci 26:1784, 1985.
25. Bill, A: The drainage of aqueous humor. Invest Ophthal 14:1, 1975.
26. Rohen, JW, Linner, E, Witmer, R: Electron microscopic studies on the trabecular meshwork in two cases of corticosteroid-glaucoma. Exp Eye Res 17:19, 1973.
27. Roll, P, Benedikt, O: Electronmicroscopic investigation of the trabecular meshwork in cortisone glaucoma. Klin Monatsbl Augenheilkd 174:421, 1979.
28. Schirru, A, Pecori-Giraldi, J, Pellegrino, N: Topical corticosteroids and vitreous dynamics in the rabbit. Acta Ophthal 51:811, 1973.
29. Virno, M, Schirru, A, Pecori-Giraldi, J, Pellegrino, N: Aqueous humor alkalosis and marked reduction in ocular ascorbic acid content following long-term topical cortisone (9_a-fluoro-16_a-methylprednisolone). Ann Ophthal 6:983, 1974.
30. Spaeth, GL: The effect of autonomic agents on the pupil and the intraocular pressure of eyes treated with dexamethasone. Br J Ophthal 64:426, 1980.
31. Kimura, R, Honda, M: Effect of orally administered hydrocortisone on the rate of aqueous flow in man. Acta Ophthal 60:584, 1982.
32. Rice, SW, Bourne, WM, Brubaker, RF: Absence of an effect of topical dexamethasone on endothelial permeability and flow of aqueous humor. Invest Ophthal Vis Sci 24:1307, 1983.
33. Podos, SM, Becker, B, Morton, WR: High myopia and primary open-angle glaucoma. Am J Ophthal 62:1039, 1966.
34. Becker, B: Diabetes mellitus and primary open-angle glaucoma. Am J Ophthal 71:1, 1971.
35. Gaston, H, Absolon, MJ, Thurtle, OA, Sattar, MA: Steroid responsiveness in connective tissue diseases. Br J Ophthal 67:487, 1983.
36. Cubey, RB: Glaucoma following the application of corticosteroid to the skin of the eyelids. Br J Dermatol 95:207, 1976.
37. Zugerman, C, Sauders, D, Levit, F: Glaucoma from topically applied steroids. Arch Dermatol 112:1326, 1976.
38. Vie, R: Glaucoma and amaurosis associated with long-term application of topical corticosteroids to the eyelids. Acta Derm Venereol 60:541, 1980.
39. Kalina, RE: Increased intraocular pressure following subconjunctival corticosteroid administration. Arch Ophthal 81:788, 1969.
40. Nozik, RA: Periocular injection of steroids. Trans Am Acad Ophthal Otol 76:695, 1972.
41. Herschler, J: Intractable intraocular hypertension induced by repository triamcinolone acetonide. Am J Ophthal 74:501, 1972.
42. Herschler, J: Increased intraocular pressure induced by repository corticosteroids. Am J Ophthal 82:90, 1976.
43. Ferry, AP, Harris, WP, Nelson, MH: Histopathologic features of subconjunctivally injected corticosteroids. Am J Ophthal 103:716, 1987.
44. Stern, JJ: Acute glaucoma during cortisone therapy. Am J Ophthal 36:389, 1953.
45. Covell, LL: Glaucoma induced by systemic steroid therapy. Am J Ophthal 45:108, 1958.
46. Godel, V, Feiler-Ofry, V, Stein, R: Systemic steroids and ocular fluid dynamics. I. Analysis of the sample as a whole. Influence of dosage and duration of therapy. Acta Ophthal 50:655, 1972.
47. Godel, V, Feiler-Ofry, V, Stein, R: Systemic steroids and ocular fluid dynamics. II. Systemic versus topical steroids. Acta Ophthal 50:664, 1972.
48. Adhikary, HP, Sells, RA, Basu, PK: Ocular complications of systemic steroid after renal transplantation and their association with HLA. Br J Ophthal 66:290, 1982.
49. Kitazawa, Y: Increased intraocular pressure induced by corticosteroids. Am J Ophthal 82:492, 1976.
50. Leibowitz, HM, Kupperman, A, Stewart, RH, Kimbrough, RL: Evaluation of dexamethasone acetate as a topical ophthalmic formulation. Am J Ophthal 86:418, 1978.
51. Brubaker, RF, Halpin, JA: Open-angle glaucoma associated with topical administration of flurandrenolide to the eye. Mayo Clin Proc 50:322, 1975.
52. Ramsell, TG, Bartholomew, RS, Walker, SR: Clinical evaluation of clobetasone butyrate: a comparative study of its effects in postoperative inflammation and on intraocular pressure. Br J Ophthal 64:43, 1980.
53. Dunne, JA, Travers, JP: Double-blind clinical trial of topical steroids in anterior uveitis. Br J Ophthal 63:762, 1979.
54. Eilon, LA, Walker, SR: Clinical evaluation of clobetasone butyrate eye drops in the treatment of anterior uveitis and its effect on intraocular pressure. Br J Ophthal 65:644, 1981.
55. Bedrossian, RH, Eriksen, SP: The treatment of ocular inflammation with medrysone. Arch Ophthal 99:184, 1969.

56. Spaeth, GL: Hydroxymethylprogesterone. An anti-inflammatory steroid without apparent effect on intraocular pressure. Arch Ophthal 75:783, 1966.
57. Dorsch, W, Thygeson, P: The clinical efficacy of medrysone, a new ophthalmic steroid. Am J Ophthal 65:74, 1968.
58. Mindel, JS, Tavitian, HO, Smith, H Jr, Walker, EC: Comparative ocular pressure elevation by medrysone, fluorometholone, and dexamethasone phosphate. Arch Ophthal 98:1577, 1980.
59. Green, K, Cheeks, L, Slagle, T, Phillips, CI: Interaction between progesterone and mifepristone on intraocular pressure in rabbits. Curr Eye Res 8:317, 1989.
60. Fairbairn, WD, Thorson, JC: Fluorometholone. Anti-inflammatory and intraocular pressure effects. Arch Ophthal 86:138, 1971.
61. Akingbehin, AO: Comparative study of the intraocular pressure effects of fluorometholone 0.1% versus dexamethasone 0.1%. Br J Ophthal 67:661, 1983.
62. Morrison, E, Archer, DB: Effect of fluorometholone (FML) on the intraocular pressure of corticosteroid responders. Br J Ophthal 68:581, 1984.
63. Stewart, RH, Kimbrough, RL: Intraocular pressure response to topically administered fluorometholone. Arch Ophthal 97:2139, 1979.
64. Kass, M, Cheetham, J, Duzman, E, Burke, PJ: The ocular hypertensive effect of 0.25% fluorometholone in corticosteroid responders. Am J Ophthal 102:159, 1986.
65. Wilhemi, E: Experimental and clinical investigation of a non-hormonal anti-inflammatory eye ointment. Ophthal Res 5:253, 1973.
66. Gieser, DK, Hodapp, E, Goldberg, I, et al: Flurbiprofen and intraocular pressure. Ann Ophthal 13:831, 1981.
67. Espildora, J, Vicuna, P, Diaz, E: Cortisone-induced glaucoma: a report on 44 affected eyes. J Fr Ophthal 4:503, 1981.

Chapter 21

GLAUCOMAS ASSOCIATED WITH INTRAOCULAR HEMORRHAGE

Intraocular hemorrhage is most commonly caused by trauma or surgery. In addition, hyphemas may occur spontaneously in association with several ocular disorders, most of which have been discussed in previous chapters. Whatever the initial cause of the intraocular hemorrhage may be, secondary intraocular pressure (IOP) elevation frequently occurs when the aqueous outflow channels become obstructed by blood in various forms. In this chapter, we will consider the mechanisms and management of the blood-induced glaucomas, as well as some specific causes of intraocular hemorrhage that are not covered in other chapters.

GLAUCOMAS ASSOCIATED WITH HYPHEMA

Blunt Trauma

A common source of hyphema, or blood in the anterior chamber, is blunt trauma. This usually results from a tear in the ciliary body, causing bleeding from the small branches of the major arterial circle.

General Features

Young age and male gender appear to be risk factors for blunt ocular trauma. In one large series, 77% of the patients with traumatic hyphemas were less than 30 years of age.[1] In another large study, the annual incidence of traumatic hyphema was significantly higher in men, and sports-related injuries were identified as a cause for a recent increase in the incidence rate.[2]

The initial clinical finding may be a microscopic hyphema, which is characterized by red blood cells circulating in the aqueous. In other cases, the quantity of blood may be sufficient to create a layered hyphema. These range in size from a small layer of blood in the inferior quadrant of the anterior chamber to a total hyphema, with the smaller hemorrhages being more common. In most cases, the blood clears within a few days, primarily through the trabecular meshwork, and the prognosis is good unless the associated trauma has caused other ocular injuries. However, complications may occur during the postinjury course, which can have devastating results.

Complications

Recurrent Hemorrhage. In 20 reported series of traumatic hyphemas, the frequency with which eyes rebled ranged from 4 to 35%, with an average of approximately 15%.[2–21] Rebleeding usually occurs during the first week after the initial injury, which is probably related to the normal lysis and retraction of the clot. Aspirin has been shown to have a detrimental effect on the frequency of rebleeding,[9,14,22] and there is a suggestion that hypotony may also increase the chances of recurrent hemorrhage.[3,5] One study found black race to be another risk factor for secondary hemorrhage.[21] Reports differ as to whether the size of the initial hyphema influences rebleeding. However, all studies agree that recurrent hemorrhage, as compared with the initial hyphema, is associated with significantly more complications and a more frequent need for surgical intervention.

Secondary Glaucoma. Although IOP elevation may occur following the initial bleed, it is more common after a recurrent hemorrhage and constitutes the most serious complication of a traumatic hyphema. The incidence of glaucoma associated with a traumatic hyphema is partly related to the size of the hemorrhage. In one study of 235 cases, glaucoma occurred in 13.5% of the eyes in which the hyphema filled less than one-half of the anterior chamber, 27% of those with a bleed involving greater than half the chamber, and 52% of the cases with a total hyphema.[17] It is important to distinguish between a total hyphema with bright red blood and an "eight-ball," or "black-ball," hyphema, which is characterized by dark reddish-black blood (Fig. 21.1), since the latter carries a more grave prognosis relative to secondary glaucoma.[4] In one series of 113 cases, elevated IOP occurred in one-third of those with a rebleed but in all cases with eight-ball hyphemas.[4]

The mechanism of pressure elevation is related to obstruction of the trabecular meshwork in most cases of traumatic hyphema. Although fresh red blood cells are known to pass through the conventional aqueous outflow system with relative ease, it appears to be the overwhelming numbers of cells, combined with plasma, fibrin, and debris, that may lead to a transient obstruction of aqueous outflow.[23] In cases of eight-ball hyphema, it is presumably the formation of a clot, occasionally with degenerated red blood cells from an associated vitreous hemorrhage, that further impedes outflow.

Sickle cell hemoglobinopathies, including sickle cell trait, increase the incidence of glaucoma in association with hyphema.[24–26] Erythrocytes in these disorders have a greater tendency to sickle in the aqueous humor,[24,25,27] and the elongated, rigid cells pass more slowly through the trabecular meshwork,[28] leading to IOP elevation even with small amounts of intracameral blood.[24,25] In addition, even moderate elevations of pressure may have a more deleterious effect on the optic nerve head in patients with sickle cell anemia, possibly because of reduced vascular perfusion.[24,25] Another mechanism of secondary open-angle glaucoma associated with sickle cell hemoglobinopathies is obstruction to aqueous outflow resulting from sickled erythrocytes in Schlemm's canal, which has been observed following blunt trauma and in one case with no antecedent trauma.[26]

Another condition that may be associated with delayed clearing of blood from the anterior chamber is diabetes. Erythrocytes from diabetic patients have decreased deformability and increased adherence, result-

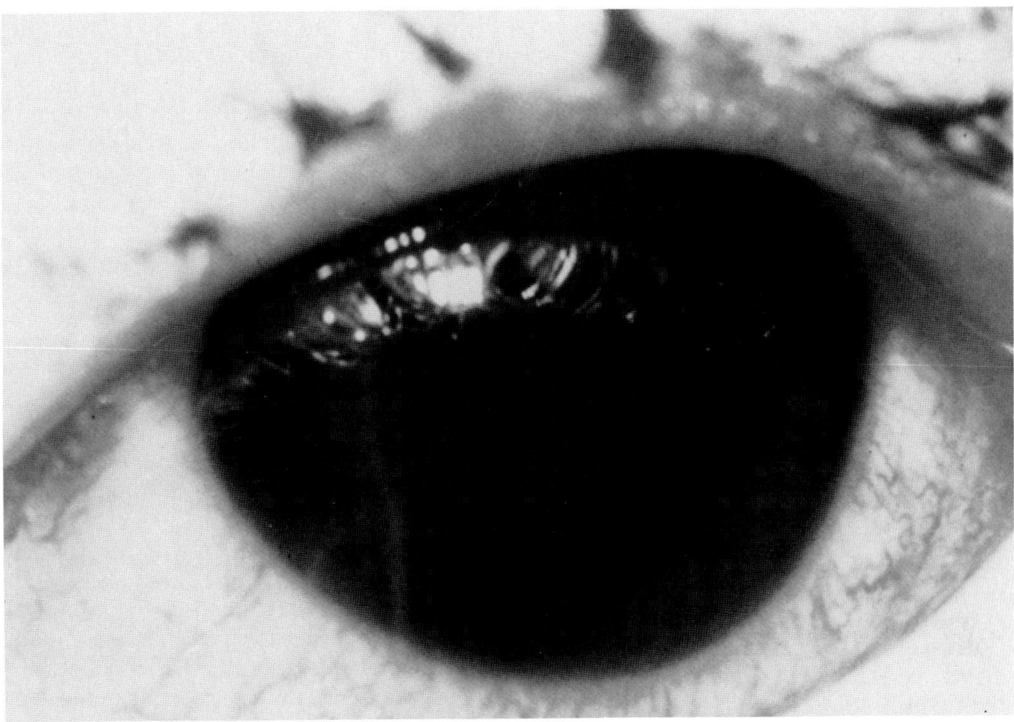

Figure 21.1. Slit-lamp view of eye with total, "eight-ball" hyphema and secondary glaucoma.

ing in delayed clearance time from the rabbit anterior chamber, as compared with red blood cells from healthy human subjects.[29]

Corneal Blood Staining. Corneal blood staining is typically the result of a prolonged, total hyphema that is usually, but not always,[30] associated with elevated IOP. This complication occurred in six of 289 patients (2%) with traumatic hyphema, all of whom had a recurrent, total hyphema.[28] The earliest pathologic event may be corneal endothelial decompensation associated with the passage of hemoglobin and hemoglobin products into the stroma.[31] The cornea may initially have a red discoloration, which was found in rabbit studies to be associated with extracellular hemoglobin particles and oxyhemoglobin.[31] The hemoglobin is apparently phagocytized by keratocytes and degraded to hemosiderin.[31,32] The cornea takes on a brownish discoloration at this stage, which is associated with methemoglobin in the stroma.[31] Clearing of the corneal blood staining begins in the peripheral and posterior stroma, apparently as a result of diffusion of hemoglobin breakdown products out of the cornea, and may take up to 2 or 3 years for total clearing.[32,33]

Management

Conservative Management of Hyphema. There is general agreement that the uncomplicated hyphema should be managed nonsurgically, with an aim toward accelerating resorption of the hyphema and minimizing rebleeding. However, opinions vary as to the best means of accomplishing these goals. A traditional approach was to admit the patient for approximately 5 days of bed rest with elevation of the head of the bed and monocular or binocular patching.[4,10] However, one study showed no significant difference between patients treated with strict bed rest and patching as compared with a group that was allowed limited activity without patching.[34] A comparison of monocular and binocular patching also revealed no difference in outcome.[35] It is reasonable, therefore, to allow limited ambulation, with a shield simply to protect the injured eye. Hospitalization is not always necessary, unless sickle cell disease or trait is present.

Acceleration of Hyphema Clearance. Various drugs have been used by some physicians to accelerate resorption of the hyphema, but none of these has proved value in this regard. Rabbit studies have not supported the efficacy of atropine,[36] pilocarpine,[36] or acetazolamide[37] for this purpose, although there is a suggestion that hyperosmotics may accelerate resorption of a clotted hyphema.[38] Intracameral tissue plasminogen activator, a clot-specific fibrinolytic agent, has been shown to accelerate the clearance of experimental hyphema in rabbits,[39] although it may also increase the risk of rebleeding.[40] Therefore, at the present time there is no drug with proved efficacy for safely accelerating hyphema resorption.

Prevention of Rebleeding. Numerous drugs have also been evaluated regarding their ability to prevent a rebleed, with conflicting results. Some investigators found that oral prednisone significantly lowered the rebleed rate,[8] while others found neither steroids[15] nor estrogen[4] to be of value in this regard. *Antifibrinolytic agents* (including *tranexamic acid*[12,13,41,42] and *aminocaproic acid*[11,21,43–47]) have been used in an effort to minimize rebleeding by delaying the natural lysis of the clot. Most reports indicate that the use of these drugs is associated with a significant reduction in rebleeds,[11,13,41–44] although some found no significant difference from placebo therapy.[12,45] Aminocaproic acid is typically given as 100 mg/kg every 4 hours up to a maximum of 30 grams/day for 5 days, which is associated with frequent side effects, including light-headedness, nausea and vomiting, and systemic hypotension. A half dose of 50 mg/kg reduced the incidence of dizziness and hypotension without adversely affecting the reduced rate of recurrent hemorrhage, but did not lower the incidence of nausea and vomiting.[46] Another reported complication is elevated IOP, associated with the accelerated clot dissolution.[47] Preliminary evidence in rabbit studies suggests that topical aminocaproic acid may be an effective alternative to systemic treatment, which may at least reduce the systemic side effects.[48,49]

The influence of hydrostatic pressure on the damaged vessels has also been studied, and one report described fewer rebleeds with medical reduction of systemic blood pressure and elevation of the head of the bed.[50] As previously noted, the use of aspirin may increase the chances of secondary hemorrhage,[9,14] and any drug that may increase the risk of bleeding should be avoided, whenever possible, for the first week after the trauma and until the hyphema has completely cleared.

Management of Associated Intraocular Pressure Elevation. *Medical treatment* of elevated IOP is occasionally needed to protect the optic nerve head and enhance the resorption of the hyphema. Pressure reduction is best accomplished with topical beta-blocker therapy. Caution should be given to the use of carbonic anhydrase inhibitors in patients with sickle cell hemoglobinopathies, since they increase the concentration of ascorbic acid in the aqueous humor, leading to more sickling in the anterior chamber.[51] Epinephrine may increase intravascular and intracameral sickling by its vasoconstrictive and subsequent deoxygenating effect, although the drug had no effect on the duration of the hyphema or percentage of sickled cells in the anterior chamber when human sickle cell thalassemia blood was injected into the anterior chamber of rabbits.[52] In the management of patients with sickle cell trait, control of the IOP during the first 24 hours was found to be associated with a good prognosis, while lack of control during that time period was associated with continued difficulty in managing the pressure.[53] Hyperbaric oxygen therapy has been shown to significantly reduce the percentage of sickled cells injected intracamerally in rabbits by raising the aqueous pO_2, which may be of value in patients with sickle cell hyphema.[54]

Surgical intervention becomes necessary when a sustained IOP elevation cannot be controlled medically and threatens to damage the optic nerve or is associated with corneal blood staining. The critical pressure level depends on the status of the optic nerve head (if this is known), with healthy discs usually tolerating pressures of 40–50 mm Hg for 5 or 6 days, while a nerve head with preexisting glaucomatous optic atrophy may undergo further damage at pressures less than 30 mm Hg within 24–48 hours. A total hyphema for more than 4 days is an additional indication for surgical intervention. As previously noted, special attention must be given to patients with sickle cell anemia or trait, since their nerve heads are especially vulnerable to damage at minimal to moderate elevations in IOP. A pressure in the mid-20s for more than 1 day may be an indication to surgically intervene in these patients.[53]

The surgical approach most often used is evacuation of the hyphema, which usually includes clotted blood, from the anterior chamber. The liquified portion of the hyphema may be removed by gentle anterior chamber washout through a paracentesis wound and the clot allowed to resorb.[55] This technique is of particular value when a sudden increase in pressure requires emergency measures to avoid irreversible loss of vision, as may occur with sickle cell disease.[56] A corneal transfixing needle has been developed for simultaneous irrigation of the anterior chamber and evacuation of a fluid hyphema.[57]

Many surgeons prefer to also remove the clot, and fibrinolytic agents such as urokinase[58,59] and fibrinolysin[60–64] have been used to facilitate clot lysis and irrigation. Other reported surgical techniques to remove the clot include cryoextraction,[65] ultrasonic emulsification and extraction,[66] and removal with vitrectomy instruments.[67–69] Viscoelastic agents, such as sodium hyaluronate, have also been used to mechanically dissect a clot from the iris and express it through a corneoscleral incision.[70,71] The 4th day after injury is said to be the optimum time for removal of the clot, because it has usually retracted from the adjacent structures.[72,73] In a histopathologic evaluation of two black-ball clots removed 4 and 7 days after traumatic total hyphemas, the surface of the clot consisted of a fibrin "pseudocapsule" with no attachment to intraocular structures and no evidence of organization (fibroblasts or new vessels) within the clot.[74]

Other surgeons have advocated a trabeculectomy and iridectomy combined with gentle irrigation of the anterior chamber.[75] The iris may prolapse into the incision during any surgical attempt to evacuate the hyphema, because of a pupillary block, necessitating an iridectomy,[76] and it has been reported that complete resorption of the hyphema may follow iridectomy alone.[77] When recurrent bleeding occurs during clot extraction, raising the IOP to 50 mm Hg for 5 minutes has been used to stop the bleeding.[69] Cyclodiathermy has also been used to control intraocular bleeding.[78]

Penetrating Injuries

Intraocular hemorrhage is also frequently associated with penetrating injuries, although secondary glaucoma is less common than with blunt trauma during the early postinjury period because of the open wound. However, IOP elevation may follow closure of the wound, especially if meticulous care is not given to reconstruction of the anterior chamber and treatment of the associated inflammation in the early postoperative period.[79]

Hyphema Associated with Intraocular Surgery

Bleeding within the eye can be a serious complication of any intraocular procedure and may occur during the operation or in the early or even late postoperative period.

During Surgery. As an intraoperative complication, bleeding is usually associated with damage to the ciliary body, as can occur when performing a cyclodialysis, filtering procedure, or iridectomy. This bleeding can usually be controlled by placing a large air bubble in the anterior chamber for a few minutes, which raises the IOP and acts as a tamponade. Direct, gentle pressure with the tip of a sponge of Gel-Foam or the application of epinephrine 1:1000 to the ciliary body for 1–2 minutes can also be helpful in stopping ciliary body bleeding. Cautery is generally avoided in these cases, although use of an intraocular, bipolar unit may be effective.

Postoperatively. Bleeding in the *early* postoperative period is usually not associated with serious sequelae and should be managed conservatively with limited activity and elevation of the head. Small hyphemas after intraocular surgery normally clear rapidly, although the time may be considerably longer in eyes with preexisting glaucoma, because of delayed passage of red blood cells through the trabecular meshwork. When a postoperative hyphema is associated with elevated IOP, conservative medical management should be instituted as required, using drugs that lower aqueous production or hyperosmotics if necessary. Surgical intervention is reserved for critical cases, although the indications may be somewhat more liberal than with a traumatic hyphema if there is danger of rupturing a corneoscleral wound or causing further atrophy to an optic nerve that has previously been damaged by glaucoma.

Hemorrhage during the *late* postoperative period may result from reopening of a uveal wound or from disruption of new vessels growing across a corneoscleral incision.[80] In a study of 58 eyes 5–10 years after cataract extraction, 12% had vessels in the inner aspects of the incision site and nearly half of these had evidence of mild intraocular hemorrhage.[81] Direct argon laser therapy may be used to treat such vessels when they can be visualized gonioscopically,[80] and transscleral Nd:YAG photocoagulation may be effective when the former fails.[82] Penetrating cyclodiathermy[83] and cryotherapy[81] are also reported to be useful in managing the intraocular hemorrhage.

Spontaneous Hyphemas

Hyphemas may also develop spontaneously in a variety of conditions, most of which have been considered in previous chapters. In some cases, the hyphema may cause or contribute to an elevation of the IOP.

Intraocular Tumors

As noted in Chapter 18, a spontaneous hyphema may occur in a child with juvenile xanthogranuloma, and intraocular hemorrhage may also be a manifestation of an ocular malignant melanoma.

Neovascularization

New blood vessels in the anterior ocular segment, which may lead to a spontaneous hyphema, are seen in neovascular glaucoma (Chapter 16) and in Fuchs' heterochromic cyclitis (Chapter 19).

Vascular Tufts at the Pupillary Margin

This condition is also referred to as neovascular tufts or iris microhemangiomas and represents yet another source of spontaneous hyphema. Slit-lamp biomicroscopy may reveal multiple vascular tufts along the pupillary margin, and fluorescein angiography of the iris is reported to demonstrate small areas of staining and leakage from the lesions.[84] One histopathologic study revealed thin-walled new vessels at the pupillary margin of the iris with a mild inflammatory cell infiltration,[85] while another report described the vascular abnormality as a hamartoma of the capillary hemangioma type.[86] The condition is typically seen in elderly individuals but may be found in young adults. Most of these patients have no systemic disease,[84] although associations with diabetes mellitus[84,87] and myotonic dystrophy[87,88] have been reported. Spontaneous hyphemas occur in a small number of these cases, occasionally causing transient IOP elevation.[89,90] Laser photocoagulation has been reported to successfully eradicate bleeding vascular tufts.[85,91] However, since it is rare to have recurrent hyphemas or permanent damage related to the transiently elevated IOP, it is best to withhold treatment until one or more recurrences of bleeding are documented.

GLAUCOMAS ASSOCIATED WITH DEGENERATED OCULAR BLOOD

Ghost Cell Glaucoma

In 1976, Campbell and co-workers[92] described a form of secondary glaucoma in which degenerated red blood cells (ghost cells) develop in the vitreous cavity and subsequently enter the anterior chamber, where they temporarily obstruct aqueous outflow.

Theories of Mechanism[92]

Having entered the vitreous cavity by one of several mechanisms (trauma, surgery, or retinal disease), fresh erythrocytes are

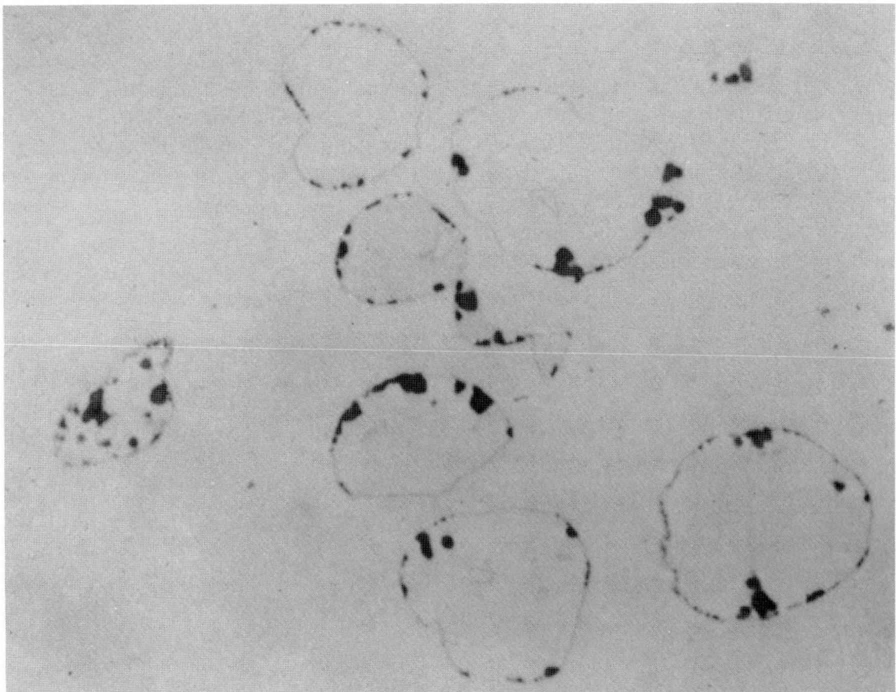

Figure 21.2. Transmission electron microscopic appearance of red blood cell ghosts from eye of patient with ghost cell glaucoma. Dark areas at cell periphery are Heinz bodies (Original magnification, ×23,000). (Courtesy of David G. Campbell, M.D.)

transformed from their typical biconcave, pliable nature to tan or khaki-colored, spherical, less pliable structures, referred to as ghost cells. Histologically, these cells have thin walls and appear hollow except for clumps of denatured hemoglobin, called Heinz bodies (Fig. 21.2). Unlike fresh red blood cells, ghost cells do not pass readily through a 5-micron Millipore filter or human trabecular meshwork. The ghost cells develop within a matter of weeks and may then remain in the vitreous cavity for many months until a disruption of the anterior hyaloid allows them to enter the anterior chamber. Once in the anterior chamber, the abnormal cells accumulate in the trabecular meshwork, where they may cause a temporary, but occasionally marked, elevation of IOP.

Specific Causes

Several situations have been described that may lead to ghost cell glaucoma.

Cataract extraction may be associated with glaucoma resulting from ghost cells in one of three ways.[93] (1) A large hyphema with vitreous hemorrhage occurs in the early postoperative period. As the hyphema clears, ghost cells, which developed in the vitreous, come forward and obstruct aqueous outflow. (2) A vitreous hemorrhage is present before cataract surgery, and disruption of the anterior hyaloid as a result of the operation allows the ghost cells to enter the anterior chamber. (3) A vitreous hemorrhage develops at some point after cataract extraction because of retinal disease, and the ghost cells develop and come forward through previously made defects in the anterior hyaloid. Ghost cell glaucoma has also been associated with intraocular lens implantation, especially when anterior chamber or iris-fixation lenses were used.[94]

Vitrectomy may lead to ghost cell glaucoma in eyes with preexisting vitreous hemorrhage if the anterior hyaloid is disrupted and the vitreous and cells are not completely removed.[95]

Vitreous hemorrhage without surgery may also lead to ghost cell glaucoma. The vitreous hemorrhage may be due to trauma or may be associated with a retinal disorder, such as diabetic retinopathy.[96,97] The traumatic cases may have associated hyphema, which may have cleared before the ghost cell glaucoma develops or which may persist and mask the actual mechanism of the glaucoma. The route of ghost cells to the anterior chamber in these phakic eyes is presumed to be a defect in the anterior hyaloid face.[96,97]

Clinical Features[92]

Depending on the number of ghost cells in the anterior chamber, the IOP ranges from normal to marked elevation with pain and corneal edema. Slit-lamp biomicroscopy reveals characteristic khaki-colored cells in the aqueous and on the corneal endothelium. If present in large quantities, the ghost cells may layer out inferiorly, creating a pseudohypopyon, which is occasionally associated with a layer of fresher red blood cells (candy-stripe sign) (Fig. 21.3). The anterior chamber angle, on gonioscopy, is typically open and may appear normal or may be covered by scant to heavy amounts of khaki-colored cells.

Differential Diagnosis

Glaucoma resulting from ghost cells may be confused with the less common hemolytic and hemosiderotic glaucomas, which are discussed below. In addition, neovascular glaucoma and glaucoma resulting from inflammation must be ruled out. Although the diagnosis is usually easily made on the basis of history and clinical features, it may be confirmed by examination of an aqueous aspirate, which reveals the typical ghost cells. This examination may be performed with phase contrast microscopy[92] or by rou-

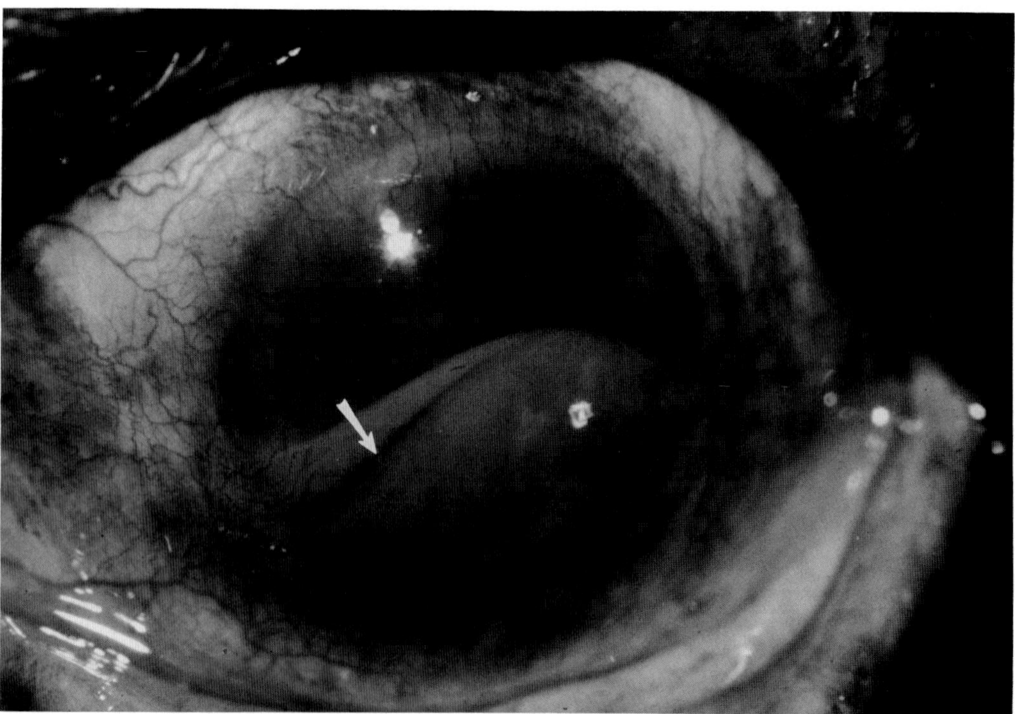

Figure 21.3. Slit-lamp view of eye with ghost cell glaucoma showing typical layered hyphema of dark (*arrow*) and light colored cells (candy-stripe sign). (Courtesy of David G. Campbell, M.D.)

tine light microscopy of a paraffin-embedded specimen stained with hematoxylin and eosin.[98]

Management

Glaucoma resulting from ghost cells is not a permanent condition but may last for months before the abnormal cells eventually clear from the anterior chamber angle. In the interim, it is often possible to control the IOP with standard antiglaucoma medication. However, other cases require surgical intervention, which usually involves removal of the ghost cells from the anterior chamber by irrigation[92] or removal of all ocular ghost cells by vitrectomy.[99]

Hemolytic Glaucoma

Fenton and Zimmerman[100] described a form of secondary glaucoma associated with intraocular hemorrhage in which macrophages ingest contents of the red blood cells and then accumulate in the trabecular meshwork, where they temporarily obstruct aqueous outflow. Clinically, numerous red-tinted blood cells are seen floating in the aqueous, and the anterior chamber angle is typically open, with reddish-brown pigment covering the trabecular meshwork.[101] Cytologic examination of the aqueous reveals *macrophages* containing golden-brown pigment,[101] and an ultrastructural study of seven eyes revealed red blood cells and macrophages with phagocytized blood and pigment in the trabecular spaces.[102] The endothelial cells of the trabecular meshwork were degenerated and also had phagocytized blood.[102] The condition is self-limiting and should be managed medically if possible. When surgical intervention is required, anterior chamber lavage has been recommended.[101]

Hemosiderotic Glaucoma

This is a rare condition in which hemoglobin from lysed red blood cells in the anterior chamber is phagocytized by endothelial cells of the trabecular meshwork. Iron in the hemoglobin subsequently causes siderosis, which is believed to produce tissue alterations in the trabecular meshwork, eventually resulting in obstruction to aqueous outflow.[103] However, an association between iron staining of the trabecular meshwork and impairment of aqueous outflow has yet to be clearly established.

SUMMARY

Red blood cells in the anterior chamber, in either a fresh or degenerated form, may lead to elevated IOP by obstructing aqueous outflow through the trabecular meshwork. The most common cause of a fresh hyphema is blunt trauma. Glaucoma may result from the primary hemorrhage but more often from a rebleed, and initial therapy is directed toward accelerating resorption of the hyphema and minimizing rebleeding. When glaucoma occurs, medical management may control the IOP until the hyphema clears, although some cases require surgical intervention, which includes removal of the blood. Other causes of fresh hyphema include spontaneous bleeding from tumors, neovascularization, or vascular tufts at the pupillary margin. The most common form of glaucoma associated with degenerated ocular blood is ghost cell glaucoma, in which erythrocytes in the vitreous degenerate to a rigid, spherical state and then enter the anterior chamber to obstruct aqueous outflow. This may follow cataract extraction, vitrectomy, or trauma. Other situations in which degenerated blood may lead to glaucoma include hemolytic glaucoma and hemosiderotic glaucoma.

References

1. Pilger, IS: Medical treatment of traumatic hyphema. Surv Ophthal 20:28, 1975.
2. Kennedy, RH, Brubaker, RF: Traumatic hyphema in a defined population. Am J Ophthal 106:123, 1988.
3. Howard, GM, Hutchinson, BT, Frederick, AR Jr: Hyphema resulting from blunt trauma. Gonioscopic, tonographic, and ophthalmoscopic observation following resolution of the hemorrhage. Trans Am Acad Ophthal Otol 69:294, 1965.
4. Spaeth, GL, Levy, PM: Traumatic hyphema: its clinical characteristics and failure of estrogens to alter its course. A double-blind study. Am J Ophthal 62:1098, 1966.
5. Milstein, BA: Traumatic hyphema: a study of 83 consecutive cases. South Med J 64:1081, 1971.
6. Giles, CL, Bromley, WG: Traumatic hyphema. A retrospective analysis from the University of

Michigan Teaching Hospitals. J Ped Ophthal 9:90, 1972.

7. Edwards, WC, Layden, WE: Traumatic hyphema. A report of 184 consecutive cases. Am J Ophthal 75:110, 1973.
8. Yasuna, E: Management of traumatic hyphema. Arch Ophthal 91:190, 1974.
9. Crawford, JS, Lewandowski, RL, Chan, W: The effect of aspirin on rebleeding in traumatic hyphema. Am J Ophthal 80:543, 1975.
10. Fritch, CD: Traumatic hyphema. Ann Ophthal 8:1223, 1976.
11. Crouch, ER Jr, Frenkel, M: Aminocaproic acid in the treatment of traumatic hyphema. Am J Ophthal 81:355, 1976.
12. Mortensen, KK, Sjølie, AK: Secondary haemorrhage following traumatic hyphaema. A comparative study of conservative and tranexamic acid treatment. Acta Ophthal 56:763, 1978.
13. Bramsen, T: Fibrinolysis and traumatic hyphaema. Acta Ophthal 57:447, 1979.
14. Gorn, RA: The detrimental effect of aspirin on hyphema rebleed. Ann Ophthal 11:351, 1979.
15. Spoor, TC, Hammer, M, Belloso, H: Traumatic hyphema. Failure of steroids to alter its course: a double-blind prospective study. Arch Ophthal 98:116, 1980.
16. Rakusin, W: Traumatic hyphema. Am J Ophthal 74:284, 1972.
17. Coles, WH: Traumatic hyphema: an analysis of 235 cases. South Med J 61:813, 1968.
18. Cassel, GH, Jeffers, JB, Jaeger, EA: Wills Eye Hospital traumatic hyphema study. Ophthal Surg 16:441, 1985.
19. Thomas, MA, Parrish, RK II, Feuer, WJ: Rebleeding after traumatic hyphema. Arch Ophthal 104:206, 1986.
20. Agapitos, PJ, Noel, L-P, Clarke, WN: Traumatic hyphema in children. Ophthalmology 94:1238, 1987.
21. Spoor, TC, Kwitko, GM, O'Grady, JM, Ramocki, JM: Traumatic hyphema in an urban population. Am J Ophthal 109:23, 1990.
22. Ganley, JP, Geiger, JM, Clemet, JR, Rigby, et al: Aspirin and recurrent hyphema after blunt ocular trauma. Am J Ophthal 96:797, 1983.
23. Sternberg, P Jr, Tripathi, RC, Tripathi, BJ, Chilcote, RR: Changes in outflow facility in experimental hyphema. Invest Ophthal Vis Sci 19:1388, 1980.
24. Goldberg, MF: The diagnosis and treatment of secondary glaucoma after hyphema in sickle cell patients. Am J Ophthal 87:43, 1979.
25. Goldberg, MF: Sickled erythrocytes, hyphema, and secondary glaucoma: 1. The diagnosis and treatment of sickled erythrocytes in human hyphemas. Ophthal Surg 10:17, 1979.
26. Friedman, AH, Halpern, BL, Friedberg, DN, et al: Transient open-angle glaucoma associated with sickle cell trait: report of 4 cases. Br J Ophthal 63:832, 1979.
27. Goldberg, MF: Sickled erythrocytes, hyphema, and secondary glaucoma: IV. The rate and percentage of sickling of erythrocytes in rabbit aqueous humor, in vitro and in vivo. Ophthal Surg 10:62, 1979.
28. Goldberg, MF, Tso, MOM: Sickled erythrocytes, hyphema, and secondary glaucoma: VII. The passage of sickled erythrocytes out of the anterior chamber of the human and monkey eye: light and electron microscopic studies. Ophthal Surg 10:89, 1979.
29. Williams, GA, Hatchell, DL, Collier, BD, Knobel, J: Clearance from the anterior chamber of RBCs from human diabetics. Arch Ophthal 102:930, 1984.
30. Beyer, TL, Hirst, LW: Corneal blood staining at low pressures. Arch Ophthal 103:654, 1985.
31. Gottsch, JD, Messmer, EP, McNair, DS, Font, RL: Corneal blood staining. An animal model. Ophthalmology 93:797, 1986.
32. McDonnell, PJ, Green, WR, Stevens, RE, et al: Blood staining of the cornea. Light microscopic and ultrastructural features. Ophthalmology 92:1668, 1985.
33. Brodrick, JD: Corneal blood staining after hyphema. Br J Ophthal 56:589, 1972.
34. Read, J, Goldberg, MF: Comparison of medical treatment of traumatic hyphema. Trans Am Acad Ophthal Otol 78:799, 1974.
35. Edwards, WC, Layden, WE: Monocular versus binocular patching in traumatic hyphema. Am J Ophthal 76:359, 1973.
36. Rose, SW, Coupal, JJ, Simmons, G, Kielar, RA: Experimental hyphema clearance in rabbits. Drug trials with 1% atropine and 2% and 4% pilocarpine. Arch Ophthal 95:1442, 1977.
37. Masket, S, Best, M: Therapy in experimental hyphema. II. Acetazolamide. Arch Ophthal 87:222, 1972.
38. Masket, S, Best, M, Fisher, LV, et al: Therapy in experimental hyphema. Arch Ophthal 85:329, 1971.
39. Lambrou, FH, Snyder, RW, Williams, GA: Use of tissue plasminogen activator in experimental hyphema. Arch Ophthal 105:995, 1987.
40. Williams, DF, Han, DP, Abrams, GW: Rebleeding in experimental traumatic hyphema treated with intraocular tissue plasminogen activator. Arch Ophthal 108:264, 1990.
41. Bramsen, T: Traumatic hyphaema treated with the antifibrinolytic drug tranexamic acid. Acta Ophthal 54:250, 1976.
42. Uusitalo, RJ, Ranta-Kemppainen, L, Tarkkanen, A: Management of traumatic hyphema in children. An analysis of 340 cases. Arch Ophthal 106:1207, 1988.
43. McGetrick, JJ, Jampol, LM, Goldberg, MF, et al:

Aminocaproic acid decreases secondary hemorrhage after traumatic hyphema. Arch Ophthal 101:1031, 1983.

44. Kutner, B, Fourman, S, Brein, K, et al: Aminocaproic acid reduces the risk of secondary hemorrhage in patients with traumatic hyphema. Arch Ophthal 105:206, 1987.
45. Kraft, SP, Christianson, MD, Crawford, JS, et al: Traumatic hyphema in children. Treatment with Epsilon-Aminocaproic acid. Ophthalmology 94:1232, 1987.
46. Palmer, DJ, Goldberg, MF, Frenkel, M, et al: A comparison of two dose regimens of epsilon aminocaproic acid in the prevention and management of secondary traumatic hyphemas. Ophthalmology 93:102, 1986.
47. Dieste, MC, Hersh, PS, Kylstra, JA, et al: Intraocular pressure increase associated with epsilon-aminocaproic acid therapy for traumatic hyphema. Am J Ophthal 106:383, 1988.
48. Allingham, RR, Williams, PB, Crouch, ER Jr, et al: Topically applied aminocaproic acid concentrates in the aqueous humor of the rabbit in therapeutic levels. Arch Ophthal 105:1421, 1987.
49. Allingham, RR, Crouch, ER Jr, Williams, PB, et al: Topical aminocaproic acid significantly reduces the incidence of secondary hemorrhage in traumatic hyphema in the rabbit model. Arch Ophthal 106:1436, 1988.
50. Macdougald, TJ: The treatment of traumatic hyphaema. Trans Ophthal Soc UK 92:815, 1972.
51. Goldberg, MF: Sickled erythrocytes, hyphema, and secondary glaucoma: V. The effect of vitamin C on erythrocyte sickling in aqueous humor. Ophthal Surg 10:70, 1979.
52. Vernot, JA, Barron, BA, Goldberg, MF: Effects of topical epinephrine on experimental sickle cell hyphema. Arch Ophthal 103:280, 1985.
53. Deutsch, TA, Weinreb, RN, Goldberg, MF: Indications for surgical management of hyphema in patients with sickle cell trait. Arch Ophthal 102:566, 1984.
54. Wallyn, CR, Jampol, LM, Goldberg, MF, Zanetti, CL: The use of hyperbaric oxygen therapy in the treatment of sickle cell hyphema. Invest Ophthal Vis Sci 26:1155, 1985.
55. Belcher, CD III, Brown, SVL, Simmons, RJ: Anterior chamber washout for traumatic hyphema. Ophthal Surg. 16:475, 1985.
56. Wax, MB, Ridley, ME, Magargal, LE: Reversal of retinal and optic disc ischemia in a patient with sickle cell trait and glaucoma secondary to traumatic hyphema. Ophthalmology 89:845, 1982.
57. Tripathi, RC: A corneal transfixing irrigation/perfusion device: a new method for evacuation of hyphema. Ophthal Surg 11:569, 1980.
58. Rakusin, W: The role of urokinase in the management of traumatic hyphaema. Ophthalmologica 167:373, 1973.
59. Leet, DM: Treatment of total hyphemas with urokinase. Am J Ophthal 84:79, 1977.
60. Oosterhuis, JA: Fibrinolysin irrigation in traumatic secondary hyphema. Ophthalmologica 155:357, 1968.
61. Podos, S, Liebman, S, Pollen, A: Treatment of experimental total hyphemas with intraocular fibrinolytic agents. Part II. Arch Ophthal 71:537, 1964.
62. Scheie, HG, Ashley, BJ Jr, Burns, DT: Treatment of total hyphema with fibrinolysin. Arch Ophthal 69:147, 1963.
63. Polychronakos, D, Razoglou, CH: Treatment of total hyphema with fibrinolysin. Ophthalmologica 154:31, 1967.
64. Horven, I: Fibrinolysis and hyphema. The effect of "thrombolysin" and "kabikinas" on clotted blood in cameral anterior of the eye in rabbits. Acta Ophthal 46:320, 1962.
65. Hill, K: Cryoextraction of total hyphema. Arch Ophthal 80:368, 1968.
66. Kelman, CD, Brooks, DL: Ultrasonic emulsification and aspiration of traumatic hyphema. A preliminary report. Am J Ophthal 71:1289, 1971.
67. McCuen, BW, Fung, WE: The role of vitrectomy instrumentation in the treatment of severe traumatic hyphema. Am J Ophthal 88:930, 1979.
68. Diddie, KR, Ernest, JT: Rotoextractor evacuation of total hyphema. Ophthal Surg 7:49, 1976.
69. Stern, WH, Mondal, KM: Vitrectomy instrumentation for surgical evacuation of total anterior chamber hyphema and control of recurrent anterior chamber hemorrhage. Ophthal Surg 10:34, 1979.
70. Sholiton, DB, Solomon, OD: Surgical management of black ball hyphema with sodium hyaluronate. Ophthal Surg 12:820, 1981.
71. Bartholomew, RS: Visoelastic evacuation of traumatic hyphaema. Br J Ophthal 71:27, 1987.
72. Sears, ML: Surgical management of black ball hyphema. Trans Am Acad Ophthal Otol 74:820, 1970.
73. Wolter, JR, Henderson, JW, Talley, TW: Histopathology of a black ball blood clot removed four days after total traumatic hyphema. J Ped Ophthal 8:15, 1971.
74. Caprioli, J, Sears, ML: The histopathology of black ball hyphema: report of two cases. Ophthal Surg 15:491, 1984.
75. Weiss, JS, Parrish, RK, Anderson, DR: Surgical therapy of traumatic hyphema. Ophthal Surg 14:343, 1983.
76. Heinze, J: The surgical management of total hyphema. Aust J Ophthal 3:20, 1975.
77. Parrish, R, Bernardino, V Jr: Iridectomy in the surgical management of eight-ball hyphema. Arch Ophthal 100:435, 1982.
78. Gilbert, HD, Smith, RE: Traumatic hyphema:

treatment of secondary hemorrhage with cyclodiathermy. Ophthal Surg 7:31, 1976.
79. Richardson, K: Acute glaucoma after trauma. In: Ocular Trauma, Freeman, H MacK, ed. Appleton-Century-Croft, New York, 1979, p. 161.
80. Bene, C, Hutchins, R, Kranias, G: Cataract wound neovascularization. An often overlooked cause of vitreous hemorrhage. Ophthalmology 96:50, 1989.
81. Watzke, RC: Intraocular hemorrhage from vascularization of the cataract incision. Ophthalmology 87:19, 1980.
82. Kramer, TR, Brown, RH, Lynch, MG, Martinez, L: Transscleral Nd:YAG photocoagulation for cataract incision vascularizaiton associated with recurrent hyphema. Am J Ophthal 107:681, 1989.
83. Lieppman, M, Goldberg, MF: The treatment of postoperative hyphema by cyclodiathermy. Surv Ophthal 26:253, 1982.
84. Cobb, B: Vascular tufts at the pupillary margin: a preliminary report on 44 patients. Trans Ophthal Soc UK 88:211, 1968.
85. Coleman, SL, Green, WR, Partz, A: Vascular tufts of pupillary margin of iris. Am J Ophthal 83:881, 1977.
86. Meades, KV, Francis, IC, Kappagoda, MB, Filipic, M: Light microscopic and electron microscopic histopathology of an iris microhaemangioma. Br J Ophthal 70:290, 1986.
87. Mason, GI: Iris neovascular tufts. Relationship to rubeosis, insulin, and hypotony. Arch Ophthal 97:2346, 1979.
88. Cobb, B, Shilling, JS, Chisholm, IH: Vascular tufts at the pupillary margin in myotonic dystrophy. Am J Ophthal 69:573, 1970.
89. Perry, HD, Mallen, FJ, Sussman, W: Microhaemangiomas of the iris with spontaneous hyphaema and acute glaucoma. Br J Ophthal 61:114, 1977.
90. Mason, GI, Ferry, AP: Bilateral spontaneous hyphema arising from iridic microhemangiomas. Ann Ophthal 11:87, 1979.
91. Hagen, AP-V, Williams, GA: Argon laser treatment of a bleeding iris vascular tuft. Am J Ophthal 101:379, 1986.
92. Campbell, DG, Simmons, RJ, Grant, WM: Ghost cells as a cause of glaucoma. Am J Ophthal 81:441, 1976.
93. Campbell, DG, Essigmann, EM: Hemolytic ghost cell glaucoma. Further studies. Arch Ophthal 97:2141, 1979.
94. Summers, CG, Lindstrom, RL: Ghost cell glaucoma following lens implantation. Am Intra-Ocular Implant Soc J 9:429, 1983.
95. Campbell, DG, Simmons, RJ, Tolentino, FI, McMeel, JW: Glaucoma occurring after closed vitrectomy. Am J Ophthal 83:63, 1977.
96. Brooks, AMV, Gillies, WE: Haemolytic glaucoma occurring in phakic eyes. Br J Ophthal 70:603, 1986.
97. Mansour, AM, Chess, J, Starita, R: Nontraumatic ghost cell glaucoma—case report. Ophthal Surg 17:34, 1986.
98. Cameron, JD, Havener, VR: Histologic confirmation of ghost cell glaucoma by routine light microscopy. Am J Ophthal 96:251, 1983.
99. Singh, H, Grand, MG: Treatment of blood-induced glaucoma by trans pars plana vitrectomy. Retina 1:255, 1981.
100. Fenton, RH, Zimmerman, LE: Hemolytic glaucoma. An unusual cause of acute open-angle secondary glaucoma. Arch Ophthal 70:236, 1963.
101. Phelps, CD, Watzke, RC: Hemolytic glaucoma. Am J Ophthal 80:690, 1975.
102. Grierson, I, Lee, WR: Further observations on the process of haemophagocytosis in the human outflow system. Graefes' Arch Ophthal 208:49, 1978.
103. Vannas, S: Hemosiderosis in eyes with secondary glaucoma after delayed intraocular hemorrhages. Acta Ophthal 38:254, 1960.

Chapter 22

GLAUCOMAS ASSOCIATED WITH OCULAR TRAUMA

CONTUSION INJURIES

General Features

Blunt injuries involving the eye are not uncommon. Young men appear to be most prone to such trauma. In a series of 205 patients with ocular contusion injuries, 85% were males and 75% were less than 30 years of age.[1] Sporting and domestic accidents accounted for nearly two-thirds of these injuries, with the remaining known causes being divided between industrial accidents and malicious acts. Among 32 patients who were hospitalized for sports-related ocular contusion, ball games were the most common cause.[2] Boxing is an especially high-risk sport for ocular trauma, which was seen in 66% of one series of 74 boxers.[3]

Clinical Findings

The anterior segment is the portion of the eye most frequently damaged by blunt trauma, and *hyphema* is the most common mode of clinical presentation, occurring in 81% of the eyes in one series.[1] The management of traumatic hyphema was discussed in Chapter 21. As the blood clears, ruptures in various structures of the anterior segment may be found (Fig. 22.1). The most common of these is *angle recession*, which is seen by gonioscopy as an irregular widening of the ciliary body band (Fig. 22.2). Histologically, this represents a tear between the longitudinal and circular muscles of the ciliary body. The reported prevalence of angle recession in eyes with traumatic hyphemas ranges from 60 to 94%.[4–8] Angle abnormalities were noted in more than half of the 32 patients with sports-related ocular contusion[2] and in 19% of the 74 boxers.[3] Other associated injuries include *iridodialysis*, a tear in the root of the iris (Fig. 22.3), and *cyclodialysis*, which is a separation of the ciliary body from the scleral spur. Patients with blunt ocular trauma may also present with iritis, cataracts, or dislocation of the lens.

Mechanisms of Glaucoma

Early Postinjury Period. A patient with a recent blunt ocular injury may present with a slightly reduced intraocular pressure (IOP). This may result from a reduction in aqueous production because of the associated iritis or possibly a temporary increase in outflow facility as a consequence of the

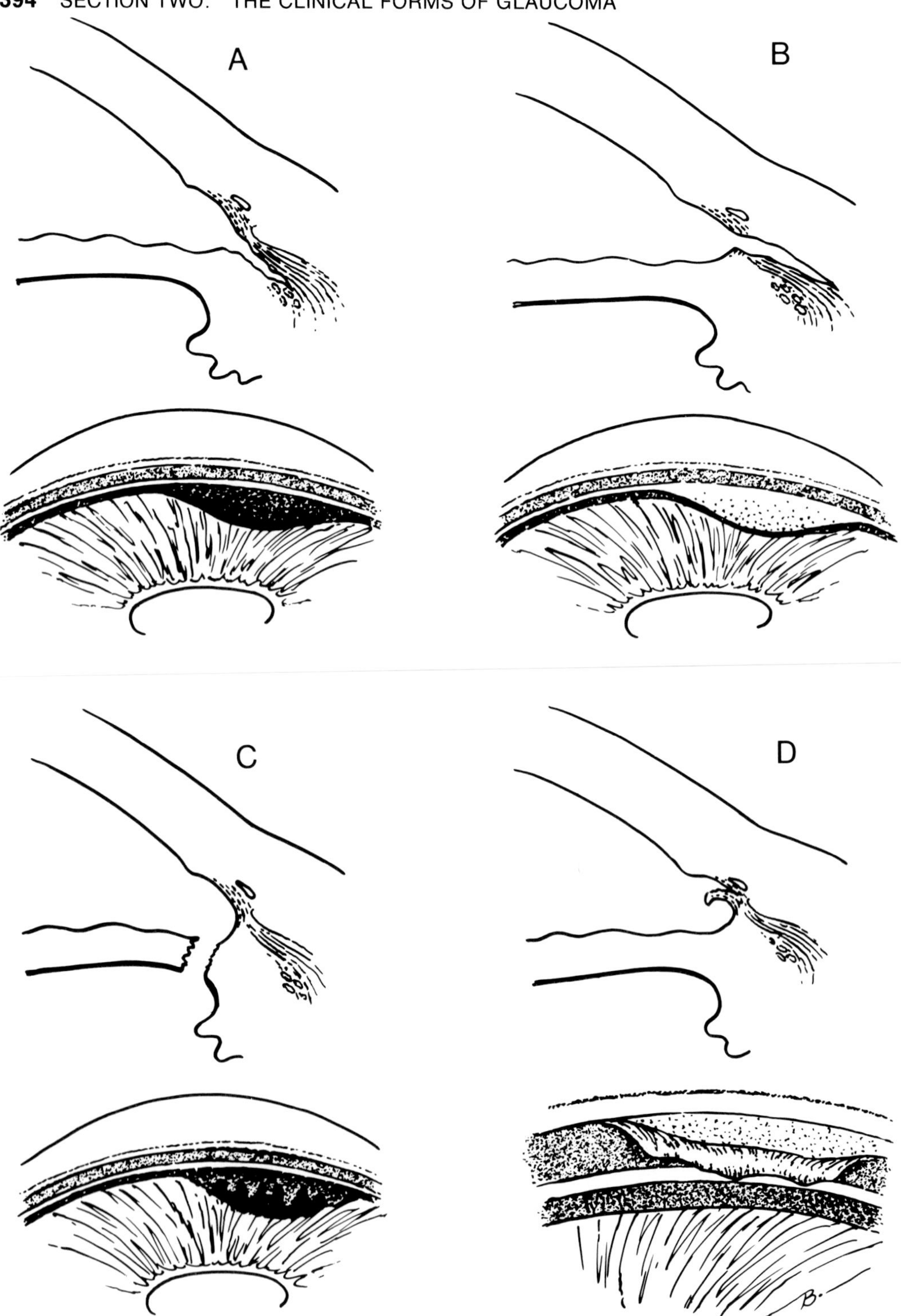

Figure 22.1. Forms of anterior chamber angle injury associated with blunt trauma, showing cross-sectional and corresponding gonioscopic appearance: **A,** Angle recession (tear between longitudinal and circular muscles of ciliary body); **B,** Cyclodialysis (separation of ciliary body from scleral spur, with widening of suprachoroidal space); **C,** Iridodialysis (tear in root of iris); and **D,** Trabecular damage (tear in anterior portion of meshwork, creating a flap that is hinged at the scleral spur).

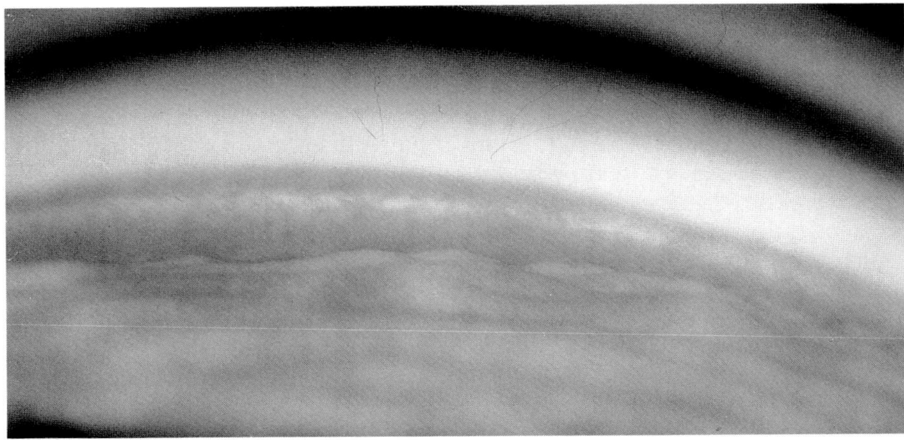

Figure 22.2. Gonioscopic view of eye with angle recession, characterized by the irregular widening of the ciliary body band. (Courtesy of L. Frank Cashwell, M.D.)

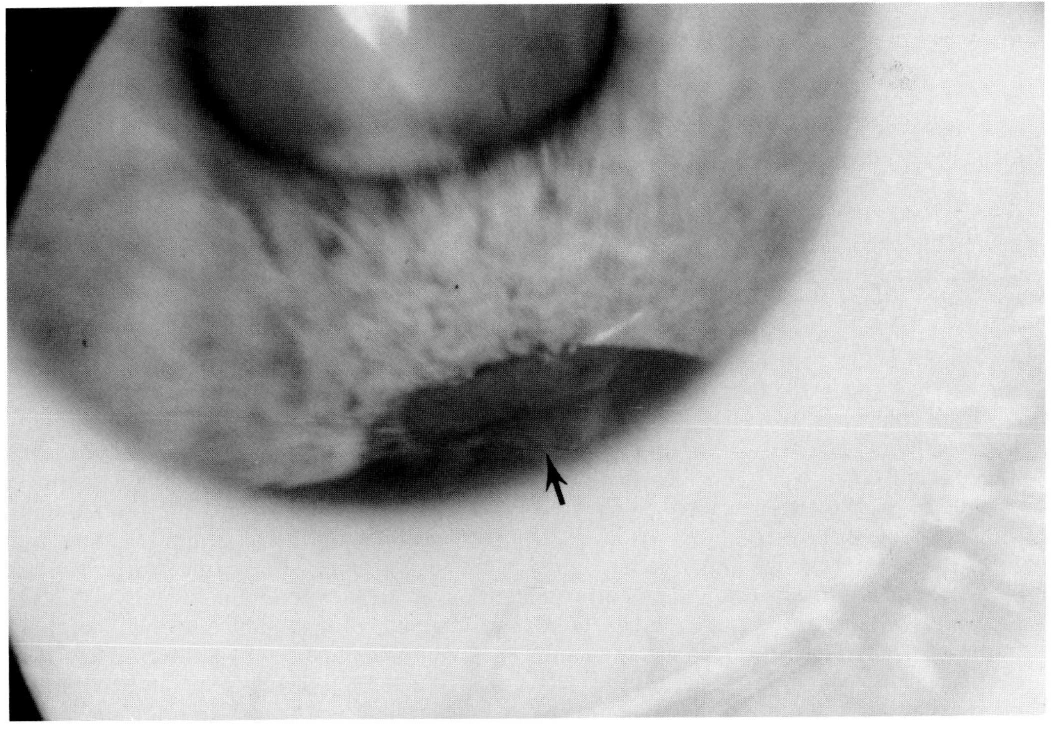

Figure 22.3. Slit-lamp view of eye with iridodialysis (*arrow*).

disruption of structures in the anterior chamber angle.

Other patients may have an elevated IOP during the early postcontusion period. In some cases, this may be a transient elevation, which lasts for one to several weeks and occurs in the absence of any other obvious damage to the eye. The anterior chamber angle is grossly normal as shown by gonioscopy, and the mechanism of the pressure rise is unknown. The secondary pressure elevation may also result from the traumatic iritis, hyphema, or dislocation of the lens, the mechanisms of which were discussed in previous chapters (19, 21, and 15, respectively). Other reported mechanisms of elevated IOP associated with blunt trauma to the eye include shallowing of the anterior chamber as a result of uveal effusion[9,10] and vitreous's filling a deep anterior chamber.[11]

Late Postinjury Period. Although the elevated IOP following blunt ocular trauma is transient in most cases, it is important to follow these patients indefinitely, since a reported 4–9% of those with angle recessions greater than 180° will eventually, often many years later, develop a chronic glaucoma.[5,7,12,13] This condition has been called *angle recession glaucoma,* although the term is somewhat of a misnomer, since the angle recession is not the actual cause of the obstruction to aqueous outflow. The clinicopathologic correlation between blunt injury to the eye and the delayed development of glaucoma was noted by Wolff and Zimmerman,[14] who suggested that the angle recession provided evidence of past injury but was not the actual cause of the glaucoma. They suggested that initial trauma to the trabecular meshwork stimulated proliferative and/or degenerative changes in the trabecular tissue, which led to obstruction of aqueous outflow. Herschler[15] supported this concept by observations of clinical cases and animal studies that revealed tears in the trabecular meshwork just posterior to Schwalbe's line, during the early posttrauma period. This produced a flap of trabecular tissue, which was hinged at the scleral spur (Fig. 22.1). With time, scarring ensued, causing the initial trabecular injury to be less apparent but also leading to chronic obstruction in portions of the aqueous outflow system.

Another mechanism of delayed IOP elevation, in addition to alterations within the trabecular meshwork, is the extension of an endothelial layer with a Descemet's-like membrane from the cornea over the anterior chamber angle.[14,16,17] Additional factors may influence which eyes with a history of blunt trauma will develop chronic secondary glaucoma. For example, the majority of eyes that eventually develop glaucoma after blunt injury appear to have an underlying predisposition to reduced aqueous outflow, as evidenced by frequent alterations of IOP in the fellow eye.[8,15,18] Among 13 patients who developed angle recession glaucoma an average of 34 years following trauma, seven had definite or suspicious glaucomatous visual field loss in the fellow eye.[18] It has also been noted that elderly patients are more susceptible to late postcontusion pressure elevation.[13]

Management of Glaucoma

Elevated IOP in the early postinjury period is best controlled medically, if possible, primarily with drugs that reduce aqueous production, such as carbonic anhydrase inhibitors and topical beta-blockers. Concomitant disorders, such as inflammation, hyphema, and dislocation of the lens, must also be managed as discussed in previous chapters. Eyes with a shallow anterior chamber and uveal effusion may respond to corticosteroids and mydriatic-cycloplegics.[9]

Chronic IOP elevation resulting from trabecular damage does not respond well to standard medical therapy. In one reported case with associated angle recession, pilocarpine caused a paradoxic pressure rise, while cycloplegics lowered the tension.[19] The authors theorized that the reduction in conventional outflow, combined with the tear in the ciliary body, may have shifted the eye to a predominantly uveoscleral mechanism of aqueous outflow, which is known to be impaired by miotics. They suggested that cycloplegics may have therapeutic value in these cases. In addition, drugs that reduce aqueous production may be more efficacious in eyes with scarring of the trabecular meshwork. Laser trabeculoplasty has not had a high success rate in this form of glaucoma, although it should usually be tried when medical therapy is ineffective, before going to filtering surgery.

Occasionally, blunt trauma may lead to chronic hypotony resulting from cyclodialysis, and application of argon laser to the cleft may correct the problem.[20]

PENETRATING INJURIES

General Features

Penetrating injuries of the eye may result from blunt force, sharp lacerations, or missiles. In a study of 453 patients, the relative frequency of these three sources of trauma was 22, 37, and 41%, respectively.[21] As with the nonpenetrating injuries, young men are most vulnerable to these types of accidents. Eighty-six percent of the patients in the above study were males, and the mean age of the entire group was 26 years.[21]

The IOP immediately after a penetrating injury is usually reduced, because of the open wound or the associated iridocyclitis. Following closure of the corneal or scleral wound, however, secondary glaucoma may develop as a result of intraocular tissue changes induced by the penetrating injury.

Mechanisms of Glaucoma

Tissue Disruption. During the early postinjury period, the IOP may be elevated because of inflammation, hyphema, or angle closure from a swollen, disrupted lens. As these conditions subside, more chronic mechanisms of secondary glaucoma may follow. In some cases, a cyclitic membrane may develop as the result of inflammatory material. This arises from the nonpigmented ciliary epithelium and organizes on a scaffold of lens, iris, anterior hyaloid, or whatever tissue may remain after the injury.[22] The membrane may lead to closure of the anterior chamber angle by forward displacement of the lens-iris diaphragm or by seclusion of the pupil with subsequent iris bombé. Failure to reform a flat anterior chamber or adequately treat the inflammation may lead to chronic pressure elevation as a result of peripheral anterior synechiae. Additional, rare causes of delayed elevation of IOP include sympathetic ophthalmia and epithelial ingrowth, which are discussed in Chapters 19 and 23, respectively.

Retained Intraocular Foreign Bodies. These bodies may be associated with the same tissue disruption and secondary glaucoma as noted above. In addition, prolonged intraocular retention of certain metallic foreign bodies may lead to delayed tissue alterations. *Siderosis* results from the intraocular retention of ferrous metal (iron) but may also be due to intraocular hemorrhage (the ionized form of iron is indistinguishable from hemosiderin). This material can cause structural alterations in tissues throughout the eye. Glaucoma may be a complication of advanced cases, although there is no proof that trabecular outflow is impaired by iron staining of the trabecular structures. Copper is also oxidized within the eye and can lead to *chalcosis,* with tissue damage that is nearly as severe as that encountered with ferrous foreign bodies. Glaucoma appears to be less common in these patients, although retinal changes may lead to visual field defects that might be confused with those of glaucoma.[23]

Management of Glaucoma

The best way to avoid loss of vision from glaucoma following penetrating ocular injuries is to minimize the development of chronic aqueous outflow obstruction by proper treatment of the initial injury. This may include removal of portions of incarcerated uveal tissue, aspiration of the lens if disrupted or swollen, anterior vitrectomy, removal of foreign bodies, meticulous closure of the wound, and reformation of the anterior chamber. In some cases it is necessary to close the wound initially and perform the intraocular surgery with vitreous instruments at a later date. In a series of 112 such patients, the final visual result was best when the vitrectomy was done within 72 hours of the injury.[22] Corticosteroid therapy to avoid cyclitic membranes and scarring in the anterior chamber angle is also important during the early postinjury period, and antibiotic therapy is required as prophylaxis against endophthalmitis.

Antiglaucoma medication may be required for control of transient pressure elevations during the early postinjury period as well as subsequent chronic secondary glaucoma, and drugs that reduce aqueous production are preferable in both situations. When medical therapy is insufficient, especially in the chronic cases, surgical intervention is indicated. Laser trabeculoplasty is usually not possible because of peripheral anterior synechiae, in which case filtering surgery should be recommended. In siderosis bulbi, removal of the intraocular foreign body by vitrectomy techniques may be beneficial in some cases.[24]

CHEMICAL BURNS

Alkali burns of the eye may produce a rapid initial rise in the IOP. This is often followed by a return to normal or subnormal pressure and then a slower, sustained elevation of tension.[25] Possible mechanisms of the early pressure rise include shrinkage of the cornea and sclera[25] and an increase in uveal blood flow.[26] The altered blood flow dynamics may be mediated by prostaglandins,[26] which may also be associated with the later IOP elevation.[25] A hypopyon may also develop and contribute to the pressure rise.

In managing the secondary glaucoma associated with an alkali burn of the cornea, topical corticosteroids may be helpful if a significant inflammatory component is present. It has been shown in rabbits that topical steroids can be used for the first week without increasing the risk of corneal melting, but not thereafter.[27] In addition, the presence of prostaglandins during the delayed pressure rise suggests that the early use of drugs that inhibit prostaglandin synthesis, such as indomethacin and imidazole, may be beneficial. Antiglaucoma agents, especially those that reduce aqueous production, are also frequently required in these cases. As with other forms of anterior uveitis, miotics usually should be avoided.

Acid burns of the cornea have been shown to cause an IOP response in rabbits similar to that seen with alkali burns.[28] A rapid tension increase, lasting up to 3 hours, is believed to result from shrinkage of the outer ocular coats, while a subsequent sustained rise is considered to be mediated by prostaglandin release.[28] Treatment of secondary glaucoma in these cases is similar to that for alkali burns.

RADIATION DAMAGE

Radiation therapy to structures near the eyes may lead to elevation of IOP.[29] The mechanism of pressure rise is not understood in all cases, although some rises result from neovascular glaucoma or intraocular hemorrhage secondary to retinal radiation damage. Medical therapy should be used when possible, although surgical intervention, such as filtering surgery or a cyclodestructive procedure, is often required, and the prognosis is generally poor.

SUMMARY

The most common form of ocular trauma that may lead to IOP elevation is blunt, or contusion, injuries. These may cause an early pressure rise as a result of iritis, hyphema, or lens dislocation, or a delayed secondary glaucoma from scarring of the damaged trabecular meshwork. Penetrating injuries may also cause an elevation of tension because of tissue disruption in the anterior chamber angle or in association with the retention of intraocular foreign bodies, such as iron and copper. In addition, either alkali or acid burns may cause a pressure rise, the mechanisms of which may include collagen shrinkage and prostaglandin release. Radiation damage is another, rare cause of secondary glaucoma.

References

1. Canavan, YM, Archer, DB: Anterior segment consequences of blunt ocular injury. Br J Ophthal 66:549, 1982.
2. Gracner, B, Kurelac, Z: Gonioscopic changes in ocular contusions sustained in sports. Klin Monatsbl Augenheilkd 186:128, 1985.
3. Giovinazzo, VJ, Yannuzzi, LA, Sorenson, JA, et al: The ocular complications of boxing. Ophthalmology 94:587, 1987.
4. Howard, GM, Hutchinson, BT, Frederick, AR: Hyphema resulting from blunt trauma. Gonioscopic, tonographic, and ophthalmoscopic observations following resolution of the hemorrhage. Trans Am Acad Ophthal Otol 69:294, 1965.
5. Blanton, FM: Anterior chamber angle recession

and secondary glaucoma. A study of the after effects of traumatic hyphemas. Arch Ophthal 72:39, 1964.

6. Tonjum, AM: Gonioscopy in traumatic hyphema. Acta Ophthal 44:650, 1966.
7. Mooney, D: Angle recession and secondary glaucoma. Br J Ophthal 57:608, 1973.
8. Spaeth, GL: Traumatic hyphema, angle recession, dexamethasone hypertension, and glaucoma. Arch Ophthal 78:714, 1967.
9. Dotan, S, Oliver, M: Shallow anterior chamber and uveal effusion after nonperforating trauma to the eye. Am J Ophthal 94:782, 1982.
10. Kutner, BN: Acute angle closure glaucoma in nonperforating blunt trauma. Arch Ophthal 106:19, 1988.
11. Samples, JR, Van Buskirk, EM: Open-angle glaucoma associated with vitreous humor filling the anterior chamber. Am J Ophthal 102:759, 1986.
12. Kaufman, JH, Tolpin, DW: Glaucoma after traumatic angle recession. A ten-year prospective study. Am J Ophthal 79:648, 1974.
13. Thiel, H-J, Aden, G, Pulhorn, G: Changes in the chamber angle following ocular contusions. Klin Monatsbl Augenheilkd 177:165, 1980.
14. Wolff, SM, Zimmerman, LE: Chronic secondary glaucoma. Associated with retrodisplacement of iris root and deepening of the anterior chamber angle secondary to contusion. Am J Ophthal 54:547, 1962.
15. Herschler, J: Trabecular damage due to blunt anterior segment injury and its relationship to traumatic glaucoma. Trans Am Acad Ophthal Otol 83:239, 1977.
16. Lauring, L: Anterior chamber glass membranes. Am J Ophthal 68:308, 1969.
17. Iwamoto, T, Witmer, R, Landolt, E: Light and electron microscopy in absolute glaucoma with pigment dispersion phenomena and contusion angle deformity. Am J Ophthal 72:420, 1971.
18. Tesluk, GC, Spaeth, GL: The occurrence of primary open-angle glaucoma in the fellow eye of patients with unilateral angle-cleavage glaucoma. Ophthalmology 92:904, 1985.
19. Bleiman, BS, Schwartz, AL: Paradoxical intraocular pressure response to pilocarpine. A proposed mechanism and treatment. Arch Ophthal 97:1305, 1979.
20. Alward, WLM, Hodapp, EA, Parel, J-M, Anderson, DR: Argon laser endophotocoagulator closure of cyclodialysis clefts. Am J Ophthal 106:748, 1988.
21. deJuan, E Jr, Sternberg, P Jr, Michels, RG: Penetrating ocular injuries. Types of injuries and visual results. Ophthalmology 90:1318, 1983.
22. Coleman, DJ: Early vitrectomy in the management of the severely traumatized eye. Am J Ophthal 93:543, 1982.
23. Rosenthal, AR, Marmor, MF, Leuenberger, P, Hopkins, JL: Chalcosis: a study of natural history. Ophthalmology 86:1956, 1979.
24. Sneed, SR, Weingeist, TA: Management of siderosis bulbi due to a retained iron-containing intraocular foreign body. Ophthalmology 97:375, 1990.
25. Paterson, CA, Pfister, RR: Intraocular pressure changes after alkali burns. Arch Ophthal 91:211, 1974.
26. Green, K, Paterson, CA, Siddiqui, A: Ocular blood flow after experimental alkali burns and prostaglandin administration. Arch Ophthal 103:569, 1985.
27. Donshik, PC, Berman, MB, Dohlman, CH, et al: Effect of topical corticosteroids on ulceration in alkali-burned corneas. Arch Ophthal 96:2117, 1978.
28. Paterson, CA, Eakins, KE, Paterson, E, et al: The ocular hypertensive response following experimental acid burns in the rabbit eye. Invest Ophthal Vis Sci 18:67, 1979.
29. Barron, A, McDonald, JE, Hughes, WF: Long-term complications of beta radiation therapy in ophthalmology. Trans Am Ophthal Soc 68:112, 1970.

Chapter 23

GLAUCOMAS FOLLOWING OCULAR SURGERY

Another large group of secondary glaucomas are those that occur as a complication of various ocular surgical procedures.

MALIGNANT (CILIARY BLOCK) GLAUCOMA

Terminology

In 1869, von Graefe[1] described a rare complication of certain ocular procedures, which was characterized by shallowing or flattening of the anterior chamber and an elevation of the intraocular pressure (IOP). He called the condition *malignant glaucoma,* because of the poor response to conventional therapy. Today, the concept of malignant glaucoma has been expanded to include a variety of clinical situations, which have the following common denominators: (1) shallowing or flattening of both the central and peripheral anterior chamber; (2) elevation of the IOP; and (3) unresponsiveness to or aggravation by miotics, but frequent relief with cycloplegic-mydriatic therapy.[2,3]

Studies regarding the mechanism of malignant glaucoma, which is considered later in this chapter, have led some authors to recommend new terms for this group of diseases. Based on the theory that obstruction of normal aqueous flow is due to apposition of the ciliary processes against the equator of the lens or the anterior hyaloid, the name *ciliary block glaucoma* was proposed.[4,5] The term *aqueous misdirection* is also commonly used to denote the concept of posterior diversion of the aqueous as a result of the ciliary block. To describe the concept that a forward shift of the lens pushes peripheral iris into the anterior chamber angle, the term *direct lens block angle closure* has also been suggested.[6] At the present time, there is no universal agreement regarding the terminology for this group of conditions, and the traditional term, malignant glaucoma, is retained for purposes of discussion in this text.

Clinical Forms

It has yet to be established whether all clinical conditions that are called malignant glaucoma should actually be included within a single disease category. Nevertheless, the following disorders have been described under that name.

Classic Malignant Glaucoma

This is the prototype and most common form of the disease group. It follows incisional surgical intervention for angle-closure glaucoma and is reported to complicate 0.6–4% of these cases.[2,3,7] Neither the type of surgery nor the level of IOP immediately prior to surgical intervention appears to be related to the postoperative development of malignant glaucoma.[3] However, partial or total closure of the anterior chamber angle at the time of surgery is associated with an increased incidence of this complication.[3] Furthermore, a primary angle-closure attack may be a predisposing factor, since malignant glaucoma, when it occurs, nearly always does so in an eye that has had an attack, even though the angle may be open preoperatively.[7] However, the condition rarely, if ever, follows a prophylactic iridectomy, when the angle is open at the time of surgery.[7] The condition usually occurs immediately after surgery but may also be seen months to years later, often corresponding to the cessation of cycloplegic therapy or the institution of miotic drops.[2,3]

Malignant Glaucoma in Aphakia

Although classic malignant glaucoma typically occurs in phakic eyes, it may persist after lens removal for treatment of the disease or develop after cataract extraction in eyes without preexisting glaucoma.[3] It is important to distinguish malignant glaucoma in aphakia from pupillary block glaucoma in aphakia,[8] which is considered later in this chapter.

Malignant Glaucoma in Pseudophakia

Malignant glaucoma may occur in association with an anterior chamber intraocular lens implant, presumably by the same mechanism as with malignant glaucoma in aphakia.[9] More recently, it has also been observed in eyes with posterior chamber implants, with or without an associated glaucoma filtering procedure.[10–13] A large posterior chamber intraocular lens optic (7 mm) in a small eye (axial length of 21.7 mm) was thought to be responsible for malignant glaucoma in one case, and caution is advised in these patients.[14]

Miotic-Induced Malignant Glaucoma

As noted above, the onset of classic malignant glaucoma may correspond to the institution of miotic therapy, suggesting a causal relationship.[15] In addition, similar clinical pictures have been described in unoperated eyes that were receiving miotic therapy[16] and in an eye treated with miotics after a filtering procedure for open-angle glaucoma.[17]

Malignant Glaucoma Associated with Inflammation

Inflammation and trauma have also been reported as precipitating factors of malignant glaucoma.[6] A form of malignant glaucoma has been reported in association with endophthalmitis secondary to fungal keratomycosis[18] and the atypical bacterium *Nocardia asteroides*.[19]

Malignant Glaucoma Associated with Retinal Disorders

Retinal detachment surgery was said to cause the "malignant glaucoma syndrome" in a patient who developed choroidal detachments after a buckling procedure.[20] The condition has also been reported in children with retinopathy of prematurity.[21]

Spontaneous Malignant Glaucoma

It has also been reported that malignant glaucoma may develop in an eye without previous surgery, miotic therapy, or other apparent cause.[22]

Theories of Mechanism

There is a lack of general agreement regarding the sequence of events responsible for the development of malignant glaucoma, although the following are the more popular theories.

Posterior Pooling of Aqueous

Shaffer[23] hypothesized that an accumulation of aqueous behind a posterior vitreous detachment causes the forward displacement of the iris-lens or iris-vitreous diaphragm, and the concept was subsequently expanded to include the pooling of aqueous within vitreous pockets. This theory has been supported by an ultrasonographic study of eyes with malignant glaucoma in aphakia, demonstrating echo-free zones in the vitreous from which aqueous was reportedly aspirated.[24] The mechanism(s) leading to the posterior diversion of aqueous is uncertain, although strong evidence supports the following possibilities.

Ciliolenticular (or ciliovitreal) Block. It has been observed in cases of malignant glaucoma that the tips of the ciliary processes rotate forward and press against the lens equator in the phakic eye, or against the anterior hyaloid in aphakia, which might create the obstruction to forward flow of aqueous (Figs. 23.1 and 23.2).[4,25] As previously noted, it was this concept that led to the proposed term "ciliary block glaucoma" as a substitute for malignant glaucoma.[4]

Anterior Hyaloid Obstruction. It has also been suggested that the anterior hyaloid may contribute to ciliolenticular block

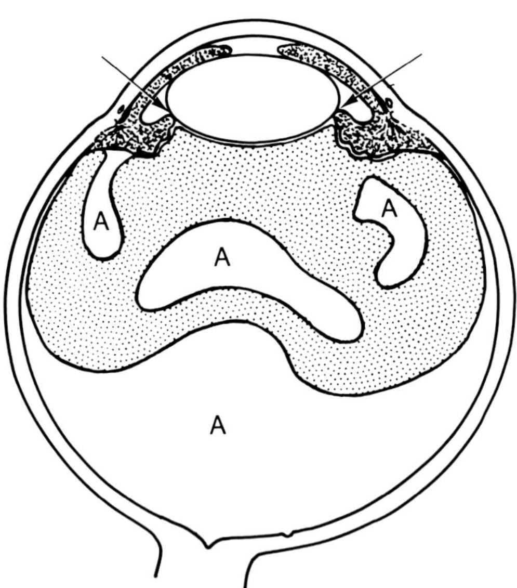

Figure 23.1. Concept of ciliolenticular block as the mechanism of malignant glaucoma. Apposition of ciliary processes to the lens equator (*arrows*) causes a posterior diversion of aqueous (*A*), which pools in and behind the vitreous with a forward shift of the lens-iris diaphragm.

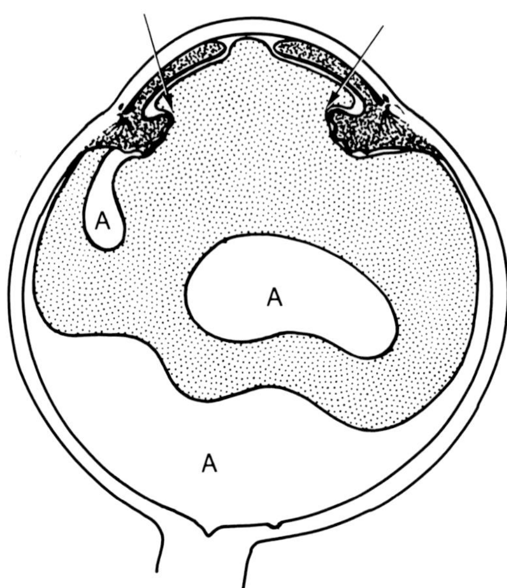

Figure 23.2. Concept of ciliovitreal block as the mechanism of malignant glaucoma in aphakia. Apposition of ciliary processes against the anterior hyaloid (*arrows*) leads to posterior diversion of aqueous (*A*), which causes a forward shift of the vitreous and iris.

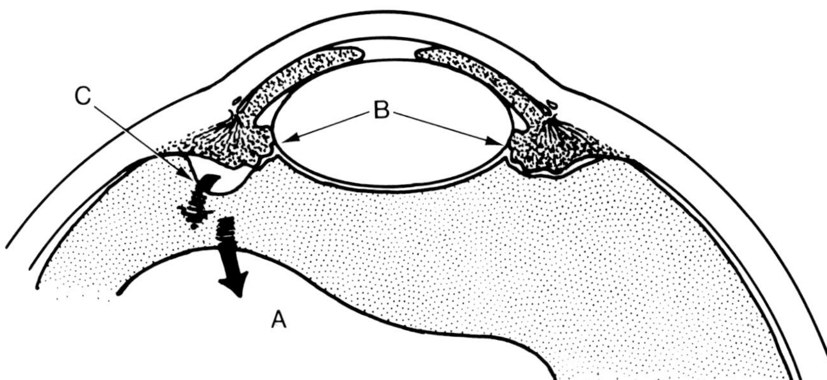

Figure 23.3. The anterior hyaloid may contribute to the ciliolenticular block (*B*), and breaks in the hyaloid near the vitreous base (*C*) may allow the aqueous (*A*) to be diverted posteriorly (*arrows*).

and that breaks in the hyaloid near the vitreous base possibly allow the posterior diversion of aqueous (Fig. 23.3).[5] However, the hyaloid breaks have a one-way valve effect, since fluid coming anteriorly closes the vitreous face against the ciliary body, preventing forward flow.[5] Some investigators have observed the ciliolenticular contact but note that the spaces between the ciliary processes are open, with vitreous visible behind them, suggesting that the obstruction to anterior aqueous flow is the anterior vitreous face, which is abnormally forward against the ciliary processes in both phakic and aphakic forms of malignant glaucoma.[3]

Perfusion studies with both animal[26] and human[27,28] eyes have shown that resistance to flow of a fluid through vitreous increases significantly with an elevation of pressure in the eye. It has been postulated that the increased resistance might be due to compression of the vitreous as well as its displacement against the ciliary body, lens, and iris, thereby reducing the available area of anterior hyaloid through which fluid could flow.[27,28] These clinical and laboratory observations support the concept that an intact anterior hyaloid may be important in preventing the forward movement of aqueous that has been trapped in or behind the vitreous.

Slackness of Lens Zonules

Chandler and Grant[29] have postulated that the forward movement of the lens-iris diaphragm in malignant glaucoma might be due to abnormal slackness or weakness of the zonules of the lens, as well as pressure from the vitreous. Others have also advocated this theory and suggested that the laxity of the zonules might be the result of severe, prolonged angle closure[7] or ciliary muscle spasm induced by surgery, miotics, inflammation, trauma, or unknown factors.[6] The concept that the lens subsequently pushes the peripheral iris into the anterior chamber angle, as noted earlier in this chapter, led to the proposed term "direct lens block angle closure."[6]

It seems very likely that malignant glaucoma is a multifactorial disorder, in which elements of all the aforementioned mechanisms may be involved to variable degrees.

Differential Diagnosis

The diagnosis of malignant glaucoma requires the exclusion of the following conditions.[3,5]

Pupillary Block Glaucoma

Pupillary block is the most difficult entity to distinguish from malignant glaucoma but must be ruled out before the latter diagnosis can be made. During slit-lamp biomicroscopy, attention should be directed to two questions. First, is there moderate depth to the central anterior chamber with bowing of the peripheral iris into the chamber angle as with pupillary block, or is the entire iris-lens

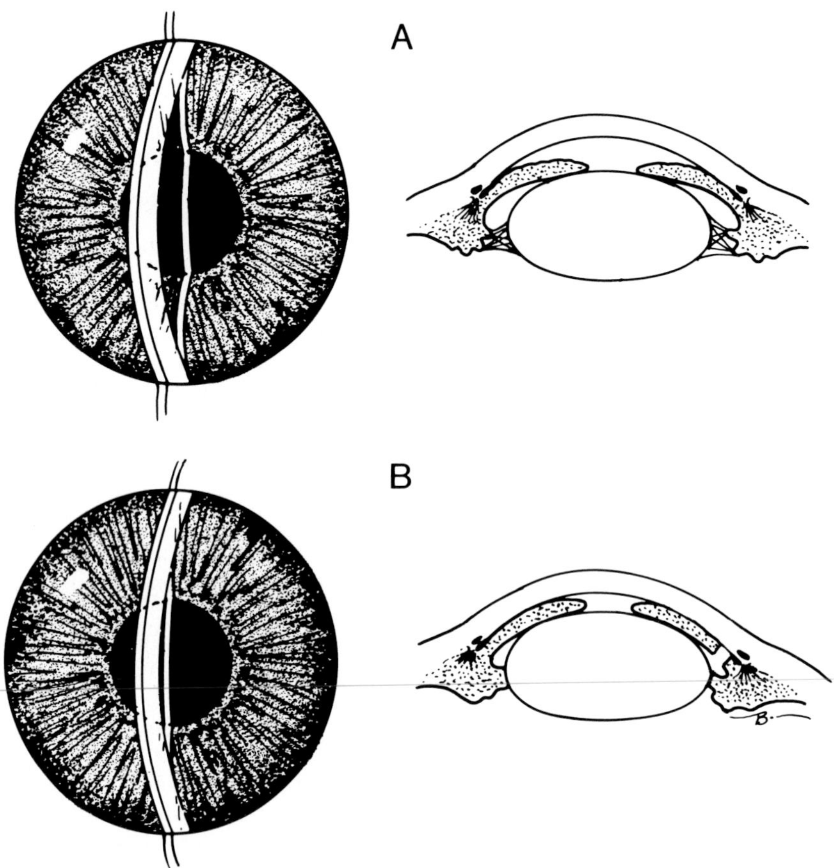

Figure 23.4. Distinctions between pupillary block glaucoma and malignant glaucoma: **A,** In pupillary block glaucoma, there is moderate depth to the central anterior chamber, with forward bowing of the peripheral iris and absence of a patent iridectomy. **B,** In malignant glaucoma, the entire lens-iris diaphragm is shifted forward with marked shallowing or loss of the central anterior chamber, and a patent peripheral iridectomy may be present.

or iris-vitreous diaphragm shifted forward with marked shallowing or loss of the central anterior chamber as with malignant glaucoma (Fig. 23.4)? Second, and probably of more diagnostic value, is a patent iridectomy present? If the iridectomy is clearly patent, a pupillary block is unlikely. However, if patency cannot be confirmed, the diagnosis of pupillary block cannot be ruled out, and one should proceed with an iridectomy.

Choroidal Detachments

Choroidal separation with serous fluid is common after glaucoma filtering procedures and might be confused with malignant glaucoma resulting from the shallow or flat anterior chamber. However, these eyes are typically hypotonous, and the light brown choroidal detachments are easily seen if there is adequate visibility of the posterior ocular segment, or otherwise they can be diagnosed by ultrasonography. Most choroidal detachments will resolve spontaneously. However, those that are persistent or massive with central touch can be approached surgically by making scleral incisions in the inferior quadrants. If a characteristic straw-colored fluid is obtained from the suprachoroidal space, the diagnosis of choroidal separation is confirmed, and the procedure is completed by reforming the anterior chamber with air and/or saline.

Suprachoroidal Hemorrhage

This may occur hours or days after ocular surgery and create shallowing or loss of the anterior chamber, which is typically associated with pain and elevated IOP. The eye is usually more inflamed than with choroidal detachment and the choroidal elevation is frequently dark reddish-brown. The surgical approach is the same as for choroidal detachments, except for the drainage of blood from the suprachoroidal space via the sclerotomies.

Management

Medical

Chandler and Grant[29] reported in 1962 that mydriatic-cycloplegic treatment was effective for malignant glaucoma, and the following year, Weiss and co-workers[30] recommended the use of hyperosmotics to combat this condition. The value of a cycloplegic may be both to pull the lens back by tightening the zonules[29] and to break a ciliary block,[5] while the presumed benefit of a hyperosmotic is to reduce the pressure exerted by the vitreous.[30] These two measures, along with a carbonic anhydrase inhibitor and/or topical beta-blocker to reduce the amount of aqueous that may be pooling posteriorly, constitute the standard medical approach to malignant glaucoma. A standard medical regimen includes the use of topical atropine four times daily, oral glycerol or intravenous mannitol, a topical beta-blocker, and oral acetazolamide or methazolamide. The patient should be maintained on atropine indefinitely after the attack is broken to prevent recurrences.

Surgical

The above medical regimen is curative in approximately half of the cases within 5 days.[2,3] If the condition persists beyond this time, surgical intervention is usually indicated. There is no clear-cut evidence as to which of several surgical approaches for malignant glaucoma is superior. In general, it is best to try one of the more conservative laser approaches first if circumstances permit. If this is not effective or feasible, the next step is either a posterior sclerotomy with air injection or an anterior vitrectomy, followed by lens removal if necessary.

Laser Techniques. Argon laser photocoagulation of the ciliary processes that can be visualized through an iridectomy, followed by medical therapy, has been reported to relieve malignant glaucoma, presumably by breaking the ciliolenticular block.[31] Other investigators have also found this approach to be effective, even without the concomitant use of cycloplegics,[32] although the latter drug should remain a standard part of the therapy for malignant glaucoma. The neodymium:YAG laser has also been effective in treating aphakic and pseudophakic malignant (ciliovitreal block) glaucoma by disrupting the anterior hyaloid face[33] or the posterior lens capsule and hyaloid face.[13]

Posterior Sclerotomy and Air Injection. A pars plana incision with aspiration of fluid from the vitreous and reformation of the anterior chamber with an air bubble (Fig. 23.5) is considered by some to be the procedure of choice for classic malignant glaucoma.[2,3,5] It has been suggested that the sclerotomy should be placed 3 mm posterior

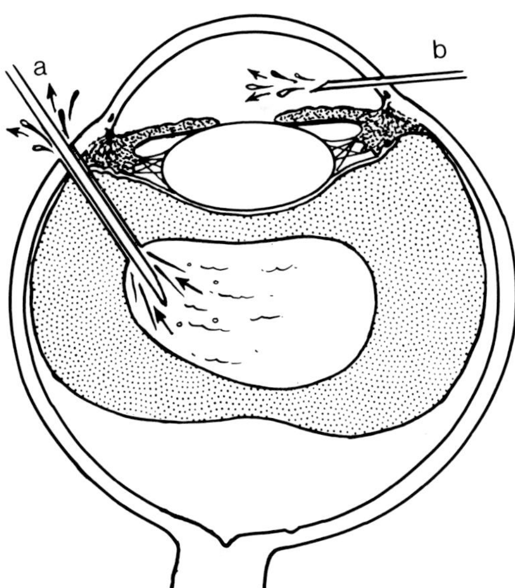

Figure 23.5. Posterior sclerotomy and air injection in the management of malignant glaucoma. Fluid is drained or aspirated from the vitreous via a pars plana incision (*a*), and the anterior chamber is deepened with air (*b*).

to the limbus to break the anterior hyaloid, thereby reducing its contribution to the blockade.[5] Postoperatively, patients are generally maintained on atropine to avoid recurrence.

Anterior Pars Plana Vitrectomy. Other surgeons prefer a careful removal of the anterior vitreous with vitrectomy instruments.[34–37] The reported results with both the posterior sclerotomy and the anterior vitrectomy techniques are favorable, while both also have a potential for serious complications. The choice in most cases will depend upon the surgeon's experience and preference.

Lens Extraction. Some surgeons favor this as the procedure of choice, while others use the approach if the posterior sclerotomy and air injection or anterior vitrectomy fails.[38] To be effective, lens extraction should be combined with an incision of the anterior hyaloid and possibly with deep incisions into fluid pockets in the vitreous.[2,3]

Other Surgical Approaches. Cyclocryotherapy has also been advocated, with the presumed mechanism being alteration in the ciliary body or vitreous.[39] Perilenticular incision of the vitreous was described by Chandler,[40] but the procedure was generally abandoned because of the significant risks involved.

Management of the Fellow Eye

When malignant glaucoma has occurred in one eye, there is a significant chance that it will develop in the fellow eye if surgery is performed following an acute angle closure attack. For this reason, it is best to do a prophylactic laser iridotomy early. However, if angle-closure glaucoma is present, every effort should be made to break the attack before surgery and, if the attack cannot be broken, mydriatic-cycloplegic therapy should be used vigorously postiridotomy and continued indefinitely.

GLAUCOMAS IN APHAKIA OR PSEUDOPHAKIA

Terminology

The terms "aphakic glaucoma" or "pseudophakic glaucoma" will occasionally be seen in the literature. They are mentioned in this text only to discourage their use, since they imply that a single form of glaucoma is associated with aphakia or pseudophakia. As will be seen in the following discussion, there are many mechanisms by which cataract extraction, with or without intraocular lens implantation, can lead to glaucoma, and it is best to refer to these glaucomas in aphakia or pseudophakia by terms that describe the particular events leading to the IOP elevation.

Incidence

The IOP may be elevated transiently in the early postoperative period or may become chronically elevated at any time after cataract surgery.

Aphakia

In the days before intraocular lens implantation, a rise in IOP during the first several days after cataract extraction was not uncommon, although the frequency of this complication undoubtedly varied according to the surgical technique. Early studies in which the corneoscleral incision was approximated with various numbers of silk or gut sutures revealed no significant difference between pre- and postoperative pressures[41] and only occasional, minor fluctuations in tonographic facilities of outflow.[42] However, in later series, in which multiple, fine sutures were used for tight wound closure, a significant IOP rise occurred in the early postoperative period in a high percentage of the eyes.[43,44]

Chronic glaucoma in aphakia was much less common than the early, transient form. In one series of 203 uncomplicated cataract extractions, secondary glaucoma occurred in 3% of the eyes.[45] However, these chronic cases posed a much greater threat to vision, as well as a much more difficult therapeutic challenge, than the eyes with transient pressure rise.

Pseudophakia

The advent of extracapsular cataract extraction and posterior chamber intraocular lens implantation has, in general, been associated with a reduced incidence of postoperative IOP complications. In one series of

373 eyes undergoing cataract surgery, those receiving intracapsular extraction and anterior chamber (133) or iris fixation (31) lenses had a late mean IOP rise of 0.8 mm Hg, while those undergoing extracapsular surgery with posterior chamber implants (209) had a mean IOP fall of 0.6 mm Hg.[46] However, the latter procedure is not without pressure complications in both the early and late postoperative periods. In eyes without preexisting glaucoma, more than half of one series had an IOP of 25 mm Hg or more 2–3 hours postoperatively,[47] while a pressure above 23 mm Hg on the first postoperative day was seen in 29% of eyes in another study.[48] Chronic secondary glaucoma was seen in 4% of eyes undergoing standard extracapsular extraction in one series[48] and in 2.1% of another large series.[49] Postoperative glaucoma also occurred in 11.3% of eyes receiving secondary anterior chamber implants.[50]

Extracapsular cataract extraction and posterior chamber intraocular lens implantation, as compared with intracapsular surgery, has also reduced, but not eliminated, IOP complications in eyes with preexisting glaucoma. In one comparative study, the former procedure was associated with a slightly more favorable pressure course, although an IOP above 21 mm Hg on the first postoperative day was seen with approximately half the eyes undergoing either operation.[51] However, late results indicate that most patients require the same medication as preoperatively, or less, to control their IOP.[52,53]

Mechanisms of Intraocular Pressure Elevation

Distortion of the Anterior Chamber Angle

Kirsch and co-workers[54,55] described the gonioscopic appearance of an internal white ridge resembling an inverted snow bank along the inner margins of the corneoscleral incision following routine cataract extraction. For approximately the first 2 weeks, the ridge typically obscures visualization of the trabecular meshwork and then gradually recedes over the next few months. There is some controversy regarding the pathogenesis of the internal ridge. Campbell and Grant[56] provided evidence that distortion of the anterior chamber angle is induced by tight corneoscleral sutures (Fig. 23.6), while Kirsch and co-workers[55] suggested that edema of the deep corneal stroma is the mechanism. Whatever the initiating factor(s) may be, the consequences of the ridge are known to include the formation of peripheral anterior synechiae, vitreous adhesions, and hyphema.[54] In addition, it is quite likely that the white ridge contributes, at least in some cases, to the early, transient pressure elevation after cataract surgery. In one study of 95 cataract extractions, early IOP rise occurred in 23% of the cases with limbal incisions but in none with corneal incisions, suggesting that distortion produced by the corneoscleral wound temporarily influences the adjacent trabecular meshwork and aqueous outflow.[57]

Influence of Alpha-Chymotrypsin

The enzyme alpha-chymotrypsin produces a selective disintegration of the lens zonules. Barraquer,[58] in 1958, demonstrated the value of the enzymatic zonulolysis in facilitating intracapsular cataract extraction, and the enzyme was commonly used for that purpose during the era of intracapsular surgery. In 1964, Kirsch[59] reported a study of 343 cataract extractions in which early, transient pressure rise occurred in 75% of the eyes in which 2–4 cc of a 1:5000 dilution of the enzyme was used, as compared with a 24% incidence of high pressures in a group without enzyme. The complication was somewhat more common in patients with preexisting open-angle glaucoma.[60] Tonographic studies showed a decrease in aqueous outflow facility,[61,62] although no abnormal parameters were noted 2–4 months postoperatively.[63] The enzyme-induced pressure response has been produced experimentally in monkeys,[64–66] and histologic studies of these eyes suggest that the pressure rise was due to an accumulation of lens zonule fragments, characterized by uniform segments of approximately 1000 Å[67] in the trabecular meshwork.[66,68]

Based on the above clinical and laboratory observations, the term *enzyme glaucoma* was often applied to those cases of early, transient IOP elevation with deep an-

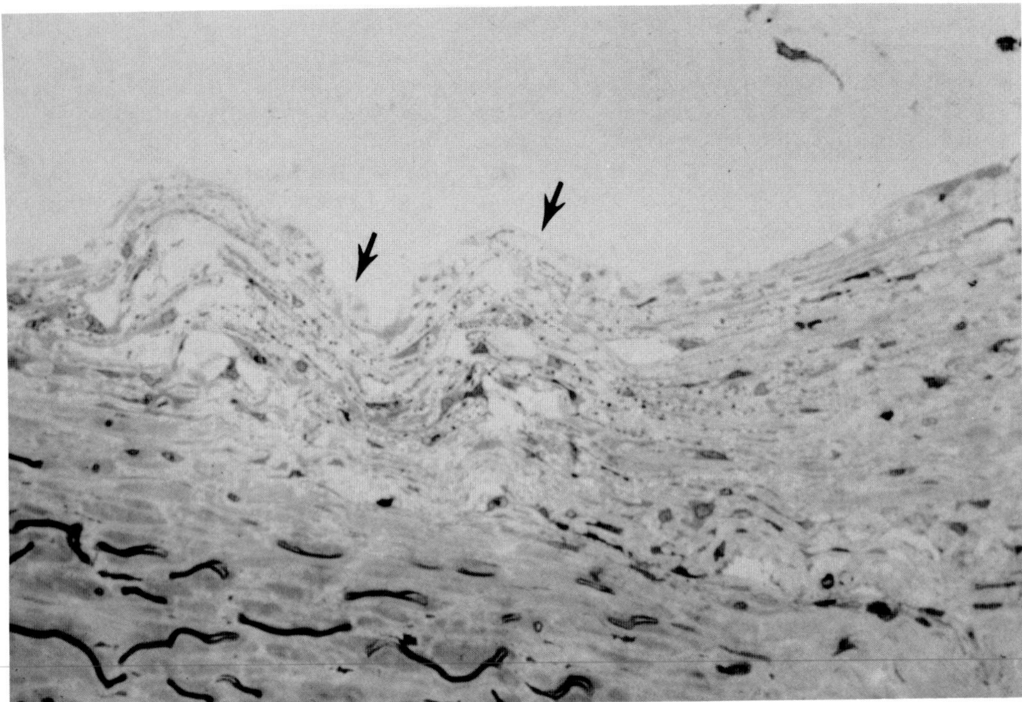

Figure 23.6. Light microscopic view of autopsy eye showing distortion of trabecular meshwork (*arrows*) resulting from placement of corneoscleral sutures as performed in routine cataract surgery. (Courtesy of David G. Campbell, M.D.)

terior chambers, in which the enzyme was used to facilitate intracapsular lens extraction. However, it is still uncertain how important the enzyme is in causing this complication of cataract surgery. Several studies noted no difference in the postoperative pressure course in groups with and without enzyme,[44,57,69] even in eyes with preexisting glaucoma.[70] It has been suggested that the volume or concentration of alpha-chymotrypsin might influence the enzyme-induced pressure response, in that eyes receiving 0.25–0.5 cc of 1:5,000–1:10,000 dilution had pressure responses similar to cases without enzyme.[69] Kirsch[71] also observed a dose relationship but still found a 55% incidence of high pressures in the early postoperative period following the use of 0.25 cc of 1:5000 alpha-chymotrypsin.

Influence of Viscoelastic Substances

To protect the corneal endothelium during certain stages of cataract extraction and intraocular lens implantation, it has become common practice to fill the anterior chamber with a viscous aqueous substitute. The viscoelastic substance most often used for this purpose is *sodium hyaluronate*. While some surgeons have noted no significant postoperative pressure rises associated with the use of sodium hyaluronate,[72,73] others have documented high pressures in the first few days after surgery.[74,75] Sodium hyaluronate injected into the anterior chamber of rabbit and monkey eyes caused marked pressure rises,[76] and perfusion in enucleated human eyes decreased the outflow facility by 65%.[77] This was not reversed by vigorous anterior chamber irrigation, but facility was restored to baseline by irrigation with hyaluronidase.[77] Clinically, aspiration of sodium hyaluronate at the end of cataract surgery did not significantly reduce the incidence or degree of postoperative IOP rise in one study.[78]

Alternative viscoelastic substances have also been evaluated. *Chondroitin sulfate* has been shown to cause minimal pressure elevation when used during lens implantation in a variety of animal eyes[79] or when injected as a 10% concentration into the anterior chamber of rabbit and monkey eyes.[76] A formulation of chondroitin sulfate and sodium hyaluronate was compared with sodium hyaluronate and found to be less advantageous during cataract surgery and to still cause IOP rises in the immediate postoperative period in many patients.[80] *Methylcellulose* 1–2% has not been found to cause a significant postoperative pressure rise in either animal[77] or human[81] eyes and appears to provide good protection of the corneal endothelium.[81] A 2% solution of hydroxypropylmethylcellulose was compared with balanced salt solution and found to have the same effect on corneal thickness with no rise in IOP.[82]

Inflammation and Hemorrhage

Transient postoperative inflammation occurs to some degree after every cataract extraction. When the inflammation is excessive, obstruction of the trabecular meshwork by inflammatory cells and fibrin may lead to IOP elevations. The inflammatory response and secondary glaucoma may be particularly prominent when lens fragments are retained in the vitreous following extracapsular cataract extraction.[83]

Intraocular lens implants increase the risk of serious postoperative uveitis, especially with anterior chamber and iris-supported lenses.[84] This may be associated with hyphema and glaucoma, which has been referred to as the "UGH" (uveitis, glaucoma, and hemorrhage) syndrome.[85,86] Uveitis was particularly common with the iris-supported lenses, apparently because of the movement of the lens against the iris and the subsequent cellular reaction.[87,88] The mechanism of inflammation and hemorrhage with anterior chamber lenses is believed to be contact of the rough posterior surface of the lens with the iris, and the degree to which this occurs is apparently related to the design and quality of the specific lens.[85,86,89] Posterior chamber lenses are least likely to induce uveitis. Fluorophotometric studies have shown that pseudophakic eyes with a posterior chamber lens and an intact posterior lens capsule have minimal alteration in the blood-aqueous barrier.[90–92] Nevertheless, the UGH syndrome after posterior chamber lens implantation has been described.[93]

In addition to the hyphema associated with uveitis, bleeding in the aqueous or vitreous compartments may be seen immediately after cataract surgery or as a late or recurring complication. One source of the late hemorrhage is new vessels in the corneoscleral wound.[94] Intraocular lens implantation may also be complicated by late or recurrent hemorrhage, which has been reported with anterior chamber,[95] iris fixation,[96] and posterior chamber implants.[97,98] The latter usually have sulcus fixation, and the mechanism in all cases is presumably an erosion into the adjacent tissue.[99] Postoperative bleeding from any source may lead to IOP elevation by the mechanisms discussed in Chapter 21, including ghost cell glaucoma from a vitreous hemorrhage.[100]

Pigment Dispersion

Variable amounts of pigment granules, primarily from the iris pigment epithelium, are dispersed into the anterior chamber with all cataract operations. If the degree of pigment dispersion is excessive, it can lead to a transient IOP elevation in either aphakic or pseudophakic eyes, with the latter occasionally leading to a chronic form of glaucoma.

Pseudophakic pigmentary glaucoma is most often associated with posterior chamber lenses.[101–104] The mechanism appears to be rubbing of the iris pigment epithelium against the periphery and haptics of the intraocular lens, leading to the dispersion of pigment granules that obstruct the trabecular meshwork, similar to the situation with phakic pigmentary glaucoma. Pigment granules on the central corneal endothelium (Krukenberg spindle) is an occasional but not consistent finding. The granules may also be seen circulating in the aqueous of the anterior chamber, especially after pupillary dilation. However, the most diagnostic finding is iris transillumination defects at the sites of contact with the implant. The iris may also have pigment granules on the stroma, and blue irides may have a grayish discoloration.[102] Gonioscopy will reveal heavy pigmentation of the trabecular meshwork.

Vitreous Filling the Anterior Chamber

Grant[105] described a mechanism of acute open-angle glaucoma in which vitreous humor fills the anterior chamber after cataract surgery. He reported that this can be cured in some cases by mydriasis to minimize pupillary block, while other eyes require miosis to draw the vitreous from the angle. Simmons[106] noted that many cases will resolve spontaneously in several months. When surgical intervention is required, an iridotomy may be curative, while other eyes will require an anterior vitrectomy.[107]

Pupillary Block

In Aphakia. This is a relatively rare complication of cataract extraction but tends to occur more commonly with round pupil extractions.[108,109] It is particularly likely to occur weeks after a transient flat anterior chamber secondary to a wound leak. The condition may also be more common following surgery for congenital cataracts, and a combination of sector and peripheral iridectomies with multiple sphincterotomies was reported to minimize this complication.[110] With modern techniques of congenital cataract surgery, such measures are probably not necessary, although a peripheral iridectomy is still advisable.

The pathogenesis of pupillary block in aphakia is believed to be an adherence between the iris and anterior vitreous face, which prevents aqueous flow into the anterior chamber either through the pupil or iridectomy. The aqueous accumulates in pools behind the iris, causing a forward shift of the iris and closure of anterior chamber angle (Fig. 23.7). The mechanism may be dependent on an intact anterior hyaloid, since fluorescein studies have shown that aqueous will flow through spontaneous openings in the vitreous face.[111] It may be possible to distinguish this condition from the much less common malignant glaucoma in aphakia by the deeper central anterior chamber and forward bowing of the peripheral iris in the former situation (Fig. 23.8), although such a distinction is often difficult.

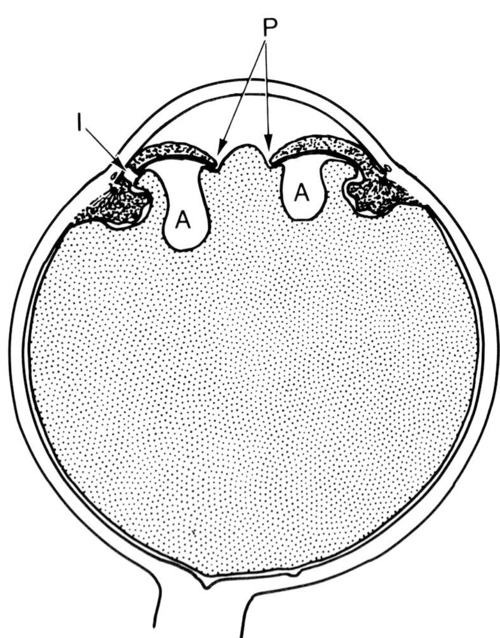

Figure 23.7. Pupillary block in aphakia. An adherence between the iris and anterior vitreous face blocks the flow of aqueous into the anterior chamber at both the pupil (*P*) and iridectomy site (*I*). The posterior accumulation of aqueous (*A*) causes forward bowing of the peripheral iris with closure of the anterior chamber angle.

In Pseudophakia. Pupillary block glaucoma in pseudophakia was once seen most often with anterior chamber[112–114] and iris-supported[115,116] lenses, although there have now been numerous reports of this complication following posterior chamber lens implantation.[112,117–120] It usually appears in the early period after surgery but may occur months or years later. Many cases are asymptomatic and are discovered during a routine postoperative examination. Some may even have a normal IOP, although peripheral anterior synechiae and chronic pressure elevation usually follow if the peripheral anterior chamber depth is not promptly restored. With anterior chamber lenses, the iris bulges forward on either side of the lens (Fig. 23.9), while the mechanism with posterior chamber lenses appears to be excessive inflammation with posterior synechiae to the intraocular lens. In either case, the situation can usually, but not always, be avoided with an adequate iridectomy.

There has been a tendency to omit peripheral iridectomies in association with extracapsular cataract extraction and posterior chamber lens implantation. This is largely based on the belief that the iridectomy is not necessary and that the additional surgical step may increase surgical complications, such as bleeding, inflammation, iridodialysis, inadvertent cutting of the lens haptic, and postoperative glare.[121,122] However, the growing number of reported cases of pupillary block in these eyes argues against this philosophy. To minimize the potential complications of peripheral iridotomy with posterior chamber lens implantation, modified iris scissors with a fine forcep tooth at the tip of each blade (iridotomy scissor-forceps) was designed to allow cutting of a small iridotomy with a single pinching, cutting motion without removing the iris from the eye.[123]

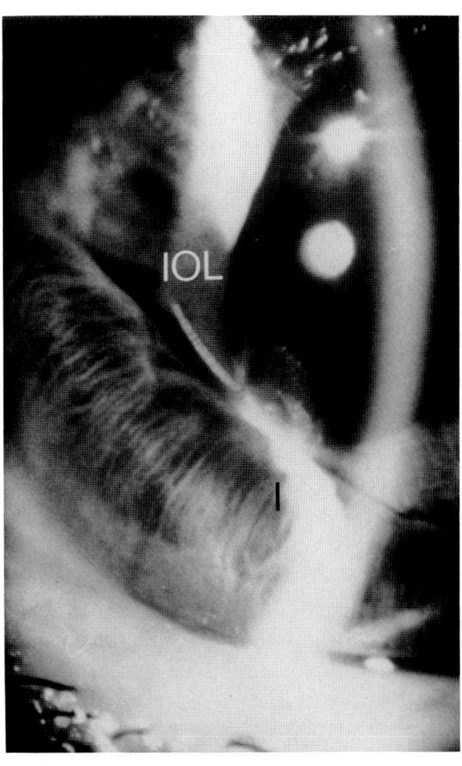

Figure 23.9. Slit-lamp view of pupillary block in pseudophakia showing forward bulging of iris (*I*) peripheral to margin of anterior chamber intraocular lens (*IOL*).

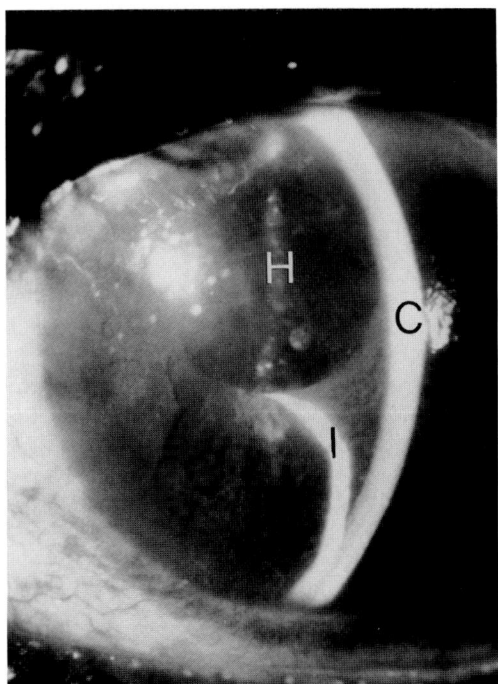

Figure 23.8. Slit-lamp view of eye with pupillary block in aphakia showing hyaloid face (*H*) well back from cornea (*C*) centrally, but peripheral anterior bowing of iris (*I*) with closure of anterior chamber angle.

Peripheral Anterior Synechiae and/or Trabecular Damage

In most cases of chronic glaucoma in aphakia or pseudophakia, peripheral anterior synechiae are present, presumably as a result of a flat anterior chamber and/or excessive inflammation in the early postoperative period. Flat anterior chambers after cataract surgery may be due to a *wound leak* with subsequent hypotony and choroidal detachments. This leads to a vicious cycle, since the choroidal detachments cause decreased aqueous production with further hypotony and also contribute to the forward shift of the iris and vitreous. To avoid the complication of peripheral anterior synechiae and chronic glaucoma, a flat anterior chamber should be corrected promptly. In one series of 203 uncomplicated cataract extractions, 47% had some degree of peripheral anterior synechiae, and all of those with secondary glaucoma had goniosynechiae in more than one-fourth of the angle.[45] In some cases, peripheral anterior synechiae may develop over the lens haptics months after the surgery and continue to progress over time.[124]

In other cases of glaucoma in aphakia or pseudophakia, the angle may be open in all quadrants and appear normal, except for variable degrees of increased pigmentation. This condition may occur in both adults and children. In one series of pediatric aphakic patients, the prevalence of chronic glaucoma was 6.1%.[125] The use of a vitrectomy instrument for aspiration, with wide excision of the posterior capsule, has been reported to reduce the incidence of this complication.[125] The mechanism of aqueous outflow obstruction in cases of chronic open-angle glaucoma in aphakia or pseudophakia is uncertain but most likely relates to alterations within the trabecular meshwork as a result of the surgery and possibly to a preexisting reduction in outflow facility.

Epithelial Ingrowth

In this condition, also referred to as *epithelial downgrowth,* an epithelial membrane grows into the eye through a penetrating wound. It extends over the posterior surface of the cornea, causing corneal edema, and also grows down across the anterior chamber angle and onto the iris, which may lead to secondary glaucoma. It is reported to occur in 0.09–0.12% of eyes after cataract surgery,[126–128] although the incidence appears to be declining with newer cataract techniques.[128] It may also occur after penetrating trauma,[129] penetrating keratoplasty,[130] and glaucoma surgery.[131]

Early in the disease process, a wound leak may be demonstrated by the Seidel test. By slit-lamp biomicroscopy, the epithelial ingrowth on the cornea is seen as a thin gray translucent or transparent membrane with a scalloped, thickened leading edge. Specular microscopy is reported to reveal a characteristic pattern of cell borders, which may have some diagnostic value.[131] The membrane on the iris is more difficult to see, but it typically causes a flattening of the stroma and can be delineated by the characteristic white burns that result from diagnostic laser photocoagulation.[132] Gonioscopy often reveals peripheral anterior synechiae, and glaucoma may be present. Cytologic evaluation of an aqueous aspirate has been described as a diagnostic aid,[133,134] although the clinical features are usually sufficient to establish the diagnosis.

A wound leak is generally believed to be the initial factor leading to epithelial ingrowth and is frequently seen at the time of diagnosis.[132,135,136] Reports differ as to whether the condition is more likely to occur with a fornix-based conjunctival flap during cataract surgery, as opposed to a limbus-based flap.[126,127] Ultrastructural studies show well-developed epithelium, resembling that of the bulbar conjunctiva, growing over the posterior cornea, anterior chamber angle, and iris.[137–140] Mechanisms that have been proposed for the glaucoma secondary to epithelial ingrowth include the growth of epithelium over the trabecular meshwork, areas of necrosis in the trabecular meshwork, peripheral anterior synechiae, pupillary block, or desquamated epithelium in the aqueous outflow system.[126,137,140,141]

Fibrous Proliferation

Two forms of this condition have been described: fibrous ingrowth and retrocorneal membranes. *Fibrous ingrowth* is the result of inadequate wound closure after intraocular surgery or penetrating trauma. It has been reported to occur in approximately one-third of eyes enucleated after cataract extraction.[142,143] The hallmark of this form of fibrous proliferation is a break in the corneal endothelium and Descemet's membrane, which allows fibroblasts to enter the anterior chamber from subepithelial connective tissue[144] or from corneal or limbal stroma.[145,146] The fibrous tissue, which is often vascularized, may grow over the corneal endothelium, anterior chamber angle, and iris, and into the vitreous cavity. Peripheral anterior synechiae are frequently seen in these cases.[146] Clinically, the condition may be difficult to distinguish from epithelial ingrowth, although it is usually less progressive and less destructive. When glaucoma is present, it may be the result of either damage from the surgery or trauma from the direct effect of the fibrous tissue in the anterior chamber angle. *Retrocorneal membranes* may result from a variety of inflammatory or traumatic insults to the cornea. Descemet's membrane is typically intact and the fibrous tissue is believed to represent metaplastic endothelial cells.[147] Glaucoma is not commonly associated but may result from the initial insult.

Melanocyte Proliferation

A proliferation of melanocytes from the iris across the trabecular meshwork and posterior surface of the cornea has also been described as a mechanism of secondary glaucoma following cataract extraction.[148]

Neodymium:YAG Laser Posterior Capsulotomy

Another cause of IOP elevation after cataract surgery, with or without intraocular lens implantation, is the use of neodymium:YAG (Nd:YAG) laser to perform a discission in the posterior lens capsule following extracapsular cataract extraction, whenever that structure becomes opacified following the initial surgery. The procedure may be associated with significant pressure elevation.[149–159] The pressure rise may be detected within the first few hours and usually returns to baseline within 1 week, although some may last for several weeks, and one large series revealed persistent pressure elevation 6 months postoperatively in 0.8% of the cases.[151] Cases have been reported in which the laser-induced pressure elevation caused progressive glaucomatous visual field loss[152] or transient loss of light perception requiring emergency paracentesis.[153] Risk factors for significant IOP elevations after Nd:YAG capsulotomy include preexisting glaucoma or a preoperative pressure above 20 mm Hg, larger capsulotomies, a sulcus rather than capsular fixed posterior chamber lens,[159] the absence of a posterior chamber lens, myopia, vitreoretinal disease, and vitreous prolapse into the anterior chamber.[160]

The mechanism of IOP elevation following Nd:YAG capsulotomy is not fully understood, although tonographic studies have shown that it is related to reduced aqueous outflow.[154] Possible causes of outflow obstruction include pupillary block resulting from forward movement of the vitreous and obstruction of the trabecular meshwork with fibrin, inflammatory cells, or debris from the capsule or cortical remnants.[157,161,162] In one case, herniated vitreous occluded a preexisting glaucoma surgical fistula, causing an acute pressure rise.[158] Pretreatment with indomethacin did not reduce the postoperative pressure rise,[163] while pretreatment with timolol[163,164] or pre- and posttreatment with apraclonidine[165] has been shown to minimize the early postoperative rise in IOP.

Anterior capsulotomies have also been evaluated in animal eyes, which produced pressure rises in all cases, presumably because of outflow obstruction by liquified cortical material.[166] In human cases, IOP elevations occurred at varying intervals after laser surgery but were usually transient.[167]

Management

Preoperative Considerations

In preparing for a cataract operation, certain considerations may help to minimize the risk of postoperative complications related to glaucoma, particularly in eyes with preexisting glaucoma. For example, in administering retrobulbar anesthesia it may be best not to include *epinephrine* in the analgesic mixture for fear of the influence this could have on perfusion of the optic nerve head.

Pressure Reducers. Many surgeons elect to reduce the vitreous volume and IOP by applying external pressure to the globe before surgery to maintain a deep anterior chamber and to minimize the potential complications of vitreous loss and expulsive hemorrhage. The external force may be accomplished by digital pressure, a rubber ball with an elastic band around the head, or a pneumatic rubber balloon (Honan intraocular pressure reducer). Each technique has the potential risk of optic atrophy or arterial occlusion from the excessive or prolonged application of pressure, and the Honan device may be the safest in this regard by allowing monitoring of the pressure in the balloon. Although the IOP does not correlate directly or linearly with the pressure in the Honan balloon, studies suggest that it is safe in normotensive eyes, especially when the instrument is set at 30 mm Hg for 5 minutes.[168] However, the induced IOP rise is a function of the initial ocular tension, and marked pressure elevations may occur in eyes with initial levels above 30 mm Hg, indicating the need for extreme caution in these cases.[168]

Selection of Intraocular Lens. As noted earlier, posterior chamber intraocular lens implantation in association with extracapsular cataract extraction, while not devoid of potential glaucoma-related complications, is generally associated with a slight reduction in postoperative IOP and is well tolerated even in eyes with advanced preexisting glaucoma. However, preoperative glaucoma or anterior chamber angle abnormalities are relative contraindications to the implantation of anterior chamber intraocular lenses. In one study of 18 normotensive eyes with angle-supported lenses, synechiae developed around the haptics in 12 cases,[169] which can lead to aqueous outflow obstruction, especially in eyes with preexisting glaucoma. In another study, anterior chamber lens implantation in eyes with preoperative peripheral anterior synechiae was associated with corneal endothelial cell loss, fibrous endothelial metaplasia, and angle cicatrization.[170] In addition, as previously discussed, anterior chamber lens implantation is associated with an increased incidence of other mechanisms of secondary glaucoma.

Intraoperative Considerations

Attention to gentle handling of tissues, hemostasis, and minimal intraocular manipulation may reduce the risk of postoperative IOP rise associated with hemorrhage or excessive inflammation or pigment dispersion. In addition, judicious use of intraocular agents such as viscoelastic substances and alpha-chymotrypsin, especially in eyes with preexisting glaucoma, may help to minimize the risk of postoperative glaucoma complications.

Another class of agents that are often injected into the eye during cataract surgery are the miotics *acetylcholine* and *carbachol,* which are used to constrict the pupil, especially after posterior chamber intraocular lens implantation. Acetylcholine, as compared with balanced salt solution, is associated with lower IOPs at 3 and 6 hours postoperatively, although the difference was not statistically significantly different at 24 hours.[171] Carbachol, on the other hand, is associated with lower postoperative pressures, as compared with either acetylcholine or balanced salt solution, at 24 hours, 2 days, and 3 days postoperatively.[172–175] Therefore, the intracameral use of carbachol may be helpful in avoiding early IOP rises, especially in eyes with preexisting glaucoma.

Early Postoperative Period

The IOP has been noted to rise within 6–7 hours after routine cataract extraction and generally returns to normal within 1 week. A modest pressure rise (e.g., less than 30 mm Hg) in an eye with a deep anterior chamber is usually of no consequence and requires no antiglaucoma therapy. However, high pressures may cause pain and occasional disruption of the corneoscleral wound. Furthermore, eyes with preexisting glaucoma and advanced glaucomatous optic atrophy may have further nerve damage with even short episodes of pressure elevation. In addition, anterior ischemic optic neuropathy has been reported to occur during these periods of elevated pressure in eyes with vulnerable optic nerve head circulation.[176] Therefore, if there is pain or a threat to the optic nerve head, cornea, or cataract incision, temporary medical measures should be employed.

A number of drugs have been evaluated for efficacy in controlling the early IOP rise in eyes with *open anterior chamber angles.* While the results are somewhat conflicting, both acetazolamide[177–179] and timolol[179–184] are generally believed to be useful in these cases. One study compared levobunolol, timolol, and betaxolol, and found the former to be the most effective of the three beta-blockers in controlling the early postcataract IOP rise.[185] Pilocarpine drops were not believed to be of value in one study,[178] although pilocarpine gel was found to be effective in another study, without significantly increasing postoperative inflammation.[186] Pilocarpine has also been shown to be effective in controlling the transient pressure rise following Nd:YAG posterior capsulotomy.[187] As previously noted, apraclonidine is particularly effective for the latter condition and may also be useful for other mechanisms of transient postcataract pressure rise.[165] Epinephrine is generally avoided because of the danger of macular edema.[188] Steroids were reported to be ineffective in one study[178] but may be helpful in controlling the pressure when inflammation is excessive. Indomethacin and aspirin have also been shown to reduce the postoperative pressure rise, presumably by inhibiting prostaglandin synthesis.[189] When uveitis and glaucoma are associated with retained lens fragments in the vitreous, pars plana vitrectomy is reported to yield good results.[83]

Uveitis, glaucoma, and *hyphema* may be managed with either mydriatics or miotics to minimize iris movement against the lens in mild cases. In more severe cases, steroids should be employed for the iritis and a carbonic anhydrase inhibitor or topical beta-blocker for the glaucoma. Argon laser photocoagulation may be effective in controlling the hemorrhage if the bleeding sites are visible.[97] Recurrent hyphema and glaucoma is usually an indication to remove the lens, although this is often difficult and can lead to significant intraoperative complications. When glaucoma secondary to blood in the anterior chamber is associated with vitreous hemorrhage, pars plana vitrectomy has been recommended.[190] *Pigment dispersion in pseudophakia* can usually be controlled medically and gradually becomes easier to manage in most cases. Removal of the lens is rarely required.

Pupillary block in aphakia may be treated initially with mydriasis to break the block, although an iridotomy is usually required.[108,109] To be effective, the iridotomy must be placed over a pocket of aqueous behind the iris, rather than an area in which the vitreous is in broad apposition to the posterior surface of the iris. The laser is particularly useful in these cases, since more than one iridotomy can be made until an aqueous pocket is found, as evidenced by a deepening of the peripheral anterior chamber. Suggested alternative surgical approaches include separating the iris from the vitreous adhesions with laser iridoplasty[191] or an iris repositor[192] and pars plana vitrectomy.[193]

Pupillary block in pseudophakia may be broken with mydriatic therapy by enlarging the pupil beyond the edges of an anterior chamber lens or by lysing posterior synechiae from a posterior chamber lens. Carbonic anhydrase inhibitors, hyperosmotics, and a topical beta-blocker may also be required as an emergency measure. The definitive treatment is an iridotomy, which is best achieved with a laser when possible. The laser may also be used to dilate the pupil.[194] Closed vitrectomy has also been used to relieve pseudophakic pupillary block.[195]

Late Postoperative Period

The majority of patients with chronic glaucoma in aphakia or pseudophakia can and should be managed medically. Miotic therapy is frequently effective, as is the use of drugs that reduce aqueous production, such as carbonic anhydrase inhibitors and topical beta-blockers. Epinephrine is usually avoided because of the danger of macular edema.[188] Surgical intervention is reserved for cases that are uncontrolled on maximum tolerable medical therapy. Laser trabeculoplasty may be effective in those cases without extensive peripheral anterior synechiae and is the initial surgical procedure of choice.[196] When strict IOP and visual acuity criteria are used to define success, no surgical procedure is highly effective for chronic glaucoma in aphakia or pseudophakia.[197] In one series of trabeculectomies in 82 aphakic eyes, less than half were successful.[198] However, other surgeons have had somewhat better results and believe that trabeculectomy is the procedure of choice if trabeculoplasty fails or is not possible.[196] The postoperative use of 5-fluorouracil has been shown to increase the success rate of filtering surgery in aphakic eyes.[199] Transscleral Nd:YAG cyclophotocoagulation has also been shown to be effective in chronic glaucoma in aphakia and pseudophakia.[200]

When *epithelial ingrowth* is present, radical surgical intervention is usually required. Maumenee[132] described a technique of excising the fistula and involved iris and destroying the epithelium on the posterior cornea with cryotherapy. Subsequent modifications have included en bloc excision of the involved chamber angle tissues,[201–203] excision of all involved tissue followed by keratoplasty,[202,203] and the use of vitrectomy instruments to remove involved iris and vitreous.[136] The implantation of a Molteno drainage device has also been shown to be effective palliative treatment for the secondary glaucoma in these cases.[204] In cases of *fibrous ingrowth,* treatment is generally confined to controlling the IOP, preferably with medications, although surgery, such as a cyclodestructive procedure, may be necessary.

GLAUCOMAS ASSOCIATED WITH PENETRATING KERATOPLASTY

Incidence

Penetrating keratoplasty, using modern techniques of tight wound closure, is complicated by a significant incidence of IOP elevation in both the early and late postoperative periods, although reported incidences vary considerably.[205–207] One study revealed a 31% incidence of early increases in IOP and a 29% incidence of late (more than 3 months) increases,[205] while another large survey had a 9% incidence of immediate postoperative glaucoma and an 18% incidence of chronic postkeratoplasty glaucoma.[207] Late, chronic glaucoma is more likely to occur in those eyes that had an early postoperative pressure rise.[206] Factors associated with glaucoma after penetrating keratoplasty are aphakia and preexisting glaucoma.[205–208] In one series, the average maximum pressure in the first week was 24 mm Hg in phakic eyes, 40 mm Hg in aphakic eyes, and 50 mm Hg in those with combined cataract extraction and keratoplasty.[209] When keratoplasty is combined with cataract extraction, the incidence of glaucoma is higher when an intracapsular extraction is used, as compared with extracapsular surgery.[210] The incidence of secondary glaucoma is also higher following repeated penetrating keratoplasty.[211] Glaucoma after corneal grafting is dangerous not only from the standpoint of glaucomatous optic atrophy but also from the high incidence of associated graft failures.[212]

Clinical Findings and Glaucoma Mechanisms

Early Postoperative Period

In some cases, the postoperative glaucoma after penetrating keratoplasty has the same pressure elevating mechanisms that are associated with other intraocular procedures, including uveitis, hemorrhage, pupillary block, and steroid-induced glaucoma.[213] However, additional mechanisms of secondary glaucoma occur early in the postoperative period, which are unique to eyes having undergone penetrating keratoplasty, especially when aphakia is also present. Two such mechanisms have been postulated.

Collapse of the trabecular meshwork may result from the loss of anterior support, because of the incision in Descemet's membrane, which may be compounded in the aphakic eye by a reduction in posterior support from the loss of zonular tension.[214,215] This hypothesis is considered to be supported by the observation that through-and-through suturing in one study was associated with better facility of outflow in autopsy eyes[214] and lower early postoperative IOP as compared with eyes with conventional suturing.[215] However, other surgeons reported less postoperative pressure rise with superficial sutures, which they believed prevented angle distortion.[216]

Compression of the anterior chamber angle may be caused by the conventional techniques of penetrating keratoplasty, causing an early postoperative IOP rise as well as subsequent chronic glaucoma resulting from peripheral anterior synechiae.[216,217] Modified techniques that may help to avoid this complication are discussed under "Management."

Late Postoperative Period

Gradual flattening of the anterior chamber several months after aphakic keratoplasty has been described.[218] This phenomenon appeared to be related to an intact anterior vitreous face, and prophylactic vitrectomy has been suggested to avoid this complication. Intraocular pressure elevation may also occur in association with graft rejection, which may require long-term steroid and antiglaucoma therapy.[219] The pigment dispersion syndrome may also be seen with pseudophakic corneal transplants, which has the unique feature of an inferior linear pigmented endothelial line, which must not be confused with an allograft reaction.[220] Another late-developing glaucoma occurs after keratoplasty for congenitally opaque corneas.[221] It is not associated with peripheral anterior synechiae, and the mechanism is unknown. Other forms of late-onset glaucoma may be due to peripheral anterior synechiae, steroid-induced glaucoma,[213] and epithelial ingrowth.[130,222]

Management

Preventive Measures

Based on a mathematical model, it has been postulated that the following factors may minimize angle compression and also improve trabecular support: (1) a donor graft that is larger than the recipient trephine; (2) looser or shorter suture bites to minimize tissue compression; (3) smaller trephine size; (4) a thinner peripheral host cornea; and (5) a larger host corneal diameter.[217,223] Reports are conflicting as to whether an oversized corneal donor graft improves outflow and reduces postkeratoplasty glaucoma. A perfusion study with autopsy eyes did not reveal an improvement in outflow,[224] and the use of 0.5 mm oversized grafts in one clinical series did not afford any protection against postoperative glaucoma.[225] However, other clinical studies indicate that oversized grafts are associated with deeper anterior chamber depths[226] and a lower incidence of progressive angle closure,[227] while other investigations of aphakic eyes revealed significantly lower postoperative pressure with oversized grafts as compared with eyes with same sized grafts.[228,229] However, oversize grafts are contraindicated in treating keratoconus, since they cause a significant increase in myopia.[230] Another technique to prevent postkeratoplasty angle-closure glaucoma is the placement of sutures near the pupillary portion of a flaccid iris to create a taut iris.[231] It has also been emphasized that glaucoma following keratoplasty can be minimized by using meticulous wound closure and extensive postoperative steroids.[232]

Treatment of Glaucoma

Medical therapy should be tried first, unless a specific, treatable condition, such as pupillary block, is apparent. However, attempts to alter the early postoperative pressure rise are frequently unsuccessful. Carbonic anhydrase inhibitors were not found to be significantly efficacious in this situation,[233,234] although they may be useful in treating the chronic glaucoma. Reported results with timolol have been conflicting,[216,234] although it does appear to have some value, especially in controlling chronic glaucoma after keratoplasty.[213] Hyperosmotic agents may be useful for the temporary control of extreme pressure elevation in the early postoperative period.[233] Miotics and epinephrine may also occasionally be of value.

Surgical therapy is indicated when either the optic nerve head or the graft is threatened by a persistent elevation of IOP. Cyclodialysis was successful in only 22 of 100 such cases in one study,[235] and another investigation found a 30% incidence of graft failure after any intraocular procedure.[236] Implantation of a Molteno drainage tube achieved IOP control of 21 mm Hg or less with one or more procedures in a series of 17 eyes, although seven had allograft rejections.[237] Cyclocryotherapy is the most commonly used surgical procedure for glaucoma following penetrating keratoplasty,[238] although this operation is not without serious potential complications, and newer cyclodestructive procedures, such as cyclophotocoagulation, may prove to be preferable.

GLAUCOMAS ASSOCIATED WITH VITREOUS AND RETINAL PROCEDURES

Glaucomas Following Pars Plana Vitrectomy

Incidence

Intraocular pressure elevation is the most common major complication following pars plana vitreous surgery.[239–244] The reported incidence of postoperative glaucoma ranges from 20 to 26%.[241–243] In a prospective study of 222 cases, an IOP rise of 5–22 mm Hg during the first 48 hours occurred in 61.3% of eyes, with a 30 mm Hg rise in 35.6%.[244]

Clinical Findings and Glaucoma Mechanisms

Most of the factors that lead to IOP elevation after pars plana vitrectomy and the management of these conditions have been considered in other chapters. It may be helpful to review these various mechanisms according to the time frame in which they occur after vitreous surgery.[242]

First Day. *Air* or long-acting gases, such as *sulfur hexafluoride* and *perfluorocarbons* (perfluoropropane and perfluoroethane), are occasionally injected into the vitreous cavity to tamponade the retina. The expansion of these gases during the early postoperative period not uncommonly leads to significant IOP elevation.[241–248] Perfluorocarbons are capable of greater expansion and longevity than is sulfur hexafluoride.[249] In one study of 10 patients receiving 0.3 ml perfluoropropane, all eyes had an immediate IOP rise, which was sufficient in four eyes to collapse the central retinal artery.[248] However, the pressure fell to baseline in 30–60 minutes and did not rise again for the subsequent 5 days.

Monitoring of IOP in the early postoperative period is important when using any long-acting gas, and attention must be given to the tonometer used. Studies with living rabbit and enucleated human eyes indicate that the Schiøtz tonometer gives falsely low readings,[250,251] which apparently is due to low scleral rigidity.[252] Pneumatic tonometry also underestimates IOP in gas-filled human autopsy eyes, while Perkins applanation tonometry gave the most accurate readings, when using a mercury manometer as a reference standard.[251] In a clinical study of 84 gas-filled eyes, the Tono-Pen gave pressure readings that were comparable to those obtained by Goldmann applanation tonometry, while pneumatic tonometry again underestimated the IOP.[253]

Occasionally, it is necessary to remove a portion of the gas to relieve extremely high IOPs.[241] Patients with a gas-filled eye should be cautioned regarding air travel, although expansion of a 0.6 ml bubble during ascent is usually compensated for by accelerated aqueous outflow without a significant IOP rise.[254,255] If the patient does notice pain or dimness of vision, the pilot should be asked to adjust the altitude to the next flight level.[255] On descent, the eye may become hypotonous, and drugs that reduce aqueous production should be avoided, since they may prolong the hypotony, leading to uveal effusion.[255]

Severe choroidal and ciliary body *hemorrhage,* the equivalent of an expulsive hemorrhage in open-eye surgery, can also cause angle closure glaucoma in the immediate postoperative period.[242]

First Week. Intraocular pressure elevation during this period most likely results from one of the following, all of which are discussed in other chapters: (1) hyphema, ghost cells, or hemolytic glaucoma (Chapter 21); (2) retained lens material with phacolytic glaucoma (Chapter 15); (3) uveitis (Chapter 19); and (4) preexisting glaucoma. Yet another cause of IOP elevation in the early postvitrectomy period is *fibrin pupillary block.*[256,257] This has been successfully treated by making holes in the fibrin pupillary membrane with argon laser[256] and by the intracameral injection of recombinant tissue plasminogen activator to dissolve the fibrin clot.[257]

Two to Four Weeks Postoperatively. At this point, the cause of newly developed glaucoma is almost invariably *neovascular glaucoma,* which is discussed in Chapter 16.

Silicone oil is occasionally used as a retinal tamponade in unusually difficult vitreoretinal procedures. The frequency with which this technique is associated with postoperative IOP elevation varies among studies, with some revealing a high percentage,[258–260] while one series showed no influence of silicone on ocular tension.[261] This discrepancy may relate to the numerous variables induced by the intraocular silicone as well as the underlying disease of the eye, which may reduce both aqueous outflow and inflow, with the resulting IOP representing a balance of the two. However, recent studies suggest that a high percentage of patients do have a transient postoperative pressure rise, with a small number retaining chronic secondary glaucoma.[262,263]

Mechanisms of IOP elevation that are directly attributable to the silicone include pupillary block[264–266] and silicone oil in the anterior chamber.[265,267] Histologic studies have shown obstruction of the trabecular meshwork by minute silicone bubbles, pigmented cells, and silicone-laden macrophages.[268,269] However, these findings are not always associated with glaucoma, possibly because of the pressure-lowering effect of ciliary body detachment by cyclitic membranes[260] or total retinal detachments.[270] Fibrous tissue has been shown to form around silicone vesicles, the retraction of which may lead to these detachments.[270]

An iridectomy may relieve not only the pupillary block mechanism but also some cases of open-angle glaucoma, by allowing the silicone to fall back into the vitreous cavity.[264–266] Since the silicone oil rises to the top of the eye, the iridectomy should be placed inferiorly, and this should be a standard part of all vitreoretinal procedures that include use of silicone. When the iridectomy does not relieve the chronic IOP elevation, antiglaucoma medications may be adequate, while other patients may require surgical intervention, including a cyclodestructive procedure and/or removal of the silicone oil.

Glaucoma Following Scleral Buckling Procedures

Scleral buckling procedures are reported to cause a transient shallowing of the anterior chamber with elevation of the IOP in 4–7% of the cases.[271] However, this is frequently asymptomatic and may go undetected unless slit-lamp biomicroscopy and tonometry are performed in the early postoperative period. Experimental studies with monkeys suggest that occlusion of the vortex veins by an encircling band or sectoral scleral indentation causes congestion and forward rotation of the ciliary body with subsequent shallowing of the anterior segment.[272] The same study showed that occlusion of the vortex veins also caused the ciliary processes to produce a protein-rich aqueous, which might further reduce outflow.[272] These changes in the early postoperative period rarely lead to serious sequelae. In fact, many eyes have reduced IOP months after retinal detachment surgery, which is due to a decrease in aqueous production.[273] However, peripheral anterior synechiae may develop with subsequent chronic glaucoma, and care must be taken, especially since reduced scleral rigidity in these patients may give falsely low IOP readings, especially with indentation tonometry.[274]

Treatment includes atropine to relieve ciliary muscle spasm and corticosteroids to reduce the inflammation and prevent synechia formation. Carbonic anhydrase inhibitors, topical beta-blockers, and epinephrine compounds may also be used when necessary for temporary pressure control. When surgical intervention is required, drainage of suprachoroidal fluid is usually the procedure of choice. A peripheral iridectomy is rarely of value in these cases.

Glaucoma Following Retinal Photocoagulation

An elevated IOP may follow extensive xenon or laser photocoagulation of the retina.[275–277] In many cases, the anterior chamber angle remains open, and the mechanism of pressure elevation in these eyes is unknown. Other patients will have a closed angle either initially or later in the course of the pressure elevation. The mechanism of angle closure is believed to be either swelling of the ciliary body[275] or an outpouring of fluid from the choroid to the vitreous with subsequent forward displacement of the lens-iris diaphragm.[276] The condition is temporary, with normal or slightly reduced pressures having been recorded after 1 month,[278] although an analysis of data from the Diabetic Retinopathy Study did not support the belief that panretinal photocoagulation may reduce IOP.[279] The pressure rise should be managed medically in the same manner described for the early pressure rise and shallow anterior chamber after scleral buckling.

SUMMARY

Malignant, or ciliary block, glaucoma occurs most often as a complication of conventional surgery for angle-closure glaucoma. The mechanism appears to be a posterior diversion of aqueous, leading to a collapse of the anterior chamber from forward vitreous displacement. Atropine is the mainstay of the medical therapy, although approximately half of the patients require surgical intervention. Another group of procedures that may be complicated by IOP elevation is cataract surgery. Causes of increased pressure during the early postoperative period include inflammation, hemorrhage, pigment dispersion, anterior chamber angle distortion, angle closure, vitreous in the anterior chamber, and the use of alpha-chymotrypsin or sodium hyaluronate. Chronic glaucoma following cataract surgery may result from peripheral anterior synechiae, trabecular meshwork damage, epithelial ingrowth, or fibrous proliferation. The implantation of an intraocular lens may induce some additional mechanisms of secondary glaucoma, associated with pupillary block, inflammation, hemorrhage, or pigment dispersion. Discission of the posterior lens capsule with a neodymium:YAG laser is yet another cause of IOP elevation in association with cataract surgery. Penetrating keratoplasty may be complicated by secondary glaucoma, with the common glaucoma mechanism being angle closure. Vitreoretinal procedures, including vitrectomy, the intravitreal injection of gas or silicone, scleral buckling, and retinal photocoagulation, may also be associated with postoperative IOP elevation.

References

1. von Graefe, A: Beitrage zur pathologie und therapie des glaucoms. Arch Fur Ophthal 15:108, 1869.
2. Chandler, PA, Simmons, RJ, Grant, WM: Malignant glaucoma. Medical and surgical treatment. Am J Ophthal 66:495, 1968.
3. Simmons, RJ: Malignant glaucoma. Br J Ophthal 56:263, 1972.
4. Weiss, DI, Shaffer, RN: Ciliary block (malignant) glaucoma. Trans Am Acad Ophthal Otol 76:450, 1972.
5. Shaffer, RN, Hoskins, HD Jr: Ciliary block (malignant) glaucoma. Ophthalmology 85:215, 1978.
6. Levene, R: A new concept of malignant glaucoma. Arch Ophthal 87:497, 1972.
7. Lowe, RF: Malignant glaucoma related to primary angle closure glaucoma. Aust J Ophthal 7:11, 1979.
8. Boke, W, Teichmann, KD: Differential diagnosis of postoperative glaucoma following iridectomy and filtering procedures. Klin Monatsbl Augenheilkd 177:545, 1980.
9. Hanish, SJ, Lamberg, RL, Gordon, JM: Malignant glaucoma following cataract extraction and intraocular lens implant. Ophthal Surg 13:713, 1982.
10. Tomey, KF, Senft, SH, Antonios, SR, et al: Aqueous misdirection and flat chamber after posterior chamber implants with and without trabeculectomy. Arch Ophthal 105:770, 1987.
11. Duy, TP, Wollensak, J: Ciliary block (malignant) glaucoma following posterior chamber lens implantation. Ophthal Surg 18:741, 1987.
12. Dickens, CJ, Shaffer, RN: The medical treatment of ciliary block glaucoma after extracapsular cataract extraction. Am J Ophthal 103:237, 1987.
13. Risco, JM, Tomey, KF, Perkins, TW: Laser capsulotomy through intraocular lens positioning holes in anterior aqueous misdirection. Arch Ophthal 107:1569, 1989.
14. Reed, JE, Thomas, JV, Lytle, RA, Simmons, RJ: Malignant glaucoma induced by an intraocular lens. Ophthal Surg 21:177, 1990.
15. Pecora, JL: Malignant glaucoma worsened by miotics in a postoperative angle-closure glaucoma patient. Ann Ophthal 11:1412, 1979.
16. Rieser, JC, Schwartz, B: Miotic-induced malignant glaucoma. Arch Ophthal 87:706, 1972.
17. Merritt, JC: Malignant glaucoma induced by miotics postoperatively in open-angle glaucoma. Arch Ophthal 95:1988, 1977.
18. Jones, BR: Principles in the management of oculomycosis. Trans Am Acad Ophthal Otol 79:15, 1975.
19. Lass, JH, Thoft, RA, Bellows, AR, Slansky, HH: Exogenous nocardia asteroids endophthalmitis associated with malignant glaucoma. Ann Ophthal 13:317, 1981.
20. Weiss, IS, Deiter, PD: Malignant glaucoma syndrome following retinal detachment surgery. Ann Ophthal 6:1099, 1974.
21. Kushner, BJ: Ciliary block glaucoma in retinopathy of prematurity. Arch Ophthal 100:1078, 1982.
22. Schwartz, AL, Anderson, DR: "Malignant glaucoma" in an eye with no antecedent operation or miotics. Arch Ophthal 93:379, 1975.
23. Shaffer, RN: The role of vitreous detachment in aphakic and malignant glaucoma. Trans Am Acad Ophthal Otol 58:217, 1954.
24. Buschmann, W, Linnert, D: Echography of the vitreous body in case of aphakia and malignant aphakic glaucoma. Klin Monatsbl Augenheilkd 168:453, 1976.
25. Lippas, J: Mechanics and treatment of malignant

glaucoma and the problem of a flat anterior chamber. Am J Ophthal 57:620, 1964.
26. Fatt, I: Hydraulic flow conductivity of the vitreous gel. Invest Ophthal Vis Sci 16:555, 1977.
27. Epstein, DL, Hashimoto, JM, Anderson, PJ, Grant, WM: Experimental perfusions through the anterior and vitreous chambers with possible relationships to malignant glaucoma. Am J Ophthal 88:1078, 1979.
28. Quigley, HA: Malignant glaucoma and fluid flow rate. Am J Ophthal 89:879, 1980.
29. Chandler, PA, Grant, WM: Mydriatic-cycloplegic treatment in malignant glaucoma. Arch Ophthal 68:353, 1962.
30. Weiss, DI, Shaffer, RN, Harrington, DO: Treatment of malignant glaucoma with intravenous mannitol infusion. Medical reformation of the anterior chamber by means of an osmotic agent: a preliminary report. Arch Ophthal 69:154, 1963.
31. Herschler, J: Laser shrinkage of the ciliary processes. A treatment for malignant (ciliary block) glaucoma. Ophthalmology 87:1155, 1980.
32. Weber, PA, Henry, MA, Kapetansky, FM, Lohman, LF: Argon laser treatment of the ciliary processes in aphakic glaucoma with flat anterior chamber. Am J Ophthal 97:82, 1984.
33. Epstein, DL, Steinert, RF, Puliafito, CA: Neodymium-YAG laser therapy to the anterior hyaloid in aphakic malignant (ciliovitreal block) glaucoma. Am J Ophthal 98:137, 1984.
34. Sugar, HS: Bilateral aphakic malignant glaucoma. Arch Ophthal 87:347, 1972.
35. Koerner, FH: Anterior pars plana vitrectomy in ciliary and iris block glaucoma. Graefe's Arch Klin Exp Ophthal 214:119, 1980.
36. Boke, W, Teichmann, K-D, Junge, W: Experiences with ciliary block (''malignant'') glaucoma. Klin Monatsbl Augenheilkd 177:407, 1980.
37. Momeda, S, Hayashi, H, Oshima, K: Anterior pars plana vitrectomy for phakic malignant glaucoma. Jap J Ophthal 27:73, 1983.
38. Bastian, A, Kohler, U: Therapy and functional results in malignant glaucoma. Klin Monatsbl Augenheilkd 161:316, 1972.
39. Benedikt, O: A new operative method for the treatment of malignant glaucoma. Klin Monatsbl Augenheilkd 170:665, 1977.
40. Chandler, PA: A new operation for malignant glaucoma: a preliminary report. Trans Am Ophthal Soc 62:408, 1964.
41. Galin, MA, Baras, I, Perry, R: Intraocular pressure following cataract extraction. Arch Ophthal 66:80, 1961.
42. Lee, P-F, Trotter, RR: Tonographic and gonioscopic studies before and after cataract extraction. Arch Ophthal 58:407, 1957.
43. Tuberville, A, Tomoda, T, Nissenkorn, I, Wood, TO: Postsurgical intraocular pressure elevation. Am Intra-Ocular Implant Soc J 9:309, 1983.
44. Rich, WJ, Radtke, ND, Cohan, BE: Early ocular hypertension after cataract extraction. Br J Ophthal 58:725, 1974.
45. Racz, P, Szilvassy, I, Pinter, E: Findings in the anterior chamber angle after cataract extraction without complication. Klin Monatsbl Augenheilkd 164:218, 1974.
46. Radius, RL, Schultz, K, Sobocinski, K, et al: Pseudophakia and intraocular pressure. Am J Ophthal 97:738, 1984.
47. Gross, JG, Meyer, DR, Robin, AL, et al: Increased intraocular pressure in the immediate postoperative period after extracapsular cataract extraction. Am J Ophthal 105:466, 1988.
48. Kooner, KS, Dulaney, DD, Zimmerman, TJ: Intraocular pressure following extracapsular cataract extraction and posterior chamber intraocular lens implantation. Ophthal Surg 19:471, 1988.
49. David, R, Tessler, Z, Yagev, R, et al: Persistently raised intraocular pressure following extracapsular cataract extraction. Br J Ophthal 74:272, 1990.
50. Kooner, KS, Dulaney, DD, Zimmerman, TJ: Intraocular pressure following secondary anterior chamber lens implantation. Ophthal Surg 19:274, 1988.
51. Vu, MT, Shields, MB: The early postoperative pressure course in glaucoma patients following cataract surgery. Ophthal Surg 19:467, 1988.
52. Handa, J, Henry, JC, Krupin, T, Keates, E: Extracapsular cataract extraction with posterior chamber lens implantation in patients with glaucoma. Arch Ophthal 105:765, 1987.
53. Kooner, KS, Dulaney, DD, Zimmerman, TJ: Intraocular pressure following ECCE and IOL implantation in patients with glaucoma. Ophthal Surg 19:570, 1988.
54. Kirsch, RE, Levine, O, Singer, JA: Ridge at internal edge of cataract incision. Arch Ophthal 94:2098, 1976.
55. Kirsch, RE, Levine, O, Singer, JA: Further studies on the ridge at the internal edge of the cataract incision. Trans Am Acad Ophthal Otol 83:224, 1977.
56. Campbell, DG, Grant, WM: Trabecular deformation and reduction of outflow facility due to cataract and penetrating keratoplasty sutures. Invest Ophthal Vis Sci (suppl):126, 1977.
57. Rothkoff, L, Biedner, B, Blumenthal, M: The effect of corneal section on early increased intraocular pressure after cataract extraction. Am J Ophthal 85:337, 1978.
58. Barraquer, J: Zonulolisis enzymatica. An Med Cirugia 34:148, 1958.
59. Kirsch, RE: Glaucoma following cataract extraction associated with use of alpha-chymotrypsin. Arch Ophthal 72:612, 1964.
60. Lantz, JM, Quigley, JH: Intraocular pressure after cataract extraction: effects of alpha chymotrypsin. Can J Ophthal 8:339, 1973.

61. Kirsch, RE: Further studies on glaucoma following cataract extraction associated with the use of alpha-chymotrypsin. Trans Am Acad Ophthal Otol 69:1011, 1965.
62. Galin, MA, Barasch, KR, Harris, LS: Enzymatic zonulolysis and intraocular pressure. Am J Ophthal 61:690, 1966.
63. Jocson, VL: Tonography and gonioscopy: before and after cataract extraction with alpha chymotrypsin. Am J Ophthal 60:318, 1965.
64. Kalvin, NH, Hamasaki, DI, Gass, JDM: Experimental glaucoma in monkeys. I. Relationship between intraocular pressure and cupping of the optic disc and cavernous atrophy of the optic nerve. Arch Ophthal 76:82, 1966.
65. Lessell, S, Kuwabara, T: Experimental alpha-chymotrypsin glaucoma. Arch Ophthal 81:853, 1969.
66. Anderson, DR: Experimental alpha chymotrypsin glaucoma studied by scanning electron microscopy. Am J Ophthal 71:470, 1971.
67. Ley, AP, Holmberg, AS, Yamashita, T: Histology of zonulolysis with alpha chymotrypsin employing light and electron microscopy. Am J Ophthal 49:67, 1960.
68. Anderson, DR: Scanning electron microscopy of zonulolysis by alpha chymotrypsin. Am J Ophthal 71:619, 1971.
69. Barraquer, J, Rutlan, J: Enzymatic zonulolysis and postoperative ocular hypertension. Am J Ophthal 63:159, 1967.
70. Gombos, GM, Oliver, M: Cataract extraction with enzymatic zonulolysis in glaucomatous eyes. Am J Ophthal 64:68, 1968.
71. Kirsch, RE: Dose relationship of alpha chymotrypsin in production of glaucoma after cataract extraction. Arch Ophthal 75:774, 1966.
72. Holmberg, SÅ, Philipson, BT: Sodium hyaluronate in cataract surgery. I. Report on the use of Healon® in two different types of intracapsular cataract surgery. Ophthalmology 91:45, 1984.
73. Holmberg, SÅ, Philipson, BT: Sodium hyaluronate in cataract surgery. II. Report on the use of Healon® in extracapsular cataract surgery using phacoemulsification. Ophthalmology 91:53, 1984.
74. Binkhorst, CD: Inflammation and intraocular pressure after the use of Healon in intraocular lens surgery. Am Intra-ocular Implant Soc J 6:340, 1980.
75. Pape, LG: Intracapsular and extracapsular technique of lens implantation with Healon. Am Intra-ocular Implant Soc J 6:342, 1980.
76. Mac Rae, SM, Edelhauser, HF, Hyndiuk, RA, et al: The effects of sodium hyaluronate, chondroitin sulfate, and methylcellulose on the corneal endothelium and intraocular pressure. Am J Ophthal 95:332, 1983.
77. Berson, FG, Patterson, MM, Epstein, DL: Obstruction of aqueous outflow by sodium hyaluronate in enucleated human eyes. Am J Ophthal 95:668, 1983.
78. Stamper, RL, DiLoreto, D, Schacknow, P: Effect of intraocular aspiration of sodium hyaluronate on postoperative intraocular pressure. Ophthal Surg 21:486, 1990.
79. Harrison, SE, Soll, DB, Shayegan, M, Clinch, T: Chondroitin sulfate: a new and effective protective agent for intraocular lens insertion. Ophthalmology 89:1254, 1982.
80. Alpar, JJ, Alpar, AJ, Baca, J, Chapman, D: Comparison of Healon and Viscoat in cataract extraction and intraocular lens implantation. Ophthal Surg 19:636, 1988.
81. Aron-Rosa, D, Cohn, HC, Aron, J-J, Bouquety, C: Methylcellulose instead of Healon® in extracapsular surgery with intraocular lens implantation. Ophthalmology 90:1235, 1983.
82. Bigar, F, Gloor, B, Schimmelpfennig, B, Thumm, D: Tolerance and safety of intraocular use of 2% hydroxypropylymethylcellulose. Klin Monatsbl Augenheilkd 193:21, 1988.
83. Hutton, WL, Snyder, WB, Vaiser, A: Management of surgically dislocated intravitreal lens fragments by pars plana vitrectomy. Ophthalmology 85:176, 1978.
84. Layden, WE: Pseudophakia and glaucoma. Ophthalmology 89:875, 1982.
85. Ellingson, FT: The uveitis-glaucoma-hyphema syndrome associated with the Mark-VII Choyce anterior chamber lens implant. Am Intra-ocular Implant Soc J 4:50, 1978.
86. Keates, RH, Ehrlich, DR: "Lenses of chance" complications of anterior chamber implants. Ophthalmology 85:408, 1978.
87. Miller, D, Doane, MG: High-speed photographic evaluation of intraocular lens movements. Am J Ophthal 97:752, 1984.
88. Sievers, H, von Domarus, D: Foreign-body reaction against intraocular lenses. Am J Ophthal 97:743, 1984.
89. Hagan, JC: A comparative study of the 91Z and other anterior chamber intraocular lenses. Am Intra-ocular Implant Soc J 10:324, 1984.
90. Liesegang, TJ, Bourne, WM, Brubaker, RF: The effect of cataract surgery on the blood-aqueous barrier. Ophthalmology 91:399, 1984.
91. Sawa, M, Sakanishi, Y, Shimizu, H: Fluorophotometric study of anterior segment barrier functions after extracapsular cataract extraction and posterior chamber intraocular lens implantation. Am J Ophthal 97:197, 1984.
92. Miyake, K, Asakura, M, Kobayashi, H: Effect of intraocular lens fixation of the blood-aqueous barrier. Am J Ophthal 98:451, 1984.
93. Percival, SPB, Das, SK: UGH syndrome after posterior chamber lens implantation. Am Intra-ocular Implant Soc J 9:200, 1983.
94. Bene, C, Hutchins, R, Kranias, G: Cataract

wound neovascularization. An often overlooked cause of vitreous hemorrhage. Ophthalmology 96:50, 1989.

95. Wiley, RG, Neville, RG, Martin, WG: Late postoperative hemorrhage following intracapsular cataract extraction with the IOLAB 91Z anterior chamber lens. Am Intra-ocular Implant Soc J 9:466, 1983.
96. Magargal, LE, Goldberg, RE, Uram, M, et al: Recurrent microhyphema in the pseudophakic eye. Ophthalmology 90:1231, 1983.
97. Pazandak, B, Johnson, S, Kratz, R, Faulkner, GD: Recurrent intraocular hemorrhage associated with posterior chamber lens implantation. Am Intra-ocular Implant Soc J 9:327, 1983.
98. Johnson, SH, Kratz, RP, Olson, PF: Iris transillumination defect and microhyphema syndrome. Am Intra-ocular Implant Soc J 10:425, 1984.
99. Apple, DJ, Craythorn, JM, Olson, RJ, et al: Anterior segment complications and neovascular glaucoma following implantation of a posterior chamber intraocular lens. Ophthalmology 91:403, 1984.
100. Summers, CG, Lindstrom, RL: Ghost cell glaucoma following lens implantation. Am Intra-ocular Implant Soc J 9:429, 1983.
101. Woodhams, JT, Lester, JC: Pigmentary dispersion glaucoma secondary to posterior chamber intra-ocular lenses. Ann Ophthal 16:852, 1984.
102. Huber, C: The gray iris syndrome. An iatrogenic form of pigmentary glaucoma. Arch Ophthal 102:397, 1984.
103. Smith, JP: Pigmentary open-angle glaucoma secondary to posterior chamber intraocular lens implantation and erosion of the iris pigment epithelium. Am Intra-ocular Implant Soc J 11:174, 1985.
104. Caplan, MB, Brown, RH, Love, LL: Pseudophakic pigmentary glaucoma. Am J Ophthal 105:320, 1988.
105. Grant, WM: Open-angle glaucoma associated with vitreous filling the anterior chamber. Trans Am Ophthal Soc 61:196, 1963.
106. Simmons, RJ: The vitreous in glaucoma. Trans Ophthal Soc UK 95:422, 1975.
107. Samples, JR, Van Buskirk, EM: Open-angle glaucoma associated with vitreous humor filling the anterior chamber. Am J Ophthal 102:759, 1986.
108. Chandler, PA: Glaucoma from pupillary block in aphakia. Arch Ophthal 67:14, 1962.
109. Chandler, PA: Glaucoma in aphakia. Trans Am Acad Ophthal Otol 67:483, 1963.
110. Chandler, PA: Surgery of congenital cataract. Trans Am Acad Ophthal Otol 72:341, 1968.
111. Zauberman, H, Yassur, Y, Sachs, U: Fluorescein pupillary flow in aphakics with intact and spontaneous openings of the vitreous face. Br J Ophthal 61:450, 1977.
112. Van Buskirk, EM: Pupillary block after intraocular lens implantation. Am J Ophthal 95:55, 1983.
113. Shrader, CE, Belcher, CD III, Thomas, JV, et al: Pupillary and iridovitreal block in pseudophakic eyes. Ophthalmology 91:831, 1984.
114. Moses, L: Complications of rigid anterior chamber implants. Ophthalmology 91:819, 1984.
115. Werner, D, Kaback, M: Pseudophakic pupillary-block glaucoma. Br J Ophthal 61:329, 1977.
116. Kielar, RA, Stambaugh, JL: Pupillary block glaucoma following intraocular lens implantation. Ophthal Surg 13:647, 1982.
117. Cohen, JS, Osher, RH, Weber, P, Faulkner, JD: Complications of extracapsular cataract surgery. The indications and risks of peripheral iridectomy. Ophthalmology 91:826, 1984.
118. Willis, DA, Stewart, RH, Kimbrough, RL: Pupillary block associated with posterior chamber lenses. Ophthal Surg 16:108, 1985.
119. Samples, JR, Bellows, AR, Rosenquist, RC, et al: Pupillary block with posterior chamber intraocular lenses. Arch Ophthal 105:335, 1987.
120. Forman, JS, Ritch, R, Dunn, MW, Szmyd, L: Pupillary block following posterior chamber lens implantation. Ophthal Laser Ther 2:85, 1987.
121. Schulze, RR, Copeland, JR: Posterior chamber intraocular lens implantation without peripheral iridectomy. A preliminary report. Ophthal Surg 13:567, 1982.
122. Simel, PF: Posterior chamber implants without iridectomy. Am Intra-ocular Implant Soc J 8:141, 1982.
123. Shields, MB: Iridotomy scissor-forceps. Am J Ophthal 99:609, 1985.
124. Van Buskirk, EM: Late onset, progressive, peripheral anterior synechiae with posterior chamber intraocular lenses. Ophthal Surg 18:115, 1987.
125. Chrousos, GA, Parks, MM, O'Neill, JF: Incidence of chronic glaucoma, retinal detachment and secondary membrane surgery in pediatric aphakic patients. Ophthalmology 91:1238, 1984.
126. Bernardino, VB, Kim, JC, Smith, TR: Epithelialization of the anterior chamber after cataract extraction. Arch Ophthal 82:742, 1969.
127. Theobald, GD, Haas, JS: Epithelial invasion of the anterior chamber following cataract extraction. Trans Am Acad Ophthal Otol 52:470, 1948.
128. Weiner, MJ, Trentacoste, J, Pon, DM, Albert, DM: Epithelial downgrowth: a 30-year clinicopathological review. Br J Ophthal 73:6, 1989.
129. Eldrup-Jørgensen, P: Epithelialization of the anterior chamber. A clinical and histopathological study of a Danish material. Acta Ophthal 47:328, 1969.
130. Sugar, A, Meyer, RF, Hood, CI: Epithelial downgrowth following penetrating keratoplasty in the aphake. Arch Ophthal 95:464, 1977.
131. Smith, RE, Parrett, C: Specular microscopy of epithelial downgrowth. Arch Ophthal 96:1222, 1978.
132. Maumenee, AE: Treatment of epithelial down-

growth and intraocular fistula following cataract extraction. Trans Am Ophthal Soc 62:153, 1964.
133. Calhoun, FP Jr: An aid to the clinical diagnosis of epithelial downgrowth into the anterior chamber following cataract extraction. Am J Ophthal 61:1055, 1966.
134. Verrey, F: Invasion epitheliale de la chambre anterieure: confirmation anatomique par l'examen cytologique de l'humeur aqueuse. Ophthalmologica 153:467, 1967.
135. Maumenee, AE, Paton, D, Morse, PH, Butner, R: Review of 40 histologically proven cases of epithelial downgrowth following cataract extraction and suggested surgical management. Am J Ophthal 69:598, 1970.
136. Stark, WJ, Michels, RG, Maumenee, AE, Cupples, H: Surgical management of epithelial ingrowth. Am J Ophthal 85:772, 1978.
137. Jensen, P, Minckler, DS, Chandler, JW: Epithelial ingrowth. Arch Ophthal 95:837, 1977.
138. Iwamoto, T, Srinivasan, BD, DeVoe, AG: Electron microscopy of epithelial downgrowth. Ann Ophthal 9:1095, 1977.
139. Zavala, EY, Binder, PS: The pathologic findings of epithelial ingrowth. Arch Ophthal 98:2007, 1980.
140. Zagorski, Z, Shrestha, HG, Lang, GK, Naumann, GOH: Secondary glaucoma due to intraocular epithelial invasion. Klin Monatsbl Augenheilkd 193:16, 1988.
141. Terry, TL, Chisholm, JF Jr, Schonberg, AL: Studies on surface-epithelium invasion of the anterior segment of the eye. Am J Ophthal 22:1083, 1939.
142. Allen, JC: Epithelial and stromal ingrowths. Am J Ophthal 65:179, 1968.
143. Bettman, JW Jr: Pathology of complications of intraocular surgery. Am J Ophthal 68:1037, 1969.
144. Swan, KC: Fibroblastic ingrowth following cataract extraction. Arch Ophthal 89:445, 1973.
145. Sherrard, ES, Rycroft, PV: Retrocorneal membranes. II. Factors influencing their growth. Br J Ophthal 51:387, 1967.
146. Friedman, AH, Henkind, P: Corneal stromal overgrowth after cataract extraction. Br J Ophthal 54:528, 1970.
147. Michels, RG, Kenyon, KR, Maumenee, AE: Retrocorneal fibrous membrane. Invest Ophthal 11:822, 1972.
148. Ueno, H, Green, WR, Kenyon, KR, Hoover, RE: Trabecular and retrocorneal proliferation of melanocytes and secondary glaucoma. Am J Ophthal 88:592, 1979.
149. Terry, AC, Stark, WJ, Maumenee, AE, Fagadau, W: Neodymium-YAG for posterior capsulotomy. Am J Ophthal 96:716, 1983.
150. Channell, MM, Beckman, H: Intraocular pressure changes after neodymium-YAG laser posterior capsulotomy. Arch Ophthal 102:1024, 1984.
151. Keates, RH, Steinert, RF, Puliafito, CA, Maxwell, SK: Long-term follow-up of Nd:YAG laser posterior capsulotomy. Am Intra-ocular Implant Soc J 10:164, 1984.
152. Kurata, F, Krupin, T, Sinclair, S, Karp, L: Progressive glaucomatous visual field loss after neodymium-YAG laser capsulotomy. Am J Ophthal 98:632, 1984.
153. Vine, AK: Ocular hypertension following Nd:YAG laser capsulotomy: a potentially blinding complication. Ophthal Surg 15:283, 1984.
154. Richter, CU, Arzeno, G, Pappas, HR, et al: Intraocular pressure elevation following Nd:YAG laser posterior capsulotomy. Ophthalmology 92:636, 1985.
155. Flohr, MJ, Robin, AL, Kelley, JS: Early complications following Q-switched neodymium:YAG laser posterior capsulotomy. Ophthalmology 92:360, 1985.
156. Stark, WJ, Worthen, D, Holladay, JT, Murray, G: Neodymium:YAG lasers. An FDA report. Ophthalmology 92:209, 1985.
157. Ruderman, JM, Mitchell, PG, Kraff, M: Pupillary block following Nd:YAG laser capsulotomy. Ophthal Surg 14:418, 1983.
158. Shrader, CE, Belcher, CD III, Thomas, JV, Simmons, RJ: Acute glaucoma following Nd:YAG laser membranotomy. Ophthal Surg 14:1015, 1983.
159. Gimbel, HV, Van Westenbrugge, JA, Sanders, DR, Raanan, MG: Effect of sulcus vs capsular fixation on YAG-induced pressure rises following posterior capsulotomy. Arch Ophthal 108:1126, 1990.
160. Schubert, HD: Vitreoretinal changes associated with rise in intraocular pressure after Nd:YAG capsulotomy. Ophthal Surg 18:19, 1987.
161. Schrems, W, Glaab-Schrems, E, Kreiglstein, GK: Rises in intraocular pressure in postcataract surgery with the Neodymium-YAG laser. Klin Monatsbl Augenheilkd 187:14, 1985.
162. Mitchell, PG, Blair, NP, Deutsch, TA, Hershey, JM: The effect of Neodymium:YAG laser shocks on the blood-aqueous barrier. Ophthalmology 94:488, 1987.
163. Van Der Sloot, D, Stilma, JS, Boen-Tan, TN, Bezemer, PD: Prevention of IOP-rise following Nd-YAG laser capsulotomy with topical Timolol and Indomethacin. Doc Ophthalmologica 70:209, 1989.
164. Migliori, ME, Beckman, H, Channell, MM: Intraocular pressure changes after Neodymium-YAG laser capsulotomy in eyes pretreated with Timolol. Arch Ophthal 105:473, 1987.
165. Pollack, IP, Brown, RH, Crandall, AS, et al: Prevention of the rise in intraocular pressure following Neodymium-YAG posterior capsulotomy using topical 1% apraclonidine. Arch Ophthal 106:754, 1988.

166. Khodadoust, AA, Arkfeld, DF, Caprioli, J, Sear, ML: Ocular effect of neodymium-YAG laser. Am J Ophthal 98:144, 1984.
167. Drews, RC: Anterior capsulotomy with the neodymium:YAG laser: results and opinions. Am Intra-ocular Implant Soc J 11:240, 1985.
168. McDonnell, PJ, Quigley, HA, Maumenee, AE, et al: The Honan intraocular pressure reducer. An experimental study. Arch Ophthal 103:422, 1985.
169. Poleski, SA, Willis, WE: Angle-supported intraocular lenses: a goniophotographic study. Ophthalmology 91:838, 1984.
170. Rowsey, JJ, Gaylor, JR: Intraocular lens disasters. Peripheral anterior synechia. Ophthalmology 87:646, 1980.
171. Hollands, RH, Drance, SM, Schulzer, M: The effect of acetylcholine on early postoperative intraocular pressure. Am J Ophthal 103:749, 1987.
172. Ruiz, RS, Rhem, MN, Prager, TC: Effects of carbachol and acetylcholine on intraocular pressure after cataract extraction. Am J Ophthal 107:7, 1989.
173. Hollands, RH, Drance, SM, Schulzer, M: The effect of intracameral carbachol on intraocular pressure after cataract extraction. Am J Ophthal 104:225, 1987.
174. Linn, DK, Zimmerman, TJ, Nardin, GF, et al: Effect of intracameral carbachol on intraocular pressure after cataract extraction. Am J Ophthal 107:133, 1989.
175. Wood, TO: Effect of carbachol on postoperative intraocular pressure. J Cat Ref Surg 14:654, 1988.
176. Hayreh, SS: Anterior ischemic optic neuropathy. IV. Occurrence after cataract extraction. Arch Ophthal 98:1410, 1980.
177. Biedner, B, Rothkoff, L, Blumenthal, M: The effect of acetazolamide on early increased intraocular pressure after cataract extraction. Am J Ophthal 83:565, 1977.
178. Bloomfield, S: Failure to prevent enzyme glaucoma. A negative report. Am J Ophthal 64:405, 1968.
179. Packer, AJ, Fraioli, AJ, Epstein, DL: The effect of timolol and acetazolamide on transient intraocular pressure elevation following cataract extraction with alpha-chymotrypsin. Ophthalmology 88:239, 1981.
180. Obstbaum, SA, Galin, MA: The effects of timolol on cataract extraction and intraocular pressure. Am J Ophthal 88:1017, 1979.
181. Haimann, MH, Phjelps, CD: Prophylactic timolol for the prevention of high intraocular pressure after cataract extraction. A randomized, prospective, double-blind trial. Ophthalmology 88:233, 1981.
182. Tilen, A, Leuenberger, AE: Effect of timolol and acetazolamide on intraocular hypertension after intracapsular lens extraction with alpha-chymotrypsin. Klin Monatsbl Augenheilkd 176:558, 1980.
183. Shields, MB, Braverman, SD: Timolol in the management of secondary glaucomas. Surv Ophthal 28:266, 1983.
184. Tomoda, T, Tuberville, AW, Wood, TO: Timolol and postoperative intraocular pressure. Am Intraocular Implant Soc J 10:180, 1984.
185. West, DR, Lischwe, TD, Thompson, VM, Ide, CH: Comparative efficacy of the β-blockers for the prevention of increased intraocular pressure after cataract extraction. Am J Ophthal 106:168, 1988.
186. Ruiz, RS, Wilson, CA, Musgrove, KH, Prager, TC: Management of increased intraocular pressure after cataract extraction. Am J Ophthal 103:487, 1987.
187. Brown, SVL, Thomas, JV, Belcher, CD III, Simmons, RJ: Effect of pilocarpine in treatment of intraocular pressure elevation following neodymium:YAG laser posterior capsulotomy. Ophthalmology 92:354, 1985.
188. Kolker, AE, Becker, B: Epinephrine maculopathy. Arch Ophthal 79:552, 1968.
189. Rich, WJCC: Prevention of postoperative ocular hypertension by prostaglandin inhibitors. Trans Ophthal Soc UK 97:268, 1977.
190. Brucker, AJ, Michels, RG, Green, WR: Pars plana vitrectomy in the management of blood-induced glaucoma with vitreous hemorrhage. Ann Ophthal 10:1427, 1978.
191. Theodossiadis, G, Kouris-Bairaktari, E, Velissaropoulos, P: Clinical and pathologic-anatomical results following the application of a mobile argon-laser beam in aphakic pupillary block glaucoma. Klin Monatsbl Augenheilkd 175:180, 1979.
192. Hitchings, RA: Acute aphakic pupil block glaucoma: an alternative surgical approach. Br J Ophthal 63:31, 1979.
193. Peyman, GA, Sanders, DR, Minatoya, H: Pars plana vitrectomy in the management of pupillary block glaucoma following irrigation and aspiration. Br J Ophthal 62:336, 1978.
194. Obstbaum, SA, Galin, MA, Barasch, KR, Baras, I: Laser photomydriasis in pseudophakic pupillary block. Am Intra-ocular Implant Soc J 7:28, 1981.
195. Mackool, RJ: Closed vitrectomy and the intraocular implant. Ophthalmology 88:414, 1981.
196. Bellows, AR, Johnstone, MA: Surgical management of chronic glaucoma in aphakia. Ophthalmology 90:807, 1983.
197. Gross, RL, Feldman, RM, Spaeth, GL, et al: Surgical therapy of chronic glaucoma in aphakia and pseudophakia. Ophthalmology 95:1195, 1988.
198. Heuer, DK, Gressel, MG, Parrish, RD II, et al: Trabeculectomy in aphakic eyes. Ophthalmology 91:1045, 1984.
199. The Fluorouracil Filtering Surgery Study Group.

Fluorouracil filtering surgery study one-year follow-up. Am J Ophthal 108:625, 1989.
200. Hampton, C, Shields, MB, Miller, KN, Blasini, M: Evaluation of a protocol for transscleral Nd:YAG cyclophotocoagulation in 100 patients. Ophthalmology 97:910, 1990.
201. Brown, SI: Treatment of advanced epithelial downgrowth. Trans Am Acad Ophthal Otol 77:618, 1973.
202. Brown, SI: Results of excision of advanced epithelial downgrowth. Ophthalmology 86:321, 1979.
203. Friedman, AH: Radical anterior segment surgery for epithelial invasion of the anterior chamber: report of three cases. Trans Am Acad Ophthal Otol 83:216, 1977.
204. Fish, LA, Heuer, DK, Baerveldt, G, et al: Molteno implantation for secondary glaucomas associated with advanced epithelial ingrowth. Ophthalmology 97:557, 1990.
205. Karesh, JW, Nirankari, VS: Factors associated with glaucoma after penetrating keratoplasty. Am J Ophthal 96:160, 1983.
206. Olson, RF, Kaufman, HE: Prognostic factors of intraocular pressure after aphakic keratoplasty. Am J Ophthal 86:510, 1978.
207. Foulks, GN: Glaucoma associated with penetrating keratoplasty. Ophthalmology 94:871, 1987.
208. Goldberg, DB, Schanzlin, DJ, Brown, SI: Incidence of increased intraocular pressure after keratoplasty. Am J Ophthal 92:372, 1981.
209. Irvine, AR, Kaufman, HE: Intraocular pressure following penetrating keratoplasty. Am J Ophthal 68:835, 1969.
210. Brightbill, FS, Stainer, GA, Hunkeler, JD: A comparison of intracapsular and extracapsular lens extraction combined with keratoplasty. Ophthalmology 90:34, 1983.
211. Robinson, CH Jr: Indications, complications and prognosis for repeat penetrating keratoplasty. Ophthal Surg 10:27, 1979.
212. Heydenreich, A: Corneal regeneration and intraocular tension. Klin Monatsbl Augenheilkd 148:500, 1966.
213. Lass, JH, Pavan-Langston, D: Timolol therapy in secondary angle-closure glaucoma post penetrating keratoplasty. Ophthalmology 86:51, 1979.
214. Zimmerman, TJ, Krupin, T, Grodzki, W, Waltman, SR: The effect of suture depth on outflow facility in penetrating keratoplasty. Arch Ophthal 96:505, 1978.
215. Zimmerman, TJ, Waltman, SR, Sachs, U, Kaufman, HE: Intraocular pressure after aphakic penetrating keratoplasty "through-and-through" suturing. Ophthal Surg 10:49, 1979.
216. Nissenkorn, I, Wood, TO: Intraocular pressure following aphakic transplants. Ann Ophthal 15:1168, 1983.
217. Olson, RJ, Kaufman, HE: A mathematical description of causative factors and prevention of elevated intraocular pressure after keratoplasty. Invest Ophthal Vis Sci 16:1085, 1977.
218. Gnad, HD: Athalamia as a late complication after keratoplasty on aphakic eyes. Br J Ophthal 64:528, 1980.
219. Polack, FM: Graft rejection and glaucoma. Am J Ophthal 101:294, 1986.
220. Insler, MS, McShrerry Zatzkis, S: Pigment dispersion syndrome in pseudophakic corneal transplants. Am J Ophthal 102:762, 1986.
221. Schanzlin, DJ, Goldberg, DB, Brown, SI: Transplantation of congenitally opaque corneas. Ophthalmology 87:1253, 1980.
222. Yamaguchi, T, Polack, FM, Valenti, J: Electron microscopic study of epithelial downgrowth after penetrating keratoplasty. Br J Ophthal 65:374, 1981.
223. Olson, RJ: Aphakic keratoplasty. Determining donor tissue size to avoid elevated intraocular pressure. Arch Ophthal 96:2274, 1978.
224. Zimmerman, TJ, Krupin, T, Grodzki, W, et al: Size of donor corneal button and outflow facility in aphakic eyes. Ann Ophthal 11:809, 1979.
225. Perl, T, Charlton, KH, Binder, PS: Disparate diameter grafting. Astigmatism, intraocular pressure, and visual acuity. Ophthalmology 88:774, 1981.
226. Heidemann, DG, Sugar, A, Meyer, RF, Musch, DC: Oversized donor grafts in penetrating keratoplasty. A randomized trial. Arch Ophthal 103:1807, 1985.
227. Foulks, GN, Perry, HD, Dohlman, CH: Oversize corneal donor grafts in penetrating keratoplasty. Ophthalmology 86:490, 1979.
228. Zimmerman, T, Olson, R, Waltman, S, Kaufman, H: Transplant size and elevated intraocular pressure. Postkeratoplasty. Arch Ophthal 96:2231, 1978.
229. Bourne, WM, Davison, JA, O'Fallon, WM: The effects of oversize donor buttons on postoperative intraocular pressure and corneal curvature in aphakic penetrating keratoplasty. Ophthalmology 89:242, 1982.
230. Perry, HD, Foulks, GN: Oversize donor buttons in corneal transplantation surgery for keratoconus. Ophthal Surg 18:751, 1987.
231. Cohen, EJ, Kenyon, KR, Dohlman, CH: Iridoplasty for prevention of post-keratoplasty angle closure and glaucoma. Ophthal Surg 13:994, 1982.
232. Thoft, RA, Gordon, JM, Dohlman, CH: Glaucoma following keratoplasty. Trans Am Acad Ophthal Otol 78:352, 1974.
233. Wood, TO, West, C, Kaufman, HE: Control of intraocular pressure in penetrating keratoplasty. Am J Ophthal 74:724, 1972.
234. Olson, RJ, Kaufman, HE, Zimmerman, TJ: Effects of timolol and daranide on elevated intrao-

cular pressure after aphakic keratoplasty. Ann Ophthal 11:1833, 1979.
235. Casey, TA, Gibbs, D: Complications in corneal grafting. Trans Ophthal Soc UK 92:517, 1972.
236. Lemp, MA, Pfister, RR, Dohlman, CG: The effect of intraocular surgery on clear corneal grafts. Am J Ophthal 70:719, 1970.
237. McDonnell, PJ, Robin, JB, Schanzlin, DJ, et al: Molteno implant for control of glaucoma in eyes after penetrating keratoplasty. Ophthalmology 95:364, 1988.
238. Binder, PS, Abel, R Jr, Kaufman, HE: Cyclocryotherapy for glaucoma after penetrating keratoplasty. Am J Ophthal 79:489, 1975.
239. Wilensky, JT, Goldberg, MF, Alward, P: Glaucoma after pars plana vitrectomy. Trans Am Acad Ophthal Otol 83:114, 1977.
240. Huamonte, FU, Peyman, GA, Goldberg, MF: Complicated retinal detachment and its management with pars plana vitrectomy. Br J Ophthal 61:754, 1977.
241. Faulborn, J, Conway, BP, Machemer, R: Surgical complications of pars plana vitreous surgery. Ophthalmology 85:116, 1978.
242. Aaberg, TM, Van Horn, DL: Late complications of pars plana vitreous surgery. Ophthalmology 85:126, 1978.
243. Ghartey, KN, Tolentino, FI, Freeman, HM, et al: Closed vitreous surgery. XVII. Results and complications of pars plana vitrectomy. Arch Ophthal 98:1248, 1980.
244. Han, DP, Lewis, H, Lambrou, FH Jr, et al: Mechanisms of intraocular pressure elevation after pars plana vitrectomy. Ophthalmology 96:1357, 1989.
245. Sabates, WI, Abrams, GW, Swanson, DE, Norton, EWD: The use of intraocular gases. The results of sulfur hexafluoride gas in retinal detachment surgery. Ophthalmology 88:447, 1981.
246. Abrams, GW, Swanson, DE, Sabates, WI: The results of sulfur hexafluoride gas in vitreous surgery. Am J Ophthal 94:165, 1982.
247. Chang, S, Lincoff, HA, Coleman, DJ, et al: Perfluorocarbon gases in vitreous surgery. Ophthalmology 92:651, 1985.
248. Coden, DJ, Freeman, WR, Weinreb, RN: Intraocular pressure response after pneumatic retinopexy. Ophthal Surg 19:667, 1988.
249. Crittenden, JJ, deJuan, E Jr, Tiedeman, J: Expansion of long-acting gas bubbles for intraocular use. Principles and practice. Arch Ophthal 103:831, 1985.
250. Aronowitz, JD, Brubaker, RF: Effect of intraocular gas on intraocular pressure. Arch Ophthal 94:1191, 1976.
251. Poliner, LS, Schoch, LH: Intraocular pressure assessment in gas-filled eyes following vitrectomy. Arch Ophthal 105:200, 1987.
252. Simone, JN, Whitacre, MM: The effect of intraocular gas and fluid volumes on intraocular pressure. Ophthalmology 97:238, 1990.
253. Hines, MW, Jost, BF, Fogelman, KL: Oculab Tono-Pen, Goldmann applanation tonometry, and pneumatic tonometry for intraocular pressure assessment in gas-filled eyes. Am J Ophthal 106:174, 1988.
254. Lincoff, H, Weinberger, D, Reppucci, V, Lincoff, A: Air travel with intraocular gas. I. The mechanisms for compensation. Arch Ophthal 107:902, 1989.
255. Lincoff, H, Weinberger, D, Stergiu, P: Air travel with intraocular gas. II. Clinical considerations. Arch Ophthal 107:907, 1989.
256. Lewis, H, Han, D, Williams, GA: Management of fibrin pupillary-block glaucoma after pars plana vitrectomy with intravitreal gas injection. Am J Ophthal 103:180, 1987.
257. Jaffe, GJ, Lewis, H, Han, DP, et al: Treatment of postvitrectomy fibrin pupillary block with tissue plasminogen activator. Am J Ophthal 108:170, 1989.
258. Okun, E: Intravitreal surgery utilizing liquid silicone. A long term follow-up. Tran Pac Coast Oto-Ophthal Soc 49:141, 1968.
259. Grey, RHB, Leaver, PK: Results of silicone oil injection in massive preretinal retraction. Trans Ophthal Soc UK 97:238, 1977.
260. Sugar, HS, Okamura, ID: Ocular findings six years after intravitreal silicone injection. Arch Ophthal 94:612, 1976.
261. Watzke, RC: Silicone retinopiesis for retinal detachment. A long-term clinical evaluation. Arch Ophthal 77:185, 1967.
262. Burk, LL, Shields, MB, Proia, AD, McCuen, B: Intraocular pressure following intravitreal silicone oil injection. Ophthal Surg 19:565, 1988.
263. de Corral, LR, Cohen, SB, Peyman, GA: Effect of intravitreal silicone oil on intraocular pressure. Ophthal Surg 18:446, 1987.
264. Ando, F: Intraocular hypertension resulting from pupillary block by silicone oil. Am J Ophthal 99:87, 1985.
265. Zborowski-Gutman, L, Treister, G, Naveh, N, et al: Acute glaucoma following vitrectomy and silicone oil injection. Br J Ophthal 71:903, 1987.
266. Beekhuis, WH, Ando, F, Zivojnovic, R, et al: Basal iridectomy at 6 o'clock in the aphakic eye treated with silicone oil: prevention of keratopathy and secondary glaucoma. Br J Ophthal 71:197, 1987.
267. Gao, R, Neubauer, L, Tang, S, Kampik, A: Silicone oil in the anterior chamber. Graefe's Arch Ophthal 227:106, 1989.
268. Rentsch, FJ: Electronmicroscopical aspects of acid compartments of the ground substance and of collagen in different cases of intravitreal tissue proliferation. Der Ophthal 2:385, 1981.

269. Ni, C, Wang, W-J, Albert, DM, Schepens, CL: Intravitreous silicone injection. Histopathologic findings in a human eye after 12 years. Arch Ophthal 101:1399, 1983.
270. Laroche, L, Pavlakis, C, Saraux, H, Orcel, L: Ocular findings following intravitreal silicone injection. Arch Ophthal 101:1422, 1983.
271. Sebestyen, JG, Schepens, CL, Rosenthal, ML: Retinal detachment and glaucoma. I. Tonometric and gonioscopic study of 160 cases. Arch Ophthal 67:736, 1962.
272. Hayreh, SS, Baines, JAB: Occlusion of the vortex veins. An experimental study. Br J Ophthal 57:217, 1973.
273. Araie, M, Sugiura, Y, Minota, K, Akazawa, K: Effects of the encircling procedure on the aqueous flow rate in retinal detachment eyes: a fluorometric study. Br J Ophthal 71:510, 1987.
274. Johnson, MW, Han, DP, Hoffman, KE: The effect of scleral buckling on ocular rigidity. Ophthalmology 97:190, 1990.
275. Mensher, JH: Anterior chamber depth alteration after retinal photocoagulation. Arch Ophthal 95:113, 1977.
276. Boulton, PE: A study of the mechanism of transient myopia following extensive Xenon Arc photocoagulation. Trans Ophthal Soc UK 93:287, 1973.
277. Blondeau, P, Pavan, PR, Phelps, CD: Acute pressure elevation following panretinal photocoagulation. Arch Ophthal 99:1239, 1981.
278. Schidte, SN: Changes in eye tension after panretinal Xenon arc and argon laser photocoagulation in normotensive diabetic eyes. Acta Ophthal 60:692, 1982.
279. Kaufman, SC, Ferris, FL III, Swartz, M, et al: Intraocular pressure following panretinal photocoagulation for diabetic retinopathy: Diabetic Retinopathy Report No. 11. Arch Ophthal 105:807, 1987.

Section Three

The Management of Glaucoma

Chapter 24

PRINCIPLES OF MEDICAL THERAPY FOR GLAUCOMA

A Classification of Antiglaucoma Drugs

The variety of medications that are used to control the intraocular pressure (IOP) in the management of glaucoma may first be classified according to the two major modes of administration: topical and systemic.

Topical Drugs

Topically-applied antiglaucoma agents constitute the first-line defense, as well as the most frequently used medications, in most cases of glaucoma. All of these drugs are thought to exert their pharmacologic effect by acting on the *autonomic nervous system*. We may, therefore, classify the topical antiglaucoma medications within the framework of this system.

There are two main subdivisions of the autonomic nervous system: the *cholinergic* (parasympathetic) and *adrenergic* (sympathetic) systems. These subsystems differ on the basis of (1) receptors and (2) postganglionic physiologic mediators (Fig. 24.1).[1] Receptors are located in the cell membrane and represent the sites at which both physiologic mediators and most pharmacologic agents interact to produce a particular cellular response. The cell membrane is composed of lipid and protein. The actual arrangement of these components is uncertain, although the "lipid-globular protein mosaic model" theory suggests that molecules of protein are embedded in a layer of lipid, with protrusion of the globular protein on either side of the membrane.[1] Although this is an oversimplification of a highly complex and poorly understood subject, it provides a conceptual basis for a discussion of drug interactions. According to this hypothesis, the extracellular side of the protein globules contains the receptors, while the intracellular side contains catalysts, which are involved in specific cellular functions in response to a physiologic mediator or drug.

Cholinergic System. It has traditionally been held that only one receptor type exists in the parasympathetic nervous system, although more recent studies have suggested

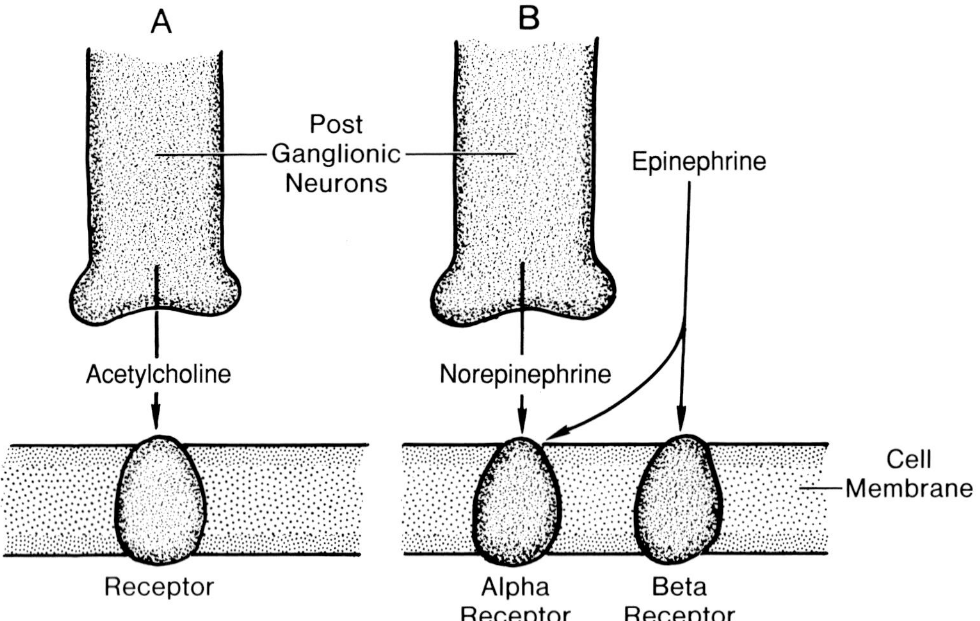

Figure 24.1. Main divisions of autonomic nervous system: **A,** Cholinergic (parasympathetic) system, mediated by acetylcholine; **B,** Adrenergic (sympathetic) system, mediated by norepinephrine and epinephrine.

the possibility of more than one cholinergic receptor.[2] Stimulation of the receptor(s) produces miosis and increased aqueous outflow. The mechanism of improved outflow facility appears to be related to contraction of the ciliary muscle.[3–5]

Acetylcholine is the postganglionic physiologic mediator of the cholinergic nervous system. It is produced in the postganglionic neuron, where it is stored and released when the membrane is polarized by increased Na^+ flux. After its release from the neuron, the mediator is rapidly inactivated by acetylcholinesterase. This enzymatic inactivation is too rapid to allow the effective use of acetylcholine as a topical drug, although it is often injected into the anterior chamber during intraocular surgery to achieve rapid miosis.

Pharmacologic agents may either simulate or antagonize the action of the physiologic mediator. Drugs that mimic the effect of acetylcholine, referred to as *parasympathomimetics* or *cholinergic stimulators* or *agonists,* may act directly by stimulating the receptor or indirectly by enhancing the action of the physiologic mediator. The direct stimulator most commonly used in the treatment of glaucoma is *pilocarpine,* while an example of the indirect stimulators is *echothiophate iodide,* which enhances the action of acetylcholine by inhibiting the cholinesterases.

Drugs that block the response of acetylcholine at the receptor are called *parasympatholytics* or *cholinergic antagonists.* This class of compounds, which includes atropine, cyclopentolate, and tropicamide, are not routinely used in the treatment of glaucoma, since the mydriasis and cycloplegia they produce may actually increase the IOP, as discussed in Chapters 9 and 10.

Adrenergic System. Two basic types of adrenergic receptors (alpha and beta) have been identified, although subdivisions are known to exist within these categories, and it is likely that there are additional receptors that have yet to be recognized. *Alpha-adrenergic receptor* stimulation produces mydriasis and vasoconstriction. The *beta-adrenergic receptors* have been further subdivided into $beta_1$ and $beta_2$ types.[6] Stimulation of $beta_1$-receptors increases cardiac contractility and lypolysis, while the beta$_2$-subsystem is related to bronchodilation and vasodepression. Both alpha- and beta-adrenergic receptors appear to influence aqueous humor dynamics, although the precise mechanisms are not fully understood. In general, the stimulation of the beta-receptors increases aqueous outflow facility, while inhibition reduces aqueous production.

There are two physiologic mediators in the sympathetic nervous system, *epinephrine* and *norepinephrine,* which are often referred to as catacholamines. Epinephrine is secreted by the adrenal glands, where it is produced from phenylalanine and tyrosine. This mediator stimulates both alpha- and beta-receptors. Norepinephrine is the postganglionic mediator and primarily stimulates the alpha-receptor. It is also secreted by the adrenal glands, where it is made from the same amino acids as epinephrine. In the postganglionic neuron, norepinephrine is produced from tyrosine alone and stored in two pools in the axon terminal. Slow release and re-uptake of the mediator constantly occur, and that which is not released is inactivated to vanillylmandelic acid by monoamine oxidase. Following massive release of the mediator by nerve stimulation, 90% is recaptured by the nerve, a small amount is inactivated by catechol-o-methyltransferase and monoamine oxidase, and the remainder enters the circulation in active form (Fig. 24.2).

The pharmacologic agents within the adrenergic system, as with the cholinergic drugs, may either mimic or inhibit the action of the physiologic mediators. The *sympathomimetics* or *adrenergic stimulators* may act either directly or indirectly on the alpha-receptors, the beta-receptors, or both. The only adrenergic stimulator that is commercially available for the chronic treatment of glaucoma is the physiologic mediator *epinephrine,* which is a direct alpha- and beta-stimulator. Recently, an analogue of clonidine, *apraclonidine,* an alpha$_2$-stimulator, has been approved and released for treating the short-term IOP elevation associated with certain glaucoma laser procedures.

Other sympathomimetics that have been evaluated for their IOP lowering effect include the direct alpha-stimulator and physiologic mediator norepinephrine, and a group of indirect alpha-stimulators, which enhance the effect of norepinephrine by: (1) stimulating its release from axon terminals; (2) increasing its release in response to nerve stimulation; (3) decreasing its re-uptake; and (4) inhibiting monoamine oxidase or catachol-o-methyltransferase. Indirect beta-stimulators, which mimic the effect of beta-adrenergic stimulation by enhancing the action of adenylate cyclase in various ways, have also been studied. In addition, another group of compounds, the adrenergic potentiators, enhance the effect of epinephrine by producing adrenergic supersensitivity.

The *sympatholytics* or *adrenergic inhibitors* compete with the catecholamines for the alpha-receptors or with epinephrine for the beta-receptors. Beta-antagonists or blockers lower the IOP by reducing aqueous production. *Timolol, betaxolol, levobunolol,* and *metipranolol* are beta-blockers that are currently available in the United States for topical therapy in the treatment of glaucoma. In addition, a number of systemic beta-blockers are available, primarily for treating cardiovascular disorders, which also have an ocular hypotensive effect.

Systemic Drugs

Carbonic anhydrase inhibitors are the only class of systemic medications that are used on a chronic basis in the treatment of glaucoma. These agents lower the IOP by reducing aqueous production. *Acetazolamide* is the prototype carbonic anhydrase inhibitor and may be administered either orally, intramuscularly, or intravenously. *Methazolamide* is another commonly used oral carbonic anhydrase inhibitor.

Hyperosmotic agents are occasionally used for the rapid reduction of severely elevated IOP on an emergency basis, although rarely for prolonged periods of time. The hypotensive mechanism of these drugs is not fully understood, although it is generally believed to be through reduction of the vitreous volume. The hyperosmotics can be administered either orally, in which case *glycerine* is the most common form, or intravenously, in which case *mannitol* is the most popular drug.

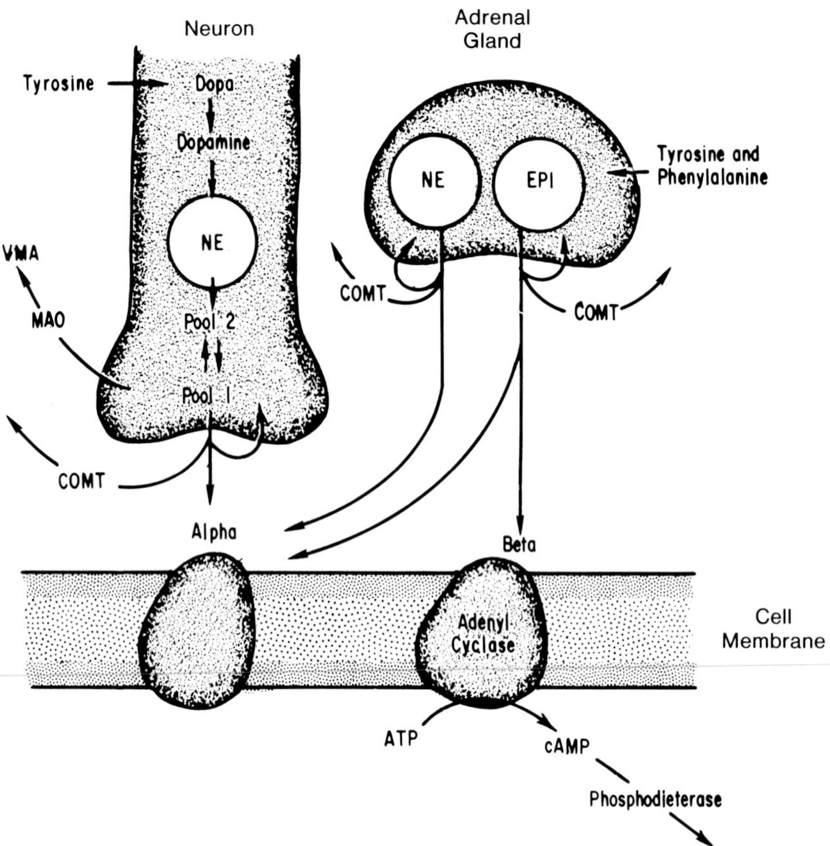

Figure 24.2. Adrenergic nervous system: Norephinephrine (*NE*) is produced in postganglionic neurons from tyrosine and in the adrenal glands from tyrosine and phenylalanine. It exists in two pools in the axon terminal, with a constant, slow release and re-uptake or inactivation to vanillylmandelic acid (*VMA*) by monoamine oxidase (*MAO*). It primarily stimulates alpha-adrenergic receptors, following which most is recaptured by the nerve, while the rest is inactivated by MAO or catechol-o-methyltransferase (*COMT*) or released in active form into the circulation. Epinephrine is produced only in the adrenal glands from tyrosine and phenylalanine and stimulates both alpha- and beta-adrenergic receptors. Beta stimulation activates the conversion of adenosine triphosphate (*ATP*) to cyclic adenosine monophosphate (*cAMP*) by the enzyme adenyl cyclase. Phosphodiesterase then inactivates cAMP.

The Pharmacokinetics of Topical Drugs

Pharmacokinetics deal with the absorption, distribution, metabolism, and elimination of an administered drug.[7] With regard to topical medications, the availability of the pharmacologic agent at the receptor site is influenced by (1) drug kinetics in the conjunctival cul-de-sac, (2) corneal penetration, and (3) the distribution and rate of drug elimination within the eye.[8]

Drug Kinetics in the Conjunctival Cul-de-sac

Following topical instillation, a medication first mixes with the tears in the cul-de-sac. The bulk of the drug is then lost through the lacrimal drainage system, while a small amount mixes with the precorneal tear film and is absorbed by the cornea. The dilution and drainage of a pharmacologic agent and the degree to which it saturates the tear film significantly influence the bioavailability of the drug.

Dilution and Drainage. The conjunctival cul-de-sac normally contains 7–9 μL of tears and has a maximum capacity of approximately 30 μL.[8] The drop size of commercial glaucoma medications ranges from 25.1 to 56.4 μL, with an average of 39 μL.[9] Therefore, up to one-half of the medication may spill out from the lids at the time of instillation. A large percentage of that which remains in the cul-de-sac then enters the lacrimal drainage system as a result of the pumping action created by blink movements. The loss rate in the tears is rapid, with the peak time occurring within the first few minutes after instillation. This loss not only reduces the amount of drug available for the pharmacologic effect within the eye but also increases the potential for systemic side effects by absorption into the systemic circulation via the nasopharyngeal mucosa. The degree to which this occurs can be influenced by nasolacrimal occlusion, which is discussed later in this chapter.

Tear Film Saturation. The precorneal tear film is a stagnant fluid layer that depends on blink movements for mixing with instilled drugs. In addition, the degree to which a drug saturates the tear film depends on the rate of drug loss in the tears, or the retention time in the conjunctival cul-de-sac. The amount of precorneal tear film saturation, in turn, determines the amount of drug available for corneal penetration and subsequent transfer to the intraocular receptor sites.

Corneal Penetration[10]

It may be helpful to think of the cornea as a lipid-water-lipid sandwich, in that the lipid content of the epithelium and endothelium is approximately 100 times greater than that of the stroma.[11] As a result of this composition, the epithelium and endothelium are readily traversed by lipid-soluble substances (i.e., compounds in a nonionized or nonelectrolyte form) but are impermeable to water-soluble agents (ionized compounds or electrolytes). This difference in permeability characteristics creates a selective barrier, in that only drugs that can exist in both a water-soluble and lipid-soluble state are able to penetrate the intact cornea. This has been referred to as the differential solubility concept.[11]

Drugs that are capable of existing in both the ionized and nonionized form include most of the weak bases, such as pilocarpine and epinephrine.[11] The two forms of the drug exist in equilibrium and, as one form penetrates a particular layer of the cornea, its concentration is replenished from the other form to maintain the equilibrium (Fig. 24.3). Quaternary ammonium compounds, such as echothiophate and carbachol, do not readily permeate the cornea. However, they are so potent that the small amount that does enter the eye is sufficient for antiglaucoma therapy.[12]

Drugs tend to concentrate in various layers of the cornea. Some of the drug may be degraded at this level, while another portion is temporarily stored in the cornea. Therefore, the cornea acts as a depot and a limiting factor for transfer of the drug to the aqueous.[8,13]

Intraocular Factors Influencing Drug Concentrations

Having penetrated the cornea, the drug must now pass through the aqueous to the appropriate structures in the anterior segment of the eye. A portion of the drug in the anterior chamber is eliminated by diffusion into the vascular system or escapes with the aqueous via the outflow system. Another percentage is bound to various ocular tissues. Both cholinergic[14,15] and adrenergic[15] drugs appear to bind to melanin in the anterior uveal tract, which prevents the drug from reaching the receptor site.[16–18] Histochemical studies show that adrenergic nerves are located close to melanocytes.[18] Some drugs, such as beta-adrenergic inhibitors, are released very slowly from the pigmented uveal tissues, accounting for the longer duration of effect in pigmented eyes.[8] Other drugs, including pilocarpine, are metabolized in the ocular tissues. It has also been suggested, based on studies with pilocarpine in pigmented and albino rabbits, that a larger amount of the topically applied drug may be metabolized in the cornea of eyes with more pigment.[19]

That small portion of the instilled drop which escapes extraocular or intraocular

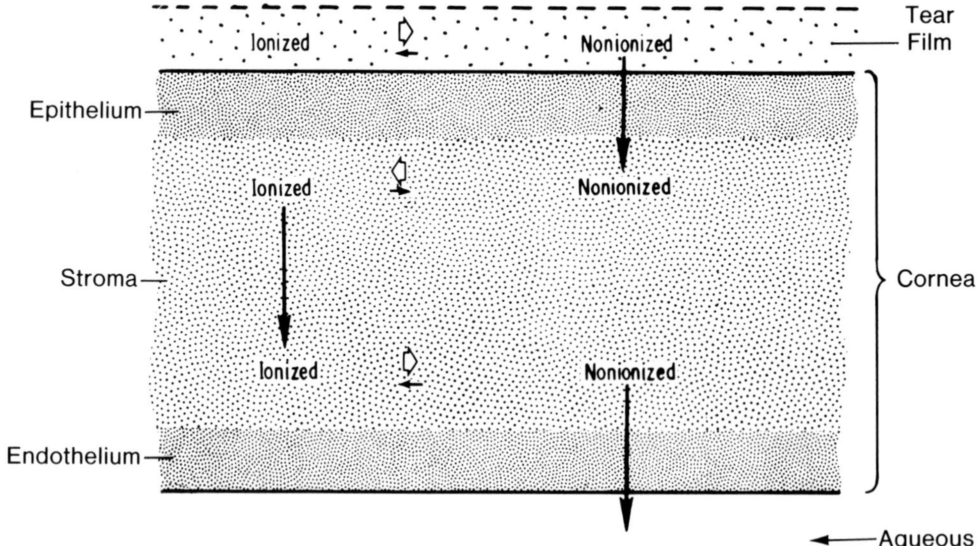

Figure 24.3. The differential solubility concept of corneal penetration. Only drugs with the potential to exist in both lipid-soluble (nonionized) and water-soluble (ionized) forms are able to penetrate the intact cornea. The two forms are in equilibrium and, as one form penetrates a particular corneal layer, its concentration is replenished from the other form to maintain the equilibrium.

elimination, tissue binding, or inactivation may finally reach the appropriate receptor, where it exerts its pharmacologic effect.

Formulations of Topical Drugs

The pharmacokinetics of a particular drug can be greatly influenced by the manner in which it is formulated. This includes the vehicle, pH, concentration, and additives of the formulation.

Vehicles

The vehicle in which a drug is delivered affects the amount of medication available for corneal penetration by influencing the rate of drug loss in the tears, the precorneal tear film saturation, and the length of time that the drug remains in contact with the cornea.[20]

Soluble Polymers. These commonly used vehicles, which include methylcellulose and polyvinyl alcohol, reduce the initial rapid drainage and prolong drug-corneal contact time. This is presumably accomplished by increasing tear viscosity, providing solution homogeneity (uniform suspension of drug particles in solution), and reducing surface tension.[21,22] However, this has only a minimal influence on enhanced drug bioavailability in the human eye.[20]

Ointments. These vehicles do significantly increase drug bioavailability by reducing loss in the tears, inhibiting dilution by the tears, providing a higher effective concentration of the drug, and increasing tissue contact time.[23–25] However, they are limited by interference with vision and aesthetic considerations.

Soluble Gels. Newer vehicles have been shown to prolong the therapeutic effect of a drug. Most of this work has been done with pilocarpine. One such vehicle is a soluble gel, described as a high-viscosity acrylic vehicle, which reportedly delivers a 24-hour pilocarpine dose following a single, nighttime application in the cul-de-sac.[26,27] It has not yet been established whether the prolonged drug action results from an increased surge in corneal absorption or a prolongation of the drug absorption phase.[20]

Emulsions and Suspensions. Another formulation that has been shown to prolong the therapeutic effect of pilocarpine is an emulsion of the drug with a polymeric material.[28] The prolonged action appears to be due to both enhanced pulse entry and a prolongation of drug release from the vehicle.[29] This results in a pilocarpine effect well in excess of 12 hours.[30]

Drugs administered in the form of suspended particles also have enhanced availability for corneal absorption because they mix less rapidly with tears and remain in the cul-de-sac longer than those administered in solutions.[12]

Liposomes. The interaction of phospholipids and water under special conditions results in concentric lipid bilayers, separated by aqueous layers. These multilamellar vesicles, called liposomes, can be reduced to smaller unilamellar structures of homogeneous size that are suitable for incorporation into topical medications.[20] A drug will concentrate in either the lipid or aqueous layer, depending upon its solubility characteristics, resulting in enhanced corneal penetration of the drug by adsorbing to the corneal surface, with direct transfer of the drug from liposomal to epithelial cell membranes.[31] Temperature-sensitive liposomes are also being evaluated, which release substances in the ocular vasculature when exposed to heat produced by an argon laser[32] or microwave.[33]

Ocular Insert Devices. A variety of solid materials have been evaluated for their ability to release a drug at a sustained rate from a location on the cornea or in the conjunctival cul-de-sac. Such a sustained release has been shown to achieve the same therapeutic effect as frequent topical applications, but with significantly less medication.[34]

Pulse Release. In one group of insert devices, the pattern of drug release is characterized by a very high initial rate that declines rapidly because of the leaching action by the tears.[20] This mode of delivery, which is also characteristic of conventional drop administration, is referred to as first-order kinetics. It has the disadvantage of transient overdosing with associated side effects, followed by a prolonged period of underdosing. Included in this group of drug delivery systems are water-soluble polymer matrices,[35,36] insoluble material,[37] and presoaked hydrophilic contact lenses[38,39] and collagen corneal shields.[40]

Rate-controlled Release.[20] To avoid the problems of first-order delivery, a second group of inserts has been developed, which deliver the drug at a controlled rate. This is referred to as zero-order kinetics, since the amount of drug delivered per unit time is independent of the amount left undelivered. Three such systems have been evaluated: (1) *diffusional systems,* in which pilocarpine is released from between two polymer membranes[41] (this is currently the only commercially available rate-controlled system and is discussed in the next chapter); (2) *osmotic systems,* in which the osmotic properties of a drug incorporated into a nonhydrophilic polymer matrix are used to achieve fairly constant drug delivery; and (3) *bioerodible systems,* which use an erodible hydrophobic matrix that does not allow leaching of the drug by the tears.

Mechanical Delivery Devices. As an alternative to the traditional drop delivery system, devices have been evaluated that mechanically transfer medication to the eye. One such device is a plastic rod with drug coated on the tip,[42–44] and another is a stiffened paper strip with medication incorporated into a water-soluble polyvinyl alcohol film at the tip.[45] In either case, the medication dissolves in the tear film when the tip is placed in the cul-de-sac. In addition to possibly being easier to administer, these devices have the potential advantage of delivering a more appropriate volume of medication and not requiring preservatives.

pH

As discussed before, the lipid:water solubility ratio (partition coefficient) of a compound influences corneal penetration. A greater degree of corneal penetration occurs when a higher concentration of nonionized (lipid-soluble) drug exists in the instilled drop.[12] The pH at which a drug is formulated influences this ratio, with weak bases (which include most antiglaucoma preparations) being absorbed through the cornea at a higher pH, while weak acids are absorbed better at a lower pH. For example, pilocarpine penetration was shown to be better at pH 6.5–7.5 than at pH 4,[46,47] although no significant difference was noted between formulations at pH 4.1 and 5.8.[48] Solution pH also affects drug stability and patient comfort upon instillation. Fortunately, most weak bases at physiologic pH 7.4 exist predominantly in the nonionized form.[12]

Concentration

Corneal penetration is enhanced by increasing the concentration of a drug up to a point. Beyond this point, the percentage of drug crossing the cornea decreases with increasing concentrations, and the greater amount of drug lost in the lacrimal drainage system increases the potential for systemic side effects. In a monkey study, topical 1% pilocarpine had a greater percentage recovered in the aqueous than did 4% or 8%.[49]

Additives

Certain additives that are used in commercial formulations, such as benzalkonium chloride, not only serve as a "preservative" by providing bacteriostatic activity but also influence corneal penetration through surface wetting properties. The latter property decreases the surface tension of nonpolar drugs, allowing them to mix more readily with the precorneal tear film, leading to enhanced corneal absorption. This is particularly important with drugs that have poor corneal penetration, such as carbachol.[50] However, such agents may also damage the corneal epithelium. Additives do not invariably prevent bacterial contamination. In seven cases of microbial keratitis, the same organism was cultured from corneal scrapings and the patient's timolol bottle,[51] emphasizing the importance of proper handling of eyedrop dispensers.

Molecular Weight

Compounds with a molecular weight greater than 500 g/mole have poor corneal absorption. However, this is not a major factor, since most ophthalmic drugs have a lower molecular weight.[10]

Drop Size

As previously noted, the drop size of commercial glaucoma medications ranges from 25.1 to 56.4 μL, with an average of 39 μL.[9] All of these may be significantly in excess of that required for effective bioavailability. A comparison of 8- and 30-μL drop volumes of 2.5% phenylephrine in neonates and infants revealed an equivalent pupillary effect but a significantly higher plasma level with the larger drop.[52]

Some Practical Aspects of Medical Therapy

When to Treat

The decision of when to initiate medical therapy varies according to the type of glaucoma being treated. The general approach is to recommend therapy whenever glaucomatous damage is documented or when the degree of IOP elevation or other risk factors is such that future damage is likely. The details of this issue, as they relate to specific forms of glaucoma, are considered in Section Two.

What to Prescribe

This decision depends not only on the type of glaucoma but also on several considerations related to the particular patient. A medication that may be effective for one form of glaucoma may be ineffective or actually counterproductive with another type. The reader must again be referred to Section Two for the details of this question as they relate to specific forms of glaucoma. In some cases, such as primary open-angle glaucoma, several medications may be potentially effective. A prospective study of 71 open-angle glaucoma patients revealed a significant reduction in IOP with the first drug used, but not with changes to stronger drugs or combination therapy.[53,54] Therefore, in selecting the initial drug it is best to try the one that is least likely to cause significant ocular and systemic side effects. This requires careful attention to the patient's medical history and physical findings, as well as a detailed understanding of potential drug-induced side effects, which are considered in subsequent chapters of Section Three. In general, the rule of thumb to follow whenever prescribing medication is to use the least amount of medication that will accomplish the desired therapeutic effect with the fewest adverse reactions.

How to Prescribe

It is almost always advisable to prescribe only one new drug at a time, so that the efficacy of each medication can be evaluated. One exception to this rule is the patient with a markedly elevated IOP that poses an immediate threat to vision. In this emergency situation, it is usually best to advance rapidly to maximum medical therapy by starting with a combination of two or more drugs and then to gradually reduce the medication, if possible, after the desired pressure level is reached. Another useful practice when prescribing a new drug in the less urgent situations is to use a *uniocular trial* of therapy, in which the untreated eye serves as a control during the trial period. This allows the physician to differentiate between drug effect and spontaneous fluctuations in IOP.

Instructing the Patient

Noncompliance. Noncompliance with recommended medical therapy is a major problem in the prevention of blindness from glaucoma. Studies have shown that glaucoma, by its very nature, fosters noncompliance.[55] In other words, most forms of glaucoma represent chronic diseases in which symptoms are mild or absent, treatment is prophylactic, and the consequences of stopping therapy are delayed, all of which are factors associated with poor patient compliance to medical therapy.[56] As a result, even studies of compliance that are based on the patient's own estimation reveal that one-third to two-thirds of the patients miss at least one treatment per month[57,58] or use their medications incorrectly.[59] Even more revealing are studies in which patient compliance is monitored by electronic devices in the medication bottle.[60] Studies with these instruments have shown that 41% of the patients omitted at least 10% of their prescribed pilocarpine treatments[61] and 15% missed more than half of their drops.[62] Many of these patients had inadequate spacing between treatments, frequent misses at noon, and long interruptions in the use of their medication.[62,63] Traditional parameters such as the IOP, pupillary diameter, patient's report or log book, and remaining medicine in bottle are all inadequate in distinguishing patients with low rates of compliance.[64] Reducing the frequency with which a medication must be taken appears to improve compliance but does not eliminate defaulting.[65,66] Efforts that have been shown to be effective in improving patient compliance include (1) educating the patient about the disease and its treatment; (2) tailoring the therapeutic regimen to the patient's daily schedule; (3) training and reinforcing the patient in the instillation of eyedrops; (4) cooperating with primary care physicians; (5) alleviating side effects; and (6) improving doctor-patient relationships.[55]

About the Disease. It is essential for the patient to be made aware of the disease and its potential seriousness without creating undue apprehension. In other words, the patient should be told: (1) that he or she has glaucoma; (2) what glaucoma is; (3) that it can lead to total, irreversible blindness; but (4) that the blindness can be prevented with proper treatment. It is not uncommon for patients who have been on antiglaucoma medications for years to be unaware that they have glaucoma or to fail to relate their disease to blindness, while others may live in daily fear that they will inevitably go blind. The time taken to correct these misconceptions is one of the most important measures in preventing blindness and improving the general well being of the patient.

Why the Medication. The patient must understand that the purpose of the medication is to lower the IOP to prevent loss of vision and that this treatment usually will not improve the present state of their visual acuity. Many patients stop using their drops because "they didn't seem to be helping."

Side Effects. It is equally important to make the patient aware of the more common side effects that they may experience with their new drug. If the patient knows what to expect and that the symptoms may lessen with time, it is hoped that this will allay the apprehension when side effects do occur and prevent the premature discontinuation of the drug.

The physician should also select a drug, especially if it is the patient's first antiglaucoma medication, that has the fewest possible potential side effects. It is usually best to begin with a weaker drug, even if it is unlikely to be sufficient, to allow the patient to adjust to the use of eyedrops before going to stronger medications with more side effects.

Administration of Eyedrops. It should not be assumed that a patient knows the proper techniques for instilling eyedrops. The inability to adequately instill a drop into the eye has been identified as a major factor in the failure of medical therapy.[67] When patients have been observed administering their drops, some were noted to flood their eye with an excess of medication, while others missed their eye altogether or contaminated the eyedropper by touching the lids or periocular tissue.[68,69] The first step in avoiding these pitfalls is to observe the patient instill the drops in the office, since some may already have a good technique. If they do not, the following is one effective method in which the patient can be instructed: (1) pinch the lower lid or pull it forward by the lashes to create a pocket; (2) place one drop in the cul-de-sac without touching the eyedropper to ocular tissues; (3) keep the lid held forward for a few seconds while the drop settles into the cul-de-sac; (4) look down while bringing the lower lid up until it touches the eye; (5) release the lid and close the eye gently while placing gentle pressure over the lacrimal sac (Fig. 24.4).[70]

The final step of *nasolacrimal occlusion* (Fig. 24.5), when performed for 5 minutes after instillation, has been shown to significantly reduce drug loss in the tears with a marked reduction in systemic drug absorption and an increase in anterior chamber concentration.[71] However, nasolacrimal occlusion was difficult for some patients, and

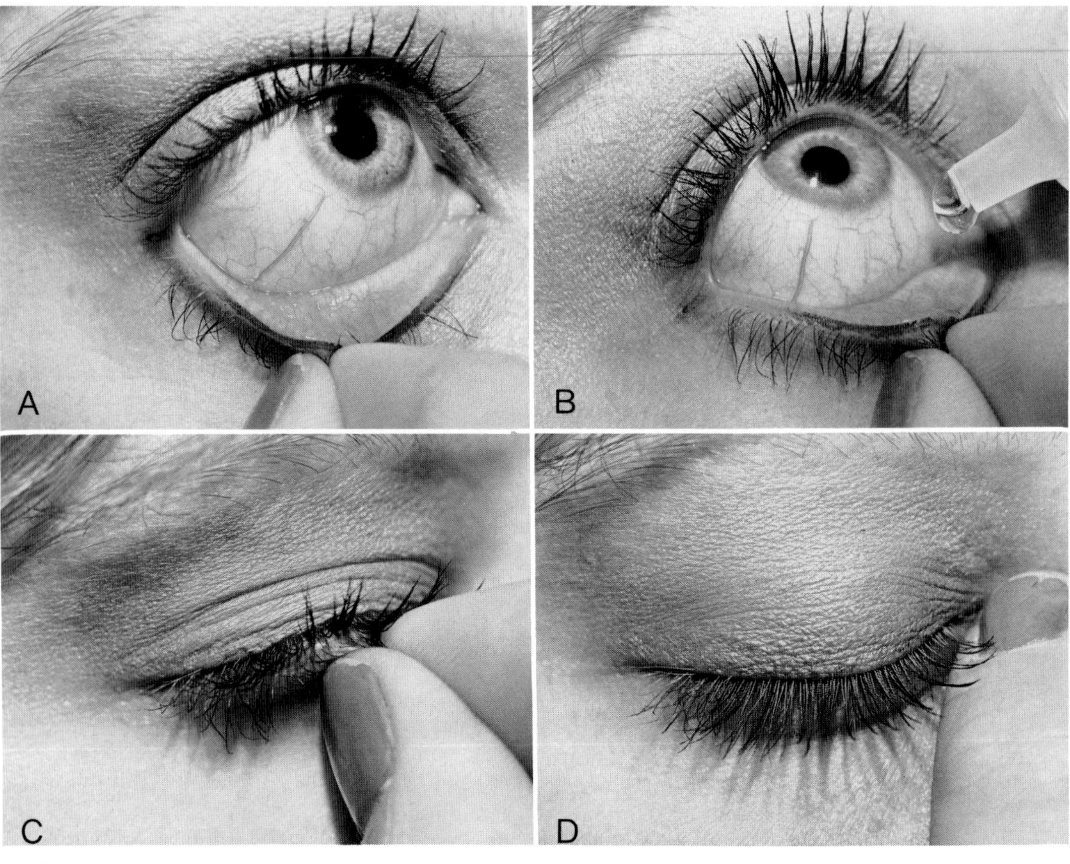

Figure 24.4. A technique for instillation of eyedrops: **A,** Pinch lower lid and pull down to create a pocket. **B,** Place one drop in pocket. **C,** Look down while bringing lower lid up to touch eye. **D,** Close eye and apply gentle pressure over lacrimal sac.

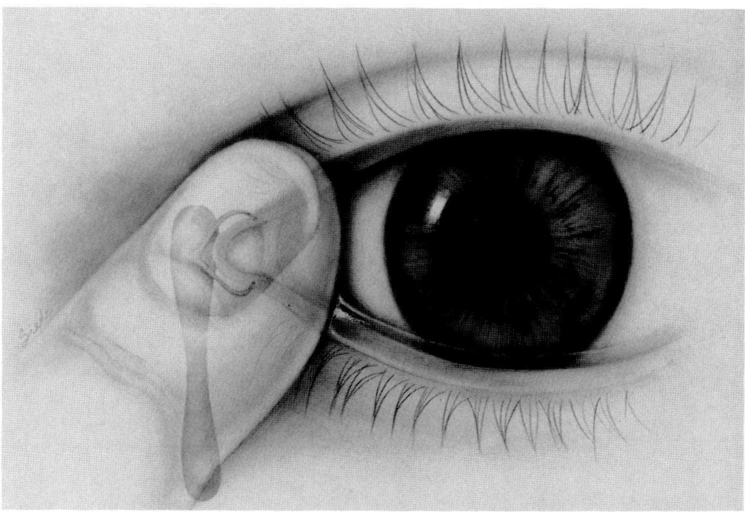

Figure 24.5. Proper placement of finger to achieve nasolacrimal occlusion. (Reprinted with permission from Zimmerman TJ, Kooner KS, Kandarakis AS, Ziegler LP: Arch Ophthal 102:551, 1984.)

gentle *eyelid closure* for 5 minutes, which minimizes lacrimal drainage by eliminating the blink movements, gave essentially the same results.[71] Punctal occlusion with silicone or collagen plugs has also been evaluated, with conflicting reports as to whether this improves drug efficacy.[72–74]

The Therapeutic Regimen. It is not enough to tell the patient to use the medication two or four times each day. Some patients may fail to space their dosages properly, while others may have such difficulty establishing a daily schedule that they become poor compliers.[62] In addition, if they are taking more than one drop at the same time of day, they may be instilling them so close together that they are diluting or washing each other from the cul-de-sac. The patient should be instructed to space the instillation of any two medications by at least 5–10 minutes. A patient may be on three different topical medications, which can be particularly complicated. This is especially true of the elderly, who constitute a large percentage of the glaucoma population, and whose impaired vision, limited motion, and failing memory significantly impair their ability to comply with prescribed therapy.[75]

To minimize these problems, the medicine bottles should first be clearly identified. Referring to the color of the top is usually best, although large labels on the bottles may also be helpful. The patient's daily routine should then be reviewed and the times of drug instillation should be selected to correspond with specific daily activities. The best times of day are usually with meals and at bedtime for a four-times-a-day medication, and a breakfast-supper or lunch-bedtime routine for twice-daily administration. The schedule should be placed on a card, which is large enough for the patient to see and which he or she can keep in a convenient location (Fig. 24.6).

Follow-up

Evaluation of Efficacy. It is obviously important to recheck the IOP within a few days or weeks of starting a new drug, depending on the urgency of the situation, to insure that the desired goal of pressure reduction has been achieved. This is best accomplished with the uniocular trial of therapy, as previously discussed. When using the fellow eye as a control, however, it must be kept in mind that most antiglaucoma drops will also cause a small consensual IOP fall in the untreated eye.[76]

Once a stable pressure reduction has been

name
date

drug/time	breakfast	lunch	supper	bedtime
pilocarpine (Green Top)	X	X	X	X
Epifrin (White Top)	X		X	
Timoptic (Yellow Top)		X		X
Diamox (Capsule)	X		X	

DAILY DRUG REMINDER

Figure 24.6. Example of drug schedule that can be used to instruct the patient in the use of glaucoma medications and to serve as a reminder for the patient. (Courtesy of Sharon Brooks, RN, McPherson Hospital, Durham, North Carolina.)

achieved, the patient is usually reevaluated every 3–4 months. It is a good practice to temporarily discontinue a drug once every several years to ensure that it is still contributing to the reduced IOP. This is especially true if the pressure is starting to rise, which may represent the development of tolerance to a drug rather than progression of the disease. Instead of simply adding more medication, the physician should first temporarily discontinue the existing medication in one eye (one drug at a time) to ensure that these are still having a significant effect on the pressure.

Patient Reinforcement. On every visit, patients should be asked about compliance with their medication and whether they are encountering any difficulties. Noncompliance should be dealt with by reviewing the seriousness of their glaucoma and the importance of treatment and by trying to find out why they are not complying. Such circumstances may include difficult daily schedules, visual or other physical limitations, or inability to afford the medication, and each must be dealt with on an individual basis. It is also important to seek out possible side effects, which patients may not relate to the treatment of their eyes but which could be adversely influencing their daily life or endangering their general health.

Contact with Family Physician. It is important to keep the primary care physician informed of the patient's ocular medication and also to keep a record from that physician as to the patient's additional medications or diseases, to avoid drug interactions or the use of medications that may be contraindicated. In addition, the family physician may help in reinforcing the importance of medical compliance and in spotting side effects.

Techniques of Patient Education

The physician is ultimately responsible for the education of his or her patient and must take the time, no matter how busy the day's schedule may be, to discuss the basic aspects of the disease and its treatment when it is first diagnosed. If it has not already been done, this is the time when a good doctor-patient relationship must be established. However, the physician rarely has time to be personally involved in all aspects of patient education and should make use of other personnel and material.

The most important ancillary individual is

the office nurse or technician. This person should be able to restate and expand upon what the physician has said, instruct the patient in the instillation of eyedrops, work out the therapeutic regimen, and provide the necessary reinforcement of these matters on each follow-up visit. That individual should also be able to answer the inevitable phone calls when patients have questions about the use of their medications or possible side effects.

Important resource materials include booklets on glaucoma, which are available from a number of health-related organizations. Videotapes have also been shown to be an effective method of patient education.[77] In some centers, classes or meetings are provided for glaucoma patients to broaden their understanding of their condition. These are usually conducted by nurses, technicians, or social workers and may incorporate lectures, videotapes, question-and-answer sessions, or group discussions.

SUMMARY

All commercially available topical antiglaucoma drugs act on the autonomic nervous system and include cholinergic stimulators and adrenergic stimulators and inhibitors, while systemic antiglaucoma agents include carbonic anhydrase inhibitors and hyperosmotics. The pharmacokinetics of topical drugs involves interaction with the tears, corneal penetration, and intraocular factors, each of which can be influenced by the vehicle, pH, concentration, and additives of the drug formulation. In prescribing medications, important questions are when to treat, what to use, and how it should be used. To improve compliance with recommended medical therapy, the patient should be told about the disease, why he or she is using the medicine, how to use the drug, and what side effects to expect. It is also important to evaluate the efficacy of the therapy initially and periodically during the treatment.

References

1. Richardson, KT: Ocular microtherapy. Membrane-controlled drug delivery. Arch Ophthal 93:74, 1975.
2. Bito, LZ, Merritt, SQ: Paradoxical ocular hypertensive effect of pilocarpine on echothiophate iodide-treated primate eyes. Invest Ophthal Vis Sci 19:371, 1980.
3. Kaufman, PL, Barany, EH: Loss of acute pilocarpine effect on outflow facility following surgical disinsertion and retrodisplacement of the ciliary muscle from the scleral spur in the cynomolgus monkey. Invest Ophthal 15:793, 1976.
4. Kaufman, PL, Barany, EH: Residual pilocarpine effects on outflow facility after ciliary muscle disinsertion in the cynomolgus monkey. Invest Ophthal 15:558, 1976.
5. Grierson, I, Lee, WR, Abraham, S: Effects of pilocarpine on the morphology of the human outflow apparatus. Br J Ophthal 62:302, 1978.
6. Lands, AM, Arnold, A, McAuliff, JP, et al: Differentiation of receptor systems activated by sympathomimetic amines. Nature 214:597, 1967.
7. Shell, JW: Pharmacokinetics of topically applied ophthalmic drugs. Surv Ophthal 26:207, 1982.
8. Mishima, S: Clinical pharmacokinetics of the eye. Proctor lecture. Invest Ophthal Vis Sci 21:504, 1981.
9. Lederer, CM Jr, Harold, RE: Drop size of commercial glaucoma medications. Am J Ophthal 101:691, 1986.
10. Benson, H: Permeability of the cornea to topically applied drugs. Arch Ophthal 91:313, 1974.
11. Havener, WH: Ocular Pharmacology, 4th ed. CV Mosby, St. Louis, 1978, pp. 19, 429.
12. Akers, MJ: Ocular bioavailability of topically applied ophthalmic drugs. Am Pharm NS23:33, 1983.
13. Mindel, JS, Smith, H, Jacobs, M, et al: Drug reservoirs in topical therapy. Invest Ophthal Vis Sci 25:346, 1984.
14. Harris, LS, Galin, MA: Effect of ocular pigmentation on hypotensive response to pilocarpine. Am J Ophthal 72:923, 1971.
15. Melikian, HE, Lieberman, TW, Leopold, IH: Ocular pigmentation and pressure and outflow responses to pilocarpine and epinephrine. Am J Ophthal 72:70, 1971.
16. Lyons, JS, Krohn, DL: Pilocarpine uptake by pigmented uveal tissue. Am J Ophthal 75:885, 1973.
17. Newsome, DA, Stern, R: Pilocarpine adsorption by serum and ocular tissues. Am J Ophthal 77:918, 1974.
18. Path, PN, Jacobowitz, D: Unequal accumulation of adrenergic drugs by pigmented and nonpigmented iris. Am J Ophthal 78:470, 1974.
19. Lee, VH-L, Hul, H-W, Robinson, JR: Corneal metabolism of pilocarpine in pigmented rabbits. Invest Ophthal Vis Sci 19:210, 1980.
20. Shell, JW: Ophthalmic drug delivery systems. Surv Ophthal 29:117, 1984.

21. Lemp, MA, Holly, FJ: Ophthalmic polymers as ocular wetting agents. Ann Ophthal 4:15, 1972.
22. Trueblood, JH, Rossomondo, RM, Carlton, WH, Wilson, LA: Corneal contact times of ophthalmic vehicles. Evaluation by microscintigraphy. Arch Ophthal 93:127, 1975.
23. Hardberger, R, Hanna, C, Boyd, CM: Effects of drug vehicles on ocular contact time. Arch Ophthal 93:42, 1975.
24. Hardberger, RE, Hanna, C, Goodart, R: Effects of drug vehicles on ocular uptake of tetracycline. Am J Ophthal 80:133, 1975.
25. Waltman, SR, Buerk, K, Foster, CS: Effects of ophthalmic ointments on intraocular penetration of topical fluorescein in rabbits and man. Am J Ophthal 78:262, 1974.
26. Mandell, AI, Stewart, RM, Kass, MA: Multiclinic evaluation of pilocarpine gel. Invest Ophthal Vis Sci (suppl) 165, 1979.
27. March, WF, Stewart, RM, Mandell, AI, Bruce, LA: Duration of effect of pilocarpine gel. Arch Ophthal 100:1270, 1982.
28. Ticho, U, Blumenthal, M, Zonis, S, et al: Piloplex, a new long-acting pilocarpine polymer salt: a long-term study. Br J Ophthal 63:45, 1979.
29. Mazor, A, Ticho, U, Rehany, U, Rose, L: Piloplex—a new long-acting polymer salt: B. Comparative study of the visual effects of pilocarpine and piloplex eyedrops. Br J Ophthal 63:48, 1979.
30. Klein, HZ, Lugo, M, Shields, MB, et al: A dose-response study of piloplex for duration of action. Am J Ophthal 99:23, 1985.
31. Schaeffer, HE, Krohn, DL: Liposomes in topical drug delivery. Invest Ophthal Vis Sci 21:220, 1982.
32. Zeimer, RC, Khoobehi, B, Niesman, MR, Magin, RL: A potential method for local drug and dye delivery in the ocular vasculature. Invest Ophthal Vis Sci 29:1179, 1988.
33. Khoobehi, B, Peyman, GA, McTurnan, WG, et al: Externally triggered release of dye and drugs from the liposomes into the eye. An in vitro and in vivo study. Ophthalmology 95:950, 1988.
34. Lerman, S, Reininger, B: Simulated sustained release pilocarpine therapy and aqueous humor dynamics. Can J Ophthal 6:14, 1971.
35. Maichuk, YF: Ophthalmic drug inserts. Invest Ophthal 14:87, 1975.
36. Katz, IM, Blackman, WM: A soluble sustained-release ophthalmic delivery unit. Am J Ophthal 83:728, 1977.
37. Leaders, FE, Hecht, G, VanHoose, M, Kellog, M: New polymers in drug delivery. Ann Ophthal 5:513, 1973.
38. Maddox, YT, Bernstein, HN: An evaluation of the bionite hydrophilic contact lens for use in a drug delivery system. Ann Ophthal 4:789, 1972.
39. Hull, DS, Edelhauser, HF, Hyndiuk, RA: Ocular penetration of prednisolone and the hydrophilic contact lens. Arch Ophthal 92:413, 1974.
40. Sawusch, MR, O'Brien, TP, Dick, JD, Gottsch, JD: Use of collagen corneal shields in the treatment of bacterial keratitis. Am J Ophthal 106:279, 1988.
41. Dohlman, CH, Pavan-Langston, D, Rose, J: A new ocular insert device for continuous constant-rate delivery of medication to the eye. Ann Ophthal 4:823, 1972.
42. Gwon, A, Borrmann, LR, Duzman, E, et al: Ophthalmic rods. New ocular drug delivery devices. Ophthalmology 93(S):82, 1986.
43. Alani, SD: The ophthalmic rod—a new ophthalmic drug delivery system I. Graefe's Arch Ophthal 228:297, 1990.
44. Alani, SD, Hammerstein, W: The ophthalmic rod—a new drug-delivery system II. Graefe's Arch Ophthal 228:302, 1990.
45. Kelly, JA, Molyneux, PD, Smith, SA, Smith, SE: Relative bioavailability of pilocarpine from a novel ophthalmic delivery system and conventional eyedrop formulations. Br J Ophthal 73:360, 1989.
46. Anderson, RA, Cowle, JB: Influence of pH on the effect of pilocarpine on aqueous dynamics. Br J Ophthal 52:607, 1968.
47. Ramer, RM, Gasset, AR: Ocular penetration of pilocarpine: the effect of pH on the ocular penetration of pilocarpine. Ann Ophthal 7:293, 1975.
48. David, R, Goldberg, L, Luntz, MH: Influence of pH on the efficacy of pilocarpine. Br J Ophthal 62:318, 1978.
49. Asseff, CF, Weisman, RL, Podos, SM, Becker, B: Ocular penetration of pilocarpine in primates. Am J Ophthal 75:212, 1973.
50. Smolen, VF, Clevenger, JM, Williams, EJ, Bergdolt, MW: Biophasic availability of ophthalmic carbachol I: Mechanisms of cationic polymer- and surfactant-promoted miotic activity. J Pharm Sci 62:958, 1973.
51. Schein, OD, Wasson, PJ, Boruchoff, SA, Kenyon, KR: Microbial keratitis associated with contaminated ocular medications. Am J Ophthal 105:361, 1988.
52. Lynch, MG, Brown, RH, Goode, SM, et al: Reduction of phenylephrine drop size in infants achieves equal dilation with decreased systemic absorption. Arch Ophthal 105:1364, 1987.
53. Begg, IS, Cottle, RW, et al: Epidemiological approach to open-angle glaucoma: 1. Control of intraocular pressure. Report of the Canadian Ocular Adverse Drug Reaction Registry Program. Can J Ophthal 23:273, 1988.
54. Begg, IS, Cottle, RW: Epidemiologic approach to open-angle glaucoma: 2. Survival analysis of adverse drug reactions. Report of the Canadian Ocular Adverse Drug Reaction Registry Program. Can J Ophthal 24:15, 1989.
55. Zimmerman, TJ, Zalta, AH: Facilitating patient compliance in glaucoma therapy. Surv Ophthal 28(suppl):252, 1983.

56. Blackwell, B: Patient compliance. N Engl J Med 289:249, 1973.
57. Bloch, S, Rosenthal, AR, Friedman, L, Caldarolla, P: Patient compliance in glaucoma. Br J Ophthal 61:531, 1977.
58. Kass, MA, Hodapp, E, Gordon, M, et al: Patient administration of eyedrops: Part I. Interview. Ann Ophthal 14:775, 1982.
59. Spaeth, GL: Visual loss in a glaucoma clinic. I. Sociological considerations. Invest Ophthal 9:73, 1970.
60. Kass, MA, Meltzer, DW, Gordon, M: A miniature compliance monitor for eyedrop medication. Arch Ophthal 102:1550, 1984.
61. Norell, SE, Granstrom, PA: Self-medication with pilocarpine among outpatients in a glaucoma clinic. Br J Ophthal 64:137, 1980.
62. Kass, MA, Meltzer, DW, Gordon, M, et al: Compliance with topical pilocarpine treatment. Am J Ophthal 101:515, 1986.
63. Granstrom, P-A: Glaucoma patients not compliant with their drug therapy: clinical and behavioural aspects. Br J Ophthal 66:464, 1982.
64. Kass, MA, Gordon, M, Meltzer, DW: Can ophthalmologists correctly identify patients defaulting from pilocarpine therapy? Am J Ophthal 101:524, 1986.
65. Kass, MA, Gordon, M, Morley, RE, et al: Compliance with topical timolol treatment. Am J Ophthal 103:188, 1987.
66. Cramer, JA, Mattson, RH, Prevey, ML, et al: How often is medication taken as prescribed? A novel assessment technique. JAMA 261:3273, 1989.
67. Winfield, AJ, Jessiman, D, Williams, A, Esakowitz, L: A study of the causes of non-compliance by patients prescribed eyedrops. Br J Ophthal 74:477, 1990.
68. Kass, MA, Hodapp, E, Gordon, M, et al: Patient administration of eyedrops: Part II. Observation. Ann Ophthal 14:889, 1982.
69. Brown, MM, Brown, GC, Spaeth, GL: Improper topical self-administration of ocular medications among patients with glaucoma. Can J Ophthal 19:2, 1984.
70. Fraunfelder, FT: Extraocular fluid dynamics: how best to apply topical ocular medication. Trans Am Ophthal Soc 74:457, 1976.
71. Zimmerman, TJ, Kooner, KS, Kandarakis, AS, Ziegler, LP: Improving the therapeutic index of topically applied ocular drugs. Arch Ophthal 102:551, 1984.
72. Huang, TC, Lee, DA: Punctal occlusion and topical medications for glaucoma. Am J Ophthal 107:151, 1989.
73. Gilbert, ML, Wilhelmus, KR, Osato, MS: Intracanalicular collagen implants enhance topical antibiotic bioavailability. Cornea 5:167, 1986.
74. Simel, DL, Simel, PJ: Does lacrimal duct occlusion decrease intraocular pressure in patients refractory to medical treatment for glaucoma? A randomized, sham-controlled, crossover trial. J Clin Epidemiol 41:859, 1988.
75. Polk, IJ: Drug compliance in the elderly. JAMA 248:1239, 1982.
76. Gibbens, MV: The consensual ophthalmotonic reaction. Br J Ophthal 72:746, 1988.
77. Rosenthal, AR, Zimmerman, JF, Tanner, J: Educating the glaucoma patient. Br J Ophthal 67:814, 1983.

Chapter 25

CHOLINERGIC STIMULATORS

Pharmacologic agents that mimic the cholinergic effects of acetylcholine are generally referred to as *parasympathomimetics, cholinergic stimulators,* or *miotics,* the latter because of their common action on the pupil. This was the first class of drugs to be used in the treatment of glaucoma, having been introduced in the 1870s. These compounds all have the same basic effect on aqueous humor dynamics and their primary clinical differences are in duration of action and severity of side effects.

PILOCARPINE

Pilocarpine is the most commonly used and the most extensively studied miotic. It is a direct-acting parasympathomimetic, although there is evidence that it may also have an indirect effect by activating choline acetyltransferase synthesis of acetylcholine.[1] The following ocular effects of pilocarpine are generally representative of all the miotics.

Mechanisms of Action

Increased Facility of Aqueous Outflow. The principal mode of intraocular pressure (IOP) reduction by pilocarpine is enhanced aqueous outflow. In eyes with open anterior chamber angles, the mechanism of this action appears to be stimulation of ciliary muscle contraction. It has been demonstrated that aqueous outflow facility can be increased by accommodation,[2] a posterior depression of the lens,[3–5] tension on the choroid,[6] or a pull on the root of the iris.[7] In each of these situations, the common action appears to be traction on the scleral spur by virtue of its attachment to the ciliary musculature. The displacement of the scleral spur leads to an increased facility of aqueous outflow, presumably by altering the configuration of the trabecular meshwork, Schlemm's canal, or both (Fig. 25.1). Pilocarpine, and the other miotics, exert a similar traction on the scleral spur by stimulating contraction of the ciliary muscle.

More direct evidence for the influence of pilocarpine-induced cyclotonia on outflow facility is that disinsertion of the ciliary muscle from the scleral spur in monkeys eliminates the effect of pilocarpine on IOP and facility of outflow.[8,9] To rule out other possible mechanisms, it was shown that the

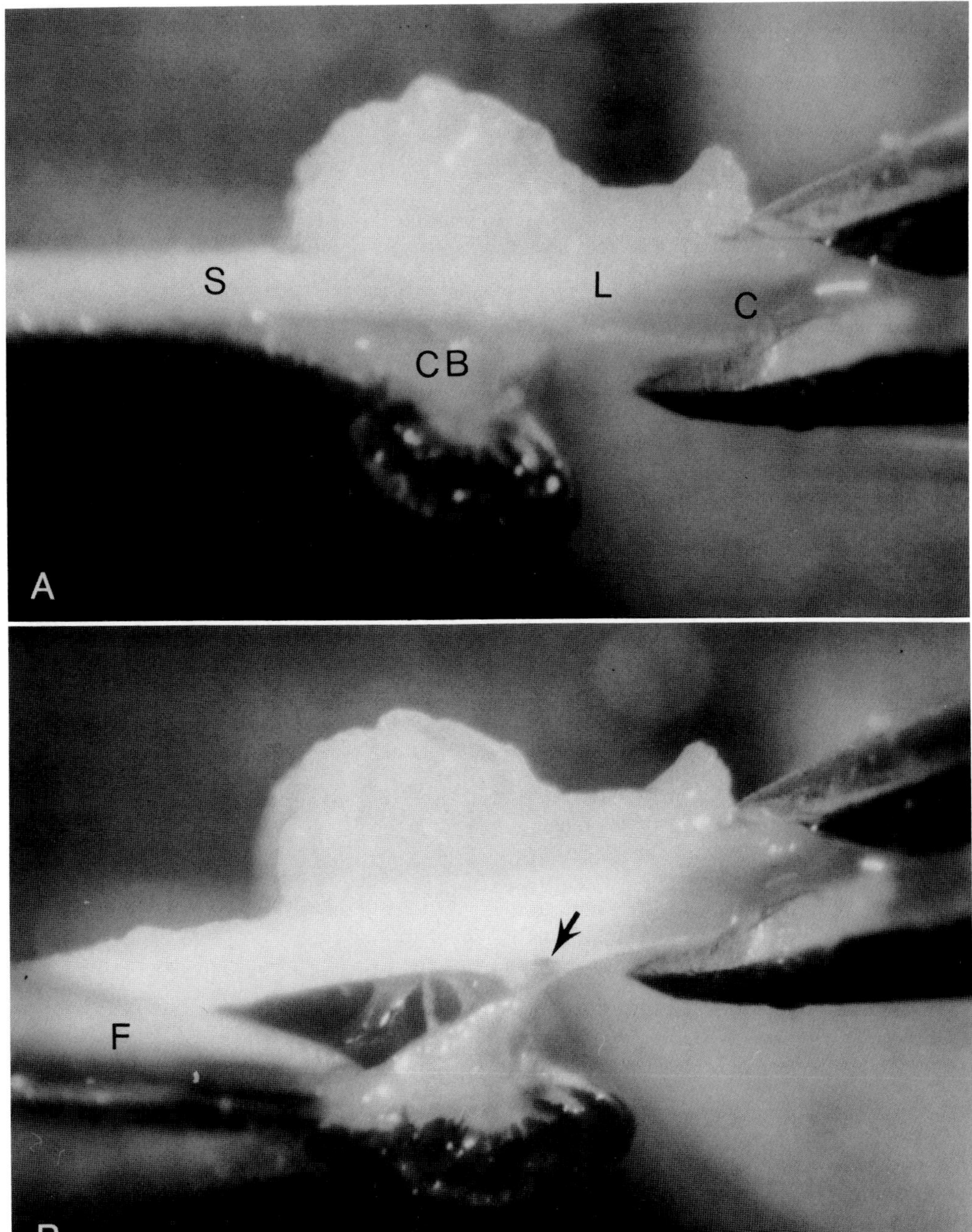

Figure 25.1. The influence of tension on the ciliary body in widening Schlemm's canal is demonstrated in a human autopsy eye: **A,** Without tension, the canal is collapsed and cannot be seen in this photo. **B,** When the ciliary body is stretched with forceps (*F*), Schlemm's canal opens (*arrow*) as a result of inward, posterior displacement of the scleral spur. A similar mechanism is believed to explain the improvement in outflow facility following cholinergic stimulation. Ciliary body (*CB*); sclera (*S*); limbus (*L*); cornea (*C*). (Courtesy of David G. Campbell, M.D.)

disinsertion neither altered conventional outflow[10] nor caused histologic changes in the ciliary muscle, trabecular meshwork, or Schlemm's canal.[11] Histologic studies of human eyes treated with pilocarpine prior to enucleation for malignant melanoma demonstrated a posterior, internal pull on the scleral spur, with widening of the trabecular spaces, distention of the endothelial meshwork, an increase in the number of giant vacuoles, and larger, more frequent pores in the inner endothelium of Schlemm's canal.[12,13] Primate studies suggest that the greater number of giant vacuoles is a result of increased aqueous flow through the outflow system, rather than a direct action of pilocarpine on the endothelium of Schlemm's canal.[14] The contractile response of ciliary muscle to pilocarpine in monkeys diminishes with age at a rate similar to that for accommodative decline.[15]

Denervation of the ciliary muscle by ciliary ganglionectomy in monkeys produces an initial supersensitivity to pilocarpine.[16] Reinnervation occurs by 6 months with return of normal accommodative response to pilocarpine,[16] although, for reasons that have yet to be explained, pilocarpine in these eyes has no effect on outflow facility.[17]

Miosis. The miotic effect of pilocarpine is useful in the short-term management of certain angle-closure glaucomas. The miosis results primarily from direct stimulation of the sphincter muscle of the iris, although significant cholinergic inhibition of the dilator muscle has also been demonstrated in the bovine eye.[18] Miosis improves outflow facility in eyes with angle-closure glaucomas by relieving pupillary block or by pulling peripheral iris from the anterior chamber angle. However, miosis does not appear to be related to the improvement of aqueous outflow facility in open-angle glaucomas, since total removal of the iris in monkeys did not alter the facility response to intravenous pilocarpine.[19]

Decreased Aqueous Production. There is some controversy as to whether the IOP-lowering effect of pilocarpine is partly related to decreased aqueous inflow. The reduction in pressure has been reported to exceed[20] and outlast[21] the improvement in outflow facility, and pilocarpine 0.1% was shown to reduce aqueous humor formation in monkey eyes.[22] Bárány[23] suggested that prolonged treatment with pilocarpine may result in subsensitivity of the ciliary muscle, with a shift in emphasis to inhibition of aqueous secretion by an unknown mechanism. In support of this therapy is the observation that acetylcholine transiently hyperpolarizes the cell membrane potential of cultured human nonpigmented ciliary epithelial cells by an action on K^+ channels.[24] There is also a suggestion from studies with rabbit iris-ciliary body tissue preparations that the cholinergic system may play a direct role in the modulation of ciliary epithelial adenylate cyclase and aqueous humor secretion.[25] However, fluorophotometric studies in humans revealed a stimulation of aqueous humor formation with pilocarpine, although this was too small to be of clinical significance.[26]

It should also be noted that pilocarpine *decreases uveoscleral outflow*.[27] This may have clinical significance in eyes with markedly reduced conventional outflow. As these eyes become increasingly dependent on unconventional drainage, pilocarpine may cause a paradoxic rise in IOP.[28] Episcleral venous pressure does not appear to be altered by pilocarpine.[20]

Administration

Ocular Penetration. The cornea is the main route by which topical pilocarpine enters the eye,[29] although this tissue may also impede ocular penetration. Studies differ somewhat as to the predominant portion of the cornea in which pilocarpine concentrates, with one suggesting the epithelium[30] and others the corneal stroma.[31,32] In any case, the drug is largely complexed or degraded in the cornea,[33] with only a small percentage entering the anterior chamber.[33–35] Selecting the optimum drug concentration, frequency of administration, and delivery system may improve the efficiency of ocular penetration.

Drug Concentration. The IOP-lowering effect of pilocarpine is dose related up to a concentration of 4%.[36–39] However, studies differ as to whether there is significant dose-response curve with single dose instillations.[36,37] Furthermore, higher concentrations of pilocarpine, such as 6%, may cause additional pressure reduction in darkly pigmented eyes.[40]

Frequency of Administration. Following topical instillation in animals, the maximum concentrations of pilocarpine in the aqueous and iris were reached in approximately 20 minutes,[32] and aqueous levels were gone in 4 hours.[34] In studies of ocular hypertensive individuals, the maximum effect on IOP occurred within 2 hours and lasted for at least 8 hours, with a reduction in IOP of approximately 20%.[37] The pressure response began to decline by the 9th hour, although there was still a 14–15% reduction at 12–15 hours after instillation.[38] To ensure adequate pressure control, standard pilocarpine drops are generally given four times daily. However, recent evidence suggests that twice-daily instillation is adequate for 2% pilocarpine followed by nasolacrimal occlusion (Thom J. Zimmerman, M.D., personal communication). Efficiency may be improved by frequent, repeated instillations[41] or by continuous infusion[42] of dilute solutions. Since these methods have obvious practical limitations for long-term therapy, efforts are being made to achieve similar results with newer drug delivery systems.

Delivery Systems. A goal of any drug therapy is to achieve the desired pharmacologic effect with the least amount of medicine. Animal and human studies suggest that the volume of pilocarpine delivered by commercial droppers is significantly in excess of that needed to produce the desired response.[43,44] The result is an initial overdosing with its associated side effects, followed by an underdosing before the next instillation. This problem can be reduced by using vehicles for drug delivery that prolong the duration of the therapeutic effectiveness, thereby decreasing the frequency of instillations and associated side effects (Table 25.1).

Soluble Polymers. As discussed in Chapter 24, soluble polymers such as methylcellulose and polyvinyl alcohol may increase corneal retention time and are commonly used in commercial preparations.[45] However, the results of clinical studies with pilocarpine in such vehicles have been conflicting. One formulation of pilocarpine in water-soluble polymers was reported to have a prolonged duration of action with improved pressure control,[46–48] although this was not confirmed by subsequent studies.[49–51]

An aqueous emulsion of pilocarpine bound to a polymer vehicle (Piloplex) was shown to be more effective in twice-daily administration than pilocarpine hydrochloride four times a day.[52–55] A single dose lowered the IOP in a dose-related fashion, with a duration of action of at least 14 hours.[56] This formulation is still under investigation.

Table 25.1
Commercial Pilocarpine Preparations*

Preparations	Brand Names	Concentrations (%)
Solutions		
Hydrochlorides	Adsorbocarpine	1, 2, 4
	Akarpine	0.5, 1, 2, 3, 4, 6
	Almocarpine	1, 2, 4
	Isopto carpine	0.25, 0.5, 1, 2, 3, 4, 6, 10
	Ocu-carpine	0.5, 1, 2, 3, 4, 6
	Pilocar	0.5, 1, 2, 3, 4, 6
	Pilokair	0.5, 1, 2, 3, 4, 6
Nitrate	P.V. carpine	1, 2, 4
Gel	Pilopine HS gel	4
Inserts	Ocusert Pilo-20	(20 μg/hr)
	Ocusert Pilo-40	(40 μg/hr)
Epinephrine combinations	E-Pilo-1, E-Pilo-2, etc. P_1E_1, P_2E_1, etc.	1, 2, 3, 4, 6 (+ epi. 1%)

* Other generic products may also be available.

Pilocarpine Gel. The equivalent of 4% pilocarpine hydrochloride in a high-viscosity acrylic vehicle (Pilopine), when applied once daily at bedtime, has been reported to produce a significant reduction in IOP for 24 hours.[57,58] It was found to be at least as effective as pilocarpine hydrochloride drops four times daily,[59,60] with less induced myopia and impaired nocturnal visual acuity than with the drops.[61] However, since the effect 12 hours after administration is greater than that at 24 hours, the physician is advised to measure the pressure 24 hours after administration before prescribing pilocarpine gel on a once-daily regimen.[57] Furthermore, 20–28% of patients have been shown to develop a subtle diffuse superficial corneal haze.[60,62] In some patients, this persisted for 2 years after the gel was discontinued.[57] The corneal haze produced no symptoms, although the long-term consequences remain unknown.[55,57]

Oily Solutions. Such solutions of pilocarpine have also been shown to have a greater degree and duration of effect on the pupil[63] and IOP[64] than the same drug in an aqueous solution.

Other Vehicles. Other drug delivery vehicles that have been shown to prolong the effect of topical pilocarpine include sodium hyaluronate,[65,66] cyanoacrylate block copolymer,[66] and poly (butylcyanoacrylate) nanoparticles.[67]

Membrane-Controlled Delivery System. Pilocarpine between two polymeric membranes provides a constant drug release of 20 micrograms per hour (Ocusert P-20) or 40 micrograms per hour (Ocusert P-40), which is roughly comparable to 1–2% and 4% pilocarpine, respectively.[68–72] The insert device is retained in the cul-de-sac (Fig. 25.2) and is effective for up to 7 days,[70,73] although both relative effectiveness[74] and duration of action[71] must be established for each patient by therapeutic trial.

This therapeutic delivery system offers distinct advantages over topical instillation of pilocarpine. The constant rate of release (zero-order delivery) provides comparable

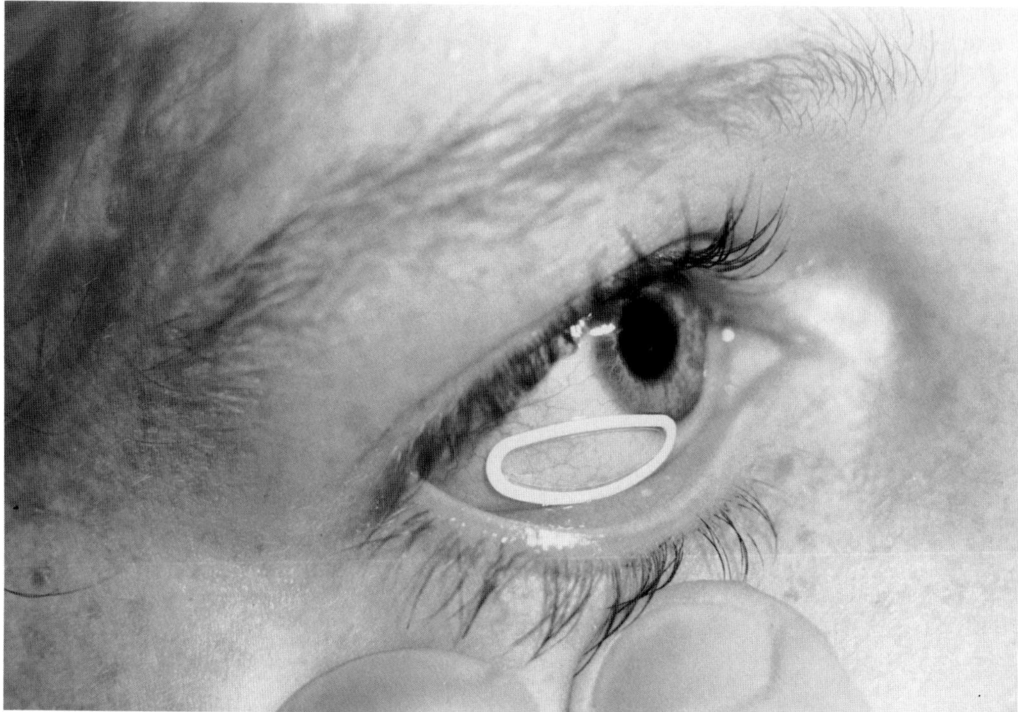

Figure 25.2. Appearance of Ocusert, a pilocarpine delivery system, in the lower cul-de-sac.

pressure control with one-fifth the amount of medicine delivered by drops,[68–75] which reduces side effects.[68,76,77] Two exceptions to this steady delivery rate are an initial period of increased drug release following insertion of the device and occasional subsequent episodes of transient increased release, which has been called the sudden leakage phenomenon.[69] Another advantage of this delivery system is that it partly levels out the diurnal curve.[78] The primary disadvantages are occasional discomfort and retention problems.[79,80]

Soluble Insert Devices. These devices impregnated with pilocarpine have been shown to provide IOP control for up to 24 hours when placed in the cul-de-sac.[81,82] A mechanical delivery device in which pilocarpine, incorporated into a water-soluble polyvinyl alcohol film on the end of a stiffened paper strip, is placed in the lower conjunctival sac, where it dissolves in the tear film, provided approximately eight-fold greater bioavailability than a conventional eyedrop formulation.[83] With further study of new designs, the ocular insert devices may become an increasingly useful form of drug delivery in the treatment of glaucoma.

Soft Contact Lenses. A soft contact lens that has been soaked in pilocarpine is reported to give longer corneal contact time,[84,85] greater aqueous drug levels,[34,86] and longer IOP control[87] than topically applied pilocarpine. However, this mode of drug delivery has not yet been recommended for general clinic use.

Injections. It has also been reported that subconjunctival injection of 0.15–0.2 ml of 4% pilocarpine achieves a more rapid and sustained miosis than does instillation of pilocarpine drops.[88] Intraocular injection of pilocarpine should be avoided, since it has been shown to cause corneal edema, presumably because of the osmotic effect of the solution.[89]

Drug Interactions

Other Miotics. When other miotics are administered in combination with pilocarpine, they not only fail to increase the pressure lowering effect but may interfere with the action of pilocarpine. *Echothiophate iodide,* a potent indirect-acting parasympathomimetic, is as effective alone as in combination with pilocarpine.[90] Furthermore, pretreating monkeys with echothiophate iodide or diisopropyl fluorophosphate, another potent indirect-acting parasympathomimetic, produced a reversible subsensitivity or insensitivity to pilocarpine.[91–95] One such study showed that pilocarpine paradoxically increased the IOP after pretreatment with echothiophate iodide, while the miotic effect of pilocarpine was only partly abolished.[96] This was thought to suggest the presence of two cholinergic receptor populations. Physostigmine (eserine), a slightly weaker indirect-acting parasympathomimetic, had no additive effect on tonographic values when added to pilocarpine therapy.[97]

Additional Antiglaucoma Medications. Epinephrine[97,98] and timolol[99] both produce additional IOP reduction when combined with pilocarpine. However, the effect of either combination is less than the additive effect of the two drugs. In one case report, epinephrine compounds apparently increased the induced myopia of pilocarpine Ocuserts.[100] Studies of a *fixed combination* of pilocarpine 2–4% and timolol 0.5% given twice daily revealed a pressure lowering effect equivalent to that of the two drugs given separately[101] and a greater effect than either pilocarpine[102] or timolol[103] given alone. Pilocarpine may also be used effectively in combination with carbonic anhydrase inhibitors or hyperosmotic agents.

Antibiotic and Corticosteroid Ointments. These medications have been shown to decrease the aqueous concentration of topically applied pilocarpine in rabbits.[104] Although this was believed to be due to the drug components rather than the ointment base, it is advisable when a drop and an ointment have been prescribed to instill the drop 5–10 minutes before the ointment.

Side Effects

Systemic Toxicity. Pilocarpine can produce systemic effects similar to those of muscarine.[105] These include diaphoresis (perspiration), stimulation of glands, and contraction of smooth muscle. The glands involved include salivary, lacrimal, gastric, pancreatic, intestinal, and mucosa of the respiratory tract. Increased bronchial secretion may result from the pilocarpine-induced decrease in pulmonary surfactant, which is responsible for the stability of the alveoli.[106] Pulmonary edema resulting from this may be fatal. Smooth muscle contraction may cause nausea, vomiting, diarrhea, and bronchospasm, the latter of which may also be fatal. Other organs in which contraction of smooth muscle may occur include the ureters, urinary bladder, gallbladder, and the capsular muscle of spleen, contraction of which may cause leukocytosis. Blood pressure and pulse may rise or fall, depending on the degree of autonomic stimulation, and high concentrations of pilocarpine may weaken myocardial contractility. Third-degree atrioventricular block was reported in an elderly patient with a history of first-degree atrioventricular block following seven hourly instillations of 2% pilocarpine.[107] Patients with *Alzheimer's disease* have reduced levels of cholinesterase in their brains, making them more sensitive to cholinergic drugs, and progressive cognitive dysfunction has been associated with topical pilocarpine therapy.[108]

Systemic toxicity is rare with the usual doses of pilocarpine used in the chronic management of glaucoma. The danger comes when large doses are given within a short period of time, as was once the practice for angle-closure glaucoma.[105] The problem is compounded by the fact that pilocarpine-induced toxicity may be confused with that of concomitant hyperosmotic therapy or of the systemic reactions to the disease itself. The antidote for systemic pilocarpine toxicity is atropine.

Ocular Side Effects. These are common with pilocarpine and can interfere with the patient's compliance to therapy.[109]

Ciliary muscle spasm may lead to a browache, which usually subsides with continued therapy. A more debilitating effect is induced myopia, which is due to shallowing of the anterior chamber, with an axial thickening and forward shift of the lens.[110–114] This is more marked in young individuals but also occurs in presbyopes.[115] Following instillation of 2% pilocarpine, the induced myopia begins in approximately 15 minutes, peaks in 45–60 minutes, and lasts for 1½–2 hours.[110,115] A statistically significant dose-related response was found for the duration, but not the magnitude, of the effects on anterior chamber depth and lens thickness.[111]

Miosis may cause dimness of vision and alterations in the visual fields as discussed in Chapter 6, especially if cataracts are present. In other patients, the smaller pupil may actually improve visual acuity, and the patients may note a decline in acuity when the medication is stopped.

Retinal detachment resulting from the use of miotics has been suspected on the basis of circumstantial evidence, although a definite cause-and-effect relationship has not been established.[116–118] These are typically rhegmatogenous detachments, and it is presumed that ciliary body contraction exerts vitreoretinal traction, which causes the retinal tears. The degree of risk appears to be related to preexisting retinal pathology[116–118] and possibly to the potency of the miotic. A vitreous hemorrhage without a detectable retinal hole or detachment has also been reported in a patient 1 day after starting pilocarpine therapy,[119] and a macular hole was reported to develop in a patient within weeks after starting therapy with 2% pilocarpine.[120]

A cataractogenic effect of pilocarpine has been suggested from observing patients on long-term uniocular miotic therapy.[121]

Corneal endothelial toxicity was dose related in in-vitro rabbit studies.[122] As previously noted, corneal edema may occur with intracameral injection of pilocarpine, although this is more likely related to the osmotic effect of the solution.[89]

Atypical band keratopathy (Fig. 25.3) has been observed in patients on long-term pilocarpine therapy,[123,124] but this was found to result from the preservative phenylmercuric nitrate,[125] which is no longer used.

Cicatricial pemphigoid has been reported to occur in patients on long-term topical glaucoma therapy.[126,127] In one survey of 111 patients with cicatricial pemphigoid, 29 (26%) had glaucoma.[126] Most of these patients have been on multiple glaucoma drops, and virtually all glaucoma medications, including pilocarpine, have been implicated. The cause-and-effect relationship of this association is uncertain, but a spectrum of drug-induced ocular pemphigoid has been proposed, ranging from a self-lim-

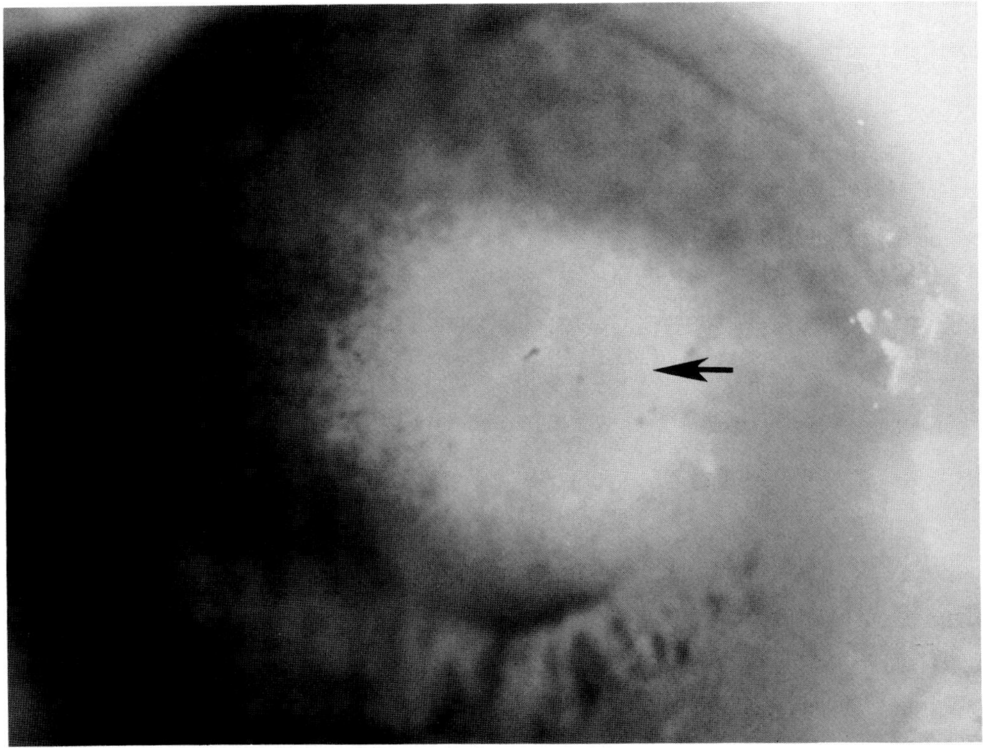

Figure 25.3. Slit-lamp view of atypical band keratopathy (*arrow*) caused by chronic use of pilocarpine with phenylmercuric nitrate as a preservative.

iting toxic form to a progressive, immunologic form.[127]

DUAL ACTION PARASYMPATHOMIMETICS

The following two drugs have both a direct and an indirect action on the parasympathetic nervous system (Table 25.2).

Carbachol

This drug produces direct motor end plate stimulation as well as an indirect parasympathomimetic effect by inhibition of acetylcholinesterase. The usual dosage of carbochal is 1.5–3.0% three times daily. A concentration of 1.5% instilled three times daily was reported to have a more potent and prolonged pressure effect than 2% pilocarpine four times a day.[128] However, carbachol causes more accommodative spasm and pain than pilocarpine.[114] Furthermore, as noted in Chapter 24, carbachol has poor corneal penetration and requires an adjuvant such as benzalkonium chloride to achieve effective aqueous levels.[129] A retrospective study of 26 open-angle glaucoma patients, uncontrolled on medical therapy that included pilocarpine, revealed that changing the miotic to carbachol had a low chance of improved long-term IOP control and an increased chance of side effects.[130]

N-demethylated carbachol is a synthetic tertiary nitrogen derivative of carbachol, which has a higher lipid solubility and better corneal penetration than the parent compound. It is less effective than 1% pilocarpine but also has fewer ocular and systemic side effects.[131]

Intracameral carabachol, which is frequently used to achieve miosis during cataract surgery, has been shown to provide better protection against early postoperative IOP rise than does intracameral acetylcholine[132] or a placebo (balanced salt solution).[132–134] It has been associated with tran-

Table 25.2
Other Commercial Miotic Preparations*

Generic Preparations	Brand Names	Concentrations (%)
Carbachol	Isopto carbachol	0.75, 1.5, 2.25, 3
Echothiophate iodide	Phospholine iodide	0.03, 0.06, 0.125, 0.25
Physostigmine sulfate	Eserine sulfate	0.25
Demecarium bromide	Humorsol	0.125, 0.25
Isoflurophate	Floropryl (gel)	0.025
Intracameral injections		
Acetylcholine chloride	Miochol	0.01 in 2 ml vial
Carbachol	Miostat	0.01 in 1.5 ml vial

* Other generic products may also be available.

sient corneal swelling in rabbits,[135] although a 1-year follow-up of cataract patients revealed no short-term or long-term adverse effects.[136]

Aceclidine

This is a synthetic ester with direct motor end plate action and weak anticholinesterase activity.[137,138] The IOP lowering[138,139] and miotic[114,139] effects are comparable to those of pilocarpine, while aceclidine has the advantage of less accommodative spasm.[114,137,140–142] The drug is available in Europe but at present is not marketed in the United States.

INDIRECT PARASYMPATHOMIMETICS

The pure inhibitors of acetylcholinesterase have traditionally been divided, somewhat arbitrarily, into two groups, designated "reversible" and "irreversible". Actually, none of these drugs is totally irreversible, and more precise definitions might be relatively "weaker" and "stronger" cholinesterase inhibitors, respectively (Table 25.2).

Physostigmine (Eserine)

This drug is a "weaker" cholinesterase inhibitor. It is administered as a 0.5% ointment, usually twice daily. As previously noted, it is not additive with pilocarpine.[97] Furthermore, as is true of all the cholinesterase inhibitors, it causes vascular congestion, which may be a disadvantage in eyes with angle-closure glaucoma.

Echothiophate Iodide

This pharmacologic agent is a strong, relatively irreversible cholinesterase inhibitor.

Mechanism of Action. Human ocular tissue contains true cholinesterase,[143] while pseudocholinesterase is found in human serum.[144] In vitro and in vivo studies of cat irides indicate that true cholinesterase is the enzyme portion related to the drug-induced alteration of the iris sphincter and is the portion primarily inhibited by echothiophate iodide.[145,146] The mechanism of improved aqueous outflow facility with this drug is presumed to be the same as that previously discussed for pilocarpine. Some eyes eventually become refractory, which appears from monkey studies to be associated with structural changes in the trabecular meshwork, Schlemm's canal, and ciliary muscle that are mediated, at least in part, by an anterior segment muscarinic receptor.[147]

Administration. In vitro studies indicated that echothiophate iodide has the same efficacy (maximum effect produced by a drug regardless of dose) as most of the other miotics.[148] Clinical trials have shown that a concentration of 0.03% echothiophate iodide has a potency (effect produced by a particular concentration) equivalent to 1–2% pilocarpine,[21] while 0.06% echothiophate iodide is comparable to 4% pilocarpine.[39] No additional IOP reduction is normally achieved with concentrations of echothiophate iodide higher than 0.06%.[39,149] Therefore, the usual dosage of echothiophate iodide is 0.03–0.06%, although higher concentrations of 0.125% or 0.25% may occasionally have an additional pressure-lowering effect in eyes with darkly pigmented irides. Echothiophate has the advantage of a prolonged duration of action, with the maximum effect occuring in 4–6 hours and a substantial residual effect present after 24 hours,[21] allowing it to be used on a twice-daily regimen.

Indications. Because of a significant cataractogenic effect, which is discussed later in this chapter, echothiophate iodide is usually reserved for treating open-angle glaucomas in aphakia or pseudophakia. In a retrospective study of such patients who were uncontrolled on medical therapy that included pilocarpine or carbachol, changing the miotic to echothiophate iodide restored long-term pressure control in a significant number of patients.[150]

Side Effects. The advantage of prolonged duration of action with echothiophate iodide therapy is significantly offset by the adverse reactions of this drug.

Systemic Toxicity. Systemic toxicity is related to cholinesterase depletion. Echothiophate iodide depletes both true cholinesterase (acetylcholinesterase), which is associated with the cell wall of red blood cells, as well as pseudocholinesterase (butyrylcholinesterase), which is a soluble form of cholinesterase found in serum. This depletion begins in the first 2 weeks of chronic therapy, peaks in 5–7 weeks, and requires several weeks to recover after discontinuing the drug.[151] Pseudocholinesterase may also be depleted in newborns whose mothers received echothiophate in late pregnancy.[152]

Pseudocholinesterase hydrolyzes succinylcholine, and prolonged respiratory paralysis can occur during general anesthesia if this muscle relaxant is used in a patient depleted of cholinesterase.[151] Local anesthetics of the ester linkage group, such as procaine and tetracaine, are also hydrolyzed by pseudocholinesterase, and depletion of the enzyme may lead to toxic reactions to these anesthetics.[153]

In addition, topical echothiophate iodide may rarely cause the parasympathomimetic reactions of diarrhea, nausea, abdominal cramps, and malaise. A case was reported in which these symptoms developed following bilateral conjunctivo-dacryocystorhinostomies with Jones' tubes in a patient on long-term treatment with echothiophate iodide.[154] The danger of increased systemic absorption after this operation should be considered with all topical medications.

Severe pancreatitis was reported in a patient with anticholinesterase insecticide intoxication, presumably resulting from increased pancreatic intraductal pressure.[155] However, in a study of 44 patients on a long-term echothiophate iodide therapy for glaucoma, serum pancreatic enzyme levels were normal.[156]

The antidote for echothiophate iodide toxicity is pralidoxime chloride (Protopam). This frees cholinesterase from the complex and prevents further inhibition but does not alter the IOP-lowering effect.[157]

A Cataractogenic Effect. As previously noted, a cataractogenic effect has been observed with the chronic use of echothiophate for the management of glaucoma.[158–160] The cataracts have been described as initially having fine anterior subcapsular vacuoles,[158,159] although nuclear and posterior subcapsular changes have also been observed.[160] The side effect appears to be dose related[160] and has not been observed in patients receiving cholinesterase inhibitor therapy for accommodative esotropia or in pesticide workers who are chronically exposed to cholinesterase-inhibiting organophosphates.[161]

The mechanism of echothiophate-induced cataracts is unclear. Experimental models have been produced in monkeys,[162–166] which reveal swollen lens fibers, reduced protein concentration, and abnormal material in the intercellular spaces.[165] It has also been suggested that mannitol, which is used as a vehicle, may contribute to the cataract formation.[167] One study suggested that atropine inhibits the cataractogenic effect in monkeys,[168] which apparently is not related to relaxation of accommodation, since echothiophate cataracts occurred in monkeys despite retrodisplacement of the ciliary muscle.[169]

Other Ocular Side Effects. A disruption of the blood-aqueous barrier may cause increased inflammation following intraocular surgery in eyes pretreated with echothiophate iodide, and it is usually advisable to discontinue the drug several weeks before such surgery. Retinal detachments may be associated with miotic therapy, as discussed previously in this chapter. Iris cysts near the pupillary margin are not uncommon in children receiving echothiophate iodide for the treatment of accommodative esotropia. As previously noted, structural alterations have been observed in the iris, ciliary muscle, ciliary processes, and trabecular meshwork of monkey eyes receiving chronic topical applications of echothiophate iodide.[170] Ocular pseudopemphigoid[171] and periorbital allergic contact dermatitis[172] have both been associated with the use of echothiophate iodide. Corneal epithelial toxicity with echothiophate iodide therapy is reported to be greater than with pilocarpine but less than with carbachol.[173]

Other Strong, Relatively Irreversible Cholinesterase Inhibitors

Diisopropyl Fluorophosphate. This drug is similar in action and side effects to echothiophate iodide but produces more intense ciliary spasm and is susceptible to contamination with water.

Demecarium. This compound is also similar to the other indirect parasympathomimetics but may be effective when echothiophate iodide has failed.

Tetraethyl Pyrophosphate. This compound was found to be comparable to other strong miotics but had the disadvantage of a considerable tendency to induce local sensitization.[174,175]

SUMMARY

The parasympathomimetics share common mechanisms of action that lead to improved aqueous outflow, either through stimulation of ciliary muscle contraction for patients with open-angle glaucoma or through the miotic effect in the treatment of angle-closure glaucoma. These drugs also share common ocular side effects, which include browache and induced myopia from ciliary muscle spasm, dimness of vision from the miosis, and a risk of retinal detachment. The most commonly used miotic is pilocarpine, which produces direct motor end plate stimulation. Another drug, carbachol, has both a direct parasympathomimetic effect as well as an indirect action through inhibition of acetylcholinesterase. Yet a third group of cholinergic stimulators has only the indirect action, of which echothiophate iodide is the most commonly used.

References

1. Mindel, JS, Kharlamb, AB: Alteration of acetylcholine synthesis by pilocarpine. Arch Ophthal 102:1546, 1984.
2. Armaly, MF, Jepson, NC: Accommodation and the dynamics of the steady-state intraocular pressure. Invest Ophthal 1:480, 1952.
3. Van Buskirk, EM, Grant, WM: Lens depression and aqueous outflow in enucleated primate eyes. Am J Ophthal 76:632, 1973.
4. Van Buskirk, EM: Changes in the facility of aqueous outflow induced by lens depression and intraocular pressure in excised human eyes. Am J Ophthal 82:736, 1978.
5. Van Buskirk, EM: The canine eye: lens depression and aqueous outflow. Invest Ophthal Vis Sci 19:789, 1980.
6. Moses, RA, Grodzki, WJ Jr: Choroid tension and facility of aqueous outflow. Invest Ophthal Vis Sci 16:1062, 1977.
7. Cairns, JE: Goniospasis: a method designed to relieve canicular blockade in primary open-angle glaucoma. Ann Ophthal 8:1417, 1976.
8. Kaufman, PL, Bárány, EH: Residual pilocarpine effects on outflow facility after ciliary muscle disinsertion in the cynomolgus monkey. Invest Ophthal 15:558, 1976.
9. Kaufman, PL, Bárány, EH: Loss of acute pilocarpine effect on outflow facility following surgical disinsertion and retrodisplacement of the ciliary muscle from the scleral spur in the cynomolgus monkey. Invest Ophthal 15:793, 1976.
10. Kaufman, PL, Bill, A, Bárány, EH: Formation and drainage of aqueous humor following iris removal and ciliary muscle disinsertion in the cynomolgus monkey. Invest Ophthal Vis Sci 16:226, 1977.
11. Lütjen-Drecoll, E, Kaufman, PL, Bárány, EH: Light and electron microscopy of the anterior chamber angle structures following surgical disinsertion of the ciliary muscle in the cynomolgus monkey. Invest Ophthal Vis Sci 16:218, 1977.
12. Grierson, I, Lee, WR, Abraham, S: Effects of pilocarpine on the morphology of the human outflow apparatus. Br J Ophthal 62:302, 1978.
13. Grierson, I, Lee, WR, Moseley, H, Abraham, S: The trabecular wall of Schlemm's canal: a study of the effects of pilocarpine by scanning electron microscopy. Br J Ophthal 63:9, 1979.
14. Grierson, I, Lee, WR, Abraham, S: The effects of topical pilocarpine on the morphology of the

outflow apparatus of the baboon (*Papio cynocephalus*). Invest Ophthal Vis Sci 18:346, 1979.

15. Lütjen-Drecoll, E, Tamm, E, Kaufman, PL: Age-related loss of morphologic responses to pilocarpine in Rhesus monkey ciliary muscle. Arch Ophthal 106:1591, 1988.
16. Erickson-Lamy, KA, Kaufman, PL: Reinnervation of primate ciliary muscle following ciliary ganglionectomy. Invest Ophthal Vis Sci 28:927, 1987.
17. Erickson-Lamy, KA, Kaufman, PL: Effect of cholinergic drugs on outflow facility after ciliary ganglionectomy. Invest Ophthal Vis Sci 29:491, 1988.
18. Suzuki, R, Oso, T, Kobayashi, S: Cholinergic inhibitory response in the bovine iris dilator muscle. Invest Ophthal Vis Sci 24:760, 1983.
19. Kaufman, PL: Aqueous humor dynamics following total iridectomy in the cynomolgus monkey. Invest Ophthal Vis Sci 18:870, 1979.
20. Gaasterland, D, Kupfer, C, Ross, K: Studies of aqueous humor dynamics in man. IV. Effects of pilocarpine upon measurements in young normal volunteers. Invest Ophthal 14:848, 1975.
21. Barsam, PC: Comparison of the effect of pilocarpine and echothiophate on intraocular pressure and outflow facility. Am J Ophthal 73:742, 1972.
22. Miichi, H, Nagataki, S: Effects of pilocarpine, salbutamol, and timolol in aqueous humor formation in cynomolgus monkeys. Invest Ophthal Vis Sci 24:1269, 1983.
23. Bárány, EH: A pharmacologist looks at medical treatment in glaucoma—in retrospect and in prospect. Ophthalmology 86:80, 1979.
24. Helbig, H, Korbmacher, C, Wohlfarth, J, et al: Effect of acetylcholine on membrane potential of cultured human nonpigmented ciliary epithelial cells. Invest Ophthal Vis Sci 30:890, 1989.
25. Jumblatt, JE, North, GT, Hackmiller, RC: Muscarinic cholinergic inhibition of adenylate cyclase in the rabbit iris—ciliary body and ciliary epithelium. Invest Ophthal Vis Sci 31:1103, 1990.
26. Nagataki, S, Brubaker, RF: Effect of pilocarpine on aqueous humor formation in human beings. Arch Ophthal 100:818, 1982.
27. Bill, A, Phillips, CI: Uveoscleral drainage of aqueous humour in human eyes. Exp Eye Res 12:275, 1971.
28. Bleiman, BS, Schwartz, AL: Paradoxical intraocular pressure response to pilocarpine. A proposed mechanism and treatment. Arch Ophthal 97:1305, 1979.
29. Doane, MB, Jensen, AD, Dohlman, CH: Penetration routes of topically applied eye medications. Am J Ophthal 85:383, 1978.
30. Sieg, JW, Robinson, JR: Mechanistic studies on transcorneal permeation of pilocarpine. J Pharm Sci 65:1816, 1976.
31. Van Hoose, MC, Leaders, FE: The role of the cornea in the biologic response to pilocarpine. Invest Ophthal 13:377, 1974.
32. Lazare, R, Horlington, M: Pilocarpine levels in the eyes of rabbits following topical application. Exp Eye Res 21:281, 1975.
33. Krohn, DL, Breitfeller, JM: Transcorneal flux of topical pilocarpine to the human aqueous. Am J Ophthal 87:50, 1979.
34. Asseff, CG, Weisman, RL, Podos, SM, Becker, B: Ocular penetration of pilocarpine in primates. Am J Ophthal 75:212, 1973.
35. Chrai, SS, Robinson, JR: Corneal permeation of topical pilocarpine nitrate in the rabbit. Am J Ophthal 77:735, 1974.
36. Harris, LS, Galin, MA: Dose response analysis of pilocarpine-induced ocular hypotension. Arch Ophthal 84:605, 2970.
37. Drance, SM, Nash, PA: The dose response of human intraocular pressure to pilocarpine. Can J Ophthal 6:9, 1971.
38. Drance, SM, Bensted, M, Schulzer, M: Pilocarpine and intraocular pressure. Duration of effectiveness of 4% and 8% pilocarpine instillation. Arch Ophthal 91:104, 1974.
39. Harris, LS: Comparison of pilocarpine and echothiophate iodide in open-angle glaucoma. Ann Ophthal 4:736, 1972.
40. Harris, LS, Galin, MA: Effect of ocular pigmentation of hypotensive response to pilocarpine. Am J Ophthal 72:923, 1971.
41. Lerman, S, Reininger, B: Simulated sustained release pilocarpine therapy and aqueous humor dynamics. Can J Ophthal 6:14, 1971.
42. Birmingham, AT, Galloway, NR, Walker, DA: Intraocular pressure reduction in chronic simple glaucoma by continuous infusion of dilute pilocarpine solution. Br J Ophthal 63:808, 1979.
43. Patton, TF, Francoeur, M: Ocular bioavailability and systemic loss of topically applied ophthalmic drugs. Am J Ophthal 85:225, 2978.
44. File, RR, Patton, TF: Topically applied pilocarpine. Human pupillary response as a function of drop size. Arch Ophthal 98:112, 1980.
45. Shell, JW: Ophthalmic drug delivery systems. Surv Ophthal 29:117, 1984.
46. Barsam, PC: The most commonly used miotic—now longer acting. Ann Ophthal 6:809, 1974.
47. Magder, H, Boyaner, D: The use of a longer acting pilocarpine in the management of chronic simple glaucoma. Can J Ophthal 9:285, 1974.
48. Sherman, SE: Clinical comparison of pilocarpine preparations in heavily pigmented eyes: an evaluation of the influence of polymer vehicles on corneal penetration, drug availability, and duration of hypotensive activity. Ann Ophthal 9:1231, 1977.
49. Quigley, HA, Pollack, IP: Intraocular pressure

control with twice-daily pilocarpine in two vehicle solutions. Ann Ophthal 9:427, 1977.
50. Green, K, Downs, SJ: Ocular penetration of pilocarpine in rabbits. Arch Ophthal 93:1165, 1975.
51. Harbin, TS Jr, Kaback, MB, Podos, SM, Becker, B: Comparative intraocular pressure effects of Adsorbocarpine and Isoptocarpine. Ann Ophthal 10:59, 1978.
52. Ticho, U, Blumenthal, M, Zonis, S, et al: Piloplex, a new long-acting pilocarpine polymer salt. A: Long-term study. Br J Ophthal 63:45, 1979.
53. Mazor, Z, Ticho, U, Rehany, U, Rose, L: Piloplex, a new long-acting pilocarpine polymer salt. B: Comparative study of the visual effects of pilocarpine and Piloplex eye drops. Br J Ophthal 63:48, 1979.
54. Ticho, U, Blumenthal, M, Zonis, S, et al: A clinical trial with Piloplex—a new long-acting pilocarpine compound: preliminary report. Ann Ophthal 11:555, 1979.
55. Duzman, E, Quinn, CA, Warman, A, Warman, R: One-month crossover trial comparing the intraocular pressure control of 3.4% piloplex twice daily with 2.0% pilocarpine four times daily. Acta Ophthal 60:613, 1982.
56. Klein, HZ, Lugo, M, Shields, MB, et al: A dose-response study of piloplex for duration of action. Am J Ophthal 99:23, 1985.
57. March, WF, Stewart, RM, Mandell, AI, Bruce, LA: Duration of effect of pilocarpine gel. Arch Ophthal 100:1270, 1982.
58. Stewart, RH, Kimbrough, RL, Smith, JP, Ward, RL: Long acting pilocarpine gel: a dose-response in ocular hypertensive subjects. Glaucoma 6:182, 1984.
59. Goldberg, I, Ashburn, FS Jr, Kass, MA, Becker, B: Efficacy and patient acceptance of pilocarpine gel. Am J Ophthal 88:843, 1979.
60. Johnson, DH, Epstein, DL, Allen, RC, et al: A one-year multicenter clinical trial of pilocarpine gel. Am J Ophthal 97:723, 1984.
61. Krause, K, Kuchle, JH, Baumgart, M: Comparative investigations of pilocarpine gel and pilocarpine eye drops. Klin Monatsbl Augenheilkd 187:178, 1985.
62. Johnson, DH, Keyon, KR, Epstein, DL, Van Buskirk, EM: Corneal changes during pilocarpine gel therapy. Am J Ophthal 101:13, 1986.
63. Smith, SA, Smith, SE, Lazare, R: An increased effect of pilocarpine on the pupil by application of the drug in oil. Br J Ophthal 62:314, 1978.
64. Bhojwani, SC, Jones, DK: Comparative study of aqueous and oily pilocarpine in the production of ocular hypotension. Br J Ophthal 65:530, 1981.
65. Camber, O, Edman, P, Gurny, R: Influence of sodium hyaluronate on the miotic effect of pilocarpine in rabbits. Curr Eye Res 6:779, 1987.
66. Cheeks, L, Green, K, Stone, RP, Riedhammer, T: Comparative effects of pilocarpine in different vehicles on pupil diameter in albino rabbits and squirrel monkeys. Curr Eye Res 8:1251, 1989.
67. Diepold, R, Kreuter, J, Himber, J, et al: Comparison of different models for the testing of pilocarpine eyedrops using conventional eyedrops and a novel depot formulation (nanoparticles). Graefe's Arch Ophthal 227:188, 1989.
68. Place, VA, Fisher, M, Herbst, S, et al: Comparative pharmacologic effects of pilocarpine administered to normal subjects by eyedrops or by ocular therapeutic systems. Am J Ophthal 80:706, 1975.
69. Lee, P-F, Shen, Y-T, Eberle, M: The long-acting Ocusert-pilocarpine system in the management of glaucoma. Invest Ophthal 14:43, 1975.
70. Quigley, HA, Pollack, IP, Harbin, TS Jr: Pilocarpine Ocuserts. Long-term clinical trials and selected pharmacodynamics. Arch Ophthal 93:771, 1975.
71. Armaly, MF, Rao, KR: The effect of pilocarpine Ocusert with different release rates on ocular pressure. Invest Ophthal 12:491, 1973.
72. Worthen, DM, Zimmerman, TJ, Wind, CA: An evaluation of the pilocarpine Ocusert. Invest Ophthal 13:296, 1974.
73. Drance, SM, Mitchell, DWA, Schultzer, M: The duration of action of pilocarpine Ocusert on intraocular pressure in man. Can J Ophthal 10:450, 1975.
74. Macoul, KL, Pavan-Langston, D: Pilocarpine Ocusert system for sustained control of ocular hypertension. Arch Ophthal 93:587, 1975.
75. Sendelbeck, L, Moore, D, Urquhart, J: Comparative distribution of pilocarpine in ocular tissues of the rabbit during administration by eyedrops or by membrane-controlled delivery systems. Am J Ophthal 80:274, 1975.
76. Brown, HS, Meltzer, G, Merrill, RC, et al: Visual effects of pilocarpine in glaucoma. Comparative study of administration by eyedrops or by ocular therapeutic systems. Arch Ophthal 94:1716, 1976.
77. Francois, J, Goes, F, Zagorski, Z: Comparative ultrasonographic study of the effect of pilocarpine 2% and Ocusert P 20 on the eye components. Am J Ophthal 86:233, 1978.
78. Fruanfelder, FT, Shell, JW, Herbst, SF: Effect of pilocarpine ocular therapeutic systems on diurnal control of intraocular pressure. Ann Ophthal 8:1031, 1976.
79. Smith, SE, Smith, SA, Friedmann, AI, Chaston, JM: Comparison of the pupillary, refractive, and hypotensive effects of Ocusert-40 and pilocarpine eyedrops in the treatment of chronic simple glaucoma. Br J Ophthal 63:228, 1979.
80. Akerblom, T, Aurell, E, Cristiansson, J, et al: A multicentre study of the effect and tolerance of Ocusert-P-40. Acta Ophthal 58:617, 1980.
81. Bensinger, R, Shin, DH, Kass, MA, et al: Pilocarpine ocular inserts. Invest Ophthal 15:1008, 1976.

82. Maichuk, YF, Erichev, VP: Soluble ophthalmic drug inserts with pilocarpine: experimental and clinical study. Glaucoma 3:239, 1981.
83. Kelly, JA, Molyneux, PD, Smith, SA, Smith, SE: Relative bioavailability of pilocarpine from a novel ophthalmic delivery system and conventional eyedrop formulations. Br J Ophthal 73:360, 1989.
84. Krohn, DL, Breitfeller, JM: Quantitation of pilocarpine flux enhancement across isolated rabbit cornea by hydrogel polymer lenses. Invest Ophthal 14:152, 1975.
85. Ruben, M, Watkins, R: Pilocarpine dispensation for the soft hydrophilic contact lens. Br J Ophthal 59:455, 1975.
86. Ramer, RM, Gasset, AR: Ocular penetration of pilocarpine: the effect of hydrophilic soft contact lenses on the ocular penetration of pilocarpine. Ann Ophthal 6:1325, 1974.
87. Podos, SM, Becker, B, Asseff, C, Hartstein, J: Pilocarpine therapy with soft contact lenses. Am J Ophthal 73:336, 1972.
88. Mehta, HK: Subconjunctival injection of pilocarpine. Trans Ophthal Soc UK 96:184, 1976.
89. Jay, JL, MacDonald, M: Effects of intraocular miotics on cultured bovine corneal endothelium. Br J Ophthal 62:815, 1978.
90. Kini, MM, Dahl, AA, Roberts, CR, et al: Echothiophate, pilocarpine, and open-angle glaucoma. Arch Ophthal 89:190, 1973.
91. Kaufman, PL, Bárány, EH: Subsensitivity to pilocarpine in primate ciliary muscle following topical anticholinesterase treatment. Invest Ophthal 14:302, 1975.
92. Kaufman, PL, Bárány, EH: Subsensitivity to pilocarpine of the aqueous outflow system in monkey eyes after topical anticholinesterase treatment. Am J Ophthal 82:883, 1976.
93. Kaufman, PL: Anticholinesterase-induced cholinergic subsensitivity in primate accommodative mechanism. Am J Ophthal 85:622, 1978.
94. Bito, LZ, Baroody, RA: Gradual changes in the sensitivity of rhesus monkey eyes to miotics and the dependence of these changes on the regimen of topical cholinesterase inhibitor treatment. Invest Ophthal Vis Sci 18:794, 1979.
95. Erickson-Lamy, KA, Polansky, JR, Kaufman, PL, Zlock, DM: Cholinergic drugs alter ciliary muscle response and receptor content. Invest Ophthal Vis Sci 28:375, 1987.
96. Bito, LZ, Mirritt, SQ: Paradoxical ocular hypertensive effect of pilocarpine on echothiophate iodide-treated primate eyes. Invest Ophthal Vis Sci 19:371, 1980.
97. Kronfeld, PC: The efficacy of combinations of ocular hypotensive drugs. A tonographic approach. Arch Ophthal 78:140, 1967.
98. Harris, LS, Mittag, TW, Galin, MA: Aqueous dynamics of pilocarpine-treated eyes. The influence of topically applied epinephrine. Arch Ophthal 86:1, 1971.
99. Knupp, JA, Shields, MB, Mandell, AI, et al: Combined timolol and epinephrine therapy for open-angle glaucoma. Surv Ophthal 28:280, 1983.
100. Duffey, RJ, Ferguson, JG: Interaction of dipivefrin and epinephrine with the pilocarpine ocular therapeutic system (Ocusert). Arch Ophthal 104:1135, 1986.
101. Söderström, MB, Wallin, Ö, Granström, P-A, Thorburn, W: Timolol-pilocarpine combined vs timolol and pilocarpine given separately. Am J Ophthal 107:465, 1989.
102. Airaksinen, PJ, Valkonen, R, Stenborg, T, et al: A double-masked study of timolol and pilocarpine combined. Am J Ophthal 104:587, 1987.
103. Maclure, GM, Vogel, R, Sturm, A, Binkowitz, B: Effect on the 24-hour diurnal curve of intraocular pressure of a fixed ratio combination of timolol 0.5% and pilocarpine 2% in patients with COAG not controlled on timolol 0.5%. Br J Ophthal 73:827, 1989.
104. Ellis, PP, Riegel, M: Influence of ophthalmic ointments on the penetration of pilocarpine drops. J Ocul Pharmacol 5:119, 1989.
105. Greco, JJ, Kelman, CD: Systemic pilocarpine toxicity in the treatment of angle closure glaucoma. Ann Ophthal 5:57, 1973.
106. Curti, PC, Renovanz, H-D: The effect of unintentional overdoses of pilocarpine on pulmonary surfactant in mice. Klin Monatsbl Augenheilkd 179:113, 1981.
107. Littman, L, Kempler, P, Rhola, M, Fenyvesi, T: Severe symptomatic atrioventricular block induced by pilocarpine eye drops. Arch Intern Med 147:586, 1987.
108. Reyes, PF, Dwyer, BA, Schwartzman, RJ, Sacchetti, T: Mental status changes induced by eye drops in dementia of the Alzheimer type. J Neurol Neurosurg Psych 50:113, 1987.
109. Granstrom, PA, Norell, S: Visual ability and drug regimen: relation to compliance with glaucoma therapy. Acta Ophthal 61:206, 1983.
110. Abramson, DH, Coleman, DJ, Forbes, M, Franzen, LA: Pilocarpine. Effect on the anterior chamber and lens thickness. Arch Ophthal 87:615, 1972.
111. Abramson, DH, Chang, S, Coleman, DJ, Smith, ME: Pilocarpine-induced lens changes. An ultrasonic biometric evaluation of dose response. Arch Ophthal 92:464, 1974.
112. Abramson, DH, Chang, S, Coleman, DJ: Pilocarpine therapy in glaucoma. Effects on anterior chamber depth and lens thickness in patients receiving long-term therapy. Arch Ophthal 94:914, 1976.
113. Pooinoosawmy, D, Nagasubramanian, S, Brown, NAP: Effect of pilocarpine on visual acuity and

on the dimensions of the cornea and anterior chamber. Br J Ophthal 60:676, 1976.
114. Francois, J, Goes, F: Ultrasonographic study of the effect of different miotics on the eye components. Ophthalmologica 175:328, 1977.
115. Abramson, DH, Franzen, LA, Coleman, DJ: Pilocarpine in the presbyope. Demonstration of an effect on the anterior chamber and lens thickness. Arch Ophthal 89:100, 1973.
116. Pape, LG, Forbes, M: Retinal detachment and miotic therapy. Am J Ophthal 85:558, 1978.
117. Beasley, H, Fraunfelder, FT: Retinal detachments and topical ocular miotics. Ophthalmology 86:95, 1979.
118. Alpar, JJ: Miotics and retinal detachment: a survey and case report. Ann Ophthal 11:395, 1979.
119. Schuman, JS, Hersh, P, Kylstra, J: Vitreous hemorrhage associated with pilocarpine. Am J Ophthal 108:333, 1989.
120. Garlikov, RS, Chenoweth, RG: Macular hole following topical pilocarpine. Ann Ophthal 7:1313, 1975.
121. Levene, RZ: Uniocular miotic therapy. Trans Am Acad Ophthal Otol 79:376, 1975.
122. Coles, WH: Pilocarpine toxicity. Effects on the rabbit corneal endothelium. Arch Ophthal 93:36, 1975.
123. Kennedy, RE, Roca, PD, Landers, PH: Atypical band keratopathy in glaucomatous patients. Am J Ophthal 72:917, 1971.
124. Brazier, DJ, Hitchings, RA: Atypical band keratopathy following long-term pilocarpine treatment. Br J Ophthal 73:294, 1989.
125. Kennedy, RE, Roca, PD, Platt, DS: Further observations on atypical band keratopathy in glaucoma patients. Trans Am Ophthal Soc LXXII:107, 1974.
126. Tauber, J, Melamed, S, Foster, CS: Glaucoma in patients with ocular cicatricial pemphigoid. Ophthalmology 96:33, 1989.
127. Fiore, PM, Jacobs, IH, Goldbert, DB: Drug-induced pemphigoid. A spectrum of diseases. Arch Ophthal 105:1660, 1987.
128. O'Brein, CS, Swan, KD: Carbaminoylcholine chloride in the treatment of glaucoma simplex. Arch Ophthal 27:253, 1942.
129. Smolen, VF, Clevenger, JM, Williams, EJ, Bergdolt, MW: Biophasic availability of ophthalmic carbachol I: Mechanisms of cationic polymer- and surfactant-promoted miotic activity. J Pharm Sci 62:958, 1973.
130. Reichert, RW, Shields, MB, Stewart, WC: Intraocular pressure response to replacing pilocarpine with carbachol. Am J Ophthal 106:747, 1988.
131. Hung, PT, Hsieh, JW, Chiou, GCY: Ocular hypotensive effects of N-demethylated carbachol on open angle glaucoma. Arch Ophthal 100:262, 1982.
132. Ruiz, RS, Rhem, MN, Prager, TC: Effects of carbachol and acetylcholine on intraocular pressure after cataract extraction. Am J Ophthal 107:7, 1989.
133. Linn, DK, Zimmerman, TJ, Nardin, GF, et al: Effect of intracameral carbachol on intraocular pressure after cataract extraction. Am J Ophthal 107:133, 1989.
134. Wood, TO: Effect of carbachol on postoperative intraocular pressure. J Cat Ref Surg 14:654, 1988.
135. Birnbaum, DB, Hull, DS, Green, K, Frey, NP: Effect of carbachol on rabbit corneal endothelium. Arch Ophthal 105:253, 1987.
136. Zimmerman, TJ, Dukar, U, Nardin, GF, et al: Carbachol dose response. Am J Ophthal 108:456, 1989.
137. Fechner, PU, Teichmann, KD, Weyrauch, W: Accommodative effects of aceclidine in the treatment of glaucoma. Am J Ophthal 79:104, 1975.
138. Drance, SM, Fairclough, M, Schulzer, M: Dose response of human intraocular pressure to aceclidine. Arch Ophthal 88:394, 1972.
139. Riegel, D, Leydhecker, W: Experiences with aceclidine in the treatment of simple glaucoma. Klin Monatsbl Augenheilkd 151:882, 1967.
140. Fechner, PU: Avoiding spasm of accommodation in the treatment of young glaucoma patients. Klin Monatsbl Augenheilkd 158:112, 1971.
141. Pilz, A, Lommatzsch, P, Ulrich, W-D: Experimentelle und klinsche Untersuchungen mit Aceclidin (Glaucostat). Ophthalmologica 168:376, 1974.
142. Erickson-Lamy, K, Schroeder, A: Dissociation between the effect of aceclidine on outflow facility and accommodation. Exp Eye Res 50:143, 1990.
143. Leopold, IH, Furman, M: Cholinesterase isoenzymes in human ocular tissue homogenates. Am J Ophthal 72:460, 1971.
144. Juul, P: Human plasma cholinesterase isoenzymes. Clin Chim Acta 19:205, 1968.
145. Harris, LS, Shimmyno, M, Mittag, TW: Cholinesterases and contractility of cat irides. Effect of echothiophate iodide. Arch Ophthal 89:49, 1973.
146. Harris, LS, Shimmyno, M, Mittag, TW: Effects of echothiophate on cholinesterases in cat irides. Arch Ophthal 91:57, 1974.
147. Lütjen-Drecoll, E, Kaufman, PL: Biomechanics of echothiophate-induced anatomic changes in monkey aqueous outflow system. Graefe's Arch Ophthal 224:564, 1986.
148. Harris, LS, Shimmyno, M, Hughes, J: Dose-response of cholinergic agonists on cat irides. Arch Ophthal 91:299, 1974.
149. Harris, LS: Dose-response analysis of echothiophate iodide. Arch Ophthal 86:502, 1971.
150. Reichert, RW, Shields, MB: Intraocular pressure response to replacing pilocarpine or carbachol with echothiophate iodide. Graefe's Arch Ophthal 229:252, 1991.

151. Ellis, PP, Esterdahl, M: Echothiophate iodide therapy in children. Effect upon blood cholinesterase levels. Arch Ophthal 77:598, 1967.
152. Birks, DA, Prior, VJ, Silk, E, Whittaker, M: Echothiophate iodide treatment of glaucoma in pregnancy. Arch Ophthal 79:283, 1968.
153. Ellis, PP, Littlejohn, K: Effects of topical anticholinesterases on procaine hydrolysis. Am J Ophthal 77:71, 1974.
154. Wood, JR, Anderson, RL, Edwards, JJ: Phospholine iodide toxicity and Jones' tubes. Ophthalmology 87:346, 1980.
155. Dressel, TD, Goodale, RL, Arneson, MA, Borner, JW: Pancreatitis as a complication of anticholinesterase insecticide intoxication. Ann Surg 189:199, 1979.
156. Friberg, TR, Thomas, JV, Dressel, TD: Serum cholinesterase, serum lipase, and serum amylase levels during long-term echothiophate iodide therapy. Am J Ophthal 91:530, 1981.
157. Lipson, ML, Holmes, JH, Ellis, PP: Oral administration of pralidoxime chloride in echothiophate iodide therapy. Arch Ophthal 82:830, 1969.
158. Axelsson, U, Holmberg, :Å The frequency of cataract after miotic therapy. Acta Ophthal 44:421, 1966.
159. Axelsson, U: Studies on echothiophate (phospholine iodide) and paraoxon (mintacol) with regard to cataractogenic effect. Acta Ophthal (suppl) 102, 1969.
160. Thoft, RA: Incidence of lens changes in patients treated with echothiophate iodide. Arch Ophthal 80:317, 1968.
161. Pietsch, RL, Bobo, CB, Finklea, JF, Vallotton, WW: Lens opacities and organophosphate cholinesterase-inhibiting agents. Am J Ophthal 73:236, 1973.
162. Kaufman, PL, Axelsson, U: Induction of subcapsular cataracts in aniridic vervet monkeys by echothiophate. Invest Ophthal 14:863, 1975.
163. Kaufman, PL, Axelsson, U, Bárány, E: Induction of subcapsular cataracts in cynomolgus monkeys by echothiophate. Arch Ophthal 95:499, 1977.
164. Albrecht, M, Bárány, E: Early lens changes in *Macaca fascicularis* monkeys under topical treatment with echothiophate or carbachol studied by slit-image photography. Invest Ophthal Vis Sci 18:179, 1979.
165. Philipson, B, Kaufman, PL, Fagerholm, P, et al: Echothiophate cataracts in monkeys. Electron microscopy and microradiography. Arch Ophthal 97:340, 1979.
166. Michon, J Jr, Kinoshita, JH: Experimental miotic cataract. II. Permeability, cation transport, and intermediary metabolism. Arch Ophthal 79:611, 1968.
167. Lazar, M, Nowakowski, J, Furman, M, Shore, B: Ocular penetration of topically applied mannitol. Am J Ophthal 70:849, 1970.
168. Kaufman, PL, Axelsson, U, Bárány, EH: Atropine inhibition of echothiophate cataractogenesis in monkeys. Arch Ophthal 95:1262, 1977.
169. Kaufman, PL, Erickson, KA, Neider, MW: Echothiophate iodide cataracts in monkeys. Occurrence despite loss of accommodation induced by retrodisplacement of ciliary muscle. Arch Ophthal 101:125, 1983.
170. Lütjen-Drecoll, E, Kaufman, PL: Echothiophate-induced structural alterations in the anterior chamber angle of the cynomolgus monkey. Invest Ophthal Vis Sci 18:918, 1979.
171. Patten, JT, Cavanagh, HD, Allansmith, MR: Induced ocular pseudopemphigoid. Am J Ophthal 82:272, 1976.
172. Mathias, CGT, Maibach, HI, Irvine, A, Adler, W: Allergic contact dermatitis to echothiophate iodide and phenylephrine. Arch Ophthal 97:286, 1979.
173. Krejci, L, Harrison, R: Antiglaucoma drug effects on corneal epithelium. A comparative study in tissue culture. Arch Ophthal 84:766, 1970.
174. Grant, WM: Miotic and antiglaucomatous activity of tetraethyl pyrophosphate in human eyes. Arch Ophthal 39:579, 1948.
175. Grant, WM: Additional experiences with tetraethyl pyrophosphate in treatment of glaucoma. Arch Ophthal 44:362, 1950.

Chapter 26

ADRENERGIC STIMULATORS

EPINEPHRINE

This direct-acting sympathomimetic stimulates both alpha- and beta-adrenergic receptors and is a standard topical drug for the chronic management of open-angle forms of glaucoma.

Mechanisms of Action

Theories regarding the mechanism of IOP reduction in response to epinephrine therapy have changed considerably in recent years. Early observations suggested that the primary action was decreased aqueous production.[1–5] However, it was subsequently noted that an improvement in aqueous outflow facility occurred after prolonged use of epinephrine.[6–7] Still more recent studies have revealed that increased outflow is an early and predominant feature of epinephrine-induced pressure reduction,[8–14] and that aqueous production is actually increased during one phase of the drug response.[15–17]

Sears and Neufeld[18–20] have proposed a unified concept for the action of epinephrine on aqueous humor dynamics, which consists of the following three phases.

Phase One: Decreased Aqueous Production. Within minutes after instillation of epinephrine, aqueous inflow is reduced, presumably because of the alpha-adrenergic effect of vasoconstriction, which reduces the ultrafiltration of plasma into the stroma of the ciliary processes. Vascular casting studies in rabbits have shown that alpha-adrenergic stimulation is associated with constriction of sphincter-like structures in the vessel lumen just as the ciliary process arterioles branch from the major arterial circle of the iris, with downstream luminal narrowing and poor ciliary process capillary filling.[21] Topical epinephrine in monkeys[22] and retrobulbar injections in rabbits[23] have both been shown to significantly reduce blood flow in the iris and ciliary body. However, this alpha-adrenergic effect on aqueous production is transient and not of sufficient magnitude to significantly influence IOP.[20]

Phase Two: Early Increase In Outflow Facility. This phase overlaps with the first and has two components. The first portion is actually a part of phase one and is believed to be an early, moderate-sized alpha-adrenergic effect on true outflow facility.[20] The second component occurs hours after administration, when the vasoconstrictor and mydriatic effects are gone, and lasts for several hours. Fluorophotometric and tonographic studies in normal[15–17] and ocular hypertensive[17] human eyes suggest that IOP reduction for at least the first several hours after topical instillation of epinephrine is associated with improved facility of outflow. These studies also revealed a slight increase in the rate of aqueous humor formation with epinephrine therapy.[15–17] This effect was not altered by the alpha-adrenergic antagonist thymoxamine,[24] although pretreatment with the beta-adrenergic antagonist timolol,[25] as well as sympathetic denervation secondary to third neuron Horner's syndrome,[26] were both associated with a decrease in aqueous inflow in response to epinephrine administration.

The mechanism of improved outflow is uncertain. Tonographic studies performed in conjunction with fluorophotometry suggest that epinephrine may increase the rate of outflow via the uveoscleral pathway.[15,17] Studies in rabbits and humans have shown that either systemic or topical indomethacin, a cyclo-oxygenase inhibitor, can inhibit the epinephrine-induced reduction of IOP, increased facility of outflow, and disruption of the blood-aqueous barrier, suggesting that endogenous production of prostaglandins may be associated with the hypotensive mechanism of topically applied epinephrine.[27–29] The mechanism of improved outflow does not appear to be mediated by the iris or ciliary body, since epinephrine and norepinephrine-induced increased facility of outflow in monkey eyes was not influenced by removal of the iris or total disinsertion of the ciliary muscle.[30,31] The increase in outflow facility associated with topical epinephrine in monkeys is blocked by timolol but not betaxolol, suggesting that the effect is mediated by beta$_2$-adrenergic receptors,[32] probably through stimulation of cyclic adenosine monophosphate (cAMP) synthesis, since the latter has been shown to mediate increased outflow facility in primates.[33] However, tissue culture studies suggest that the action of epinephrine on human trabecular endothelium is mediated through both alpha- and beta-adrenergic receptors and intimately involves the cytoskeletal system of the cells.[34]

Phase Three: Late Increase In Outflow Facility. This phase is believed to occur weeks to months after continued administration of epinephrine. The mechanism is uncertain but may be related to glycosaminoglycans metabolism in the trabecular meshwork.[18,20] This is consistent with the observation that epinephrine activates lysosomal hyaluronidase in the rabbit iris.[35] Other possible causes of the long-term effect include supersensitivity to topical epinephrine, which has been noted with chronic use of the drug,[36] or the gradual release of the agent from pigment-binding sites.

Administration

Concentrations. Studies have shown that the pressure lowering effect of epinephrine is proportional to the concentration of free base (or active form of the drug) within the range of 0.25–1%,[18] and that 2% may have some additional efficacy over the 1% concentration.[5] It has also been shown that topical epinephrine may be an effective ocular hypotensive drug in concentrations as low as 0.06%.[37] Standard commercial preparations are available in concentrations of 0.5%, 1%, and 2%.

Frequency of Administration. Twice-daily instillation provides a continuous pressure-lowering effect in most cases. However, a question that needs further study is whether more frequent administration (e.g., four times daily) might maximize the early effect of decreased aqueous production.

Table 26.1
Commercial Adrenergic Stimulators*

Generic Preparations	Brand Names	Concentrations (%)
Epinephrine HCl	Epifrin	0.25, 0.5, 1, 2
	Glaucon	0.5, 1, 2
Epinephryl borate	Epinal	0.25, 0.5, 1
	Eppy/N	0.5, 1, 2
Epinephrine bitartrate	Epitrate	2 (1.1 free base)
Dipivefrin HCl	Propine	0.1
Pilocarpine/epinephrine	E-Pilo-1, E-Pilo-2, etc.	1, 2, 3, 4, 6(pilo + 1(epi)
	P_1E_1, P_2E_1, etc.	
Apraclonidine HCl	Iopidine	1

*Other generic epinephrine products may also be available.

Standard Formulations. Standard commercial preparations are available in three salt forms: hydrochloride, borate, and bitartrate (Table 26.1). No significant difference has been found in the pressure-lowering efficacy of these three preparations,[10] although the drugs may differ slightly with regard to side effects.

Epinephrine hydrochloride has the advantage of stability and is available in all three concentrations (0.5%, 1%, and 2%) of the free base. It has the disadvantage of irritation upon instillation because of a low pH of approximately 3.5.

Epinephryl borate is a complex of boric acid and epinephrine and causes less irritation because of a higher pH of 7.4.[38] It is also available in 0.5%, 1%, and 2% concentrations of free base.

Epinephrine bitartrate also has the disadvantage of irritation with instillation because of a low pH. In addition, the stated concentration of some commercial preparations is higher than that of the free base of epinephrine. This salt form has been tested in rabbits in a polymeric matrix, which releases the drug osmotically at a rate of 1–4 micrograms of free base per hour over a 12-hour period.[39] This form of drug delivery provided IOP control equivalent to that of the drug in drop form but with considerably less total medication and without reducing the tear film pH.

Dipivefrin

Dipivefrin, or dipivalyl epinephrine (DPE), is a modification of epinephrine in which two pivalic acid groups are added to the parent drug.[40–42] The new compound is significantly more lipophilic than epinephrine, which increases the corneal penetration 17-fold.[43] In addition, dipivefrin is a prodrug, which is a drug that undergoes biotransformation before exhibiting its pharmacologic effect. The compound is hydrolyzed to epinephrine after absorption into the eye,[44] with the majority of the hydrolysis occurring in the cornea.[45] The enzymatic conversion of dipivefrin by esterases releases the pivalic acid, which is not metabolized in the eye but is rapidly eliminated without apparent sequestration in ocular tissues.[46] Preliminary rabbit studies suggested that echothiophate iodide inhibits the hydrolysis of dipivefrin,[47] consistent with the in vitro observation that echothiophate is a competitive, reversible inhibitor of the soluble corneal dipivefrin esterases.[48] However, subsequent studies indicated that the lack of hypotensive effect with dipivefrin in rabbits is due to an ocular hypertensive response to echothiophate,[49] that cholinesterase inhibitors do not affect the conversion of dipivefrin to epinephrine,[50] and that the combination of dipivefrin and echothiophate is an effective form of therapy in humans.[51]

Clinical trials indicate that the pressure-lowering effect of 0.1% dipivefrin is somewhere between that of 1% and 2% epinephrine.[52–55] Dipivefrin has the advantage over standard epinephrine formulations of less systemic toxicity, especially with regard to the cardiovascular side effects.[56] Advantages with regard to ocular toxicity include less burning and irritation with instillation[57] and the elimination of hydrophilic contact lens discoloration.[58] However, external ocular toxicity, including large bulbar conjunctival follicles, may occur with prolonged use of dipivefrin.[59–62] Once the drug is converted to epinephrine within the eye, it presumably has the same intraocular complications as other forms of epinephrine.

Adrenergic Supersensitivity

Another method for enhancing the effect of epinephrine is to increase the sensitivity of ocular tissues to the drug. This has been accomplished with both 6-hydroxydopamine and guanethidine, although neither drug is commercially available in the United States.

6-Hydroxydopamine. This compound produces a "chemical sympathectomy" by causing temporary degeneration of axon terminals.[63–66] The result is a transient increase in outflow facility resulting from an initial release of norepinephrine, and a more sustained effect on IOP reduction when given with epinephrine therapy by enhancing the action of exogenous epinephrine. A similar effect has been demonstrated in rabbits with alpha-methyl-para-tyrosine, an inhibitor of norepinephrine synthesis.[67,68] These drugs produce both an alpha- and beta-adrenergic supersensitivity, although the latter appears to be the predominant effect with 6-hydroxydopamine.[63–65]

Clinical trials have shown a significant IOP reduction in most patients.[69] However, a practical disadvantage of 6-hydroxydopamine is the need for subconjunctival or iontophoretic administration at weekly to monthly intervals.[70,71] Furthermore, both 6-hydroxydopamine and alpha-methyl-para-tyrosine cause a subsensitivity to cholinergic drugs in rabbits.[67,68]

Guanethidine. This drug is a postganglionic adrenergic antagonist that creates an adrenergic supersensitivity by depleting stores of catecholamines.[72] It may lower the IOP when given alone, presumably by an effect on both aqueous production and outflow,[73] but is particularly effective when used in combination with epinephrine.[74,75] Clinical trials with such a combined drop have revealed significant, sustained reductions in IOP.[76–84] The IOP-lowering effect is reportedly equal to or better than that of epinephrine alone,[84,85] pilocarpine,[85] or timolol.[86] However, one study revealed a biphasic response in which a phase of elevated IOP occurred as a result of increased aqueous production.[87] Furthermore, guanethidine is reported to cause soreness, conjunctival hyperemia, corneal epithelial changes, lid edema, and ptosis in some patients.[88] The effect of ptosis by topical guanethidine has actually been used to treat thyrotoxic lid retraction.[72,89,90] However, the combination drops are said to be generally well tolerated,[76–82] and the side effects can be reduced by using lower concentrations of guanethidine, although this also reduces the pressure-lowering efficacy.[91]

Drug Interactions

Miotics and Carbonic Anhydrase Inhibitors. When an epinephrine compound and a miotic are given in combination therapy, the reduction in IOP is usually significantly greater than the effect of either drug given alone. This fact is used in some commercial preparations that combine epinephrine and pilocarpine in a single formulation. Epinephrine also provides additional IOP reduction in most cases when added to carbonic anhydrase inhibitor therapy. Furthermore, the combination of epinephrine, a miotic, and a carbonic anhydrase inhibitor is often an effective regimen when any two of the three drugs alone is insufficient.

Beta-Adrenergic Inhibitors. The interaction between epinephrine and beta-adrenergic blockers is less clear-cut than with the drugs noted above. Since epinephrine stimulates and beta-blockers inhibit beta-adrenergic receptors, it might be anticipated that one drug would interfere with the action of the other. Clinical studies suggest that this does occur to a degree, although some additive effect on IOP may be achieved with simultaneous use of the two drugs.[92–94]

When timolol, a nonselective beta-adrenergic inhibitor, is given to eyes pretreated with epinephrine, there is a significant additional pressure reduction for the first few weeks, after which the pressure-lowering effect of the combined regimen is only slightly greater than with timolol alone.[95–99]

When the reverse sequence is followed and epinephrine therapy is added to eyes already receiving timolol, an additional reduction in IOP is usually small or absent.[95–101] Continued therapy with either epinephrine[102,103] or dipivefrin,[98,101,104] in combination with timolol, provides a small additional IOP reduction in the magnitude of 1–3 mm Hg over that achieved with timolol alone. One study suggested that this combined effect might be enhanced by separating the administration of the two drugs by several hours rather than several minutes.[102] However, a subsequent study revealed no difference between these two treatment plans.[105] Pretreatment with topical epinephrine has also been shown to decrease the systemic concentration of timolol,[106] suggesting that it may be best to give the epinephrine first when using both drugs within a short time period of each other.

Based on the above observations, Thomas and Epstein[95] postulated a model for the influence of the adrenergic system on aqueous humor dynamics. Stimulation of beta-adrenergic receptors in the inflow system is believed to increase aqueous production. Assuming that this system has a "resting tone," inhibition by timolol would reduce aqueous production as well as block the influence of epinephrine on inflow. Stimulation of beta-adrenergic receptors in the outflow system is believed to increase aqueous outflow, as supported by tonographic and fluorophotometric studies.[15–17] This system presumably has no resting tone, since timolol therapy alone does not alter outflow. However, timolol does block the effect of epinephrine on outflow, which most likely explains the minimal additional effect of adding epinephrine to timolol therapy.

Studies with betaxolol, a cardioselective, $beta_1$ adrenergic inhibitor, suggest that the effect of epinephrine on aqueous outflow is mediated through $beta_2$ adrenergic receptors, since the addition of either epinephrine hydrochloride[107] or dipivefrin[108] to betaxolol has a greater additional pressure-lowering effect than the addition of either drug to timolol.

Studies have also shown that the ocular hypotensive effect of topical epinephrine is reduced by treatment with oral timolol[109] or oral or topical indomethacin, a cyclo-oxygenase inhibitor.[27–29]

Side Effects

Side effects are common with the topical administration of standard epinephrine preparations. It may be helpful to think of these in three categories: systemic, extraocular, and intraocular.

Systemic Toxicity. These adverse reactions include elevated blood pressure, tachycardia, arrhythmias, headaches, tremor, nervousness, and anxiety. As previously noted, dipivefrin is not converted to active epinephrine until it enters the eye, and therefore it is associated with fewer systemic effects than the standard forms of epinephrine, even though the systemic absorption is 55–65% of the topically applied dose for both drugs.[110]

Extraocular Reactions. Side effects involving the lids and external portion of the eye constitute the most common adverse reactions encountered with topical epinephrine therapy.

Burning. Burning on instillation is practically universal with the hydrochloride and bitartrate preparations but may be minimized with the use of epinephryl borate or dipivefrin.

Reactive Hyperemia. This reaction occurs with all forms of epinephrine. The patient often fails to associate this with use of the drug, since the initial vasoconstrictive effect of epinephrine tends to whiten the conjunctiva, and the hyperemia appears later (Fig. 26.1).

Adrenochrome Pigmentation. Oxidation and polymerization of epinephrine converts the drug to adrenochrome, a pigment of the melanin family, which may be deposited in several ocular structures. In the lower conjunctiva, it forms small, round deposits, which are usually asymptomatic[111] (Fig. 26.2), while deposits in the upper conjunctiva tend to be branching or "staghorn" in shape (Fig. 26.3) and may abrade the cornea.[112–114] Electron microscopic analysis suggests that this material is not typical melanin but a related pigment.[115] When IOP elevation and bullous keratopathy are present, adrenochrome may deposit in the superficial cornea, producing a so-called

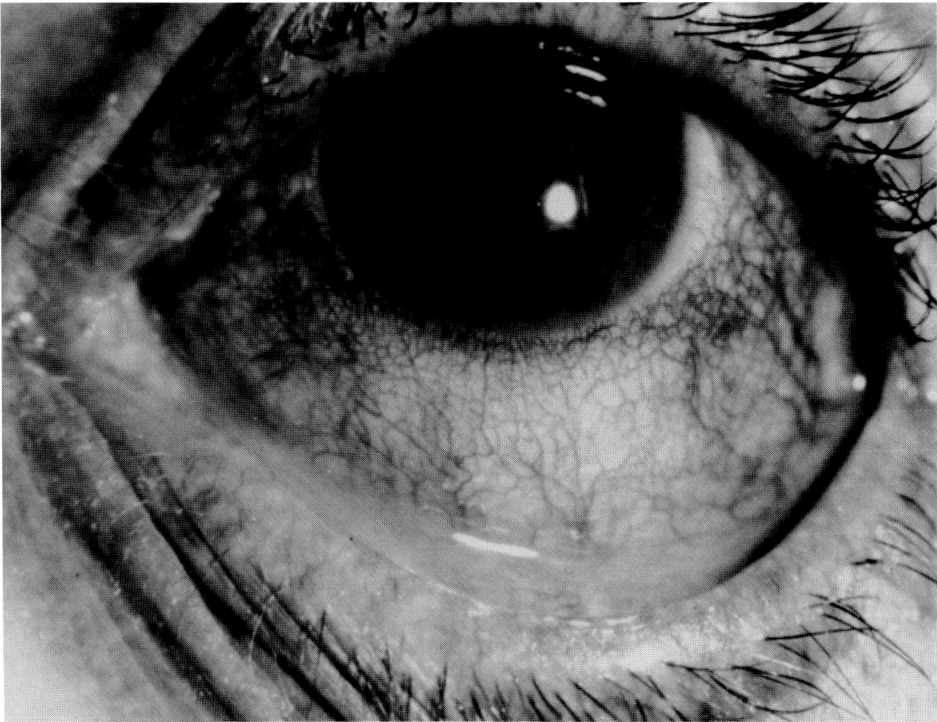

Figure 26.1. Diffuse conjunctival reactive hyperemia as a complication of chronic topical epinephrine therapy. (Reprinted with permission from Bigger JF: Ann Ophthal 11:183, 1979.)

"black cornea" (Fig. 26.4).[116–121] Adrenochrome may also deposit in the lacrimal sac[122] or nasolacrimal duct.[123,124] It has been reported to stain a senile scleral plaque, giving the appearance of a malignant melanoma.[125] It may also discolor soft contact lenses,[126,127] which, as previously noted, is reported not to occur with dipivefrin.[58]

Miscellaneous. Other less common extraocular reactions include tearing, photophobia, blurred vision, epidermalization of the lacrimal punctum,[128] and madarosis (loss of eyelashes).[129] An association with ocular pemphigoid has been suggested,[130,131] although a clear cause-and-effect relationship has not been established. In an evaluation of 17 glaucoma patients with ocular cicatricial pemphigoid, eight were receiving dipivefrin, although each of these was on one or more other topical glaucoma medications.[132] True allergic reactions with topical epinephrine are not common. Epinephrine has also been shown to cause shedding of latent ocular herpes simplex virus in rabbits.[133]

Intraocular Reactions. While less common than the extraocular side effects, the intraocular reactions generally have more serious consequences. With regard to dipivefrin, it should be anticipated that the intraocular reactions will be the same as with other forms of epinephrine, since it becomes the active drug after entering the eye.

Mydriasis. This reaction is a standard, although somewhat variable, response to epinephrine. It is usually of no consequence but may precipitate angle-closure glaucoma in the predisposed eye, and it is clearly contraindicated in such cases before an iridotomy has been performed.

Epinephrine Maculopathy. This is a form of cystoid macular edema, which occurs in some aphakic eyes receiving topical epinephrine.[134,135] A fluorescein angiographic study of 128 consecutive eyes revealed macular edema in 28% of those receiving epinephrine and in 13% of those not

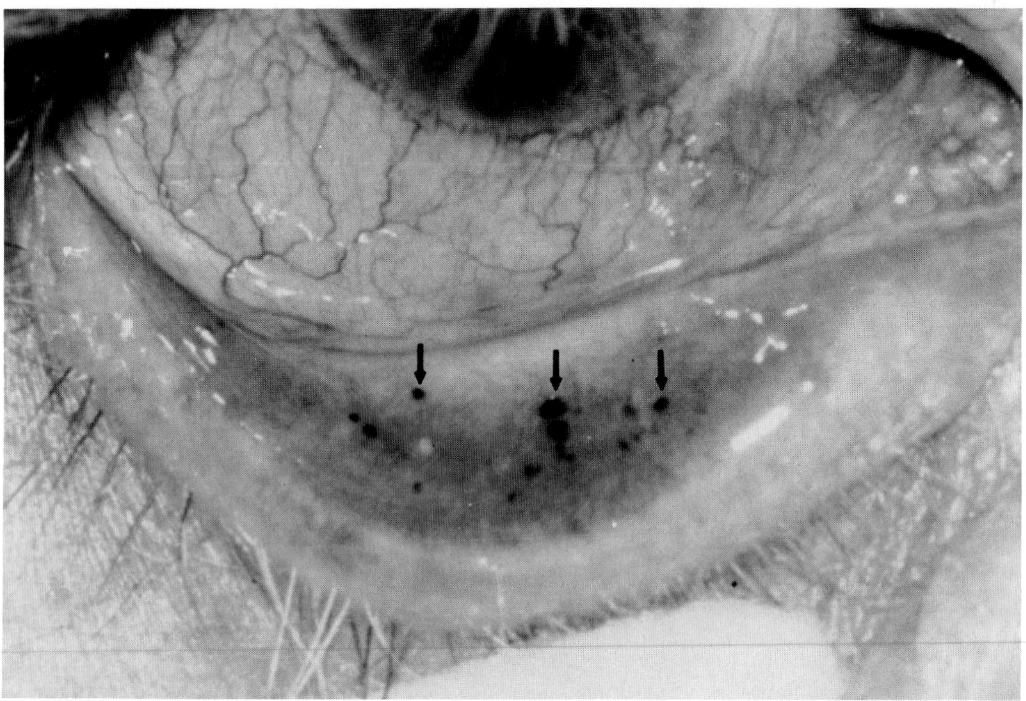

Figure 26.2. Adrenochrome deposits (*arrows*) of the lower palpebral conjunctiva in patient on chronic topical epinephrine therapy showing small, round configuration, which is typical of this location. (Reprinted with permission from Cashwell LF, Shields MB, Reed JW: Arch Ophthal 95:514, 1977.)

on the drug.[136] The pathogenesis of epinephrine maculopathy may be related to the epinephrine-induced synthesis of prostaglandins,[137] which leads to a disruption of the blood-ocular barrier.[28,138] Epinephrine maculopathy is usually reversible, at least with early discontinuation of the drug, and is probably dose related.

Corneal Endothelial Damage. Such damage has been observed with intracameral injection of epinephrine 1:1000 in rabbit[139,140] and monkey[139] eyes, but not with a 1:5000 concentration.[139] Decreased endothelial cell counts have also been reported in glaucoma patients after prolonged use of topical epinephrine.[141]

Ocular Hypoxia. It has been suggested that epinephrine might reduce optic nerve head perfusion by causing vasoconstriction of the adrenergically-innervated vessels behind the lamina cribrosa, and that this might particularly be a problem in the unprotected fellow eye during uniocular treatment with epinephrine.[142] The lens appears to serve as a barrier to posterior diffusion of epinephrine, since aphakic eyes, following topical epinephrine therapy, have significantly more labeled epinephrine in the choroid and, to a lesser degree, in the retina and optic nerve than do phakic eyes.[143] Aphakic eyes also have an attenuated epinephrine effect in the anterior segment with a potentiation of vasoconstriction in the posterior pole.[144] However, retrobulbar injection of epinephrine in phakic or aphakic rabbit eyes did not alter optic nerve or ocular blood flow.[145] It has also been shown that topical epinephrine causes a decrease in anterior chamber PO_2,[146] which might have clinical significance in some situations, such as neovascular glaucoma.

Apraclonidine

Apraclonidine hydrochloride is a para-amino derivative of clonidine hydrochlo-

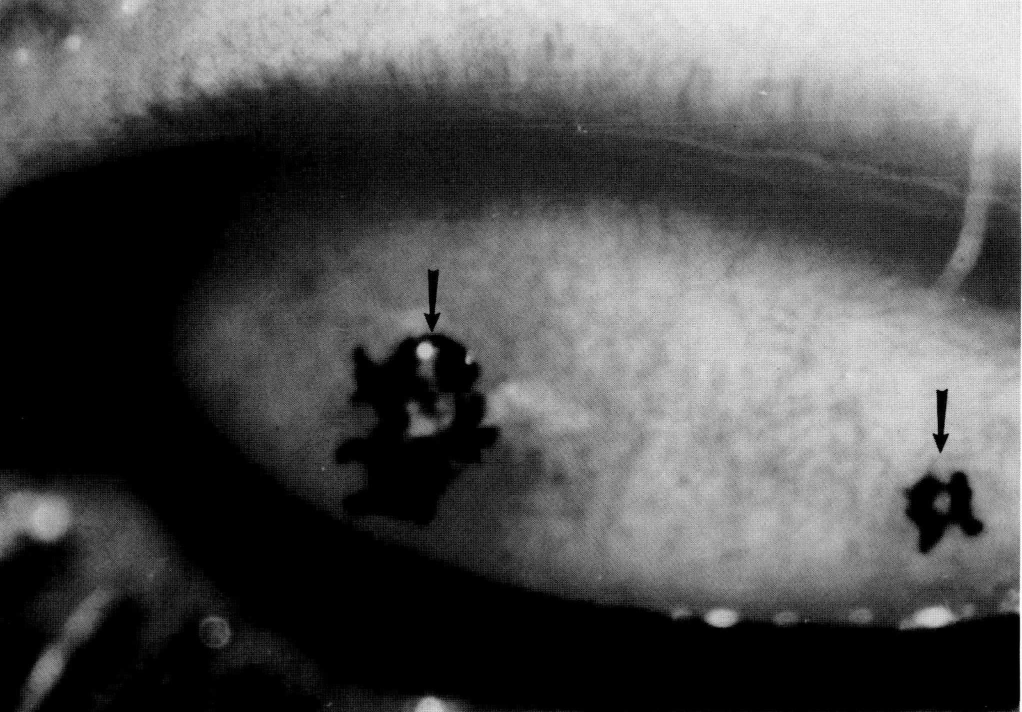

Figure 26.3. "Staghorn"-shaped adrenochrome deposits (*arrows*) of the upper palpebral conjunctiva caused by chronic topical epinephrine, typical of the complication in this location. (Reprinted with permission from Cashwell LF, Shields, MB, Reed JW: Arch Ophthal 95:514, 1977.)

ride, an alpha$_2$-adrenergic agonist that is used clinically as a potent systemic antihypertensive agent. Topical 1% apraclonidine, or para-aminoclonidine, recently became available commercially in the United States for the treatment of short-term IOP elevation, especially in association with anterior segment laser procedures.

The Parent Compound

Clonidine is believed to exert its systemic hypotensive effect by activation of central alpha$_2$-adrenergic receptors and reduction of sympathetic outflow from the brain. It has also been shown to lower the IOP following systemic or topical administration.[147–150] The mechanism of pressure reduction, as suggested by fluorophotometric studies in human eyes, is reduced aqueous production,[151] which may be due to constriction of afferent vessels in the ciliary processes.[152] The clinical value of clonidine as an ocular hypotensive agent is limited by the fact that it penetrates the blood-brain barrier, even with topical administration, occasionally causing significant systemic hypotensive episodes. Topical clonidine 0.125% was shown to reduce ocular perfusion pressure by a decrease in systemic blood pressure as well as a local perfusion pressure-reducing effect.[153]

Mechanisms of Action

Apraclonidine has the advantage over clonidine of minimal blood-brain barrier penetration, thereby reducing the cardiovascular side effects.[154] As with clonidine, fluorophotometric studies suggest that apraclonidine lowers the IOP by reducing aqueous production with little, if any, effect on blood-aqueous barrier permeability.[155] However, apraclonidine was also found to increase prostaglandin levels in the aqueous humor of rabbits, and flurbiprofen, an inhib-

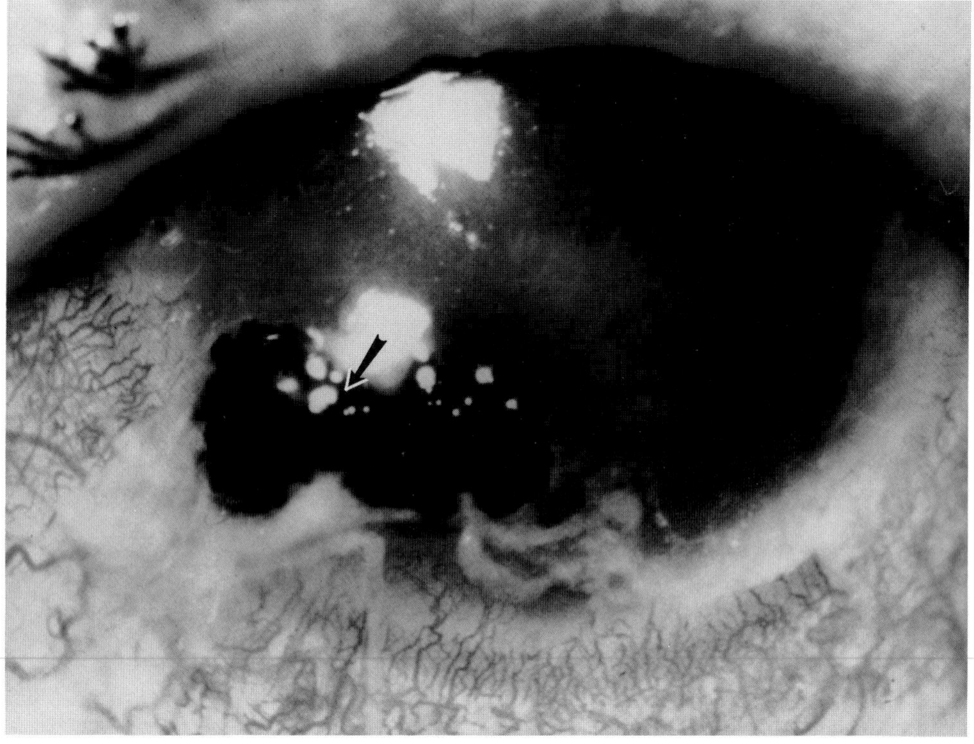

Figure 26.4. "Black cornea" adrenochrome deposition (*arrow*) in patient with bullous keratopathy and chronic topical epinephrine therapy. (Reprinted with permission from Cashwell LF, Shields MB, Reed JW: Arch Ophthal 95:514, 1977; and courtesy of David Donaldson, M.D.)

itor of prostaglandin synthesis, blocked the ocular hypotensive effect of the drug in monkeys.[156] Since prostaglandins presumably lower IOP by increasing uveoscleral outflow, this may be another mechanism of apraclonidine-induced pressure reduction.

Efficacy Studies

Apraclonidine 0.25% and 0.5% given twice daily for 1 week were equally effective, with an average IOP reduction of 27%, which was significantly more than that achieved with a 0.125% concentration.[157] A comparison of 0.5% and 1% apraclonidine showed no significant difference in pressure-lowering efficacy in either normotensive or ocular hypertensive subjects.[158] Studies with 1% apraclonidine indicate that a single dose lowers the mean IOP a maximum of 37%[159] and that this is maintained for at least 1 month of twice-daily therapy.[160] No significant contralateral IOP effect was seen with 0.25% or 0.5% apraclonidine.[154]

Clinical Indications

The main value of apraclonidine appears to be the ability to minimize short-term IOP elevations. In rabbits treated with laser irradiation of the iris, apraclonidine prevented the IOP rise and significantly reduced the aqueous protein elevation, but it did not affect the increase in prostaglandins.[161] In clinical studies, apraclonidine has been shown to be highly effective in minimizing the transient IOP rise following several anterior segment laser procedures, specifically trabeculoplasty,[162] iridotomy,[162–164] and capsulotomy.[164,165] A standard protocol is to instill one drop of 1% apraclonidine in the eye scheduled for laser surgery approximately 1 hour before the procedure and a second drop immediately after the operation. Apraclonidine has also been reported to be useful in treating acute angle-closure glaucoma.[166] It was also shown to produce a significant additional IOP lowering when added twice daily to eyes already receiving timolol therapy during a 3-week study,[167] although the efficacy of apraclonidine in the chronic management of glaucoma has yet to be established.

Side Effects

Several studies have confirmed the lack of effect of apraclonidine on blood pressure and pulse.[154,157–160] However, systemic side effects that have been identified include a transient dry nose or dry mouth, which was reported by 30–50% of patients.[157,160] A case of syncope and chest tightness 10 minutes after receiving one drop of 1% apraclonidine has also been reported.[168] Ocular side effects that have been reported include eyelid retraction, mydriasis, and conjunctival blanching.[157,159] A significant decrease in conjunctival oxygen tension has been observed 1 and 3 hours after instillation of 1% apraclonidine,[169] although the clinical significance of this has yet to be established.

Investigational Alpha-Adrenergic Stimulators

Norepinephrine

The postganglionic physiologic mediator of the adrenergic nervous system, norepinephrine, has had limited clinical usefulness because of instability. However, newer, more stable preparations have led to a reevaluation of the drug. Concentrations of 2–4%, given twice daily, significantly lowered the IOP, presumably by an alpha-induced increase in outflow facility, without causing beta-induced side effects, such as tachycardia.[170,171] Rabbit studies revealed an early mydriasis and rise in IOP[172,173] before the pressure reduction occurs.[172]

The ocular effects of norepinephrine can be potentiated by bilateral cervical ganglionectomy,[173] monoamine oxidase inhibitors (pargyline or pheniprazone),[174] or protriptyline,[175] which potentiates adrenergic activity by blocking catecholamine uptake into postganglionic neurons. A prodrug, norepinephrine dipivalylate, has been shown to produce a significant and prolonged dose-related reduction of IOP in human subjects.[176] Norepinephrine is also limited by adaptation, or the development of subsensitivity, which was suppressed in rabbits' eyes by treatment with flurbiprofen, an inhibitor of prostaglandin synthesis.[177]

Pargyline

The monoamine oxidase inhibitor pargyline is an indirect alpha-adrenergic stimulator used in the treatment of systemic hypertension.[178] It has been shown to lower the IOP in rabbits by decreasing aqueous production,[178,179] provided the adrenergic nervous system is intact.[180] Topical pargyline 0.5% significantly lowered the pressure in open-angle glaucoma patients, without affecting the pupil.[181]

Investigational Beta-Adrenergic Stimulators

Isoproterenol

Isoproterenol is a direct beta-adrenergic stimulator. The racemic form, dl-isoproterenol, reduces IOP in humans but causes tachycardia with palpitation and weakness, which is an l-isomer effect.[182,183] D-isoproterenol also reduces the IOP in rabbits[183,184] without causing tachycardia, vasoconstriction, or mydriasis.[183] However, d-isoproterenol does not appear to have the same pressure effect in human eyes.[184] The mechanism of IOP reduction is unknown but is apparently unrelated to aqueous production.[185]

Forskolin

This diterpene derivative of the plant *Coleus forskohlii* stimulates adenylate cyclase activity, without interacting with cell surface receptors, to increase intracellular levels of cyclic AMP,[186] which in turn may enhance norepinephrine release at intraocular synapses.[187] Forskolin has been shown to lower IOP in rabbits, monkeys, and humans.[186,188,189] Tolerance developed by the 3rd day in monkeys[188] but was not seen after 15 days with rabbits.[186] According to several studies, the mechanism of IOP lowering is reduced aqueous production,[186,188,190,191] which may be related to an increase in the permeability of the blood-aqueous barrier.[192] However, a fluorophotometric study in normal volunteers revealed no statistically significant effect of forskolin on aqueous production during the day or night.[193] Forskolin has a specific affinity for melanin granules, which may delay the onset but prolong the duration of the ocular hypotensive effect.[194]

Cholera Toxin

Cholera toxin, a specific, irreversible activator of adenylate cyclase, stimulates cyclic AMP production in the anterior uvea[195,196] and scleral-trabecular ring[196] in rabbits, with a subsequent reduction in IOP. The mechanism of pressure lowering is uncertain, with one study indicating decreased aqueous flow[195] and another suggesting increased outflow facility.[196] Ultracytochemistry studies suggest that the cell-surface receptors that mediate the action on aqueous production are likely located in the apical plasma membranes of the ciliary epithelium.[197] Fine structural studies of rabbit ciliary processes after treatment with cholera toxin revealed capillary dilation and stromal edema with no significant damage to the epithelial layers.[198]

Terbutaline

The selective beta$_2$-adrenergic stimulator terbutaline, used in the treatment of bronchial asthma, has been shown to inhibit induced IOP elevation in rabbits.[199] The effect is less than that of timolol or pilocarpine but more than that of epinephrine or clonidine.[199] Tolerance develops after a few days, which is prevented by concomitant treatment with diclofenac, a potent nonsteroidal antiinflammatory drug.[200] Ibuterol, a prodrug of terbutaline, was significantly more efficacious than the parent compound in rabbit studies.[201]

Salbutamol

Salbutamol is another selective beta$_2$-adrenergic agonist. It has been shown to lower IOP in human eyes, associated with an increase in both the rate of aqueous production and tonographic facility of outflow.[202] The latter was calculated to be due to an increase in uveoscleral outflow.

Pirbuterol

This active sympathomimetic bronchodilator has a high affinity for beta$_2$-adrenergic receptors and has been shown to lower IOP in rabbits, presumably by activating adenylate cyclase.[203]

Investigational Nonspecific Adrenergic Agents

Vanadate

Topical administration of 1% vanadate lowered the IOP in rabbits, associated with a significant decrease in aqueous humor flow.[204,205] Possible mechanisms of reduced flow are inhibition of ciliary epithelium (Na^+K^+) ATPase or stimulation of adenylate cyclase,[206] although the anterior uveal content of vanadate at the time of IOP reduction was too small for these actions, and other cellular mechanisms are considered likely.[207]

Nylidrin

The nonspecific adrenergic agent nylidrin hydrochloride lowered IOP in rabbits and monkeys, apparently by increasing uveoscleral outflow.[208] Although purported to be a sympathomimetic amine, it has a complex mode of action, which may include a partial agonist action on beta$_1$-adrenergic receptors but an antagonist action on beta$_2$-receptors.[203]

SUMMARY

Epinephrine is the only adrenergic stimulator commercially available for the chronic treatment of glaucoma. Acting at both the alpha- and beta-receptors, it lowers IOP through a complex system that primarily involves improved aqueous outflow. Side effects occur in three categories: systemic (e.g., elevated blood pressure, tachycardia, and tremor); extraocular (e.g., irritation, reactive hyperemia, and adrenochrome pigmentation); and intraocular (e.g., mydriasis and cystoid macular edema in aphakia). Another adrenergic stimulator, apraclonidine, is an alpha$_2$-agonist that is commercially available for short-term pressure control, especially in association with certain laser procedures. Other adrenergic stimulators that are under investigation for the treatment of glaucoma include alpha-adrenergic stimulators, such as norepinephrine and clonidine, beta-adrenergic stimulators, including isoproterenol and forskolin, and nonspecific adrenergic agents.

References

1. Goldmann, H: L'origine de l'hypertension oculaire dans le glaucome primitif. Ann Ocul (Paris) 184:1086, 1951.
2. Weekers, R, Prijot, E, Gustin, J: Recent advances and future prospects in the medical treatment of ocular hypertension. Br J Ophthal 38:742, 1954.
3. Weekers, R, Delmarcelle, Y, Gustin, J: Treatment of ocular hypertension by adrenalin and diverse sympathomimetic amines. Am J Ophthal 40:666, 1955.
4. Becker, B, Ley, AP: Epinephrine and acetazolamide in the therapy of the chronic glaucomas. Am J Ophthal 45:639, 1958.
5. Garner, LL, Johnstone, WW, Ballintine, EJ, Carroll, ME: Effect of 2% levo-rotary epinephrine on the intraocular pressure of the glaucomatous eye. Arch Ophthal 62:230, 1959.
6. Becker, B, Pettit, TH, Gay, AJ: Topical epinephrine therapy of open-angle glaucoma. Arch Ophthal 66:219, 1961.
7. Ballintine, EJ, Garner, LL: Improvement of the coefficient of outflow in glaucomatous eyes. Prolonged local treatment with epinephrine. Arch Ophthal 66:314, 1961.
8. Kronfeld, PC: Dose-effect relationships as an aid in the evaluation of ocular hypotensive drugs. Invest Ophthal 3:258, 1964.
9. Krill, AE, Newell, FW, Novak, M: Early and long-term effects of levo-epinephrine on ocular tension and outflow. Am J Ophthal 59:833, 1965.
10. Criswick, VG, Drance, SM: Comparative study of four different epinephrine salts on intraocular pressure. Arch Ophthal 75:768, 1966.
11. Richards, JSF, Drance, SM: The effect of 2% epinephrine on aqueous dynamics in the human eye. Can J Ophthal 2:259, 1967.
12. Kronfeld, PC: Early effects of single and repeated doses of L-epinephrine in man. Am J Ophthal 72:1058, 1971.
13. Vannas, S, Linkova, M: Adrenalin therapy in glaucoma. Acta Ophthalmologica XX Meeting of Nordic Ophthalmologists 1971, p. 39.
14. Green, K, Padgett, D: Effect of various drugs on pseudofacility and aqueous humor formation in the rabbit eye. Exp Eye Res 28:239, 1979.
15. Townsend, DJ, Brubaker, RF: Immediate effect of epinephrine on aqueous formation in the normal human eye as measured by fluorophotometry. Invest Ophthal Vis Sci 19:256, 1980.
16. Nagataki, S, Brubaker, RF: Early effect of epinephrine on aqueous formation in the normal human eye. Ophthalmology 88:278, 1981.
17. Schenker, HI, Yablonski, ME, Podos, SM, Linder, L: Fluorophotometric study of epinephrine and timolol in human subjects. Arch Ophthal 99:1212, 1981.
18. Sears, ML: The mechanism of action of adrenergic drugs in glaucoma. Invest Ophthal 5:115, 1966.
19. Sears, ML, Neufeld, AH: Adrenergic modulation of the outflow of aqueous humor. Invest Ophthal 14:83, 1975.
20. Sears, ML: Autonomic Nervous System: Adrenergic Agonists. In: Handbook of Experimental Pharmacology, vol. 69, Sears, ML, ed. Springer-Verlag, Berlin, 1984.
21. Van Buskirk, EM: The ciliary vasculature and its perturbation with drugs and surgery. Trans Am Ophthal Soc 86:794, 1988.
22. Alm, A: The effect of topical l-epinephrine on regional ocular blood flow in monkeys. Invest Ophthal Vis Sci 19:487, 1980.
23. Jay, WM, Aziz, MZ, Green, K: Further studies on the effect of retrobulbar epinephrine injection on ocular and optic nerve blood flow. Curr Eye Res 5:63, 1986.
24. Lee, DA, Brubaker, RF, Nagataki, S: Acute effect of thymoxamine on aqueous humor formation in the epinephrine-treated normal eye as measured by fluorophotometry. Invest Ophthal Vis Sci 24:165, 1983.
25. Higgins, RG, Brubaker, RF: Acute effect of epinephrine on aqueous humor formation in the timolol-treated normal eye as measured by fluorophotometry. Invest Ophthal Vis Sci 19:420, 1980.
26. Wentworth, WO, Brubaker, RF: Aqueous humor dynamics in a series of patients with third neuron Horner's syndrome. Am J Ophthal 92:407, 1981.
27. Camras, CB, Feldman, SG, Podos, SM, et al: Inhibition of the epinephrine-induced reduction of intraocular pressure by systemic indomethacin in humans. Am J Ophthal 100:169, 1985.
28. Miyake, K, Miyake, Y, Kuratomi, R: Long-term effects of topically applied epinephrine on the blood-ocular barrier in humans. Arch Ophthal 105:1360, 1987.
29. Anderson, L, Wilson, WS: Inhibition by indomethacin of the increased facility of outflow induced by adrenaline. Exp Eye Res 50:119, 1990.
30. Kaufman, PL, Barany, EH: Adrenergic drug effects on aqueous outflow facility following ciliary muscle retrodisplacement in the cynomolgus monkey. Invest Ophthal Vis Sci 20:644, 1981.
31. Kaufman, PL: Epinephrine, norepinephrine, and isoproterenol dose—outflow facility response relationships in cynomolgus monkey eyes with and without ciliary muscle retrodisplacement. Acta Ophthal 64:356, 1986.

32. Robinson, JC, Kaufman, PL: Effects and interactions of epinephrine, norepinephrine, timolol, and betaxolol on outflow facility in the cynomolgus monkey. Am J Ophthal 109:189, 1990.
33. Neufeld, AH, Sears, ML: Adenosine 3[1],5[1]-monophosphate analogue increases the outflow facility of the primate eye. Invest Ophthal 14:688, 1975.
34. Tripathi, BJ, Tripathi, RC: Effect of epinephrine in vitro on the morphology, phagocytosis, and mitotic activity of human trabecular endothelium. Exp Eye Res 39:731, 1984.
35. Hayasaka, S, Sears, M: Effects of epinephrine, indomethacin, acetylsalicylic acid, dexamethasone, and cyclic AMP on the in vitro activity of lysosomal hyaluronidase from the rabbit iris. Invest Ophthal Vis Sci 17:1109, 1978.
36. Flach, AJ, Kramer, SG: Supersensitivity to topical epinephrine after long-term epinephrine therapy. Arch Ophthal 98:482, 1980.
37. Harris, LS, Galin, MA, Lerner, R: The influence of low dose L-epinephrine on intraocular pressure. Ann Ophthal 2:253, 1970.
38. Vaughan, D, Shaffer, R, Riegelman, S: A new stabilized form of epinephrine for the treatment of open-angle glaucoma. Arch Ophthal 66:232, 1961.
39. Birss, SA, Longwell, A, Heckbert, S, Keller, N: Ocular hypotensive efficacy of topical epinephrine in normotensive and hypertensive rabbits: continuous drug delivery vs eyedrops. Ann Ophthal 10:1045, 1978.
40. Kaback, MB, Podos, SM, Hargin, TS Jr, et al: The effects of dipivalyl epinephrine on the eye. Am J Ophthal 81:768, 1976.
41. Bigger, JF: Dipivefrin and glaucoma. Pers Ophthal 4:87, 1980.
42. Adamek, R: New perspectives in glaucoma therapy with epinephrine and epinephrine derivatives. Klin Monatsbl Augenheilkd 176:978, 1980.
43. Mandell, AI, Stentz, F, Kitabchi, AE: Dipivalyl epinephrine: a new pro-drug in the treatment of glaucoma. Ophthalmology 85:268, 1978.
44. Wei, C-P, Anderson, JA, Leopold, I: Ocular absorption and metabolism of topically applied epinephrine and dipivalyl ester of epinephrine. Invest Ophthal Vis Sci 17:315, 1978.
45. Anderson, JA, Davis, WL, Wei, C-P: Site of ocular hydrolysis of a prodrug, dipivefrin, and a comparison of its ocular metabolism with that of the parent compound, epinephrine. Invest Ophthal Vis Sci 19:817, 1980.
46. Tamaru, RD, Davis, WL, Anderson, JA: Comparison of ocular disposition of free pivalic acid and pivalic acid esterified in dipivefrin. Arch Ophthal 101:1127, 1983.
47. Abramovsky, I, Mindel, JS: Dipivefrin and echothiophate. Contraindications to combined use. Arch Ophthal 97:1937, 1979.
48. Anderson, JA, Richman, JB, Mindel, JS: Effects of echothiophate on enzymatic hydrolysis of dipivefrin. Arch Ophthal 102:913, 1984.
49. Mindel, JS, Koenigsberg, AM, Kharlamb, AB, et al: The effect of echothiophate on the biphasic response of rabbit ocular pressure to dipivefrin. Arch Ophthal 100:147, 1982.
50. Mindel, JS, Cohen, G, Barker, LA, Lewis, DE: Enzymatic and nonenzymatic hydrolysis of D,L-dipivefrin. Arch Ophthal 102:457, 1984.
51. Mindel, JS, Yablonski, ME, Tavitian, HO, et al: Dipivefrin and echothiophate. Efficacy of combined use in human beings. Arch Ophthal 99:1583, 1981.
52. Kass, MA, Mandell, AI, Goldberg, I, et al: Dipivefrin and epinephrine treatment of elevated intraocular pressure. A comparative study. Arch Ophthal 97:1865, 1979.
53. Kohn, AN, Moss, AP, Hargett, NA, et al: Clinical comparison of dipivalyl epinephrine and epinephrine in the the treatment of glaucoma. Am J Ophthal 87:196, 1979.
54. Bischoff, P: Clinical studies conducted with a new epinephrine derivative for the treatment of glaucoma (dipivalyl epinephrine). Klin Monatsbl Augenheilkd 172:565, 1978.
55. Krieglstein, GK, Leydhecker, W: The dose-response relationships of dipivalyl epinephrine in open-angle glaucoma. Graefe's Arch Ophthal 205:141, 1978.
56. Kerr, CR, Hass, I, Drance, SM, et al: Cardiovascular effects of epinephrine and dipivalyl epinephrine applied topically to the eye in patients with glaucoma. Br J Ophthal 66:109, 1982.
57. Yablonski, ME, Shin, DH, Kolker, AE, et al: Dipivefrin use in patients with intolerance to topically applied epinephrine. Arch Ophthal 95:2157, 1977.
58. Newton, MJ, Nesburn, AB: Lack of hydrophilic lens discoloration in patients using dipivalyl epinephrine for glaucoma. Am J Ophthal 87:193, 1979.
59. Theodore, JA, Leibowitz, HM: External ocular toxicity of dipivalyl epinephrine. Am J Ophthal 88:1013, 1979.
60. Wandel, T, Spinak, M: Toxicity of dipivalyl epinephrine. Ophthalmology 88:259, 1981.
61. Liesegang, TJ: Bulbar conjunctival follicles associated with dipivefrin therapy. Ophthalmology 92:228, 1985.
62. Coleiro, JA, Sigurdsson, H, Lockyer, JA: Follicular conjunctivitis on dipivefrin therapy for glaucoma. Eye 2:440, 1988.
63. Holland, MG: Treatment of glaucoma by chemical sympathectomy with 6-hydroxydopamine. Trans Am Acad Ophthal Otol 76:437, 1972.
64. Holland, MG, Wei, C-P: Epinephrine dose-response characteristics of glaucomatous human eyes following chemical sympathectomy with 6-hydroxydopamine. Ann Ophthal 5:633, 1973.

65. Holland, MG, Wei, C-P: Chemical sympathectomy in glaucoma therapy: an investigation of alpha and beta adrenergic supersensitivity. Ann Ophthal 5:783, 1973.
66. Diamond, JG: 6-hydroxydopamine in treatment of open-angle glaucoma. Arch Ophthal 94:41, 1976.
67. Colasanti, BK, Kosa, JE, Trotter, RR: Responsiveness of the rabbit eye to adrenergic and cholinergic agonists after treatment with 6-hydroxydopamine or alpha-methyl-para-tyrosine. Part I—Pupillary changes. Ann Ophthal 10:1067, 1978.
68. Colasanti, BK, Trotter, RR: Responsiveness of the rabbit eye to adrenergic and cholinergic agonists after treatment with 6-hydroxydopamine or alpha-methyl-para-tyrosine. Part II—Intraocular pressure changes. Ann Ophthal 10:1209, 1978.
69. Talusan, E, Schwartz, B, Mandell, AI, et al: 6-Hydroxydopamine in the treatment of open-angle glaucoma. Am J Ophthal 92:792, 1981.
70. Kitazawa, Y, Nose, H, Horie, T: Chemical sympathectomy with 6-hydroxydopamine in the treatment of primary open-angle glaucoma. Am J Ophthal 79:98, 1975.
71. Watanabe, H, Levene, RZ, Bernstein, MR: 6-Hydroxydopamine therapy in glaucoma. Trans Am Acad Ophthal Otol 83:69, 1977.
72. Sneddon, JM, Turner, P: The interactions of local guanethidine and sympathomimetic amines in the human eye. Arch Ophthal 81:622, 1969.
73. Bonomi, L, Di Comite, P: Outflow facility after guanethidine sulfate administration. Arch Ophthal 78:337, 1967.
74. Crombie, AL: Adrenergic supersensitization as a therapeutic tool in glaucoma. Trans Ophthal Soc UK 94:570, 1974.
75. Jones, DEP, Norton, DA, Harvey, J, Davies, DJG: Effect of adrenaline and guanethidine in reducing intraocular pressure in rabbits' eyes. Br J Ophthal 59:304, 1975.
76. Nagasubramanian, S, Tripathi, RC, Poinoosawmy, D, Gloster, J: Low concentration guanethidine and adrenaline therapy of glaucoma. A preliminary report. Trans Ophthal Soc UK 96:179, 1976.
77. Mills, KB, Ridgway, AEA: A double blind comparison of guanethidine-and-adrenaline drops with 1% adrenaline alone in chronic simple glaucoma. Br J Ophthal 62:320, 1978.
78. Hoyng, PhFJ, Dake, CL: The combination of guanethidine 3% and adrenaline 0.5% in 1 eyedrop (GA) in glaucoma treatment. Br J Ophthal 63:56, 1979.
79. Romano, J, Patterson, G: Evaluation of a 5% guanethidine and 0.5% adrenaline mixture (Ganda 5.05) and of a 3% guanethidine and 0.5% adrenaline mixture (Ganda 3.05) in the treatment of open-angle glaucoma. Br J Ophthal 63:52, 1979.
80. Jones, DEP, Norton, DA, Davies, DJG: Control of glaucoma by reduced dosage guanethidine-adrenaline formulation. Br J Ophthal 63:813, 1979.
81. Hoyng, PhFJ, Dake, CL: Maintenance therapy of glaucoma patients with guanethidine (3%) and adrenaline (0.5%) once daily. Graefe's Arch Ophthal 214:269, 1980.
82. Van Husen, H: A combination of 1% guanethidine and 0.2% epinephrine in drop form to lower IOP in open angle glaucoma. Klin Monatsbl Augenheilkd 177:622, 1980.
83. Murray, A, Glover, D, Hitchings, R: Low-dose combined guanethidine 1% and adrenaline 0.5% in the treatment of chronic simple glaucoma: a prospective study. Br J Ophthal 65:533, 1981.
84. Hitchings, RA, Glover, D: Adrenaline 1% combined with guanethidine 1% versus adrenaline 1%: a randomised prospective double-blind cross-over study. Br J Ophthal 66:247, 1982.
85. Romano, JH, Nagasubramanian, S, Poinoosawmy, D: Double-masked cross-over comparison of Ganda 1.02 (guanethidine 1% and adrenaline 0.2% mixture) with gutt. adrenaline 1% (Simplene 1%) and with pilocarpine 1% (Sno-Pilo 1%). Br J Ophthal 65:50, 1981.
86. Heilmann, K: Course of intraocular pressure during long-term treatment with a combination of guanethidine and epinephrine. Klin Monatsbl Augenheilkd 183:17, 1983.
87. Hoyng, PhFJ, Dake, CL: The aqueous humor dynamics and the biphasic response in intraocular pressure induced by guanethidine and adrenaline in the glaucomatous eye. Graefe's Arch Ophthal 214:263, 1980.
88. Gloster, J: Guanethidine and glaucoma. Trans Ophthal Soc UK 94:573, 1974.
89. Asregadoo, ER: Guanethidine ophthalmic solution 5%. Use in the treatment of endocrine exophthalmos. Arch Ophthal 84:21, 1970.
90. Riley, FC, Moyer, NJ: Experimental Horner's syndrome: a pupillographic evaluation of guanethidine-induced adrenergic blockade in humans. Am J Ophthal 69:442, 1970.
91. Urner-Bloch, U, Aeschlimann, JE, Gloor, BP: Treatment of chronic simple glaucoma with an adrenaline/guanethidine combination at three different dosages (comparative double-blind study). Graefe's Arch Ophthal 213:175, 1980.
92. Keates, EU: Evaluation of timolol maleate combination therapy in chronic open-angle glaucoma. Am J Ophthal 88:565, 1979.
93. Smith, RJ, Nagasubramanian, S, Watkins, R, Poinoosawmy, D: Addition of timolol maleate to routine medical therapy: a clinical trial. Br J Ophthal 64:779, 1980.
94. Nielsen, NV, Eriksen, JS: Timolol in maintenance treatment of ocular hypertension and glaucoma. Acta Ophthal 57:1070, 1979.
95. Thomas, JV, Epstein, DL: Timolol and epineph-

rine in primary open angle glaucoma. Transient additive effect. Arch Ophthal 99:91, 1981.
96. Thomas, JV, Epstein, DL: Study of the additive effect of timolol and epinephrine in lowering intraocular pressure. Br J Ophthal 65:596, 1981.
97. Goldberg, I, Ashburn, FS Jr, Palmberg, PF, et al: Timolol and epinephrine. A clinical study of ocular interactions. Arch Ophthal 98:484, 1980.
98. Keates, EC, Stone, RA: Safety and effectiveness of concomitant administration of dipivefrin and timolol maleate. Am J Ophthal 91:243, 1981.
99. Ohrstrom, A, Pandolfi, M: Regulation of intraocular pressure and pupil size by beta-blockers and epinephrine. Arch Ophthal 98:2182, 1980.
100. Ohrstrom, A, Kattstrom, O: Interaction of timolol and adrenaline. Br J Ophthal 65:53, 1981.
101. Knupp, JA, Shields, MB, Mandell, AI, et al: Combined timolol and epinephrine therapy for open angle glaucoma. Surv Ophthal 28(suppl):280, 1983.
102. Cyrlin, MS, Thomas, JV, Epstein, DL: Additive effect of epinephrine to timolol therapy in primary open angle glaucoma. Arch Ophthal 100:414, 1982.
103. Korey, MS, Hodapp, E, Kass, MA, et al: Timolol and epinephrine. Long-term evaluation of concurrent administration. Arch Ophthal 100:742, 1982.
104. Ober, M, Scharrer, A: The effect of timolol and dipivalyl-epinephrine in the treatment of the elevated intraocular pressure. Graefe's Arch Ophthal 213:273, 1980.
105. Tsoy, EA, Meekins, BB, Shields, MB: Comparison of two treatment schedules for combined timolol and dipivefrin therapy. Am J Ophthal 102:320, 1986.
106. Urtti, A, Kyyronen, K: Ophthalmic epinephrine, phenylephrine, and pilocarpine affect the systemic absorption of ocularly applied timolol. J Ocul Pharmacol 5:127, 1989.
107. Allen, RC, Epstein, DL: Additive effect of betaxolol and epinephrine in primary open angle glaucoma. Arch Ophthal 104:1178, 1986.
108. Weinreb, RN, Ritch, R, Kushner, FH: Effect of adding betaxolol to dipivefrin therapy. Am J Ophthal 101:196, 1986.
109. Ohrstrom, A: Dose response of oral timolol combined with adrenaline. Br J Ophthal 66:242, 1982.
110. Anderson, JA: Systemic absorption of topical ocularly applied epinephrine and dipivefrin. Arch Ophthal 98:350, 1980.
111. Corwin, ME, Spencer, WH: Conjunctival melanin depositions. A side-effect of topical epinephrine therapy. Arch Ophthal 69:73, 1963.
112. Veirs, ER, McGrew, JC: Ocular complications from topical epinephrine therapy of glaucoma. EENT Monthly 42:46, 1963.
113. Cashwell, LF, Shields, MB, Reed, JW: Adrenochrome pigmentation. Arch Ophthal 95:514, 1977.
114. Pardos, GJ, Krachmer, JH, Mannis, MJ: Persistent corneal erosion secondary to tarsal adrenochrome deposit. Am J Ophthal 90:870, 1980.
115. Pau, H, Schmitt-Graeff, A: Pigmented deposits into conjunctiva after local application of epinephrine. Graefe's Arch Ophthal 216:69, 1981.
116. Reinecke, RD, Kuwabara, T: Corneal deposits secondary to topical epinephrine. Arch Ophthal 70:170, 1963.
117. Krejci, L, Harrison, R: Corneal pigment deposits from topically administered epinephrine. Experimental production. Arch Ophthal 82:836, 1969.
118. Green, WR, Kaufer, GJ, Dubroff, S: Black cornea. A complication of topical use of epinephrine. Ophthalmologica 154:88, 1967.
119. Cleasby, G, Donaldson, DD: Epinephrine pigmentation of the cornea. Arch Ophthal 78:74, 1967.
120. Madge, GE, Geeraets, WJ, Guerry, DP III: Black cornea secondary to topical epinephrine. Am J Ophthal 71:402, 1971.
121. McCarthy, RW, LeBlanc, R: A 'black cornea' secondary to topical epinephrine. Can J Ophthal 11:336, 1976.
122. Barishak, R, Romano, A, Stein, R: Obstruction of lacrimal sac caused by topical epinephrine. Ophthalmologica 159:373, 1969.
123. Spaeth, GL: Nasolacrimal duct obstruction caused by topical epinephrine. Arch Ophthal 77:355, 1967.
124. Bradbury, JA, Rennie, IG, Parsons, MA: Adrenaline dacryolith: detection by ultrasound examination of the nasolacrimal duct. Br J Ophthal 72:935, 1988.
125. Soong, HK, McKenney, MJ, Wolter, JR: Adrenochrome staining of senile plaque resembling malignant melanoma. Am J Ophthal 101:380, 1986.
126. Sugar, J: Adrenochrome pigmentation of hydrophilic lenses. Arch Ophthal 91:11, 1974.
127. Miller, D, Brooks, SM, Mobilia, E: Adrenochrome staining of soft contact lenses. Ann Ophthal 8:65, 1976.
128. Romano, A, Barishak, R, Stein, R: Obstruction of lacrimal puncta caused by topical epinephrine. Ophthalmologica 166:301, 1973.
129. Kass, MA, Stamper, RL, Becker, B: Madarosis in chronic epinephrine therapy. Arch Ophthal 88:429, 1972.
130. Kristensen, EB, Norn, MS: Benign mucous membrane pemphigoid. 1. Secretion of mucus and tears. Acta Ophthal 52:266, 1974.
131. Fiore, PM, Jacobs, IH, Goldberg, DB: Drug-induced pemphigoid. A spectrum of diseases. Arch Ophthal 105:1660, 1987.
132. Tauber, J, Melamed, S, Foster, CS: Glaucoma in

patients with ocular-cicatricial pemphigoid. Ophthalmology 96:33, 1989.

133. Kwon, BS, Gangarosa, LP Sr, Green, K, Hill, JM: Kinetics of ocular herpes simplex virus shedding induced by epinephrine iontophoresis. Invest Ophthal Vis Sci 22:818, 1982.
134. Kolker, AE, Becker, B: Epinephrine maculopathy. Arch Ophthal 79:552, 1968.
135. Michels, RG, Maumenee, AE: Cystoid macular edema associated with topically applied epinephrine in aphakic eyes. Am J Ophthal 80:379, 1975.
136. Thomas, JV, Gragoudas, ES, Blair, NP, Lapus, JV: Correlation of epinephrine use and macular edema in aphakic glaucomatous eyes. Arch Ophthal 96:625, 1978.
137. Miyake, K, Shirasawa, E, Hikita, M, et al: Synthesis of prostaglandin E in rabbit eyes with topically applied epinephrine. Invest Ophthal Vis Sci 29:332, 1988.
138. Miyake, K, Kayazawa, F, Manabe, R, Miyake, Y: Indomethacin and the epinephrine-induced breakdown of the blood-ocular barrier in rabbits. Invest Ophthal Vis Sci 28:482, 1987.
139. Hull, DS, Chemotti, T, Edelhauser, HF, et al: Effect of epinephrine on the corneal endothelium. Am J Ophthal 79:245, 1975.
140. Edelhauser, HF, Hyndiuk, RA, Zeeb, A, Schultz, RO: Corneal edema and the intraocular use of epinephrine. Am J Ophthal 93:327, 1982.
141. Waltman, SR, Yarian, D, Hart, W Jr, Becker, B: Corneal endothelial changes with long-term topical epinephrine therapy. Arch Ophthal 95:1357, 1977.
142. Kramer, SG: Considerations on epinephrine therapy in glaucoma. Ann Ophthal 10:1077, 1978.
143. Kramer, SG: Epinephrine distribution after topical administration to phakic and aphakic eyes. Trans Am Ophthal Soc 78:947, 1980.
144. Morgan, TR, Mirate, DJ, Bowman, K, Green, K: Topical epinephrine and regional ocular blood flow in aphakic eyes of rabbits. Arch Ophthal 101:112, 1983.
145. Jay, WM, Aziz, MZ, Green, K: The effect of retrobulbar epinephrine injection on ocular and optic nerve blood flow. Curr Eye Res 4:55, 1985.
146. Stefansson, E, Robinson, D, Wolbarsht, ML, et al: Effect of epinephrine on PO_2 in anterior chamber. Arch Ophthal 101:636, 1983.
147. Harrison, R, Kaufmann, CS: Clonidine. Effects of a topically administered solution on intraocular pressure and blood pressure in open-angle glaucoma. Arch Ophthal 95:1368, 1977.
148. Hodapp, E, Kolker, AE, Kass, MA, et al: The effect of topical clonidine on intraocular pressure. Arch Ophthal 99:1208, 1981.
149. Petursson, G, Cole, R, Hanna, C: Treatment of glaucoma using minidrops of clonidine. Arch Ophthal 102:1180, 1984.
150. Krieglstein, GK, Langham, ME, Leydhecker, W: The peripheral and central neural actions of clonidine in normal and glaucomatous eyes. Invest Ophthal Vis Sci 17:149, 1978.
151. Lee, DA, Topper, JE, Brubaker, RF: Effect of clonidine on aqueous humor flow in normal human eyes. Exp Eye Res 38:239, 1984.
152. Macri, FJ, Cevario, SJ: Clonidine. Effects on aqueous humor formation and intraocular pressure. Arch Ophthal 96:2111, 1978.
153. Marquardt, R, Pillunat, LE, Stodtmeister, R: Ocular hemodynamics following local application of clonidine. Klin Monatsbl Augenheilkd 193:637, 1988.
154. Coleman, AL, Robin, AL, Pollack, IP, et al: Cardiovascular and intraocular pressure effects and plasma concentrations of apraclonidine. Arch Ophthal 108:1264, 1990.
155. Gharagozloo, NZ, Relf, SJ, Brubaker, RF: Aqueous flow is reduced by the alpha-adrenergic agonist, apraclonidine hydrochloride (ALO 2145). Ophthalmology 95:1217, 1988.
156. Wang, R-F, Camras, CB, Podos, SM, et al: The role of prostaglandins in the para-aminoclonidine-induced reduction of intraocular pressure. Trans Am Ophthal Soc 87:94, 1989.
157. Jampel, HD, Robin, AL, Quigley, HA, Pollack, IP: Apraclonidine. A one-week dose-response study. Arch Ophthal 106:1069, 1988.
158. Abrams, DA, Robin, AL, Crandall, AS, et al: A limited comparison of apraclonidine's dose response in subjects with normal or increased intraocular pressure. Am J Ophthal 108:230, 1989.
159. Robin, AL: Short-term effects of unilateral 1% apraclonidine therapy. Arch Ophthal 106:912, 1988.
160. Abrams, DA, Robin, AL, Pollack, IP, et al: The safety and efficacy of topical 1% ALO 2145 (p-aminoclonidine hydrochloride) in normal volunteers. Arch Ophthal 105:1205, 1987.
161. Sugiyama, K, Kitazawa, Y, Kawai, K: Apraclonidine effects on ocular responses to YAG laser irradiation to the rabbit iris. Invest Ophthal Vis Sci 31:708, 1990.
162. Brown, RH, Stewart, RH, Lynch, MG, et al: ALO 2145 reduces the intraocular pressure elevation after anterior segment laser surgery. Ophthalmology 95:378, 1988.
163. Kitazawa, Y, Taniguchi, T, Sugiyama, K: Use of apraclonidine to reduce acute intraocular pressure rise following Q-switched Nd:YAG laser iridotomy. Ophthal Surg 20:49, 1989.
164. Sridharrao, B, Badrinath, SS: Efficacy and safety of apraclonidine in patients undergoing anterior segment laser surgery. Br J Ophthal 73:884, 1989.
165. Pollack, IP, Brown, RH, Crandall, AS, et al: Prevention of the rise in intraocular pressure following neodymium-YAG posterior capsulotomy using topical 1% apraclonidine. Arch Ophthal 106:754, 1988.

166. Krawitz, PL, Podos, SM: Use of apraclonidine in the treatment of acute angle closure glaucoma. Arch Ophthal 108:1208, 1990.
167. Morrison, JC, Robin, AL: Adjunctive glaucoma therapy. A comparison of apraclonidine to dipivefrin when added to timolol maleate. Ophthalmology 96:3, 1989.
168. King, MH, Richards, DW: Near syncope and chest tightness after administration of apraclonidine before argon laser iridotomy. Am J Ophthal 110:308, 1990.
169. Serdahl, CL, Galustian, J, Lewis, RA: The effects of apraclonidine on conjunctival oxygen tension. Arch Ophthal 107:1777, 1989.
170. Pollack, IP, Rossi, H: Norepinephrine in treatment of ocular hypertension and glaucoma. Arch Ophthal 93:173, 1975.
171. Pollack, IP: Effect of l-norepinephrine and adrenergic potentiators on the aqueous humor dynamics of man. Am J Ophthal 76:641, 1973.
172. Potter, DE, Rowland, JM: Adrenergic drugs and intraocular pressure: effects of selective beta-adrenergic agonists. Exp Eye Res 27:615, 1978.
173. Waitzman, MB, Woods, WD, Cheek, WV: Effects of prostaglandins and norepinephrine on ocular pressure and pupil size in rabbits following bilateral cervical ganglionectomy. Invest Ophthal Vis Sci 18:52, 1979.
174. Colansanti, BK, Barany, EH: Potentiation of the mydriatic effect of norepinephrine in the rabbit after monoamine oxidase inhibition. Invest Ophthal Vis Sci 18:200, 1979.
175. Kitazawa, Y: Topical adrenergic potentiators in primary open-angle glaucoma. Am J Ophthal 74:588, 1972.
176. Stewart, RH, Kimbrough, RL, Martin, PA, et al: Norepinephrine dipivalylate dose-response in ocular hypertensive subjects. Ann Ophthal 13:1279, 1981.
177. Duffin, RM, Christensen, RE, Bergamini, MVW: Suppression of adrenergic adaptation in the eye with a prostaglandin synthesis inhibitor. Invest Ophthal Vis Sci 21:756, 1981.
178. Zeller, EA, Shoch, D, Cooperman, SG, Schnipper, RI: Enzymology of the refractory media of the eye. IX. On the role of monoamine oxidase in the regulation of aqueous humor dynamics of the rabbit eye. Invest Ophthal 6:618, 1967.
179. Zeller, EA, Shoch, D, Czerner, TB, et al: Enzymology of the refractory media of the eye. X. Effects of topically administered bradykinin, amine releasers, and pargyline on aqueous humor dynamics. Invest Ophthal 10:274, 1971.
180. Bausher, LP: Identification of A and B forms of monoamine oxidase in the iris-ciliary body, superior cervical ganglion, and pineal gland of albino rabbits. Invest Ophthal 15:529, 1976.
181. Mehra, KS, Roy, PN, Singh, R: Pargyline drops in glaucoma. Arch Ophthal 92:453, 1974.
182. Ross, RA, Drance, SM: Effects of topically applied isoproterenol on aqueous dynamics in man. Arch Ophthal 83:39, 1970.
183. Seidehamel, RJ, Dungan, KW, Hickey, TE: Specific hypotensive and antihypertensive ocular effects of d-isoproterenol in rabbits. Am J Ophthal 79:1018, 1975.
184. Kass, MA, Reid, TW, Neufeld, AH, et al: The effect of d-isoproterenol on intraocular pressure of the rabbit, monkey, and man. Invest Ophthal 15:113, 1976.
185. Brubaker, RF, Gaasterland, D: The effect of isoproterenol on aqueous humor formation in humans. Invest Ophthal Vis Sci 25:357, 1984.
186. Caprioli, J, Sears, M, Bausher, L, et al: Forskolin lowers intraocular pressure by reducing aqueous inflow. Invest Ophthal Vis Sci 25:268, 1984.
187. Jumblatt, JE, North, GT: Potentiation of sympathetic neurosecretion by forskolin and cyclic AMP in the rabbit iris-ciliary body. Curr Eye Res 5:495, 1986.
188. Lee, P-Y, Podos, SM, Mittag, T, Severin, C: Effect of topically applied forskolin on aqueous humor dynamics in cynomolgus monkey. Invest Ophthal Vis Sci 25:1206, 1984.
189. Badian, M, Dabrowski, J, Grigoleit, H-G, et al: Effect of forskolin-eyedrops on the intraocular pressure of healthy male subjects. Klin Monatsbl Augenheilkd 185:522, 1984.
190. Caprioli, J, Sears, M: Combined effect of forskolin and acetazolamide on intraocular pressure and aqueous flow in rabbit eyes. Exp Eye Res 39:47, 1984.
191. Burstein, NL, Sears, ML, Mead, A: Aqueous flow in human eyes is reduced by forskolin, a potent adenylate cyclase activator. Exp Eye Res 39:745, 1984.
192. Bartels, SP, Lee, SR, Neufeld, AH: The effects of forskolin on cyclic AMP, intraocular pressure and aqueous humor formation in rabbits. Curr Eye Res 6:307, 1987.
193. Brubaker, RF, Carlson, KH, Kullerstrand, LJ, McLaren, JW: Topical forskolin (Colforsin) and aqueous flow in humans. Arch Ophthal 105:637, 1987.
194. Shibata, T, Mishima, H, Kurokawa, T: Ocular pigmentation and intraocular pressure response to forskolin. Curr Eye Res 7:667, 1988.
195. Gregory, D, Sears, M, Bausher, L, et al: Intraocular pressure and aqueous flow are decreased by cholera toxin. Invest Ophthal Vis Sci 20:371, 1981.
196. Bartels, SP, Roth, HO, Neufeld, AH: Effects of intravitreal cholera toxin on adenosine 3′,5′-monophosphate, intraocular pressure, and outflow facility in rabbits. Invest Ophthal Vis Sci 20:410, 1981.
197. Mishima, H, Sears, M, Bausher, L, Gregory, D: Ultracytochemistry of cholera-toxin binding sites

in ciliary processes. Cell Tissue Res 223:241, 1982.

198. Mishima, H, Bausher, L, Sears, M, et al: Fine structural studies of ciliary processes after treatment with cholera toxin or its B subunit. Graefe's Arch Ophthal 219:272, 1982.
199. Bonomi, L, Perfetti, S, Bellucci, R, Massa, F: Effects of terbutaline on experimentally induced ocular hypertension in the rabbit. Glaucoma 4:134, 1982.
200. Bonomi, L, Perfetti, S, Bellucci, R, et al: Prevention by diclofenac of the subsensitivity to the IOP-lowering effect of terbutaline. Glaucoma 6:241, 1984.
201. Bonomi, L, Perfetti, S, Bellucci, R, et al: Intraocular pressure lowering effect of ibuterol in the rabbit. Glaucoma 6:216, 1984.
202. Coakes, RL, Siah, PB: Effects of adrenergic drugs on aqueous humour dynamics in the normal human eye. I. Salbutamol. Br J Ophthal 68:393, 1984.
203. Mittag, TW, Tormay, A, Messenger, M, Podos, SM: Ocular hypotension in the rabbit. Receptor mechanisms of pirbuterol and nylidrin. Invest Ophthal Vis Sci 26:163, 1985.
204. Krupin, T, Becker, B, Podos, SM: Topica vanadate lowers intraocular pressure in rabbits. Invest Ophthal Vis Sci 19:1360, 1980.
205. Podos, SM, Lee, P-Y, Severin, C, Mittag, T: The effect of vanadate on aqueous humor dynamics in cynomolgus monkeys. Invest Ophthal Vis Sci 25:359, 1984.
206. Becker, B: Vanadate and aqueous humor dynamics. Invest Ophthal Vis Sci 19:1156, 1980.
207. Mittag, TW, Serle, JB, Podos, SM, et al: Vanadate effects on ocular pressure, (Na^+, K^+) ATPase and adenylate cyclase in rabbit eyes. Invest Ophthal Vis Sci 25:1335, 1984.
208. Sobel, L, Serle, JB, Podos, SM, et al: Topical nylidrin and aqueous humor dynamics in rabbits and monkeys. Arch Ophthal 101:1281, 1983.

Chapter 27

ADRENERGIC INHIBITORS

BETA-ADRENERGIC INHIBITORS

Early Experience

Beta-adrenergic inhibitors or antagonists, or "beta-blockers" as they are commonly called, are the most frequently used class of drugs for the treatment of glaucoma. The first commercially available beta-blocker was *propranolol,* which was introduced in 1967 for the treatment of cardiac arrhythmias, angina pectoris, and systemic hypertension. The drug was also found to reduce intraocular pressure (IOP) when given orally,[1–5] topically,[6,7] or intravenously.[8]

Early experience with beta-adrenergic antagonists, however, revealed adverse reactions that limited the usefulness of many of these compounds as topical antiglaucoma agents. Propranolol, as well as several other beta-blockers, were found to cause corneal anesthesia, as a result of membrane stabilizing activity,[6] and reduced tear production.[9] The latter side effect is particularly a problem with another systemic beta-blocking agent, *practolol,* which causes a severe dry eye syndrome in some patients, possibly through an immunologic mechanism,[10] occasionally associated with subconjunctival fibrosis, corneal ulcers, and a skin rash.[10–12] Other beta-blockers were found to have carcinogenicity in test animals.[13]

Timolol

Early Studies

Timolol maleate is a nonselective, $beta_1$- and $beta_2$-adrenergic antagonist. It was found in preliminary trials to have none of the adverse reactions described above for some beta-blockers.[14,15] Rabbit studies revealed an IOP-lowering effect in both the treated[16,17] and fellow, untreated eye.[17] Single doses in human volunteers effectively lowered the IOP in normotensive individuals[14] as well as patients with primary open-angle glaucoma,[18,19] and a small hypotensive effect was again noted in the fellow, untreated eye.[20] Short-term, multiple-dose trials with open-angle glaucoma patients demonstrated a sustained reduction in IOP.[21–24] Comparative studies showed the IOP lowering efficacy of timolol to be greater than that of epinephrine[22,25] and equal to or slightly weaker than various concentrations of combined epinephrine and guanethidine.[26] When compared with pilocarpine, timolol had an equivalent or slightly greater IOP-lowering effect.[27–31] In one comparative study, echothiophate iodide was preferred over timolol in the treatment of glaucoma in aphakia.[32]

Mechanisms of Action

Tonographic[33,34] and fluorophotometric[35–37] studies in humans, as well as research with cats[38] and monkeys,[39,40] all indicate that timolol lowers the IOP primarily, if not exclusively, by reducing aqueous humor production. This effect is not seen in sleeping human subjects, presumably because aqueous production is minimal during sleep.[37] Primate studies suggest that the degree of effect on aqueous flow in the fellow, untreated eye is dose related.[40]

The influence of timolol on inflow presumably represents a direct action on the ciliary processes, either on the nonpigmented epithelium to decrease secretion or on local capillary perfusion to reduce ultrafiltration.[41,42] The possibility of a direct action by beta-adrenergic agents on the formation of aqueous humor is supported by the identification of beta-adrenergic receptors,[43] predominantly of the $beta_2$ subtype,[44–48] in both animal[43,45–47] and human[44,48] ciliary processes.

To explain the mechanism by which an adrenergic antagonist might reduce aqueous production, it is necessary to postulate a physiologic, sympathetic "resting tone" in the ciliary process receptors that are associated with the formation of aqueous humor.[41,42] Animal studies have supported the concept that adrenergic innervation participates in the IOP-lowering action of timolol,[49] although this was not substantiated in a human study in which sympathetic denervation from postganglionic Horner's syndrome affected neither flow nor pressure.[50] However, the possibility remains that tone could arise from catecholamines brought to the tissue by the circulation.[42]

The influence of timolol on aqueous humor formation may be related to inhibition of catecholamine-stimulated synthesis of cyclic AMP, which has been demonstrated in rabbit studies.[51] Although the duration of this effect is shorter than that of the IOP reduction, it may be that pigment binding of the drug provides a slow-release depot, which helps maintain the concentration of timolol for a prolonged effect.[52]

It does not appear that timolol significantly influences the blood-aqueous barrier. Simultaneous bilateral fluorescein angiography of the iris revealed no effect of timolol on dye leakage.[53] Topical application of timolol is associated with a significant increase in aqueous humor protein,[54] although the normal ratio of albumin to IgG[55] and of the different molecular weight classes of protein[56] are not altered, suggesting that this finding is a result of reduced aqueous humor flow and not a change in permeability of the blood-aqueous barrier. It also appears that the timolol mechanism is not prostaglandin-mediated, since it is not altered by concurrent systemic or topical indomethacin therapy.[57,58]

There is some evidence that timolol may reduce aqueous humor formation by a mechanism other than beta-adrenergic blockade. In a study with rabbit eyes, there was a suggestion that timolol might act as a dopaminergic antagonist to lower blood flow to the ciliary body.[59] However, metoclopramide, a dopamine-2 antagonist, did not affect the ocular hypotensive action of timolol in normal human volunteers.[60]

Most studies indicate that timolol has little, if any, influence on outflow facility.[33,34] A theoretic explanation for this is that, unlike the system related to aqueous inflow, there may be no sympathetic resting tone associated with aqueous outflow. This assumption may not be entirely correct, however, since topical timolol was associated with a small myopic shift in one human study, suggesting that sympathetic innervation is involved in the resting tone of the ciliary muscle.[61] In addition, some tonographic studies have shown a small increase in outflow,[62] and beta-adrenergic receptors, primarily of the $beta_2$ subtype, have been demonstrated in human trabecular meshwork.[63,64] However, a histologic study of the outflow apparatus in human eyes, treated with timolol before enucleation for malignant melanoma, revealed no morphologic changes suggestive of a pressure-lowering action by the drug.[65]

Administration

Concentrations. Timolol maleate is commercially available in 0.25% and 0.5% concentrations (Table 27.1). Early experience with primary open-angle glaucoma patients indicated that the maximum IOP-lowering effect is achieved with 0.5% timolol.[14,18] However, in other studies the 0.25% concentration was equally as or more efficacious than the 0.5%, although the latter provided a somewhat longer duration of action.[66,67] One investigation revealed that adequate IOP control could be achieved in more than half the patients with 0.1% timolol,[68] and another showed that even a 0.008% concentration had a definite but minimal ocular hypotensive effect.[69] Prodrugs of timolol have been evaluated in rabbits with the indication that the therapeutic index, as determined by the ratio of aqueous to plasma concentrations, may improve 15-fold over standard preparations.[70,71] Individuals with darker irides appear to require higher concentrations of timolol.[72] In one study, timolol had a significant ocular hypotensive effect 1 hour after instillation in patients with blue irides but no effect in brown-eyed patients, which may relate to early pigment binding.[73]

Frequency of Administration. Good corneal penetration of timolol has been demonstrated in rabbit[74] and human[75,76] eyes, with peak aqueous humor concentrations in human eyes occurring within the first 1–2 hours. The IOP-lowering effect peaks approximately 2 hours after administration[14,18] and lasts for at least 24 hours.[19] The optimum frequency of administration in most cases is twice daily, although once-a-day treatment has been shown to be adequate in many cases.[77,78] When timolol is discontinued following long-term therapy, aqueous flow does not increase significantly until the 4th day and the IOP until 14 days later.[79]

Long-Term Efficacy

Numerous long-term studies have confirmed the continued efficacy of chronic timolol therapy for many patients.[80–87] In a significant number of cases, however, the pressure responsiveness to timolol will decrease with continued administration. This occurs in two phases, which Boger[88] has called the "short-term 'escape' and long-term 'drift.' "

Short-Term "Escape." Many patients will experience a dramatic reduction in IOP with the initiation of timolol therapy. However, the pressure nearly always rises during the next few days to plateau finally at a maintenance level.[27,89–91] The 1-hour IOP response to timolol does not predict which patients will have a significant loss of responsiveness 3–4 weeks later.[91] It has been demonstrated that the number of beta-receptors in ocular tissues increases during the first few days of timolol therapy,[92] which may explain this "escape" phenomenon.

Long-Term "Drift." Once the IOP has leveled off following the initiation of timolol therapy, control will be maintained in most cases. However, some patients will have a slow decline in pressure response to timolol, usually beginning 3 months to a year after starting treatment.[62,80–87] Fluorophotometric studies indicate that aqueous flow

Table 27.1
Commercial Topical Beta-Blockers*

Generic Preparations	Brand Name	Concentrations (%)
Timolol maleate	Timoptic	0.25, 0.5
Betaxolol HCl	Betoptic	0.5
	Betoptic S*	0.25
Levobunolol HCl	Betagan	0.25, 0.5
Metipranolol HCl	OptiPranolol	0.3

* Suspension.

is higher in most patients following 1 year of timolol therapy as compared with the value 1 week after initiating treatment.[93] Some patients will regain responsiveness to timolol after a "washout" period. In one study of 39 eyes showing a long-term drift with 0.5% timolol, 23 eyes received dipivefrin (a prodrug of epinephrine) during a 30- or 60-day "timolol holiday," and the remainder received artificial tears in place of the timolol.[94] When the timolol was reinstituted, the dipivefrin-treated group had a mean IOP decrease of 8.2 mm Hg, compared with 3.9 in the nondipivefrin-treated group, and the response to timolol was more prolonged in eyes treated for 60 days with dipivefrin.

Drug Interactions

Long-term, multiple-drug studies have shown that timolol will cause additional lowering of IOP in many cases when added to maximum tolerable antiglaucoma therapy.[95–97] More specifically, the combined effect of timolol and a *miotic*[98–101] or timolol and a *carbonic anhydrase inhibitor*[98,100,101–105] is, for most patients, significantly greater than the effect of either medication alone, although less than the arithmetic sum of the effects of the individual drugs. Evaluations of a *combined timolol-pilocarpine* formulation indicate that twice-daily administration provides IOP reduction that is equivalent to timolol twice daily and pilocarpine three times daily given separately[106] and significantly greater than either drug given alone.[107–109]

The combination of timolol and an *epinephrine* compound, on the other hand, has less clinical value. This subject was reviewed in the previous chapter, with the conclusion that, while a statistically significant additional pressure reduction may occur when one drug is added to the other, the amount of this reduction is usually very small, with considerable variation from one patient to the next.[110,111] Therefore, the efficacy in each individual case must be confirmed by a uniocular therapeutic trial before chronic therapy with this combination of drugs is prescribed. Combined therapy with timolol and an epinephrine-guanethidine formulation was shown to have greater IOP-lowering efficacy than the epinephrine-guanethidine combination or timolol alone.[112]

Another important clinical question is the efficacy and safety of combined topical timolol and *oral beta-blockers*. In general, topical timolol will produce additional IOP reduction, without altering pulse or blood pressure, in patients pretreated with oral timolol,[113,114] propranolol,[115] alprenolol,[114] or metaprolol,[114] although the IOP-lowering efficacy of topical timolol appears to diminish with increasing dosages of the oral beta-blocker.[115]

Clinical Indications

Although timolol was originally evaluated and approved for the treatment of primary open-angle glaucoma, it has subsequently been found to lower the IOP in essentially all forms of glaucoma.[116,117] Since it lowers the IOP by reducing aqueous production and does not alter the pupil, it is helpful in situations in which conventional aqueous outflow cannot be improved medically and in which miosis or mydriasis is not desirable. Timolol is reported to help control glaucoma in aphakia during the early postoperative period[118–121] as well as in chronic cases.[62,117,122] The drug has also been found to control secondary angle-closure glaucoma after penetrating keratoplasty,[123] and following an iridectomy for angle-closure glaucoma when the pressure elevation persisted postoperatively.[124]

Timolol therapy in children is not always successful but is often useful. The incidence of side effects in the pediatric group is similar to those in the adult population, although experience with the very young is still limited, and extreme caution must be exercised.[125–128]

Another possible indication that has been evaluated for timolol is IOP reduction in ocular hypertensives to prevent the development of glaucomatous damage. In one study, timolol therapy was found to be significantly protective against visual field and optic nerve head damage,[129] while another study showed that timolol lowered the IOP approximately 5 mm Hg below that of an untreated control group but altered neither the pressure curve over time[130] nor the differential light sensitivity in tested meridia.[131]

Side Effects

As previously noted, early clinical experience suggested that adverse ocular and systemic reactions are unusually low with topical timolol therapy. Specifically, the drug does not affect the pupillary size[132] or accommodation and rarely causes burning or conjunctival hyperemia. However, continued experience has disclosed side effects, some of which can have serious consequences.

Ocular toxicity is uncommon with timolol therapy, although allergic and toxic reactions have been reported. Ocular cicatricial pemphigoid has been reported in patients receiving topical timolol.[133,134] In most of these cases the patient was also receiving additional glaucoma medications, although a small number were being treated with timolol alone when the pemphigoid was diagnosed. Burning and conjunctival hyperemia may occasionally occur and are frequently associated with superficial punctate keratopathy and corneal anesthesia.[135–139] Timolol does not affect corneal sensation in most patients, although a small subgroup may have markedly diminished corneal sensitivity.[138,139] Corneal epithelial erosions were reported in two patients wearing gas-permeable contact lenses soon after starting topical timolol therapy, and the combination of timolol and a contact lens in rabbits caused marked alterations in corneal epithelium and endothelium.[140] Animal studies have also suggested that topical timolol inhibits corneal epithelial wound healing.[141,142] One rabbit study showed ultrastructural corneal endothelial changes following topical timolol therapy for one month,[142] although most human and animal investigations have revealed no toxicity of topical timolol therapy to the corneal endothelium.[143–145]

Tear production may be reduced in some cases, although this is usually of no consequence unless the patient has low baseline tear flow.[146–148] Reduced central visual acuity has been noted in some patients on timolol therapy.[135–137] In some cases this may be due to a change in the refractive error or the pupillary diameter associated with discontinuation of miotic therapy, while the cause in other patients is not clear.

Topical timolol therapy has been shown to promote the recurrent shedding of latent herpes simplex virus type 1 induced by epinephrine in both a mouse[149] and rabbit[150] model. A study of cat eyes suggests that topical timolol does not cause a clinically or statistically significant decrease in anterior chamber oxygen tension.[151]

Systemic toxicity has been reported more often than ocular reactions and constitutes the more significant adverse effects of topical timolol therapy. Measurable plasma levels of timolol are present within 8 minutes or less of topical application,[152] and punctal occlusion after instillation of the drug significantly reduces plasma timolol levels,[153] which may help to minimize these side effects.

Cardiovascular. Blockade of beta$_1$-adrenergic receptors slows the pulse rate and weakens myocardial contractility. In most healthy patients, these effects are of no consequence. However, a potential for serious complications exists in patients with preexisting conditions such as sinus bradycardia, greater than first-degree heart block, and congestive heart failure. Topical timolol therapy has been associated with severe bradycardia, arrhythmias, heart failure, and syncope.[135–137,154–156]

Even healthy individuals may be at risk under certain circumstances, such as the stress of surgery[157] or heavy exercise.[158,159] In the latter situation, timolol has been shown to affect maximal heart rate and time to exhaustion.[158,159] The induced bradycardia may also be more pronounced when timolol is used concomitantly with other drugs, such as quinidine[160] or the calcium antagonist verapamil.[161]

Respiratory. Blockade of beta$_2$-adrenergic receptors produces contraction of bronchial smooth muscle, which may cause bronchospasm and airway obstruction, especially in asthmatics.[135,137,154,156,162–165] Thirteen cases of death in status asthmaticus following initiation of timolol therapy had been reported to the National Registry of Drug-Induced Ocular Side Effects by 1984.[165] Dyspnea[154,166] and apneic spells[167] have also been reported. These may be more common in young children, and caution must be taken by nursing mothers, since high levels of timolol were found in the milk of a mother receiving topical timolol.[168]

Central Nervous System Effects. This may be the most common class of systemic reactions to timolol therapy and includes depression, anxiety, confusion, dysarthria, hallucinations, lightheadedness, drowsiness, weakness, fatigue, tranquilization, dissociative behavior, disorientation, and emotional lability.[135–137,154,169]

Other Systemic Reactions. Other reactions that have been reported in association with timolol therapy include gastrointestinal distress (nausea, diarrhea, and cramping),[135,137,154] dermatologic disorders (maculopapular rash, alopecia, and hives),[137,154,170] and sexual impotence.[135,136] Since these observations were made in a predominantly elderly population, it is difficult to confirm a cause-and-effect relationship in all cases. However, of greater concern with timolol therapy is the exacerbation of myasthenia gravis[171,172] and the altered response to hypoglycemic episodes in diabetic patients, which may mask the awareness of the attack.[173]

Oral beta-blockers are known to adversely alter plasma lipid profiles, and 0.5% topical timolol twice daily for 2 months, without nasolacrimal occlusion, has been shown to decrease plasma high-density lipoprotein cholesterol levels of a magnitude that has been estimated to increase the risk of coronary artery disease by 21%.[174]

Betaxolol

Betaxolol hydrochloride is a cardioselective, $beta_1$-adrenergic antagonist. The mechanism of ocular hypotension appears to be the same as that for timolol, with reduction of aqueous humor production but no effect on outflow resistance or pupillary diameter.[175]

Efficacy

In preliminary clinical trials, betaxolol provided a significant reduction in IOP when evaluated alone[176] or in contrast to a placebo.[177–179] When compared with timolol at 0.25% and 0.5% concentrations, the magnitude of IOP reduction is usually slightly less with betaxolol, and there may be a greater need for adjunctive therapy than with timolol.[180–182] In one study of 153 glaucoma patients who were controlled on timolol, the half who were switched to betaxolol, in a masked and random fashion, had a significant increase in IOP.[183]

Drug Interactions

As with other beta-blockers, betaxolol usually provides significant additional IOP reduction when added to miotic or carbonic anhydrase inhibitor therapy.[184] However, the interaction with epinephrine compounds may differ somewhat from that of timolol and other nonselective beta-blockers. In both monkey[185] and human[186] studies, adding epinephrine to established betaxolol therapy was associated with a significant additional lowering of IOP and a significant increase in the outflow facility, which was not seen when adding epinephrine to timolol-treated eyes. In addition, adding betaxolol in open-angle glaucoma patients already on dipivefrin therapy resulted in a mean additional IOP reduction of 3.6 mm Hg at 4 weeks.[187] The additive effect of epinephrine compounds when used in conjunction with betaxolol may represent a $beta_2$ effect on outflow, which is blocked by nonselective beta-blockers but not by cardioselective $beta_1$-antagonists. However, since the nonselective beta-blockers have a greater IOP-lowering effect than betaxolol, when either is used alone, the net effect of combined therapy with epinephrine and either a nonselective or cardioselective beta-blocker is often the same.

Side Effects

Betaxolol is similar to the other topical beta-blockers in having a low incidence of ocular side effects, although the original formulation with a 0.5% concentration caused more burning with instillation than the other commercial beta-blockers.[180] However, a newer ophthalmic delivery vehicle with 0.25% betaxolol, formulated as a suspension, has the same IOP-lowering efficacy as the 0.5% preparation, with significantly less discomfort (Table 27.1).[188] As with other beta-blockers, betaxolol may reduce corneal sensitivity in a small number of patients.[139] One case of aphakic cystoid macular edema has been reported secondary to betaxolol therapy.[189]

With regard to adverse systemic reactions, the advantage of betaxolol over timolol is the absence of beta$_2$-adrenergic inhibition, which minimizes the risk of respiratory side effects. The drug does not cause a decrease in airflow in most patients with proved airway disease,[190–194] although exceptions to this have been reported.[194–197] While oral administration of the beta$_1$-blocker has been reported to significantly inhibit exercise tachycardia,[198] this is less common with topical betaxolol therapy[199,200] and may be less than with topical timolol.[199] However, cardiovascular side effects have been reported with topical betaxolol therapy, including arrhythmia,[195] bradycardia,[195] sinus arrest,[201] and decompensation of congestive heart failure.[202] With regard to central nervous system side effects, there may be less risk for this with betaxolol than with timolol therapy,[203] although such complications have been reported in association with betaxolol therapy.[204]

Levobunolol

Levobunolol (l-bunolol) is an analog of propranolol with potent nonselective beta$_1$- and beta$_2$-adrenergic antagonism. It presumably has the same mechanism of IOP reduction as timolol, although one tonographic study suggested that it may also increase aqueous outflow.[205] In preliminary short-term studies, the onset of an ocular hypotensive effect occurred within the first hour after instillation, peaked at 2 hours, and lasted up to 24 hours.[206] Concentrations of 0.3% and 0.6% levobunolol provided significant IOP reductions up to 4 hours, while the effect of 1% and 2% concentrations persisted at 12 hours.[207] However, in a 3-month comparison with the vehicle, 0.5% and 1% concentrations of levobunolol produced similar average pressure reductions.[208] Levobunolol is commercially available in concentrations of 0.25% and 0.5% (Table 27.1).

In comparative short-term and long-term clinical studies, levobunolol was equivalent to timolol with regard to ocular hypotensive efficacy and side effects when the two drugs were administered twice daily in commercial formulations.[206,209–217] It was also shown to be equivalent to the nonselective beta-blocker metipranolol[218] but had significantly greater pressure-lowering efficacy than betaxolol in a 3-month study.[219]

Levobunolol is effective with once-daily administration in a high percentage of patients,[220] with the 0.25% concentration providing adequate control in most of these cases.[221] When compared in 0.5% concentrations, once-daily levobunolol or timolol provided IOP control in 72% and 64% of patients, respectively.[222] In commercial bottles, a drop of levobunolol is significantly larger than that of timolol, which appears to be due to both the dispensing system and the increased viscosity of levobunolol.[223] However, the drop size does not appear to influence the efficacy or safety of the drug.[224]

Levobunolol has been found to be effective in controlling the early postoperative IOP rise following extracapsular cataract extraction[225,226] and laser posterior capsulotomy.[226] It has also been shown to provide additional IOP reduction when added to dipivefrin, with efficacy and safety comparable to concomitant timolol and dipivefrin therapy.[227]

Metipranolol

This nonselective beta-blocker is commercially available in a 0.3% concentration (Table 27.1). Comparative studies have shown that it is comparable to timolol[228,229] and levobunolol[218] with regard to efficacy and safety. However, one study revealed more bronchoconstriction in asthmatic patients than with timolol or carteolol.[230] As with other topical beta-blockers, metipranolol may cause a brief corneal anesthesia in some patients.[231] One study showed metipranolol to be effective in controlling IOP elevation after cataract surgery.[232] A fixed combination of metipranolol 0.1% and pilocarpine 2% was found to have better IOP-lowering efficacy than either drug used alone.[233]

Other Topical Beta-Blockers

The following beta-blockers have also been evaluated for their ocular hypotensive

Table 27.2
Commercial Oral Beta Blockers*

Generic Preparations	Brand Name	With Diuretic Antihypertensive
Acebutolol HCl	Sectral	
Atenolol	Tenormin	Tenoretic
Carteolol HCl	Cartrol	
Labetalol HCl	Normodyne	Normozide
Metoprolol tartrate	Lopressor	Lopressor HCT
Nadolol	Corgard	Corzide
Penbutolol sulfate	Levatol	
Pindolol	Visken	
Propranolol HCl	Inderal	Inderide
Timolol maleate	Blocadren	Timolide

* Other generic products may also be available.

effect. None are currently available in the United States for topical therapy at the time of this publication. However, several are available in oral form for treatment of cardiovascular and other systemic disorders, which may also influence the IOP (Table 27.2).

Carteolol

Carteolol is a nonselective beta-adrenergic antagonist with intrinsic sympathomimetic activity. The latter feature produces an early, transient adrenergic agonist response that is not found in the other beta-blockers described above. Studies with systemic beta-blockers indicate that intrinsic sympathomimetic activity does not interfere with the therapeutic benefits of beta-blockers,[234] and it was hoped that this activity in carteolol might actually protect against the adverse reactions of beta-antagonism. Preliminary studies showed the ocular hypotensive efficacy and duration of action to be comparable to those of timolol.[235] This has been confirmed in most subsequent studies, although no reduction in systemic side effects has been observed,[236–239] and one study showed that timolol 0.5% caused a significantly greater reduction in IOP at 12 hours after instillation than did carteolol 2%.[240] Another study indicated that 1% and 2% concentrations of carteolol have comparable pressure-lowering efficacy.[241] The only advantage of carteolol that has been demonstrated thus far is less ocular irritation as compared with timolol.[236,237] While other adverse reactions appear to be comparable, one study revealed a significant drop in ciliary systolic perfusion pressure, which was not seen with timolol or betaxolol.[242]

D-timolol

Previous reference to timolol in this chapter has been to l-timolol (or the S-enantiomer), which is the stereoisomer form of the drug and that which is currently used in the treatment of glaucoma. More recent research with d-timolol (the R-enantiomer) reveals that this is a significantly less potent beta-adrenergic antagonist with regard to both IOP reduction and systemic effects.[243–245] However, it does have some beneficial ocular hypotensive effect and may prove to have clinical value due to the reduction in systemic side effects.[244,245]

Atenolol

Atenolol is a selective beta$_1$-adrenergic antagonist with no intrinsic sympathomimetic or membrane-stabilizing properties.[246,247] Oral atenolol (25–100 mg) provided significant IOP reduction when compared with a placebo,[248,249] and an oral dose of 50 mg had a better pressure-lowering effect than did 40 mg of propranolol[250] or 500 mg of acetazolamide.[251] Topical administration of 2% atenolol was comparable to 2% pilocarpine,[252] and 4% atenolol was more effective than 1% epinephrine.[253] However, a long-term study showed that the initial pressure control gradually wore off in some patients.[254]

Metoprolol

Metoprolol is a cardioselective beta$_1$-adrenergic antagonist which, like betaxolol, has been shown to reduce IOP without the adverse respiratory side effects of the nonselective beta-blockers.[255,256] Significant aqueous humor concentrations are achieved with oral administration,[257] and prolonged ocular hypotensive action has been demonstrated with both oral administration of 100-mg tablets or topical instillation of 1–5% metoprolol.[255] The topical administration is well tolerated except for transient burning, and the ocular hypotensive effect persists in most cases, except for an early, partial loss of the initial pressure reduction.[258,259] Metoprolol 3% was similar to pilocarpine 2–4% in lowering IOP in one study[260] and was roughly equivalent to the ocular hypotensive effect of timolol in another evaluation.[261]

Pindolol

Pindolol is a potent beta-adrenergic antagonist with an intrinsic sympathomimetic effect, and it is reported to provide a good ocular hypotensive effect.[262–264] Pindolol 0.5–1% has been shown to provide prolonged IOP reduction without significant ocular or systemic side effects,[263,264] although reports are conflicting regarding the influence of pindolol on corneal anesthesia.[262,265] Comparisons with timolol revealed no significant differences in the ocular hypotensive action of the two drugs.[266–268]

Nadolol

Nadolol is a nonselective beta-blocker with no intrinsic sympathomimetic action. Oral administration of nadolol 10–80 mg daily has been shown to cause a significant, dose-related reduction in IOP.[269] A significant IOP lowering for 24 hours was achieved with 40 mg once daily[270] and with 10 or 20 mg twice daily.[271] Nadolol 20 mg daily was equivalent to topical timolol 0.25% twice daily,[272,273] and nadolol 40 or 80 mg daily had an ocular hypotensive effect comparable to that of timolol 0.5% twice daily.[273] However, the oral medication caused a significantly greater reduction in heart rate[269,272,273] and blood pressure.[269,272] Topical preparations also produce a significant dose-dependent IOP reduction, which lasts more than 9 hours with the higher concentrations of 1–2%.[274] When compared with the ocular hypotensive effect of timolol, however, nadolol is much less effective with continued use.[275] This may be due to poor corneal penetration, and the prodrug analogue of nadolol, diacetyl nadolol, was found to be as effective as timolol in lowering the IOP up to 8 hours with less efficacy thereafter.[276] However, diacetyl nadolol 2% had a lower incidence of tolerance than timolol 0.5% during a 3-month study.[277]

Befunolol

Befunolol 0.25% and 0.5% was reported to provide good IOP reduction during a 3-month study,[278] with no significant diminution of effect during a 1-year follow-up.[279] In a preliminary study, changing from timolol 0.5% to befunolol 0.5% therapy was associated with a significant additional decrease in IOP.[280]

Penbutolol

Penbutolol[281] has also been evaluated as a topical antiglaucoma agent, with encouraging preliminary results, and it is likely that additional beta-adrenergic inhibitors will appear in the near future as this exciting field of pharmacology continues to expand.

Alpha-Adrenergic Inhibitors

Thymoxamine

Thymoxamine hydrochloride competes with norepinephrine for alpha-adrenergic receptors. As a result, it produces miosis by inhibiting the dilator muscle of the iris, without influencing the ciliary muscle-induced facility of aqueous outflow.[282] It also has no effect on the rate of aqueous humor formation, IOP, or anterior chamber volume.[283] This provides several potential clinical applications for the drug, most of which have been considered in previous chapters. (At the present time, however, the drug is not commercially available in the United States.)

Reversal of Mydriasis. Thymoxamine 0.1% can reverse the mydriatic effect of phenylephrine 2.5% within 1 hour in most patients[284] and of ephedrine 0.5%, but not when the latter is combined with homotropine 0.5%.[285] Because it does not cause shallowing of the anterior chamber or ciliary spasm, it provides safe, rapid reversal of the effects of an adrenergic mydriatic drug. Intraocular administration of 0.2–0.5 ml of thymoxamine 0.01% or 0.02% was effective in reversing phenylephrine or epinephrine mydriasis in cataract surgery and other intraocular procedures with no corneal endothelial damage.[286]

Management of Angle-Closure Glaucoma. Thymoxamine has the advantages of (1) causing miosis despite pressure-induced ischemia of the iris sphincter and (2) not increasing the posterior vector force of the iris, which might aggravate the pupillary block. In a study of patients with acute angle-closure glaucoma, 0.5% thymoxamine was administered every minute for five times and then every 15 minutes for 2–3 hours. The attacks were broken in all cases, except those with peripheral anterior synechiae or prolonged angle closure.[287]

Differentiating Angle-Closure Glaucoma from Open-Angle Glaucoma with Narrow Angles. Since thymoxamine produces miosis without affecting the ciliary muscle-controlled facility of outflow, it will break an angle-closure attack but have no effect on open-angle glaucoma.[288] It has been demonstrated that this property of thymoxamine can be used as a diagnostic adjunct to gonioscopy in distinguishing between angle-closure glaucoma and open-angle glaucoma with narrow angles.[289]

Management of Pigmentary Glaucoma. One theory for the mechanism of pigment dispersion in pigmentary glaucoma, as discussed in Section Two, is contact between the iris pigment epithelium and packets of lens zonules. It has been suggested that miosis without cyclotonia, as produced by thymoxamine, theoretically provides the optimum means of minimizing this effect.[290]

Management of Eyelid Retraction. Thymoxamine 0.5% causes a substantial narrowing of the palpebral fissure in many patients with eyelid retraction, especially cases secondary to thyroid disease, and it has been suggested that this may have value in the diagnosis of thyroid eye disease and possibly in the medical treatment of eyelid retraction.[291]

Prazosin

This postsynaptic alpha-adrenergic antagonist is used as an oral medication to lower blood pressure and produce peripheral vasodilation. Rabbit studies have shown that topical administration of 0.001% to 0.1% prazosin causes a dose-related lowering of IOP by reducing aqueous humor formation.[292,293]

Corynanthine

This selective alpha$_1$-adrenergic antagonist produced IOP reduction in animals without altering conventional outflow facility or the rate of aqueous humor flow.[294] It was postulated that the mechanism of pressure reduction might be an increase in uveoscleral outflow. In a clinical trial, a single dose of corynanthine 1% had no IOP-lowering effect, while 2% and 5% concentrations did lower the IOP, although a 3-week study with the 2% did not reveal a sustained pressure reduction.[295]

Dapiprazole

This alpha-adrenergic blocking agent was evaluated in human volunteers and was found to produce miosis and IOP reduction.[296] Higher concentrations of 1–2% caused transient conjunctival hyperemia and ptosis, while lower doses of 0.25% had loss of effectiveness with time. Intermediate strengths may prove to have some value.

Alpha- and Beta-Adrenergic Inhibitors

Labetalol

This is a combined alpha- and beta-adrenergic blocking agent, which has been shown to produce a significant, dose-related IOP reduction in rabbits,[297–299] although it has a poor ocular hypotensive effect in human eyes.[299,300]

SUMMARY

Beta-adrenergic inhibitors lower the IOP by reducing aqueous production. The drugs in this class differ primarily with regard to IOP-lowering efficacy and relative ocular and systemic side effects. Timolol, a potent $beta_1$- and $beta_2$-adrenergic antagonist, has a profound ocular hypotensive action with few ocular side effects, but a potential for serious systemic adverse reactions, especially on the cardiovascular ($beta_1$) and pulmonary ($beta_2$) systems. Betaxolol, a cardioselective $beta_1$-blocker, is slightly less effective than timolol in lowering IOP but has the advantage of a reduced potential for pulmonary side effects. Levobunolol and metipranolol, both nonselective beta-adrenergic inhibitors, are similar to timolol in ocular hypotensive efficacy and incidence of side effects. Many other beta-blockers are also being evaluated for the treatment of glaucoma. Alpha-adrenergic antagonists produce miosis by inhibiting the dilator muscle of the iris. Some of these drugs, such as thymoxamine, have no direct effect on aqueous humor dynamics, while others also have some ocular hypotensive action.

References

1. Wettrell, K, Pandolfi, M: Effect of oral administration of various beta-blocking agents on the intraocular pressure in healthy volunteers. Exp Eye Res 21:451, 1975.
2. Pandolfi, M, Ohrstrom, A: Treatment of ocular hypertension with oral beta-adrenergic blocking agents. Acta Ophthal 52:464, 1974.
3. Wettrell, K, Pandolfi, M: Early dose response analysis of ocular hypotensive effects of propranolol in patients with ocular hypertension. Br J Ophthal 60:680, 1976.
4. Wettrell, K, Pandolfi, M: Propranolol vs acetazolamide. A long-term double-masked study of the effect on intraocular pressure and blood pressure. Arch Ophthal 97:280, 1979.
5. Ohrstrom, A, Pandolfi, M: Long-term treatment of glaucoma with systemic propranolol. Am J Ophthal 86:340, 1978.
6. Musini, A, Fabbri, B, Bergamaschi, M, et al: Comparison of the effect of propranolol, lignocaine, and other drugs on normal and raised intraocular pressure in man. Am J Ophthal 72:773, 1971.
7. Maerte, HJ, Merkle, W: Long-term treatment of glaucoma with propranolol ophthalmic solution. Klin Monatsbl Augenheilkd 177:437, 1980.
8. Takats, I, Szilvassy, I, Kerek, A: Intraocular pressure and circulation of aqueous humour in rabbit eyes following intravenous administration of propranolol (Inderal®). Graefe's Arch Ophthal 185:331, 1972.
9. Cubey, RB, Taylor, SH: Ocular reaction to propranolol and resolution on continued treatment with a different beta-blocking drug. Br Med J 4:327, 1975.
10. Garner, A, Rahi, AHS: Practolol and ocular toxicity. Antibodies in serum and tears. Br J Ophthal 60:684, 1976.
11. Rahi, AHS, Chapman, CM, Garner, A, Wright, P: Pathology of practolol-induced ocular toxicity. Br J Ophthal 60:312, 1976.
12. Skegg, DCG, Doll, R: Frequency of eye complaints and rashes among patients receiving practolol and propranolol. Lancet 2:475, 1977.
13. Status report on beta-blockers. FDA Drug Bulletin 8:13, 1978.
14. Katz, IM, Hubbard, WA, Getson, AJ, Gould, AL: Intraocular pressure decrease in normal volunteers following timolol ophthalmic solution. Invest Ophthal 15:489, 1976.
15. Zimmerman, TJ: Timolol maleate—a new glaucoma medication? Invest Ophthal Vis Sci 16:687, 1977.
16. Vareilles, P, Silverstone, D, Plazonnet, B, et al: Comparison of the effects of timolol and other adrenergic agents on intraocular pressure in the rabbit. Invest Ophthal Vis Sci 16:987, 1977.
17. Radius, RL, Diamond, GR, Pollack, IP, Langham, ME: Timolol. A new drug for management of chronic simple glaucoma. Arch Ophthal 96:1003, 1978.
18. Zimmerman, TJ, Kaufman, HE: Timolol. A beta-adrenergic blocking agent for the treatment of glaucoma. Arch Ophthal 95:601, 1977.
19. Zimmerman, TJ, Kaufman, HE: Timolol: dose response and duration of action. Arch Ophthal 95:605, 1977.
20. Spinelli, D, Montanari, P, Vigasio, F, Cormanni, V: Effects of timolol maleate on untreated contralateral eye. J Fr Ophthal 5:153, 1982.
21. Ritch, R, Hargett, NA, Podos, SM: The effect of 1.5% timolol maleate on intraocular pressure. Acta Ophthal 56:6, 1978.
22. Moss, AP, Ritch, R, Hargett, NA, et al: A comparison of the effects of timolol and epinephrine on intraocular pressure. Am J Ophthal 86:489, 1978.
23. Zimmerman, TJ, Kass, MA, Yablonski, ME, Becker, B: Timolol maleate. Efficacy and safety. Arch Ophthal 97:656, 1979.
24. LeBlanc, RP, Krip, G: Timolol—Canadian multicenter study. Ophthalmology 88:244, 1981.
25. Sonntag, JR, Brindley, GO, Shields, MB, et al: Timolol and epinephrine. Comparison of efficacy and side effects. Arch Ophthal 97:273, 1979.

26. Hoyng, PFJ, Verbey, NLJ: Timolol vs guanethidine-epinephrine formulations in the treatment of glaucoma. An open clinical trial. Arch Ophthal 102:1788, 1984.
27. Boger, WP III, Steinert, RF, Puliafito, CA, Pavan-Langston, D: Clinical trial comparing timolol ophthalmic solution to pilocarpine in open-angle glaucoma. Am J Ophthal 86:8, 1978.
28. Hass, I, Drance, SM: Comparison between pilocarpine and timolol on diurnal pressures in open-angle glaucoma. Arch Ophthal 98:480, 1980.
29. Merté, HJ, Merkle, W: Experiences in a double-blind study with different concentrations of timolol and pilocarpine. Klin Monatsbl Augenheilkd 177:443, 1980.
30. Calissendorff, B, Maren, N, Wettrell, K, Ostberg, A: Timolol versus pilocarpine separately or combined with acetazolamide—effects on intraocular pressure. Acta Ophthal 58:624, 1980.
31. Merté, H-J, Merkle, W: Experiences in a double-blind study with different concentrations of timolol and pilocarpine. Klin Monatsbl Augenheilkd 177:443, 1980.
32. Christakis, C, Mangouritsas, N: Comparative studies of the pressure-lowering effect of timolol and phospholine iodide. Klin Monatsbl Augenheilkd 179:197, 1981.
33. Zimmerman, TJ, Harbin, R, Pett, M, Kaufman, HE: Timolol and facility of outflow. Invest Ophthal Vis Sci 16:623, 1977.
34. Sonntag, JR, Brindley, GO, Shields, MB: Effect of timolol therapy on outflow facility. Invest Ophthal Vis Sci 17:293, 1978.
35. Coakes, RL, Brubaker, RF: The mechanism of timolol in lowering intraocular pressure in the normal eye. Arch Ophthal 96:2045, 1978.
36. Yablonski, ME, Zimmerman, TJ, Waltman, SR, Becker, B: A fluorophotometric study of the effect of topical timolol on aqueous humor dynamics. Exp Eye Res 27:135, 1978.
37. Topper, JE, Brubaker, RF: Effects of timolol, epinephrine, and acetazolamide on aqueous flow during sleep. Invest Ophthal Vis Sci 26:1315, 1985.
38. Liu, HK, Chiou, GCY, Garg, LC: Ocular hypotensive effects of timolol in cat eyes. Arch Ophthal 98:1467, 1980.
39. Miichi, H, Nagataki, S: Effects of pilocarpine, salbutamol, and timolol on aqueous humor formation in cynomolgus monkeys. Invest Ophthal Vis Sci 24:1269, 1983.
40. Bartels, SP: Aqueous humor flow measured with fluorophotometry in timolol-treated primates. Invest Ophthal Vis Sci 29:1498, 1988.
41. Neufeld, AH: Experimental studies on the mechanism of action of timolol. Surv Ophthal 23:363, 1979.
42. Neufeld, AH, Bartels, SP, Liu, JHK: Laboratory and clinical studies on the mechanism of action of timolol. Surv Ophthal 28:286, 1983.
43. Bromberg, BB, Gregory, DS, Sears, ML: Beta-adrenergic receptors in ciliary processes of the rabbit. Invest Ophthal Vis Sci 19:203, 1980.
44. Nathanson, JA: Human ciliary process adrenergic receptor: pharmacological characterization. Invest Ophthal Vis Sci 21:798, 1981.
45. Trope, GE, Clark, B: Beta adrenergic receptors in pigmented ciliary processes. Br J Ophthal 66:788, 1982.
46. Trope, GE, Clark, B: Binding potencies of 2 new $beta_2$ specific blockers to beta receptors in the ciliary processes and the possible relevance of these drugs to intraocular pressure control. Br J Ophthal 68:245, 1984.
47. Schmitt, CJ, Gross, DM, Share, NN: Beta-adrenergic receptor subtypes in iris-ciliary body of rabbits. Graefe's Arch Ophthal 221:167, 1984.
48. Wax, MB, Molinoff, PB: Distribution and properties of β-adrenergic receptors in human iris-ciliary body. Invest Ophthal Vis Sci 28:420, 1987.
49. Liu, JHK, Bartels, SP, Neufeld, AH: Effects of timolol on intraocular pressure following ocular adrenergic denervation. Curr Eye Res 3:1113, 1984.
50. Wentworth, WO, Brubaker, RF: Aqueous humor dynamics in a series of patients with third neuron Horner's syndrome. Am J Ophthal 92:407, 1981.
51. Bartels, SP, Roth, O, Jumblatt, MM, Neufeld, AH: Pharmacological effects of topical timolol in the rabbit eye. Invest Ophthal Vis Sci 19:1189, 1980.
52. Bartels, SP, Liu, JHK, Neufeld, AH: Decreased beta-adrenergic responsiveness in cornea and iris-ciliary body following topical timolol or epinephrine in albino and pigmented rabbits. Invest Ophthal Vis Sci 24:718, 1983.
53. Airaksinen, PJ, Alanko, HI: Vascular effects on timolol and pilocarpine in the iris. A simultaneous bilateral fluorescein angiographic study. Acta Ophthal 61:195, 1983.
54. Beardsley, TL, Shields, MB: Effect of timolol on aqueous humor protein concentration in humans. Am J Ophthal 95:448, 1983.
55. Stur, M, Grabner, G, Dorda, W, Zehetbauer, G: The effect of timolol on the concentrations of albumin and IgG in the aqueous humor of the human eye. Am J Ophthal 96:726, 1983.
56. Stur, M, Grabner, G, Huber-Spitzy, V, et al: Effect of timolol on aqueous humor protein concentration in the human eye. Arch Ophthal 104:899, 1986.
57. Lichter, M, Feldman, F, Clark, L, Cohen, MM: Effect of indomethacin on the ocular hypotensive action of timolol maleate. Am J Ophthal 98:79, 1984.
58. Goldberg, HS, Feldman, F, Cohen, MM, Clark, L: Effect of topical indomethacin and timolol ma-

leate on intraocular pressure in normal subjects. Am J Ophthal 99:576, 1985.
59. Wantenabe, K, Chiou, GCY: Action mechanism of timolol to lower the intraocular pressure in rabbits. Ophthal Res 15:160, 1983.
60. Mekki, QA, Turner, P: Dopamine-2 receptor blockade does not affect the ocular hypotensive action of timolol. Br J Ophthal 72:598, 1988.
61. Gilmartin, B, Hogan, RE, Thompson, SM: The effect of timolol maleate on tonic accommodation, tonic vergence, and pupil diameter. Invest Ophthal Vis Sci 25:763, 1984.
62. Lin, L-L, Galin, MA, Ostbaum, SA, Katz, I: Longterm timolol therapy. Surv Ophthal 23:377, 1979.
63. Wax, MB, Molinoff, PB, Alvarado, J, Polansky, J: Characterization of β-adrenergic receptors in cultured human trabecular cells and in human trabecular meshwork. Invest Ophthal Vis Sci 30:51, 1989.
64. Jampel, HD, Lynch, MG, Brown, RH, et al: β-adrenergic receptors in human trabecular meshwork. Identification and autoradiographic localization. Invest Ophthal Vis Sci 28:772, 1987.
65. McMenamin, PG, Lee, WR, Grierson, I, Grindle, FCJ: Giant vacuoles in the lining endothelium of the human Schlemm's canal after topical timolol maleate. Invest Ophthal Vis Sci 24:339, 1983.
66. Collignon-Brach, J, Weekers, R: Timolol. Etude clinique. J Fr Ophthal 2:603, 1979.
67. Mills, KB: Blind randomised non-crossover long-term trial comparing topical timolol 0.25% with timolol 0.5% in the treatment of simple chronic glaucoma. Br J Ophthal 67:216, 1983.
68. Dausch, D, Schad, K: Are 0.1% timolol-maleate eyedrops suitable for treating chronic glaucoma? Klin Monatsbl Augenheilkd 180:141, 1982.
69. Mottow-Lippa, LS, Lippa, EA, Naidoff, MA, et al: 0.008% timolol ophthalmic solution. A minimal-effect dose in a normal volunteer model. Arch Ophthal 108:61, 1990.
70. Chang, S-C, Bundgaard, H, Buur, A, Lee, VHL: Low dose O-butyryl timolol improves the therapeutic index of timolol in the pigmented rabbit. Invest Ophthal Vis Sci 29:626, 1988.
71. Potter, DE, Shumate, DJ, Bundgaard, H, Lee, VHL: Ocular and cardiac β-antagonism by timolol prodrugs, timolol and levobunolol. Curr Eye Res 7:755, 1988.
72. Katz, IM, Berger, ET: Effects of iris pigmentation on response of ocular pressure to timolol. Surv Ophthal 23:395, 1979.
73. Salminen, L, Imre, G, Huupponen, R: The effect of ocular pigmentation on intraocular pressure response to timolol. Acta Ophthal 63 (suppl):15, 1985.
74. Schmitt, CJ, Lotti, VJ, LeDouarec, JC: Penetration of timolol into the rabbit eye. Measurements after ocular instillation and intravenous injection. Arch Ophthal 98:547, 1980.
75. Phillips, CI, Bartholomew, RS, Kazi, G, et al: Penetration of timolol eye drops into human aqueous humour. Br J Ophthal 65:593, 1981.
76. Phillips, CI, Bartholomew, RS, Levy, AM, et al: Penetration of timolol eye drops into human aqueous humour: the first hour. Br J Ophthal 69:217, 1985.
77. Soll, DB: Evaluation of timolol in chronic open-angle glaucoma. Once a day vs twice a day. Arch Ophthal 98:2178, 1980.
78. Yalon, M, Urinowsky, E, Rothkoff, L, et al: Frequency of timolol administration. Am J Ophthal 92:526, 1981.
79. Schlecht, LP, Brubaker, RF: The effects of withdrawal of timolol in chronically treated glaucoma patients. Ophthalmology 95:1212, 1988.
80. Krieglstein, GK: A follow-up study on the intraocular pressure response of timolol eye drops. Klin Monatsbl Augenheilkd 175:627, 1979.
81. Merte, HJ, Merkle, W: Results of long-term treatment of glaucoma with timolol ophthalmic solution. Klin Monatsbl Augenheilkd 177:562, 1980.
82. Steinert, RF, Thomas, JV, Boger, WP III: Long-term drift and continued efficacy after multiyear timolol therapy. Arch Ophthal 99:100, 1981.
83. Plan, CH, Boulmier, A: Long-term treatment of chronic glaucoma with timolol drops: results after four years. J Fr Ophthal 4:751, 1981.
84. Airaksinen, PJ, Valle, O, Takki, KK, Klemetti, A: Timolol treatment of chronic open-angle glaucoma and ocular hypertension. A 2.5-year multicenter study. Graefe's Arch Ophthal 219:68, 1982.
85. Blika, S, Saunte, E: Timolol maleate in the treatment of glaucoma simplex and glaucoma capsulare. A three-year followup study. Acta Ophthal 60:967, 1982.
86. Maclure, GM: Chronic open angle glaucoma treated with timolol. A four year study. Trans Ophthal Soc UK 103:78, 1983.
87. LeBlanc, RP, Saheb, NE, Krip, G: Timolol: long-term Canadian multicentre study. Can J Ophthal 20:128, 1985.
88. Boger, WP III: Shortterm "escape" and longterm "drift." The dissipation effects of the beta adrenergic blocking agents. Surv Ophthal 28:235, 1983.
89. Boger, WP III, Puliafito, CA, Steinert, RF, Langston, DP: Long-term experience with timolol ophthalmic solution in patients with open-angle glaucoma. Ophthalmology 85:259, 1978.
90. Oksala, A, Salminen, L: Tachyphylaxis in timolol therapy for chronic glaucoma. Klin Monatsbl Augenheilkd 177:451, 1980.
91. Krupin, T, Singer, PR, Perlmutter, J, et al: One-hour intraocular pressure response to timolol.

Lack of correlation with long-term response. Arch Ophthal 99:840, 1981.
92. Neufeld, AH, Zawistowski, KA, Page, ED, Bromberg, BB: Influences on the density of beta-adrenergic receptors in the cornea and iris-ciliary body of the rabbit. Invest Ophthal Vis Sci 17:1069, 1978.
93. Brubaker, RF, Nagataki, S, Bourne, WM: Effect of chronically administered timolol on aqueous humor flow in patients with glaucoma. Ophthalmology 89:280, 1982.
94. Gandolfi, SA: Restoring sensitivity to timolol after long-term drift in primary open-angle glaucoma. Invest Ophthal Vis Sci 31:354, 1990.
95. Ashburn, FS Jr, Gillespie, JE, Kass, MA, Becker, B: Timolol plus maximum tolerated antiglaucoma therapy: a one-year follow-up study. Surv Ophthal 23:389, 1979.
96. Sonty, S, Schwartz, B: The additive effect of timolol on open angle glaucoma patients on maximal medical therapy. Surv Ophthal 23:381, 1979.
97. Zimmerman, TJ, Gillespie, JE, Kass, MA, et al: Timolol plus maximum-tolerated antiglaucoma therapy. Arch Ophthal 97:278, 1979.
98. Keates, EU: Evaluation of timolol maleate combination therapy in chronic open-angle glaucoma. Am J Ophthal 88:565, 1979.
99. Smith, RJ, Nagasubramanian, S, Watkins, R, Poinoosawmy, D: Addition of timolol maleate to routine medical therapy. A clinical trial. Br J Ophthal 64:779, 1980.
100. Nielsen, NV, Eriksen, JS: Timolol in maintenance treatment of ocular hypertension and glaucoma. Acta Ophthal 57:1070, 1979.
101. Kass, MA: Efficacy of combining timolol with other antiglaucoma medications. Surv Ophthal 28:274, 1983.
102. Scharrer, A, Ober, M: Timolol and acetazolamide in the treatment of increased intraocular pressure. Graefe's Arch Ophthal 212:129, 1979.
103. Berson, FG, Epstein, DL: Separate and combined effects of timolol maleate and acetazolamide in open-angle glaucoma. Am J Ophthal 92:788, 1981.
104. Dailey, RA, Brubaker, RF, Bourne, WM: The effects of timolol maleate and acetazolamide on the rate of aqueous formation in normal human subjects. Am J Ophthal 93:232, 1982.
105. Kass, MA, Korey, M, Gordon, M, Becker, B: Timolol and acetazolamide. A study of concurrent administration. Arch Ophthal 100:941, 1982.
106. Söderstrom, MB, Wallin, Ö, Granström, P-A, Thorburn, W: Timolol-pilocarpine combined vs timolol and pilocarpine given separately. Am J Ophthal 107:465, 1989.
107. Schnarr, K-D, Merte, H-J: Effectivity and tolerance of an active substance combination of timolol and pilocarpine—a pilot study. Klin Monatsbl Augenheilkd 191:436, 1987.
108. Maclure, GM, Vogel, R, Sturm, A, Binkowitz, B: Effect on the 24-hour diurnal curve of intraocular pressure of a fixed ratio combination of timolol 0.5% and pilocarpine 2% in patients with COAG not controlled on timolol 0.5%. Br J Ophthal 73:827, 1989.
109. Airaksinen, PJ, Valkonen, R, Stenborg, T, et al: A double-masked study of timolol and pilocarpine combined. Am J Ophthal 104:587, 1987.
110. Alexander, DW, Berson, FG, Epstein, DL: A clinical trial of timolol and epinephrine in the treatment of primary open-angle glaucoma. Ophthalmology 95:247, 1988.
111. Tsoy, EA, Meekins, BB, Shields, MB: Comparison of two treatment schedules for combined timolol and dipivefrin therapy. Am J Ophthal 102:320, 1986.
112. Pfeiffer, N, Grehn, F: Treatment of primary open-angle glaucoma by a combination of timolol 0.5% and epinephrine 0.5% plus guanethidine 3%. Klin Monatsbl Augenheilkd 194:161, 1989.
113. Batchelor, ED, O'Day, DM, Shand, DG, Wood, AJ: Interaction of topical and oral timolol in glaucoma. Ophthalmology 86:60, 1979.
114. Maren, N, Alvan, G, Calissendorff, BM, et al: Additive intraocular pressure reducing effect of topical timolol during systemic beta-blockade. Acta Ophthal 60:16, 1982.
115. Blondeau, P, Coté, M, Tétrault, L: Effect of timolol eye drops in subjects receiving systemic propranolol therapy. Can J Ophthal 18:18, 1983.
116. Wilson, RP, Kanal, N, Spaeth, GL: Timolol: its effectiveness in different types of glaucoma. Ophthalmology 86:43, 1979.
117. Zimmerman, TJ, Canale, P: Timolol—further observations. Ophthalmology 86:166, 1979.
118. Obstbaum, SA, Galin, MA: The effects of timolol on cataract extraction and intraocular pressure. Am J Ophthal 88:1017, 1979.
119. Haimann, MH, Phelps, CD: Prophylactic timolol for the prevention of high intraocular pressure after cataract extraction. A randomized, prospective, double-blind trial. Ophthalmology 88:233, 1981.
120. Sierpinski-Bart, J, Neumann, E: Timolol in early ocular hypertension following cataract extraction. Glaucoma 3:234, 1981.
121. Shields, MB, Braverman, SD: Timolol in the management of secondary glaucomas. Surv Ophthal 28:266, 1983.
122. Steinbach, P-D: Pressure-lowering effect of timolol in various forms of glaucoma. Klin Monatsbl Augenheilkd 176:844, 1980.
123. Lass, JH, Pavan-Langston, D: Timolol therapy in secondary angle-closure glaucoma post penetrating keratoplasty. Ophthalmology 86:51, 1979.
124. Phillips, CI: Timolol in operated closed-angle glaucoma. Br J Ophthal 64:240, 1980.
125. McMahon, CD, Hetherington, J Jr, Hoskins, HD

Jr, Shaffer, RN: Timolol and pediatric glaucomas. Ophthalmology 88:249, 1981.
126. Boger, WP III, Walton, DS: Timolol in uncontrolled childhood glaucomas. Ophthalmology 88:253, 1981.
127. Zimmerman, TJ, Kooner, KS, Morgan, KS: Safety and efficacy of timolol in pediatric glaucoma. Surv Ophthal 28:262, 1983.
128. Hoskins, HD Jr, Hetherington, J Jr, Magee, SD, et al: Clinical experience with timolol in childhood glaucoma. Arch Ophthal 103:1163, 1985.
129. Epstein, DL, Krug, JH Jr, Hertzmark, E, et al: A long-term clinical trial of timolol therapy versus no treatment in the management of glaucoma suspects. Ophthalmology 96:1460, 1989.
130. Chauhan, BC, Drance, SM, Douglas, GR: The time-course of intraocular pressure in timolol-treated and untreated glaucoma suspects. Am J Ophthal 107:471, 1989.
131. Chauhan, BC, Drance, SM, Douglas, GR: The effect of long-term intraocular pressure reduction on the differential light sensitivity in glaucoma suspects. Invest Ophthal Vis Sci 29:1478, 1988.
132. Johnson, SH, Brubaker, RF, Trautman, JC: Absence of an effect of timolol on the pupil. Invest Ophthal Vis Sci 17:924, 1978.
133. Tauber, J, Melamed, S, Foster, CS: Glaucoma in patients with ocular cicatricial pemphigoid. Ophthalmology 96:33, 1989.
134. Fiore, PM, Jacobs, IH, Goldberg, DB: Drug-induced pemphigoid. A spectrum of diseases. Arch Ophthal 105:1660, 1987.
135. McMahon, CD, Shaffer, RN, Hoskins, HD Jr, Hetherington, J Jr: Adverse effects experienced by patients taking timolol. Am J Ophthal 88:736, 1979.
136. Wilson, RP, Spaeth, GL, Poryzees, E: The place of timolol in the practice of ophthalmology. Ophthalmology 87:451, 1980.
137. Van Buskirk, EM: Adverse reactions from timolol administration. Ophthalmology 87:447, 1980.
138. Van Buskirk, EM: Corneal anesthesia after timolol maleate therapy. Am J Ophthal 88:739, 1979.
139. Weissman, SS, Asbell, PA: Effects of topical timolol (0.5%) and betaxolol (0.5%) on corneal sensitivity. Br J Ophthal 74:409, 1990.
140. Arthur, BW, Hay, GJ, Wasan, SM, Willis, WE: Ultrastructural effects of topical timolol on the rabbit cornea. Outcome alone and in conjunction with a gas permeable contact lens. Arch Ophthal 101:1607, 1983.
141. Nork, TM, Holly, FJ, Hayes, J, et al: Timolol inhibits corneal epithelial wound healing in rabbits and monkeys. Arch Ophthal 102:1224, 1984.
142. Liu, GS, Basu, PK, Trope, GE: Ultrastructural changes of the rabbit corneal epithelium and endothelium after timoptic treatment. Graefe's Arch Ophthal 225:325, 1987.
143. Brubaker, RF, Coakes, RL, Bourne, WM: Effect of timolol on the permeability of corneal endothelium. Ophthalmology 86:108, 1979.
144. Staatz, WD, Radius, RL, Van Horn, DL, Schultz, RO: Effects of timolol on bovine corneal endothelial cultures. Arch Ophthal 99:660, 1981.
145. Alanko, HI, Airaksinen, PJ: Effects of topical timolol on corneal endothelial cell morphology in vivo. Am J Ophthal 96:615, 1983.
146. Nielsen, NV, Eriksen, JS: Timolol. Transitory manifestations of dry eyes in long term treatment. Acta Ophthal 57:418, 1979.
147. Bonomi, L, Zavarise, G, Noya, E, Michieletto, S: Effects of timolol maleate on tear flow in human eyes. Graefe's Arch Ophthal 213:19, 1980.
148. Coakes, RL, Mackie, IA, Seal, DV: Effects of long-term treatment with timolol on lacrimal gland function. Br J Ophthal 65:603, 1981.
149. Harwick, J, Romanowski, E, Araullo-Cruz, T, Gordon, YJ: Timolol promotes reactivation of latent HSV-1 in the mouse iontophoresis model. Invest Ophthal Vis Sci 28:580, 1987.
150. Hill, JM, Shimomura, Y, Dudley, JB, et al: Timolol induces HSV-1 ocular shedding in the latently infected rabbit. Invest Ophthal Vis Sci 28:585, 1987.
151. Pakalnis, VA, Rustgi, AK, Stefansson, E, et al: The effect of timolol on anterior-chamber oxygenation. Ann Ophthal 19:298, 1987.
152. Kaila, T, Salminen, L, Huupponen, R: Systemic absorption of topically applied ocular timolol. J Ocul Pharmacol 1:79, 1985.
153. Passo, MS, Palmer, EA, Van Buskirk, EM: Plasma Timolol in glaucoma patients. Ophthalmology 91:1361, 1984.
154. Fraunfelder, FT: Interim report: national registry of possible drug-induced ocular side effects. Ophthalmology 87:87, 1980.
155. Flammer, J, Barth, D: Cardiovascular effects of local timolol therapy. Klin Monatsbl Augenheilkd 176:561, 1980.
156. Nelson, WL, Fraunfelder, FT, Sills, JM, et al: Adverse respiratory and cardiovascular events attributed to timolol ophthalmic solution, 1978–1985. Am J Ophthal 102:606, 1986.
157. Caprioli, J, Sears, ML: Caution on the preoperative use of topical timolol. Am J Ophthal 95:561, 1983.
158. Doyle, WJ, Weber, PA, Meeks, RH: Effect of topical timolol maleate on exercise performance. Arch Ophthal 102:1517, 1984.
159. Leier, CV, Baker, ND, Weber, PA: Cardiovascular effects of ophthalmic timolol. Ann Intern Med 104:197, 1986.
160. Dinai, Y, Sharir, M, Naveh, N, Halkin, H: Bradycardia induced by interaction between quinidine and ophthalmic timolol. Ann Intern Med 103:890, 1985.
161. Pringle, SD, MacEwen, CJ: Severe bradycardia

due to interaction of timolol eye drops and verapamil. Br Med J 294:155, 1987.
162. Jones, FL Jr, Ekberg, NL: Exacerbation of asthma by timolol. N Engl J Med 301:270, 1979.
163. Holtmann, HW, Holle, JP, Glanzer, K: Alteration of bronchial flow resistance due to timolol 0.25% in bronchial asthma. Klin Monatsbl Augenheilkd 176:441, 1980.
164. Schoene, RB, Martin, TR, Charan, NB, French, CL: Timolol-induced bronchospasm in asthmatic bronchitis. JAMA 245:1460, 1981.
165. Van Buskirk, EM, Fraunfelder, FT: Ocular beta-blockers and systemic effects. Am J Ophthal 98:623, 1984.
166. Burnstine, RA, Felton, JL, Ginther, WH: Cardiorespiratory reaction to timolol maleate in a pediatric patient: a case report. Ann Ophthal 14:905, 1982.
167. Olson, RJ, Bromberg, BB, Zimmerman, TJ: Apneic spells associated with timolol therapy in a neonate. Am J Ophthal 88:120, 1979.
168. Lustgarten, JS, Podos, SM: Topical timolol and the nursing mother. Arch Ophthal 101:1381, 1983.
169. Coyle, JT: Timoptic and depression. J Ocul Therap Surg Nov-Dec:311, 1983.
170. Fraunfelder, FT, Meyer, SM, Menacker, SJ: Alopecia possibly secondary to topical ophthalmic β-blockers. JAMA 263:1493, 1990.
171. Shaivitz, SA: Timolol and myasthenia gravis. JAMA 252:1611, 1979.
172. Coppeto, JR: Timolol-associated myasthenia gravis. Am J Ophthal 98:244, 1984.
173. Velde, TM, Kaiser, FE: Ophthalmic timolol treatment causing altered hypoglycemic response in a diabetic patient. Arch Intern Med 143:1627, 1983.
174. Coleman, AL, Diehl, DLC, Jampel, HD, et al: Topical timolol decreases plasma high-density lipoprotein cholesterol level. Arch Ophthal 108:1260, 1990.
175. Reiss, GR, Brubaker, RF: The mechanism of betaxolol, a new ocular hypotensive agent. Ophthalmology 90:1369, 1983.
176. Berrospi, R, Leibowitz, HM: Betaxolol. A new beta-adrenergic blocking agent for treatment of glaucoma. Arch Ophthal 100:943, 1982.
177. Radius, RL: Use of betaxolol in the reduction of elevated intraocular pressure. Arch Ophthal 101:898, 1983.
178. Caldwell, DR, Salisbury, CR, Guzek, JP: Effects of topical betaxolol in ocular hypertensive patients. Arch Ophthal 102:539, 1984.
179. Feghali, JG, Kaufman, PL: Decreased intraocular pressure in the hypertensive human eye with betaxolol, a β_1-adrenergic antagonist. Am J Ophthal 100:777, 1985.
180. Berry, DP, Van Buskirk, EM, Shields, MB: Betaxolol and timolol. A comparison of efficacy and side effects. Arch Ophthal 102:42, 1984.
181. Stewart, RH, Kimbrough, RL, Ward, RL: Betaxolol vs timolol. A six-month double-blind comparison. Arch Ophthal 104:46, 1986.
182. Allen, RC, Hertzmark, E, Walker, AM, Epstein, DL: A double-masked comparison of betaxolol vs timolol in the treatment of open-angle glaucoma. Am J Ophthal 101:535, 1986.
183. Vogel, R, Tipping, R, Kulaga, SF Jr, et al: Changing therapy from timolol to betaxolol. Effect on intraocular pressure in selected patients with glaucoma. Arch Ophthal 107:1303, 1989.
184. Smith, JP, Weeks, RH, Newland, EF, Ward, RL: Betaxolol and acetazolamide. Combined ocular hypotensive effect. Arch Ophthal 102:1794, 1984.
185. Robinson, JC, Kaufman, PL: Effects and interactions of epinephrine, norepinephrine, timolol, and betaxolol on outflow facility in the cynomolgus monkey. Am J Ophthal 109:189, 1990.
186. Allen, RC, Epstein, DL: Additive effect of betaxolol and epinephrine in primary open angle glaucoma. Arch Ophthal 104:1178, 1986.
187. Weinreb, RN, Ritch, R, Kushner, FH: Effect of adding betaxolol to dipivefrin therapy. Am J Ophthal 101:196, 1986.
188. Weinreb, RN, Caldwell, DR, Goode, SM, et al: A double-masked three-month comparison between 0.25% betaxolol suspension and 0.5% betaxolol ophthalmic solution. Am J Ophthal 110:189, 1990.
189. Hesse, RJ, Swan, JL II: Aphakic cystoid macular edema secondary to betaxolol therapy. Ophthal Surg 19:562, 1988.
190. Schoene, RB, Abuan, T, Ward, RL, Beasley, CH: Effects of topical betaxolol, timolol, and placebo on pulmonary function in asthmatic bronchitis. Am J Ophthal 97:86, 1984.
191. Van Buskirk, EM, Weinreb, RN, Berry, DP, et al: Betaxolol in patients with glaucoma and asthma. Am J Ophthal 101:531, 1986.
192. Ofner, S, Smith, TJ: Betaxolol in chronic obstructive pulmonary disease. J Ocular Pharmacol 3:171, 1987.
193. Bleckmann, H, Dorow, P: Treatment of patients with glaucoma and obstructive airway diseases with betaxolol and placebo eye drops. Klin Monatsbl Augenheilkd 191:199, 1987.
194. Weinreb, RN, Van Buskirk, EM, Cherniack, R, Drake, MM: Long-term betaxolol therapy in glaucoma patients with pulmonary disease. Am J Ophthal 106:162, 1988.
195. Nelson, WL, Kuritsky, JN: Early postmarketing surveillance of betaxolol hydrochloride, September 1985-September 1986. Am J Ophthal 103:592, 1987.
196. Roholt, PC: Betaxolol and restrictive airway disease. Arch Ophthal 105:1172, 1987.
197. Harris, LS, Greenstein, SH, Bloom, AF: Respiratory difficulties with betaxolol. Am J Ophthal 102:274, 1986.
198. Cadigan, PJ, London, DR, Pentecost, BL, et al:

Cardiovascular effects of single oral doses of the new beta-adrenoceptor blocking agent betaxolol (SL 75212) in healthy volunteers. Br J Clin Pharmacol 9:569, 1980.

199. Atkins, JM, Pugh, BR Jr, Timewell, RM: Cardiovascular effects of topical beta-blockers during exercise. Am J Ophthal 99:173, 1985.

200. Dickstein, K, Hapnes, R, Aarsland, T, et al: Comparison of topical timolol vs betaxolol on cardiopulmonary exercise performance in healthy volunteers. Acta Ophthal 66:463, 1988.

201. Zabel, RW, MacDonald, IM: Sinus arrest associated with betaxolol ophthalmic drops. Am J Ophthal 104:431, 1987.

202. Ball, S: Congestive heart failure from betaxolol. Arch Ophthal 105:320, 1987.

203. Lynch, MG, Whitson, JT, Brown, RH, et al: Topical β-blocker therapy and central nervous system side effects. A preliminary study comparing betaxolol and timolol. Arch Ophthal 106:908, 1988.

204. Orlando, RG: Clinical depression associated with betaxolol. Am J Ophthal 102:275, 1986.

205. Calugaru, M: The effect of topically applied levobunolol on the trabecular outflow of aqueous humor in open-angle glaucoma. Klin Monatsbl Augenheilkd 194:164, 1989.

206. Duzman, E, Ober, M, Scharrer, A, Leopold, IH: A clinical evaluation of the effects of topically applied levobunolol and timolol on increased intraocular pressure. Am J Ophthal 94:318, 1982.

207. Partamian, LG, Kass, MA, Gordon, M: A dose-response study of the effect of levobunolol on ocular hypertension. Am J Ophthal 95:229, 1983.

208. Bensinger, RE, Keates, EU, Gofman, JD, et al: Levobunolol. A three-month efficacy study in the treatment of glaucoma and ocular hypertension. Arch Ophthal 103:375, 1985.

209. Cinotti, A, Cinotti, D, Grant, W, et al: Levobunolol vs timolol for open-angle glaucoma and ocular hypertension. Am J Ophthal 99:11, 1985.

210. Long, D, Zimmerman, T, Spaeth, G, et al: Minimum concentration of levobunolol required to control intraocular pressure in patients with primary open-angle glaucoma or ocular hypertension. Am J Ophthal 99:18, 1985.

211. Berson, FG, Cohen, HB, Foerster, RJ, et al: Levobunolol compared with timolol for the long-term control of elevated intraocular pressure. Arch Ophthal 103:379, 1985.

212. Stryz, JR, Merte, HJ: A one-year comparison of 0.5% and 1.0% levobunolol with 0.5% timolol eye drops in the treatment of open-angle glaucoma. Klin Monatsbl Augenheilkd 187:537, 1985.

213. Freyler, H, Novack, GD, Menapace, R, et al: Comparison of ocular hypotensive efficacy and safety of levobunolol and timolol. Klin Monatsbl Augenheilkd 193:257, 1988.

214. Boozman, FW III, Carriker, R, Foerster, R, et al: Long-term evaluation of 0.25% levobunolol and timolol for therapy for elevated intraocular pressure. Arch Ophthal 106:614, 1988.

215. Berson, FG, Cinotti, A, Cohen, H, et al: Levobunolol. A beta-adrenoceptor antagonist effective in the long-term treatment of glaucoma. Ophthalmology 92:1271, 1985.

216. Geyer, O, Lazar, M, Novack, GD, et al: Levobunolol compared with timolol: a four-year study. Br J Ophthal 72:892, 1988.

217. The Levobunolol Study Group: levobunolol. A four-year study of efficacy and safety in glaucoma treatment. Ophthalmology 96:642, 1989.

218. Krieglstein, GK, Novack, GD, Voepel, E, et al: Levobunolol and metipranolol: comparative ocular hypotensive efficacy, safety, and comfort. Br J Ophthal 71:250, 1987.

219. Long, DA, Johns, GE, Mullen, RS, et al: Levobunolol and betaxolol. A double-masked controlled comparison of efficacy and safety in patients with elevated intraocular pressure. Ophthalmology 95:735, 1988.

220. Rakofsky, SI, Melamed, S, Cohen, JS, et al: A comparison of the ocular hypotensive efficacy of once-daily and twice-daily levobunolol treatment. Ophthalmology 96:8, 1989.

221. Wandel, T, Fishman, D, Novack, GD, et al: Ocular hypotensive efficacy of 0.25% levobunolol instilled once daily. Ophthalmology 95:252, 1988.

222. Wandel, T, Charap, AD, Lewis, RA, et al: Glaucoma treatment with once-daily levobunolol. Am J Ophthal 101:298, 1986.

223. Schwartz, JS, Christensen, RE, Lee, DA: Comparison of timolol maleate and levobunolol: doses and volume per bottle. Arch Ophthal 107:17, 1989.

224. Charap, AD, Shin, DH, Petursson, G, et al: Effect of varying drop size on the efficacy and safety of a topical beta blocker. Ann Ophthal 21:351, 1989.

225. West, DR, Lischwe, D, Thompson, VM, Ide, CH: Comparative efficacy of the β-blockers for the prevention of increased intraocular pressure after cataract extraction. Am J Ophthal 106:168, 1988.

226. Silverstone, DE, Novack, GD, Kelley, EP, Chen, KS: Prophylactic treatment of intraocular pressure elevations after neodymium:YAG laser posterior capsulotomies and extracapsular cataract extractions with levobunolol. Ophthalmology 95:713, 1988.

227. Allen, RC, Robin, AL, Long, D, et al: A combination of levobunolol and dipivefrin for the treatment of glaucoma. Arch Ophthal 106:904, 1988.

228. Kruse, W: Metipranolol—a new beta-receptor blocking agent. Klin Monatsbl Augenheilkd 182:582, 1983.

229. Merte, HJ, Stryz, JR, Mertz, M: Comparative studies on initial pressure reduction using meti-

pranolol 0.3% and timolol 0.25% in eyes with open-angle glaucoma. Klin Monatsbl Augenheilkd 182:286, 1983.
230. Le Jeunne, CL, Hughues, FC, Dufier, JL, et al: Bronchial and cardiovascular effects of ocular topical β-antagonists in asthmatic subjects: comparison of timolol, carteolol, and metipranolol. J Clin Pharmacol 29:97, 1989.
231. Draeger, J, Schneider, B, Winter, R: The local anesthetic action of metipranolol as compared to timolol. Klin Monatsbl Augenheilkd 182:210, 1983.
232. Schmitz Valckenberg, P: The use of metipranolol to prevent elevation of intraocular pressure after cataract extraction. Klin Monatsbl Augenheilkd 182:150, 1983.
233. Scharrer, A, Ober, M: Fixed combination of metipranolol 0.1% and pilocarpine 2% compared with the individual drugs in glaucoma therapy. A controlled, randomized clinical study for intraindividual comparison of efficacy and tolerance. Klin Monatsbl Augenheilkd 189:450, 1986.
234. Frishman, WH, Kostis, J: The significance of intrinsic sympathomimetic activity in beta-adrenoceptor blocking drugs. Cardiovasc Rev Rep 3:503, 1982.
235. Kitazawa, Y, Azuma, I, Takase, M: Evaluation of the effect of carteolol eyedrops for primary open-angle glaucoma and ocular hypertension. Igaku No Ayumi 127:859, 1983.
236. Negishi, C, Kanai, A, Nakajima, A, et al: Ocular effects of beta-blocking agent carteolol on healthy volunteers and glaucoma patients. Jap J Ophthal 25:464, 1981.
237. Scoville, B, Mueller, B, White, BG, Krieglstein, GK: A double-masked comparison of carteolol and timolol in ocular hypertension. Am J Ophthal 105:150, 1988.
238. Brazier, DJ, Smith, SE: Ocular and cardiovascular response to topical carteolol 2% and timolol 0.5% in healthy volunteers. Br J Ophthal 72:101, 1988.
239. Stewart, WC, Shields, MB, Allen, RC, et al: A three-month comparison of 1% and 2% carteolol and 0.5% timolol in open-angle glaucoma. Graefe's Arch Ophthal 229:258, 1991.
240. Duff, GR, Newcombe, RG: The 12-hour control of intraocular pressure on carteolol 2% twice daily. Br J Ophthal 72:890, 1988.
241. Duff, GR: A double-masked crossover study comparing the effects of carteolol 1% and 2% on intra-ocular pressure. Acta Ophthal 65:618, 1987.
242. Pillunat, L, Stodtmeister, R: Effect of different antiglaucomatous drugs on ocular perfusion pressures. J Ocular Pharmacol 4:231, 1988.
243. Liu, JHK, Bartels, SP, Neufeld, AH: Effects of l- and d-timolol on cyclic AMP synthesis and intraocular pressure in water-loaded, albino and pigmented rabbits. Invest Ophthal Vis Sci 24:1276, 1983.
244. Keates, EU, Stone, R: The effect of d-timolol on intraocular pressure in patients with ocular hypertension. Am J Ophthal 98:73, 1984.
245. Share, NN, Lotti, VJ, Gautheron, P, et al: R-Enantiomer of timolol: a potential selective ocular antihypertensive agent. Graefe's Arch Ophthal 221:234, 1984.
246. Wettrell, K, Pandolfi, M: Effect of topical atenolol on intraocular pressure. Br J Ophthal 61:334, 1977.
247. Elliot, MJ, Cullen, PM, Phillips, CI: Ocular hypotensive effect of atenolol (Tenormin, ICI). A new beta-adrenergic blocker. Br J Ophthal 59:296, 1975.
248. Stenkula, E, Wettrell, K: A dose-response study of oral atenolol administered once daily in patients with raised intra-ocular pressure. Graefe's Arch Ophthal 218:96, 1982.
249. Tutton, MK, Smith, RJH: Comparison of ocular hypotensive effects of 3 dosages of oral antenolol. Br J Ophthal 67:664, 1983.
250. MacDonald, MJ, Cullen, PM, Phillips, CI: Atenolol versus propranolol. A comparison of ocular hypotensive effect of an oral dose. Br J Ophthal 60:789, 1976.
251. MacDonald, MJ, Gore, SM, Cullen, PM, Phillips, CI: Comparison of ocular hypotensive effects of acetazolamide and atenolol. Br J Ophthal 61:345, 1977.
252. Wettrell, K, Wilke, K, Pandolfi, M: Topical atenolol versus pilocarpine: a double-blind study of the effect on ocular tension. Br J Ophthal 62:292, 1978.
253. Phillips, CI, Gore, SM, Gunn, PM: Atenolol versus adrenaline eye drops and an evaluation of these two combined. Br J Ophthal 62:296, 1978.
254. Brenkman, RF: Long-term hypotensive effect of atenolol 4% eyedrops. Br J Ophthal 62:287, 1978.
255. Alm, A, Wickstrom, CP: Effects of systemic and topical administration of metoprolol on intraocular pressure in healthy subjects. Acta Ophthal 58:740, 1980.
256. Urner-Bloch, U, Bucheli, J, Elta, H, et al: Clinical trials of various glaucoma drugs acting on the adrenergic system. Klin Monatsbl Augenheilkd 176:555, 1980.
257. Calissendorff, B: Aqueous humour concentration of metoprolol after oral administration. Acta Ophthal 65:721, 1987.
258. Bucheli, J, Aeschlimann, J, Gloor, B: The influence of metoprolol eye drops on intraocular pressure. Klin Monatsbl Augenheilkd 177:146, 1980.
259. Krieglstein, GK: The long-term ocular and systemic effects of topically applied metoprolol tartrate in glaucoma and ocular hypertension. Acta Ophthal 59:15, 1981.
260. Nielsen, PG, Ahrendt, N, Buhl, H, Byrn, E: Met-

oprolol eyedrops 3%, a short-term comparison with pilocarpine and a five-month follow-up study. Acta Ophthal 60:347, 1982.

261. Collignon-Brach, J, Weekers, R: Comparative clinical study of metoprolol and timolol. J Fr Ophthal 4:275, 1981.

262. Bonomi, L, Steindler, P: Effect of pindolol on intraocular pressure. Br J Ophthal 59:301, 1975.

263. Dausch, D, Gorlich, W, Honegger, H: Is pindolol suitable for the treatment of glaucoma? Klin Monatsbl Augenheilkd 184:536, 1984.

264. Smith, RJH, Blamires, T, Nagasubramanian, S, et al: Addition of pindolol to routine medical therapy: a clinical trial. Br J Ophthal 66:102, 1982.

265. Huuppone, R, Salminen, L: Transient corneal anaesthesia after topical pindolol in rabbits. Acta Ophthal 63:19, 1985.

266. Andréasson, S, Møller Jensen, K: Effect of pindolol on intraocular pressure in glaucoma: pilot study and a randomised comparison with timolol. Br J Ophthal 67:228, 1983.

267. Dausch, D, Gorlich, W, Honegger, H: Clinical suitability of pindolol eye drops for the treatment of chronic open-angle glaucoma. Klin Monatsbl Augenheilkd 184:539, 1984.

268. Flammer, J, Robert, Y, Gloor, B: Influence of pindolol and timolol treatment on the visual fields of glaucoma patients. J Ocular Pharmacol 2:305, 1986.

269. Williamson, J, Atta, HR, Kennedy, PA, Muir, JG: Effect of orally administered nadolol on the intraocular pressure in normal volunteers. Br J Ophthal 69:38, 1985.

270. Rennie, IG, Smerdon, DL: The effect of a once-daily oral dose of nadolol on intraocular pressure in normal volunteers. Am J Ophthal 100:445, 1985.

271. Duff, GR: The effect of twice daily nadolol on intraocular pressure. Am J Ophthal 104:343, 1987.

272. Duff, GR, Watt, AH, Graham, PA: A comparison of the effects of oral nadolol and topical timolol on intraocular pressure, blood pressure, and heart rate. Br J Ophthal 71:698, 1987.

273. Williamson, J, Young, JDH, Atta, H, et al: Comparative efficacy of orally and topically administered β blockers for chronic simple glaucoma. Br J Ophthal 69:41, 1985.

274. Krieglstein, GK: Nadolol eye drops in glaucoma and ocular hypertension: a controlled clinical study of dose response and duration of action. Graefe's Arch Ophthal 217:309, 1981.

275. Krieglstein, GK, Mohamed, J: The comparative multiple-dose intraocular pressure responses of nadolol and timolol in glaucoma and ocular hypertension. Acta Ophthal 60:284, 1982.

276. Duzman, E, Chen, C-C, Anderson, J, et al: Diacetyl derivative of nadolol. I. Ocular pharmacology and short-term ocular hypotensive effect in glaucomatous eyes. Arch Ophthal 100:1916, 1982.

277. Duzman, E, Rosen, N, Lazar, M: Diacetyl nadolol: 3-month ocular hypotensive effect in glaucomatous eyes. Br J Ophthal 67:668, 1983.

278. Merte, HJ, Stryz, JR: Initial experience with the beta-blocker befunolol in the treatment of open angle glaucoma. Klin Monatsbl Augenheilkd 184:55, 1984.

279. Merte, HJ, Stryz, JR: Further experience with the beta-blocker befunolol in treatment of open-angle glaucoma over a period of one year. Klin Monatsbl Augenheilkd 184:316, 1984.

280. Tanaka, Y, Nakaya, H, Yamada, Y, Nakamura, Y: Therapeutic results obtained in patients with glaucoma with alteration from 0.5% timolol eye solution to 0.5% befunolol eye solution. Folia Ophthal Jap 36:741, 1985.

281. Krieglstein, GK, Gramer, E, Leydhecker, W: The ocular responses of oral administration of penbutolol in the glaucomatous patient. Acta Ophthal 58:608, 1980.

282. Wand, M, Grant, WM: Thymoxamine hydrochloride: an alpha-adrenergic blocker. Surv Ophthal 25:75, 1980.

283. Lee, DA, Brubaker, RF, Nagataki, S: Effect of thymoxamine on aqueous humor formation in the normal human eye as measured by fluorophotometry. Invest Ophthal Vis Sci 21:805, 1981.

284. Relf, SJ, Ghargozloo, NZ, Skuta, GL, et al: Thymoxamine reverses phenylephrine-induced mydriasis. Am J Ophthal 106:251, 1988.

285. Small, S, Stewart-Jones, JH, Turner, P: Influence of thymoxamine on changes in pupil diameter and accommodation produced by homatropine and ephedrine. Br J Ophthal 60:132, 1978.

286. Grehn, F, Fleig, T, Schwarzmüller, E: Thymoxamine: a miotic for intraocular use. Graefe's Arch Ophthal 224:174, 1986.

287. Halasa, AH, Rutkowski, PC: Thymoxamine therapy for angle-closure glaucoma. Arch Ophthal 90:177, 1973.

288. Wand, M, Grant, WM: Thymoxamine hydrochloride: effects on the facility of outflow and intraocular pressure. Invest Ophthal 15:400, 1976.

289. Wand, M, Grant, WM: Thymoxamine test: differentiating angle-closure glaucoma from open-angle glaucoma with narrow angles. Arch Ophthal 96:1009, 1978.

290. Campbell, DG: Pigmentary dispersion and glaucoma. A new theory. Arch Ophthal 97:1667, 1979.

291. Dixon, RS, Anderson, RL, Hatt, MU: The use of thymoxamine in eyelid retraction. Arch Ophthal 97:2147, 1979.

292. Smith, BR, Murray, DL, Leopold, IH: Influence of topically applied prazosin on the intraocular pressure of experimental animals. Arch Ophthal 97:1933, 1979.

293. Krupin, T, Feitl, M, Becker, B: Effect of prazosin

on aqueous humor dynamics in rabbits. Arch Ophthal 98:1639, 1980.

294. Serle, JB, Stein, AJ, Podos, SM, Severin, CH: Corynanthine and aqueous humor dynamics in rabbits and monkeys. Arch Ophthal 102:1385, 1984.
295. Serle, JB, Podos, SM, Lustgarten, JS, et al: The effect of corynanthine on intraocular pressure in clinical trials. Ophthalmology 92:977, 1985.
296. Iuglio, N: Ocular effects of topical application of dapiprazole in man. Glaucoma 6:110, 1984.
297. Leopold, IH, Murray, DL: Ocular hypotensive action of labetalol. Am J Ophthal 88:427, 1979.
298. Murray, DL, Podos, SM, Wei, C-P, Leopold, IH: Ocular effects in normal rabbits of topically applied labetalol. A combined alpha- and beta-adrenergic antagonist. Arch Ophthal 97:723, 1979.
299. Bonomi, L, Perfetti, S, Bellucci, R, et al: Ocular hypotensive action of labetalol in rabbit and human eyes. Graefe's Arch Ophthal 217:175, 1981.
300. Krieglstein, GK, Kontić, D: Nadolol and labetalol. Comparative efficacy of two beta-blocking agents in glaucoma. Graefe's Arch Ophthal 216:313, 1981.

Chapter 28

CARBONIC ANHYDRASE INHIBITORS

The carbonic anhydrase inhibitors are at present the only class of drugs that are commonly used as systemically-administered agents in the long-term management of glaucoma. The prototype, acetazolamide, was introduced as an ocular hypotensive drug in 1954,[1] and most of our understanding of the carbonic anhydrase inhibitors comes from experience with this compound. Other commercially available members of the drug class include methazolamide, dichlorphenamide, and ethoxzolamide. The carbonic anhydrase inhibitors all share the same basic mechanisms of action and have side effects that essentially differ only in degree. Therefore, these aspects are first considered collectively before discussing unique features of the individual compounds.

Mechanisms of Action

Carbonic Anhydrase

Carbonic anhydrase (CA) is an enzyme that is responsible for the catalytic hydration of CO_2 and dehydration of H_2CO_3:

$$CO_2 + H_2O \overset{CA}{\rightleftarrows} H_2CO_3 \rightleftarrows HCO_3^- + H^+$$

The enzyme exists in several isoenzyme forms throughout the body, but in the ciliary processes of human eyes it is almost purely CA II (formerly called type C).[2–4] Histochemical studies of animal and human eyes have revealed carbonic anhydrase in the pigmented and nonpigmented epithelium of the ciliary body, most prominently in the basal and lateral membranes.[5,6] Clear-cut regional differences have been observed in the nonpigmented ciliary epithelium of human and monkey eyes, which coincide with morphologic indicators of secretory activity.[6] Theories as to how carbonic anhydrase relates to aqueous production were discussed in Chapter 2. The most likely explanation is that it helps to maintain a pH that is optimum for the enzymes involved in ion transport.

Carbonic Anhydrase Inhibition

The carbonic anhydrase inhibitors belong to the sulfonamide class of drugs. They have an active moiety, which is identical to carbonic acid and complimentary to carbonic anhydrase, that interferes with the function of the enzyme. The failure of acetazolamide to decrease IOP in patients with carbonic anhydrase type II deficiency suggests that it is this isozyme that the drug inhibits.[7]

The carbonic anhydrase inhibitors lower IOP by reducing aqueous humor formation. One fluorophotometric study indicated that acetazolamide decreases flow in the human eye by 27%.[8] Another fluorophotometric study of intravenous carbonic anhydrase inhibitors in rabbits suggested that the initial reduction in aqueous flow may result from a contraction of the uveal volume as a result of vasoconstriction, which may be induced by the base content of the injected solution, followed by a more gradual decrease in flow caused by the direct effect of the drug on aqueous humor formation.[9] The mechanism by which a reduction in aqueous production is accomplished is uncertain, but the following theories have been considered.

Ion transport associated with secretion of aqueous humor may be altered by the inhibition of carbonic anhydrase, possibly by creation of a local acid environment.[10] The principal ion that appears to be affected by carbonic anhydrase inhibitors differs according to the animal model being studied[10–12] and has not been established in human eyes.

Metabolic acidosis is known to reduce IOP and has been proposed as the mechanism of action for carbonic anhydrase inhibitors.[13] However, studies have shown that the ocular hypotensive effect of these drugs is neither time-related to the metabolic acidosis[14] nor dependent upon alterations of pH in the blood[15–17] or aqueous.[17] Nevertheless, strong carbonic anhydrase inhibitors, which do create a metabolic acidosis, may exert an additional pressure-lowering effect by this mechanism. It has also been suggested that acetazolamide-induced acidosis may improve visual function in glaucoma patients by increasing blood flow to the optic nerve, since visual field improvement has been documented following administration of the drug, independent of a change in perfusion pressure.[18]

Other Observations. An *adrenergic effect* of carbonic anhydrase inhibitors has also been considered, since the action of acetazolamide in dogs was found to be altered by adrenalectomy or adrenergic blocking agents.[19] In human eyes, the rate of aqueous formation was reduced 33% by timolol alone, 27% by acetazolamide therapy, and 44% by the combination of the two drugs.[8]

The *diuretic effect* of the carbonic anhydrase inhibitors is not a factor in the reduction of IOP.[20,21] Furthermore, although acetazolamide was shown to reduce the venous pressure of the cat eye, which paralleled the IOP fall,[22] ocular blood flow does not appear to be involved in the pressure-lowering action of this drug,[23] aside from the possible transient effect on uveal volume noted above.[9] Whole-blood levels of zinc, a component of carbonic anhydrase, are increased in patients receiving carbonic anhydrase inhibitors, suggesting that the drug induces synthesis of the enzyme.[24]

Carbonic anhydrase has also been demonstrated in the *retina*[4] and appears to be related to fluid movement from the retina toward the choroid.[25] Acetazolamide has been shown to increase the rate of subretinal fluid absorption in experimental retinal detachment,[26] to increase the adhesion between retina and pigment epithelium,[27] and to treat chronic macular edema in patients with retinal pigment epithelial cell disease,[28,29] although not macular edema associated with primary retinal vascular diseases.[28]

Administration

Routes of Delivery. At the present time, the carbonic anhydrase inhibitors that are commercially available are effective only when given orally, intramuscularly, or intravenously. However, current research, which is discussed at the end of this chapter, offers the possibility in the near future of topical carbonic anhydrase inhibitors.

The Dose-Response Curve. This curve for carbonic anhydrase inhibitors is very restricted, in that aqueous production is not significantly reduced until more than 90% of the carbonic anhydrase activity is inhibited.[30] For this reason, it is important that the drug not be used in inadequate doses.[31] However, it may be that some of the dosages in common use exceed that required for maximum benefit, which is considered in the discussion of the individual carbonic anhydrase inhibitors.

Distribution and Metabolism. Carbonic anhydrase inhibitors are not distributed randomly throughout the body fluids but have a preferential affinity for certain tissues, including the iris and ciliary processes.[32] The drugs are not metabolized but are excreted unchanged in the urine.

Side Effects

Side effects are common with carbonic anhydrase inhibitor therapy and frequently necessitate discontinuation of the drugs. *Paresthesias* of the fingers, toes, and around the mouth are a common side effect, and *urinary frequency* from the diuretic action is experienced by nearly all patients initially. However, both of these effects are usually transient and of no serious consequence.

Serum Electrolyte Imbalances

Serum electrolyte imbalances may create more debilitating problems:

Metabolic acidosis, associated with bicarbonate depletion, occurs with the higher dosages of carbonic anhydrase inhibitors and should be avoided in patients with hepatic insufficiency, renal failure, adrenocortical insufficiency, hyperchloremic acidosis, depressed sodium or potassium levels, or severe pulmonary obstruction.[33] The risk in patients with liver disease was reemphasized in a case report of a patient with cirrhosis who developed hepatic encephalopathy as a result of ammonia intoxication within days after starting acetazolamide therapy.[34] It has also been reemphasized that the metabolic acidosis of carbonic anhydrase inhibitor therapy is especially common among elderly patients.[35]

A symptom complex of malaise, fatigue, weight loss, anorexia, depression and decreased libido is not uncommon in patients on carbonic anhydrase inhibitor therapy.[36,37] It has been correlated with the degree of metabolic acidosis, and preliminary experience suggests that treatment with sodium bicarbonate[36] or sodium acetate[38] may help to minimize this situation. It has also been reported that combined therapy with a carbonic anhydrase inhibitor and aspirin may cause serious acid-base imbalance and salicylate intoxication.[39]

Potassium depletion may occur during the initial phase of carbonic anhydrase inhibitor therapy, as a result of increased urinary excretion, especially if diuresis is brisk, and is the apparent explanation for the frequent paresthesias. However, this is normally transient[40] and does not lead to significant hypokalemia unless it is given concomitantly with chlorothiazide diuretics, digitalis, corticosteroids, or ACTH, or in patients with hepatic cirrhosis. Potassium supplement is indicated only when significant hypokalemia is documented.[41]

Serum sodium and chloride may also be transiently reduced, the latter occurring primarily with dichlorphenamide.

Gastrointestinal Symptoms

Gastrointestinal symptoms are also very common and include vague abdominal discomfort, a peculiar metallic taste, nausea, and diarrhea. These symptoms do not appear to be related to any serum chemical change, and the cause is unknown. Taking the medication with meals may help to reduce the symptoms in some cases.[36]

Sulfonamide-Related Reactions

The following side effects are common to the sulfonamide group of drugs, of which the carbonic anhydrase inhibitors are members.

Renal calculi formation has been shown to be increased in patients receiving acetazolamide,[42] and this is probably the most common serious adverse reaction associated with carbonic anhydrase inhibitor therapy. The precise mechanism is unknown, but there may be an association with reduced excretion of urinary citrate[43] or magnesium,[44] since both are believed to help keep calcium salts in solution. An alkaline urine is also known to predispose to precipitation of calcium salts, and this has been proposed as the mechanism of urolithiasis associated with carbonic anhydrase inhibitor therapy.[45,46] However, it has been shown that the urinary pH returns to pretreatment levels once the initial acetazolamide-induced bicarbonate diuresis subsides,[47] and some patients with renal stones during acetazolamide therapy may actually have an acidic urine.[48] Renal colic may also be associated with carbonic anhydrase inhibitor therapy and may rarely be associated with hematuria or anuria.[49]

Blood dyscrasias are rare, but thrombocytopenia, agranulocytosis, aplastic anemia, and neutropenia have been reported with acetazolamide or methazolamide therapy.[50–54] The National Registry of Drug-Induced Ocular Side Effects received 79 case reports, as of 1985, of suspected hematologic reactions to carbonic anhydrase inhibitor therapy, of which 26 were fatal.[53] The authors of that report recommended that, in addition to warning the patient to report a persistent sore throat, fever, fatigue, pallor, easy bruising, epistaxis, purpura, or jaundice, a complete blood count should be obtained before initiating therapy and every 6 months thereafter. The latter recommendation led to considerable controversy within the ophthalmic community. A survey revealed that the vast majority of ophthalmologists who responded do not routinely monitor blood counts of patients on carbonic anhydrase inhibitor therapy, and the authors of that report suggested that routine blood monitoring is of questionable value because of the idiosyncratic, non-dose-related nature of the dyscrasias and the variability of their onset.[54]

There is clearly a division of opinion on this issue, although an editorial on the subject provided a well-balanced perspective.[55] The authors began by noting that agranulocytosis and thrombocytopenia are nearly always acute in onset with initial clinical features of acute bacterial infection and bleeding, respectively. They cannot be predicted by monitoring blood cell counts and are completely reversible upon cessation of the drug. On the other hand, aplastic anemia typically has a delayed, insidious onset and is frequently fatal. Most cases occur within less than 6 months of initiating therapy, and some patients have been known to recover after stopping the drug. To be most effective, blood cell counts (hematocrit, white blood cell count, and platelet count) should be obtained initially and every 2 months for the first 6 months. However, it is estimated that this would cost approximately $1.5 million for each life saved from aplastic anemia. The authors conclude that "a physician should not be regarded as negligent if he or she does not routinely monitor blood cell counts" but that "a physician who does so cannot be accused of thoughtlessly squandering health resources."[55]

Other sulfonamide-related side effects include exfoliative dermatitis, hypersensitive nephropathy, and acute myopia.[44] The latter is the only ocular reaction commonly associated with carbonic anhydrase inhibitor therapy, and it is idiosyncratic and transient. Ultrasonography of a patient with induced myopia associated with sulfamethoxazole therapy revealed shallowing of the anterior chamber without thickening of the lens, suggesting that swelling of the ciliary body might cause forward movement of the lens-iris diaphragm.[56]

Other Adverse Reactions

Other adverse reactions that have been reported in association with carbonic anhydrase inhibitor therapy include elevated blood uric acid,[44] hirsutism,[57] and a transient (30-minute) elevation of cerebral blood flow and cerebrospinal fluid pressure.[44] Teratogenic effects have been observed in rats[58] and in one human case, although the mother was also on the anticholinergic dicyclomine during weeks 8–12 of pregnancy.[59] Caution during pregnancy is advised. It has also been noted that an oral hypoglycemic agent, acetohexamide, was inadvertently substituted for acetazolamide because of the similar names.[60]

The adverse reactions noted above for the carbonic anhydrase inhibitors appear to be more frequent and debilitating in the older age population, with patients 40 years of age or less having a significantly higher incidence of long-term tolerance.[61] Measures that may help to reduce the side effects, as previously noted, include supplemental alkali therapy and taking the medication with meals. It has also been noted that some patients who cannot tolerate one form of carbonic anhydrase inhibitor will do better with another agent or with a lower dose of the drug.[62]

SPECIFIC CARBONIC ANHYDRASE INHIBITORS (Table 28.1)

Acetazolamide

As previously noted, acetazolamide is the prototype of the carbonic anhydrase inhibi-

Table 28.1
Commercial Carbonic Anhydrase Inhibitors*

Generic Preparations	Brand Names	Strengths (mg)
Acetazolamide	Ak-Zol	250
	Diamox, tablets	125, 250
	Diamox Sequels	500
	Diamox, parenteral	500/vial
Methazolamide	Neptazane	25, 50
Dichlorphenamide	Daranide	50

* Other generic products may also be available.

tors, and most of the preceding information in this chapter was based on experience with this drug.

Administration. The traditional oral dosage for long-term therapy in adults is 250 mg in tablet form every 6 hours or one 500-mg sustained release capsule twice a day. However, a single dose study showed that 63 mg gave the maximum effect on the IOP.[63] In the same study, 250 mg gave a slightly longer duration of action, but 500 mg had no advantage. However, in a study of open-angle glaucoma patients, uncontrolled on maximum topical therapy, there was a consistent, positive dose response to acetazolamide 125, 250, and 500 mg tablets and acetazolamide 500 and 1000 mg sustained-release capsules.[64] A daily 500-mg sustained-release capsule was shown to provide a substantial pressure-lowering effect for at least 23 hours, although one capsule twice a day was more effective than the daily dose in controlling the pressure.[65] Twice-daily 500-mg sustained-release capsules is equivalent to one 250-mg tablet every 6 hours.[65,66] The analgesic diflunisal, 500 mg twice daily, has been shown to increase total plasma concentrations and the IOP-lowering effect of acetazolamide, when the two drugs are given concomitantly.[67] The recommended dose of acetazolamide for children is 5–10 mg/kg of body weight every 4–6 hours.[68]

In tablet form, the ocular hypotensive effect peaks in 2 hours and lasts up to 6 hours, while that of the capsule peaks in 8 hours and persists beyond 12 hours. For more rapid action, the drug may be given intravenously, which provides a peak effect in 15 minutes and a duration of 4 hours. A useful routine for emergency situations, such as acute angle-closure glaucoma, is to give 250 mg intramuscularly and 250 mg intravenously.

Metabolic acidosis is greater with intravenous injections of acetazolamide than with oral administration.[13] However, the acidosis associated with chronic oral therapy is such that the reduced serum carbon dioxide level is said to be a useful indicator of compliance with acetazolamide therapy.[69] An oral drug delivery system has been investigated, which releases acetazolamide at a rate of 15 mg/hour and is reported to cause fewer side effects.[70]

Advantages. The main advantage of acetazolamide over the other carbonic anhydrase inhibitors is that more is known about the drug, by virtue of greater laboratory and clinical experience. In one study, acetazolamide sustained-release capsules, given twice daily, were found in a crossover, randomized study to be better tolerated than four-times-a-day dosages of methazolamide 50 mg (which was the next best tolerated), ethoxzolamide 125 mg, acetazolamide 250 mg, or dichlorphenamide 50 mg.[71] Generic acetazolamide tablets are commercially available and have been shown to be comparable to the brand-name acetazolamide in IOP reduction and blood levels of the drug, while providing a significant cost savings.[72]

Methazolamide

Administration. Although methazolamide has been recommended in dosages up to 100 mg three times daily,[68] studies suggest that considerably less is needed in most cases to provide the desired therapeutic effect.[73–76] A dose of 25 mg twice daily was found to produce significant IOP reduction without metabolic acidosis.[73,74] Studies differ as to whether higher doses of methazolamide produce additional pressure reduction,[74,75] but a 500-mg sustained release capsule of acetazolamide was shown to have a greater ocular hypotensive effect than either 25 or 50 mg of methazolamide.[74] A suggested regimen for the titrated use of carbonic anhydrase inhibitor therapy is to begin with methazolamide 25 mg twice a day, advancing to 50 mg of methazolamide twice daily if necessary, and finally to the acetazolamide 500-mg sustained release capsule twice a day as required to achieve the desired effect.[77]

Advantages. The main advantage of methazolamide is that the drug can be used in smaller dosages, which causes fewer side effects. This is due to low protein binding, which allows the drug to diffuse more readily into tissue and thereby be more active on a weight basis in reducing aqueous production.[73,74] It also has a significantly longer plasma half-life than acetazolamide. In addition, there is evidence that methazolamide causes significantly fewer renal side effects,[43,78] although renal stone formation during methazolamide therapy has been reported.[79,80]

Dichlorphenamide

The recommended dosage of this carbonic anhydrase inhibitor is 25–100 mg three times a day. Its greater potency is probably due to a double molecular configuration resembling carbonic acid. The drug causes less metabolic acidosis, as a result of increased chloride excretion, but often has sustained diuresis with chronic use.[68]

Ethoxzolamide

This carbonic anhydrase inhibitor is given in a dosage of 125 mg every 6 hours and is similar in action and side effects to acetazolamide.[68]

TOPICAL CARBONIC ANHYDRASE INHIBITORS

With the numerous and significant side effects associated with oral and parenteral administration of carbonic anhydrase inhibitors, there is an obvious need for topical forms of these drugs that would concentrate the effect in the eye and reduce adverse system reactions. Early experience with acetazolamide revealed that it did not exert an ocular hypotensive effect when given topically or subconjunctivally.[21] This was initially thought to indicate that an effect on carbonic anhydrase in the blood is necessary for the action of carbonic anhydrase inhibitors on aqueous humor formation. However, more recently it has been learned that limited ocular penetration, resulting in an insufficient amount of drug reaching the ciliary body, is the primary explanation for the poor topical response. This observation has led to a considerable amount of investigation into new vehicles and forms of carbonic anhydrase inhibitors to enhance the topical delivery of these drugs.

In rabbits, topical administration of acetazolamide has been shown to blunt a water-induced ocular hypertensive response,[81,82] and both acetazolamide and methazolamide, delivered topically by high-water-content soft contact lenses, produced significant IOP reduction in albino rabbits.[83] In vitro studies of human and rabbit cornea revealed similar permeability to methazolamide and ethoxzolamide, although in vivo studies showed that topical methazolamide produced markedly higher aqueous concentrations in rabbit than in human eyes.[84] This discrepancy was thought possibly to be due to a relatively greater blinking rate and tear turnover and a lower corneal/conjunctival area in humans. In any case, it further emphasized the need for new forms of carbonic anhydrase inhibitors for topical delivery.

Newer carbonic anhydrase inhibitors, which combine certain elements of water- and lipid-solubility to enhance corneal penetration, have been shown to effectively lower aqueous production and IOP in rabbits. Examples of such drugs include *trifluoromethazolamide,* a halogenated derivative of methazolamide,[85] *6-hydroxyethoxzolamide,* an analogue of ethoxzolamide,[86] and L-645,151, which is also structurally related to ethoxzolamide.[87] Clinical experience with another ethoxzolamide analogue, *aminozolamide* gel, revealed a significant lowering of IOP,[88] but which lasted only about 8 hours and was associated with a high incidence of bulbar injection and follicular conjunctivitis.[89]

The largest amount of research that has been done to date with topical carbonic anhydrase inhibitors has been with *MK-927,* the hydrochloride salt of an amino-substituted heteroaromatic sulfonamide. Topical MK-927 has been shown to lower the IOP in normotensive rabbits[90] and glaucomatous monkeys.[91] Three drops of 2% MK-927, administered within 70 minutes, produced significant IOP reduction in both normal volunteers[92] and patients with primary open-angle glaucoma or ocular hypertension,[93] with no contralateral effect in either group. Dose response studies indicate that 0.125% and 0.5% MK-927 have little or no effect on IOP, while a 1% concentration produces a significantly greater pressure reduction than a placebo for up to 6 hours, and the 2% preparation causes further lowering of IOP with a duration of 8 hours.[94,95] However, even 2% MK-927 has less ocular hypotensive activity than systemic agents such as methazolamide, which may relate to the additional effect of metabolic acidosis with the oral compounds,[94] and there is considerable variability in peak response to single doses within individual patients.[95] L-671,152, a water-soluble carbonic anhydrase that is structurally similar to MK-927, has been shown to be a more potent inhibitor of human erythrocyte CA II than MK-927 and to have a greater and more prolonged ocular hypotensive effect in rabbits and monkeys than does MK-927.[96]

While the ideal topical carbonic anhydrase inhibitor has yet to be found, continued research in this area promises the addition of such drugs to our medical armamentarium within the near future.

SUMMARY

Carbonic anhydrase inhibitors lower IOP by reducing aqueous production, probably through an alteration in ion transport associated with secretion of aqueous humor. The numerous systemic side effects of the carbonic anhydrase inhibitors include diuresis, paresthesias, malaise, anorexia, serum electrolyte imbalances, gastrointestinal upset, renal calculi, and blood dyscrasias. The drugs in this class, which differ primarily only in degree of side effects, include acetazolamide, methazolamide, dichlorphenamide, and ethoxzolamide. These drugs are at present limited to systemic administration, although research with new preparations suggests the possibility of effective topical forms.

References

1. Becker, B: Decrease in intraocular pressure in man by a carbonic anhydrase inhibitor, Diamox. Am J Ophthal 37:13, 1954.
2. Dobbs, PC, Epstein, DL, Anderson, PF: Identification of isoenzyme C as the principal carbonic anhydrase in human ciliary processes. Invest Ophthal Vis Sci 18:867, 1979.
3. Wistrand, PJ, Garg, LC: Evidence of a high-activity C type of carbonic anhydrase in human ciliary processes. Invest Ophthal Vis Sci 18:802, 1979.
4. Wistrand, PJ, Schenholm, M, Lönnerholm, G: Carbonic anhydrase isoenzymes CA I and CA II in the human eye. Invest Ophthal Vis Sci 27:419, 1986.
5. Lutgen-Drecoll, E, Lonnerholm, G: Carbonic anhydrase distribution in the rabbit eye by light and electron microscopy. Invest Ophthal Vis Sci 21:782, 1981.
6. Lutjen-Drecoll, E, Lonnerholm, G, Eichhorn, M: Carbonic anhydrase distribution in the human and monkey eye by light and electron microscopy. Graefe's Arch Ophthal 220:285, 1983.
7. Krupin, T, Sly, WS, Whyte, MP, Dodgson, SJ: Failure of acetazolamide to decrease intraocular pressure in patients with carbonic anhydrase II deficiency. Am J Ophthal 99:396, 1985.
8. Dailey, RA, Brubaker, RF, Bourne, WM: The effects of timolol maleate and acetazolamide on the rate of aqueous formation in normal human subjects. Am J Ophthal 93:232, 1982.
9. Yablonski, ME, Hayashi, M, Cook, DJ, et al: Fluorophotometric study of intravenous carbonic anhydrase inhibitors in rabbits. Invest Ophthal Vis Sci 28:2076, 1987.
10. Berggren, L: Direct observation of secretory pumping in vitro of the rabbit eye ciliary processes. Influence of ion milieu and carbonic anhydrase inhibition. Invest Ophthal 3:266, 1964.
11. Maren, TH: The rates of movement of Na^+, Cl^-, and HCO_3^- from plasma to posterior chamber: effect of acetazolamide and relation to the treatment of glaucoma. Invest Ophthal 15:356, 1976.
12. Holland, MG, Gipson, CC: Chloride ion transport in the isolated ciliary body. Invest Ophthal 9:20, 1970.
13. Bietti, G, Virno, M, Pecori-Giraldi, J, Pellegrino, N: Acetazolamide, metabolic acidosis, and intraocular pressure. Am J Ophthal 80:360, 1975.

14. Soser, M, Ogriseg, M, Kessler, B, Zirm, H: New findings concerning changes in intraocular pressure and blood acidosis after peroral application of acetazolamide. Klin Monatsbl Augenheilkd 176:88, 1980.
15. Benedikt, O, Zirm, M, Harnoncourt, K: Relations between metabolic acidosis and intraocular pressure after inhibition of carbonic anhydrase with acetazolamide. Graefe's Arch Ophthal 190:247, 1974.
16. Friedman, Z, Krupin, T, Becker, B: Ocular and systemic effects of acetazolamide in nephrectomized rabbits. Invest Ophthal Vis Sci 23:209, 1982.
17. Mehra, KS: Relationship of pH of aqueous and blood with acetazolamide. Ann Ophthal 11:63, 1979.
18. Flammer, J, Drance, SM: Effect of acetazolamide on the differential threshold. Arch Ophthal 101:1378, 1983.
19. Thomas, RP, Riley, MW: Acetazolamide and ocular tension. Notes concerning the mechanism of action. Am J Ophthal 60:241, 1965.
20. Peczon, JD, Grant, WM: Diuretic drugs in glaucoma. Am J Ophthal 66:680, 1968.
21. Becker, B: The mechanism of the fall in intraocular pressure induced by the carbonic anhydrase inhibitor, Diamox. Am J Ophthal 39:177, 1955.
22. Macri, FJ: Acetazolamide and the venous pressure of the eye. Arch Ophthal 63:953, 1960.
23. Bill, A: Effects of acetazolamide and carotid occlusion on the ocular blood flow in unanesthetized rabbits. Invest Ophthal 13:954, 1974.
24. Walker, AM, Arrigg, C, Hertzmark, E, Epstein, DL: Carbonic anhydrase inhibitors induce elevations in human whole-blood zinc levels. Arch Ophthal 102:1785, 1984.
25. Tsuboi, S, Pederson, J: Experimental retinal detachment: X. Effect of acetazolamide on vitreous fluorescein disappearance. Arch Ophthal 103:1557, 1985.
26. Marmor, MF, Negi, A: Pharmacologic modifications of subretinal fluid absorption in the rabbit eye. Arch Ophthal 104:1674, 1986.
27. Marmor, MF, Maack, T: Enhancement of retinal adhesion and subretinal fluid resorption by acetazolamide. Invest Ophthal Vis Sci 23:121, 1982.
28. Cox, SN, Hay, E, Bird, AC: Treatment of chronic macular edema with acetazolamide. Arch Ophthal 106:1190, 1988.
29. Fishman, GA, Gilbert, LD, Fiscella, RG, et al: Acetazolamide for treatment of chronic macular edema in retinitis pigmentosa. Arch Ophthal 107:1445, 1989.
30. Friedenwald, JS: Current studies on acetazolamide (Diamox) and aqueous humor flow. Am J Ophthal 40:139, 1955.
31. Becker, B: Misuse of acetazolamide. Am J Ophthal 43:799, 1957.
32. Goren, SB, Newell, FW, O'Toole, JJ: The localization of Diamox-S^{35} in the rabbit eye. Am J Ophthal 51:87, 1961.
33. Block, ER, Rostand, RA: Carbonic anhydrase inhibition in glaucoma: hazard or benefit for the chronic lunger? Surv Ophthal 23:169, 1978.
34. Margo, CE: Acetazolamide and advanced liver disease. Am J Ophthal 101:611, 1986.
35. Heller, I, Halevy, J, Cohen, S, Theodor, E: Significant metabolic acidosis induced by acetazolamide: not a rare complication. Arch Intern Med 145:1815, 1985.
36. Epstein, DL, Grant, WM: Carbonic anhydrase inhibitor side effects. Serum chemical analysis. Arch Ophthal 95:1378, 1977.
37. Wallace, TR, Fraunfelder, FT, Petursson, GJ, Epstein, DL: Decreased libido—a side effect of carbonic anhydrase inhibitor. Ann Ophthal 11:1563, 1979.
38. Arrigg, CA, Epstein, DL, Giovanoni, R, Grant, WM: The influence of supplemental sodium acetate on carbonic anhydrase inhibitor-induced side effects. Arch Ophthal 99:1969, 1981.
39. Anderson, CJ, Kaufman, PL, Sturm, RJ: Toxicity of combined therapy with carbonic anhydrase inhibitors and aspirin. Am J Ophthal 86:516, 1978.
40. Spaeth, GL: Potassium, acetazolamide, and intraocular pressure. Arch Ophthal 78:578, 1967.
41. Critchlow, AS, Freeborn, SF, Roddie, RA: Potassium supplements during treatment of glaucoma with acetazolamide. Br Med J 289:21, 1984.
42. Kass, MA, Kolker, AE, Gordon, M, et al: Acetazolamide and urolithiasis. Ophthalmology 88:261, 1981.
43. Constant, MA, Becker, B: The effect of carbonic anhydrase inhibitors on urinary excretion of citrate by humans. Am J Ophthal 49:929, 1960.
44. Grant, WM: Antiglaucoma drugs: problems with carbonic anhydrase inhibitors. In: Symposium on Ocular Therapy, vol. 6, Leopold, IH, ed. CV Mosby, St. Louis, 1972, p. 19.
45. Simpson, DP: Effect of acetazolamide on citrate excretion in the dog. Am J Physiol 206:883, 1964.
46. Kondo, T, Sakaue, E, Koyama, S, et al: Urolithiasis during treatment of carbonic anhydrase inhibitors. Folia Ophthal Jap 19:576, 1968.
47. Parfitt, AM: Acetazolamide and renal stone formation. Lancet 2:153, 1970.
48. Persky, L, Chambers, D, Potts, A: Calculus formation and ureteral colic following acetazolamide (Diamox) therapy. JAMA 161:1625, 1956.
49. Charron, RC, Feldman, F: Acetazolamide therapy with renal complications. Can J Ophthal 9:282, 1974.
50. Wisch, N, Fischbein, FI, Siegel, R, et al: Aplastic anemia resulting from the use of carbonic anhydrase inhibitors. Am J Ophthal 75:130, 1973.
51. Gangitano, JL, Foster, SH, Contro, RM: Nonfatal methazolamide-induced aplastic anemia. Am J Ophthal 86:138, 1978.

52. Werblin, TP, Pollack, IP, Liss, RA: Blood dyscrasias in patients using methazolamide (Neptazane) for glaucoma. Ophthalmology 87:350, 1980.
53. Fraundfelder, FT, Meyer, SM, Bagby, GC Jr, Dreis, MW: Hematologic reactions to carbonic anhydrase inhibitors. Am J Ophthal 100:79, 1985.
54. Mogk, LG, Cyrlin, MN: Blood dyscrasias and carbonic anhydrase inhibitors. Ophthalmology 95:768, 1988.
55. Zimran, A, Beutler, E: Can the risk of acetazolamide-induced aplastic anemia be decreased by periodic monitoring of blood cell counts? Am J Ophthal 104:654, 1987.
56. Bovino, JA, Marcus, DF: The mechanism of transient myopia induced by sulfonamide therapy. Am J Ophthal 94:99, 1982.
57. Weiss, IS: Hirsutism after chronic administration of acetazolamide. Am J Ophthal 78:327, 1974.
58. Maren, TH: Teratology and carbonic anhydrase inhibition. Arch Ophthal 85:1, 1971.
59. Worsham, GF, Beckman, EN, Mitchell, EH: Sacrococcygeal teratoma in a neonate. JAMA 240:251, 1978.
60. Hargett, NA, Ritch, R, Mardirossian, J, et al: Inadvertent substitution of acetohexamide for acetazolamide. Am J Ophthal 84:580, 1977.
61. Shrader, CE, Thomas, JV, Simmons, RJ: Relationship of patient age and tolerance to carbonic anhydrase inhibitors. Am J Ophthal 96:730, 1983.
62. Lichter, PR: Reducing side effects of carbonic anhydrase inhibitors. Ophthalmology 88:266, 1981.
63. Friedland, BR, Mallonee, J, Anderson, DR: Short-term dose response characteristics of acetazolamide in man. Arch Ophthal 95:1809, 1977.
64. Lichter, PR, Musch, DC, Medzihradsky, F, Standardi, CL: Intraocular pressure effects of carbonic anhydrase inhibitors in primary open-angle glaucoma. Am J Ophthal 107:11, 1989.
65. Berson, FG, Epstein, DL, Grant, WM, et al: Acetazolamide dosage forms in the treatment of glaucoma. Arch Ophthal 98:1051, 1980.
66. Joyce, PW, Mills, KB, Richardson, T, Mawer, GE: Equivalence of conventional and sustained release oral dosage formulations of acetazolamide in primary open angle glaucoma. Br J Clin Pharmacol 27:597, 1989.
67. Yablonski, ME, Maren, TH, Hayashi, M, et al: Enhancement of the ocular hypotensive effect of acetazolamide by diflunisal. Am J Ophthal 106:332, 1988.
68. Havener, WH: Ocular Pharmacology, 4th ed. CV Mosby, St. Louis, 1978, p.475.
69. Alward, PD, Wilensky, JT: Determination of acetazolamide compliance in patients with glaucoma. Arch Ophthal 99:1973, 1981.
70. Theeuwes, F, Bayne, W, McGuire, J: Gastrointestinal therapeutic system for acetazolamide. Efficacy and side effects. Arch Ophthal 96:2219, 1978.
71. Lichter, PR, Newman, LP, Wheeler, NC, Beall, OV: Patient tolerance to carbonic anhydrase inhibitors. Am J Ophthal 85:495, 1978.
72. Ellis, PP, Price, PK, Kelmenson, R, Rendi, MA: Effectiveness of generic acetazolamide. Arch Ophthal 100:1920, 1982.
73. Maren, TH, Haywood, JR, Chapman, SK, Zimmerman, TJ: The pharmacology of methazolamide in relation to the treatment of glaucoma. Invest Ophthal Vis Sci 16:730, 1977.
74. Stone, RA, Zimmerman, TJ, Shin, DH, et al: Low-dose methazolamide and intraocular pressure. Am J Ophthal 83:674, 1977.
75. Dahlen, K, Epstein, DL, Grant, WM, et al: A repeated dose-response study of methazolamide in glaucoma. Arch Ophthal 96:2214, 1978.
76. Merkle, W: Effect of methazolamide on the intraocular pressure of patients with open-angle glaucoma. Klin Monatsbl Augenheilkd 176:181, 1980.
77. Zimmerman, TJ: Acetazolamide and methazolamide. Ann Ophthal 10:509, 1978.
78. Becker, B: Use of methazolamide (Neptazane) in the therapy of glaucoma. Comparison with acetazolamide (Diamox). Am J Ophthal 49:1307, 1960.
79. Ellis, PP: Urinary calculi with methazolamide therapy. Doc Ophthal 34:137, 1973.
80. Shields, MB, Simmons, RJ: Urinary calculus during methazolamide therapy. Am J Ophthal 81:622, 1976.
81. Stein, A, Pinke, R, Krupin, T, et al: The effect of topically administered carbonic anhydrase inhibitors on aqueous humor dynamics in rabbits. Am J Ophthal 95:222, 1983.
82. Flach, AJ, Peterson, JS, Seligmann, KA: Local ocular hypotensive effect of topically applied acetazolamide. Am J Ophthal 98:66, 1984.
83. Friedman, Z, Allen, RC, Raph, SM: Topical acetazolamide and methazolamide delivered by contact lenses. Arch Ophthal 103:963, 1985.
84. Edelhauser, HF, Maren, TH: Permeability of human cornea and sclera to sulfonamide carbonic anhydrase inhibitors. Arch Ophthal 106:1110, 1988.
85. Bar-Ilan, A, Pessah, NI, Maren, TH: The effects of carbonic anhydrase inhibitors on aqueous humor chemistry and dynamics. Invest Ophthal Vis Sci 25:1198, 1984.
86. Lewis, RA, Schoenwald, RD, Eller, MG, et al: Ethoxzolamide analogue gel. A topical carbonic anhydrase inhibitor. Arch Ophthal 102:1821, 1984.
87. Bar-Ilan, A, Pessah, NI, Maren, TH: Ocular penetration and hypotensive activity of the topically applied carbonic anhydrase inhibitor L-645,151. J Ocular Pharmacol 2:109, 1986.
88. Lewis, RA, Schoenwald, RD, Barfknecht, CF, Phelps, CD: Aminozolamide gel. A trial of a topical carbonic anhydrase inhibitor in ocular hypertension. Arch Ophthal 104:842, 1986.
89. Kalina, PH, Shetlar, DJ, Lewis, RA, et al: 6-amino-2-benzothiazolesulfonamide. The effect of a

topical carbonic anhydrase inhibitor on aqueous humor formation in the normal human eye. Ophthalmology 95:772, 1988.
90. Sugrue, MF, Gautheron, P, Grove, J, et al: MK-927: a topically effective ocular hypotensive carbonic anhydrase (CA) inhibitor in rabbits. Invest Ophthal Vis Sci (suppl) 29:81, 1988.
91. Wang, RF, Serle, JB, Podos, SM, Sugrue, MF: The effect of MK-927, a topical carbonic anhydrase inhibitor, on IOP in glaucomatous monkeys. Curr Eye Res 9:163, 1990.
92. Lippa, EA, von Denffer, HA, Hofmann, HM, Brunner-Ferber, FL: Local tolerance and activity of MK-927, a novel topical carbonic anhydrase inhibitor. Arch Ophthal 106:1694, 1988.
93. Bron, AM, Lippa, EA, Hofmann, HM, et al: MK-927: a topically effective carbonic anhydrase inhibitor in patients. Arch Ophthal 107:1143, 1989.
94. Higginbotham, EJ, Kass, MA, Lippa, EA, et al: MK-927: a topical carbonic anhydrase inhibitor. Dose response and duration of action. Arch Ophthal 108:65, 1990.
95. Serle, JB, Lustgarten, JS, Lippa, EA, et al: MK-927, a topical carbonic anhydrase inhibitor. Dose response and reproducibility. Arch Ophthal 108:838, 1990.
96. Sugrue, MF, Mallorga, P, Schwam, H, et al: A comparison of L-671,152 and MK-927, two topically effective ocular hypotensive carbonic anhydrase inhibitors, in experimental animals. Curr Eye Res 9:607, 1990.

Chapter 29

HYPEROSMOTIC AGENTS

The drugs discussed in this chapter represent another class of compounds that may be administered systemically (orally or intravenously) for the control of elevated intraocular pressure (IOP). Unlike the carbonic anhydrase inhibitors, however, the use of these medications is generally limited to short-term, emergency situations, such as acute angle-closure glaucoma or secondary glaucomas with dangerously high pressures. Another clinical use for hyperosmotic agents is the reduction of vitreous volume as a prophylactic measure prior to some intraocular surgical procedures. The mechanisms of action and the side effects of the drugs within this class of compounds are similar, with some notable exceptions, and these features are discussed collectively before considering specific aspects of the individual agents.

MECHANISMS OF ACTION

Reduced Vitreous Volume

As noted above, one action of the hyperosmotic agents is reduction of vitreous volume. It is this effect that is generally believed to be responsible for lowering the IOP. This concept is supported by rabbit studies, which demonstrated a reduction in vitreous body weight of approximately 3–4% with various hyperosmotic agents.[1] The mechanism of vitreous shrinkage is commonly considered to be an osmotic gradient between the blood and ocular tissues, which initially pulls fluid from the eye.

With time, a variable amount of the hyperosmotic agent may enter the eye, depending upon the permeability of the blood-ocular barriers to the drug and the size of the drug molecules. As the compound is cleared from the systemic circulation, there may be a reversal of the osmotic gradient in some cases, resulting in a transient rise in IOP.

Hypothalamic-Neural Theory

Some studies have shown that changes in IOP and serum osmolarity do not always correlate,[2–5] and it may be that additional factors are involved in the ocular hypotensive effect of hyperosmotics. One alternative theory is that osmotic agents (both hyperosmotics and hypo-osmotics) influence the IOP through the central nervous system.

It has been observed that human eyes with optic nerve lesions do not manifest the usual elevation in IOP after water drinking.[6] Unilateral optic nerve transection in rabbits and monkeys also was associated with a reduced ocular hypertensive response to hypo-osmotics, as well as a diminished IOP-lowering effect with hyperosmotic agents.[2,7,8] These observations raised the possibility that the influence of osmotic agents on the IOP is mediated through the optic nerve.[2,6–8]

Additional studies suggested that the central nervous system effect of osmotic agents on IOP might originate in the hypothalamus. Phenobarbital, which has a depressant effect on the hypothalamus, lowers the IOP in rabbits, presumably by inhibition of aqueous humor formation, and this action was shown to be reduced by optic nerve transection.[9] Furthermore, pretreatment with phenobarbital prevented the ocular hypotensive response to hyperosmotic agents in rabbits with intact optic nerves.[10] In addition, the injection of osmotic agents into the third ventricle of rabbits altered the IOP without affecting serum osmolarity, and this effect was eliminated by optic nerve transection.[11] Bilateral lesions in the supraoptic nuclei (an area of the hypothalamus near the optic tracts that is known to be related to water balance) abolished the IOP response to hypo-osmotics in rabbits.[12]

The above observations are believed to support the theory that osmotic agents exert their influence on IOP through the central nervous system, possibly originating in the hypothalamus and mediated by efferent fibers in the optic nerve.[2,6,7,8,10] The exact mechanism of pressure reduction is uncertain, although preliminary evidence suggests a decrease in aqueous production.[10]

However, other reported studies have challenged the hypothalamic-neural theory. Ventriculocisternal perfusion of a hypo-osmotic solution in rabbits did not influence the IOP,[13] nor did unilateral optic nerve transection in rabbits alter the IOP response to osmotic agents.[14,15] An alternative explanation that has been proposed for the diminished IOP response to osmotic agents in eyes with optic atrophy is that an associated reduction in the retinal vasculature decreases the available route of fluid movement from the eye.[14] There is clearly a need for further investigation of this question.

Altered Ciliary Epithelium

It has been observed in monkey studies that intra-arterial injections of hyperosmotic agents cause a breakdown of the blood-aqueous barrier associated with destruction of the nonpigmented ciliary epithelium.[16–19] However, similar changes do not occur following intravenous administration,[16,17] and it is unlikely that this is part of the ocular hypotensive effect associated with clinical hyperosmotic therapy.

SIDE EFFECTS

Side effects with hyperosmotic therapy are common and can be serious,[20] or even fatal.[21,22] The magnitude of these adverse reactions varies with the specific agent and mode of administration.

Nausea and Vomiting. Nausea and vomiting are frequently encountered, especially with the oral (liquid) agents, presumably because of the heavy sweet taste. This is transient and usually of no consequence but can be a problem if the vomiting occurs during surgery or leads to loss of the medication. The nausea can be minimized by serving the medication with ice and a tart flavoring.

Diuresis. Diuresis is a standard response to hyperosmotic therapy and is particularly a problem with the use of intravenous agents. In some cases, massive diuresis during surgery may necessitate the use of an indwelling catheter.

Other Reactions. Other reactions that may occur with all hyperosmotics but that are worse with intravenous agents include headache, backache, giddiness, diarrhea, confusion and disorientation,[20] chills and fever, cardiovascular overload, intracranial hemorrhage,[21] pulmonary edema, acidemia, and renal insufficiency.[22]

SPECIFIC HYPEROSMOTIC AGENTS (TABLE 29.1)

Oral Agents

Glycerol. Glycerol, or glycerine, is administered as a liquid in a dosage of 1–1.5 g/kg of body weight of a 50% solution.[23,24] The ocular hypotensive effect occurs within 10 minutes of administration, peaks in 30 minutes, and lasts for approximately 5 hours.[23,24] Glycerol is distributed throughout the extracellular body fluids and has poor ocular penetration, which enhances the osmotic gradient effect and allows effective repeated administrations.[23] In addition, the drug is metabolized, which causes less diuresis and increased safety. However, the caloric content of 4.32 kilocalories per

Table 29.1
Commercial Hyperosmotic Agents*

Generic Preparations	Brand Names	Concentrations (%)
Oral agents		
Glycerine	Glyrol	75
	Osmoglyn	50
Isosorbide	Ismotic	45
Intravenous agents		
Mannitol	Osmitrol	5,10,15,20
Urea	Ureaphil	40 g/150 ml

* Other generic products may also be available.

gram[24] and the osmotic diuresis with resultant dehydration can cause problems with repeated administration in diabetics.[25]

Isosorbide. Isosorbide is another oral hyperosmotic agent, which became commercially available in 1980. Numerous studies have confirmed the ocular hypotensive efficacy of this agent.[26–32] The drug has an advantage over glycerol in that 95% is excreted unchanged in the urine,[26] which eliminates the caloric problem.[28] Other side effects are also reported to be less with isosorbide than with other hyperosmotics.[26–31] The recommended dosage is 1.5 g/kg of body weight of a 50% solution, which produces a peak ocular hypotensive effect in 1–3 hours and lasts for 3–5 hours.[31] As in the case of glycerol, it may also be given in repeated doses. It should be noted that isosorbide dinitrate (Isordil), an organic nitrate used in the treatment of angina pectoris, has a similar name, and care must be taken to avoid confusing these two drugs.[33]

Other Oral Drugs. Other oral drugs that have been found to be effective as hyperosmotic agents in lowering the IOP include glycine,[34] sodium lactate,[35] propylene glycol,[36] and ethyl alcohol, although the latter is effective only in large doses.[37]

Intravenous Agents

These drugs generally produce a greater ocular hypotensive effect than do oral hyperosmotics. They may be indicated when the oral agents are thought to be insufficient or when they cannot be taken for reasons such as nausea.

Mannitol. Mannitol is reported to have an ocular hypotensive effect equivalent to[38] or greater than[39] that of urea and is said to be more efficacious than glycerol.[39] In one study, intravenous mannitol and oral isosorbide produced equivalent pressure reduction at 30 and 60 minutes, although mannitol was more effective in maintaining the reduction.[27] The drug is distributed in the extracellular fluid compartments and has poor ocular penetration.[23] Although it is rapidly excreted unmetabolized in the urine, the transient rise in blood volume requires caution in patients with poor cardiac output. In general, side effects are infrequent but may include headache, angina-like chest pain,[38] and an anaphylactic reaction.[40] Death has been reported in a patient who developed pulmonary edema, acidemia, and anuria following mannitol therapy, and special caution is advised in patients with compromised renal function.[22]

A dosage of 2 g/kg of body weight of a 20% solution, given intravenously in 30 minutes, has been suggested.[23] However, it may be that significantly lower doses are equally effective. In one study of patients prior to cataract surgery, 100 ml of 20% mannitol given over 20 minutes had the same effect on magnitude of IOP reduction and deepening of the anterior chamber as 200 ml of the same solution, although the latter had a more rapid and sustained ocular hypotensive effect.[41] The onset of action is in 20–60 minutes, and the duration varies from 2 to 6 hours.[23,38,41]

Urea. Urea may be slightly less effective than mannitol, because it diffuses more freely throughout the body water and eventually penetrates into the eye.[23] In addition, urea has the significant disadvantage of causing tissue necrosis if it extravasates during intravenous administration.[20] Death from a subdural hematoma has occurred following urea administration for systemic hypertension.[21]

Glycerol[42–44] and glycerol with sorbitol[43,44] have also been given intravenously, and preliminary experience suggests that these may prove valuable as intravenous hyperosmotic agents.

SUMMARY

The systemic administration of a hyperosmotic agent is occasionally used as a short-term or emergency method of lowering the IOP. The ocular hypotensive mechanism is not fully understood but probably relates primarily to a reduction in vitreous volume. Side effects can be serious and include nausea and vomiting, diuresis, headache, disorientation, and cardiovascular overload. Specific hyperosmotic agents may be given orally, as with glycerol and isosorbide, or intravenously, as with mannitol and urea.

References

1. Robbins, R, Galin, MA: Effect of osmotic agents on the vitreous body. Arch Ophthal 82:694, 1969.
2. Podos, SM, Krupin, T, Becker, B: Effect of small-dose hyperosmotic injections on intraocular pressure of small animals and man when optic nerves are transected and intact. Am J Ophthal 71:898, 1971.
3. Ramsell, JT, Ellis, PP, Paterson, CA: Intraocular pressure changes during hemodialysis. Am J Ophthal 72:926, 1971.
4. Olsen, T, Schmitz, O, Hansen, HE: Influence of hemodialysis on corneal thickness and intraocular pressure. Klin Monatsbl Augenheilkd 181:25, 1982.
5. Goldberg, DB, Mannarino, AP, Greco, JA: Intraocular pressure and ocular pain during hemodialysis. J Ocul Ther Surg 3:246, 1984.
6. Riise, D, Simonsen, SE: Intraocular pressure in unilateral optic nerve lesion. Acta Ophthal 47:750, 1969.
7. Krupin, T, Podos, SM, Becker, B: Effect of optic nerve transection on osmotic alterations of intraocular pressure. Am J Ophthalmol 70:214, 1970.
8. Krupin, T, Podos, SM, Lehman, RAW, Becker, B: Effects of optic nerve transection on intraocular pressure in monkeys. Arch Ophthal 84:668, 1970.
9. Becker, B, Krupin, T, Podos, SM: Phenobarbital and aqueous humor dynamics: effect in rabbits with intact and transected optic nerves. Am J Ophthal 70:686, 1970.
10. Podos, SM, Krupin, T, Becker, B: Mechanism of intraocular pressure response after optic nerve transection. Am J Ophthal 72:79, 1971.
11. Krupin, T, Podos, SM, Becker, B: Alteration of intraocular pressure after third ventricle injections of osmotic agents. Am J Ophthal 76:948, 1973.
12. Cox, CE, Fitzgerald, CR, King, RL: A preliminary report on the supraoptic nucleus and control of intraocular pressure. Invest Ophthal 14:26, 1975.
13. Liu, JHK, Neufeld, AH: Study of central regulation of intraocular pressure using ventriculocisternal perfusion. Invest Ophthal Vis Sci 26:136, 1985.
14. Serafano, DM, Brubaker, RF: Intraocular pressure after optic nerve transection. Invest Ophthal Vis Sci 17:68, 1978.
15. Lam, K-W, Shihab, Z, Fu, Y-A, Lee, P-F: The effect of optic nerve transection upon the hypotensive action of ascorbate and mannitol. Ann Ophthal 12:1102, 1980.
16. Laties, AM, Rapoport, S: The blood-ocular barriers under osmotic stress. Studies on the freeze-dried eye. Arch Ophthal 94:1086, 1976.
17. Shabo, AL, Maxwell, DS, Kreiger, AE: Structural alterations in the ciliary process and the blood-aqueous barrier of the monkey after systemic urea injections. Am J Ophthal 81:162, 1976.
18. Okisaka, S, Kuwabara, T, Rapoport, SI: Effect of hyperosmotic agents on the ciliary epithelium and trabecular meshwork. Invest Ophthal 15:617, 1976.
19. Gaasterland, DE, Barranger, JA, Rapoport, SI, et al: Long-term ocular effects of osmotic modification of the blood-brain barrier in monkeys. I. Clinical examinations; aqueous ascorbate and protein. Invest Ophthal Vis Sci 24:153, 1983.
20. Tarter, RC, Linn, JC Jr: A clinical study of the use of intravenous urea in glaucoma. Am J Ophthal 52:323, 1961.
21. Marshall, S, Hinman, F Jr: Subdural hematoma following administration of urea for diagnosis of hypertension. JAMA 182:813, 1962.
22. Grabie, MT, Gipstein, RM, Adams, DA, Hepner, GW: Contraindications for mannitol in aphakic glaucoma. Am J Ophthal 91:265, 1981.
23. Havener, WH: Ocular Pharmacology, 4th ed. CV Mosby, St. Louis, 1978, p. 440.
24. Virno, M, Cantore, P, Bietti, C, Bucci, MG: Oral glycerol in ophthalmology. A valuable new method for the reduction of intraocular pressure. Am J Ophthal 55:1133, 1963.
25. Oakley, DE, Ellis, PP: Glycerol and hyperosmolar nonketotic coma. Am J Ophthal 81:469, 1976.
26. Barry, KG, Khoury, AH, Brooks, MH: Mannitol and isosorbide. Sequential effects on intraocular pressure, serum osmolality, sodium, and solids in normal subjects. Arch Ophthal 81:695, 1969.
28. Krupin, T, Kolker, AE, Becker, B: A comparison

of isosorbide and glycerol for cataract surgery. Am J Ophthal 69:737, 1970.
29. Wisznia, KI, Lazar, M, Leopold, IH: Oral isosorbide and intraocular pressure. Am J Ophthal 70:630, 1970.
30. Mehra, KS, Singh, R, Char, JN, Rajyashree, K: Lowering of intraocular tension. Effects of isosorbide and glycerin. Arch Ophthal 85:167, 1971.
31. Mehra, KS, Singh, R: Lowering of intraocular pressure by isosorbide. Effects of different doses of drug. Arch Ophthal 86:623, 1971.
32. Wood, TO, Waltman, SR, West, C, Kaufman, HE: Effect of isosorbide on intraocular pressure after penetrating keratoplasty. Am J Ophthal 75:221, 1973.
33. Buckley, EG, Shields, MB: Isosorbide and isosorbide dinitrate. Am J Ophthal 89:457, 1980.
34. Fox, SL, Kranta, JC Jr: The use of glycine in the reduction of intraocular pressure. EENT Monthly 51:469, 1972.
35. Chiang, TS, Stocks, SA, Jones, C, Thomas, RP: The ocular hypotensive effect of sodium lactate in rabbits. Arch Ophthal 86:566, 1971.
36. Bietti, G: Recent experimental, clinical, and therapeutic research on the problems of intraocular pressure and glaucoma. Am J Ophthal 73:475, 1972.
37. Obstbaum, SA, Podos, SM, Kolker, AE: Low-dose oral alcohol and intraocular pressure. Am J Ophthal 76:926, 1973.
38. Smith, EW, Drance, SM: Reduction of human intraocular pressure with intravenous mannitol. Arch Ophthal 68:734, 1962.
39. Vucicevic, AM, Tark, E III, Ahmad, S: Echographic studies of osmotic agents. Ann Ophthal 11:1331, 1979.
40. Spaeth, GL, Spaeth, EB, Spaeth, PG, Lucier, AC: Anaphylactic reaction to mannitol. Arch Ophthal 78:583, 1967.
41. O'Keeffe, M, Nabil, M: The use of mannitol in intraocular surgery. Ophthal Surg 14:55, 1983.
42. Holtmann, HW: Experiences with glycerin infusions for intra-ocular pressure-lowering. Klin Monatsbl Augenheilkd 161:322, 1972.
43. Masiakowski, J, Warchalowska, D, Orlowski, WJ: Effect of osmotic agents on intraocular pressure. I. Survey of pharmacological possibilities. Klin Oczna 43:365, 1973.
44. Bartkowska-Orlowska, M, Orlowski, WJ, Warchalowska, D, Masiakowski, J: Effect of osmotic agents on intraocular pressure. II. Intravenous administration of glycerol and glycerol with sorbitol under experimental conditions. Klin Oczna 43:371, 1973.

Chapter 30

CANNABINOIDS, PROSTAGLANDINS, AND OTHER INVESTIGATIONAL ANTIGLAUCOMA DRUGS

The classes of drugs discussed in the preceding five chapters provide effective intraocular pressure (IOP) control for the majority of glaucoma patients. However, because of intolerable side effects and lack of efficacy in some cases, these drugs are not always able to prevent progressive glaucomatous damage. Therefore, there is a need to continue the search for new and better antiglaucoma medications. Much of this work at present is being done with new forms of drugs from the classes that were discussed in the previous chapters. In addition, research is being conducted with the following groups of drugs.

CANNABINOIDS

In 1971, Hepler and Frank[1] reported that smoking a marihuana cigarette caused a significant reduction in the IOP. Animal and human studies have subsequently shown that several derivatives of *tetrahydrocannabinol* (THC), the primary class of active ingredients in marihuana, effectively lower the IOP when given orally[2–6] or intravenously,[7–10] while the reported effects of topical cannabinoids have been conflicting.[2,11–17] These observations have stimulated the search for cannabinoids that would be suitable for the long-term management of glaucoma. To date, these studies have yielded the following data.

Mechanism of Action

It was once thought that smoking marihuana might lower the IOP indirectly by the drug-induced relaxation effect.[18] However, extensive animal studies have confirmed a direct ocular hypotensive effect. The local effect may be primarily due to vasodilation of the efferent vessels in the anterior uvea, which reduces the ultrafiltration pressure for aqueous humor formation.[10,19,20] This action was reported to be inhibited by ganglionectomy,[9,21] beta-adrenergic blockers,[21] or vasodilators.[22] Biochemical studies in rabbits suggest that the ocular hypotensive mechanism of marihuana-derived material is not mediated through adenylate cyclase, ATPase, or substance P but possibly through modification of the surface membrane glycoprotein residues on the ciliary epithelium.[23]

The IOP reduction is also associated with increased facility of outflow,[9,10,19] which is said to be blocked by ganglionectomy[9,21] or alpha-adrenergic antagonists.[20,21] In another study, however, surgical removal of all autonomic input in cats did not alter the ocular hypotensive effect of delta^9-THC.[24] The cannabinoids have also been shown to stimulate monoamine oxidase activity, which could possibly be related to the influence of these compounds on the IOP.[25] Other reported actions associated with cannabinoid therapy include increased aqueous protein[10] and antagonism of the in vivo ocular production of prostaglandin from arachidonic acid.[26] Delta^9-THC produced ocular hypotension and miosis in rabbits when given intravenously but not when administered into the cerebral ventricles, suggesting that the action of cannabinoids on IOP does not originate in the central nervous system.[27]

Side Effects

Although marihuana and many of the cannabinoids are known to be highly effective in lowering the IOP, the numerous side effects of all the compounds thus far tested in humans seriously limit their general usefulness in the long-term management of glaucoma.[4,28,29] The best known of these adverse reactions is the altered mental status, which has been observed during trial therapy with inhalation of marihuana[30] and with oral administration of THC derivatives.[4,5]

Ocular side effects associated with marihuana inhalation include conjunctival hyperemia, a slight miosis, and reduced tear production.[28,29,31,32] Individuals who had used marihuana chronically for 10 years or more but had abstained for at least 3 hours prior to testing had increased basal lacrimation, decreased dark adaptation, decreased color-match limits, decreased Snellen acuity, and slightly increased IOP as compared with matched nonuser controls.[33]

From the standpoint of controlling glaucoma, the most disturbing adverse reaction is systemic hypotension, which has been observed with use of oral[4,5] and intravenous[8] cannabinoids as well as marihuana inhalation.[30] If the drop in blood pressure is found to be associated with reduced perfusion of the optic nerve head, the cannabinoids could be lowering the IOP without protecting against progressive glaucomatous optic atrophy.[4,34] Even with topical administration, systemic hypotension may be a problem. Animal studies suggest that topical cannabinoid therapy reduces the IOP by a systemic mechanism,[13] and trials with glaucoma patients revealed occasional systemic hypotension.[14] Smoking marihuana, regardless of THC content, has also been shown to cause a substantially greater respiratory burden of carbon monoxide and tar than smoking a similar quantity of tobacco.[35]

Before a cannabinoid can be recommended for the management of glaucoma, one must be found that dissociates the ocular and systemic side effects from the ocular hypotensive action. Preliminary experience suggests that the cannabinoid cannabigerol may possess such properties,[36] and further study of these compounds appears to be warranted.

It has also been shown that aqueous extractions of other plants, including tobacco, cabbage, and lettuce, contain components with potent IOP-lowering activity in rabbits, which may provide alternatives to marihuana derivatives in the management of glaucoma.[37]

PROSTAGLANDINS

Prostaglandins (PGs) are ubiquitous local hormones that represent part of the family of arachidonic acid derivatives, or *eicosanoids*. In most tissues of the body, release of arachidonic acid results in the complex *arachidonic acid cascade*, in which a cyclooxygenase pathway leads to the synthesis of stable PGs and labile products such as thromboxane A_2 and prostacyclin, while a lipoxygenase pathway leads to the production of leukotrienes. Prostaglandins, of which there are several types (e.g., A, B, D, E, and F plus numerous subsets), and other eicosanoids are produced in small amounts in conjunction with physiologic processes and in larger amounts in association with pathologic events. The latter include ocular inflammation and hypertension, which were the focus of early PG research. However, more recent studies indicate that smaller amounts of PGs may actually moderate the inflammatory response and lower the IOP, which has led to the investigation of the use of these agents in the medical management of glaucoma.[38,39]

Initial Studies

In rabbits, topical application of 25–200 μg of PGs caused an initial rise in IOP, followed by pressure reduction for 15–20 hours, whereas a 5-μg dose produced the hypotension without an initial rise.[40] Daily or twice-daily administration of various PGs has been shown to maintain a sustained IOP reduction in rabbits, cats, and monkeys.[41–45] Other arachidonic acid metabolites have also been shown to lower the IOP in rabbits.[46,47] In preliminary human studies, topical application of the tromethamine salt of prostaglandin type $F_{2\alpha}$ ($PGF_{2\alpha}$) produced significant dose-related IOP reduction in normotensive volunteers but was associated with ocular irritation, conjunctival hyperemia, and headaches.[48,49] However, the lipid-soluble ester of $PGF_{2\alpha}$, which has better corneal penetration and can be used in lower doses than the salt, also had a significant dose-related ocular hypotensive effect in both normal volunteers[50,51] and open-angle glaucoma patients[52] without serious side effects.

Mechanisms of Action

In most studies, the ocular hypotensive effect of PGs does not appear to be explained by reduced aqueous production, reduced episcleral venous pressure, or increased conventional aqueous outflow.[50,53–56] This leads to the hypothesis that the mechanism of IOP reduction is *improved uveoscleral outflow*, which has been supported by the observation that pilocarpine antagonized the $PGF_{2\alpha}$-induced ocular hypotension in monkeys.[57] The effect on uveoscleral outflow appears to be the mechanism of action for the various types of PGs,[56] although one study with topical PGD_2 in rabbits suggested that reduced flow was the main hypotensive mechanism.[58] Adrenergic antagonists were reported to block the PG-induced increase in total outflow facility,[20] although the addition of topical $PGF_{2\alpha}$ to open-angle glaucoma patients uncontrolled on timolol alone led to further significant IOP reduction.[59] Neither indomethacin nor sympathectomy altered the ocular hypertensive effect of PGs, suggesting that the mechanism does not involve de novo synthesis of prostaglandin or release of endogenous norepinephrine.[40] One study suggested that the ocular hypotensive mechanism is not mediated by the $PGF_{2\alpha}$-sensitive receptor.[60] It has also been shown that PGs have minimal influence on the ocular hypotensive effect of marihuana-derived materials.[61]

Side Effects

The intraocular inflammatory effects of aqueous cell and flare and miosis, which result from the administration of large doses of PGs, are not seen in animal or human eyes in the doses associated with the ocular hypotensive response.[41–45,48–52,62,63] Furthermore, the absorptive transport systems of the ciliary processes appear to prevent topically applied PGs and other eicosanoids from causing retinal toxicity.[38] Extraocular irritation has been more of a problem in human studies with the salt of $PGF_{2\alpha}$,[48,49] although, as previously noted, this is significantly reduced by using the lipid-soluble ester of the compound.[50–52] It has also been shown that the ocular hypotensive effect of PGD_2 may be separated from the inflammatory effect on the conjunctiva by using a selective PGD_2-sensitive receptor agonist.[64] With regard to systemic side effects, the amount of PG entering the circulation from the low doses of its ester required to lower the IOP is a small fraction of the amount of endogenous PGs normally released from virtually all tissues of the body.[39]

OTHER INVESTIGATIONAL DRUGS

A wide variety of additional agents have been evaluated for their influence on aqueous humor dynamics. The following are some of those that may one day provide a new class of drugs for the management of glaucoma.

Valinomycin. Valinomycin, a cyclic peptide that increases the permeability of the mitochondrial membrane to potassium, caused a significant IOP reduction in rabbits and monkeys, although side effects included transient corneal edema and increased aqueous protein.[65]

Atriopeptins. Atriopeptins, a group of polypeptides secreted by cardiac myocytes in response to fluid overload, have been shown to have receptors coupled to the activation of guanylate cyclase in rabbit ciliary processes.[66]

Neuropeptide Y. Neuropeptide Y, which is also abundant in ciliary processes, has been shown in rabbit studies to inhibit adenylate cyclase[67] and to modulate iris dilator muscle action.[68]

Antazoline. Antazoline, an antihistamine of the ethylenediamine class, reduced the IOP when given topically to rabbits, apparently by means of decreased aqueous production.[69]

Ethacrynic Acid. Ethacrynic acid, a sulfhydryl-reactive diuretic, increased aqueous outflow when perfused into the anterior chamber of living monkey eyes and enucleated calf eyes.[70]

Spironolactone. Spironolactone, a synthetic steroidal aldosterone antagonist with potassium-sparing diuretic-antihypertensive activity, produced significant IOP reduction in glaucoma patients, which persisted 2 weeks after termination of the treatment.[71]

Tetrahydrocortisol. Tetrahydrocortisol, a metabolite of cortisol, lowered the IOP in rabbits with dexamethasone-induced ocular hypertension.[72]

Angiotensin-Converting Enzyme Inhibitor. Angiotensin-converting enzyme inhibitor in a new topical formulation has been shown to lower the IOP in dogs and humans with ocular hypertension or open-angle glaucoma.[73]

Organic Nitrates. Organic nitrates, such as intravenous nitroglycerin or oral isosorbide dinitrate, have been reported to lower IOP in glaucoma and nonglaucoma patients.[74]

Melatonin. Melatonin, a hormone produced by the pineal gland with a well-characterized circadian rhythm, was shown to lower the IOP in normal volunteers.[75]

Calcium Channel Blockers. Calcium channel blockers, which produce vasodilation by inhibiting the entrance of calcium ions into vascular smooth muscle cells and which are used in the management of coronary heart disease, have been shown to have ocular hypotensive activity,[76] which lasted up to 10 hours in human volunteers.[77]

Demeclocycline, Tetracycline. Demeclocycline, tetracycline, and other tetracycline derivatives were shown to lower the IOP in rabbits, which appears to be related to reduced aqueous humor production.[78]

Haloperidol. Haloperidol, a dopaminergic antagonist used as an antipsychotic, was found to be equivalent or superior to timolol in suppressing artificially elevated IOP in rabbits.[79,80] The mechanism of action was believed to be reduction of aqueous humor production by lowering of blood flow to the ciliary body.

Direct Optic Nerve Head Protectors

All of the drugs previously discussed indirectly protect the optic nerve head from progressive glaucomatous atrophy by lowering the IOP. An alternative approach would be to give a medication that directly protects the nerve head from the effects of the elevated pressure. This might be particularly desirable in cases of low-tension glaucoma, where maximum medical therapy and even surgery are often unable to lower the IOP sufficiently to stop the progressive glaucomatous damage.

In 1948, McGuire[81] reported the use of bishydroxycoumarin (Dicumarol) to protect the optic nerve head by improving vascular perfusion. However, other investigators could not confirm his findings.[82] Subsequently, diphenylhydantoin (Dilantin)[83] and phosphatide complexes[84] were also reported to directly protect the optic nerve head from progressive glaucomatous damage in preliminary studies. Although none of these observations has been confirmed, all of them do represent important potential approaches to glaucoma therapy that clearly deserve further investigation.

SUMMARY

In addition to continued research with the drug groups discussed in the preceding chapters, other classes of compounds are also being studied for possible use in the treatment of glaucoma. Cannabinoids effectively lower the IOP by an uncertain mechanism, although the lack of a drug form that dissociates this action from the systemic side effects has limited the usefulness of these agents. Low doses of prostaglandins have been shown to exert significant ocular hypotensive action, probably by means of increasing uveoscleral outflow. Preliminary experience with several additional classes of drugs offers promise of other new ocular hypotensive agents as well as drugs that may protect the optic nerve from the effects of ocular tension.

References

1. Hepler, RS, Frank, IR: Marihuana smoking and intraocular pressure. JAMA 217:1392, 1971.
2. Green, K, Kim, K: Acute dose response of intraocular pressure to topical and oral cannabinoids. Proc Soc Exp Biol Med 154:228, 1977.
3. Newell, FW, Stark, P, Jay, WM, Schanzlin, DJ: Nabilone: a pressure-reducing synthetic benzopyran in open-angle glaucoma. Ophthalmology 86:156, 1979.
4. Tiedeman, JS, Shields, MB, Weber, PA, et al: Effect of synthetic cannabinoids on elevated intraocular pressure. Ophthalmology 88:270, 1981.
5. Merritt, JC, McKinnon, S, Armstrong, JR, et al: Oral delta^9-tetrahydrocannabinol in heterogeneous glaucomas. Ann Ophthal 12:947, 1980.
6. Weber, PA, Bianchine, JR, Howes, JF: Nabitan hydrochloride: ocular hypotensive effect in normal human volunteers. Glaucoma 3:163, 1981.
7. Purnell, WD, Gregg, JM: Delta^9-tetrahydrocannabinol, euphoria and intraocular pressure in man. Ann Ophthal 7:921, 1975.
8. Cooler, P, Gregg, JM: Effect of delta^9-tetrahydrocannabinol on intraocular pressure in humans. South Med J 70:951, 1977.
9. Green, K, Kim, K: Mediation of ocular tetrahydrocannabinol effects by adrenergic nervous system. Exp Eye Res 23:443, 1976.
10. Green, K, Pederson, JE: Effect of delta^1-tetrahydrocannabinol on aqueous dynamics and ciliary body permeability in the rabbit. Exp Eye Res 15:499, 1973.
11. Green, K, Kim, K, Wynn, H, Shimp, RG: Intraocular pressure, organ weights and the chronic use of cannabinoid derivatives in rabbits for one year. Exp Eye Res 25:465, 1977.
12. Green, K, Bigger, JF, Kim, K, Bowman, K: Cannabinoid penetration and chronic effects in the eye. Exp Eye Res 24:197, 1977.
13. Merritt, JC, Peiffer, RL, McKinnon, SM, et al: Topical delta^9-tetrahydrocannabinol on intraocular pressure in dogs. Glaucoma 3:13, 1981.
14. Merritt, JC, Olsen, JL, Armstrong, JR, McKinnon, SM: Topical delta^9-tetrahydrocannabinol in hypertensive glaucomas. J Pharm Pharmacol 33:40, 1981.
15. Merritt, JG, Whitaker, R, Page, CJ, et al: Topical delta^8-tetrahydrocannabinol as a potential glaucoma agent. Glaucoma 4:253, 1982.
16. Green, K, Roth, M: Ocular effects of topical administration of delta^9-tetrahydrocannabinol in man. Arch Ophthal 100:265, 1982.
17. Jay, WM, Green, K: Multiple-drop study of topically applied 1% delta^9-tetrahydrocannabinol in human eyes. Arch Ophthal 101:591, 1983.
18. Flom, MC, Adams, AJ, Jones, RT: Marijuana smoking and reduced pressure in human eyes: drug action or epiphenomenon? Invest Ophthal 14:52, 1975.
19. Green, K, Wynn, H, Padgett, D: Effects of delta^9-tetrahydrocannabinol on ocular blood flow and aqueous humor formation. Exp Eye Res 26:65, 1978.
20. Green, K, Kim, K: Interaction of adrenergic antagonists with prostaglandin E_2 and tetrahydrocannabinol in the eye. Invest Ophthal 15:102, 1976.
21. Green, K, Bigger, JF, Kim, K, Bowman, K: Cannabinoid action on the eye as mediated through the central nervous system and local adrenergic activity. Exp Eye Res 24:189, 1977.
22. Green, K, Kim, K: Papaverine and verapamil interaction with prostaglandin E_2 and delta^9-tetrahydrocannabinol in the eye. Exp Eye Res 24:207, 1977.
23. Green, K, Cheeks, K, Mittag, T, et al: Marihuana-derived material: biochemical studies of the ocular responses. Curr Eye Res 4:631, 1985.
24. Colasanti, BK, Powell, SR: Effect of delta^9-tetrahydrocannabinol on intraocular pressure after removal of autonomic input. J Ocul Pharm 1:47, 1985.
25. Gawienowski, AM, Chatterjee, D, Anderson, PJ, et al: Effect of delta^9-tetrahydrocannabinol on monoamine oxidase activity in bovine eye tissues, in vitro. Invest Ophthal Vis Sci 22:482, 1982.
26. Green, K, Podos, SM: Anatagonism of arachidonic acid-induced ocular effects by delta^1-tetrahydrocannabinol. Invest Ophthal 13:422, 1974.
27. Liu, JHK, Dacus, AC: Central nervous system and peripheral mechanisms in ocular hypotensive effect of cannabinoids. Arch Ophthal 105:245, 1987.
28. Green, K: Marihuana and the eye. Invest Ophthal 14:261, 1975.

29. Green, K, Roth, M: Marijuana in the medical management of glaucoma. Pers Ophthal 4:101, 1980.
30. Merritt, JC, Crawford, WJ, Alexander, PC, et al: Effect of marihuana on intraocular and blood pressure in glaucoma. Ophthalmology 87:222, 1980.
31. Hepler, RS, Frank, IM, Ungerleider, JT: Pupillary constriction after marijuana smoking. Am J Ophthal 74:1185, 1972.
32. Brown, B, Adams, AJ, Haegerstrom-Portnoy, G, et al: Pupil size after use of marijuana and alcohol. Am J Ophthal 83:350, 1977.
33. Dawson, WW, Jimenez-Antillon, CF, Perez, JM, Zeskind, JA: Marijuana and vision—after ten years' use in Costa Rica. Invest Ophthal Vis Sci 16:689, 1977.
34. Gaasterland, DE: Efficacy in glaucoma treatment—the potential of marijuana. Ann Ophthal 12:448, 1980.
35. Wu, T-C, Tashkin, DP, Djahed, B, Rose, JE: Pulmonary hazards of smoking marijuana as compared with tobacco. N Engl J Med 318:347, 1988.
36. Colasanti, BK, Craig, CR, Allara, RD: Intraocular pressure, ocular toxicity and neurotoxicity after administration of cannabinol or cannabigerol. Exp Eye Res 39:251, 1984.
37. Deutsch, HM, Green, K, Zalkow, LH: Water soluble high molecular weight components from plants with potent intraocular pressure lowering activity. Curr Eye Res 6:733, 1987.
38. Bito, LZ: Prostaglandins and other eicosanoids: their ocular transport, pharmacokinetics, and therapeutic effects. Trans Ophthal Soc UK 105:162, 1986.
39. Bito, LZ: Prostaglandins. Old concepts and new perspectives (editorial). Arch Ophthal 105:1036, 1987.
40. Camras, CB, Bito, LZ, Eakins, KE: Reduction of intraocular pressure by prostaglandins applied topically to the eyes of conscious rabbits. Invest Ophthal Vis Sci 16:1125, 1977.
41. Stern, FA, Bito, LZ: Comparison of the hypotensive and other ocular effects of prostaglandins E_2 and $F_{2\text{-alpha}}$ on cat and rhesus monkey eyes. Invest Ophthal Vis Sci 22:588, 1982.
42. Bito, LZ, Draga, A, Blanco, J, Camras, CB: Long-term maintenance of reduced intraocular pressure by daily or twice daily topical application of prostaglandins to cat or rhesus monkey eyes. Invest Ophthal Vis Sci 24:312, 1983.
43. Bito, LZ, Srinivasan, BD, Baroody, RA, Schubert, H: Noninvasive observations on eyes of cats after long-term maintenance of reduced intraocular pressure by topical application of prostaglandin E_2. Invest Ophthal Vis Sci 24:376, 1983.
44. Camras, CB, Podos, SM, Rosenthal, JS, et al: Multiple dosing of prostaglandin $F_{2\alpha}$ or epinephrine on cynomolgus monkey eyes. I. Aqueous humor dynamics. Invest Ophthal Vis Sci 28:463, 1987.
45. Kulkarni, PS, Srinivasan, BD: Prostaglandins E_3 and D_3 lower intraocular pressure. Invest Ophthal Vis Sci 26:1178, 1985.
46. Hoyng, PFJ, de Jong, N: Iloprost®, a stable prostacyclin analog, reduces intraocular pressure. Invest Ophthal Vis Sci 28:470, 1987.
47. Masferrer, JL, Dunn, MW, Schwartzman, ML: 12(R)-hydroxyeicosatetraenoic acid, an endogenous corneal arachidonate metabolite, lowers intraocular pressure in rabbits. Invest Ophthal Vis Sci 31:535, 1990.
48. Giuffre, G: The effects of prostaglandin $F_{2\text{-alpha}}$ in the human eye. Graefe's Arch Ophthal 222:139, 1985.
49. Lee, P-Y, Shao, H, Xu, L, Qu, C-K: The effect of prostaglandin $F_{2\alpha}$ on intraocular pressure in normotensive human subjects. Invest Ophthal Vis Sci 29:1474, 1988.
50. Kerstetter, JR, Brubaker, RF, Wilson, SE, Kullerstrand, LJ: Prostaglandin $F_{2\alpha}$-1-isopropylester lowers intraocular pressure without decreasing aqueous humor flow. Am J Ophthal 105:30, 1988.
51. Villumsen, J, Alm, A: Prostaglandin $F_{2\alpha}$-isopropylester eye drops: effects in normal human eyes. Br J Ophthal 73:419, 1989.
52. Villumsen, J, Alm, A, Söderström, M: Prostaglandin $F_{2\alpha}$-isopropylester eye drops: effect on intraocular pressure in open-angle glaucoma. Br J Ophthal 73:975, 1989.
53. Lee, P-Y, Podos, SM, Severin, C: Effect of prostaglandin $F_{2\text{-alpha}}$ on aqueous humor dynamics of rabbit, cat, and monkey. Invest Ophthal Vis Sci 25:1087, 1984.
54. Moses, RA, Parkison, G, Snower, DP: Prostaglandin E_2 effect on the facility of outflow in the rabbit eye. Ann Ophthal 13:721, 1981.
55. Crawford, K, Kaufman, PL, Gabelt, B'AT: Effects of topical $PGF_{2\alpha}$ on aqueous humor dynamics in cynomolgus monkeys. Curr Eye Res 6:1035, 1987.
56. Hayashi, M, Yablonski, ME, Bito, LZ: Eicosanoids as a new class of ocular hypotensive agents. 2. Comparison of the apparent mechanism of the ocular hypotensive effects of A and F type prostaglandins. Invest Ophthal Vis Sci 28:1639, 1987.
57. Crawford, K, Kaufman, PL: Pilocarpine antagonizes prostaglandin $F_{2\alpha}$-induced ocular hypotension in monkeys. Evidence for enhancement of uveoscleral outflow by prostaglandin $F_{2\alpha}$. Arch Ophthal 105:1112, 1987.
58. Goh, Y, Araie, M, Nakajima, M, et al: Effect of topical prostaglandin D_2 on the aqueous humor dynamics in rabbits. Graefe's Arch Ophthal 227:476, 1989.
59. Villumsen, J, Alm, A: The effect of adding prostaglandin $F_{2\alpha}$-isopropylester to timolol in patients with open angle glaucoma. Arch Ophthal 108:1102, 1990.
60. Woodward, DF, Burke, JA, Williams, LS, et al:

Prostaglandin $F_{2\alpha}$ effects on intraocular pressure negatively correlate with FP-receptor stimulation. Invest Ophthal Vis Sci 30:1838, 1989.

61. Green, K, Cheeks, KE, Watkins, L, et al: Prostaglandin involvement in the responses of the rabbit eye to water-soluble marihuana-derived material. Curr Eye Res 6:337, 1987.
62. Camras, CB, Bhuyan, KC, Podos, SM, et al: Multiple dosing of prostaglandin $F_{2\alpha}$ or epinephrine on cynomolgus monkey eyes. II. Slit-lamp biomicroscopy, aqueous humor analysis, and fluorescein angiography. Invest Ophthal Vis Sci 28:921, 1987.
63. Camras, CB, Friedman, AH, Rodrigues, MM, et al: Multiple dosing of prostaglandin $F_{2\alpha}$ or epinephrine on cynomolgus monkey eyes. III. Histopathology. Invest Ophthal Vis Sci 29:1428, 1988.
64. Woodward, DF, Hawley, SB, Williams, LS, et al: Studies on the ocular pharmacology of prostaglandin D_2. Invest Ophthal Vis Sci 31:138, 1990.
65. Lee, P-F, Lam, K-W: The effect of valinomycin on intraocular pressure. Ann Ophthal 5:33, 1973.
66. Nathanson, JA: Atriopeptin-activated guanylate cyclase in the anterior segment. Identification, localization, and effects of atriopeptins on IOP. Invest Ophthal Vis Sci 28:1357, 1987.
67. Cepelik, J, Hynie, S: Inhibitory effects of neuropeptide Y on adenylate cyclase of rabbit ciliary processes. Curr Eye Res 9:121, 1990.
68. Piccone, M, Littzi, J, Krupin, T, et al: Effects of neuropeptide Y on the isolated rabbit iris dilator muscle. Invest Ophthal Vis Sci 29:330, 1988.
69. Krupin, T, Silverstein, B, Feitl, M, et al: The effect of H_1-blocking antihistamines on intraocular pressure in rabbits. Ophthalmology 87:1167, 1980.
70. Epstein, DL, Freddo, TF, Bassett-Chu, S, et al: Influence of ethacrynic acid on outflow facility in the monkey and calf eye. Invest Ophthal Vis Sci 28:2067, 1987.
71. Witzmann, R: The effect of spironolactone on intraocular pressure in glaucoma patients. Klin Monatsbl Augenheilkd 176:445, 1980.
72. Southren, AL, l'Hommedieu, D, Gordon, GG, Weinstein, BI: Intraocular hypotensive effect of a topically applied cortisol metabolite: 3α, 5β-tetrahydrocortisol. Invest Ophthal Vis Sci 28:901, 1987.
73. Constad, WH, Fiore, P, Samson, C, Cinotti, AA: Use of an angiotensin converting enzyme inhibitor in ocular hypertension and primary open-angle glaucoma. Am J Ophthal 105:674, 1988.
74. Wizemann, A, Wizemann, V: The use of organic nitrates to lower intraocular pressure in outpatient and surgical treatment. Klin Monatsbl Augenheilkd 177:292, 1980.
75. Samples, JR, Krause, G, Lewy, AJ: Effect of melatonin on intraocular pressure. Curr Eye Res 7:649, 1988.
76. Monica, ML, Hesse, RJ, Messerli, FH: The effect of a calcium-channel blocking agent on intraocular pressure. Am J Ophthal 96:814, 1983.
77. Abelson, MB, Gilbert, CM, Smith, LM: Sustained reduction of intraocular pressure in humans with the calcium channel blocker verapamil. Am J Ophthal 105:155, 1988.
78. Wallace, I, Krupin, T, Stone, RA, Moolchandani, J: The ocular hypotensive effects of demeclocycline, tetracycline and other tetracycline derivatives. Invest Ophthal Vis Sci 30:1594, 1989.
79. Chiou, GCY: Ocular hypotensive actions of haloperidol, a dopaminergic antagonist. Arch Ophthal 102:143, 1984.
80. Chiou, GCY: Treatment of ocular hypertension and glaucoma with dopamine antagonists. Ophthal Res 16:129, 1984.
81. McGuire, WP: The effect of dicumarol on the visual fields in glaucoma. A preliminary report. Trans Am Ophthal Soc 84:96, 1948.
82. Shields, MB, Wadsworth, JAC: An evaluation of anticoagulation in glaucoma therapy. Ann Ophthal 9:1115, 1977.
83. Becker, B, Stamper, RL, Asseff, C, Podos, SM: Effect of diphenylhydantoin on glaucomatous field loss: a preliminary report. Trans Am Acad Ophthal Otol 76:412, 1972.
84. Hruby, K, Weiss, H: Therapeutic utilization of phosphatide complexes in ophthalmology. Ophthal Digest June:9, 1976.

Chapter 31

ANATOMIC PRINCIPLES OF GLAUCOMA SURGERY

All laser and incisional surgical procedures for glaucoma are designed to reduce the intraocular pressure (IOP) by either increasing the rate of aqueous humor outflow or reducing aqueous production. Therefore, the involved anatomy is the anterior ocular structures related to aqueous outflow and the portions of the ciliary body associated with aqueous inflow. To properly perform any of the operations that make up the armamentarium of glaucoma surgery, the surgeon must be familiar with both the internal (gonioscopic) and external aspects of these structures. In this chapter we will consider these portions of the ocular anatomy as they relate to glaucoma surgery.

AN OVERVIEW OF THE ANATOMY

The structures involved in aqueous humor dynamics (i.e., of aqueous production and aqueous outflow) lie in immediate proximity to each other in the periphery of the anterior ocular segment. The interrelationship among these structures was considered in Chapter 2 with a stepwise construction of a schematic model and is summarized here.

At the junction between the cornea and the sclera is the transitional zone of connective tissue known as the *limbus*. On the inner surface of the limbus, extending for 360°, is a depression, referred to as the scleral sulcus. The anterior margin of this sulcus slopes gradually into the peripheral cornea, while the posterior margin contains a lip of connective tissue, called the *scleral spur*. This spur might be thought of as the dividing point between the structures of aqueous outflow anteriorly and those of aqueous production posteriorly. The *trabecular meshwork* attaches, in part, to the anterior side of the scleral spur and extends forward to blend into the sloping anterior wall of the scleral sulcus, which converts that structure into *Schlemm's canal*. The bulk of aqueous humor in the anterior chamber flows through the trabecular meshwork to Schlemm's canal, from whence it leaves the eye via intrascleral channels and episcleral veins.

The *ciliary body* attaches to the posterior portion of the scleral spur. This is actually the only firm attachment of the ciliary body, with the remaining surfaces between the sclera and the ciliary body creating a potential space, referred to as the supraciliary space. The *ciliary processes,* the actual site of aqueous production, occupy the innermost and anteriormost portion of the ciliary body. The *iris* inserts into the ciliary body just anterior to the ciliary processes. Therefore, a peripheral iridectomy will often allow visualization of the ciliary processes, as during glaucoma filtering surgery. The insertion of the iris is usually such that a portion of the anterior ciliary body remains gonioscopically visible between the iris root and scleral spur. This is referred to as the ciliary body band. The remainder of the trabecular meshwork (i.e., that which does not attach to the scleral spur) attaches to this band and to the peripheral iris.

INTERNAL ANATOMY (FIG. 31.1)

Ciliary Body

Most of the ciliary body is located posterior to the iris and cannot be visualized directly except in unusual circumstances, such as with marked iris retraction or absence of portions of the iris. The anterior 2–3 mm of the ciliary body, the *pars plicata*, is thicker and contains the radial ridges of the ciliary processes. The latter are the site of aqueous production and the target of cyclodestructive procedures. In those unusual circumstances in which they can be visualized directly (cycloscopy), direct treatment with laser transpupillary cyclophotocoagulation may be possible. In most cases, however, an indirect, transscleral route must be used for the cyclodestructive element, requiring the use of external landmarks, which are discussed later in this chapter. The posterior 4 mm of the ciliary body is the thinner *pars plana*, which must also be approached by using external landmarks.

Gonioscopic Anatomy

The following structures in the anterior chamber can be visualized by gonioscopic examination and are involved in a number of laser and incisional glaucoma surgical procedures.

The Iris. The iris is the posteriormost structure of the anterior chamber angle. It is helpful to remember that the peripheral portion of the iris is thinner than the more central iris, which, among other reasons, makes it the preferred site for a laser iridotomy. Other anatomic considerations related to optimum laser iridotomy sites are iris crypts, or thinner areas of stroma that may be easier to penetrate, and areas of increased pigmentation, such as freckles, which may improve the absorption of laser energy in lightly pigmented eyes when using argon laser.

The Ciliary Body Band. The ciliary body band is located just anterior to the root of the iris and typically has a dark gray or brown appearance as shown by gonioscopic examination. The width of this band varies

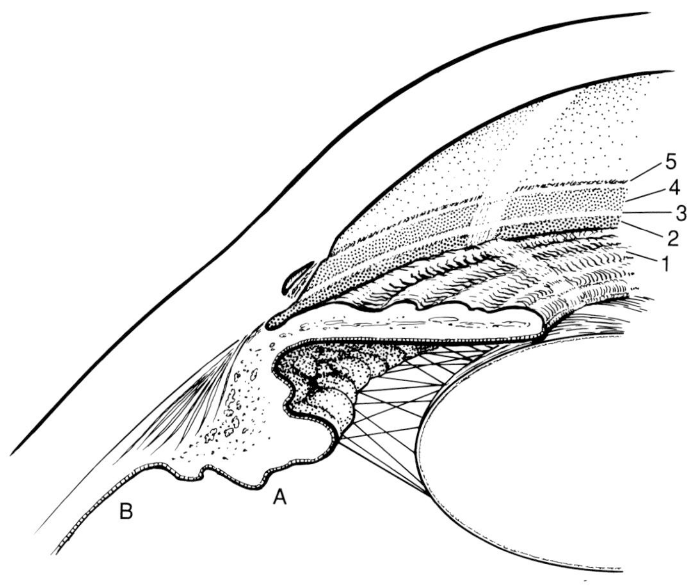

Figure 31.1. Internal anatomy. The ciliary body is located just posterior to the iris and is divided into the pars plicata (*A*) and the pars plana (*B*). The remaining internal structures can be seen via gonioscopy and include: *1*, iris; *2*, ciliary body band; *3*, scleral spur; *4*, trabecular meshwork; and *5*, Schwalbe's line.

considerably from one patient to the next, with myopes often having a wide band and hyperopes a narrow band. Care must be taken to avoid confusing this pigmented band with the trabecular meshwork in patients with lightly pigmented trabecular meshwork, especially during laser trabeculoplasty. The patient will usually let the surgeon know when this mistake is made, since the ciliary body contains nerve endings and is sensitive to the application of laser energy.

The Scleral Spur. The scleral spur is seen gonioscopically as a sharp, white line just anterior to the ciliary body band. However, in some patients the visualization of the spur may be obscured to variable degrees by iris processes or heavy pigment dispersion. This is the principal site of surgery with a cyclodialysis procedure, in which the ciliary body is separated from the scleral spur. In the early stages of neovascular glaucoma, new vessels may be seen extending across the scleral spur from the iris and ciliary body to the trabecular meshwork, where they may be amenable to treatment with goniophotocoagulation.

Trabecular Meshwork. Just anterior to the scleral spur is the functional portion of the trabecular meshwork (i.e., that portion adjacent to Schlemm's canal), through which the aqueous humor flows. This portion of the meshwork is demarcated gonioscopically by the presence of variable amounts of pigment. Since this pigment is carried to the meshwork from uveal tissue by the aqueous humor flow, it typically is light colored in young individuals and varies considerably among individuals later in life according to the amount of pigment dispersion. In some pathologic states, such as the pigment dispersion syndrome and exfoliation syndrome, the meshwork is extremely heavily pigmented. It is this pigmented portion of the trabecular meshwork to which the laser energy should be applied during laser trabeculoplasty. However, it should be kept in mind that another less pigmented portion of the meshwork lies just anterior to the functional, pigmented portion. In performing laser trabeculoplasty, it has been found that overlapping the laser beam between the pigmented and nonpigmented portions of the meshwork (i.e., along the anterior border of the pigmented portion) may help to reduce the complications of transient postoperative IOP rise and peripheral anterior synechia formation.

Schwalbe's Line. Schwalbe's line is the anteriormost structure in the anterior chamber angle and represents the junction between the nonpigmented portion of the trabecular meshwork and the peripheral cornea, where it is seen as a small ridge. This is an important landmark when performing a goniotomy, since the incision is made just posterior to this line. The structure may be difficult to visualize gonioscopically unless there has been a moderate degree of pigment dispersion, in which case there may be a build-up of pigment along the anterior side of the ridge, especially inferiorly. Care must be taken to avoid confusing this pigmented line with the trabecular meshwork when performing laser trabeculoplasty. In other cases in which there is minimal pigmentation, it is often helpful to establish the location of Schwalbe's line gonioscopically to help in determining the depth of the peripheral anterior chamber. A fine beam of light from the slit lamp can be seen reflecting from both the anterior and posterior surfaces of the peripheral cornea. As the clear portion of the peripheral cornea approaches Schwalbe's line, it is replaced externally by opaque limbal tissue, which causes the two beams to converge at Schwalbe's line, providing a useful way of determining the location of this structure.

EXTERNAL ANATOMY (FIG. 31.2)

Anterior Limbus

On the external surface of the eye, the anterior boundary of the limbus is defined as the termination of Bowman's membrane, which is approximately 0.5 mm anterior to the insertion of the conjunctiva and Tenon's capsule. This has been referred to as the *corneolimbal junction,* or the apparent or anterior limbus. It is important to note that the conjunctiva inserts more anteriorly in the superior and inferior quadrants. Consequently, the limbus is wider in these quadrants, ranging between 1 and 1.5 mm, and gradually tapers to the narrowest width in the nasal and temporal quadrants, where the

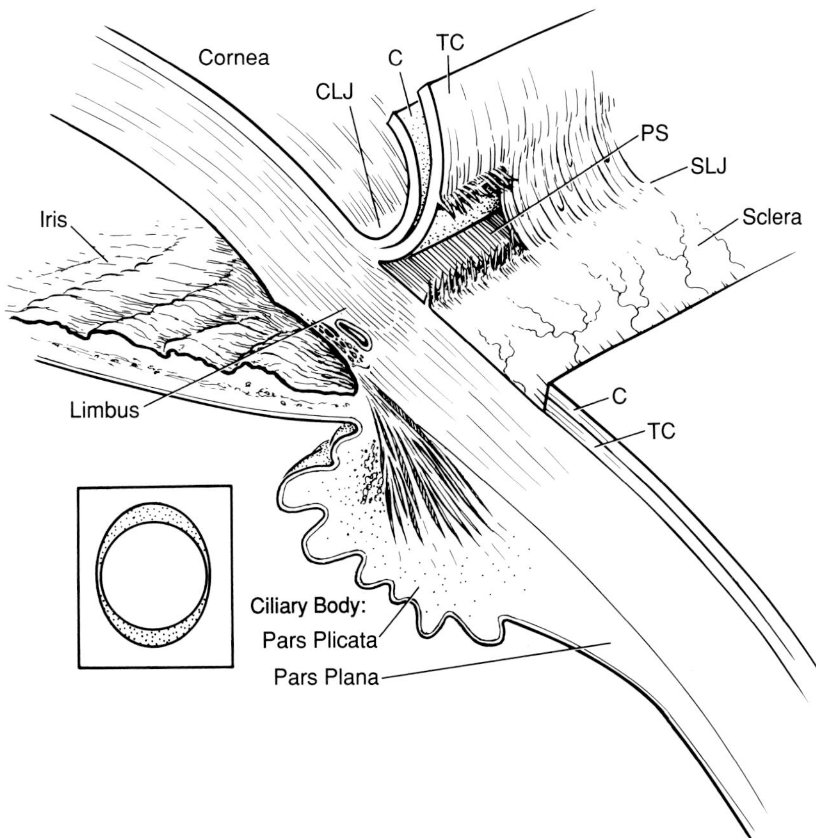

Figure 31.2. External anatomy. The limbus is bounded externally by the sclerolimbal junction (*SLJ*) posteriorly and the corneolimbal junction (*CLJ*) anteriorly. The width of the limbus varies from a maximum superiorly to a minimum on the sides (*inset*) as a result of the relative insertion of the conjunctiva (*C*). Tenon's capsule (*TC*) is firmly attached to limbal connective tissue approximately 0.5 mm behind the conjunctival insertion, creating a potential space (*PS*). Cyclodestructive procedures should be placed over the pars plicata, usually 1–2 mm posterior to the corneolimbal junction, while a posterior sclerotomy should be made through the pars plana, approximately 3–4 mm posterior to the corneolimbal junction.

range is between 0.3 and 0.5 mm.[1] In performing glaucoma filtering surgery, some surgeons choose to take advantage of the wider areas of the limbus by placing the surgical site at the 12 o'clock position. When performing surgery that involves the ciliary body, such as a cyclodestructive procedure or a pars plana incision, it is also important to remember that these structures are slightly more posterior in relation to the apparent limbus in the superior and inferior quadrants.

Conjunctiva and Tenon's Capsule

The conjunctiva and Tenon's capsule cover the limbus. The adhesions between conjunctiva and Tenon's capsule are moderately firm, so that sharp dissection is usually required when dissecting between these two structures, as is done in some techniques of preparing the conjunctival flap for glaucoma filtering surgery. The adhesion between Tenon's capsule and the underlying limbus and sclera is less firm, and these structures can often be separated with blunt dissection. However, Tenon's capsule is firmly attached to the connective tissue of the limbus approximately 0.5 mm posterior to the insertion of the conjunctiva, which creates a potential space between the anterior conjunctiva/Tenon's capsule tissue and the limbal connective tissue. When preparing a limbus-based conjunctival flap, it is necessary to dissect this adherence between the capsule and limbal tissue in order to adequately expose the limbus.

Posterior Limbus

When the conjunctiva and Tenon's capsule are reflected, the posterior boundary of the limbus is now visible. This has been referred to as the *sclerolimbal junction* or the surgical or posterior limbus. It is identified as the junction of the opaque, white sclera posteriorly and the translucent, bluish-gray limbus anteriorly. This boundary of the limbus is more useful than the corneolimbal junction in glaucoma surgery because it helps to identify the location of the deeper structures of the anterior chamber angle. The scleral spur is located just posterior to the sclerolimbal junction, and Schlemm's canal, therefore, would be found just anterior to this landmark. In performing a trabeculotomy ab externo, a radial, scratch incision across the sclerolimbal junction should reveal Schlemm's canal in the posterior portion of the gray zone. In performing a trabeculectomy or other filtering procedure, a circumferential incision at the corneolimbal junction enters the anterior chamber just in front of the trabecular meshwork. By extending the dissection posteriorly to the sclerolimbal junction, a flap of deep-limbal tissue is created that can be reflected to expose the anterior chamber angle structures and excised along the scleral spur. If by mistake the latter incision is made more posteriorly, brisk bleeding from the ciliary body may occur.

The anterior ciliary arteries enter the ciliary body behind the scleral spur in locations corresponding to the positions of the rectus muscle tendons. These vessels should be avoided during surgery, when possible, to avoid excessive bleeding. Since the ciliary body usually cannot be visualized internally, external landmarks must be used when performing surgical procedures associated with these structures. In performing cyclodestructive procedures, which involves the pars plicata, it has been suggested that the destructive element (e.g., the cryoprobe) should be placed 2–3 mm behind the corneolimbal junction, allowing for the previously discussed variation in this landmark.[1] However, more recent experience with transscleral cyclophotocoagulation suggests that a placement of the laser beam 1–1.5 mm behind the corneolimbal junction is most likely to treat the pars plicata.[2] When making a pars plana incision, as during a posterior sclerotomy for malignant glaucoma or when draining a suprachoroidal detachment or hemorrhage, the incision should be made 3–4 mm behind the corneolimbal junction.

SUMMARY

Laser and incisional surgical procedures for glaucoma are directed at the anatomic structures associated with aqueous inflow (i.e., the ciliary body) and aqueous outflow (i.e., the iris and the trabecular meshwork and related outflow pathways). For successful glaucoma surgery, it is necessary to be familiar with these structures by means of direct internal visualization through slit-lamp and gonioscopic examination, as well as by means of their relationship to the external aspects of the limbal connective tissue and the overlying conjunctiva and Tenon's capsule.

References

1. Sugar, HS: Surgical anatomy for glaucoma. Surv Ophthal 13:143, 1968.
2. Hampton, C, Shields, MB: Transscleral neodymium:YAG cyclophotocoagulation: a histologic study of human autopsy eyes. Arch Ophthal 106:1121, 1988.

Chapter 32

PRINCIPLES OF LASER SURGERY FOR GLAUCOMA

The introduction of laser therapy was undoubtedly the most significant advance in the surgical treatment of glaucoma during the 1980s, and there is promise of ever-increasing technological advances and surgical applications as we enter the 1990s. However, the concept of using light energy to alter the structure of intraocular tissues actually preceded the development of laser technology. Meyer-Schwickerath,[1] beginning in the late 1940s, pioneered this field of ocular surgery, first using focused sunlight and later the xenon-arc photocoagulator. Although the latter technique proved useful for certain retinal disorders, xenon-arc photocoagulation for glaucoma never gained clinical acceptance.

In 1960, Maiman[2] produced the first laser, using a ruby crystal. However, it was not until the development of the continuous wave argon laser, near the end of that decade, that the virtual explosion of laser applications for ocular diseases began. After several years of investigative work in the early 1970s, clinicians began applying laser energy to treat various forms of glaucoma, and today it is the most commonly used mode of glaucoma surgery.

In this chapter, we will briefly review the physical and biologic aspects of laser therapy. The application of these principles to the treatment of specific forms of glaucoma is considered in subsequent chapters.

BASIC PRINCIPLES OF LASERS[3–6]

Albert Einstein speculated that atoms, under certain conditions, could absorb light or other radiation and then be stimulated to emit the borrowed energy. His theory formed the basis of *Light Amplification by Stimulated Emission of Radiation* (laser).

When atoms absorb energy, called "pumping," they are "excited" from a lower to a higher energy level. If more atoms are in the excited than in the unexcited state, "population inversion" exists. Under such circumstances, photons with an energy equal to the difference between the two levels of excitation have an enhanced probability of stimulating the atoms to decay back to their lower energy level by emitting photons, a process called "stimulated emission." The emitted photons stimulate the emission of more photons, leading to a chain reaction.

If the system described above is enclosed between two mirrors, the photons will bounce back and forth, creating multiple stimulated emissions of light, or "light amplification." The mirrors are said to form a "cavity," which, in addition to amplifying the light, creates a parallel beam and acts as a resonator to limit the number of wavelengths. When the light amplification is sufficient, some photons are allowed to leave

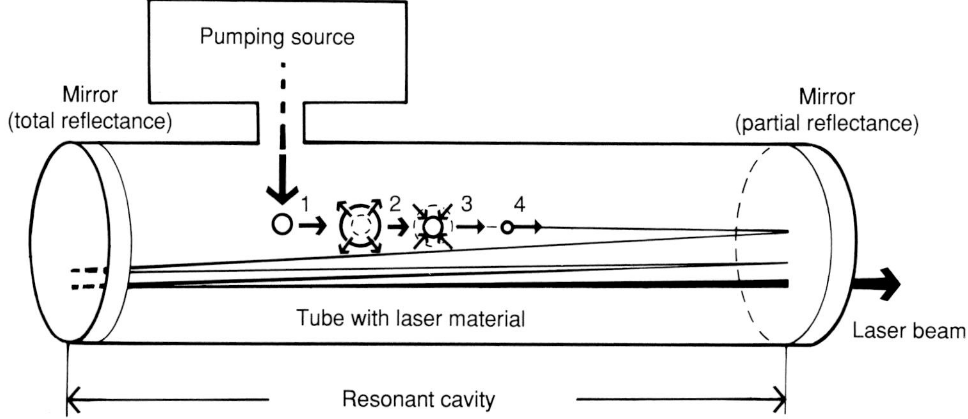

Figure 32.1. Schematic of laser system. Laser material is placed in a tube between two mirrors. When an energy source is pumped into the tube, atoms in the laser material (*1*) are excited to a higher energy level (*2*). In the excited state, atoms have an enhanced probability of being stimulated by photons to decay back to the lower energy level (*3*) by emitting photons (*4*). The emitted photons bounce between the mirrors, stimulating other excited atoms, until sufficient light amplification is achieved, at which time the light is allowed to leave the cavity as a laser beam.

the cavity in the form of a laser beam (Fig. 32.1).

The laser beam can be delivered as a "continuous wave" or in a "pulsed mode." In the latter situation, the energy is concentrated and delivered in a very short period of time, which can be accomplished in one of two ways. With one technique, "Q-switching," light is not allowed to travel back and forth in the cavity until maximum population inversion is reached. This is accomplished with either an electronic shutter or misalignment of the mirrors. When the shutter is opened or the mirrors are aligned, stimulated emission and light amplification occur suddenly, and the energy is released in a pulse of a few to tens of nanoseconds. In the other form of pulsed delivery, called "mode-locking," the energy is also released after achieving maximum population inversion, but different modes of light are synchronized, creating peaks of energy, which are emitted in tens of nanoseconds as a chain of pulses, each of which lasts a few tens of picoseconds. To provide some appreciation for the brevity of these exposures, it has been noted that the ratio between the duration of a Q-switched laser pulse and a conventional continuous wave argon laser exposure is roughly the same as the ratio between the argon exposure and a human lifetime![7]

PROPERTIES OF LASER ENERGY

Light emitted by a laser differs from normal "white" light in the following ways:

Coherence

Unlike the photons in a light bulb, which are emitted randomly, the resonator effect of the laser cavity causes the photons to be synchronized or coherent (i.e., in phase with each other in time and space).

Collimation

Since light amplification occurs only for photons that are aligned with the mirrors, a nearly parallel beam is produced, as opposed to the diverging beam of an incandescent lamp. Although limited divergence occurs with all laser beams, it is minimal enough to provide a small focal spot when the light is delivered through an optical system.

Monochromacy

Since the photons are emitted as a result of the release of energy between two defined levels of the atom, the resulting light has a narrow range of wavelengths.

High Intensity

The light amplification of a laser can produce a beam with significantly more intensity than the sun.

LASER-INDUCED TISSUE INTERACTIONS

The tissue effects produced by laser surgery are of three types: thermal, ionizing, and photochemical.[8]

Thermal Effects

In this situation, the target tissue is heated by absorption of laser energy to temperatures high enough to induce chemical changes that produce local inflammation and scarring (*photocoagulation*) or to vaporize intracellular and extracellular fluids, producing an incision in the tissue (*photovaporization*). Factors influencing the laser thermal effect include: (1) wavelength of the incident light; (2) duration of exposure; and (3) amount of light energy per area of exposure. Melanin, the pigment of most target tissues in glaucoma laser surgery, has a peak absorption in the blue-green portion of the visible spectrum. Therefore, lasers with wavelengths between 400–600 nm are most useful for these procedures, and the argon laser is the prototype photocoagulator.

The heat generated by the absorption of laser energy is dissipated by the surrounding tissue. A short exposure time and a high energy level/area reduce heat conduction, which causes tissue temperatures to reach the critical boiling point, producing gas bubbles with tissue disruption and photovaporization through a microexplosion. This reaction can be used to create holes in ocular tissues, as with laser iridotomy. At lower energy levels, photocoagulation may produce contraction of collagen, which is the mechanism of pupilloplasty and iridoplasty, and possibly of laser trabeculoplasty.

Ionizing Effects

If very intense laser energy is focused onto a very small area for a very short period of time, a reaction occurs that is independent of pigment absorption and is referred to as *photodisruption*. An instantaneous electric field is generated, which literally strips electrons from target atoms, producing a gaseous state, called "plasma."[7] As ionized atoms of a plasma recombine with free electrons, photons with a wide range of energies are emitted, producing a spark of incoherent white light. Associated shock and pressure waves create additional mechanical damage to target tissues, resulting in a reaction that can disrupt both pigmented and nonpigmented structures. Thermal effects are also involved in the mechanism of photodisruption.[9]

Neodymium:YAG lasers are the most commonly used photodisruptor. The pulse may be Q-switched or mode-locked, both of which have been shown to produce the same size rupture in polyethylene membranes.[9] The laser's main clinical use has been for the disruption, or cutting, of relatively transparent anterior segment structures, most notably the posterior lens capsule. In glaucoma surgery its primary use is for creating iridotomies, although an additional application is the reestablishment of filtering procedures by cutting scar tissue in the fistula. Neodymium:YAG lasers can also be used in a pulsed thermal or continuous wave mode for transscleral cyclophotocoagulation.

Photochemical Effects

The target tissue can be volatilized by short-pulsed ultraviolet radiation (*photoablation*), while tumor tissue can be photosensitized with hematoporphyrin and selectively destroyed with red laser light of a specific wavelength (*photodynamic therapy* or *photoradiation*).

LASER DELIVERY SYSTEMS

Most laser units use a slit-lamp biomicroscope, in which a system of fiberoptics and/or mirrors in an articulated arm directs the laser beam from the laser tube, through the slit lamp, and into the patient's eye (Fig. 32.2). Various types of contact lenses are normally used during laser surgery with slit-lamp delivery. Some contain mirrors to di-

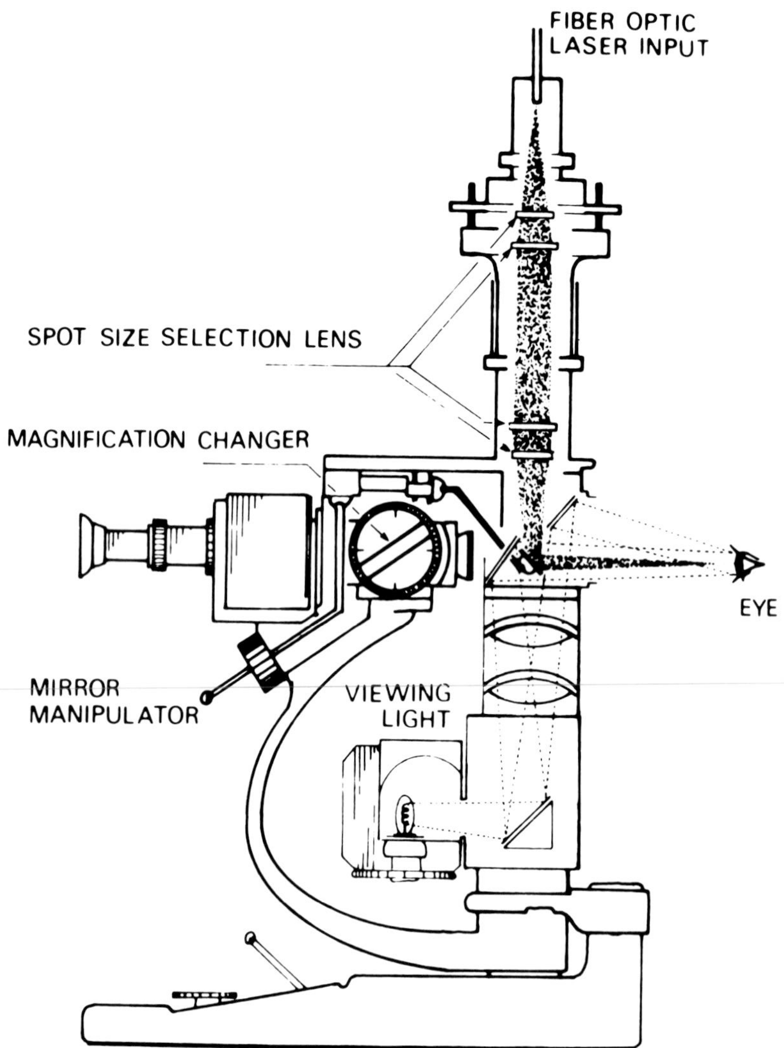

Figure 32.2. Schematic of slit-lamp delivery system for ophthalmic lasers. Laser light enters the slit-lamp through a fiberoptic or system of mirrors and is reflected by mirrors in the slit lamp into the patient's eye. (Reprinted with permission from Sliney D, Wolbarsht M: Safety with Lasers and Other Optical Sources. A Comprehensive Handbook. New York, London, Plenum Press, 1980.)

rect the laser beam into the anterior chamber angle, while others incorporate convex lenses to concentrate the light energy on the iris. For lasers within the visual spectrum, an aiming beam of attenuated laser energy can be used to allow positioning and focusing of the laser beam on the target tissue. For lasers with wavelengths outside the visual spectrum, an additional laser such as the helium-neon is used as the aiming beam. A foot pedal or finger trigger is used to release the full laser energy, producing the tissue alteration.

Other laser delivery systems use contact probes attached to the fiberoptics, allowing application of laser energy to the ocular tissues either by placing the probe externally on the eye or by aiming directly at internal ocular structures with the probe tip in the eye. The variables on the control units of most laser systems include spot size (usually expressed in microns), exposure duration (expressed in tenths of seconds, milliseconds, microseconds, or nanoseconds), and energy (joules or millijoules) or power (energy multiplied by duration in seconds, expressed as watts or milliwatts).

SPECIFIC LASERS FOR GLAUCOMA SURGERY

Lasers differ primarily according to the medium in which the atoms exist that produce the stimulated emission of photons. The media in the lasers used most commonly for glaucoma surgery are argon and neodymium, although experience with many other lasers has also been reported.

Argon Lasers (Fig. 32.3)

The medium in these instruments is argon gas, which is pumped by an electrical discharge. The wavelengths are in the blue (488 nm) and green (514 nm) portions of the visible spectrum, which is optimum for absorption by melanin. Most argon lasers operate in the continuous wave mode and have maximum power levels of 2–6 watts. However, units are also available that produce pulses of approximately 100 microseconds with powers of 20–50 watts. The latter instruments achieve full power only as needed, which reduces heat build-up and improves energy efficiency. The short duration and high energy levels of pulsed argon lasers may have an advantage in the creation of iridotomies, since, unlike continuous wave laser energy, which causes coagulative necrosis around the central defect, the pulsed energy vaporizes iris tissue with less destruction to the surrounding area.

Neodymium:YAG Lasers (Fig. 32.4)

In these instruments, the neodymium atoms are embedded in a crystal of yttrium-aluminum-garnet (YAG) and are pumped by

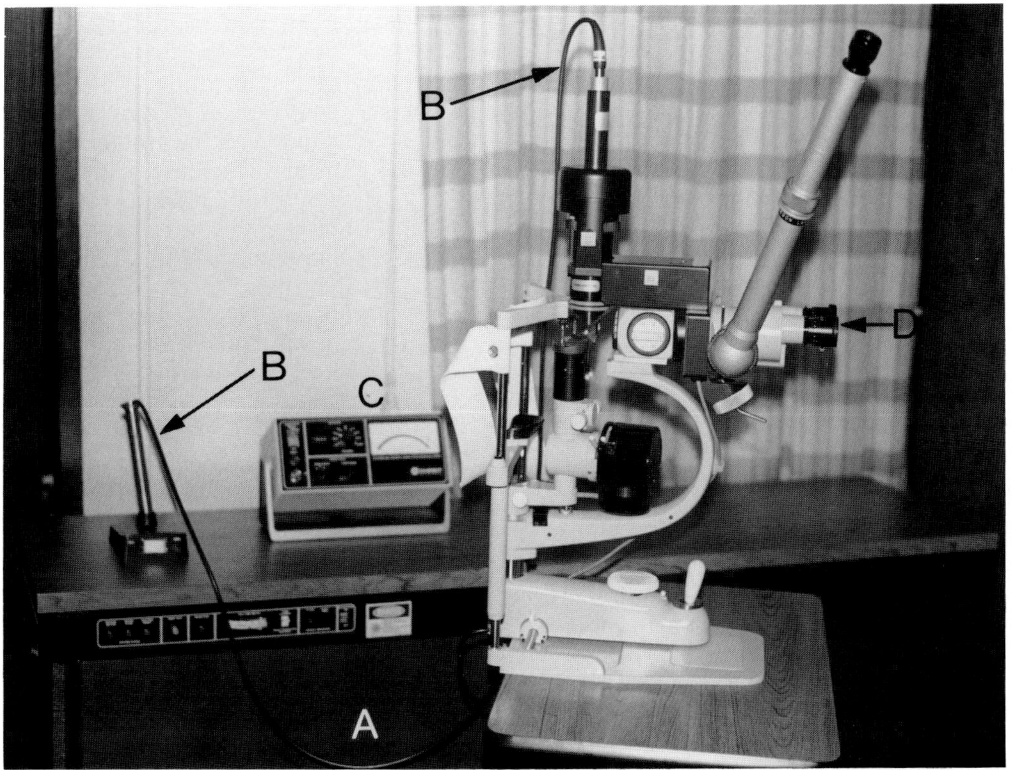

Figure 32.3. Continuous wave argon laser: housing for laser tube (*A*); laser fiberoptic (*B*); control panel (*C*); slit lamp (*D*).

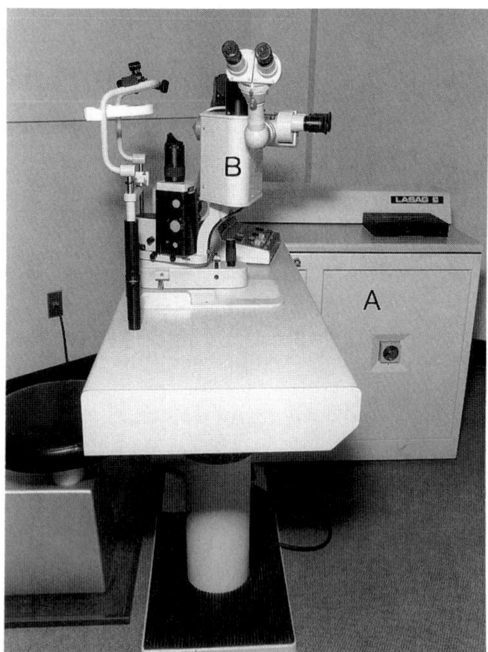

Figure 32.4. Neodymium:YAG laser: housing for laser tube (*A*); slit-lamp delivery system (*B*).

a xenon flash lamp. The laser wavelength is in the near-infrared (1064 nm) range, although it can be made a visible-light emitter by means of frequency doubling or an ultraviolet emitter by means of frequency tripling.[8] Neodymium:YAG lasers can be operated in the continuous wave mode to provide a photocoagulation effect, but they are more commonly used with pulsed delivery, using either Q-switching or mode-locking, to allow photodisruption of nonpigmented tissues.

Other Lasers

Many new lasers are being developed and evaluated for ocular surgery. Among these are the *dye lasers*, which are capable of producing monochromatic wavelengths at relatively high output powers through a large range of the visible spectrum. This allows the selection of a wavelength that would be most highly absorbed by the target tissue, thereby minimizing the transmittal of laser energy through the ocular media.[10] *Carbon dioxide lasers* in the infrared spectrum (10,600 nm) have been used in the continuous wave mode to cut tissue by means of vaporization with very little coagulation necrosis, while *eximer lasers* in the ultraviolet range (193 and 248 nm) are being evaluated in the pulsed mode to cut tissue with no visible necrosis. The *ruby laser* in the visible spectrum (694 nm) can produce photoablation with high-energy pulses, and the *krypton laser* in the yellow-red wavelength can be used for photocoagulation. As previously noted, the *helium-neon laser* in the red wavelength is used as an aiming beam in many laser systems that operate at nonvisible wavelengths.[8]

LASER SAFETY

The properties of laser energy, while providing an ideal tool for the surgical manipulation of tissues, also pose serious hazards, including electrical shock, direct laser burns, explosions, and fires. However, probably the most common and serious health hazard is accidental exposure of the retina, either directly or from reflected laser light.

The following classification of lasers is generally accepted regarding hazards:[11]

- Class I — Do not emit hazardous levels.
- Class II — Visible-light lasers that are safe for momentary viewing but should not be stared into continuously. An example is the aiming beam of ophthalmic lasers.
- Class III — Unsafe for even momentary viewing, requiring procedural controls and safety equipment.
- Class IV — Also pose a significant fire and skin hazard. Most therapeutic laser beams used in ocular surgery are in this class.

During glaucoma laser surgery, the patient has the greatest risk of injury from accidental exposure of the retina or lens. Techniques for avoiding these complications during specific laser procedures are discussed in subsequent chapters. The risk to the corneal endothelium has been evaluated with specular microscopy 1 year after laser trabeculoplasty or iridotomy, which showed a significant increase in cell size in one study[12] but no statistically significant changes in another study.[13]

The surgeon is protected during each exposure of therapeutic laser energy by a filter that is built into the delivery system. Aside from the patient, therefore, the individuals at greatest risk of retinal burns are other personnel in the laser room during the treatment, whose eyes may be exposed to reflected laser light. One study with argon lasers and various contact lenses indicated that the operator is not exposed to hazardous levels through the slit lamp, but that a hazard can exist for a bystander at the side of the slit lamp who is exposed to unattenuated back reflections of the treatment beam within 1 meter of the contact lens.[14] To minimize this hazard, only antireflective coated contact lenses should be used, ancillary personnel should wear protective goggles or look away from the laser when it is in use, and access to the laser room should be limited to necessary individuals during the treatment.

SUMMARY

Lasers operate on the principle that excited atoms can be stimulated to emit photons, resulting in a markedly amplified light that possesses the unique properties of coherence, collimation, monochromacy, and high intensity. The nature of this light allows precise alteration of tissues by means of thermal effects (photocoagulation and photovaporization), ionizing effects (photodisruption), and photochemical effects (photoablation and photodynamic therapy or photoradiation). These tissue interactions, especially photocoagulation and photodisruption, are used in a wide variety of glaucoma surgical procedures.

References

1. Meyer-Schwickerath, G: Light Coagulation (translated by Drance, SM). CV Mosby, St. Louis, 1960.
2. Maiman, TH: Stimulated optical radiation in ruby. Nature 187:493, 1960.
3. L'Esperance, FA Jr: Ophthalmic Lasers. Photocoagulation, Photoradiation, and Surgery, 2nd ed. CV Mosby, St. Louis, 1983.
4. Belcher, CD, Thomas, JV, Simmons, RJ: Photocoagulation in Glaucoma and Anterior Segment Disease. Williams and Wilkins, Baltimore, 1984.
5. Schwartz, L, Spaeth, G, Brown, G: Laser Therapy of the Anterior Segment. A Practical Approach. Slack Inc., Thorofare, 1984.
6. Peyman, GA, Raichand, M, Zeimer, RC: Ocular effects of various laser wavelengths. Surv Ophthal 28:391, 1984.
7. Mainster, MA, Sliney, DH, Belcher, CD III, Buzney, SM: Laser photodisruptors. Damage mechanisms, instrument design and safety. Ophthalmology 90:973, 1983.
8. Council on Scientific Affairs: Lasers in medicine and surgery. JAMA 256:900, 1986.
9. Vogel, A, Hentschel, W, Holzfuss, J, Lauterborn, W: Cavitation bubble dynamics and acoustic transient generation in ocular surgery with pulsed Neodymium:YAG lasers. Ophthalmology 93:1259, 1986.
10. L'Esperance, FA Jr: Clinical photocoagulation with the organic dye laser. A preliminary communication. Arch Ophthal 103:1312, 1985.
11. Sliney, D, Wolbarsht, M: Safety with Lasers and Other Optical Sources. A Comprehensive Handbook. Plenum Press, New York, 1980.
12. Hong, C, Kitazawa, Y, Tanishima, T: Influence of argon laser treatment of glaucoma on corneal endothelium. Jap J Ophthal 27:567, 1983.
13. Thoming, C, Van Buskirk, EM, Samples, JR: The corneal endothelium after laser therapy for glaucoma. Am J Ophthal 103:518, 1987.
14. Sliney, DH, Mainster, MA: Potential laser hazards to the clinician during photocoagulation. Am J Ophthal 103:758, 1987.

Chapter 33

PRINCIPLES OF INCISIONAL SURGERY

A division between laser surgery for glaucoma and the more traditional glaucoma operations is becoming more and more artificial. The latter surgical category was originally distinguished by the term "conventional surgery", although laser techniques have now become the more conventional forms of surgery for glaucoma, prompting the need to reconsider our terminology. "Invasive surgery" is not a satisfactory alternative, since invading the eye with a laser beam can cause just as much tissue alteration as invading it with a knife. The term "incisional surgery", as used in this text, is not fully satisfactory either, since some of the newer laser procedures include incisional techniques. The fact is that, as laser technology continues to expand, the day will undoubtedly come when all glaucoma surgery will include laser instruments. For these reasons, the chapters that follow combine laser and incisional procedures under general surgical categories, and this chapter, while it pertains primarily to incisional techniques, actually relates to both disciplines of glaucoma surgery.

WOUND HEALING

The incision of any tissue is followed by a complex process that attempts to heal the wound. The desire in most operations is to achieve complete, strong wound healing. However, for the glaucoma surgeon who is performing a filtering procedure, excessive wound healing can be a detriment, leading to failure of the operation. In this chapter we will consider some general aspects of wound healing, while specifics related to filtering surgery and measures to prevent excessive scarring are discussed in Chapter 36.

It may help to think of the complex, and only partly understood, process of wound healing in four phases: (1) clot phase; (2) proliferative phase; (3) granulation phase; (4) collagen phase.

Clot Phase

Almost immediately after a tissue incision, blood vessels constrict and leak blood cells and plasma proteins, which include fibrinogen, fibronectin, and plasminogen. Under the influence of certain tissue factors, these blood elements clot to form a gel-like fibrin-fibronectin matrix.[1]

Proliferative Phase

Inflammatory cells, including monocytes and macrophages, along with fibroblasts and new capillaries, migrate into the clot. In a rabbit model of filtering surgery, fibroblasts were seen to migrate from episcleral tissue, epimysium of the superior rectus, and subconjunctival connective tissue,[2] and in a monkey model they were proliferating along the walls of the limbal fistula by day 6.[3] Using the incorporation of tritiated thymidine as a marker of cell division to study the time course of cellular proliferation following filtering surgery in monkeys, incorporation was detected as early as 24 hours postoperatively, peaked in 5 days, and returned to baseline by day 11.[4]

Granulation Phase

As the fibrin-fibronectin clot is degraded by inflammatory cells, the fibroblasts begin to synthesize fibronectin, interstitial collagens, and glycosaminoglycans to form young fibrovascular connective tissue, or granulation tissue.[1] In the rabbit model, granulation tissue was seen in the fistula by the 3rd day,[2] while in the monkey model it was lining the fistula by at least day 10.[3]

Collagen Phase

Procollagen is synthesized intracellularly by fibroblasts and is then secreted into the extracellular spaces, where it undergoes biochemical transformation into tropocollagen. The tropocollagen molecules aggregate into immature soluble collagen fibrils, which then undergo cross-linking to form mature collagen. Blood vessels are eventually partly reabsorbed and fibroblasts largely disappear, leaving a dense collagenous scar with scattered fibroblasts and blood vessels.[1]

ANESTHESIA

While most laser procedures require only topical anesthesia, incisional surgery and some glaucoma laser operations require local anesthesia. Some surgeons prefer general anesthesia, although this usually is reserved for children or adults in whom cooperation or other considerations do not permit surgery under local anesthesia.

Local Anesthesia

Commonly used injectable anesthetics include *lidocaine*, *bupivacaine*, and *mepivacaine*. When compared on the basis of induced lid akinesia, these three agents were found to be similar with regard to onset (less than 6 minutes) and depth of anesthesia, while bupivacaine had the longest duration of effect (up to 6 hours, compared with 90 minutes for mepivacaine and 15–30 minutes for lidocaine).[5] In an evaluation of combined agents, 0.5% bupivacaine, 2% lidocaine, and 1:100,000 epinephrine were more effective in producing lid and globe akinesia than bupivacaine alone or the two anesthetics without epinephrine.[6] Bupivacaine alone was slower in producing anesthesia but was more effective in producing akinesia than the two anesthetics combined without epinephrine. The three combinations were similar with regard to frequency of pain during a 30-minute operation and the need for analgesia 6 hours postoperatively.

Epinephrine may enhance the effect of local anesthetics, presumably by minimizing systemic spread from the injection site by its vasoconstrictive action. However, it may also impose an additional risk in glaucomatous eyes by reducing vascular perfusion to an already compromised optic nerve head. Another supplement to local anesthesia that does appear to be safe and effective is *hyaluronidase*, which serves to improve local tissue spread within the injection site by breaking down the connective tissue ground substances.

While retrobulbar and orbicularis anesthesia are traditionally given as separate injections, it has been shown that the retrobulbar injection alone provides adequate facial akinesia in the vast majority of cases,[7] and this has also been my experience. For the retrobulbar injection, an Atkinson needle has the advantages of being short and blunt, both of which help avoid retrobulbar hemorrhage. An injection of 3–5 cc of a 50-50 mixture of 0.75% bupivacaine and 2–4% lidocaine with hyaluronidase usually provides adequate anesthesia and akinesia. Firm pressure to the globe for 30 seconds after the injection may also help to minimize retrobulbar hemorrhage by tamponading any small bleeding vessel.

Adjuncts to Local Anesthesia

Although general anesthesia is not commonly used in glaucoma surgery, it is advisable to routinely use the assistance of an anesthesiologist or anesthetist to monitor the patient's vital signs and provide adjunctive medications as required. The latter may include short-acting analgesics, such as fentanyl citrate, and short-acting central nervous system depressants, such as midazolam HCl, for sedation. In addition, ultrashort-acting barbiturate anesthetics, such as methohexital sodium (Brevitol), can be administered intravenously to provide a few minutes of sleep while the retrobulbar injection is being given.

INSTRUMENTS

The instruments used in incisional glaucoma surgery vary considerably from one procedure to the next as well as among surgeons, and the subject is beyond the scope of this book. However, it may be helpful to consider some of the basic principles.

Hemostasis

As noted earlier in this chapter, bleeding is the first step in the wound healing process, which can lead to excessive, detrimental scarring, especially in glaucoma filtering surgery. Therefore, it is desirable in all surgical procedures to minimize bleeding. This is first done, of course, by trying to avoid large vessels, such as the anterior ciliary arteries near the insertions of the rectus muscles. When bleeding does occur, it should be continuously flushed from the surgical site with a gentle stream of balanced salt solution. Small bleeders may eventually close spontaneously, although most require cauterization. An ideal cautery unit for glaucoma surgery is the small-diameter, wet-field, bipolar instrument used for intraocular diathermy. This provides adequate cauterization of episcleral bleeders without excessive tissue charring or contraction and can also be used at lower energy levels to cauterize intraocular bleeding, as from the ciliary body or iris.

Tissue Handling

Most glaucoma surgery is performed on the extraocular tissues of the anterior ocular segment. Gentle handling of these tissues is essential to avoid tearing the conjunctiva or cutting more tissue than necessary, which can also increase the risks of excessive scarring. In this regard, it is helpful to use smooth-tipped forceps to grasp the conjunctiva firmly without piercing or tearing it. When dissecting conjunctiva, it is best to use a blunt dissecting instrument when possible and cut tissue with scissors or a blade only when necessary. Details regarding specific instruments for the various surgical procedures is provided in the following chapters that deal with those operations.

Suturing

To minimize excessive inflammatory reaction and subsequent scarring, it is important to select suture material with the least tendency to induce tissue reaction. For corneoscleral suturing, 9-0 or 10-0 nylon on a fine, cutting needle may be the most satisfactory. For the conjunctiva, however, polyglycolic acid or polygalactin sutures are nearly as nonreactive as nylon and have the advantage of biodegradation. It is also important to use a needle that will not tear or leave a large hole in the conjunctiva. Fine, tapered, noncutting needles are available on the fine, biodegradable sutures, and they are excellent for all conjunctival work.

SUMMARY

The wound healing process following the incision of a tissue includes clot formation, cellular proliferation, granulation tissue formation, and the synthesis and maturation of collagen. Most incisional glaucoma surgery is performed under local anesthesia, with agents such as lidocaine and bupivacaine. Epinephrine, as a supplement, is usually avoided because of the risk to the optic nerve head, although hyaluronidase may be useful as a tissue spreading factor. In selecting the optimum instruments for incisional glaucoma surgery, consideration should be given to adequate hemostasis, gentle wound handling, and the proper suture and needle for wound closure.

References

1. Skuta, GL, Parrish, RK II: Wound healing in glaucoma filtering surgery. Surv Ophthal 32:149, 1987.
2. Miller, MH, Grierson, I, Unger, WI, Hitchings, RA:

Wound healing in an animal model of glaucoma fistulizing surgery in the rabbit. Ophthal Surg 20:350, 1989.

3. Desjardins, DC, Parrish, RK II, Folberg, R, et al: Wound healing after filtering surgery in owl monkeys. Arch Ophthal 104:1835, 1986.
4. Jampel, HD, McGuigan, LJB, Dunkelberger, GR, et al: Cellular proliferation after experimental glaucoma filtration surgery. Arch Ophthal 106:89, 1988.
5. Parrish, RK II, Spaeth, GL, Poryzees, EM, Hargens, CW: Evaluation of local anesthetic agents using a new force-sensitive lid speculum. Ophthal Surg 14:575, 1983.
6. Vettese, T, Breslin, CW: Retrobulbar anesthesia for cataract surgery: comparison of bupivacaine and bupivacaine/lidocaine combinations. Can J Ophthal 20:131, 1985.
7. Martin, SR, Baker, SS, Muenzler, WS: Retrobulbar anesthesia and orbicularis akinesia. Ophthal Surg 17:232, 1986.

Chapter 34

SURGERY OF THE ANTERIOR CHAMBER ANGLE

In this chapter we will consider the laser and incisional operations that are designed to reduce the intraocular pressure (IOP) through increased aqueous outflow by treating specific structures within the anterior chamber angle.

LASER TRABECULOPLASTY

Historical Background

In 1961, Zweng and Flocks[1] introduced the concept of applying light energy to the anterior chamber angle for the treatment of glaucoma. Using the xenon arc photocoagulator of Meyer-Schwickerath, they selectively coagulated the filtration angles of cats, dogs, and monkeys and reported subsequent lowering of the IOP. Histopathologic examination of the treated tissue revealed fragmentation of the trabecular lamellae, atrophy of ciliary muscle, and destruction of ciliary processes. However, little more was said about this technique until more than a decade later, when several investigators revived the concept by using the light energy of the laser. Yet another decade of investigative work would elapse before the operation would achieve widespread clinical popularity.

In the early 1970s, reports began to appear from several parts of the world, most notably from Krasnov[2] in Russia, Hager[3] in Germany, Demailly and associates[4] in France, and Worthen and Wickham[5] in the United States, regarding attempts to improve aqueous outflow by puncturing holes in the trabecular meshwork with laser energy. Although trabecular perforations were achieved, they eventually closed in most cases as a result of fibrosis, and IOP reduction was usually temporary. The value of laser treatment to the trabecular meshwork came under further question when, in 1975, Gaasterland and Kupfer[6] reported that experimental glaucoma could be produced by applying argon laser energy to the meshwork of rhesus monkeys. However, the following year Ticho and Zauberman[7] noted that long-term reduction in IOP occurred in some patients despite the lack of permanent trabecular openings. This led to a new concept in laser trabecular therapy in which lower energy levels were used to photocoagulate, rather than to penetrate, portions of the meshwork. In 1979, Wise and Witter[8] described the first successful protocol of what has become known as laser trabeculoplasty. Their preliminary work was corroborated in 1981,[9–11] and in less than 5 years laser trabeculoplasty became the most commonly performed operation for glaucoma.

Theories of Mechanism

Tonographic studies indicate that laser trabeculoplasty reduces IOP by improving the facility of outflow,[12–16] while fluorophotometric investigations show no significant influence on aqueous production.[14,17,18] Although fluorescein leakage into the anterior chamber, suggesting a breakdown in the blood-aqueous barrier, is seen during the first week after trabeculoplasty, it is gone within 1 month and does not seem to be a factor in the long-term effect of this procedure.[19]

The mechanism of improved aqueous outflow facility by laser trabeculoplasty is uncertain. Wise and Witter[8] originally postulated that the thermal energy produced by pigment absorption of laser light caused shrinkage of collagen in the trabecular lamellae. They believed that the subsequent shortening of the treated meshwork might enlarge existing spaces between two treatment sites or expand Schlemm's canal by pulling the meshwork centrally. While this is still the most popular theory, laboratory studies have suggested alternative or additional mechanisms of action.

Electron microscopic evaluations of trabecular meshwork from human eyes, obtained hours to weeks after trabeculoplasty, revealed disruption of trabecular beams, fibrinous material, and necrosis of occasional cells, followed by shrinkage of the collagenous components of the meshwork.[20,21] Surviving endothelial cells near the laser lesions showed phagocytic and migratory activity.[21] Specimens obtained several months after therapy had partial or total occlusion of intertrabecular spaces by a monocellular layer.[20,21]

Studies with monkeys have provided observations similar to those noted in humans, with some additional insight into the mechanism of laser trabeculoplasty. Within the first few hours there is disruption of the trabecular beams and coagulative necrosis with accumulation of debris in the juxtacanalicular region.[22] Surviving trabecular endothelial cells are noted to have increased phagocytic activity with removal of tissue debris[22] and increased cell division.[23] By 1 month, the treated regions are flat with collapsed beams and are covered with corneal endothelium.[24] The latter is more likely to occur when the laser energy is applied to the anterior portion of the trabecular meshwork.[25] Perfusion with ferritin shows lack of flow through the treated meshwork, with diversion of flow through the adjacent nonlasered meshwork, which becomes structurally altered to compensate for the overload of flow.[26] It has also been suggested that concomitant collagen degeneration and loss of trabecular cells may widen the intertrabecular spaces with improved outflow.[27]

Studies of human autopsy eyes treated with laser trabeculoplasty revealed a significant reduction in the trabecular cell density and an alteration of radioactive sulfate incorporation into the extracellular matrix of lasered eyes.[28] The authors postulated that laser trabeculoplasty eliminates some trabecular cells, which may stimulate the remaining cells to produce a different composition of extracellular matrix with less outflow-obstructing properties. Studies with a human corneoscleral explant organ culture system indicate that laser trabeculoplasty causes an early trabecular endothelial cell division in the anterior meshwork, with migration of the new cells to repopulate the burn sites over the next few weeks.[29,30]

While the precise mechanism of laser trabeculoplasty remains only partly understood, it appears to include, as postulated by Van Buskirk,[31] a complex interaction of mechanical, cellular, and biochemical properties.

Techniques

Instrumentation

The continuous-wave argon laser unit is the standard instrument for laser trabeculoplasty. It is customarily operated in the blue-green, biochromatic wavelength spectrum (454.5–528.7 nm). When compared with the use of green, monochromatic laser light (514.5 nm), no differences were noted in the postoperative IOP course or incidence of complications.[32,33] A krypton laser, with red (647.1 nm) or yellow (568.2 nm) wavelengths, was also effective in preliminary trials of laser trabeculoplasty,[34] although one comparative study showed the argon laser to be significantly more effective.[33] Preliminary experience with the neodymium:YAG laser in the thermal mode revealed tissue responses in monkey eyes that were similar but deeper into the meshwork than those produced by argon laser,[27] while tonographic studies in a clinical trial revealed increased outflow correlating with the fall in IOP.[16]

A contact lens with a mirror for visualization of the anterior chamber angle (gonioprism) is used in trabeculoplasty. As with all contact lenses for laser application, it should have an antireflection coating on the front surface. A standard Goldmann-type three-mirror lens, in which one mirror is inclined at 59° for gonioscopy, or a single-mirror gonioscopy lens can be used. However, both have the slight disadvantage of requiring rotation of the lens to view all quadrants of the anterior chamber angle. This objection can be eliminated by use of the Thorpe four-mirror gonioscopy lens, in which all mirrors are inclined at 62°, or the Ritch trabeculoplasty laser lens, in which two mirrors are inclined at 59° for viewing the inferior quadrants and two at 64° for the superior angle (Fig. 34.1).[35,36] In the latter lens, a 17-diopter plano-convex button lens over two mirrors provides 1.4× magnification, reducing a 50-micron laser spot to 35 microns, which may be particularly useful, since a 50-micron spot size with most argon lasers produces a burn in excess of 70 microns.[37]

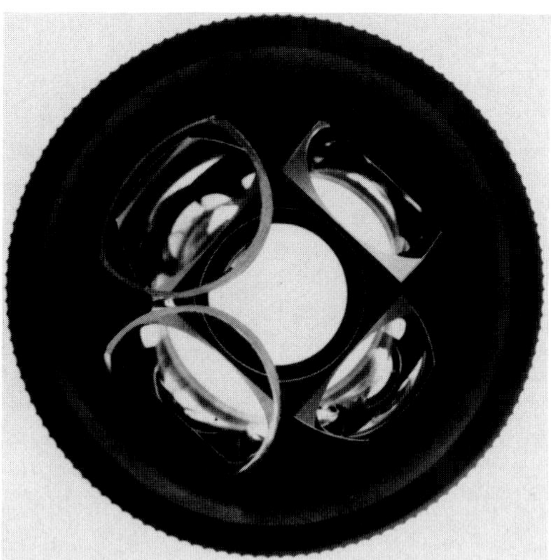

Figure 34.1. Ritch trabeculoplasty laser lens. (Reprinted with permission from Ritch R: Ophthal Surg 16:331, 1985.)

Gonioscopic Considerations

Successful laser trabeculoplasty requires accurate identification and treatment of the trabecular meshwork. Therefore, the surgeon must have a detailed knowledge of the anterior chamber angle anatomy and its many variations. The basic aspects of this subject were covered in Chapters 3 and 31, and we shall now consider some additional features that are pertinent to laser trabeculoplasty.

Two variations of the anterior chamber angle that may interfere with accurate laser application to the trabecular meshwork are (1) the degree of pigmentation and (2) the width of the chamber angle. With regard to pigmentation, some angles are so diffusely pigmented from the ciliary body band to Schwalbe's line that the exact location of the meshwork is obscured (Fig. 34.2). This is usually most marked in the inferior quadrants, and a careful inspection of all quadrants before starting treatment will usually disclose the position of the meshwork in some areas, which can then be used as a guide in locating the meshwork in the remainder of the angle. At the opposite extreme, the trabecular meshwork in some angles is so lightly pigmented that it is hard to see (Fig. 34.3). In some cases, iris processes, which normally extend to the meshwork, may be a useful indicator. Identification of the ciliary body band or Schwalbe's line may also help determine the relative position of the meshwork.

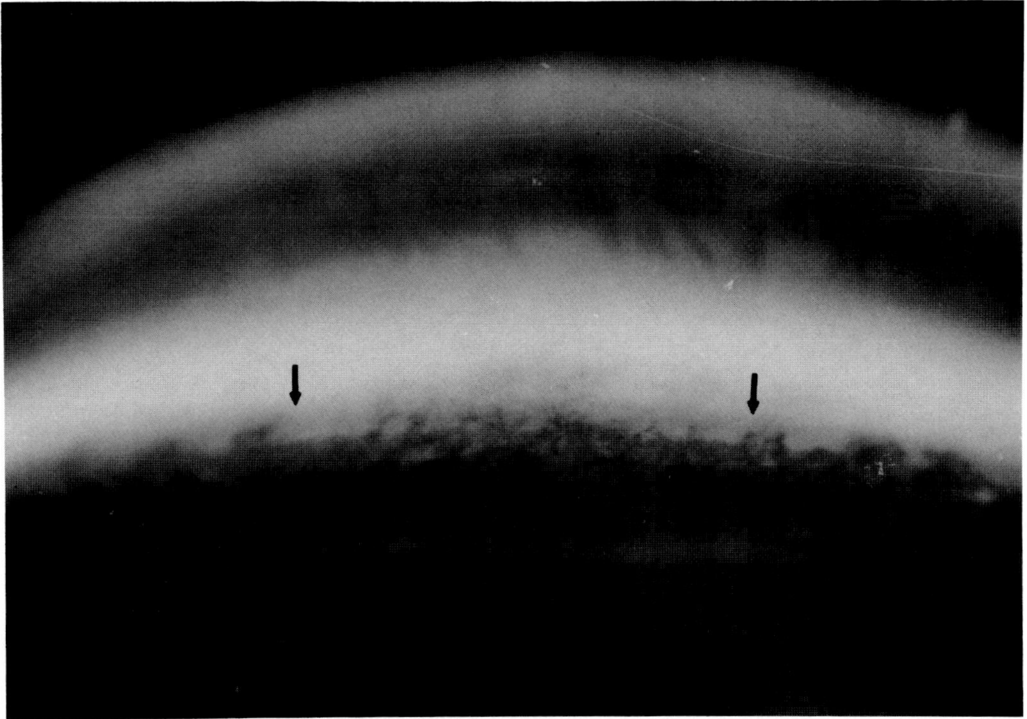

Figure 34.2. Gonioscopic view of wide open anterior chamber angle, in which heavy pigmentation interferes with precise location of the trabecular meshwork (*arrows*).

A narrow anterior chamber angle can lead to improper placement of the laser burns or may prohibit performing trabeculoplasty. If visualization of the meshwork is obscured by peripheral iris, a heavily pigmentated Schwalbe's line may be mistaken for the meshwork. Rotating the contact lens horizontally or vertically in relation to the eye, by asking the patient to look in the direction of the mirror being used, often provides a deeper view into the angle, enhancing visualization of the meshwork. Care must be taken with this maneuver not to distort the size and shape of the aiming beam. If positioning of the contact lens is not sufficient to expose the meshwork, it may be possible to deepen the chamber angle by applying low-energy laser burns to the peripheral iris, a technique called iridoplasty or gonioplasty. If the angle is still too narrow, a laser iridotomy should be performed, and the trabeculoplasty should be done at a later date. The techniques of iridoplasty and iridotomy are discussed in the next chapter.

Basic Protocol

The original protocol of Wise and Witter[8] has remained the standard approach to laser trabeculoplasty, against which variations in technique have been evaluated. A 25× magnification in the slit-lamp delivery system usually provides an optimum balance between detail and field of view. Argon laser settings of 0.1-second duration exposure and 50-micron beam diameter have remained constant through most variations in protocol. One study compared durations of 0.2 to 0.1 seconds and found no advantage to the former.[38] The most commonly used power levels range between 700 and 1500 milliwatts (mW). One study evaluated powers ranging from 100 mW to 1000 mW and found that powers of more than 500 mW gave the maximum success rates.[39] The power should be adjusted to produce a depigmentation spot or a small gas bubble at the treatment site (Fig. 34.4). This response is influenced by the amount of pigment in the trabecular meshwork. With a heavily

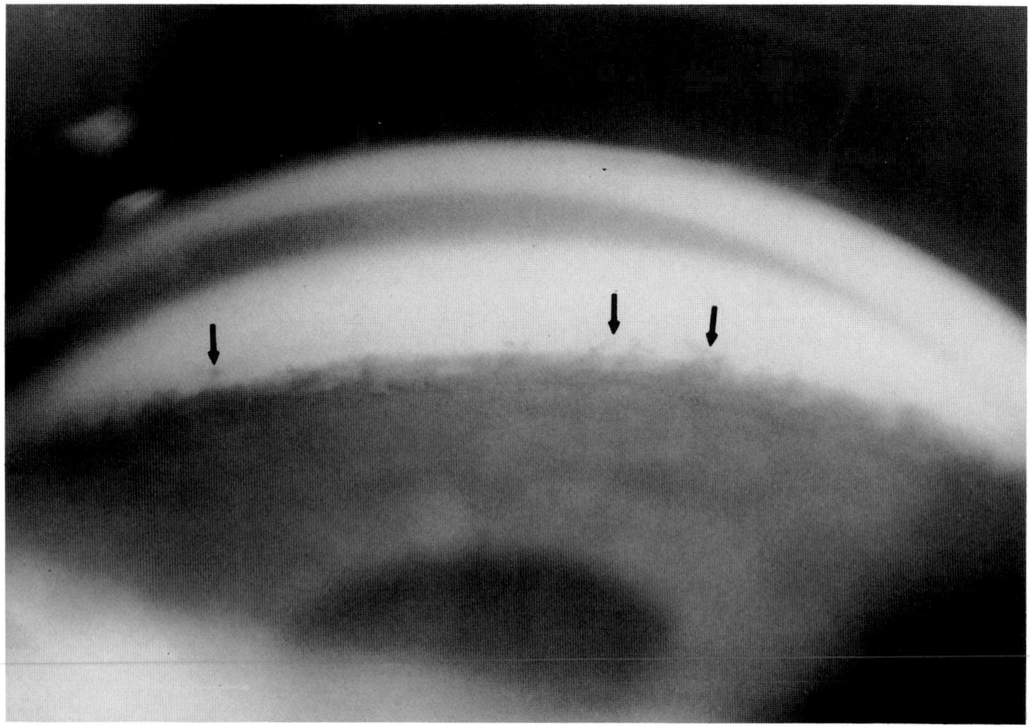

Figure 34.3. Gonioscopic view of wide open anterior chamber angle, in which scant pigmentation hampers identification of trabecular meshwork. In this case, iris processes (*arrows*) help determine the position of the meshwork.

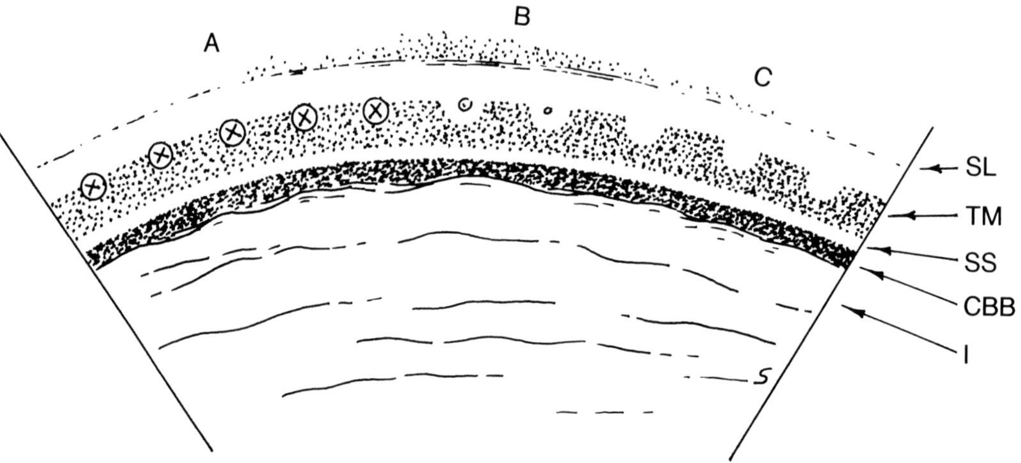

Figure 34.4. Placement of laser burns (*A*) along anterior portion of trabecular meshwork (*TM*). Desired visual result is depigmentation of the treatment site (*B,C*) and/or a small gas bubble (*B*). Schwalbe's line (*SL*), scleral spur (*SS*), ciliary body band (*CBB*), iris (*I*).

pigmented meshwork, a lower power level may be sufficient, while lightly pigmented meshworks require higher levels.

Originally, laser burns were applied onto or immediately posterior to the pigmented band of the trabecular meshwork, with approximately 100 applications evenly spaced around the full 360° of the meshwork.[8] However, complications associated with this basic protocol have led to variations in technique. We will first consider the complications and then the variations in technique that have been used to minimize them.

Complications

Transient IOP elevation. Transient IOP elevation in the immediate postoperative period is the most serious early complication of laser trabeculoplasty.[40–45] In most cases, the pressure rise is mild and lasts less than 24 hours, causing no long-term problems. However, in some patients the elevation is marked and sustained and can lead to further loss of vision, especially in eyes with advanced visual field loss before trabeculoplasty. The IOP rise occurs within 2 hours after treatment in most cases, although some eyes may not develop an increase until 4–7 hours after therapy.[43,44] Therefore, the 1-hour posttreatment pressure check is essential, and eyes with advanced damage may require close observation during the first 24 hours.

The main patient characteristic associated with the transient pressure rise is meshwork pigmentation.[45] Two patients with exfoliation syndrome had a delayed IOP rise during the first postlaser month, associated with inflammatory precipitates on the trabecular meshwork.[46] It should also be noted that eyes with active inflammation are at a high risk of marked IOP rise after laser trabeculoplasty, and the operation is contraindicated in these eyes.

Histopathologic studies suggest that the mechanism of posttrabeculoplasty pressure rise is an inflammatory reaction, with fibrinous material and tissue debris in the meshwork.[20,22,47,48]

Iritis. Iritis is a common early postoperative complication but is usually mild and transient and easily controlled with a brief postoperative course of topical corticosteroids.

Late Structural Alterations. The formation of *peripheral anterior synechiae* is also common.[49] These are typically small and tented, corresponding to the location of the laser applications. One study of corneal endothelium after laser trabeculoplasty revealed a significant increase in cell size,[50] while another showed no statistically significant changes.[51]

Late effect on glaucoma. The most serious late posttrabeculoplasty complication is, at the present time, more theoretical than real. As previously described, histopathologic studies show changes in the trabecular meshwork, including an endothelial layer over the inner surface (Fig. 34.5), which could eventually lead to an increase in resistance to aqueous outflow.[20,21,24,25] Whether the glaucoma in eyes treated with laser trabeculoplasty will one day become more difficult to control, as a result of these structural changes, is a question that awaits studies with longer periods of follow-up. There has also been concern that laser trabeculoplasty might interfere with the success rate of subsequent filtering surgery, although this did not appear to be the case in one study.[52]

Variations in Technique

Operative Measures

The parameters evaluated most extensively have been the total number of laser applications and the amount of trabecular meshwork that is treated. Applying 25 burns to 90° of the meshwork appears to be less effective than protocols with larger amounts of treatment.[53,54] However, the application of 50 burns to either 180° or 360° was found to have an effect on IOP reduction similar to that of treatment of 100 burns to 360° of the meshwork.[54–56] A two-stage protocol, in which treatment of the full 360° circumference is divided into two sessions 1 month apart, gave the same reduction in IOP as the full treatment in one session.[57] With this technique, most of the pressure reduction is achieved with the first stage of therapy, although some patients may have minimal benefit from stage one and yet a substantial pressure reduction after stage two of ther-

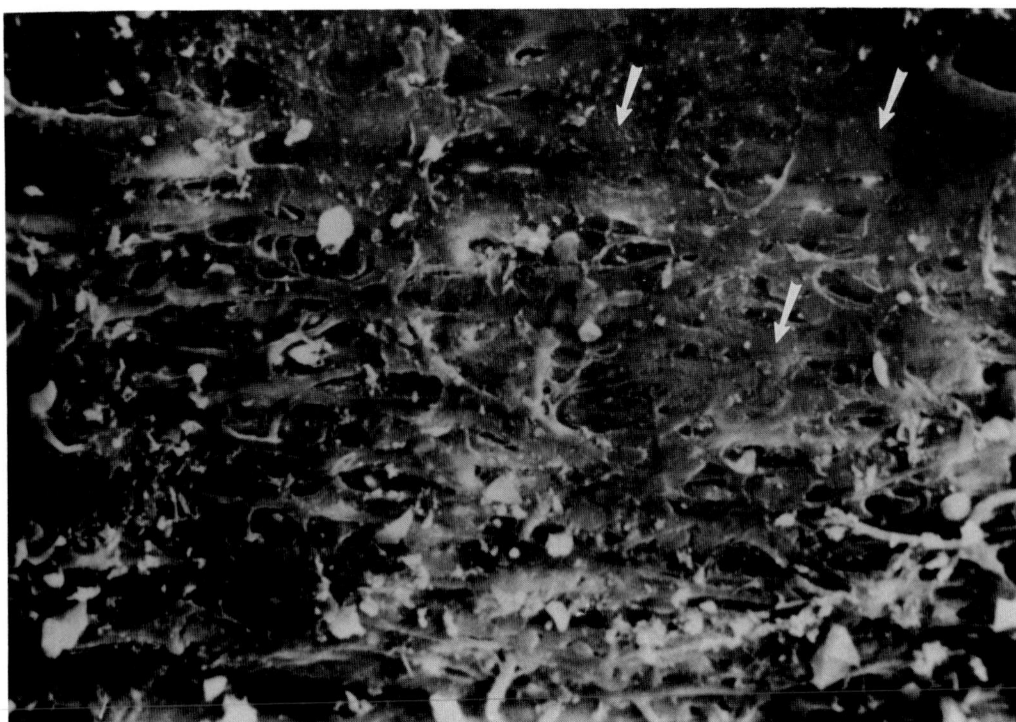

Figure 34.5. Scanning electron microscopic view of trabeculectomy specimen from eye with failed argon laser trabeculoplasty showing endothelial growth over portions of the intertrabecular spaces (*arrows*).

apy.[58] The main advantage of the lower number of laser applications during a single session is a reduction in the transient IOP rise during the immediate postoperative period.[40,41,54–59] It has also been shown that power settings in the higher ranges of 800 mW or more are associated with a higher incidence of IOP rise[60,61] and peripheral anterior synechiae formation.[49]

Another variation in technique that appears to minimize the complication of early posttreatment pressure rise is the placement of the laser applications along the anterior portion of the pigmented meshwork (Fig. 34.6).[54,56,59] An anterior placement of the laser burns also reduces the complication of peripheral anterior synechiae formation.[49,62] However, it may increase the potential complication of cellular proliferation from the corneal endothelium over the trabecular meshwork.[25] One investigator reported success with laser applications to the ciliary body band, rather than the trabecular meshwork, to open Schlemm's canal by putting traction on the scleral spur.[63]

Pharmacologic Measures

Topical *corticosteroids* are believed to reduce the mild anterior uveitis that follows laser trabeculoplasty. A preparation such as 1% prednisolone four times daily is usually prescribed for the first 4–7 days after treatment in addition to preoperative antiglaucoma medications.

One drop of 4% pilocarpine immediately after the procedure was shown to be effective in minimizing the IOP rise.[64] Subsequently, however, topical application of the alpha$_2$-adrenergic agonist 1% *apraclonidine* 1 hour before and immediately after laser trabeculoplasty was shown to have a marked effect on minimizing the postoperative pressure rise.[65] This has now become a standard part of laser trabeculoplasty for most surgeons. So profound is the benefit of apraclonidine that two sessions of 180°

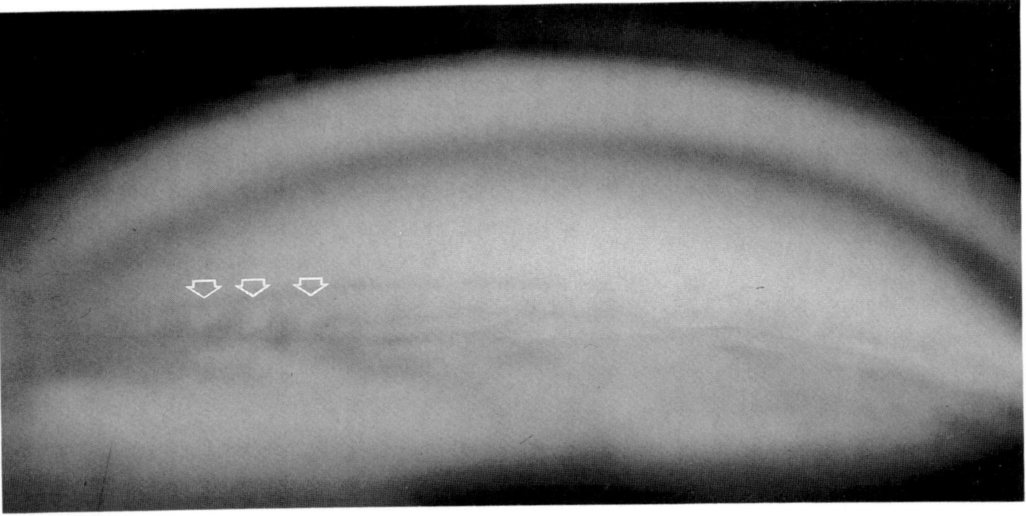

Figure 34.6. Gonioscopic view of depigmentation sites (*arrows*) along anterior margin of trabecular meshwork immediately after argon laser trabeculoplasty.

treatment each may no longer be necessary to avoid the transient IOP rise.

Acetazolamide has also been shown to reduce the IOP rise following laser trabeculoplasty.[66] However, neither corticosteroids[67] nor the prostaglandin synthetase inhibitors indomethacin[68–70] or flurbiprofen[71] significantly influenced the postoperative IOP. One study actually showed that patients receiving topical indomethacin had higher pressures after 1 month than those receiving a placebo.[69] Prostaglandin synthetase inhibitors also appear to have no influence on the postoperative iritis.[68,72]

Results

Short-Term IOP Control

Most reports show that useful IOP reduction is achieved in approximately 85% of eyes treated with laser trabeculoplasty.[8–11,13,40,73] Some eyes may have a pressure drop within the first few hours after treatment, although days or weeks are usually required to achieve the full response to trabeculoplasty, with further pressure reduction rarely occurring beyond 1 month. The magnitude of the final pressure reduction averages 6–9 mm Hg, which is usually not sufficient to allow discontinuation of all medical therapy, although the medication can occasionally be reduced or eliminated.[74] Trabeculoplasty has also been shown to reduce the diurnal pressure curve by approximately 25%.[75]

Factors Influencing IOP Response

Many factors influence the IOP response to laser trabeculoplasty. Eyes with higher *pretreatment pressures* tend to have a greater fall in IOP.[76] Despite this fact, a pretreatment pressure higher than 30 mm Hg has been associated with a higher frequency of failures,[73,77] while eyes with "normal" tensions may obtain useful pressure reduction after trabeculoplasty.[78–80]

Another significant factor is the *type of glaucoma*. A particularly favorable response is obtained with primary open-angle glaucoma, exfoliation syndrome, and pigmentary glaucoma.[12,73,76,77,81–83] Success in the latter two conditions is most likely related to the favorable influence of increased trabecular meshwork pigmentation.[84] In pigmentary glaucoma, younger patients appear to have a more sustained pressure reduction than older patients with the same condition.[83] Other forms of glaucoma that respond to laser trabeculoplasty, although less well than those noted above, include open-angle glaucoma in aphakia and angle-closure glaucoma after an iridotomy.[81] While eyes that have had multiple operations generally do not do well with trabeculoplasty,[82] those with a single failed trabeculectomy may obtain useful pressure reduction after laser therapy.[85] Other forms of glaucoma that do not respond well to laser trabeculoplasty include glaucoma associated with uveitis, angle recession glaucoma, and congenital or juvenile glaucoma.[81,82,86]

Some investigators believe that young *age* has an unfavorable influence on the results of laser trabeculoplasty,[73,87] although no effect of age was seen in another study.[77] As previously noted, young patients with pigmentary glaucoma appear to do better than older patients with the same condition.[83] Black versus white race does not appear to influence the results of laser trabeculoplasty.[88]

Long-Term IOP Control

A major question regarding the results of laser trabeculoplasty is how long the IOP reduction will last. While short-term studies of up to 1 year have not shown a significant loss of pressure-lowering effect, studies with 3–10 year follow-up have revealed a gradual rise in IOP with loss of control in approximately 10% each postoperative year.[89–93] As a result, it can be anticipated that approximately half of the patients will have lost the benefit of the initial trabeculoplasty by 5 years following the surgery.

Repeat Trabeculoplasty

If a successful IOP reduction is never achieved following 360° laser trabeculoplasty, further laser therapy is generally not thought to be indicated. However, if an initial good response to treatment, lasting for approximately a year or more, is followed by a return to higher pressures, there may be value in repeating the surgery. Most studies have shown a much lower success rate with repeat trabeculoplasty than with the initial treatment, in the range of one-third to one-half,[94–99] although one investigation team reported success in 8 of 11 eyes with greater than 1 year follow-up.[100] Some studies have noted a higher incidence of transient pressure rise following repeat laser trabeculoplasty,[94,95] and it is probably advisable to perform these in two stages of 180° each.

Indications

Laser trabeculoplasty may be indicated in the treatment of those forms of open-angle glaucoma in which favorable responses have been reported, including primary open-angle glaucoma, the exfoliation syndrome, pigmentary glaucoma, and glaucoma in aphakia or pseudophakia. During the first decade of experience with laser trabeculoplasty, the procedure was used as a supplement to maximum tolerable medical therapy and studies have shown it to be effective in this regard.[40,101] The rationale for this approach was based not only on the risk of early postoperative complications, especially the transient pressure rise, but also on the concern that eyes treated with laser trabeculoplasty may eventually become more difficult to control than if they had been left on medical therapy. The histopathologic studies showing proliferation of a cellular layer over the trabecular meshwork have given reason to seriously consider this theoretical complication.[20,21,24,25] Nevertheless, preliminary, short-term studies of laser trabeculoplasty as primary therapy for open-angle glaucoma suggest that the procedure may be safe and effective as initial treatment for glaucoma.[102–106] In a multicenter clinical trial (The Glaucoma Laser Trial), 271 patients with newly diagnosed primary open-angle glaucoma were randomized into initial laser trabeculoplasty in one eye and timolol 0.5% in the other eye, with the same stepped regimen of additional medical therapy in either eye as required.[106] During the first 2 years of follow-up, the laser treated eyes had a slightly lower mean IOP of 1–2 mm Hg, although more than half of these eyes eventually required the addition of one or more medications. Long-term studies of many years are needed before laser trabeculoplasty can be advocated as a replacement for available medical therapy in the initial treatment of glaucoma. Laser trabeculoplasty has also been compared with trabeculectomy in a prospective, randomized study and was shown to be less effective than filtering surgery in permanently reducing the IOP to normal.[107]

TRABECULOTOMY

The basic principle of this operation is the creation of an opening in the trabecular meshwork to establish direct communication between the anterior chamber and Schlemm's canal. It is generally performed with incisional surgical techniques, although laser techniques are also being evaluated.

Incisional Trabeculotomy

In 1960, Burian[108] and Smith[109] independently described techniques for incising the trabecular meshwork from an ab externo approach. The procedure was modified by Harms and Dannheim,[110] who reported success in adults as well as children, although the primary interest has been with the latter.

Basic Technique (Fig. 34.7)

The following technique, described by McPherson,[111] encompasses aspects of the procedures developed by Allen and Burian[112] and Harms and Dannheim.[110]

A conjunctival flap is prepared in the same manner as used for filtering surgery (Chapter 36), and a 2 × 4 mm limbus-based, partial-thickness scleral flap is dissected. A radial incision is made across the sclerolimbal junction until Schlemm's canal is entered. To confirm the identity of the canal, a nylon suture may be threaded into one of the cut ends and observed gonioscopically to ensure that the suture is in the canal. Alternatively, the exposed portion of the suture may be bent anteriorly or posteriorly, noting whether it returns to a position parallel to the canal when released. Failure to do so suggests that a false passage may have been created into the anterior chamber or supraciliary space.

One arm of a McPherson trabeculotome is threaded into Schlemm's canal, using the other, parallel arm as a guide. The trabeculotome is then rotated so that the arm within the canal tears through trabecular meshwork into the anterior chamber. The same procedure is then performed on the other side of the radial incision.

The scleral and conjunctival flaps are closed in the same manner as for filtering procedures. Postoperative care includes the use of topical antibiotics and steroids. A low dose of pilocarpine may also be useful by keeping the cut edges of trabecular meshwork separated, and the pupil can be dilated once daily with phenylephrine to avoid posterior synechiae.

Complications

If Schlemm's canal is not properly identified, a false passage may be created either into the anterior chamber or the supraciliary space. The latter may result in the creation of a cyclodialysis and possible hyphema. If Schlemm's canal cannot be identified, the procedure can be converted to a trabeculectomy. When the probe is rotated into the anterior chamber, it may strip Descemet's membrane if it is too far anterior, or damage the iris or lens if it is too far posterior. As with all intraocular glaucoma procedures, postoperative bleeding and infection are potential complications.

Variations

Combined Trabeculotomy-Trabeculectomy. If Schlemm's canal cannot be located with certainty, which is not uncommon in highly buphthalmic eyes, it is possible to convert the procedure to a trabeculectomy by removing a block of deep limbal tissue beneath the scleral flap. In addition, the two procedures can be combined by first performing the trabeculotomy and then creating the fistula beneath the scleral flap. In some situations (such as the Sturge-Weber syndrome) in which the exact mechanism of the glaucoma is uncertain (see Chapter 18), the combined procedure may offer the best chance of success.[113] A similar combined technique has been suggested for late-onset congenital glaucoma in which a 2 × 2 mm block of tissue beneath the scleral flap is excised, but without penetrating the trabecular meshwork.[114] This procedure was reported to be successful in all of seven eyes, five of which had diffuse filtering blebs.

Electrocautery. This technique has been used in modified trabeculotomies by insulating all sides of the probe except that exposed to the trabecular meshwork.[115–117] By burning an opening in the meshwork, it is thought that fibrotic closure of the severed

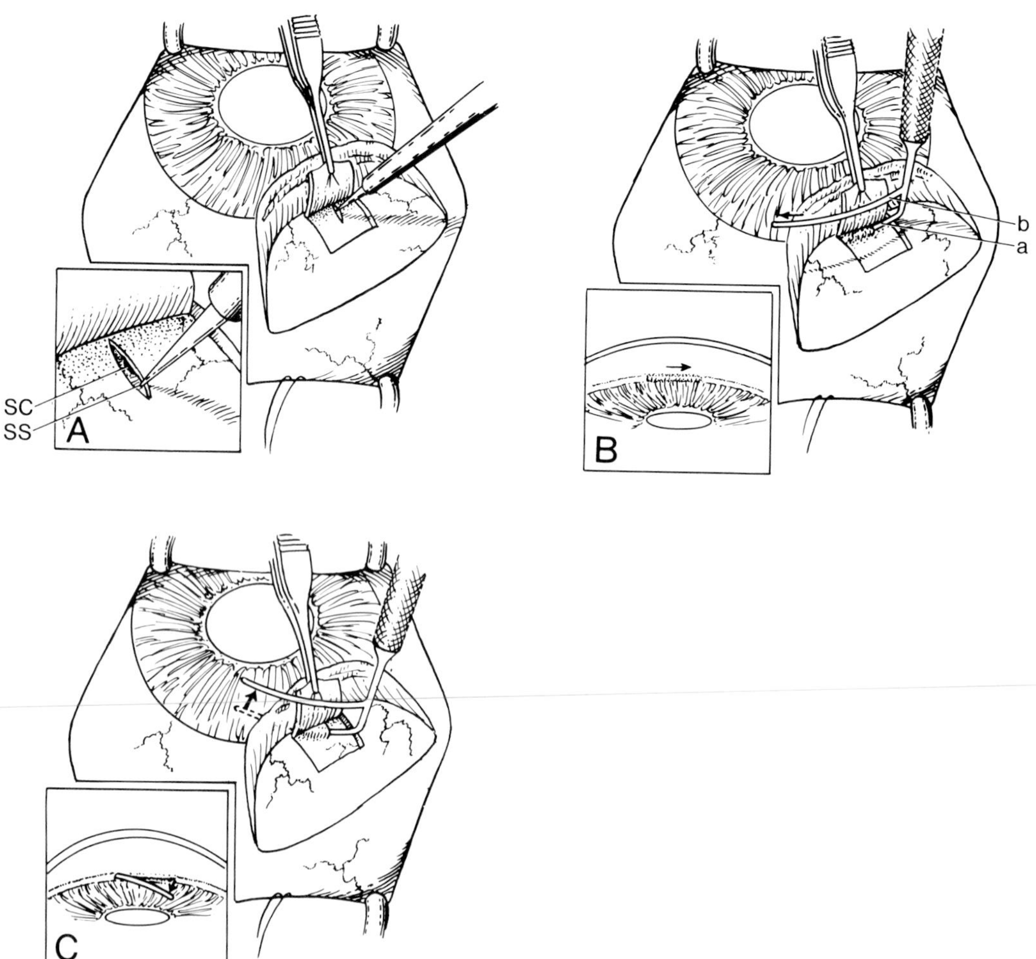

Figure 34.7. Trabeculotomy: **A,** Beneath a partial-thickness scleral flap, a radial incision is made across the sclerolimbal junction until Schlemm's canal (*SC*) is identified just anterior to the circumferential fibers of scleral spur (*SS*). **B,** The internal arm (*a*) of a trabeculotome is threaded into Schlemm's canal, using the external, parallel arm (*b*) as a guide; inset shows the gonioscopic appearance of the internal arm as it moves through the canal (*arrow*). **C,** The trabeculotome is rotated (*arrows*), causing the internal arm to tear through the trabecular meshwork into the anterior chamber.

edges is avoided. Success has been reported with this technique in patients with primary open-angle glaucoma as well as congenital glaucoma.[117] A similar approach has also been described in which electrical discharges are used to create holes in the trabecular meshwork.[118]

Miscellaneous Variations. Other experimental types of trabeculotomy use aqueous veins to localize Schlemm's canal by threading a probe through a large vein and into the canal[119] or by forcing air into a vein, which causes multiple ruptures in the meshwork.[120] An instrument has also been developed, the trabeculectome, that excises a strip of trabecular meshwork as it is pulled along the anterior chamber angle by a probe in Schlemm's canal.[121]

Laser Trabeculotomy

As noted at the outset of this chapter, the earliest efforts to treat glaucoma with the application of laser energy to the trabecular meshwork were attempts to puncture holes through the trabecular meshwork into Schlemm's canal.[2–5,7] This approach lost popularity because of early failures and the subsequent enthusiasm for laser trabeculoplasty, although advances in the technology of pulsed lasers have led to a reevaluation of laser trabeculopuncture, or trabeculotomy.

In laboratory studies with monkeys, the Q-switched ruby laser did not produce persistent penetration to Schlemm's canal.[122] With Q-switched neodymium:YAG lasers, holes were created in the trabecular meshwork but were soon sealed by proliferation of corneal endothelium and scar tissue.[123,124] Laboratory studies with human ocular tissue have shown that pulsed neodymium:YAG lasers at energy levels between 3 and 6 mJ can produce discrete lesions into Schlemm's canal with minimal damage to adjacent structures.[125,126] In human autopsy eyes, energy levels of 30 mJ produced openings in the trabecular meshwork of approximately 100 microns in diameter.[127] Similar treatment in four human eyes within 18 hours of enucleation produced irregular craters of 150–300 microns in the meshwork, with denudation of endothelial cells and deposition of debris in the adjacent trabecular and corneal tissues.[128]

Preliminary clinical experience with laser trabeculotomy has provided variable results. In one series of eight eyes of six patients with juvenile glaucoma, pressure control was achieved in six eyes (75%) with a mean follow-up of 6 months.[129] The most effective technique in this study was to make two confluent trabeculotomies of 1 clock hour each in extent. However, another study of 69 eyes of 61 patients with open-angle glaucoma had a success rate of only 46% 1 year after treatment.[130] Further study of this surgical procedure appears to be indicated.

GONIOTOMY

In 1938, Barkan[131] described an operation for congenital glaucoma in which an incision in the anterior chamber angle was believed to reduce obstruction to aqueous outflow caused by a membrane across the trabecular meshwork. Although the presence of a true membrane has never been established, the operation is effective in a high percentage of cases, presumably by means of incising whatever abnormal tissue is responsible for the outflow obstruction, and it is still preferred by many pediatric glaucoma surgeons. Subsequent modifications of the basic technique may also be useful for other forms of glaucoma in both children and adults. It should be noted that this operation differs primarily from trabeculotomy in that only a portion of the internal trabecular tissue is incised.

Basic Technique (Fig. 34.8)[131]

The procedure can be performed with a binocular head loupe, although the operating microscope provides better visualization.[132] The patient's head is rotated away from the side of the surgery and the operative eye is slightly abducted. A surgical goniolens is then placed over the nasal cornea, leaving 2–3 mm of temporal cornea exposed for the knife entry. Fixation of the globe is essential, and this can be accomplished with locking forceps, which are held by an assistant.

The goniotomy knife penetrates the cornea 1 mm anterior to the limbus at 10 o'clock in the right eye or 4 o'clock in the left eye. The blade is passed across the anterior chamber to a point in the chamber angle 180° from the entry site. The shaft of the knife is tapered to maintain a watertight seal. Numerous modifications of Barkan's goniotomy knife have been described, including attached fiberoptics for intraocular illumination.[133] Another modification is to use a 23- or 25-gauge disposable needle as the knife on a syringe containing sodium hyaluronic acid.[134]

Using the tip of the goniotomy blade, the angle tissue is incised posterior to Schwalbe's line for approximately one-third of the angle circumference. The intent is to incise only the abnormal layer of tissue in front of the trabecular meshwork, and this is best judged by observing the development of a white line as the cut edge of tissue retracts posteriorly and sclera is seen through intact trabecular meshwork.

The knife is then withdrawn, taking care not to injure adjacent ocular structures, and

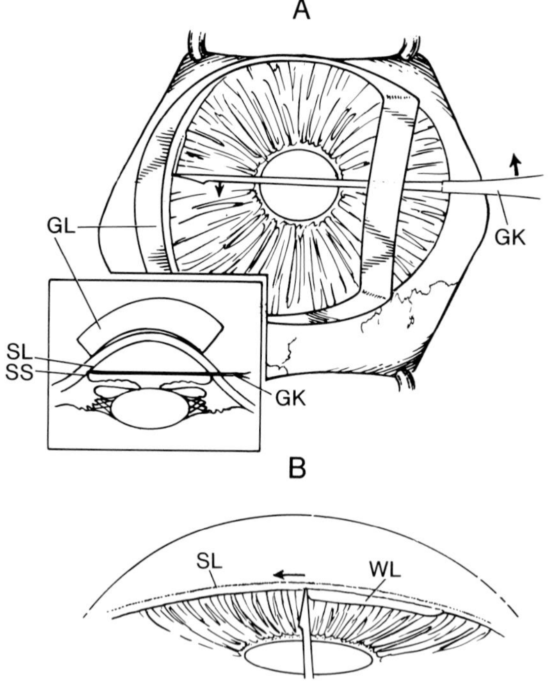

Figure 34.8. Goniotomy: **A,** With a surgical goniolens (*GL*) positioned on the cornea, a goniotomy knife (*GK*) is inserted through peripheral cornea and passed across the anterior chamber to the angle in the opposite quadrant. **B,** Under direct gonioscopic visualization, angle tissue is excised between Schwalbe's line (*SL*) and scleral spur (*SS*) for approximately one-third of the chamber angle circumference. This creates a white line (*WL*) as the cut edge of tissue retracts from the incision. *Arrows* indicate the direction of knife movement during incision of angle tissue.

the anterior chamber is deepened with air or a balanced salt solution. In one study of seven infants treated with two simultaneous goniotomies in one eye and a single goniotomy in the fellow eye, no significant differences were noted in the results.[135] If bilateral surgery is needed, it has been suggested that both procedures can be done at the same operation,[136] although these should be done with different sets of instruments. Postoperative management consists of topical antibiotics, a miotic, and topical steroids.

Complications

Intraoperative Complications. Placement of the incision is critical in performing a goniotomy. If the incision is too posterior, bleeding from the ciliary body may occur, while an incision that is too anterior will have no effect. Iridodialysis or cyclodialysis may also be created inadvertently during a goniotomy procedure.[136]

Shallowing or loss of the anterior chamber during the operation prevents adequate visualization of the angle and increases the risk of damage to ocular structures. If this occurs, the knife should be withdrawn and the chamber deepened with balanced salt solution or sodium hyaluronate through the entry site.

As with any operation under general anesthesia, the risks of the anesthesia must also be considered. In a series of 401 goniotomies under general anesthesia, the most serious complication was cardiopulmonary arrest, which occurred in 1.8%.[136]

Postoperative Complications. A moderate hyphema is common after goniotomy but rarely leads to serious sequelae. In 401 goniotomies, postoperative bleeding was reported in 0.6%, but useful vision was lost in only one case.[136] Postoperative infection is rare.

Permanent visual impairment following surgery for glaucoma in children may have an anatomic basis but is more often due to amblyopia and large refractive errors.[137] An important aspect of the postoperative management is to anticipate these causes of reduced vision and treat them appropriately.

Variations

Goniopuncture. Scheie[138,139] described a form of filtering surgery that used the goniotomy technique and was designed primarily for children in whom standard goniotomies had failed. In this procedure, saline is first injected beneath Tenon's capsule near the inferior limbus to create a bleb. The blade of a Scheie needle-knife is then passed through the peripheral cornea just below the horizontal plane and diagonally across the anterior chamber to the inferior angle. The trabecular meshwork and limbal tissue are penetrated with the tip of the blade until it is visible in the sub-Tenon's bleb. The knife is then removed and the anterior chamber is deepened with saline.

Goniodiathermy. A disadvantage of goniopuncture is that the limbal incision tends to scar closed. To avoid this, a technique was developed in which an intraocular diathermy probe is introduced into the goniopuncture tract to cause a gaping of the wound edges. Preliminary experience in rabbits was believed to be encouraging.[140]

Direct Goniotomy. When corneal clouding prevents visualization for standard goniotomy, it has been suggested that the goniotomy might be performed directly through a 60° limbal incision.[141] However, most surgeons prefer a trabeculotomy in these cases.

Trabeculodialysis. In this modification of the goniotomy technique, the trabecular meshwork is scraped from the scleral sulcus with the flat side of a goniotomy blade.[142] This technique is especially useful in *glaucoma associated with inflammation,* presumably because the trabecular tissue is friable and easily scraped away in these cases.[142–144] A histologic study has shown that this operation works by establishing a communication between the anterior chamber and Schlemm's canal.[144] In one series of 23 children or young adults with glaucoma secondary to anterior uveitis, trabeculodialysis controlled the IOP in 60% of the cases.[145]

Laser Goniotomy. By applying laser energy with a neodymium:YAG laser anterior to the insertion of the iris in patients with developmental glaucomas, it was possible to separate the iris tissue from the trabecular band. This technique improved the IOP control in seven of eight eyes with primary juvenile glaucoma.[146] In another study of 10 children with bilateral, symmetrical congenital glaucoma, one eye was treated with incisional goniotomy under general anesthesia and the other with laser goniotomy under chloral hydrate sedation, with similar pressure results.[147]

Results and Comparison of Trabeculotomy and Goniotomy

Opinions differ regarding the procedure of choice for the management of congenital glaucoma. Many pediatric glaucoma surgeons prefer the time-honored goniotomy, using trabeculotomy only in cases with marked corneal clouding or after repeated goniotomy failures. Reported success with goniotomy ranges from approximately 80 to 90%, although in one-third to one-half of the eyes, the procedure must be repeated one or more times.[148–151] A less favorable outcome is usually seen when the disease is detected either at birth or later in childhood, or if there is a very high IOP or marked buphthalmos.

Other surgeons prefer trabeculotomy as the initial procedure for most cases of primary congenital glaucoma. The reported success rates with this operation are basically the same as with goniotomy, although it may be that fewer repeat procedures are required with trabeculotomy than with goniotomy.[148,152–158] The same factors appear to influence the outcome of trabeculotomies as were noted above for goniotomy.

Advocates of goniotomy point out that it is anatomically more precise, with less surgical trauma to adjacent tissues,[159] while those who prefer trabeculotomy as a primary procedure note that it is not dependent on a clear cornea.[160] Since childhood glaucoma surgery is not performed frequently by most surgeons, there is advantage in having one procedure that can be used for all cases. In addition, with the trabeculotomy technique it is possible to determine whether or not Schlemm's canal is present and to convert immediately to a filtering procedure if necessary. However, in the final analysis the two surgical approaches appear to provide equally good results in the hands of experienced surgeons.[161]

CYCLODIALYSIS

Cyclodialysis as an operation for glaucoma was described by Heine[162] in 1905.

It has been employed as an alternative to filtering surgery, especially in aphakic eyes or in combination with cataract extraction. However, the procedure has lost popularity in recent years because of unpredictable results and newer, alternative surgical techniques.

Theories of Mechanism

Cyclodialysis involves the separation of the ciliary body from the scleral spur, which creates a direct communication between the anterior chamber and the suprachoroidal space. Most studies suggest that this lowers the IOP by means of an increase in pressure-dependent uveoscleral outflow.[163–167] However, it has also been proposed that reduced aqueous production, as a result of altered ciliary body anatomy, is the principal mode of ocular hypotension.[168,169] It may be that both mechanisms are involved in a successful cyclodialysis procedure. This was suggested by an intraocular manometric study of a glaucoma patient before and after cyclodialysis, which revealed both improved outflow and reduced aqueous production.[170]

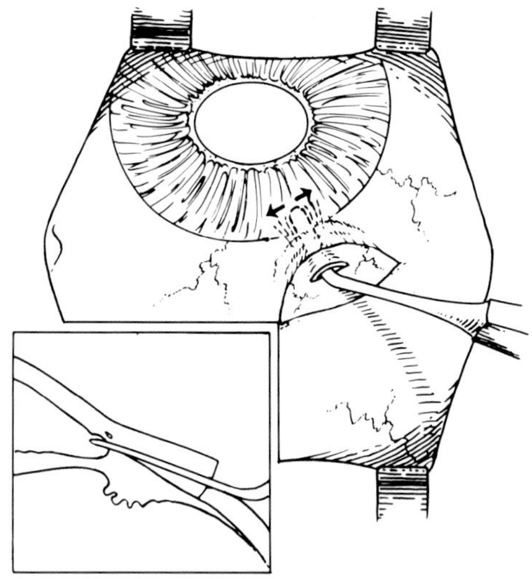

Figure 34.9. Cyclodialysis: A cyclodialysis spatula is passed through a full-thickness scleral incision and the suprachoridal space until it enters the anterior chamber. With lateral movements of the spatula tip (*arrows*), approximately one-third of the ciliary body is separated from the scleral spur.

Basic Technique[162,171]

An incision is made through conjunctiva and Tenon's capsule approximately 8 mm from the corneolimbal junction, usually in a superior quadrant between the insertions of two rectus muscles. A 3–4 mm full-thickness scleral incision, 4–6 mm from the anatomic limbus, is then made parallel to the limbus.

A cyclodialysis spatula is inserted through the scleral incision and into the supraciliary space. Staying close to the inner scleral surface, the spatula is advanced until the tip enters the anterior chamber. Lateral movements of the spatula tip are then made to either side of the entry point to separate about one-third of the ciliary body from the scleral spur (Fig. 34.9). After withdrawal of the spatula, only the conjunctiva is closed.

Variations

Variations of Basic Technique. An alternative technique is to create the cyclodialysis with multiple forward thrusts of the spatula, by which up to one-half of the ciliary body can be disinserted.[172] The injection of air[173,174] or sodium hyaluronate[175] into the anterior chamber has been advocated as a means of holding the cleft open during the early postoperative period. Modifications of the cyclodialysis spatula include a rounded, shorter handle, to facilitate use under the operating microscope,[176] a shorter blade with a blunt tip for increased safety,[176] and a fiberoptic tip, to facilitate visualization within the supraciliary space and anterior chamber.[177]

Implants. Implants (or setons) of various material have been inserted into the cyclodialysis cleft to keep it open,[170,178–181] although no evidence of lasting success has been provided for any of these techniques.

Iridocycloretraction. Krasnov[182] described a technique for the treatment of chronic angle-closure glaucoma in which two or three scleral pedicles are folded forward into a cyclodialysis cleft to keep the angle open. A modification of this technique, using a single scleral pedicle, was designed to maintain a patent cyclodialysis cleft in aphakic eyes.[183] Reports concerning the usefulness of the latter procedure are conflicting.[183,184] In another modification, called "filtering iridocycloretraction," two limbal-based scleral strips are inserted into the anterior chamber and supraciliary space in eyes with chronic angle-closure glaucoma to widen the anterior chamber angle and maintain communication between both the subconjunctival and suprachoroidal spaces.[185]

Laser Cyclodialysis. A cyclodialysis technique has been evaluated in monkey eyes by directing the argon laser beam between the ciliary body band and root of the iris.[186] A subsequent clinical trial of 52 eyes in 36 patients with open-angle glaucoma revealed a success rate of 73% after a 1-year follow-up.[187]

Postoperative Management

Postoperative management includes topical antibiotics and corticosteroids. In addition, the use of a miotic has been recommended to keep the cyclodialysis cleft open through traction on the longitudinal ciliary muscle.[163]

Complications[171,172]

Intraoperative Complications. *Hemorrhage* is a frequent complication during a cyclodialysis procedure. The risk may be minimized by making a more anterior scleral incision, avoiding anterior ciliary arteries, and keeping the cyclodialysis spatula close to the sclera to avoid perforating the ciliary body. When brisk bleeding does occur, it can usually be stopped by placing a large air bubble in the anterior chamber for several minutes. *Improper position of the spatula* can cause several complications. If the cyclodialysis spatula is too far anterior as it enters the anterior chamber, it may strip Descemet's membrane or otherwise damage the cornea. A position that is too posterior may tear the ciliary body or iris, injure the lens, or rupture the hyaloid face and possibly cause vitreous loss.

Postoperative Complications. *Hypotony* is a common postoperative complication of cyclodialysis. Penetrating cyclodiathermy or cyclocryotherapy to "wall off" the cleft may correct the problem, but the results are highly unpredictable. The application of argon laser energy into the cyclodialysis cleft may lead to closure of the cleft. In one report, settings of 0.2 seconds, 100 microns, 500–600 milliwatts, and approximately 50 exposures produced a successful result.[188] Closure of the cyclodialysis cleft with sutures has also been described.[189,190] Failure to control the IOP is usually associated with *closure of the cyclodialysis cleft*, which may result from hemorrhage, excessive inflammation, or an inadequate initial cleft. As previously noted, the risk of this complication can be reduced by the use of miotics, which presumably keeps the cyclodialysis cleft open by traction of the ciliary musculature. A complication of cyclodialysis that may occur at any time after surgery is a sudden, marked rise in the IOP.[191] This is thought to be associated with closure of the cleft and can be reversed, in some cases, with the use of miotics.

GONIOSYNECHIALYSIS

Campbell and Vela[192] have reported successful preliminary experience with a procedure for synechial angle-closure glaucoma. The technique involves deepening the anterior chamber with sodium hyaluronate and separating the synechiae from the trabecular meshwork with an irrigating cyclodialysis spatula under direct gonioscopic visualization (Fig. 34.10). The procedure has also been employed during penetrating keratoplasty, using a dental mirror to visualize the anterior chamber angle.[193] The primary value of the procedure is thought to be for patients in whom the synechiae have not been present for a prolonged period of time. In one series of 15 patients with synechial angle-closure glaucoma, goniosynechialysis alone (5 cases) or in combination with other surgical procedures (10) was associated with a reduction in mean IOP from 40 to 14 mm Hg.[194] It has also been reported that successful goniosynechialysis was achieved in 5 of 7 patients with a Q-switched neodymium:YAG laser.[195]

GONIOPHOTOCOAGULATION

Simmons and associates[196,197] described a form of laser treatment for use in the early, open-angle stages of neovascular glaucoma.

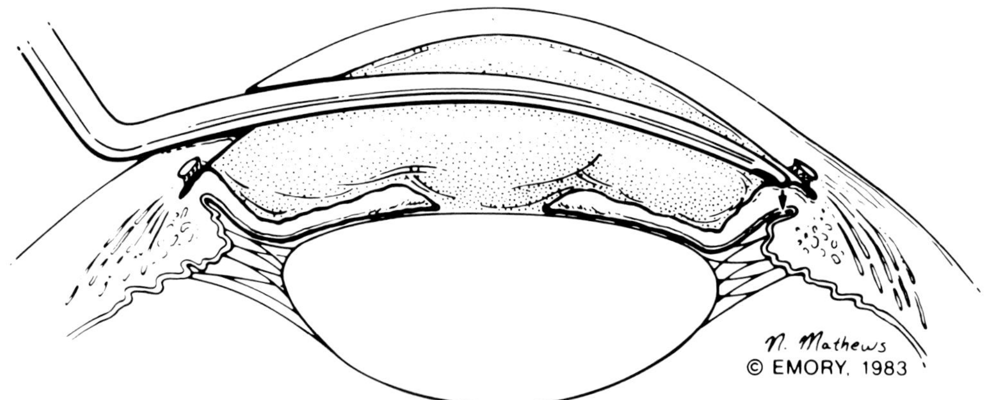

Figure 34.10. Goniosynechialysis: After deepening the anterior chamber with sodium hyaluronate, an irrigating cyclodialysis spatula is used to separate synechiae from the trabecular meshwork with an anterior-to-posterior movement. (Reprinted from Campbell DG and Vela A: Ophthalmology 91:1052, 1984, with permission.)

The purpose of the procedure is to eliminate new vessels in the anterior chamber angle by direct laser photocoagulation. The technique involves the application of argon laser energy to the vessels as they cross the scleral spur to arborize on the trabecular meshwork. The customary laser settings are 0.2 seconds exposure, 150 microns spot size, and an energy level that is sufficient to blanch and constrict the vessels (usually 100–800 milliwatts).[197]

This technique is most effective when used in the preglaucoma, or rubeosis, stage of the disease to prevent progression of angle neovascularization with subsequent angle closure and intractable glaucoma. It may be used in conjunction with panretinal photocoagulation, especially when the latter has not been successful, or when the retinal therapy is not possible or advisable. However, in the more advanced, florid open-angle stage of neovascular glaucoma, goniophotocoagulation must be used with caution, since it may cause hemorrhage or accelerated closure of the anterior chamber angle.

SUMMARY

Laser trabeculoplasty involves the application of evenly spaced photocoagulation burns to all or part of the trabecular meshwork. In the majority of cases, this leads to lowering of IOP through improvement of aqueous outflow by mechanisms that are not fully understood. The most serious known complication is an early, transient rise in ocular tension. A significant number of patients lose the ocular hypotensive effect with time, and repeated trabeculoplasty is less effective than the initial procedure.

Incisional trabeculotomy is an ab externo procedure in which trabecular meshwork is incised to establish communication between the anterior chamber and Schlemm's canal. Laser trabeculotomy is being evaluated as an alternative approach in which meshwork is punctured ab interno with pulsed laser energy. Goniotomy is an ab interno procedure in which abnormal tissue in the anterior chamber angle is incised. Incisional trabeculotomy and goniotomy are the primary surgical procedures for congenital and some other developmental glaucomas, although variations of the basic techniques may be useful for additional types of glaucoma in both children and adults.

Cyclodialysis involves the separation of the ciliary body from the scleral spur, which apparently lowers IOP primarily by increasing uveoscleral outflow. Other surgical procedures of the anterior chamber angle include goniosynechialysis for synechial angle-closure glaucoma and goniophotocoagulation for neovascular glaucoma.

References

1. Zweng, HC, Flocks, M: Experimental photocoagulation of the anterior chamber angle. A preliminary report. Am J Ophthal 52:163, 1961.
2. Krasnov, MM: Laser puncture of the anterior chamber angle in glaucoma. Vestn Oftal 3:27, 1972.
3. Hager, H: Besondere mikrochirurgische Eingriffe. II. Erste Erfahrungen mit der Argon-lasergerat 800. Klin Monatsbl Augenheilkd 163:437, 1973.
4. Demailly, P, Haut, J, Bonnet-Boutier, M: Trabeculotomie au laser a l'argon (note preliminaire). Bull Soc Ophthal Fr 73:259, 1973.
5. Worthen, DM, Wickham, MG: Argon laser trabeculotomy. Trans Am Acad Ophthal Otol 78:371, 1974.
6. Gaasterland, D, Kupfer, C: Experimental glaucoma in the rhesus monkey. Invest Ophthal 14:455, 1975.
7. Ticho, U, Zauberman, H: Argon laser application to angle structures in the glaucomas. Arch Ophthal 94:61, 1976.
8. Wise, JB, Witter, SL: Argon laser therapy for open-angle glaucoma. A pilot study. Arch Ophthal 97:319, 1979.
9. Wise, JB: Long-term control of adult open angle glaucoma by argon laser treatment. Ophthalmology 88:197, 1981.
10. Schwartz, AL, Whitten, ME, Bleiman, B, Martin, D: Argon laser trabecular surgery in uncontrolled phakic open angle glaucoma. Ophthalmology 88:203, 1981.
11. Wilensky, JT, Jampol, LM: Laser therapy for open angle glaucoma. Ophthalmology 88:213, 1981.
12. Pohjanpelto, P: Argon laser treatment of the anterior chamber angle for increased intraocular pressure. Acta Ophthal 59:211, 1981.
13. Lichter, PR: Argon laser trabeculoplasty. Trans Am Ophthal Soc 80:288, 1982.
14. Brubaker, RF, Liesegang, TJ: Effect of trabecular photocoagulation on the aqueous humor dynamics of the human eye. Am J Ophthal 96:139, 1983.
15. Merte, H-J, Denffer, H, Hirsch, B: Tonographic findings following argon laser trabeculoplasty. Klin Monatsbl Augenheilkd 186:220, 1985.
16. Schrems, W, Sold, J, Krieglstein, GK, Leydhecker, W: Tonographic response of laser trabeculoplasty in chronic glaucoma. Klin Monatsbl Augenheilkd 187:170, 1985.
17. Araie, M, Yamamoto, T, Shirato, S, Kitazawa, Y: Effects of laser trabeculoplasty on the human aqueous humor dynamics: a fluorophotometric study. Ann Ophthal 16:540, 1984.
18. Yablonski, ME, Cook, DJ, Gray, J: A fluorophotometric study of the effect of argon laser trabeculoplasty on aqueous humor dynamics. Am J Ophthal 99:579, 1985.
19. Feller, DB, Weinreb, RN: Breakdown and reestablishment of blood-aqueous barrier with laser trabeculoplasty. Arch Ophthal 102:537, 1984.
20. Rodrigues, MM, Spaeth, GL, Donohoo, P: Electron microscopy of argon laser therapy in phakic open-angle glaucoma. Ophthalmology 89:198, 1982.
21. Alexander, RA, Grierson, I, Church, WH: The effect of argon laser trabeculoplasty upon the normal human trabecular meshwork. Graefe's Arch Ophthal 227:72, 1989.
22. Melamed, S, Pei, J, Epstein, DL: Short-term effect of argon laser trabeculoplasty in monkeys. Arch Ophthal 103:1546, 1985.
23. Dueker, DK, Norberg, M, Johnson, DH, et al: Stimulation of cell division by argon and Nd:YAG laser trabeculoplasty in cynomolgus monkeys. Invest Ophthal Vis Sci 31:115, 1990.
24. Melamed, S, Pei, J, Epstein, DL: Delayed response to argon laser trabeculoplasty in monkeys. Morphological and morphometric analysis. Arch Ophthal 104:1078, 1986.
25. van der Zypen, E, Fankhauser, F: Ultrastructural changes of the trabecular meshwork of the monkey (*Macaca speciosa*) following irradiation with argon laser light. Graefe's Arch Ophthal 221:249, 1984.
26. Melamed, S, Epstein, DL: Alterations of aqueous humour outflow following argon laser trabeculoplasty in monkeys. Br J Ophthal 71:776, 1987.
27. Van der Zypen, E, Fankhauser, F, England, C, Kwasniewska, S: Morphology of the trabecular meshwork within monkey (*Macaca speciosa*) eyes after irradiation with the free-running Nd:YAG laser. Ophthalmology 94:171, 1987.
28. Van Buskirk, EM, Pond, V, Rosenquist, RC, Acott, TS: Argon laser trabeculoplasty. Studies of mechanism of action. Ophthalmology 91:1005, 1984.
29. Bylsma, SS, Samples, JR, Acott, TS, Van Buskirk, EM: Trabecular cell division after argon laser trabeculoplasty. Arch Ophthal 106:544, 1988.
30. Acott, TS, Samples, JR, Bradley, JMB, et al: Trabecular repopulation by anterior trabecular meshwork cells after laser trabeculoplasty. Am J Ophthal 107:1, 1989.
31. Van Buskirk, EM: Pathophysiology of laser trabeculoplasty. Surv Ophthal 33:264, 1989.
32. Smith, J: Argon laser trabeculoplasty: comparison of bichromatic and monochromatic wavelengths. Ophthalmology 91:355, 1984.
33. Makabe, R: Comparison of krypton and argon laser trabeculoplasty. Klin Monatsbl Augenheilkd 189:118, 1986.
34. Spurny, RC, Lederer, CM Jr: Krypton laser trabeculoplasty. A clinical report. Arch Ophthal 102:1626, 1984.

35. Dieckert, JP, Mainster, MA, Ho, PC: Contact lenses for laser applications. Ophthalmology Instrument and Book Supplement 55, 1983.
36. Ritch, R: A new lens for argon laser trabeculoplasty. Ophthal Surg 16:331, 1985.
37. Wise, JB: Errors in laser spot size in laser trabeculoplasty. Ophthalmology 91:186, 1984.
38. Blondeau, P, Roberge, JF, Asselin, Y: Long-term results of low power, long duration laser trabeculoplasty. Am J Ophthal 104:339, 1987.
39. Rouhiainen, H, Terasvirta, M: The laser power needed for optimum results in argon laser trabeculoplasty. Acta Ophthal 64:254, 1986.
40. Thomas, JV, Simmons, RJ, Belcher, CD III: Argon laser trabeculoplasty in the presurgical glaucoma patient. Ophthalmology 89:187, 1982.
41. Weinreb, RN, Ruderman, J, Juster, R, Zweig, K: Immediate intraocular pressure response to argon laser trabeculoplasty. Am J Ophthal 95:279, 1983.
42. Hoskins, HD Jr, Hetherington, J Jr, Minckler, DS, et al: Complications of laser trabeculoplasty. Ophthalmology 90:796, 1983.
43. Krupin, T, Kolker, AE, Kass, MA, Becker, B: Intraocular pressure the day of argon laser trabeculoplasty in primary open-angle glaucoma. Ophthalmology 91:361, 1984.
44. Frucht, J, Bishara, S, Ticho, U: Early intraocular pressure response following laser trabeculoplasty. Br J Ophthal 69:771, 1985.
45. Glaucoma Laser Trial Research Group: The glaucoma laser trial. 1. Acute effects of argon laser trabeculoplasty on intraocular pressure. Arch Ophthal 107:1135, 1989.
46. Fiore, PM, Melamed, S, Epstein, DL: Trabecular precipitates and elevated intraocular pressure following argon laser trabeculoplasty. Ophthal Surg 20:697, 1989.
47. Greenidge, KC, Rodrigues, MM, Spaeth, GL, et al: Acute intraocular pressure elevation after argon laser trabeculoplasty and iridectomy: a clinicopathologic study. Ophthal Surg 15:105, 1984.
48. Koss, MC, March, WF, Nordquist, RE, Gherezghiher, T: Acute intraocular pressure elevation produced by argon laser trabeculoplasty in the cynomolgus monkey. Arch Ophthal 102:1699, 1984.
49. Rouhiainen, HJ, Teräsvirta, ME, Tuovinen, EJ: Peripheral anterior synechiae formation after trabeculoplasty. Arch Ophthal 106:189, 1988.
50. Hong, C, Kitazawa, Y, Tanishima, T: Influence of argon laser treatment of glaucoma on corneal endothelium. Jap J Ophthal 27:567, 1983.
51. Traverso, C, Cohen, EJ, Groden, LR, et al: Central corneal endothelial cell density after argon laser trabeculoplasty. Arch Ophthal 102:1322, 1984.
52. Schoenlebe, DB, Bellows, AR, Hutchinson, BT: Failed laser trabeculoplasty requiring surgery in open-angle glaucoma. Ophthal Surg 18:796, 1987.
53. Wilensky, JT, Weinreb, RN: Low-dose trabeculoplasty. Am J Ophthal 95:423, 1983.
54. Schwartz, LW, Spaeth, GL, Traverso, C, Greenidge, KC: Variation of techniques on the results of argon laser trabeculoplasty. Ophthalmology 90:781, 1983.
55. Weinreb, RN, Ruderman, J, Juster, R, Wilensky, JT: Influence of the number of laser burns administered on the early results of argon laser trabeculoplasty. Am J Ophthal 95:287, 1983.
56. Lustgarten, J, Podos, SM, Ritch, R, et al: Laser trabeculoplasty. A prospective study of treatment variables. Arch Ophthal 102:517, 1984.
57. Heijl, A: One- and two-session laser trabeculoplasty. A randomized, prospective study. Acta Ophthal 62:715, 1984.
58. Klein, HZ, Shields, MB, Earnest, JT: Two-stage argon laser trabeculoplasty in open-angle glaucoma. Am J Ophthal 99:392, 1985.
59. Kitazawa, Y, Yamamoto, T, Shirato, S, Eguchi, S: Argon laser trabeculoplasty: methods and results. Klin Monatsbl Augenheilkd 184:274, 1984.
60. Rouhiainen, HJ, Teräsvirta, ME, Tuovinen, EJ: Laser power and postoperative intraocular pressure increase in argon laser trabeculoplasty. Arch Ophthal 105:1352, 1987.
61. Rosenblatt, MA, Luntz, MH: Intraocular pressure rise after argon laser trabeculoplasty. Br J Ophthal 71:772, 1987.
62. Traverso, CE, Greenidge, KC, Spaeth, GL: Formation of peripheral anterior synechiae following argon laser trabeculoplasty. A prospective study to determine relationship to position of laser burns. Arch Ophthal 102:861, 1984.
63. Payer, H: Circular argon laser coagulation of the ciliary band to lower pressure in open-angle glaucoma. Klin Monatsbl Augenheilkd 187:334, 1985.
64. Ofner, S, Samples, JR, Van Buskirk, EM: Pilocarpine and the increase in intraocular pressure after trabeculoplasty. Am J Ophthal 97:647, 1984.
65. Robin, AL, Pollack, IP, House, B, Enger, C: Effects of ALO 2145 on intraocular pressure following argon laser trabeculoplasty. Arch Ophthal 105:646, 1987.
66. Metcalfe, TW, Etchells, DE: Prevention of the immediate intraocular pressure rise following argon laser trabeculoplasty. Br J Ophthal 73:612, 1989.
67. Ruderman, JM, Zweig, KO, Wilensky, JT, Weinreb, RN: Effects of corticosteroid pretreatment on argon laser trabeculoplasty. Am J Ophthal 96:84, 1983.
68. Pappas, HR, Berry, DP, Partamian, L, et al: Topical indomethacin therapy before argon laser trabeculoplasty. Am J Ophthal 99:571, 1985.
69. Gelfand, YA, Wolpert, W: Effects of topical indomethacin pretreatment on argon laser trabecu-

loplasty: a randomised, double-masked study on black South Africans. Br J Ophthal 69:668, 1985.

70. Tuulonen, A: The effect of topical indomethacin on acute pressure elevation of laser trabeculoplasty in capsular glaucoma. Acta Ophthal 63:245, 1985.
71. Weinreb, RN, Robin, AL, Baerveldt, G, et al: Flurbiprofen pretreatment in argon laser trabeculoplasty for primary open-angle glaucoma. Arch Ophthal 102:1629, 1984.
72. Hotchkiss, ML, Robin, AL, Pollack, IP, Quigley, HA: Nonsteroidal anti-inflammatory agents after argon laser trabeculoplasty. A trial with flurbiprofen and indomethacin. Ophthalmology 91:969, 1984.
73. Forbes, M, Bansal, RK: Argon laser goniophotocoagulation of the trabecular meshwork in open-angle glaucoma. Trans Am Ophthal Soc 76:257, 1981.
74. Pollack, IP, Robin, AL, Sax, H: The effect of argon laser trabeculoplasty on the medical control of primary open-angle glaucoma. Ophthalmology 90:785, 1983.
75. Greenidge, KC, Spaeth, GL, Fiol-Silva, Z: Effect of argon laser trabeculoplasty on the glaucomatous diurnal curve. Ophthalmology 90:800, 1983.
76. Brooks, AMV, Gillies, WE: Do any factors predict a favourable response to laser trabeculoplasty? Aust J Ophthal 12:149, 1984.
77. Tuulonen, AN, Airaksinen, J, Kuulasmaa, K: Factors influencing the outcome of laser trabeculoplasty. Am J Ophthal 99:388, 1985.
78. Strasser, G, Stelzer, R: Laser trabeculoplasty in low-tension glaucoma. Klin Monatsbl Augenheilkd 183:507, 1983.
79. Schwartz, AL, Perman, KI, Whitten, M: Argon laser trabeculoplasty in progressive low-tension glaucoma. Ann Ophthal 16:560, 1984.
80. Sharpe, ED, Simmons, RJ: Argon laser trabeculoplasty as a means of decreasing intraocular pressure from "normal" levels in glaucomatous eyes. Am J Ophthal 99:704, 1985.
81. Robin, AL, Pollack IP: Argon laser trabeculoplasty in secondary forms of open-angle glaucoma. Arch Ophthal 101:382, 1983.
82. Lieberman, MF, Hoskins, HD Jr, Hetherington, J Jr: Laser trabeculoplasty and the glaucomas. Ophthalmology 90:790, 1983.
83. Lunde, MW: Argon laser trabeculoplasty in pigmentary dispersion syndrome with glaucoma. Am J Ophthal 96:721, 1983.
84. Rouhiaine, HJ, Teräsvirta, ME, Tuovinen, EJ: The effect of some treatment variables on the results of trabeculoplasty. Arch Ophthal 106:611, 1988.
85. Fellman, RL, Starita, RJ, Spaeth, GL, Poryzees, EM: Argon laser trabeculoplasty following failed trabeculectomy. Ophthal Surg 15:195, 1984.
86. Wilensky, JT, Weinreb, RN: Early and late failures of argon laser trabeculoplasty. Arch Ophthal 101:895, 1983.
87. Safran, MJ, Robin, AL, Pollack, IP: Argon laser trabeculoplasty in younger patients with primary open-angle glaucoma. Am J Ophthal 97:292, 1984.
88. Krupin, T, Patkin, R, Kurata, FK, et al: Argon laser trabeculoplasty in black and white patients with primary open-angle glaucoma. Ophthalmology 93:811, 1986.
89. Grinich, NP, Van Buskirk, EM, Samples, JR: Three-year efficacy of argon laser trabeculoplasty. Ophthalmology 94:858, 1987.
90. Schwartz, AL, Kopelman, J: Four-year experience with argon laser trabecular surgery in uncontrolled open-angle glaucoma. Ophthalmology 90:771, 1983.
91. Tuulonen, A, Niva, A-K, Alanko, HI: A controlled five-year follow-up study of laser trabeculoplasty as primary therapy for open-angle glaucoma. Am J Ophthal 104:334, 1987.
92. Shingleton, BJ, Richter, CU, Bellows, AR, et al: Long-term efficacy of argon laser trabeculoplasty. Ophthalmology 94:1513, 1987.
93. Ticho, U, Nesher, R: Laser trabeculoplasty in glaucoma. Ten-year evaluation. Arch Ophthal 107:844, 1989.
94. Starita, RJ, Fellman, RL, Spaeth, GL, Poryzees, E: The effect of repeating full-circumference argon laser trabeculoplasty. Ophthal Surg 15:41, 1984.
95. Brown, SVL, Thomas, JV, Simmons, RJ: Laser trabeculoplasty re-treatment. Am J Ophthal 99:8, 1985.
96. Richter, CU, Shingleton, BJ, Bellows, AR, et al: Retreatment with argon laser trabeculoplasty. Ophthalmology 94:1085, 1987.
97. Messner, D, Siegel, LI, Kass, MA, et al: Repeat argon laser trabeculoplasty. Am J Ophthal 103:113, 1987.
98. Grayson, DK, Camras, CB, Podos, SM, Lustgarten, JS: Long-term reduction of intraocular pressure after repeat argon laser trabeculoplasty. Am J Ophthal 106:312, 1988.
99. Weber, PA, Burton, GD, Epitropoulos, AT: Laser trabeculoplasty retreatment. Ophthal Surg 20:702, 1989.
100. Jorizzo, PA, Samples, JR, Van Buskirk, EM: The effect of repeat argon laser trabeculoplasty. Am J Ophthal 106:682, 1988.
101. Sherwood, MB, Lattimer, J, Hitchings, RA: Laser trabeculoplasty as supplementary treatment for primary open angle glaucoma. Br J Ophthal 71:188, 1987.
102. Thomas, JV, El-Mofty, A, Hamdy, EE, Simmons, RJ: Argon laser trabeculoplasty as initial therapy for glaucoma. Arch Ophthal 102:702, 1984.
103. Rosenthal, AR, Chaudhuri, PR, Chiapella, AP: Laser trabeculoplasty primary therapy in open-

angle glaucoma. A preliminary report. Arch Ophthal 102:699, 1984.

104. Migdal, C, Hitchings, R: Primary therapy for chronic simple glaucoma. The role of argon laser trabeculoplasty. Trans Ophthal Soc UK 104:62, 1984.

105. Tuulonen, A, Koponen, J, Alanko, HI, Airaksinen, PJ: Laser trabeculoplasty versus medication treatment as primary therapy for glaucoma. Acta Ophthal 67:275, 1989.

106. The Glaucoma Laser Trial Research Group. The glaucoma laser trial (GLT). 2. Results of argon laser trabeculoplasty versus topical medicines. Ophthalmology 97:1403, 1990.

107. Watson, PG, Allen, ED, Graham, CM, et al: Argon laser trabeculoplasty or trabeculectomy. A prospective randomised block study. Trans Ophthal Soc UK 104:55, 1984.

108. Burian, HM: A case of Marfan's syndrome with bilateral glaucoma. With description of a new type of operation for developmental glaucoma (trabeculotomy ab externo). Am J Ophthal 50:1187, 1960.

109. Smith, R: A new technique for opening the canal of Schlemm. Preliminary report. Br J Ophthal 44:370, 1960.

110. Harms, H, Dannheim, R: Trabeculotomy results and problems. In: Microsurgery in Glaucoma, MacKensen, C, ed. Karger, Basel, 1970, p. 121.

111. McPherson, SD Jr: Results of external trabeculotomy. Am J Ophthal 76:918, 1973.

112. Allen, L, Burian, HM: Trabeculotomy ab externo. Am J Ophthal 53:19, 1962.

113. Board, RJ, Shields, MB: Combined trabeculotomy-trabeculectomy for the management of glaucoma associated with Sturge-Weber syndrome. Ophthal Surg 12:813, 1981.

114. Rothkoff, L, Blumenthal, M, Biedner, B: Trabeculotomy in late onset congenital glaucoma. Br J Ophthal 63:38, 1979.

115. Moses, RA: Electrocautery puncture of the trabecular meshwork in enucleated human eyes. Am J Ophthal 72:1094, 1971.

116. Maselli, E, Sirellini, M, Pruneri, F, Galantino, G: Diathermo-trabeculotomy ab externo. A new technique for opening the canal of Schlemm. Br J Ophthal 59:516, 1975.

117. Maselli, E, Galantino, G, Pruneri, F, Sirellini, M: Diathermo-trabeculotomy ab externo: indications and long-term results. Br J Ophthal 61:675, 1977.

118. Hager, H, Hauck, W, Heppke, G, Hoffmann, F, Resewitz, E-P: Experimental principles of trabecular-electro-puncture (TEP). Graefe's Arch Ophthal 185:95, 1972.

119. Bonnet, M, Schiffer, H-P: On trabeculotomy ab externo. Localisation of the canal of Schlemm by passing a catheter through an aqueous vein. Klin Monatsbl Augenheilkd 161:563, 1972.

120. Jocson, VL: Air trabeculotomy. Am J Ophthal 79:107, 1975.

121. Skjaerpe, F: Selective trabeculectomy. A report of a new surgical method for open angle glaucoma. Acta Ophthal 61:714, 1983.

122. Gaasterland, DE, Bonney, CH III, Rodrigues, MM, Kuwabara, T: Long-term effects of Q-switched ruby laser on monkey anterior chamber angle. Invest Ophthal Vis Sci 26:129, 1985.

123. Van der Zypen, E, Fankhauser, F: The ultrastructural features of laser trabeculopuncture and cyclodialysis. Ophthalmologica 179:189, 1979.

124. Melamed, S, Pei, J, Puliafito, CA, Epstein, DL: Q-switched neodymium-YAG laser trabeculopuncture in monkeys. Arch Ophthal 103:129, 1985.

125. Dutton, GN, Cameron, SA, Allan, D, Thomas, R: Parameters for neodymium-YAG laser trabeculotomy: an in-vitro study. Br J Ophthal 71:782, 1987.

126. Dutton, GN, Allan, D, Cameron, SA: Pulsed neodymium-YAG laser trabeculotomy: energy requirements and replicability. Br J Ophthal 73:177, 1989.

127. Venkatesh, S, Lee, WR, Guthrie, S, et al: An in-vitro morphological study of Q-switched neodymium/YAG laser trabeculotomy. Br J Ophthal 70:89, 1986.

128. Lee, WR, Dutton, GN, Cameron, SA: Short-pulsed neodymium-YAG laser trabeculotomy. An in vivo morphological study in the human eye. Invest Ophthal Vis Sci 29:1698, 1988.

129. Melamed, S, Latina, MA, Epstein, DL: Neodymium:YAG laser trabeculopuncture in juvenile open-angle glaucoma. Ophthalmology 94:163, 1987.

130. Del Priore, LV, Robin, AL, Pollack, IP: Long-term follow-up of neodymium:YAG laser angle surgery for open-angle glaucoma. Ophthalmology 95:277, 1988.

131. Barkan, O: Technic of goniotomy. Arch Ophthal 19:217, 1938.

132. Draeger, J: New microsurgical techniques to improve chamber angle surgery. Glaucoma 2:403, 1980.

133. Amoils, SP, Simmons, RJ: Goniotomy with intraocular illumination. A preliminary report. Arch Ophthal 80:488, 1968.

134. Hodapp, E, Heuer, DK: A simple technique for goniotomy. Am J Ophthal 102:537, 1986.

135. Catalano, RA, King, RA, Calhoun, JH, Sargent, RA: One versus two simultaneous goniotomies as the initial surgical procedure for primary infantile glaucoma. J Ped Ophthal Strab 26:9, 1989.

136. Litinsky, SM, Shaffer, RN, Hetherington, J, Hoskins, HD: Operative complications of goniotomy. Trans Am Acad Ophthal Otol 83:78, 1977.

137. Biglan, AW, Hiles, DA: The visual results follow-

ing infantile glaucoma surgery. J Ped Ophthal Strab 16:377, 1979.

138. Scheie, HG: Goniopuncture—a new filtering operation for glaucoma. Arch Ophthal 44:761, 1950.
139. Scheie, HG: Goniopuncture: an evaluation after eleven years. Arch Ophthal 65:38, 1961.
140. Kozart, DM, Cameron, JD: Goniodiathermy: experimental studies on ab interno filtration. Ann Ophthal 10:1597, 1978.
141. Fernandez, JL, Galin, MA: Technique of direct goniotomy. Arch Ophthal 90:305, 1973.
142. Haas, J: Goniotomy in Aphakia, Welsh, R, ed. In: The Second Report on Cataract Surgery. Miami Educational Press, Miami, Fla., 1971, p. 551.
143. Hoskins, HD, Hetherington, J Jr, Shaffer, RN: Surgical management of the inflammatory glaucomas. Pers Ophthal 1:173, 1977.
144. Herschler, J, Davis, B: Modified goniotomy for inflammatory glaucoma. Histologic evidence for the mechanism of pressure reduction. Arch Ophthal 98:684, 1980.
145. Kanski, JJ, McAllister, JA: Trabeculodialysis for inflammatory glaucoma in children and young adults. Ophthalmology 92:927, 1985.
146. Yumita, A, Shirato, S, Yamamoto, T, Kitazawa, Y: Goniotomy with Q-switched Nd-YAG laser in juvenile developmental glaucoma: a preliminary report. Jap J Ophthal 28:349, 1984.
147. Senft, SH, Tomey, KF, Traverso, CE: Neodymium-YAG laser goniotomy vs surgical goniotomy. A preliminary study in paired eyes. Arch Ophthal 107:1773, 1989.
148. Promesberger, H, Busse, H, Mewe, L: Findings and surgical therapy in congenital glaucoma. Klin Monatsbl Augenheilkd 176:186, 1980.
149. Broughton, WL, Parks, MM: An analysis of treatment of congenital glaucoma by goniotomy. Am J Ophthal 91:566, 1981.
150. Draeger, J, Wirt, H, Von Domarus, D: Long-term results after goniotomy. Klin Monatsbl Augenheilkd 180:264, 1982.
151. Francois, J, Van Oye, R, Mendoza, A, De Sutter, E: Goniotomy for congenital glaucoma. J Fr Ophthal 5:661, 1982.
152. McPherson, SD Jr, McFarland, D: External trabeculotomy for developmental glaucoma. Ophthalmology 87:302, 1980.
153. Luntz, MH, Livingston, DG: Trabeculotomy ab externo and trabeculectomy in congenital and adult-onset glaucoma. Am J Ophthal 83:174, 1977.
154. Gregersen, E, Kessing, SVV: Congenital glaucoma before and after the introduction of microsurgery. Results of "macrosurgery" 1943–1963 and of microsurgery (trabeculotomy/ectomy) 1970–1974. Acta Ophthal 55:422, 1977.
155. Luntz, MH: Congenital, infantile, and juvenile glaucoma. Ophthalmology 86:793, 1979.
156. Dannheim, R, Haas, H: Visual acuity and intraocular pressure after surgery in congenital glaucoma. Klin Monatsbl Augenheilkd 177:296, 1980.
157. Quigley, HA: Childhood glaucoma. Results with trabeculotomy and study of reversible cupping. Ophthalmology 89:219, 1982.
158. McPherson, SD Jr, Berry, DP: Goniotomy vs external trabeculotomy for developmental glaucoma. Am J Ophthal 95:427, 1983.
159. Hoskins, HD Jr, Shaffer, RN, Hetherington, J: Goniotomy vs trabeculotomy. J Ped Ophthal Strab 21:153, 1984.
160. Luntz, MH: The advantages of trabeculotomy over goniotomy. J Ped Ophthal Strab 2:150, 1984.
161. Anderson, DR: Trabeculotomy compared to goniotomy for glaucoma in children. Ophthalmology 90:805, 1983.
162. Heine, L: Die Cyklodialyse, eine neue Glaucomoperation. Deutsche Med Wehnschr 31:825, 1905.
163. Barkan, O: Cyclodialysis: its mode of action. Histologic observations in a case of glaucoma in which both eyes were successfully treated by cyclodialysis. Arch Ophthal 43:793, 1950.
164. Bill, A: The routes for bulk drainage of aqueous humour in rabbits with and without cyclodialysis. Doc Ophthal 20:157, 1966.
165. Pederson, JE, Gaasterland, DE, MacLellan, HM: Experimental ciliochoroidal detachment. Effect on intraocular pressure and aqueous humor flow. Arch Ophthal 97:536, 1979.
166. Suguro, K, Toris, CB, Pederson, JE: Uveoscleral outflow following cyclodialysis in the monkey eye using a fluorescent tracer. Invest Ophthal Vis Sci 26:810, 1985.
167. Toris, CB, Pederson, JE: Effect of intraocular pressure on uveoscleral outflow following cyclodialysis in the monkey eye. Invest Ophthal Vis Sci 26:1745, 1985.
168. Auricchio, G: Considerations on mechanism of action of cyclodialysis. Boll Ocul 35:401, 1956.
169. Chandler, PA, Maumenee, AE: A major cause of hypotony. Trans Am Acad Ophthal Otol 52:563, 1961.
170. Gills, JP Jr, Paterson, CA, Paterson, ME: Action of cyclodialysis utilizing an implant studied by manometry in a human eye. Exp Eye Res 6:75, 1967.
171. Ascher, KW: Some details of the technique of cyclodialysis. Am J Ophthal 50:1207, 1960.
172. O'Brien, CS, Weih, J: Cyclodialysis. Arch Ophthal 42:606, 1949.
173. Haisten, MW, Guyton, JS: Cyclodialysis with air injection: technique and results in ninety-four consecutive operations. Arch Ophthal 590:507, 1958.
174. Miller, RD, Nisbet, RM: Cyclodialysis with air injection in black patients. Ophthal Surg 12:92, 1981.

175. Alpar, JJ: Sodium hyaluronate (Healon®) in cyclodialysis. CLAOJ 11:201, 1985.
176. Simmons, RJ, Kimbrough, RL: A modified cyclodialysis spatula. Ophthal Surg 10:67, 1979.
177. Cohen, SW, Banko, W, Nath, S: A fiber-optics cyclodialysis spatula. Ophthal Surg 10:74, 1979.
178. Gills, JP: Cyclodialysis implants in human eyes. Am J Ophthal 61:841, 1966.
179. Streeten, BW, Belkowitz, M: Experimental hypotony with silastic. Arch Ophthal 78:503, 1967.
180. Richards, RD: Long-term results of gonioplasty. Am J Ophthal 70:715, 1970.
181. Portney, GL: Silicone elastomer implantation cyclodialysis. A negative report. Arch Ophthal 89:10, 1973.
182. Krasnov, MM: Iridocyclo-retraction in narrow-angle glaucoma. Br J Ophthal 55:389, 1971.
183. Aviner, Z: Modified Krasnov's iridocycloretraction for aphakic glaucoma. Ann Ophthal 7:859, 1975.
184. Sugar, HS: Experiences with some modifications of cyclodialysis for aphakic glaucoma. Ann Ophthal 9:1045, 1977.
185. Nesterov, AP, Kolesnikova, LN: Filtering iridocycloretraction in chronic closed-angle glaucoma. Am J Ophthal 99:340, 1985.
186. Mizukawa, A: Histopathological study on argon laser cyclodialysis of cynomolgus monkey eyes. Folia Ophthal Jap 35:526, 1984.
187. Mizukawa, A, Okisaka, S, Taketani, P: Argon laser cyclodialysis for open angle glaucoma. Folia Ophthal Jap 36:750, 1985.
188. Partamian, LG: Treatment of a cyclodialysis cleft with argon laser photocoagulation in a patient with a shallow anterior chamber. Am J Ophthal 99:5, 1985.
189. Best, W, Hartwig, H: Traumatic cyclodialysis and its treatment. Klin Monatsbl Augenheilkd 170:917, 1977.
190. Tate, GW Jr, Lynn, JR: A new technique for the surgical repair of cyclodialysis induced hypotony. Ann Ophthal 10:1261, 1978.
191. Wagdi, SF, Simmons, RJ: Acute glaucoma from unrecognized closure of surgical cyclodialysis cleft. Glaucoma 3:287, 1981.
192. Campbell, DG, Vela, A: Modern goniosynechialysis for the treatment of synechial angle-closure glaucoma. Ophthalmology 91:1052, 1984.
193. Weiss, JS, Waring, GO III: Dental mirror for goniosynechialysis during penetrating keratoplasty. Am J Ophthal 100:331, 1985.
194. Shingleton, BJ, Chang, MA, Bellows, AR, Thomas, JV: Surgical goniosynechialysis for angle-closure glaucoma. Ophthalmology 97:551, 1990.
195. Senn, P, Kopp, B: Nd:YAG laser goniosynechialysis in angle-closure glaucoma. Klin Monatsbl Augenheilkd 196:210, 1990.
196. Simmons, RJ, Dueker, DK, Kimbrough, RL, Aiello, LM: Goniophotocoagulation for neovascular glaucoma. Trans Am Acad Ophthal Otol 83:80, 1977.
197. Simmons, RJ, Deppermann, SR, Dueker, DK: The role of goniophotocoagulation in neovascularization of the anterior chamber angle. Ophthalmology 87:79, 1980.

Chapter 35

SURGERY OF THE IRIS

LASER IRIDOTOMY

Historical Background

Meyer-Schwickerath,[1] in 1956, first reported the use of light energy to create a hole in the iris. Using the xenon arc photocoagulator, he and others found that a peripheral iridotomy could be produced but that the amount of heat required damaged the cornea and lens.[1,2] With the introduction of lasers in the 1960s, investigation of this treatment modality continued, primarily with ruby lasers.[3–7] However, as with laser trabeculoplasty, it was not until the advent of argon laser technology in the 1970s that laser iridotomy became clinically practical. By the mid-1970s, several reports of successful argon laser iridotomy appeared in the literature,[8–11] and by the end of that decade, laser iridotomy had replaced incisional iridectomy as the surgical procedure of choice for angle-closure glaucomas. During the 1980s, continued study of laser iridotomy techniques led to the popular use of the neodymium:YAG (Nd:YAG) laser for this operation.

Techniques

Instrumentation

Several different types of *lasers* and surgical techniques can be used to create an iridotomy. The unit most commonly used in the early days of laser surgery was the continuous-wave argon laser.[8–17] Other lasers that have also been shown to be effective for creating iridotomies include the pulsed argon laser[13,16,18,19] and the krypton laser.[20] However, the pulsed Nd:YAG laser has gained in popularity[21–28] and is probably the most commonly used unit today for laser iridotomies. A portable Nd:YAG laser has been shown to be effective for use in remote geographic areas.[29] The relative merits of the argon and Nd:YAG laser iridotomies are considered later in this chapter.

A *contact lens* is helpful in performing a laser iridotomy, since it (1) keeps the lids separated, (2) minimizes corneal epithelial burns by acting as a heat sink, and (3) provides some control of eye movement. In addition, convex-surfaced contact lenses have been designed to increase the power density on the iris.[30–32] The most commonly used is

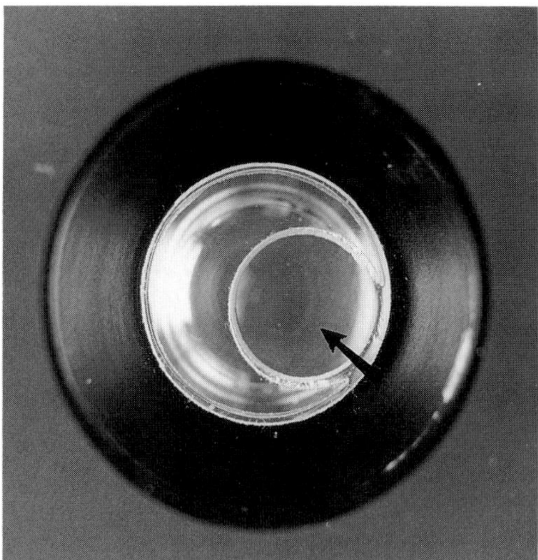

Figure 35.1. Abraham contact lens with planoconvex button (*arrow*) bonded to front surface for laser iridotomy.

the Abraham iridotomy lens, which has a +66 diopter planoconvex button bonded to the front surface of the contact lens (Fig. 35.1).[30] This lens doubles the laser beam diameter at the level of the cornea, while reducing it to approximately one-half the original size on the iris, which reduces the power density at the cornea to one-fourth the original level and increases it on the iris by a factor of 4. Another contact lens, the Wise iridotomy-sphincterotomy lens, has a 103-diopter optical button decentered 2.5 mm, which further reduces the iris focal spot and increases the energy density.[32] These principles have their greatest application with the argon laser, although the same contact lenses are also useful with the Nd:YAG laser.

With all lasers and contact lenses, a high magnification (e.g., 40×) should be used in the slit-lamp delivery system.

Preoperative Medication

Topical *pilocarpine* should be instilled prior to the procedure to maximally thin and stretch the peripheral iris. If the patient presents with an acute attack of angle-closure glaucoma, it is best to break the attack medically if possible and maintain the patient on medication to allow clearance of any corneal edema and to facilitate constriction of the pupil. If significant iritis persists after breaking the attack, it may be advisable to use topical steroids for 24–48 hours before proceeding with the laser surgery. However, if the attack does not respond to medical therapy, laser iridotomy (or iridoplasty or pupilloplasty, as discussed later in this chapter) may be effective in breaking the attack.[33]

In nearly all cases, only topical anesthesia, such as proparacaine 0.5%, is required. Only rarely is a retrobulbar injection needed for a patient with nystagmus or who is uncooperative. It has become a standard practice among many surgeons to also instill a drop of 1% *apraclonidine* 1 hour before the procedure and immediately after the surgery to reduce the risk of a postoperative intraocular pressure (IOP) rise.[34]

Selecting the Treatment Site

Any quadrant of the iris can be used to create the laser iridotomy, although the superior iris is preferable in most cases, since it places the iridotomy beneath the upper lid. The 12 o'clock position is usually avoided, since gas bubbles may collect in that area and interfere with completion of the procedure. The superior nasal quadrant has the advantage of directing the laser beam toward the nasal periphery of the retina. One exception to the selection of a superior iris quadrant is the patient with silicone oil in an aphakic eye, in which case the iridotomy should be placed inferiorly to avoid blockage by the oil, which rises to the top of the eye.

Whichever quadrant is used, the slit lamp should always be positioned so that the laser beam is directed away from the macula. The iridotomy is usually placed between the middle and peripheral thirds of the iris. However, if this is not feasible because of peripheral corneal haze or close proximity between peripheral iris and cornea, a more central location can be used, as long as it is peripheral to the sphincter muscle.

Several features of the iris may facilitate creation of the iridotomy. An area of thin iris or a large crypt is usually easier to penetrate. In lightly pigmented eyes, a local area of increased pigmentation, such as a frec-

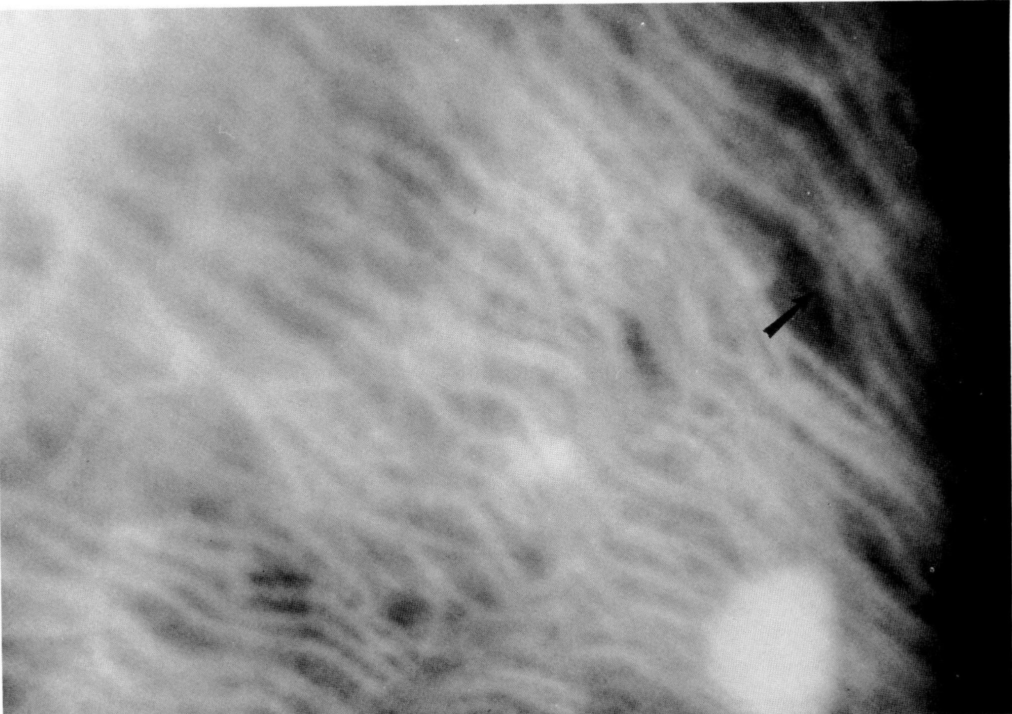

Figure 35.2. Slit-lamp view of light blue iris showing white collagen strands, which are difficult to penetrate with argon laser energy and should be avoided when possible by selecting an area where they are separated (*arrow*).

kle, may improve absorption of argon laser energy. In addition, the radially arranged white collagen strands in the stroma can be very difficult to penetrate with argon laser, and it is helpful to select a treatment site where two strands are more widely separated (Fig. 35.2).[35]

Iridotomy with Continuous-Wave Argon Laser

Several basic techniques have been advocated for producing iridotomies with the continuous-wave argon laser. The "hump" technique involves first creating a localized elevation of the iris with a large-diameter, low-energy burn, and then penetrating the hump with small, intense burns.[36] In the "drumhead" technique, large-diameter, low-energy burns are placed around the intended treatment site to put the iris on stretch, and that area is then penetrated with small, high-energy burns.[14,37] A third approach goes directly to penetrating burns.[13,16,17] The latter technique may be modified by using multiple short-duration burns.[38,39] However, none of these approaches is ideal for all situations, and it is best to tailor the iridotomy technique primarily according to the color of the iris. For irides of all colors, the laser settings are first selected for the iris stroma and then adjusted for the pigment epithelium.

Medium Brown Iris. This is the easiest iris to penetrate with continuous-wave argon laser, and the following method represents one technique in these patients.

A "straight" approach is employed for medium brown irides, with laser settings of 0.1–0.2 second duration, 50 microns spot size, and 700–1500 (average, 1000) milliwatts (mW). The first application usually produces a deep crater in the iris stroma. A gas bubble, which usually floats up away from the treatment site, may also be created (Fig. 35.3). If the bubble does not move, it can be dislodged by penetrating it with the next laser application or by placing the beam adjacent to the bubble. A cluster of

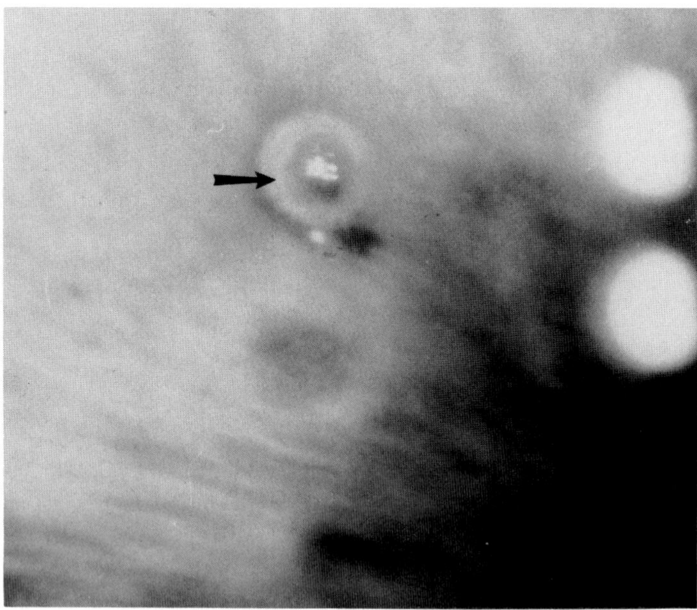

Figure 35.3. Gas bubble (*arrow*) produced during creation of argon laser iridotomy.

several contiguous burns is used to produce a stromal crater of approximately 500 microns in diameter. Additional laser applications are then placed in the bed of the crater until the pigment epithelial layer is reached, as evidenced by a cloud of pigment (Fig. 35.4).

When most of the stroma has been eliminated and only pigment epithelium remains, the laser intensity should be reduced (e.g., 100 microns and 500–700 mW, or 50 microns and 200–600 mW) to clean away the remaining tissue. The same settings can be used for irides of other colors, since the pigment epithelial layer is similar in all eyes. Higher-intensity burns at this stage of the treatment may dislodge adjacent pigment epithelium, creating a so-called "cascade phenomenon," which causes further obstruction of the iridotomy. This technique for the medium brown iris normally takes 30–60 laser applications to create a patent iridotomy.

Dark Brown Iris. A laser iridotomy is more difficult to achieve in these eyes, partly because of the thick, dense stroma. Standard penetrating burns described above often produce a black char in the stromal crater, making the site resistant to further penetration. One way to minimize this complication and achieve a patent iridotomy in the dark brown iris is to use multiple, short-duration burns, or the "chipping" technique.[36,38,40] The important feature of this modification is the short exposure time of 0.02–0.05 second, with standard settings of 50 microns and 700–1500 mW. With this approach, minute fragments of stroma are "chipped away," often requiring 200–300 applications to penetrate the stroma. Once the pigment epithelial layer is reached, the settings should be changed to the lower intensity level described for the medium brown iris to complete the procedure.

Blue Iris. These eyes can be difficult because the lightly pigmented stroma does not absorb laser light sufficiently to produce a burn through this portion of the iris. The pigment epithelium near the treatment site may be dislodged, leaving intact stroma that is impermeable to aqueous flow. Some surgeons prefer a two-stage approach, in which settings of 500 microns and 200–300 mW are first used to create a local tan-colored area of increased stromal density, followed by penetration burns of 50 microns, 500–700 mW, and 0.1 second to create a full-thickness hole in the stroma.[41] Others have suggested a direct approach, using settings of 50 microns, 1000–1500 mW, and a prolonged duration of 0.5 seconds to burn a

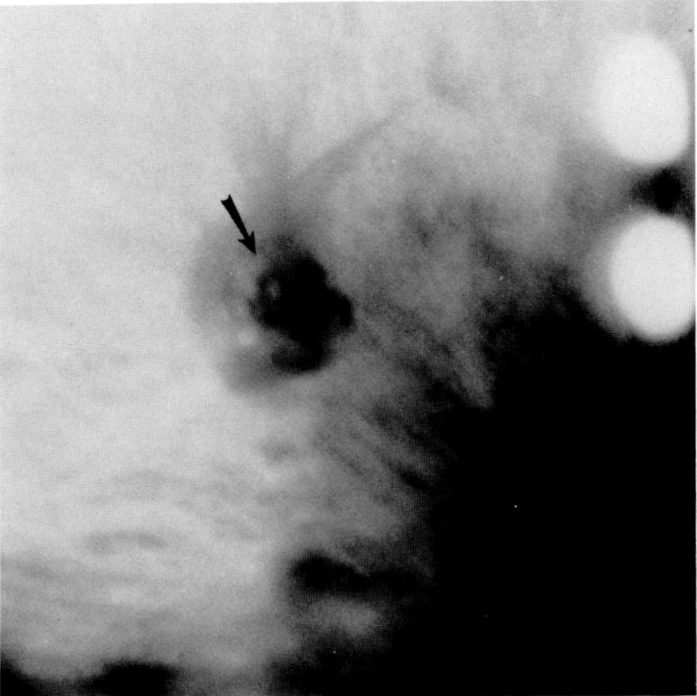

Figure 35.4. Pigment cloud (*arrow*) released from pigment epithelium when it has been perforated during creation of laser iridotomy.

hole through the stroma in two to three applications.[35,40] With either technique, the settings should then be changed to those described for the medium brown iris to penetrate or remove the remaining pigment epithelium from the iridotomy site.

Iridotomy with Pulsed Lasers

Pulsed Neodymium:YAG Laser. As previously noted, this has now become the most commonly used technique for laser iridotomy. The extremely high energy levels and short exposure times of these lasers electromechanically disrupt tissue, independent of pigment absorption and the thermal effect. As a result, they are particularly useful in creating iridotomies in light blue irides but are effective in all eyes. The technique usually involves simultaneous perforation of the iris stroma and pigment epithelium with energy levels in the range of 5–15 millijoules (mJ).[21–28] The pulse duration is fixed for each instrument, in the range of 12 nanoseconds, but the number of pulses per burst can be adjusted in most units, with surgeons generally preferring one to three pulses per burst. The spot size is also fixed, although some units provide a choice between a single focal point or multiple focal points, with the latter creating a larger lesion. Since the wavelength of the Nd:YAG laser is beyond the visible spectrum, a helium-neon laser beam is used for focusing on the iris. With instruments that allow a selected separation between the focal points of the two laser beams, the setting should be such that they are coincident when performing a laser iridotomy.

The standard technique involves selecting an iris site using the same criteria as for argon laser iridotomy, although it is often possible to place the iridotomy more peripherally with the Nd:YAG laser. The latter is desirable, among other reasons, to avoid injuring the lens. When selecting the treatment site, attention should be given to avoiding any apparent iris vessels, since these are more likely to bleed with Nd:YAG than with argon laser surgery. It is often possible to create a patent iridotomy with a single laser application and rarely with more

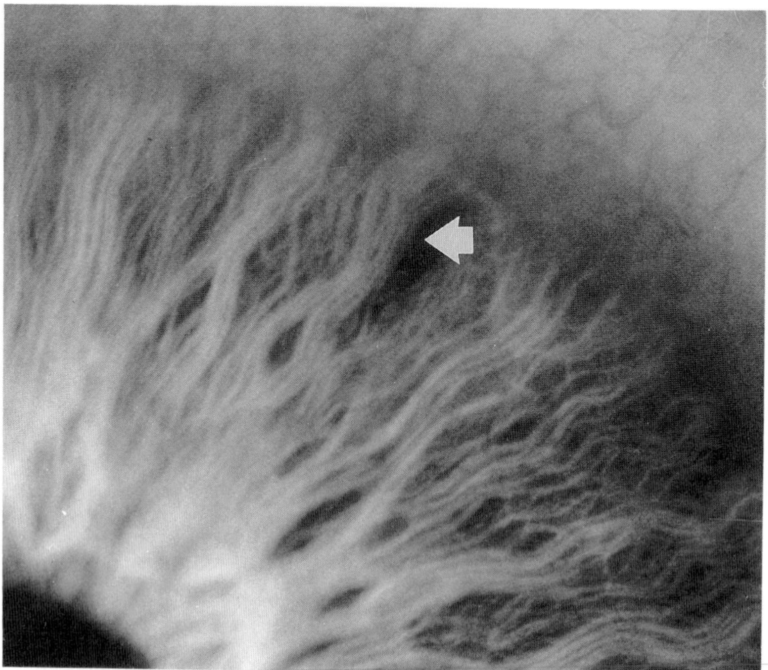

Figure 35.5. Typical appearance of peripheral iridotomy created with a neodymium:YAG laser (*arrow*).

than two or three, especially in blue or light brown eyes. However, these may be smaller than an argon laser iridotomy (Fig. 35.5), and it is often advisable to create more than one iridotomy.

Several variations in technique have been described. One employs both the argon and Nd:YAG lasers by first creating a stromal crater with short-duration argon laser burns and then penetrating the iris with low-energy, single-pulse Nd:YAG applications.[42,43] This has an advantage of minimizing bleeding by first coagulating iris vessels. It is also useful in eyes with thick, dark iris stroma, in which the Nd:YAG laser energy may cause considerable disruption and dispersion of stromal tissue before penetrating the iris. Another technique involves multiple low-energy (1.0–1.7 mJ) applications in a line across the radial iris fibers to create an iridotomy of larger, more controllable size.[44] The investigator believed that this technique was safer than a similar approach with the argon laser or the standard higher-energy Nd:YAG technique.[45] Iridotomies have also been created experimentally with the transscleral application of longer duration, thermal Nd:YAG laser burns via a fiberoptic system.[46]

Other Pulsed Lasers. The pulsed *argon* laser, which emits laser energy in a chain of very short pulses rather than in a continuous wave, vaporizes the absorbing tissue with minimal heat loss and destruction to the surrounding area. These features provide some advantage over continuous-wave argon lasers for producing iridotomies in that more energy is used in penetrating the iris, with less distortion and disruption of surrounding tissue.[18]

The basic technique is similar to that for continuous-wave argon laser iridotomy, with the straight or chipping method being used in most cases. However, the settings differ considerably for the pulsed argon laser unit. The perforating mode is employed, and the power setting is 20–25 watts. The usual parameters are 50 microns, 0.2 second, and 300 pulses/second, adjusted according to tissue response (the individual pulse is fixed at 128 microseconds). With these settings, the number of exposures to achieve an iridotomy varies from 2 to 250, depending on the type of iris.[18]

A Q-switched ruby laser was found in monkey studies to be suitable for creating iridotomies,[47] and dye lasers have been used clinically to produce iridotomies with a single pulse.[48]

Comparison of Argon and Neodymium:YAG Laser Iridotomies

Histologic studies have shown that iridotomies created with an argon laser have more extensive early edema and tissue destruction at the margins of the treatment,[18,19] as compared with those with Nd:YAG laser, in which the lesions are more circumscribed with limited tissue alterations at the margins.[26,28] However, freeze-frame analysis of high-speed cinematography in ox eyes showed particles traveling more than 8 mm from the Nd:YAG treatment site at speeds in excess of 20 K/h,[27] and the shock waves affected the trabecular meshwork and corneal endothelium of monkey eyes when the Nd:YAG was within 0.8 mm of the limbus.[49]

In clinical comparisons of the two surgical approaches, the Nd:YAG laser iridotomies had the disadvantage of frequent bleeding, although this usually stops spontaneously or with pressure to the eye by the contact lens and rarely leads to significant complications.[23,24,50,51] On the other hand, disadvantages of argon laser iridotomy include more iritis, pupillary distortion, and late closure of the iridotomy. In one study of 33 eyes in which an iridotomy could not be created with the argon laser, a patent iridotomy was achieved in all eyes with the Nd:YAG laser in single sessions.[52] In general, neodymium:YAG laser iridotomies require considerably fewer total applications with a marked reduction in total energy delivery as compared with argon laser iridotomies.

Prevention and Management of Complications

As with laser trabeculoplasty, a transient IOP rise and a mild anterior uveitis are common early postoperative complications. Other potential complications include closure of the iridotomy, corneal damage, hyphema, cataract formation, and retinal burns.

Transient IOP Rise. This is one of the most common serious complications in the early period after either argon[53] or Nd:YAG[54] laser iridotomies. Studies in rabbits suggest that this is related to a release of prostaglandin[55] and prostaglandin-like substances[56] into the aqueous with a breakdown in the blood-aqueous barrier and an accumulation of blood plasma and fibrin in the anterior chamber angle.[57–59] A histopathologic study in monkey eyes revealed a rapid accumulation of particulate debris in the angle,[60] which may also contribute to the transient pressure elevation. Clinically, the risk of transient IOP rise appears to be related to the total energy delivered but not to the presence of chronic angle-closure glaucoma.[54] As previously noted, one drop of 1% apraclonidine 1 hour before and immediately after the laser surgery has a profound effect on minimizing this complication.[34] Topical clonidine has also been shown to be effective,[61] but it has a greater risk of systemic hypotension than its para-amino derivative, apraclonidine.

Anterior Uveitis. Some degree of transient iritis occurs in all eyes, which is undoubtedly associated with the blood-aqueous barrier breakdown noted in animal studies.[57–59] Topical steroids for the first 3–5 postoperative days are sufficient to control this mild complication in the majority of cases. However, an occasional eye may have a marked inflammation, sometimes occurring days or weeks after the procedure, and a hypopyon has been reported following laser iridotomy.[62] A case of prolonged iritis with transient cystoid macular edema has also been described.[63]

Closure of Iridotomy. The iridotomy may close during the first few weeks, especially with argon laser iridotomy, as a result of accumulation of pigment granules and debris. Therefore, it is advisable to continue pilocarpine for the first 4–6 postoperative weeks. If the iridotomy remains patent, it is usually safe to stop the miotic after this time, unless it is needed to control a chronic pressure elevation. It has been suggested that a mydriatic provocative test should be employed after stopping the miotic to confirm the functional reliability of the iridotomy.[17] Late closure is rare with Nd:YAG laser iridotomies. In one series of 200 cases,

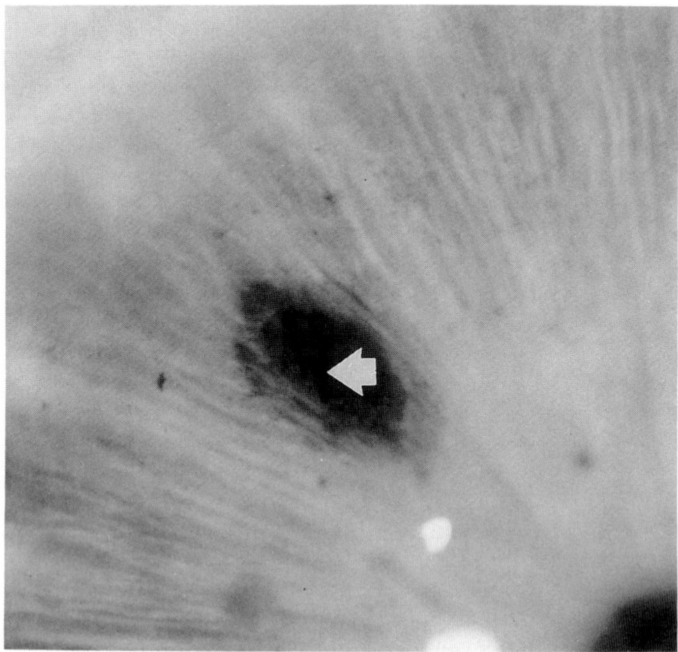

Figure 35.6. Argon laser iridotomy with patency demonstrated by visualization of anterior lens capsule (*arrow*).

the two late closures were both in eyes with preexisting chronic uveitis.[64]

The minimum diameter of a laser iridotomy that is needed to prevent further attacks of angle-closure glaucoma has yet to be determined and probably differs from one patient to the next. One case has been reported in which angle closure recurred despite a patent 75-micron iridotomy, suggesting that this is too small for at least certain eyes.[65] A minimum diameter of 150–200 microns has been recommended.[65] In some eyes, the laser iridotomy spontaneously enlarges over months or years,[66] although this should not be relied upon in borderline situations, in which case the opening should be further enlarged.

Patency of the iridotomy is best confirmed by visualizing anterior lens capsule or vitreous face through the opening (Fig. 35.6). Transillumination can also be used, although this is sometimes misleading, especially with a blue iris, in which dislodged pigment epithelium can produce a transillumination defect despite an intact overlying stroma, which is impermeable to aqueous flow.

Corneal Damage. Focal epithelial and endothelial burns of the cornea are not uncommon when larger amounts of laser energy are used, although these usually heal quickly with no apparent sequelae. In monkey eyes, laser iridotomy was not associated with significant endothelial cell damage.[67] Specular microscopy and pachymetry revealed no significant difference in the endothelial cell count or corneal thickness after laser iridotomy in two studies,[68,69] although a significant increase in endothelial cell size was noted in a third investigation.[70] Generalized corneal decompensation was reported in five eyes of three patients after argon laser iridotomy, and factors that might have predisposed to this complication included episodes of angle-closure glaucoma with pressure elevations and inflammation, cornea guttata, diabetes, and the need for multiple treatments requiring high laser energy.[71]

Hyphema. As previously noted, a small amount of bleeding from the iridotomy site is common following Nd:YAG laser iridotomy but is rarely of serious consequence.[21–25] Persistent bleeding from the treatment site can usually be stopped by applying pressure to the eye with the contact lens for a few seconds to a minute. Hyphemas are uncommon after argon laser iridotomies but may occur,[72,73] especially in eyes with rubeosis iridis or uveitis.

Cataract Formation. Focal anterior lens opacities are common beneath an iridotomy produced with an argon laser.[23,25,74] Most of these are nonprogressive, although reduced visual acuity resulting from cataract progression has been documented.[74] The rate of progression is similar to that following incisional surgical iridectomy,[17] and a clear cause-and-effect relationship between either surgical approach and cataracts has not been established. Lens changes are much less common with Nd:YAG laser iridotomies,[23–25] although capsular damage[75] with rare cataract formation[76] has been reported. In two rabbit studies, no lens damage was seen with either argon or Nd:YAG laser iridotomies, even when additional laser applications were placed through patent iridotomies.[77,78] However, a monkey study suggested a threshold for lens damage, with no damage at 6 mJ or less and one to two pulses per burst, but local damage with higher energies or three pulses per burst.[79]

Retinal Burns. Most visual function studies have shown no adverse effect from argon laser iridotomy,[80] and the same is presumably true for Nd:YAG laser iridotomy. However, one study did reveal static perimetric and fluorescein angiographic evidence of focal retinal damage in the quadrant of treatment 6 months after argon laser iridotomy.[81] Retinal damage is best minimized by always aiming the laser beam toward peripheral retina. Failure to do so may result in serious retinal burns, and acute, permanent loss of vision has been reported as a result of inadvertent foveal photocoagulation during laser iridotomy.[82] The risk is reduced but not eliminated by the use of an Abraham lens.[83] One case of temporary bilateral serous choroidal and nonrhegmatogenous retinal detachment following Nd:YAG laser iridotomy has also been reported.[84]

A case of malignant glaucoma has also been reported following a laser iridotomy for acute angle-closure glaucoma.[85]

INCISIONAL IRIDECTOMY

Laser Iridotomy vs Incisional Iridectomy

The incisional surgical iridectomy is one of the safest, most effective operations for glaucoma. For the laser iridotomy to replace it as the procedure of choice, therefore, significant advantages had to be demonstrated. Long-term follow-up studies have shown that laser iridotomies are comparable to the incisional procedures in terms of efficacy and safety.[17,86,87] In addition, the laser approach has the advantages of: (1) being an outpatient procedure; (2) eliminating the need for retrobulbar anesthesia; (3) reducing surgical complications, such as wound leak, hyphema, and endophthalmitis; (4) shortening postoperative recovery time; and (5) lowering costs. These advantages have led to a significant increase in the annual rate of laser iridotomies as compared with incisional iridectomies before the laser was in common use, which is thought to represent an improvement in the quality of care.[88]

For the reasons noted above, laser iridotomy has become the procedure of choice for most cases of angle-closure glaucoma. However, there are situations when the incisional approach is still required. Some patients are unable to sit at the slit lamp or are unable to cooperate sufficiently for laser therapy. At other times, the cornea may be too cloudy or the iris too close to the cornea to allow laser iridotomy. There is also the rare case in which a patent iridotomy cannot be achieved with laser treatment or in which the opening repeatedly closes postoperatively. The latter is particularly common in eyes with marked uveitis. For these reasons, the surgeon must still be familiar with the time-honored procedure of incisional iridectomy.

Techniques

Peripheral Iridectomy

The most commonly used incisional approach in the surgical treatment of angle-closure glaucoma is the peripheral iridectomy.

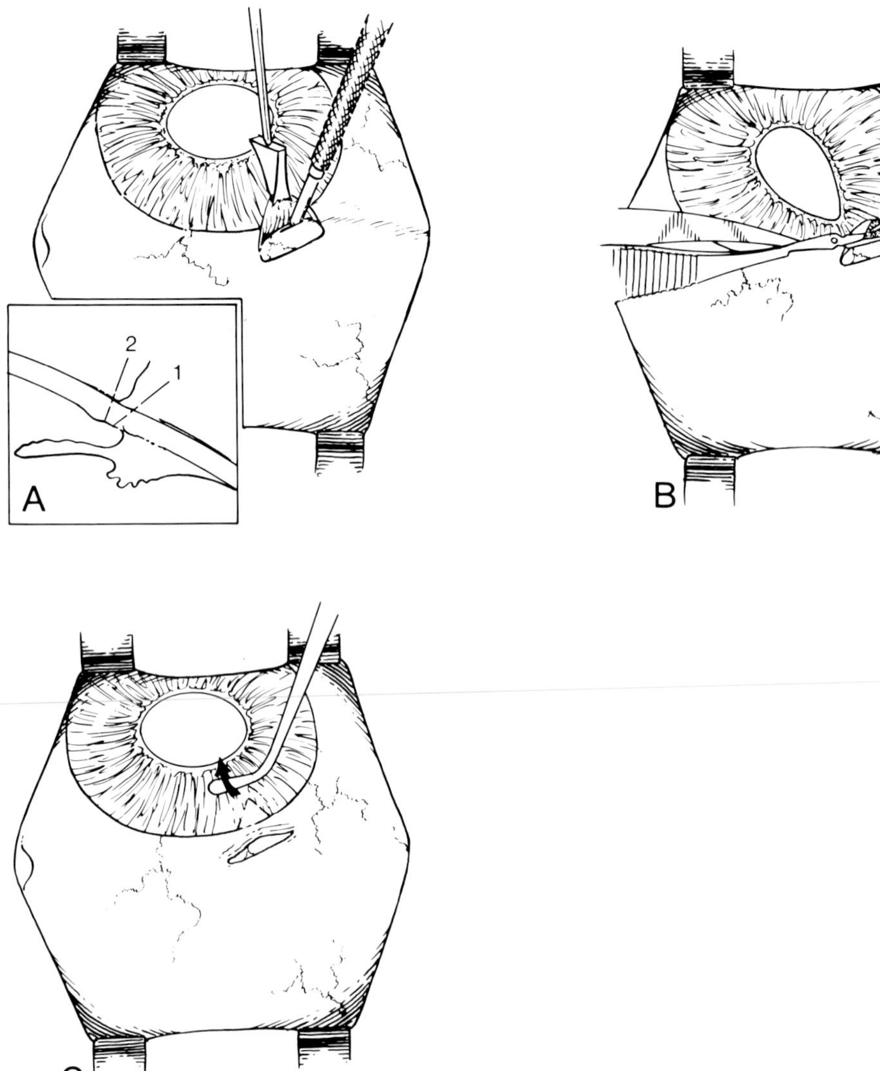

Figure 35.7. Peripheral iridectomy. **A,** Incision into anterior chamber may be placed (*1*) behind the corneolimbal junction or (*2*) in peripheral cornea (note the slant of each incision). **B,** Peripheral iris is grasped with forceps and excised with iris scissors. **C,** Remaining iris is reposited by a gentle stroking action across the cornea (*arrow*).

Basic Technique (Fig. 35.7). In the technique described by Chandler,[89] a small conjunctival flap is prepared in one of the superior quadrants with either a fornix or limbus base. A 3–4 mm incision is made into the anterior chamber, beginning approximately 1–1.5 mm behind the corneolimbal junction.

If the iris prolapses, it is lifted up with iris forceps and a small section is excised using iris scissors that are held parallel to the limbus. If the iris does not spontaneously come through the limbal opening, a slight pressure on the posterior margin of the incision may cause the prolapse. Factors that may prevent the peripheral iris from prolapsing through the limbal incision include: (1) inaccurate placement of the incision; (2) a hypotonous eye; (3) peripheral anterior synechiae; (4) a hole elsewhere in the iris; and (5) ciliary-iridial processes (attachments between the posterior, peripheral iris and the ciliary body).

When iris prolapse cannot be achieved, the iris is grasped with forceps and brought up through the incision to make the iridectomy. The iris is then reposited by a gentle stroking action across the cornea in a direction away from the incision, using a blunt instrument such as a muscle hook.

In closing the wound, a single suture may be placed through both the limbal wound and conjunctiva if a fornix-based flap was used. With a limbus-based flap, closure of the conjunctiva alone may be sufficient, if the limbal incision was beveled slightly to achieve spontaneous apposition.

Modifications. Some surgeons prefer to make the incision into the anterior chamber through *clear cornea* adjacent to the corneolimbal junction.[90–92] The main advantage is that the undamaged conjunctiva remains available for future filtering surgery if required. The incision is usually placed perpendicular to the limbus in order to reach peripheral iris (Fig. 35.7), and suture closure is generally necessary. However, some surgeons believe that suturing is not essential,[90] especially if the incision is beveled posteriorly.[92]

Another modification of the peripheral iridectomy is *transfixation,* in which the anterior chamber is entered at the limbus with a narrow cataract knife. Several incisions in the iris are then made as the blade is passed across the anterior segment of the eye (Fig. 35.8). This approach has been favored by some surgeons for the management of iris bombé in an inflamed eye, in the hope that it would reduce the danger of hemorrhage. However, one study showed that a conventional peripheral iridectomy does not have a greater incidence of bleeding.[93] The nonincisional laser approach is generally preferable to either of these techniques in this situation.

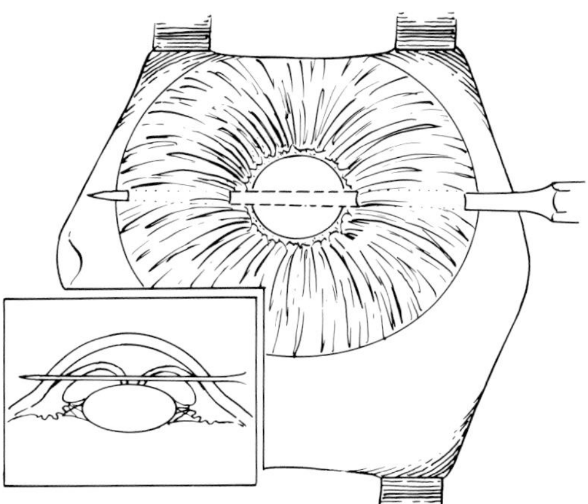

Figure 35.8. Transfixation. Multiple iridotomies are created as a narrow cataract knife is passed across the anterior segment.

Sector Iridectomy

Some surgeons believe that there are times when a sector iridectomy has advantages over a peripheral iridectomy. Such situations might include (1) the need for the larger optical opening, (2) the facilitation of future cataract extraction, and (3) the suspicion of retinal disease. In the technique described by King and Wadsworth,[94] a larger limbal incision is required so that the iris can be grasped within 1–2 mm of the pupillary margin and brought well out through the wound. A radial cut is then made across the iris at one side of the exposed portion, the iris is torn at its root, and a second incision is made across the other side of the exposed tissue. This creates a truly basal iridectomy. An alternative approach is to grasp midperipheral iris, withdraw it until the pupillary margin is exposed, and excise the tissue with a single cut.

Prevention and Management of Complications

Intraoperative Complications

Hemorrhage. Cut edges of the iris normally do not bleed. However, hemorrhage may occur, especially if inflammation or neovascularization is present. To minimize bleeding in these situations, the use of bipolar cauterization of the iris surface before cutting the iridectomy has been suggested.[95,96] Iris scissors have also been described in which insulation and an electric current allow simultaneous cutting and cauterization of the iris.[97] Brisk bleeding is especially likely to occur if the ciliary body is inadvertently cut. Hemorrhage from either iris or ciliary body can usually be stopped by placing a large air bubble in the anterior chamber for several minutes.

Incomplete Iridectomy. It is not uncommon to cut only the stroma of the iris, leaving intact pigment epithelium, which prevents a successful operation. This complication should be avoided at the time of surgery by checking the iridectomy specimen for the presence of the dark pigment epithelium and by noting transillumination through the iridectomy if there is any doubt as to its patency. If the complication is discovered postoperatively, it is best managed by penetrating the epithelial layer with the argon laser.[98,99] A low energy setting of 300–400 mW with a 100-micron spot size and a 0.1-second duration of exposure is sufficient in most cases, and the pigment epithelium is usually eliminated with a few applications.

Injury to the Lens. Injury to the lens or disruption of the lens zonules with possible dislocation of the lens and vitreous loss should be avoided by gentle surgical manipulation. Intralenticular hemorrhage has also been reported as a rare complication of iridectomy.[100]

Postoperative Complications

Elevated Intraocular Pressure. If the anterior chamber is flat, *malignant (ciliary block) glaucoma* should be considered. In one series of 155 eyes, only one such case was encountered.[101] The management of this situation is discussed in Chapter 23. An incomplete iridectomy is another cause of high pressure and a flat anterior chamber, and it can be managed as described above with the argon laser. A formed anterior chamber with an elevated pressure suggests that chronic obstruction of the trabecular meshwork may be present. The latter should initially be managed with antiglaucoma medications, although laser trabeculoplasty or a filtering procedure may be required if medical therapy is inadequate.

Hyphemas. Hyphemas should be handled conservatively with elevation of the head and limited activity.

Cataracts. The frequency with which peripheral iridectomies lead to cataract formation is somewhat controversial. However, several studies indicate that some degree of lenticular opacity occurs in up to half of the cases with an acute angle-closure glaucoma attack and in one-third of the eyes treated prophylactically.[101–105] The mechanism of this complication is uncertain, although the frequency increases with age.

Endophthalmitis. As with any intraocular procedure, infection is a potential complication.

LASER PERIPHERAL IRIDOPLASTY

There are occasions when a laser iridotomy is either technically impossible or is ineffective. Such situations include angle-closure glaucomas with persistent corneal edema,[33] nanophthalmos,[106] and angle closure as a result of ciliary body edema of various causes, including retinal detachment surgery.[107] In these cases, the application of low-energy laser burns to the peripheral stroma, which is also referred to as gonioplasty or peripheral iris retraction, may deepen the peripheral anterior chamber by causing contraction and retraction of the peripheral iris (Fig. 35.9). In addition, this technique can be used to deepen the anterior chamber angle to facilitate laser trabeculoplasty.

Suggested settings for peripheral iridoplasty are 500 microns, 0.5 second, and 150–200 mW.[33] The power should be in-

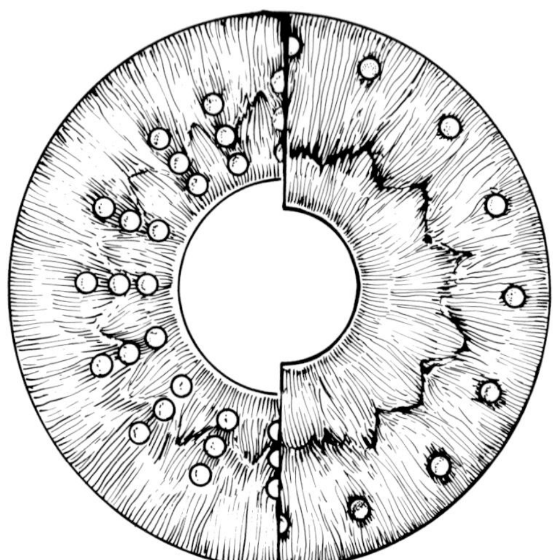

Figure 35.9. Laser peripheral iridoplasty (*right*) deepens the anterior chamber angle with low-energy contraction burns to the peripheral iris, while laser pupilloplasty (*left*) dilates the pupil with low-energy contraction burns to the more central iris.

creased if no contraction is produced, but reduced if pigment liberation is produced by the laser application. Approximately 10 burns are applied to peripheral iris in each quadrant, and additional applications can be placed in a row adjacent to the first burns if necessary.

LASER PUPILLOPLASTY

An alternative treatment for pupillary block when a laser iridotomy is not possible, as with a cloudy cornea, is laser pupilloplasty. It is an especially useful technique for pupillary block glaucoma in aphakia or pseudophakia.[108–110] By peaking the pupil in one quadrant, the iris may be retracted beyond the point of apposition with the lens or intraocular lens implant, thereby reestablishing communication between the anterior and posterior chambers. This usually works only when the amount of lens-iris contact is minimal, since the degree of pupillary retraction is small. When pupilloplasty is not effective, combined therapy with peripheral iridoplasty may be effective.[33]

Suggested settings for laser pupilloplasty are 200–500 microns, 0.2–0.5 second, and approximately 200 mW.[33] Several rows of laser energy are applied to the sphincter portion of the iris in one quadrant, starting at the pupillary border and working peripherally (Fig. 35.9). The contraction of stroma with each application tents the pupil in the direction of the treatment site, and the applications are continued until the block is broken as evidenced by a deepening of the anterior chamber. Pupilloplasty has also been used to dilate a chronically constricted pupil, although the amount of dilation is usually small and often temporary, and the procedure may be complicated by a significant IOP rise.

IRIS SPHINCTEROTOMY

A technique has also been described in which the pupil can be enlarged, reshaped, or repositioned by making a linear cut across the iris with an argon laser set at 0.01–0.05 second, 50 microns, and 1.5 watts, allowing the intrinsic tension of the iris to spread the cut apart.[111]

SUMMARY

Laser iridotomies have become the procedure of choice for the surgical management of angle-closure glaucomas and can be achieved with either continuous-wave or pulsed lasers. Techniques vary with the type of laser and the color of the iris. Complications include transient IOP elevation, uveitis, and burns of the cornea, lens, or retina. There are some situations in which laser iridotomies are not possible to achieve, in which case incisional iridectomies are still required. Laser energy can also be used to treat certain types of angle-closure glaucoma by mechanically flattening the peripheral iris (iridoplasty or gonioplasty) or dilating the pupil (pupilloplasty). Sphincterotomy is yet another iris procedure that can be performed with lasers.

References

1. Meyer-Schwickerath, G: Erfahrungen mit der Lichtokoagulation der Netzhaut und der Iris. Doc Ophthal 10:91, 1956.
2. Hogan, MF, Schwartz, A: Experimental photocoagulation of the iris of guinea pigs. Am J Ophthal 49:629, 1960.
3. Flocks, M, Zweng, HC: Laser coagulation of ocular tissues. Arch Ophthal 72:604, 1964.
4. Snyder, WB: Laser coagulation of the anterior segment. Arch Ophthal 77:93, 1967.
5. Hallman, VL, Perkins, ES, Watts, GK, et al: Laser irradiation of the anterior segment of the eye. I. Rabbit eyes. Exp Eye Res 7:481, 1968.
6. Hallman, VL, Perkins, ES, Watts, GK, et al: Laser irradiation of the anterior segment of the eye. II. Monkey eyes. Exp Eye Res 8:1, 1969.
7. Perkins, ES: Laser iridotomy for secondary glaucoma. Trans Ophthal Soc UK 91:777, 1971.
8. Khuri, CH: Argon laser iridectomies. Am J Ophthal 76:490, 1973.
9. L'Esperance, FA Jr, James, WA Jr: Argon laser photocoagulation of iris abnormalities. Trans Am Acad Ophthal Otol 79:321, 1975.
10. Abraham, RK, Miller, GL: Outpatient argon laser iridectomy for angle closure glaucoma: a two-year study. Trans Am Acad Ophthal Otol 79:529, 1975.
11. Anderson, DR, Forster, RK, Lewis, ML: Laser iridotomy for aphakic pupillary block. Arch Ophthal 93:343, 1975.
12. Pollack, IP, Patz, A: Argon laser iridotomy: an experimental and clinical study. Ophthal Surg 7:22, 1976.
13. Pollack, IP: Use of argon laser energy to produce

iridotomies. Trans Am Ophthal Soc LXXVII:674, 1979.

14. Podos, SM, Kels, BD, Moss, AP, et al: Continuous wave argon laser iridectomy in angle-closure glaucoma. Am J Ophthal 88:836, 1979.
15. Yassur, Y, Melamed, S, Cohen, S, Ben-Sira, I: Laser iridotomy in closed-angle glaucoma. Arch Ophthal 97:1920, 1979.
16. Pollack, IP: Use of argon laser energy to produce iridotomies. Ophthal Surg 11:506, 1980.
17. Quigley, HA: Long-term follow-up of laser iridotomy. Ophthalmology 88:218, 1981.
18. Schwartz, LW, Rodrigues, MM, Spaeth, GL, et al: Argon laser iridotomy in the treatment of patients with primary angle-closure or pupillary block glaucoma: a clinicopathologic study. Ophthalmology 85:294, 1978.
19. Rodrigues, MM, Streeten, B, Spaeth, GL, Schwartz, LW: Argon laser iridotomy or primary angle closure or pupillary block glaucoma. Arch Ophthal 96:2222, 1978.
20. Yassur, Y, David, R, Rosenblatt, I, Marmour, U: Iridotomy with red krypton laser. Br J Ophthal 70:295, 1986.
21. Latina, MA, Puliafito, CA, Steinert, RR, Epstein, DL: Experimental iridotomy with the Q-switched neodymium-YAG laser. Arch Ophthal 102:1211, 1984.
22. Klapper, RM: Q-switched neodymium:YAG laser iridotomy. Ophthalmology 91:1017, 1984.
23. Robin, AL, Pollack IP: A comparison of neodymium:YAG and argon laser iridotomies. Ophthalmology 91:1011, 1984.
24. McAllister, JA, Schwartz, LW, Moster, M, Spaeth, GL: Laser peripheral iridectomy comparing Q-switched neodymium YAG with argon. Trans Ophthal Soc UK 104:67, 1984.
25. Pollack, IP, Robin, AL, Dragon, DM, et al: Use of the neodymium:YAG laser to create iridotomies in monkeys and humans. Trans Am Ophthal Soc LXXXII:307, 1984.
26. Rodrigues, MM, Spaeth, GL, Moster, M, et al: Histopathology of neodymium:YAG laser iridectomy in humans. Ophthalmology 92:1696, 1985.
27. Vernon, SA, Cheng, H: Freeze frame analysis on high speed cinematography of Nd/YAG laser explosions in ocular tissues. Br J Ophthal 70:321, 1986.
28. Goldberg, MF, Tso, MOM, Mirolovich, M: Histopathological characteristics of neodymium-YAG laser iridotomy in the human eye. Br J Ophthal 71:623, 1987.
29. Robin, AL, Arkell, S, Gilbert, SM, et al: Q-switched neodymium-YAG laser iridotomy. A field trial with a portable laser system. Arch Ophthal 104:526, 1986.
30. Abraham, RK: Protocol for single-session argon laser iridectomy for angle-closure glaucoma. Int Ophthal Clin 21:145, 1981.
31. Schirmer, KE: Argon laser surgery of the iris, optimized by contact lenses. Arch Ophthal 101:1130, 1983.
32. Wise, JB, Munnerlyn, CR, Erickson, PJ: A high-efficiency laser iridotomy-sphincterotomy lens. Am J Ophthal 101:546, 1986.
33. Ritch, R: Argon laser treatment for medically unresponsive attacks of angle-closure glaucoma. Am J Ophthal 94:197, 1982.
34. Robin, AL, Pollack, IP, deFaller, JM: Effects of topical ALO 2145 (p-aminoclonidine hydrochloride) on the acute intraocular pressure rise after argon laser iridotomy. Arch Ophthal 105:1208, 1987.
35. Hoskins, HD, Migliazzo, CV: Laser iridectomy—a technique for blue irises. Ophthal Surg 15:488, 1984.
36. Abraham, RK: Procedure for outpatient argon laser iridectomies for angle closure glaucoma. Int Ophthal Clin 16:1, 1976.
37. Harrad, RA, Stannard, KP, Shilling, JS: Argon laser iridotomy. Br J Ophthal 69:368, 1985.
38. Yamamoto, T, Shirato, S, Kitazawa, Y: Argon laser iridotomy in angle-closure glaucoma: a comparison of two methods. Jap J Ophthal 26:387, 1982.
39. Mandelkorn, RM, Mendelsohn, AD, Olander, KW, Zimmerman, TJ: Short exposure times in argon laser iridotomy. Ophthal Surg 12:805, 1981.
40. Kolker, AE: Techniques of argon laser iridectomy. Trans Am Ophthal Soc 82:303, 1984.
41. Stetz, D, Smith, H Jr, Ritch, R: A simplified technique for laser iridectomy in blue irides. Am J Ophthal 96:249, 1983.
42. Damerow, A, Utermann, D: Combined thermal-photodisruptive iridotomy with the argon and Nd:YAG laser. Klin Monatsbl Augenheilkd 195:61, 1989.
43. Goins, K, Schmeisser, E, Smith, T: Argon laser pretreatment in Nd:YAG iridotomy. Ophthal Surg 21:497, 1990.
44. Wise, JB: Large iridotomies by the linear incision technique using the neodymium:YAG laser at low energy levels. A study using cynomolgus monkeys. Ophthalmology 94:82, 1987.
45. Wise, JB: Low-energy linear-incision neodymium:YAG laser iridotomy versus linear-incision argon laser iridotomy. A prospective clinical investigation. Ophthalmology 94:1531, 1987.
46. Rol, P, Kwasniewska, S, van der Zypen, E, Fankhauser, F: Transscleral iridotomy using a neodymium:YAG laser operated both with standard equipment and an optical fiber system—a preliminary report: Part 1—Optical system and biomicroscopic results. Ophthal Surg 18:176, 1987.
47. Bonney, CH, Gassterland, DE: Low-energy, Q-switched ruby laser iridotomies in *Macaca mulatta*. Invest Ophthal Vis Sci 18:278, 1979.
48. Bass, MS, Cleary, CV, Perkins, ES, Wheeler,

CB: Single treatment laser iridotomy. Br J Ophthal 63:29, 1979.
49. Richardson, TM, Brown, SV, Thomas, JV, Simmons, RJ: Shock-wave effect on anterior segment structures following experimental neodymium:YAG laser iridectomy. Ophthalmology 92:1387, 1985.
50. Moster, MR, Schwartz, LW, Spaeth, GL, et al: Laser iridectomy: a controlled study comparing argon and neodymium:YAG. Ophthalmology 93:20, 1986.
51. Del Priore, LV, Robin, AL, Pollack, IP: Neodymium:YAG and argon laser iridotomy. Long-term follow-up in a prospective, randomized clinical trial. Ophthalmology 95:1207, 1988.
52. Robin, AL, Pollack, IP: Q-switched neodymium-YAG laser iridotomy in patients in whom the argon laser fails. Arch Ophthal 104:531, 1986.
53. Krupin, T, Stone, RA, Cohen, BH, et al: Acute intraocular pressure response to argon laser iridotomy. Ophthalmology 92:922, 1985.
54. Taniguchi, T, Rho, SH, Gotoh, Y, Kitazawa, Y: Intraocular pressure rise following Q-switched neodymium:YAG laser iridotomy. Ophthal Laser Ther 2:99, 1987.
55. Gailitis, R, Peyman, GA, Pulido, J, et al: Prostaglandin release following Nd:YAG iridotomy in rabbits. Ophthal Surg 17:467, 1986.
56. Weinreb, RN, Weaver, D, Mitchell, MD: Prostanoids in rabbit aqueous humor: effect of laser photocoagulation of the iris. Invest Ophthal Vis Sci 26:1087, 1985.
57. Sanders, DR, Joondeph, B, Hutchins, R, et al: Studies on the blood-aqueous barrier after argon laser photocoagulation of the iris. Ophthalmology 90:169, 1983.
58. Schrems, W, van Dorp, HP, Wendel, M, Krieglstein, GK: The effect of YAG laser iridotomy on the blood-aqueous barrier in the rabbit. Graefe's Arch Ophthal 221:179, 1984.
59. Tawara, A, Inomata, H: Histological study on transient ocular hypertension after laser iridotomy in rabbits. Graefe's Arch Ophthal 225:114, 1987.
60. Robin, AL, Pollack, IP, Quigley, HA, et al: Histologic studies of angle structures after laser iridotomy in primates. Arch Ophthal 100:1665, 1982.
61. Kitazawa, Y, Sugiyama, K, Taniguchi, T: The prevention of an acute rise in intraocular pressure following Q-switched Nd:YAG laser iridotomy with clonidine. Graefe's Arch Ophthal 227:13, 1989.
62. Cohen, JS, Bibler, L, Tucker, D: Hypopyon following laser iridotomy. Ophthal Surg 15:604, 1984.
63. Choplin, NT, Bene, CH: Cystoid macular edema following laser iridotomy. Ann Ophthal 15:172, 1983.
64. Schwartz, LW, Moster, MR, Spaeth, GL, et al: Neodymium-YAG laser iridectomies in glaucoma associated with closed or occludable angles. Am J Ophthal 102:41, 1986.
65. Brainard, JO, Landers, JH, Shock, JP: Recurrent angle closure glaucoma following a patent 75-micron laser iridotomy: a case report. Ophthal Surg 13:1030, 1982.
66. Sachs, SW, Schwartz, B: Enlargement of laser iridotomies over time. Br J Ophthal 68:570, 1984.
67. Hirst, LW, Robin, AL, Sherman, S, et al: Corneal endothelial changes after argon-laser iridotomy and panretinal photocoagulation. Am J Ophthal 93:473, 1982.
68. Smith, J, Whitted, P: Corneal endothelial changes after argon laser iridotomy. Am J Ophthal 98:153, 1984.
69. Panek, WC, Lee, DA, Christensen, RE: Effects of argon laser iridotomy on the corneal endothelium. Am J Ophthal 105:395, 1988.
70. Hong, C, Kitazawa, Y, Tanishima, T: Influence of argon laser treatment of glaucoma on corneal endothelium. Jap J Ophthal 27:567, 1983.
71. Schwartz, AL, Martin, NF, Weber, PA: Corneal decompensation after argon laser iridectomy. Arch Ophthal 106:1572, 1988.
72. Hodes, BL, Bentivegna, JF, Weyer, NJ: Hyphema complicating laser iridotomy. Arch Ophthal 100:924, 1982.
73. Rubin, L, Arnett, J, Ritch, R: Delayed hyphema after argon laser iridectomy. Ophthal Surg 15:852, 1984.
74. Yamamoti, T, Shirato, S, Kitazawa, Y: Treatment of primary angle-closure glaucoma by argon laser iridotomy: a long-term follow-up. Jap J Ophthal 29:1, 1985.
75. Welch, DB, Apple, DJ, Mendelsohn, AD, et al: Lens injury following iridotomy with a Q-switched neodymium-YAG laser. Arch Ophthal 104:123, 1986.
76. Berger, CM, Lee, DA, Christensen, RE: Anterior lens capsule perforation and zonular rupture after Nd:YAG laser iridotomy. Am J Ophthal 107:674, 1989.
77. Seedor, JA, Greenidge, KC, Dunn, MW: Neodymium:YAG laser iridectomy and acute cataract formation in the rabbit. Ophthal Surg 17:478, 1986.
78. Higginbotham, EJ, Ogura, Y: Lens clarity after argon and neodymium-YAG laser iridotomy in the rabbit. Arch Ophthal 105:540, 1987.
79. Gaasterland, DE, Rodrigues, MM, Thomas, G: Threshold for lens damage during Q-switched Nd:YAG laser iridectomy. A study of rhesus monkey eyes. Ophthalmology 92:1616, 1985.
80. Anderson, DR, Knighton, RW, Feuer, WJ: Evaluation of phototoxic retinal damage after argon laser iridotomy. Am J Ophthal 107:398, 1989.
81. Karmon, G, Savir, H: Retinal damage after argon laser iridotomy. Am J Ophthal 101:554, 1986.

82. Berger, BB: Foveal photocoagulation from laser iridotomy. Ophthalmology 91:1029, 1984.
83. Bongard, B, Pederson, JE: Retinal burns from experimental laser iridotomy. Ophthal Surg 16:42, 1985.
84. Karjalainen, K, Laatikainen, L, Raitta, C: Bilateral nonrhegmatogenous retinal detachment following neodymium-YAG laser iridotomies. Arch Ophthal 104:1134, 1986.
85. Brooks, AMV, Harper, CA, Gillies, WE: Occurrence of malignant glaucoma after laser iridotomy. Br J Ophthal 73:617, 1989.
86. Robin, A, Pollack IP: Argon laser peripheral iridotomies in the treatment of primary angle closure glaucoma. Long-term follow-up. Arch Ophthal 100:919, 1982.
87. Go, F-J, Yamamoto, T, Kitazawa, Y: Argon laser iridotomy and surgical iridectomy in treatment of primary angle-closure glaucoma. Jap J Ophthal 28:36, 1984.
88. Rivera, AH, Brown, RH, Anderson, DR: Laser iridotomy vs surgical iridectomy. Have the indications changed? Arch Ophthal 103:1350, 1985.
89. Chandler, PA: Peripheral iridectomy. Arch Ophthal 72:804, 1964.
90. Weene, LE: Self-sealing incision for peripheral iridectomy. Ophthal Surg 9:64, 1978.
91. Freeman, LB, Ridgway, AEA: Peripheral iridectomy via a corneal section: a follow-up study. Ophthal Surg 10:53, 1979.
92. Ahmad, N: Transcorneal peripheral iridectomy. Ophthal Surg 11:124, 1980.
93. Curran, RE: Surgical management of iris bombé. Arch Ophthal 90:464, 1973.
94. King, JH, Wadsworth, JAC: An Atlas of Ophthalmic Surgery, 2nd ed. JB Lippincott, Philadelphia, 1970, p. 416.
95. Kass, MA, Hersh, SB, Albert, DM: Experimental iridectomy with bipolar microcautery. Am J Ophthal 81:451, 1976.
96. Hersh, SB, Kass, MA: Iridectomy in rubeosis iridis. Ophthal Surg 7:19, 1976.
97. Hashmi, MS, McCarthy, JP: Cauterising iris scissors. Br J Ophthal 63:754, 1979.
98. Snyder, WB, Vaiser, A, Hutton, WL: Laser iridectomy. Trans Am Acad Ophthal Otol 79:381, 1975.
99. Tessler, HH, Peyman, GA, Huamonte, F, Menachof, I: Argon laser iridotomy in incomplete peripheral iridectomy. Am J Ophthal 79:1051, 1975.
100. Feibel, RM, Bigger, JF, Smith, ME: Intralenticular hemorrhage following iridectomy. Arch Ophthal 87:36, 1972.
101. Go, F-J, Kitazawa, Y: Complications of peripheral iridectomy in primary angle-closure glaucoma. Jap J Ophthal 25:222, 1981.
102. Sugar, HS: Cataract formation and refractive changes after surgery for angle-closure glaucoma. Am J Ophthal 69:747, 1970.
103. Floman, N, Berson, D, Landau, L: Peripheral iridectomy in closed angle glaucoma—late complications. Br J Ophthal 61:101, 1977.
104. Godel, V, Regenbogen, L: Cataractogenic factors in patients with primary angle-closure glaucoma after peripheral iridectomy. Am J Ophthal 83:180, 1977.
105. Krupin, T, Mitchell, KB, Johnson, MF, Becker, B: The long-term effects of iridectomy for primary acute angle-closure glaucoma. Am J Ophthal 86:506, 1978.
106. Kimbrough, RL, Trempe, CS, Brockhurst, RJ, Simmons, RJ: Angle-closure glaucoma in nanophthalmos. Am J Ophthal 88:572, 1979.
107. Burton, TC, Folk, JC: Laser iris retraction for angle-closure glaucoma after retinal detachment surgery. Ophthalmology 95:742, 1988.
108. Patti, JC, Cinotti, AA: Iris photocoagulation therapy of aphakic pupillary block. Arch Ophthal 93:347, 1975.
109. Theodossiadis, G: A new argon-laser-approach for the management of aphakic pupillary block. Klin Monatsbl Augenheilkd 169:153, 1976.
110. Theodossiadis, GP: Pupilloplasty in aphakic and pseudophakic pupillary block glaucoma. Trans Ophthal Soc UK 104:137, 1985.
111. Wise, JB: Iris sphincterotomy, iridotomy, and synechiotomy by linear incision with the argon laser. Ophthalmology 92:641, 1985.

Chapter 36

FILTERING SURGERY

The incisional operation most frequently used for open-angle forms of glaucoma, especially in adults, is commonly referred to as a filtering procedure. Although a number of variations for this surgical procedure have been described, all filtering operations share the same basic mechanism of action and general surgical principles. We will first consider these aspects and then discuss specific filtration techniques and potential complications.

MECHANISMS OF ACTION

Drainage Fistula

The basic mechanism of all filtering procedures is the creation of an opening, or *fistula,* at the limbus, which allows aqueous humor to drain from the anterior chamber, thereby circumventing the pathologic obstruction to outflow. The aqueous flows directly or indirectly into subconjunctival spaces and is then removed by one or more routes.

Filtering Bleb

Most, but not all, successful glaucoma filtering procedures are characterized by an elevation of the conjunctiva at the surgical site, which is commonly referred to as a *filtering bleb*. The clinical appearance of these blebs varies considerably with regard to diameter, elevation, and vascularity. The blebs that are most often associated with good intraocular pressure (IOP) control are avascular with numerous microcysts in the epithelium and are either low and diffuse or more circumscribed and elevated (Fig. 36.1).[1,2]

The histologic appearance of both functioning and failed filtering blebs consists of normal epithelium with no encircling-type junctions between the cells that would limit fluid flow.[2] The subepithelial connective tissue correlates better with bleb status, in that functioning blebs have loosely arranged tissue with histologically clear spaces, while the failed blebs have dense collagenous connective tissue.[2]

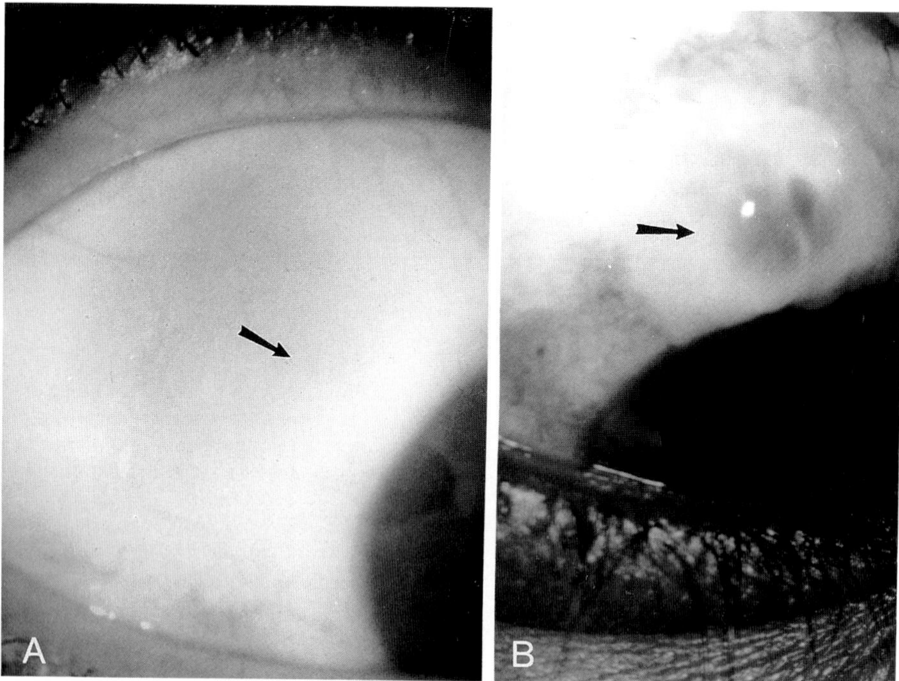

Figure 36.1. Types of functioning filtering blebs: **A,** Low, diffuse bleb (*arrow*). **B,** Discrete, elevated bleb. Note that both are avascular.

Routes of Aqueous Drainage

Studies have suggested that aqueous in the filtering bleb usually filters through the conjunctiva[3] and mixes with the tear film[4,5] or is absorbed by vascular[3] or perivascular[6] conjunctival tissue. Less commonly, a filtering procedure may be associated with IOP control in the absence of an apparent filtering bleb. This is more common when the fistula is covered by a partial-thickness scleral flap, and suggested mechanisms of aqueous drainage in these cases include flow through (1) lymphatic vessels near the scarred margins of the surgical area, (2) atypical, newly incorporated aqueous veins, and (3) normal aqueous veins.[3,6]

GENERAL FEATURES OF FILTERING SURGERY

The various types of filtering surgery differ primarily according to the method used to create the drainage fistula. The other aspects of the operation, as well as the postoperative care, are basically the same for all filtering procedures and will be discussed first before considering specific fistulizing techniques.

Limbal Stab Incision

Some surgeons first make a beveled incision into the anterior chamber at the limbus, usually in the inferior-temporal quadrant, as a route for injecting fluid at the end of the procedure. This can be done with a Wheeler or similar knife, with the cutting edge facing the anterior chamber angle. The tip of the blade is rotated toward the angle during the withdrawal, to widen the inner portion of the incision (Fig. 36.2).

Preparation of the Conjunctival Flap

Preparation of the conjunctival flap is a critical step in all filtering procedures, since the most common cause of failure is scarring of the filtering bleb. While techniques differ among surgeons, all agree that meticulous detail with minimal tissue damage and bleeding is essential.

Position of the Flap. Some surgeons elect to make the flap at the 12 o'clock position to take advantage of the wider limbus in

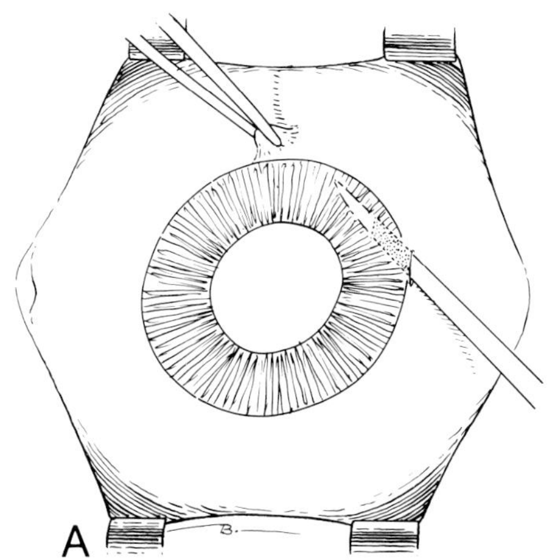

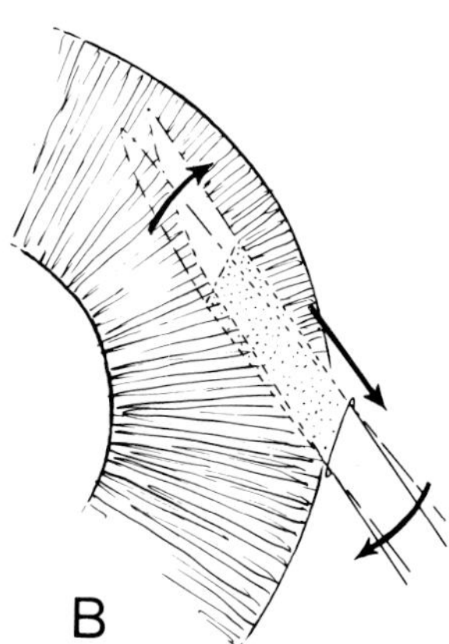

Figure 36.2. Limbal stab incision: **A,** Entry at limbus with cutting edge of blade facing the anterior chamber angle. **B,** Rotation of knife tip toward the angle during withdrawal.

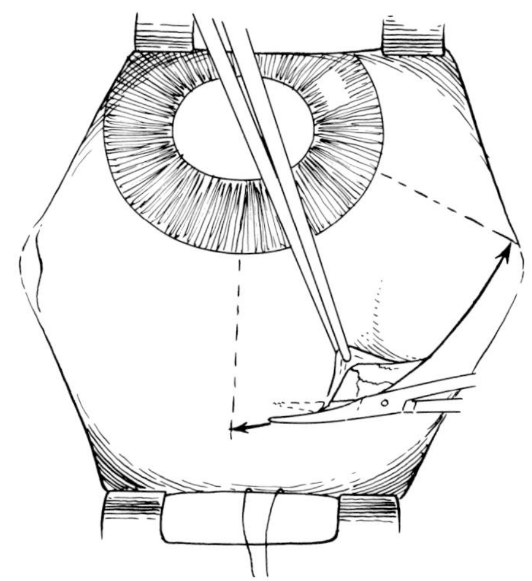

Figure 36.3. Incision through conjunctiva in preparation of a limbus-based conjunctival flap.

this area. Others prefer one of the superior quadrants, leaving the adjacent quadrant available for future surgery if required. Rarely, in cases of previous failed filtering surgery or when other ocular surgery has resulted in scarring of conjunctiva in the superior quadrants, an inferior quadrant may be used.

Limbus- vs Fornix-Based Flap. Conjunctival flaps for glaucoma filtering surgery have traditionally been limbus-based (i.e., with the initial incision in the fornix) (Fig. 36.3), although some surgeons prefer a fornix-based flap, particularly in association with a trabeculectomy.[7,8] Several studies have been described that compared limbus- and fornix-based conjunctival flaps in association with trabeculectomy, and all have reported comparable success rates.[9–13] However, one study found slightly better postoperative IOP control with the limbus-based flap,[11] while another found more diffuse blebs with the fornix-based flaps.[12] Surgeons differ on this aspect of filtering surgery, with some preferring the relative ease and improved surgical exposure of the fornix-based flap, while others prefer the tighter wound closure and possibly lower pressures achieved with the limbus-based flaps.

Management of Tenon's Capsule. There is also some controversy regarding the value of removing all or a portion of Tenon's capsule in the area of the conjunctival flap. Two studies revealed no difference in postoperative IOP control between eyes with excision of the capsular tissue and those in which it was left partly or totally intact.[14,15] For this reason, many surgeons routinely dissect between Tenon's capsule and episclera when preparing the conjunctival flap, making no attempt to remove the capsular tissue from the conjunctiva. However, others will excise variable portions of Tenon's capsule when it appears to be unusually thick, as in young patients. This can be accomplished by dissecting between the con-

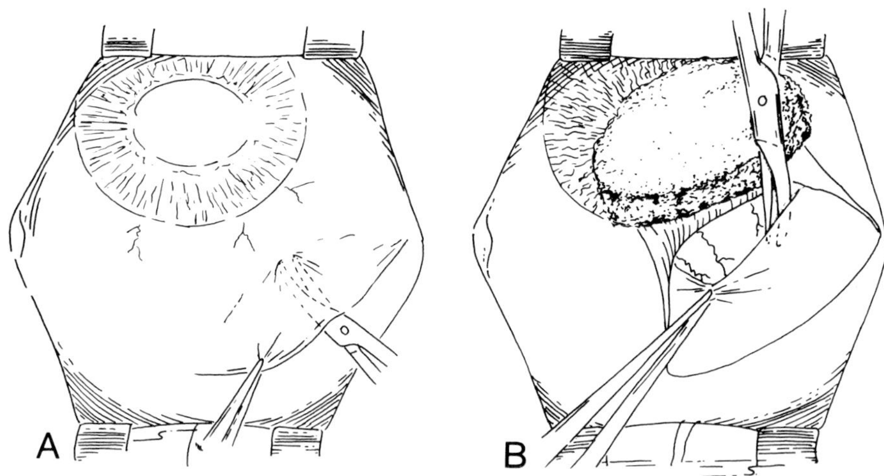

Figure 36.4. Total tenonectomy: **A,** Blunt and sharp dissection between conjunctiva and Tenon's capsule, observing closure of blades through the conjunctiva to avoid creating a buttonhole. **B,** Dissection of Tenon's capsule from episclera, beginning with incision near limbus and extending back to site of initial conjunctival incision where the capsule is excised.

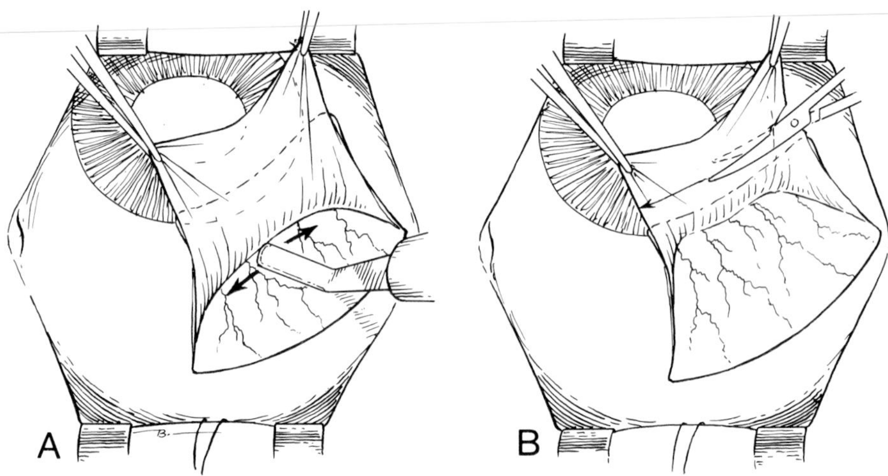

Figure 36.5. Partial tenonectomy: **A,** Blunt dissection of Tenon's capsule from episclera. **B,** Excision of the portion of Tenon's capsule that can be stripped from conjunctiva. (Reprinted from Shields MB: Ophthal Surg 11:498, 1980, by permission.)

junctiva and Tenon's capsule and then excising the capsule from the episclera (Fig. 36.4). An alternative approach is to dissect Tenon's capsule from underlying episclera, strip a portion of the capsule from the conjunctiva with gentle traction, and then excise the exposed portion of capsular tissue (Fig. 36.5). With all techniques, blunt dissection is used whenever possible to avoid bleeding, and sharp dissection is used when required. Gentle handling of the conjunctiva is essential at all times, and conjunctival forceps have been designed to grasp the conjunctiva firmly without tearing it.[16]

Fistulizing Procedure. During the fistulizing procedure, it is important to keep the conjunctival flap moist and to minimize handling of the tissue. This can be conveniently accomplished by reflecting the flap over the cornea with a moist Gelfoam sponge (Fig.

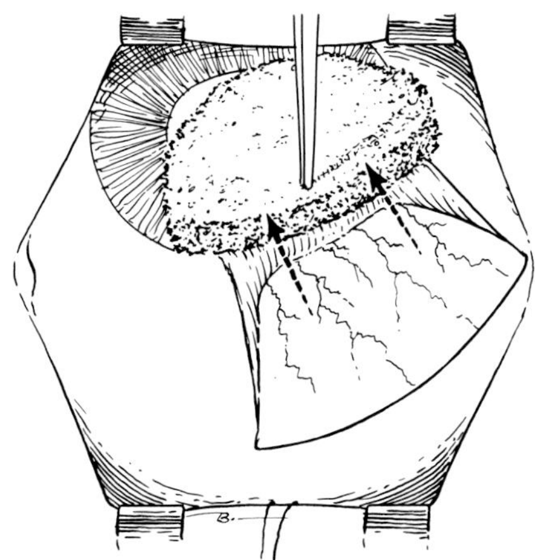

Figure 36.6. Retraction of conjunctival flap over cornea with moist Gelfoam sponge. (Reprinted from Ophthal Surg 11:498, 1980, by permission.)

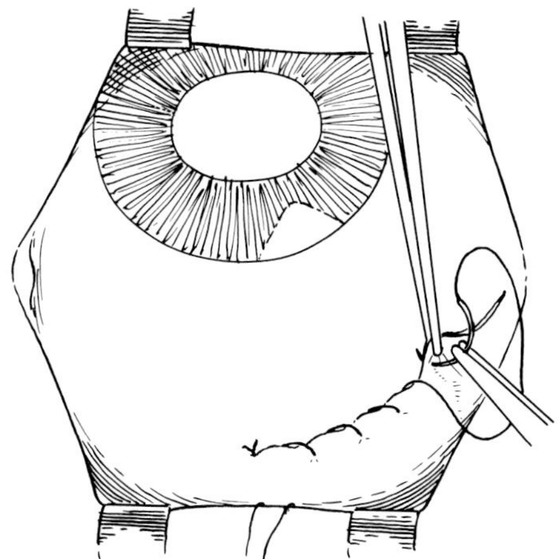

Figure 36.7. Closure of conjunctival flap with running suture. (Reprinted from Ophthal Surg 11:498, 1980, by permission.)

36.6). A Weck-Cel surgical spear with the tip cut off may also be used to gently retract the flap.[17]

Peripheral Iridectomy

A peripheral iridectomy is a routine part of all standard filtering procedures and is usually made after the fistula has been prepared. However, if the iris prolapses into the limbal wound, it is generally best to make the iridectomy and then complete the fistula. A large iridectomy is desirable to avoid obstruction of the fistula by the peripheral iris.[18]

Closure of the Conjunctival Flap

Tight wound closure is also a critical aspect of any filtering procedure, since a leaking wound may lead to a persistently flat anterior chamber and failure of the filtering bleb to develop properly. A fine suture, such as 10-0 nylon or absorbable polyglycolic acid or polyglactin, on a tapered, wire needle is desirable since it produces minimal tissue reaction. For closure of a limbus-based flap, a running suture with close bites provides the tightest closure (Fig. 36.7). A running suture can also be placed along the limbus for fornix-based flaps, although some surgeons find it adequate to use a single, interrupted suture at either end of the flap, which pulls the conjunctiva tightly over peripheral cornea.[8] Some surgeons prefer to further enhance the integrity of the wound closure by suturing Tenon's capsule and conjunctiva separately.

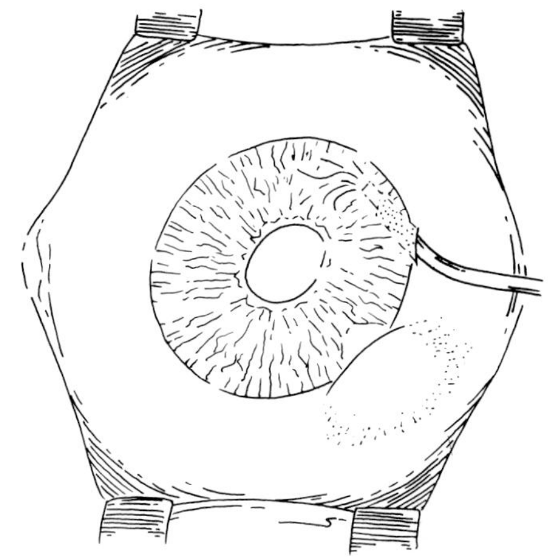

Figure 36.8. Injection of balanced salt solution into anterior chamber, with elevation of conjunctival flap.

Injection of Fluid

If a limbal stab incision was made at the outset, as previously described, the final step in the filtering operation is to inject a balanced salt solution into the anterior chamber via that incision (Fig. 36.8). This should deepen the anterior chamber and create a sustained elevation of the conjunctival flap, thereby demonstrating patency of the fistula and watertight closure of the conjunctival incision. The relative merits of injecting alternative substances into the anterior chamber during filtering surgery are discussed later in this chapter under "Prevention and Management of Complications".

Postoperative Management

Topical mydriatic-cycloplegic and antibiotic therapy should be used routinely for the first 2–3 weeks. In addition, most surgeons prefer to use a topical corticosteroid to reduce scar formation of the filtering bleb. Other drugs that may reduce scarring of the filtering bleb are discussed later in this chapter under "Prevention and Management of Complications".

FISTULIZING TECHNIQUES

There are two basic types of fistulas: (1) those that extend through the full thickness of the limbal tissue, and (2) those that are covered by a partial-thickness scleral flap. In addition, efforts have been made to maintain patency of the fistula by implanting various materials (setons) in the opening.

Full-Thickness Fistulas

The original type of limbal fistula, and one that many surgeons still employ in certain situations, involves creation of a direct opening through the full thickness of the limbal tissue. The fistula may be created by a variety of techniques.

Sclerectomy

In 1906, LaGrange[19] described a technique in which a full-thickness limbal incision is made, and a piece of tissue is then excised from the anterior lip of the wound to create a limbal fistula. Holth[20] modified this procedure 3 years later by performing the sclerectomy with a punch. Subsequent surgical variations have included excision of tissue from both the anterior and posterior lips of the circumferential incision[21,22] or from the lateral lip of a radial incision.[23] However, the sclerectomy technique most often discussed in recent literature is the *posterior lip sclerectomy*, described by Iliff and Haas.[24]

Technique (Fig. 36.9). A scratch incision is begun just behind the insertion of the conjunctival flap in an area of sclera that has been lightly cauterized. The incision is beveled inward at an angle of approximately 75° to the limbal surface and is continued until the anterior chamber is entered. Scissors are then used to widen the incision to about 5 mm.

A sclerectomy punch, such as a 1.5-mm Holth punch, is used to excise full-thickness limbal tissue from the posterior lip of the incision, creating a fistula of approximately 1 × 3 mm. Care must be taken to avoid cutting into the ciliary body, which can lead to significant bleeding.

Modifications. This technique may be modified slightly by applying light cautery to the posterior margins of the sclerectomy, which further enlarges the fistula and may help to inhibit postoperative scarring.[25] Sclerectomy punches have also been modified. One popular instrument is the Gass sclerectomy punch, which is a guillotine-type punch designed to excise a 1.5-mm semicircle of tissue.[26] The latter instrument has been further modified by rotating the opening of the punch 45° away from the handle to facilitate better visualization under the operating microscope.[27]

Trephination

In 1909, Elliot[28] and Fergus[29] both described a glaucoma filtering procedure in which the fistula is created with a small trephine placed just behind the corneolimbal junction. Elliot[30] later modified the technique by splitting the peripheral cornea and placing the trephine more anteriorly (sclerocorneal trephining). However, this modification produced a thinner filtering bleb with a greater chance of late infection, and Sugar[31] advocated a return to the original, more posterior placement of the trephine, which he called limboscleral trephination (or trepanation). The subsequent experience of Sugar[32] and others has supported the merit of this technique.

Technique (Fig. 36.10). A 1.5- or 2.0-mm trephine blade is placed over the limbus just behind the corneolimbal junction. The

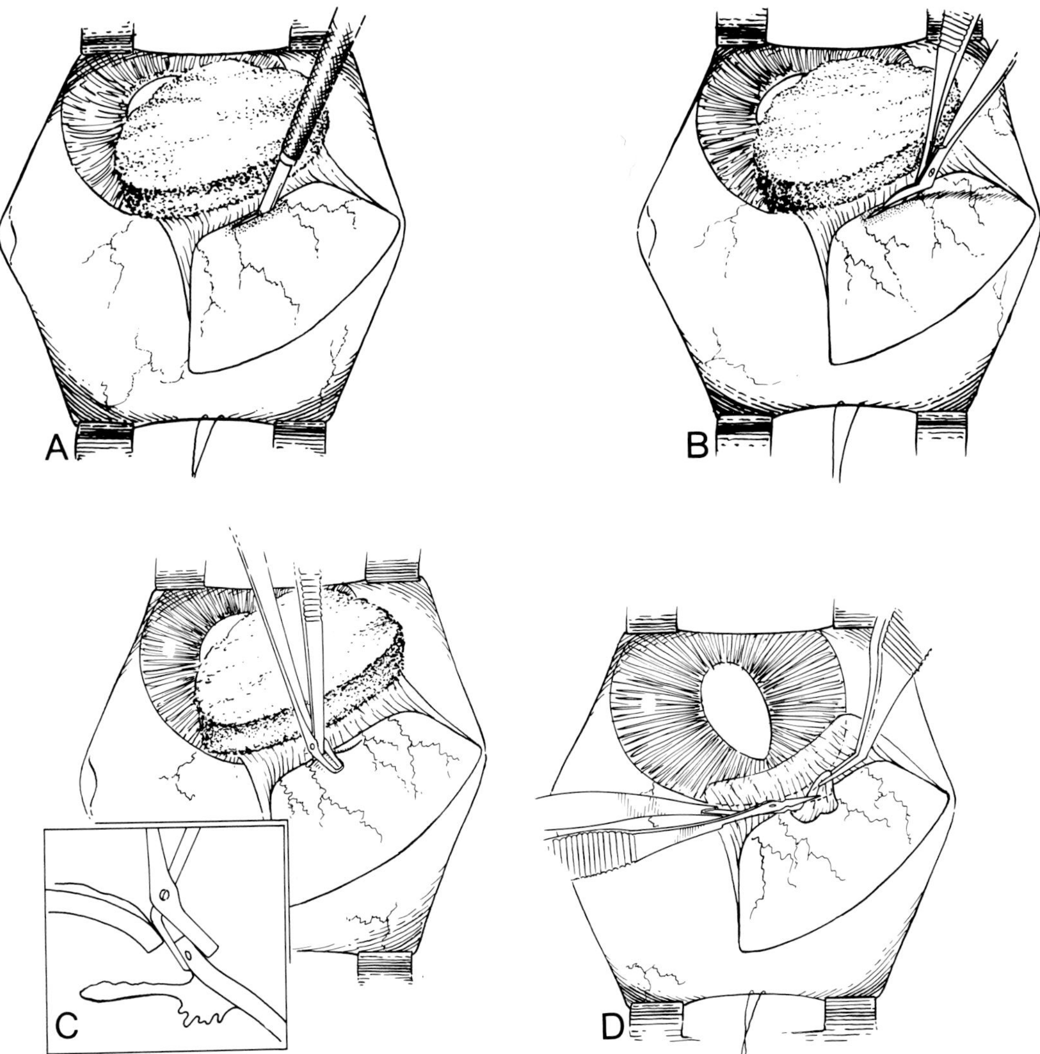

Figure 36.9. Posterior lip sclerectomy: **A,** Beveled incision into anterior chamber. **B,** Enlargement of limbal incision with scissors. **C,** Excision of full-thickness tissue from posterior lip of incision with sclerectomy punch. **D,** Peripheral iridectomy created, as for all standard filtering procedures. (Portions reprinted from Ophthal Surg 11:498, 1980, by permission.)

trephine is tilted forward so that the anterior edge of the blade enters the anterior chamber first. Entry into the anterior chamber is usually indicated by a movement of the upper pupillary margin toward the trephine. The trephine button, which is hinged on the scleral side and may rotate forward as a result of prolapse of the iris, is excised by cutting across the hinge with scissors. As with other filtering procedures, care must be taken to avoid cutting into the ciliary body.

Thermal Sclerostomy (Scheie Procedure)

Preziosi,[33] in 1924, described a filtering technique in which a limbal fistula was created by entering the anterior chamber angle with an electrocautery instrument. Scheie[34] later described a procedure that also used cautery but differed from the Preziosi operation in that a limbal scratch incision was first made, and the cautery was then used

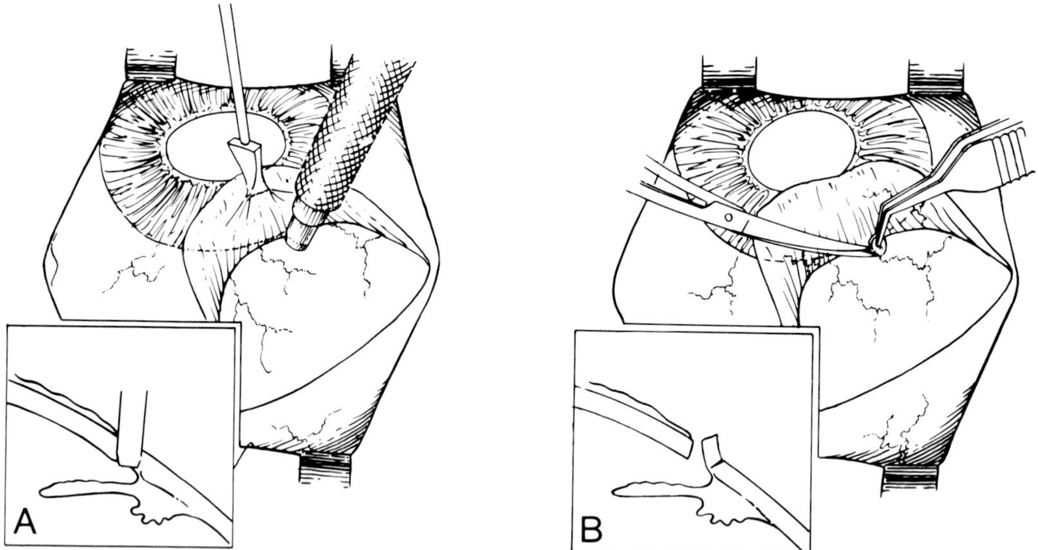

Figure 36.10. Limboscleral trephination: **A,** Trephine button partly excised by tilting the trephine anteriorly. **B,** Completion of excision by cutting posterior attachment with scissors.

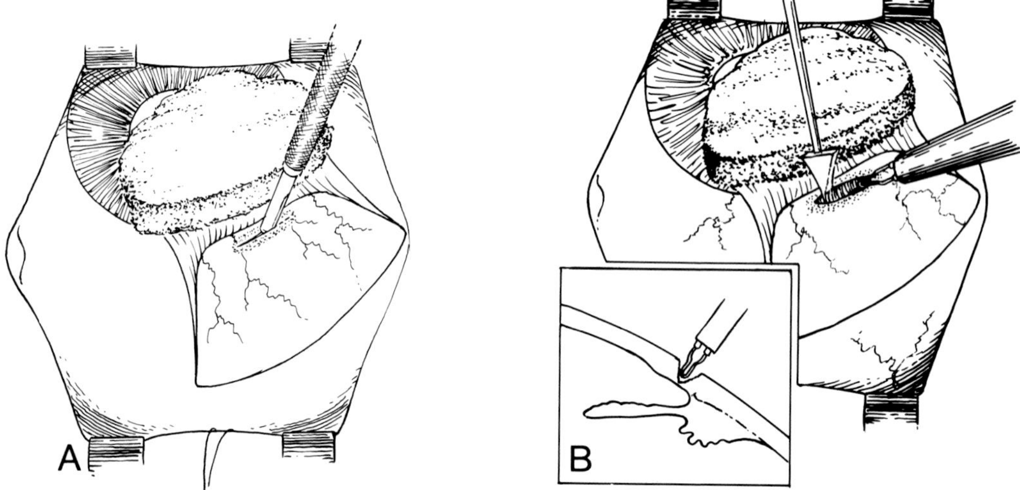

Figure 36.11. Thermal sclerostomy: **A,** Limbal incision created (may initially be partial- or full-thickness). **B,** Application of cautery to the lips of the incision to separate the wound edges. The partial-thickness incision is then extended into the anterior chamber and cautery is applied to the depths of the wound.

to retract the wound edges, thereby creating the fistula.

Technique (Fig. 36.11). Light cautery is applied to the sclera in a 1 × 5-mm area behind the corneolimbal junction. A 5-mm limbal scratch incision is then made through the cauterized area, perpendicular to the scleral surface, and cautery is applied to the lips of the incision until the wound edges separate by at least 1 mm.

The escape of aqueous from the limbal incision may interfere with the application of cautery, and this can be partly avoided by stopping the initial scratch incision just before it enters the anterior chamber, applying cautery, and then completing the incision.[35] In addition, bipolar cautery can be used effectively in the wet field. Another modification is to place a temporary suture across the fistula to avoid an early flat anterior chamber.[36]

Iridencleisis

This procedure differs from the other forms of full-thickness filtering surgery in that a wedge of iris is incarcerated into the limbal incision in an effort to maintain a patent channel for aqueous outflow. This was once a popular procedure, but it lost favor partly because of the suspicion that the associated incidence of sympathetic ophthalmia was higher than with other filtering procedures. Although this fear has not been substantiated, the operation never regained popularity.

Laser Sclerostomy (Ab Externo)

Full-thickness limbal fistulas have also been produced with lasers in animal and human eyes by preparing a conjunctival flap and perforating the limbus from the external side with laser energy.[37]

Internal Sclerostomy

In addition to creating full-thickness fistulas with laser energy from the external approach, lasers and other instruments are being evaluated to create sclerostomies ab interno (i.e., from the anterior chamber to the subconjunctival space). The main theoretical advantage of this technique is that it requires no dissection of the conjunctiva, which is elevated with a fluid injection over the surgical site, thereby reducing the risk of scarring and bleb failure. The first such attempt was made with a Q-switched neodymium:YAG laser, focused into the anterior chamber angle through a special gonioprism, which has been shown to be effective but requires very high levels of energy.[38–40] Subsequent efforts have used a contact laser probe, the tip of which is introduced into the anterior chamber via a limbal incision 180° from the sclerostomy site (Fig. 36.12). The tip is passed across the anterior chamber to the trabecular meshwork, where the sclerostomy is created. This technique has been evaluated with continuous-wave neodymium:YAG lasers,[41–44] high-energy argon blue-green laser,[45,46] and excimer lasers.[47] One study compared internal sclerostomy using the neodymium:YAG contact laser with thermal sclerostomy in rabbits and found a greater success rate with the former, apparently resulting from less conjunctival scarring.[42] Similar internal sclerostomies have also been successfully performed with an automated trephine,[48,49] and it is likely that other instruments and techniques will be evaluated in the future as this promising approach to glaucoma filtering surgery evolves.

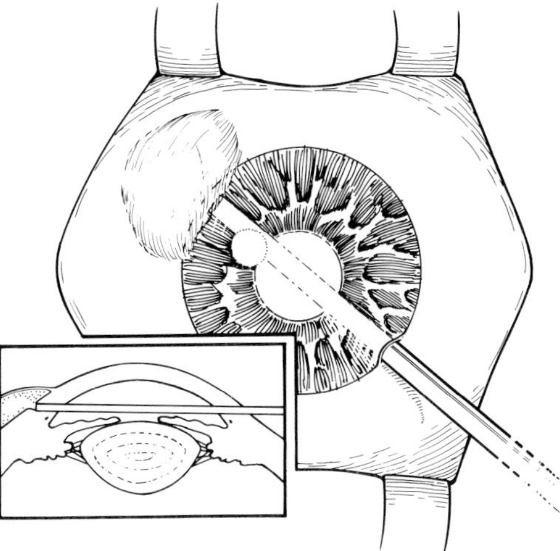

Figure 36.12. Internal sclerostomy: A laser fiberoptic probe tip or automated trephine is inserted into the anterior chamber through a limbal stab incision and is used to create a full-thickness fistula beneath elevated conjunctiva 180° from the entry site.

Partial-Thickness Fistulas (Trabeculectomy)

Standard full-thickness filtering procedures may be complicated by excessive aqueous filtration, which can lead to a prolonged flat anterior chamber, associated with corneal decompensation, synechiae formation, and cataracts. In addition, the filtering blebs often become very thin and may rupture, creating the danger of endoph-

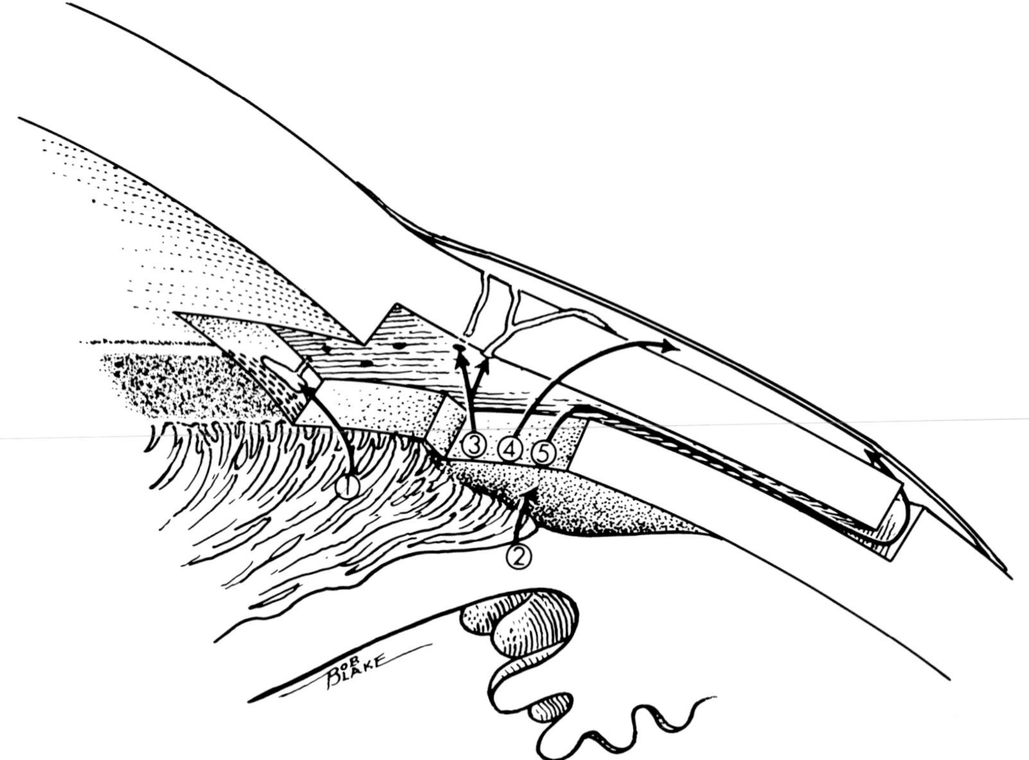

Figure 36.13. Possible routes of aqueous humor flow associated with a trabeculectomy: (*1*) Aqueous flow into cut ends of Schlemm's canal (rare); (*2*) Cyclodialysis (if tissue is dissected posterior to scleral spur); (*3*) Filtration through outlet channels in scleral flap; (*4*) Filtration through connective tissue substance of scleral flap; (*5*) Filtration around the margins of the scleral flap.

thalmitis. One attempt to minimize these complications has been to place a partial-thickness scleral flap over the fistula. This concept was suggested by Sugar[50] in 1961 but was popularized by the 1968 report of Cairns.[51] Both authors referred to the technique as a *trabeculectomy*.

Theories of Mechanism (Fig. 36.13)

It was originally thought that aqueous might flow into the cut ends of Schlemm's canal.[51] However, subsequent studies showed fibrotic closure of the canal at its cut ends in monkey[52] and human[53] eyes, and the presence of Schlemm's canal in the "trabeculectomy" specimen did not correlate with the outcome of the procedure.[54–56] Furthermore, the majority of successful cases have a filtering bleb,[57] indicating that external filtration is the principal mode of IOP reduction.

Whether the route of external filtration is primarily through or around the partial-thickness scleral flap remains a matter of controversy. While the outer layers of limbus and anterior sclera do not differ ultrastructurally from the inner layers in a way that might predispose to increased passage of aqueous,[58] perfusion studies of human autopsy eyes, in which a trabeculectomy was created and the margins of the scleral flap were sealed with adhesive, did show a significant flow through the scleral flap.[59] However, fluorescein angiographic studies of eyes with successful trabeculectomies showed the primary route of external filtration to be around the margins of the scleral flap.[60] Therefore, it may be that external filtration occurs by either route, depending on how tightly the scleral flap is sutured. Other possible mechanisms of IOP reduction by trabeculectomy include cyclodialysis[52] or aqueous outflow through newly developed aqueous veins, lymphatic vessels, or normal aqueous veins.[61,62]

Basic Trabeculectomy Technique (Fig. 36.14)

The margins of a 5 × 5-mm scleral flap, adjacent to the corneolimbal junction, are outlined with half-thickness scleral incisions. It is helpful to apply light cautery before making the incisions to minimize bleeding. A half-thickness lamellar flap, hinged at the limbus, is then raised until at least 1 mm of the bluish-gray zone is exposed.

The anterior chamber is entered with a knife just behind the hinge of the scleral flap, and the incision is widened with scissors to approximately 4 mm. Radial incisions are then extended posteriorly on either end of the initial incision for 1 mm, and the 1 × 4-mm block of tissue is reflected until the angle structures can be visualized, and the tissue is excised with scissors along the scleral spur.

After making the iridectomy, the scleral flap is then approximated. Some surgeons prefer to approximate the flap loosely with two sutures at the posterior corners to promote filtration around the margins of the scleral flap, while others use additional sutures for tighter closure, hoping that aqueous will filter through the flap.

Modifications in Technique

The numerous variations of the guarded filtering procedure that have been reported primarily involve modifications in the scleral flap or in the fistulizing technique.

Variations in the Scleral Flap. Rather than making a square flap, some surgeons prefer a triangular[63,64] or semicircular[65] shape. There is no apparent advantage of one shape over another with regard to long-term success, although the triangular flap has the advantages of requiring less dissection and allowing closure with a single suture at the posterior apex. Some surgeons attempt to influence the degree of postoperative filtration by modifying the scleral flap. For example, it has been suggested that the thickness of the flap correlates with the final IOP, in that thinner flaps provide greater filtration and lower pressures.[66] Other variations in surgical technique attempt to enhance filtration around the flap by applying light cautery to the lateral margins,[60] omitting all sutures for the scleral flap,[67] or excising the distal 2 mm of the flap.[67] Other surgeons use releasable sutures for the scleral flap or suture the flap tightly and cut sutures postoperatively with argon laser,[68] both of which have the advantage of maintaining a deeper anterior chamber during the early postoperative period.

Variations in the Fistulizing Technique. Watson[69,70] modified Cairn's basic technique by starting the dissection of the tissue block posteriorly over ciliary body, separating it from the underlying structure, and excising it at Schwalbe's line. Other techniques that have been used to create the subscleral fistula include trephinations,[65,71,72] sclerectomies,[73–75] thermal sclerostomies,[76–78] and sclerostomies with a carbon dioxide laser.[79]

Krasnov[80] describes a procedure, called *sinusotomy,* in which a strip of sclera is excised to expose a portion of Schlemm's canal. It is not clear whether the benefit of this operation is from relieving obstruction of the scleral outlet channels or from relieving the collapse of Schlemm's canal,[81,82] or whether it is just another filtration technique. A similar technique, called *nonpenetrating trabeculectomy,* carries the subscleral dissection of deep limbal tissue down to Schlemm's canal but leaves the trabecular meshwork intact.[83] This is believed to be especially advantageous in aphakic eyes and is also reported to have fewer postoper-

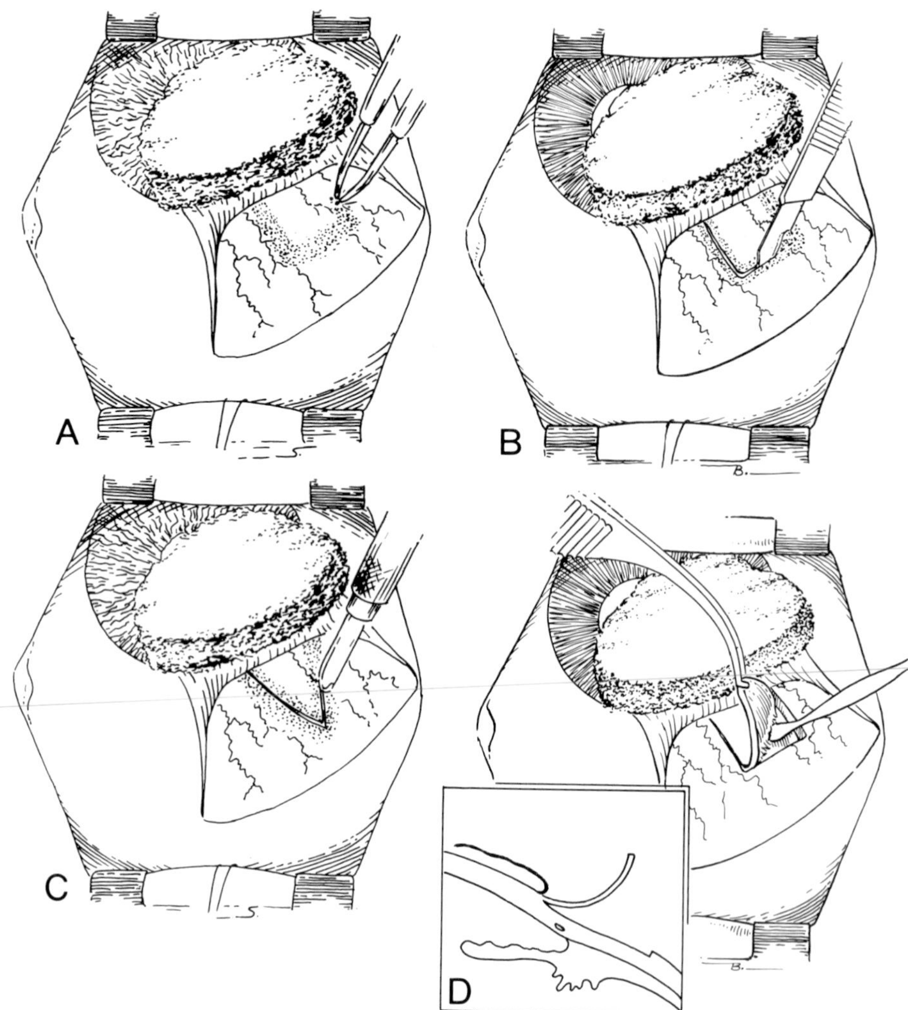

Figure 36.14. Trabeculectomy: **A,** Cauterization of area intended for margins of scleral flap. **B,** Margins of scleral flap outlined by partial-thickness incisions. **C,** Triangular scleral flap as an alternative technique. **D,** Dissection of scleral flap.

ative complications than a standard trabeculectomy in the phakic eye.[84] The technique has been modified by using the neodymium:YAG laser postoperatively to perforate the meshwork at the surgical site.[85,86]

Modifications for Neovascular Glaucoma. One variation includes excision of a large trabecular segment, partial nonpenetrating cyclodiathermy in the scleral bed, and partial ablation of abnormal iris vessels with a wide sector iridectomy.[87] Another technique uses bipolar cautery to directly treat vessels in the anterior chamber angle and the ciliary processes in the area of the filtering surgery.[88] The carbon dioxide laser is thought by some surgeons to be particularly useful for creating the fistula in eyes with neovascular glaucoma, since it also cauterizes any neovascular tissue in the corneoscleral angle.[89] Another surgical approach for this disorder is a pars plana filtering procedure combined with a lensectomy and vitrectomy. This was successful in only 50% of the eyes in one series,[90] although success rates with other techniques are not much better when dealing with neovascular glaucoma. Setons have also been used for this disorder and are discussed later in this chapter.

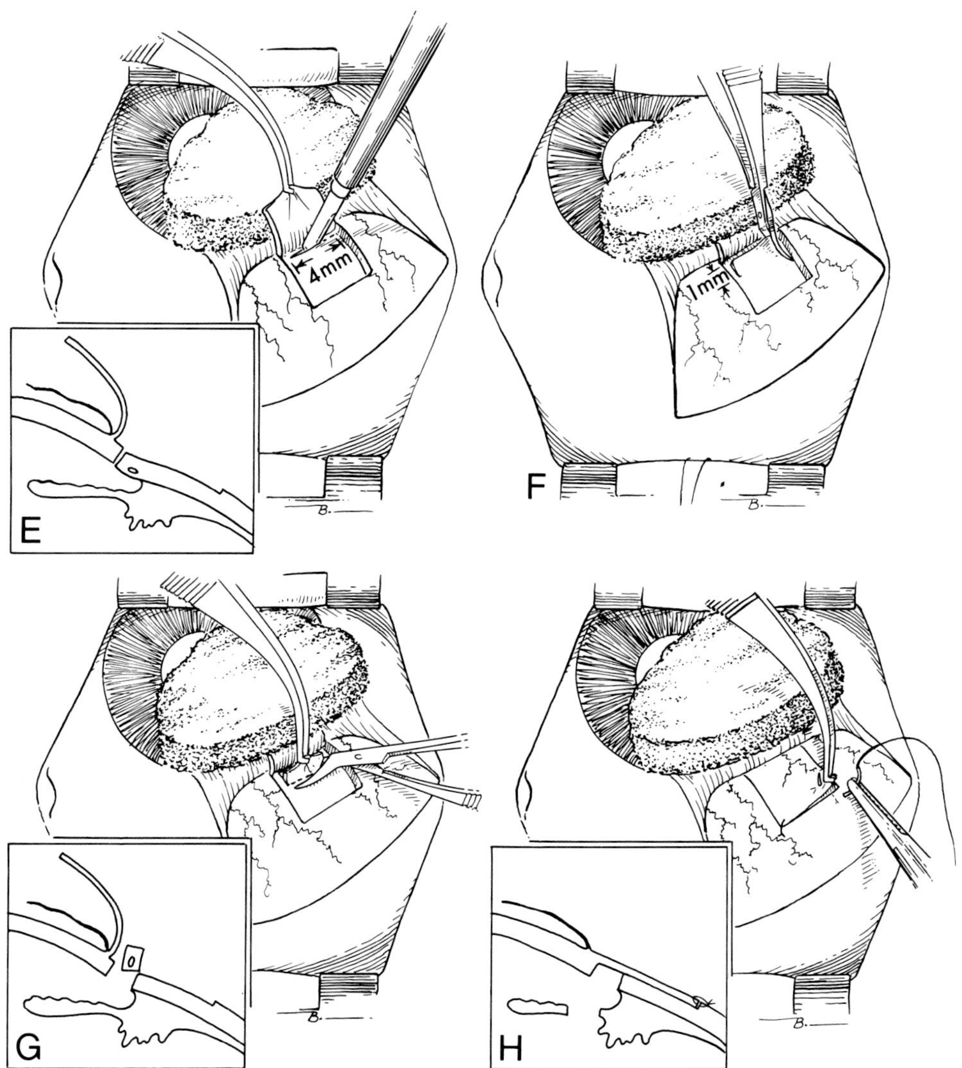

Figure 36.14. (*Continued*) **E,** Anterior chamber entered just behind the hinge of the scleral flap. **F,** Completion of anterior and lateral margins of deep limbal incision with scissors. **G,** Flap of deep limbal tissue excised by cutting along scleral spur. **H,** Approximation of scleral flap. (Portions reprinted from Shields MB: Ophthal Surg 11:498, 1980, by permission.)

Modifications for Glaucoma in Aphakia. The fornix-based conjunctival flap, as previously discussed,[7–9] is particularly useful in eyes that have had previous intraocular surgery, especially when a fornix-based conjunctival flap was used during a cataract procedure. The conjunctiva in these eyes is usually tightly scarred down to episclera near the limbus, making preparation of a limbus-based flap difficult. When using a fornix-based flap, it is probably best to suture the lateral margins of the scleral flap to promote drainage posteriorly. An anterior vitrectomy may also be required if loose vitreous is in the anterior chamber or presents at the iridectomy site. As previously noted, nonpenetrating trabeculectomy has also been advocated for glaucoma in aphakia.[83]

Implant (Seton) Procedures

In an attempt to maintain patency of the drainage fistula in either full-thickness or partial-thickness filtering operations, a wide variety of foreign materials have been placed in the fistula. Although these have been uniformly unsuccessful over the years, continued research with newer designs is beginning to show promise.

Tubes

The success of newer implant operations appears to be due, at least in part, to the concept of aqueous drainage through patent translimbal tubes. Animal studies have shown that catheters can maintain flow from the anterior chamber to a subconjunctival space for at least 6 months after implantation.[91] Success has been reported in humans using strips of hydrogel with parallel capillary channels,[92] and with silicone[93] and Teflon[94] tubes. However, the vast majority of these eventually fail because of fibrosis around the external end of the tube, and long-term success seems to require a mechanical subconjunctival reservoir into which the tube can drain. Such reservoirs may be an acrylic plate on the sclera (Molteno implant)[95] or an encircling scleral band.[96,97] The most extensively reported experience has been with the Molteno implant (Fig. 36.15), which has been shown to be useful in resistant cases of glaucoma,[98,99] especially neovascular glaucoma[100] and chronic glaucoma in aphakia,[101] as well as glaucomas associated with epithelial downgrowth,[102] glaucoma in eyes after penetrating keratoplasty,[103] and developmental glaucomas.[104] A technique has also been described (aqueous-venous shunt) in which a microsize collagen or silicone tube is inserted into the anterior chamber and then connected with the lumen of the extraocular portion of a vortex vein.[105]

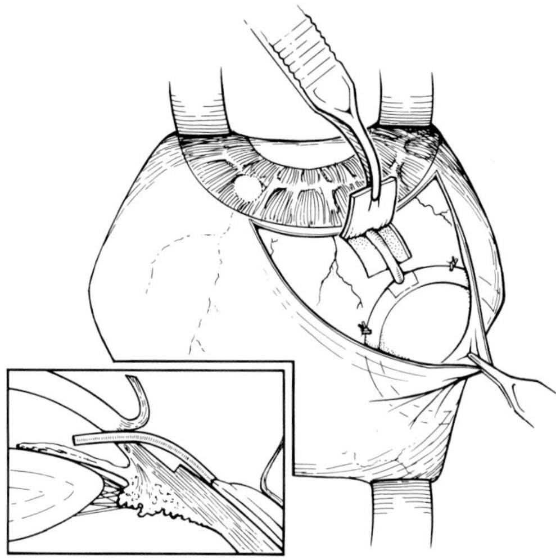

Figure 36.15. Molteno implant: A silicone tube is inserted into the anterior chamber via a limbal stab incision and is connected to a subconjunctival acrylic plate that is attached to the sclera near the equator.

Valves

Another disadvantage of open tubes, in addition to closure by subconjunctival fibrosis, is excessive drainage during the early postoperative period, leading to hypotony. One attempt to avoid this complication has been the creation of tubes with valves that allow one-way flow from the anterior chamber and that open at a predetermined IOP level. One such valve (Krupin-Denver valve) is composed of an internal Supramid tube cemented to an external (subconjunctival) Silastic tube.[106] The valve effect is created by making slits in the closed external end of the Silastic tube. Preliminary experience with this valve was encouraging,[107,108] although fibrosis again eventually closed the subconjunctival portion of the valve,[109] which led to failure in most cases. New techniques are currently being evaluated, in which the valve is directed into a reservoir, similar to those mentioned above for drainage tubes.[110–112] A valve has also been described for temporary insertion into the anterior chamber with drainage into the conjunctival cul-de-sac for control of transient IOP elevation.[113]

PREVENTION AND MANAGEMENT OF COMPLICATIONS

The following complications may occur with any filtering procedure, although some operations and techniques appear to provide certain advantages over others. We will first consider the complications in general and then compare the merits of the various filtering procedures. It is helpful to think of these complications in three phases: intraoperative, early postoperative, and late postoperative.

Intraoperative Complications

Tearing or Buttonholing the Conjunctival Flap

The conjunctiva may be inadvertently torn or cut during preparation or closure of the flap. This complication can be minimized by gentle handling of the tissues as outlined earlier in this chapter. When it does occur, it may be possible to close the defect using fine suture on a round, tapered needle. Nylon suture has been used for this purpose,[114] although 10-0 polyglycolic acid or polyglactin has the advantage of being absorbable. With small holes the tissue can be puckered together with a figure-of-eight or mattress suture, while a large tear may require a running suture. Tissue adhesive[115] and light bipolar cautery may also be used to close small holes, but these methods are less reliable than suturing.

Hemorrhage

Episcleral bleeding is particularly common in glaucoma patients who have been on long-term antiglaucoma medication. It can be managed with irrigation or light cautery and should be under control before the anterior chamber is entered. Once inside the eye, inadvertent cutting of the ciliary body may cause brisk bleeding. Cauterization is difficult in these cases, although the intraocular, bipolar units at a low temperature setting are usually effective. Alternative management involves gentle, sustained pressure over the fistula with a sponge or a large air bubble in the anterior chamber. A choroidal, or expulsive, hemorrhage is a particularly devastating complication that usually results from sudden reduction in the IOP with rupture of a large choroidal vessel. The most important step in the management of these cases is immediate closure of the fistula. Some surgeons will make a scleral incision in the inferior temporal quadrant to allow the blood to drain from this site until it stops spontaneously, although the value of this approach has not been substantiated. Hemorrhage into the lens has also been reported as a rare complication of glaucoma surgery.[116]

Choroidal Effusion

This complication may occur during glaucoma filtering surgery, especially in eyes with prominent episcleral vessels, as in cases of Sturge-Weber syndrome.[117] The suprachoroidal fluid in these cases contains very little protein (18% of plasma concentration), suggesting that a pressure differential drives fluid and small molecules from choroidal capillaries into extravascular spaces.[118] This complication is usually recognized by a sudden shallowing of the anterior chamber during the operation or by the rotation of ciliary processes through the iridectomy and into the surgical fistula. If severe, it can be managed by making a scleral incision to release the suprachoroidal fluid.[117]

Other Intraoperative Complications

Vitreous loss may occur during creation of the fistula or iridectomy, as a result of rupture of the lens zonules and hyaloid membrane, which usually results from excessive manipulation. The vitreous should be removed from the surgical site with sponges and scissors or a vitrectomy instrument. *Lens injury* may remain limited to the surgical site if it is small, while larger injuries may cause gradual widespread extension or acute cataract formation, occasionally with severe uveitis.[119] *Stripping of Descemet's membrane* during glaucoma surgery with subsequent corneal edema has also been reported.[120]

Early Postoperative Complications

During the first several days after a filtering procedure, the complications most often facing the surgeon are either excessive filtration with hypotony and a flat anterior chamber or inadequate filtration with an elevated IOP.

Hypotony and Flat Anterior Chamber

A low, often unrecordable, IOP is common during the early postoperative period and is typically associated with a shallow anterior chamber. The anterior chamber is usually shallowest on postoperative day 2 or 3 and gradually deepens over the next 2 weeks.[121] It is important to distinguish between a *shallow anterior chamber* with iridocorneal touch and a *flat anterior chamber* with cornea-lens touch, since the manage-

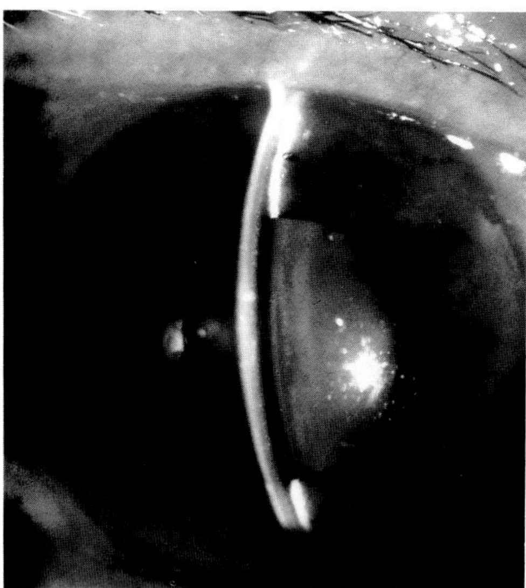

Figure 36.16. Slit-lamp appearance of shallow anterior chamber in early postoperative period following a trabeculectomy, showing iridocorneal touch with separation between cornea and lens. (Reprinted from Stewart WC, Shields MB: Am J Ophthal 106:41, 1988, by permission).

ment and prognosis differ significantly.[122] In the former situation, the cornea is typically clear and the iris stroma has not been flattened by the gentle touch with the cornea (Fig. 36.16). The anterior chamber in these eyes deepens spontaneously with time and requires no special management beyond the usual postoperative care. The prolonged shallow anterior chamber may be associated with a reduced corneal endothelial cell count[123] and some synechiae formation,[124] although these do not appear to adversely influence the long-term surgical result. However, with a flat anterior chamber the cornea is swollen and the iris stroma is flattened, and these eyes require immediate postoperative management to avoid a poor surgical result.

As in all cases, the best way to deal with a potential complication is to take steps to avoid it. Careful wound closure, as discussed earlier in this chapter, is one such step toward avoiding a flat anterior chamber. Another measure that has been evaluated is the injection of *sodium hyaluronate* into the anterior chamber. Most studies have shown that this does not reduce the incidence of flat anterior chambers when injected at the end of the filtering procedure,[125,126] although there is preliminary evidence that deepening the anterior chamber with sodium hyaluronate at the beginning of the operation and maintaining the chamber depth throughout the procedure may result in deeper chambers postoperatively.[127]

When hypotony and a flat anterior chamber do occur, the first step is to determine the cause and then take the appropriate steps to correct it. We will now consider those causes and how they can be managed.

Conjunctival Defect. If there is an obvious hole in the conjunctival flap or a leak at the wound edge, it may be possible to achieve spontaneous closure with a pressure patch (Fig. 36.17). A fusiform-shaped cottonball can be placed over the lid in the area of the fistula and held in place with the gauze pads to act as a tamponade. If this type of pressure dressing is used, the patient should be kept awake, with the fellow eye open and looking straight ahead, since the Bell's phenomenon of sleep may place the tamponade over the center of the cornea. Examination several hours later (the pressure patch is usually left on from morning until evening) often reveals closure of the defect and reformation of the anterior chamber. However, if the leaking defect persists, a scleral shell tamponade (Simmons shell) may be effective.[128] With this technique, the tamponade portion of the shell is placed over the defective area (Fig. 36.18) and secured with a tight pressure dressing. The dressing should be changed daily with examination of the eye through the shell, but the shell can be left in place for 3 days, which gives the defect more time to heal. If this is also not successful, cyanoacrylate tissue adhesive,[115] possibly covered by a collagen shield,[129] may be effective. Other cases may require suturing of the defect[114] or, when the defect is large, it may be necessary to develop a new conjunctival flap from tissue posterior to the defect.[130]

Excessive Filtration. In other cases, there may be no apparent conjunctival defect or wound leak, but filtration may simply be excessive as a result of a large fistula or an exceptionally large filtering bleb. It is in

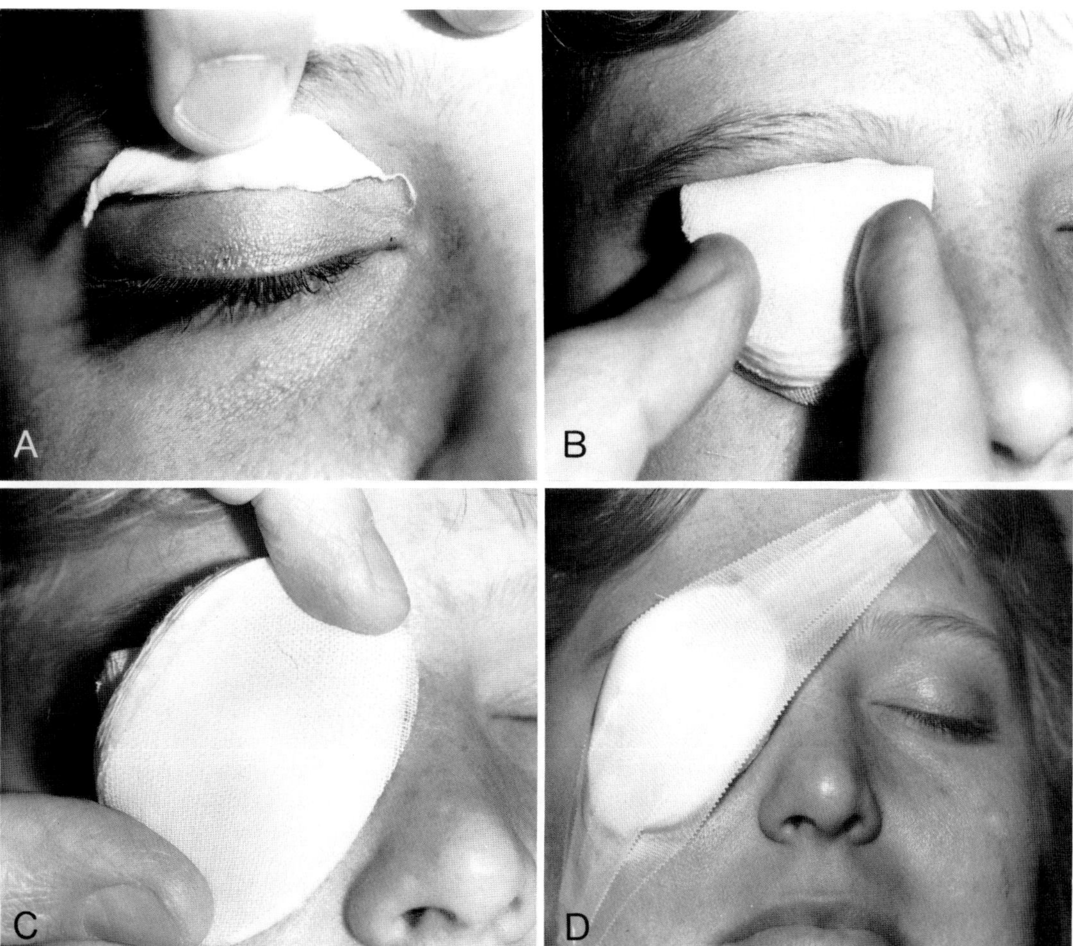

Figure 36.17. Pressure patch technique for eye with flat anterior chamber resulting from excessive filtration in early postoperative period: **A,** Fusiform-shaped cotton ball placed over upper lid in location corresponding to surgical fistula. **B,** Folded eye pad placed just below brow. **C,** Second, open eye pad positioned. **D,** Multiple strips of tape applied with moderate tension.

this regard that trabeculectomies are thought to offer one advantage, since the protective scleral flap minimizes excessive filtration. An alternative approach that has been used for preventing the early flat anterior chamber, especially with full-thickness filtering surgery, is the use of the Simmons shell, in which case the plastic tamponade may be temporarily sutured over the filtering bleb.[128] Other surgeons have suggested placing a temporary suture across a full-thickness fistula to help control the early rate of filtration.[36] Some surgeons choose to further enhance the protective aspect of a trabeculectomy by using additional nylon sutures for the scleral flap, which can be cut postoperatively with a laser if filtration is inadequate,[68,131] or by securing the scleral flap with a releasable suture.[132]

If the situation requires further corrective measures (i.e., if the anterior chamber remains flat with corneal decompensation), the first step is usually firm patching of the eye, as described above, often with the addition of the Simmons shell. If the chamber depth cannot be maintained after several days, and especially if corneal decompensation is present, surgical intervention is usu-

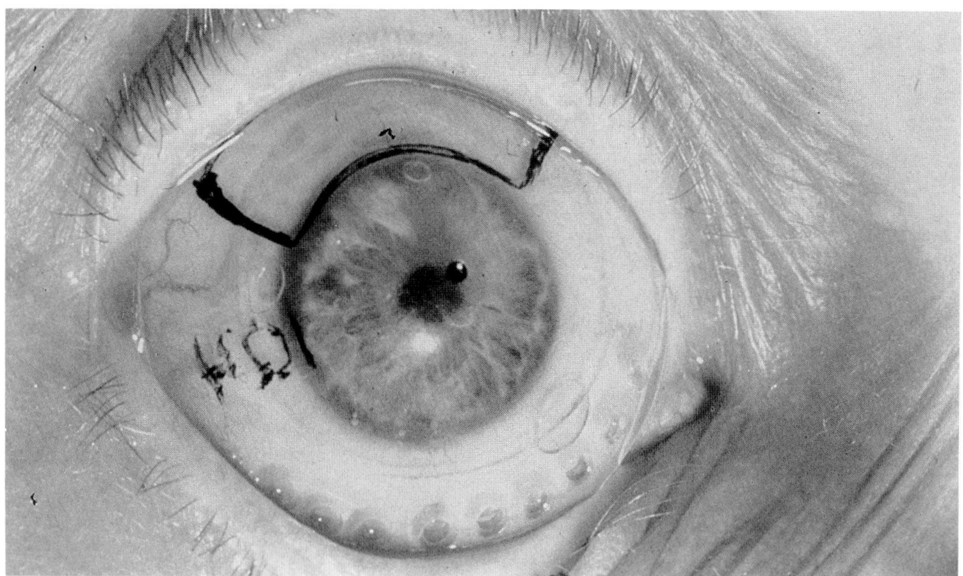

Figure 36.18. Simmons shell with tamponade positioned over surgical site prior to application of pressure patch for management of filtering bleb with leak or excessive filtration. (Courtesy of Richard J. Simmons, M.D.)

ally indicated. It may be sufficient to deepen the anterior chamber with balanced salt solution, a large air bubble,[133] or sodium hyaluronate.[134] However, if large choroidal detachments are present, these should be drained.[135]

Choroidal Detachments. Fluid commonly collects in the suprachoroidal space in hypotonous eyes. Hypotony is generally thought to contribute to the mechanism of choroidal detachments, although additional factors, such as inflammation and venous congestion, also appear to be important.[136] The detachment apparently prolongs the hypotony by further reducing aqueous production and possibly by increasing uveoscleral outflow. In most cases of hypotony and flat anterior chamber, a *serous choroidal detachment* is present, with the characteristic smooth, dome-shaped elevation of the peripheral fundus. The fluid in the detachments is high in protein (67% of plasma concentration), suggesting that a pressure differential causes fluid with small and medium-sized protein molecules to pass from choroidal capillaries to extravascular spaces.[118,137] Less commonly, the capillary membrane may rupture, leading to a *hemorrhagic choroidal detachment*.[118] This condition is more often associated with pain, IOP elevation, a flat anterior chamber, and massive choroidal detachments with central contact, and it is discussed later in this section.

Most serous choroidal detachments resolve spontaneously along with the normal rise in IOP during the first few postoperative days or weeks. It is usually necessary to drain them only when they are associated with a persistent flat anterior chamber or if a choroidal hemorrhage is suspected. The technique involves draining the suprachoroidal fluid through sclerotomies in the two inferior quadrants and deepening the anterior chamber with a balanced salt solution.

Much less commonly, a *serous retinal detachment* may occur after glaucoma filtering surgery, presumably by a mechanism similar to that for choroidal detachments. These usually resolve spontaneously.

Elevated IOP and Flat Anterior Chamber

A pressure rise during the early postoperative period may be associated with either a flat or deep anterior chamber. A flat anterior chamber suggests (1) malignant (ciliary block) glaucoma, (2) an incomplete iridectomy with pupillary block, or (3) a delayed suprachoroidal hemorrhage. The diagnosis and management of these conditions was considered in Chapter 23, and the following are a few additional details regarding the delayed hemorrhage.

Delayed suprachoroidal hemorrhages. Delayed suprachoroidal hemorrhages following filtering surgery typically present during the first few postoperative days with severe pain, occasional nausea, and a marked reduction in vision. The IOP is usually, but not always, elevated, the anterior chamber is shallow or flat, and large choroidal detachments, often with central touch, are present. The complication is uncommon (2% or less in most large series), but the incidence goes up considerably with certain risk factors, especially aphakia and vitrectomy.[138–141] In one series of 305 filtering procedures, the overall incidence of delayed suprachoroidal hemorrhage was 1.6%, but this rose to 13% in aphakic eyes and to 33% in aphakic, vitrectomized eyes.[140] These patients often do poorly, but the prognosis can be significantly improved by prompt drainage of the suprachoroidal blood and reformation of the anterior chamber.[142,143] Opinions differ regarding the benefit of vitrectomy in the surgical management of these complications, although good results have been reported with modified vitreoretinal approaches.[144,145]

Elevated IOP and Deep Anterior Chamber

An elevated IOP with a deep anterior chamber indicates inadequate filtration resulting from (1) obstruction of the fistula by iris, ciliary processes, lens, or vitreous, or (2) an absent or poorly functioning filtering bleb. Chances of the former complication may be minimized during surgery by making an adequate fistula and iridectomy and by avoiding excessive surgical manipulation. When faced with a high pressure and deep anterior chamber, the possibility of obstruction of the fistula should first be evaluated by gonioscopy. If iris or ciliary processes are obstructing the fistula, it may be possible to retract the tissue with the application of low-energy argon laser therapy. If the internal obstruction cannot be eliminated, it is usually necessary to resume antiglaucoma medication and possibly to revise the procedure or repeat it at a later date. If fistula obstruction is not found, attention must then be given to bleb failure, which is by far the more common of the two complications.

Bleb Failure. The most common cause of failure in glaucoma filtering surgery is scarring of the filtering bleb.[146] The increased amount of collagen in the failed blebs suggests that proliferation of fibroblasts with the associated production of collagen and glycosaminoglycans is important in the response to filtering surgery.[2] However, as discussed in Chapter 33, wound healing is a complex process with several phases, and it is likely that bleb failure in filtering surgery involves many of these factors as well as certain characteristics of the glaucomatous eye.

Aqueous humor normally slows or fails to support the growth of conjunctival fibroblasts in tissue culture.[147–149] A possible explanation is that aqueous contains an inhibitory factor for fibroblast proliferation. Cell culture studies have shown that the high concentration of *ascorbic acid* normally present in aqueous humor is cytotoxic to dividing human Tenon's capsule fibroblasts, which may contribute to the development of a successful filtering bleb.[150] However, aqueous obtained shortly after intraocular surgery[149] or mixed with 20% desiccated embryo extract[151] does promote proliferation of fibroblasts. Secondary aqueous humor has also been shown to stimulate the proliferation of cultured corneal endothelial cells,[152] and the aqueous humor of rabbits stimulates DNA synthesis of cultured rabbit Tenon's capsule fibroblasts, which is reduced by boiling and proteolytic enzymes.[153] In addition, aqueous humor has chemoattractant activity for ocular fibroblasts, but this activity is significantly greater in eyes that have previously failed glaucoma surgery.[154] Therefore, it may be that alterations in aqueous humor content in some glaucoma patients influence bleb failure.

Modulation of Wound Healing. Considerable attention has been given to measures, primarily in the form of drugs, that may prevent bleb failure by modulating the wound healing process. The first of these to be used clinically were the *corticosteroids*. Rabbit studies have shown that topical dexamethasone prolongs the duration of a functioning filtering bleb,[155] and clinical studies have confirmed the efficacy of topical corticosteroids, although no additional benefit is achieved with system steroids.[156] It has also been suggested that subconjunctival triamcinolone before filtering surgery may improve the success rate.[157] However, despite these efforts, the incidence of bleb failure remains high with certain types of glaucoma (e.g., glaucomas in aphakia and pseudophakia and neovascular glaucoma), which has prompted the search for additional agents to modify wound healing.

5-Fluorouracil (5-FU) is the drug that has been studied most extensively. This pyrimidine analogue antimetabolite, which blocks DNA synthesis through the inhibition of thymidylate synthesis, has been shown to inhibit fibroblast proliferation in cell cultures.[158] The subconjunctival injection of 5-FU after filtering surgery significantly improved bleb formation in monkeys[159] and improved the rate of success in difficult clinical cases.[160,161] A subsequent multicenter, randomized clinical trial of 213 patients with glaucoma in aphakia or pseudophakia or a previous failed filter in a phakic eye confirmed the ability of 5-FU to improve the success rate of filtering surgery in these high risk cases.[162] However, the protocol required twice-daily subconjunctival injections of 5 mg 5-FU for 7 days and then once-daily injections for 7 more days. In addition, significant complications included conjunctival wound leaks and corneal epithelial defects. Therefore, efforts have been made to find lower effective doses, alternative delivery systems, and alternative agents.

Success has been reported with daily injections of 5 mg 5-FU for 7–14 days,[163,164] which probably represents the most common range of dosages in current use. The treatment is believed to be most effective if started prophylactically on the first postoperative day, although success has been reported with starting 3–15 days postoperatively when signs of impending bleb failure are noted.[165] With regard to *alternative delivery systems*, topical 5-FU delayed bleb scarring in animal models but had too much corneal toxicity.[166] Iontophoresis was also effective in rabbits[167] but has questionable clinical application. Subconjunctival implants that provide a controlled release of 5-FU have also been evaluated. Collagen implants were not considered to be suitable because they incite a granulomatous inflammatory reaction,[168] but bioerodible polymers look promising.[169] Liposomes may also prolong the subconjunctival drug availability.[170,171]

Alternative agents that have been evaluated as antiproliferative drugs include cytosine arabinoside,[172] bleomycin,[172] doxorubicin,[158] 5-fluorouridine 5′-monophosphate,[170] mitomycin-c,[173] fluoroorotate,[171] heparin,[174] taxol,[175] cytochalasin B,[175] colchicine,[175] and immunotoxins.[176] Beta-irradiation was also shown to inhibit fibroblast proliferation in tissue culture[177] and to delay wound healing in rabbits,[178] but it was not effective clinically in improving the results of trabeculectomies.[179] In addition to drugs that influence fibroblast proliferation, agents have also been evaluated that alter other phases of the wound healing process. For example, tissue plasminogen activator, which causes localized fibrinolysis,[180] and beta-aminoproprionitrile[181,182] and D-penicillamine,[155,181] which inhibit cross-linking of collagen, have shown promise in animal studies. In the future, it is likely that combinations of agents will be administered according to the various phases of the wound healing process in an effort to prevent bleb failure.

Management of the Failing Bleb. The filtering bleb in these cases is typically low to flat and heavily vascularized, with no microcysts (Fig. 36.19). The operation is doomed to failure unless immediate, aggressive steps are taken. The first is to increase corticosteroid therapy, such as drops every 1–2 hours, occasionally with the addition of subconjunctival steroids. As previously noted, 5-FU may also be effective even if started several days after the surgery.[165]

Intermittent application of *digital pressure* should also be used in an attempt to expand the subconjunctival space by forcing aqueous into it (Fig. 36.20). If the digital pressure lowers the tension and expands the bleb, the patient may be instructed to perform the procedure at home several times

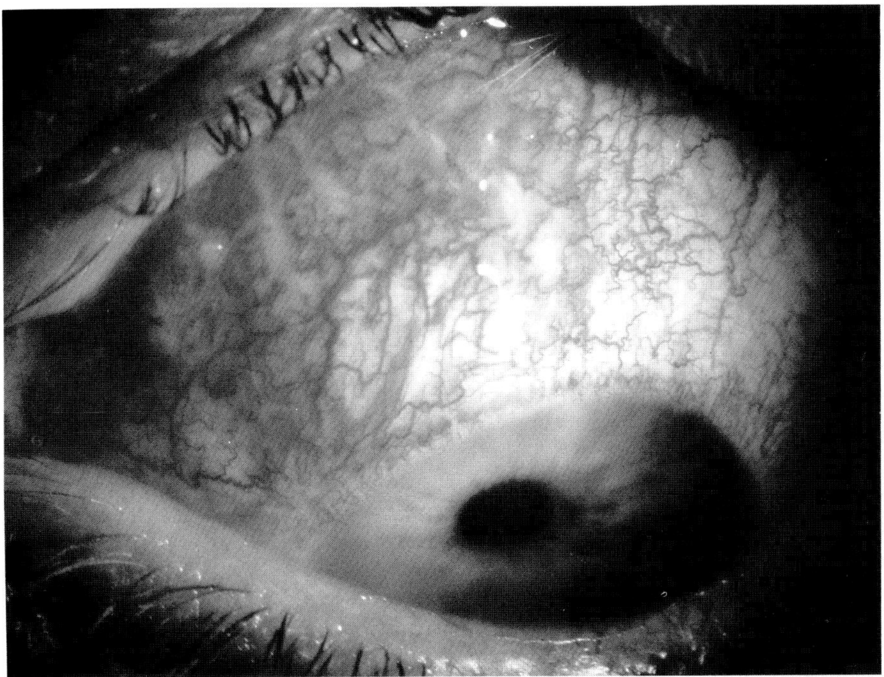

Figure 36.19. Typical appearance of a failing filtering bleb characterized by a low to flat, heavily vascularized conjunctiva.

each day. A modification of digital pressure, especially following trabeculectomy, involves pressing an anesthetic-moistened applicator beside the edge of the scleral flap.[183] The application of therapeutic ultrasound to the surgical site has also been reported to restore failing filtering blebs.[184] A case was also reported in which a subconjunctival injection of tissue plasminogen activator restored a bleb that was failing as a result of a dense hemorrhagic clot beneath the bleb.[185]

When these measures fail, glaucoma medications should be resumed. Revision of a flat, vascularized bleb has a low chance of success but can be tried. In most cases, a repeat filtering procedure with postoperative 5-FU is eventually required.

Encapsulated Filtering Bleb. These blebs, which have also been called Tenon's capsule cysts[186] and high bleb phase,[187] are characterized by a highly elevated, smooth-domed bleb with large vessels, but intervening avascular spaces and no microcysts (Fig. 36.21). Movement of the conjunctiva reveals a second, stationary set of vessels beneath the conjunctiva, which is in the layer of fibrous tissue that lines the bleb. It is important to distinguish this type of bleb from the typical failing bleb, as previously discussed. Both are associated with an elevated IOP and deep anterior chamber in the early postoperative period, but the prognosis and management differ significantly.

Encapsulated blebs are common, occuring in 10–14% of reported series.[186–188] These observations were made in the 1980s, raising the question as to whether treatment modalities that became popular during that time, such as beta-adrenergic inhibitors and argon laser trabeculoplasty, might be responsible for the apparent increase in this complication. One study suggested that long-term glaucoma therapy is associated with increased inflammation of the conjunctiva and Tenon's capsule following filtering surgery,[189] but no clear cause-and-effect relationship has been established between any glaucoma drug and encapsulated blebs. Reports are conflicting regarding the influence of argon laser trabeculoplasty.[190,191]

The encapsulated bleb usually appears during the first postoperative month. In managing them, it is important to be aware

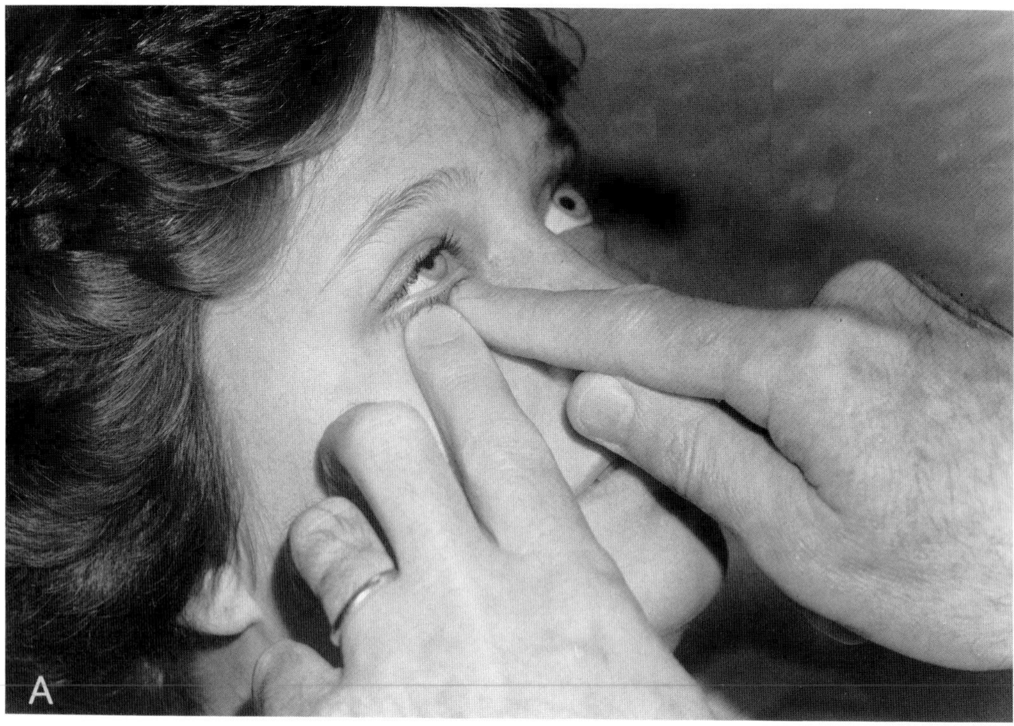

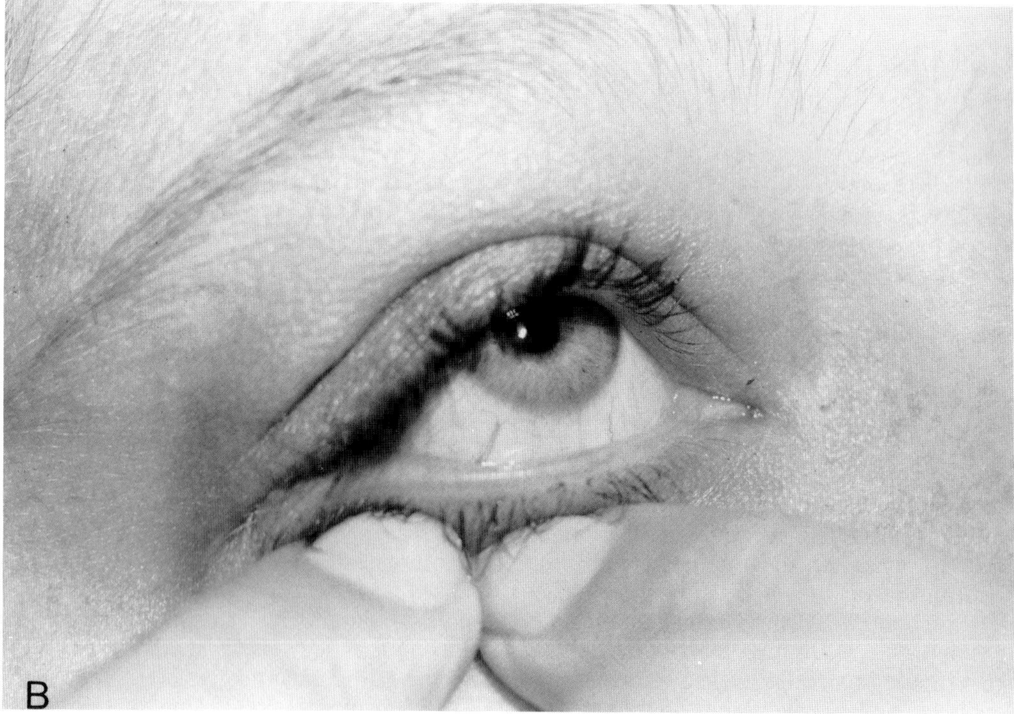

Figure 36.20. Digital pressure for eye with failing filtering bleb: **A,** Application of pressure by physician. **B,** Application of pressure by patient.

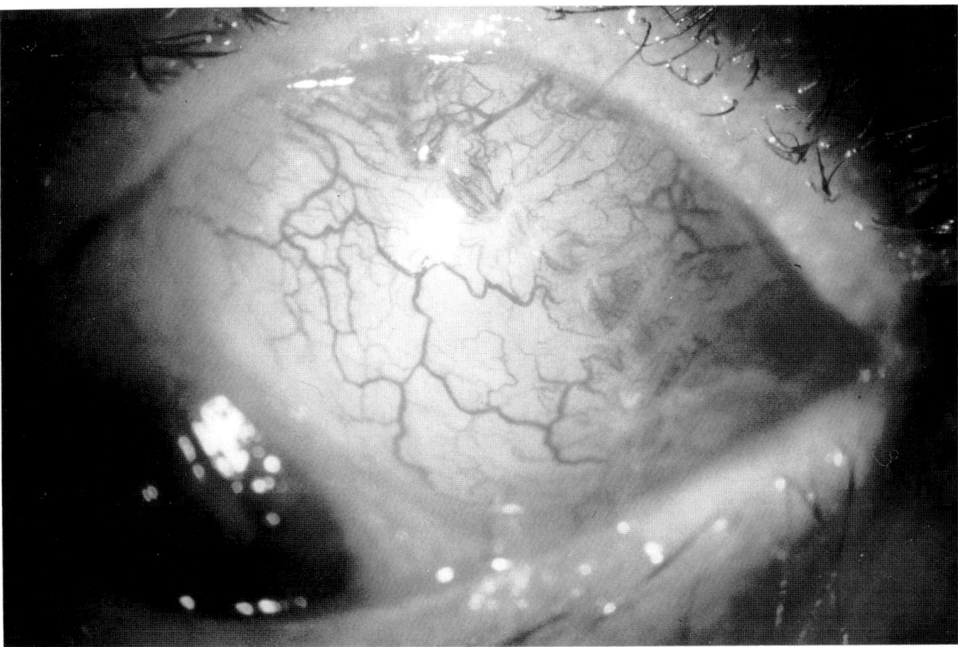

Figure 36.21. Typical appearance of an encapsulated bleb, characterized by an elevated, smooth-domed conjunctiva with large vessels but intervening avascular areas and no microcysts.

that most will begin functioning well within another few months. It is generally agreed that the mainstay of treatment is to resume glaucoma medication until the improvement occurs.[192] However, opinions differ as to whether steroids and digital pressure should be used. One study suggested that prolonged steroid therapy may actually increase the incidence of encapsulated blebs,[193] and it has been postulated that digital pressure may further reduce aqueous flow through the encapsulated bleb by compressing the subconjunctival layer of tissue.[187] Those blebs that fail to respond to conservative medical management may be restored surgically. One such technique is called *needling,* in which a needle (e.g., 25 gauge) is passed beneath the conjunctiva about 10 mm from the bleb, is used to balloon up the conjunctiva, and is then used to puncture and incise the fibrous episcleral tissue.[194,195] A more involved, but possibly more definitive, technique is to dissect the conjunctiva from the mound of fibrous tissue, completely excise the latter, and resuture the conjunctiva.[196] The success rate of either technique may be enhanced by the adjunctive use of 5-FU.[195]

Other Early Postoperative Complications

Uveitis and hyphema. Uveitis and hyphema may also occur during the early postoperative period. The former is treated with topical corticosteroids and mydriatics and the latter is managed conservatively with elevation of the head and limited activity.

Dellen. Dellen adjacent to large filtering blebs may occur during the early or late postoperative period. Most heal uneventfully with tear film replacements, although some may progress to corneal ulcers.[197]

Loss of a Small Central Island. Loss of a small central island of vision may occur after glaucoma filtering surgery. Most studies have shown this to be uncommon,[198–200] although one found it to be a considerable risk.[201] Nevertheless, a small central island is generally not considered to contraindicate glaucoma filtering surgery.[199,200]

Late Postoperative Complications

Late Failure of Filtration

The most common late complication of any filtering procedure is eventual failure to maintain a low IOP. This may develop within months to years after an initially successful operation. It is hard to predict, based on the appearance of the bleb, which cases will ultimately fail, although persistent inflammation, as well as pre- and postoperative factors that predispose to an inflammatory response, appear to play an important role.[202]

The mechanism of failure may be closure of the fistula,[203] although it is more commonly related to scarring and cyst-like formation within the bleb.[196,201,204] A histopathologic study of failed blebs revealed a marked inflammatory response, abundant fibroblasts, and deposition of new collagen within the first few months after surgery.[202] In those eyes that failed in the later postoperative period, a hypocellular capsule of fibrous tissue lined by a thick layer of fibrin was seen beneath relatively normal conjunctiva and Tenon's capsule.[202]

These cases rarely respond to digital pressure or pharmacologic agents to suppress inflammation or fibrosis. When the pressure cannot be controlled medically and the bleb appears to be encapsulated, it may be possible to revise the bleb with the surgical techniques previously described.[194–196] Transconjunctival argon laser photocoagulation has also been used to remove visible subconjunctival pigmented tissue in full-thickness filtering procedures,[205] and a Q-switched neodymium:YAG laser was successful in cutting episcleral fibrous tissue through the conjunctiva in a failed trabeculectomy.[206]

When gonioscopic evaluation suggests that the procedure has failed as a result of closure of the fistula by membranous tissue, it may be possible to reestablish patency by incising the tissue with a knife or needle from an ab interno approach.[203] However, the advent of laser therapy has now made it possible in most cases to remove the obstructing element with noninvasive surgery. Argon laser treatment has been effective for this purpose when the membrane is pigmented,[207,208] while pulsed neodymium:YAG lasers have been used successfully to eliminate nonpigmented tissue from the fistula[209,210] or to loosen or penetrate the scleral flap through the fistula.[211]

When the above measures are not effective in reestablishing a failed filtering procedure, it is usually necessary to repeat the operation in another quadrant, followed postoperatively with 5-FU.[162]

A Leaking Filtering Bleb

A bleb wall that has become too thin may rupture, leading to loss of the anterior chamber and possible endophthalmitis. The defects are usually small, and the Seidel test is often helpful in confirming the leak. In some cases the defect can be closed with tissue adhesive, although pressure patching with a Simmons shell[212,213] or a collagen shield[214] may be more effective. When these measures fail, surgical revision by creation of a new conjunctival flap from tissue posterior to the defect may be required. Histologic examination of 10 leaking filtering blebs revealed an epithelial tract running from the surface of the bleb to the episclera in eight cases, and it was suggested that the bleb should be excised before bringing down the new flap to prevent epithelial downgrowth.[215]

Endophthalmitis

Endophthalmitis is usually associated with a thin-walled filtering bleb,[216] which is more common with full-thickness procedures, although it has also been reported following trabeculectomies.[217] One study found the incidence of endophthalmitis to be the same between thermal sclerostomy and trabeculectomy.[218] The risk of endophthalmitis in eyes with filtering blebs makes it imperative that any evidence of external infection, such as conjunctivitis, be treated aggressively. Eyes with very thin blebs require especially close observation for the possibility of rupture and subsequent endophthalmitis. Some surgeons elect to use prophylactic topical antibiotics in these cases, although the value of this has not been established.

When bacterial endophthalmitis does develop in association with a ruptured filtering bleb, the majority of cases are caused by virulent organisms such as gram-negative rods and streptococci, which require prompt, aggressive management.[219] For bacterial postoperative endophthalmitis in general, a recommended approach is to establish the diagnosis with aqueous and vitreous aspirates and then to begin treatment with high-dose, broad-spectrum parenteral and periocular antibiotics, such as gentamicin and cefazolin and therapeutic vitrectomy with intravitreal antibiotics such as vancomycin and gentamicin, adjusting the treatment if necessary, according to culture and sensitivity results. Periocular and systemic corticosteroids should also be used.[219–222]

Cataracts

Cataracts are reported to occur in approximately one-third of eyes after filtering surgery.[198,223–225] The mechanism of this complication is uncertain, but possible factors include (1) patient age, (2) duration of miotic therapy, (3) surgical manipulation, (4) postoperative iritis, (5) prolonged flat anterior chamber, and (6) nutritional changes.

Other Late Postoperative Complications

Overhanging Filtering Blebs. In some cases, a large bleb may be gradually massaged downward over the cornea by the lid movements (Fig. 36.22). In some cases these can be reduced by applying argon laser energy to the bleb,[226] while others require incisional surgical correction by lifting the bleb from the cornea with an iris spatula, excising it near the limbus, and suturing the free edges.[227]

Spontaneous Hyphema. Spontaneous hyphema may occur weeks to years after filtering surgery.[228] The bleeding may come from one of the cut ends of Schlemm's canal[229] or from abnormal vessels near the internal portion of the fistula.[230] Bimanual bipolar diathermy has been suggested to treat bleeding from the anterior chamber angle,[231] although argon laser photocoagulation may be more effective in these cases.

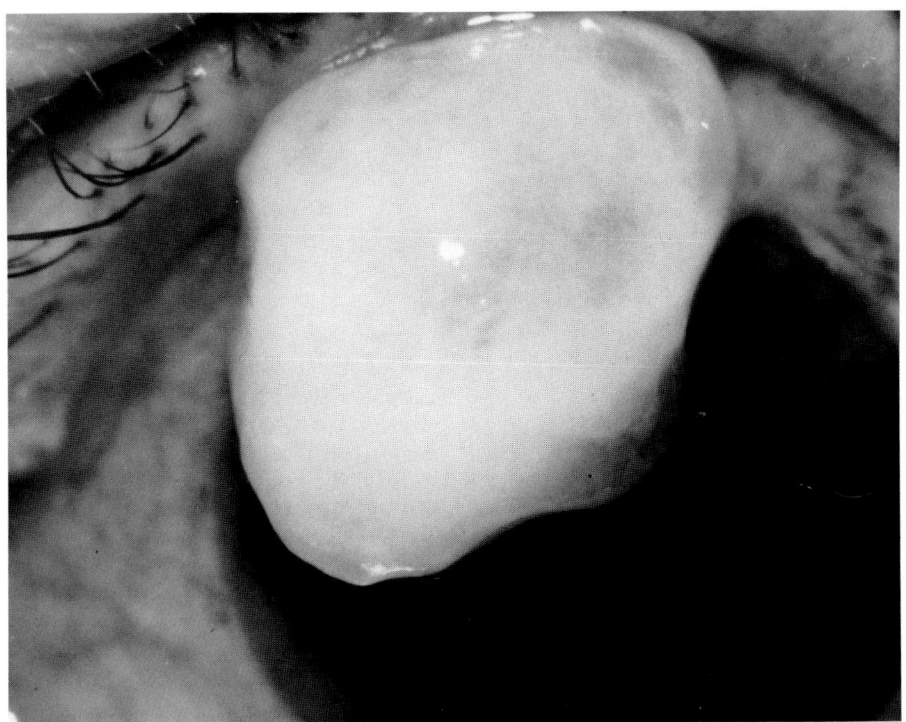

Figure 36.22. Excessive filtering bleb extending over cornea as a late complication of glaucoma filtering surgery.

Hypotony and Ciliochoroidal Detachment. These conditions may occur at any time after a filtering procedure.[232–234] Some may be chronic and recurrent,[233] and inflammation is frequently present.[233,234] Other apparent risk factors include drugs that can incite ocular inflammation and aqueous suppressants.[232,233] Management in these cases involves discontinuation of the responsible drugs and aggressive antiinflammatory therapy.[232–234] Cataracts are common with this condition and cataract extraction may be associated with resolution of the choroidal detachments.[233]

Tearing of the retinal pigment epithelium has been reported as a sequela of hypotony and choroidal or serous retinal detachment after glaucoma surgery.[235]

Staphyloma. A staphyloma has been reported as a late complication of trabeculectomy.[236]

Eyelid Changes. Upper eyelid retraction after glaucoma filtering surgery was described in two patients and was thought to result from the adrenergic effect of aqueous humor on Mueller's muscle.[237] Ptosis has also been reported following glaucoma surgery and may be related to surgical trauma to the levator muscle and adjacent tissue.[238,239]

Sympathetic Ophthalmia. This is a rare complication following glaucoma surgery. Studies suggest that it is not related to the type of operation, but rather to the preoperative condition of the eye, in that it occurs more commonly when operating on a blind, painful eye.[240]

COMPARISON OF FILTERING PROCEDURES

While most surgeons today prefer some form of trabeculectomy, there is no universal agreement regarding the filtering procedure of choice. Favorable results have been reported with both full-thickness and partial-thickness procedures. In comparing these operations, it is necessary to consider both control of the glaucoma and the rate of complications.

Full-Thickness Procedures

Glaucoma Control. With regard to control of progressive glaucomatous damage, with or without additional antiglaucoma medication, good results have been reported with each of the standard full-thickness filtering procedures (i.e., sclerectomy,[21–24] trephination,[30–32,241] and thermal sclerostomy[34–36,242]). The reported success rates for all of these operations generally range between 75 and 95%. However, one study suggested that thermal sclerostomy, despite its simplicity in concept, may be more difficult for the novice surgeon to perform effectively, as compared with a posterior lip sclerectomy.[224] This may relate to the experience required to make an adequate fistula with cautery.

Complications. A more significant difference between full-thickness filtering procedures may be seen when analyzing the complication rates of the different techniques. As previously noted, filtering procedures with a large fistula, such as trephination, may be associated with a higher incidence of complications, including prolonged flat anterior chambers in the early postoperative period and bleb leakage with possible endophthalmitis in the late period after surgery. Nevertheless, when all aspects of glaucoma control and complication rates are considered together, it is not possible to demonstrate clear-cut superiority for any one full-thickness glaucoma filtering procedure.

Trabeculectomy vs Full-Thickness Procedures

Glaucoma Control. Numerous studies have been reported regarding experience with the various forms of trabeculectomy. In general, these studies all indicate successful glaucoma control in the range of that reported for full-thickness filtering procedures, but with a variable reduction in the incidence of complications.[51,57,63–77,243–253] Studies that have specifically compared trabeculectomies and full-thickness operations have also shown comparable glaucoma control,[254,255] although some surveys suggested slightly better IOP control with full-thickness procedures.[60,256–260]

It is generally thought that glaucoma control among *black patients* is poorer than in white populations for most filtering procedures, although this has not been substantiated in all studies. With regard to trabeculectomies in black individuals, the reported success rates have mostly been in the same range as those for white patients,[261–264] although some series have revealed less than 75% success with standard trabeculectomies.[67,265] Some surgeons have noted improved pressure control in black patients when the trabeculectomy technique is modified to enhance filtration around the scleral flap.[67,266] Comparative studies of trabeculectomies and full-thickness filtering procedures within black populations have given conflicting results.[260,267–269]

It is reasonably well-established that *children* do worse with filtering procedures in general,[270] including trabeculectomies.[271–273] One study found no evidence that trabeculectomy is better than other procedures for advanced pediatric glaucomas.[274]

Aphakia is another factor that has an adverse influence on all filtering procedures, including trabeculectomies.[275,276] As previously discussed, however, the postoperative use of 5-FU appears to significantly improve the success rate in these cases.[162]

Complications. Virtually all studies agree that complication rates are lower with trabeculectomies as compared with full-thickness filtering procedures. As a result, most surgeons at present prefer a trabeculectomy for the majority of their patients, although a full-thickness procedure is still preferred by some when an especially low IOP is needed or when a trabeculectomy has failed.

SUMMARY

Glaucoma filtering procedures lower the IOP by providing a limbal fistula through which aqueous humor drains into a subconjunctival space and subsequently filters through the conjunctiva to the tear film or is absorbed by surrounding tissues. The standard filtering techniques use common principles with regard to preparation of the conjunctival flap and the iridectomy. They differ primarily according to the method of creating the fistula, with the two main variations being a full-thickness fistula and a guarded fistula beneath a partial-thickness scleral flap. An alternative approach under evaluation involves creation of a full-thickness fistula ab interno without dissection of a conjunctival flap. Complications may be encountered during filtering operations (e.g., tearing the conjunctival flap, hemorrhage, and choroidal effusion) as well as in the early postoperative period (e.g., hypotony, pressure elevation, uveitis, and hemorrhage) or late postoperative course (e.g., bleb failure, bleb leak, endophthalmitis, and cataracts). Considerable attention has been given to the modulation of wound healing to minimize bleb failure. In general, the guarded techniques have fewer complications, while the full-thickness procedures may provide slightly greater IOP reduction.

References

1. Migdal, C, Hitchings, R: The developing bleb: effect of topical antiprostaglandins on the outcome of glaucoma fistulising surgery. Br J Ophthal 67:655, 1983.
2. Addicks, EM, Quigley, HA, Green, WR, Robin, AL: Histologic characteristics of filtering blebs in glaucomatous eyes. Arch Ophthal 101:795, 1983.
3. Benedikt, O: The effect of filtering operations. Klin Monatsbl Augenheilkd 170:10, 1977.
4. Kronfeld, PC: The chemical demonstration of transconjunctival passage of aqueous after antiglaucomatous operations. Am J Ophthal 35:38, 1952.
5. Galin, MA, Baras, I, McLean, JM: How does a filtering bleb work? Trans Am Acad Ophthal Otol 69:1082, 1965.
6. Teng, CC, Chi, HH, Katzin, HM: Histology and mechanism of filtering operations. Am J Ophthal 47:16, 1959.
7. Luntz, MH: Trabeculectomy using a fornix-based conjunctival flap and tightly sutured scleral flap. Ophthalmology 87:985, 1980.
8. Faggioni, R: Trabeculectomy with conjunctival flap in the fornix: 12 months' follow-up. Klin Monatsbl Augenheilkd 182:385, 1983.
9. Shuster, JN, Krupin, T, Kolker, AE, Becker, B: Limbus- v fornix-based conjunctival flap in trabeculectomy. A long-term randomized study. Arch Ophthal 102:361, 1984.
10. Traverso, CE, Tomey, KF, Antonios, S: Limbal- vs fornix-based conjunctival trabeculectomy flaps. Am J Ophthal 104:28, 1987.
11. Reichert, R, Stewart, W, Shields, MB: Limbus-based versus fornix-based conjunctival flaps in trabeculectomy. Ophthal Surg 18:672, 1987.
12. Agbeja, AM, Dutton, GN: Conjunctival incisions for trabeculectomy and their relationship to the type of bleb formation. A preliminary study. Eye 1:738, 1987.

13. Grehn, F, Mauthe, S, Pfeiffer, N: Limbus-based versus fornix-based conjunctival flap in filtering surgery. A randomized prospective study. Internat Ophthal 13:139, 1989.
14. Kapetansky, FM: Trabeculectomy, or trabeculectomy plus tenectomy: a comparative study. Glaucoma 2:451, 1980.
15. Miller, KN, Blasini, M, Shields, MB: Total vs partial tenonectomy with trabeculectomy. Am J Ophthal 3:323, 1991.
16. Shields, MB: Conjunctival forceps for glaucoma filtering surgery. Am J Ophthal 104:666, 1987.
17. Rainin, EA: Limbal-based conjunctival flap retractor. Ann Ophthal 7:599, 1975.
18. Freedman, J: Iridectomy technique in trabeculectomy. Ophthal Surg 9:45, 1978.
19. LaGrange, F: Iridectomie et sclerectomie combinees dans le traitement du glaucome chronique. Procede nouveau pour l'etablissement de la cicatrice filtrante (1). Arch d'Opht 26:481, 1906.
20. Holth, S: Sclerectomie avec la pince emporte-piece dans le glaucome, de preference apres incision a la pique. Ann d'Ocul 142:1, 1909.
21. Berens, C: Iridocorneosclerectomy for glaucoma. Am J Ophthal 19:470, 1936.
22. McPherson, SD Jr, McCurdy, D: Anterior posterior lip sclerectomy. Proc Ann Staff Conf, McPherson Hosp 13:19, 1974.
23. Gershen, HJ: Lateral lip sclerectomy. Arch Ophthal 86:534, 1971.
24. Iliff, CE, Haas, JS: Posterior lip sclerectomy. Am J Ophthal 54:688, 1962.
25. Regan, EF: Scleral cautery with iridectomy—an experimental study. Trans Am Ophthal Soc 61:219, 1963.
26. Gass, JDM: Anterior lip sclerectomy. A microsurgical technique for filtering operation for control of glaucoma. Ann Ophthal 2:355, 1970.
27. Henry, JC, Krupin, T, Wax, MB, Feitl, ME: A modified scleral punch for filtration surgery. Am J Ophthal 108:740, 1989.
28. Elliot, RH: A preliminary note on a new operative procedure for the establishment of a filtering cicatrix in the treatment of glaucoma. Ophthalmoscope 7:804, 1909.
29. Fergus, F: Treatment of glaucoma by trephining. Br Med J 2:983, 1909.
30. Elliot, RH: Sclero-Corneal Trephining in the Operative Treatment of Glaucoma. George Pulman and Sons, London, 1913.
31. Sugar, HS: Limboscleral trephination. Am J Ophthal 52:29, 1961.
32. Sugar, HS: Limboscleral trepanation. Eleven years' experience. Arch Ophthal 85:703, 1971.
33. Preziosi, CL: The electro-cautery in the treatment of glaucoma. Br J Ophthal 8:414, 1924.
34. Scheie, HG: Retraction of scleral wound edges as a fistulizing procedure for glaucoma. Am J Ophthal 45:220, 1958.
35. Viswanathan, B, Brown, IAR: Peripheral iridectomy with scleral cautery for glaucoma. Arch Ophthal 93:34, 1975.
36. Shaffer, RN, Hetherington, J Jr, Hoskins, HD Jr: Guarded thermal sclerostomy. Am J Ophthal 72:769, 1971.
37. Litwin, RL: Successful argon laser sclerostomy for glaucoma. Ophthal Surg 10:22, 1979.
38. March, WF, Gherezghiher, T, Koss, MC, Nordquist, RE: Experimental YAG laser sclerostomy. Arch Ophthal 102:1834, 1984.
39. March, WF, Gherezghiher, R, Koss, MC, et al: Histologic study of a neodymium-YAG laser sclerostomy. Arch Ophthal 103:860, 1985.
40. Gherezghiher, T, March, WF, Koss, MC, Nordquist, RE: Neodymium-YAG laser sclerostomy in primates. Arch Ophthal 103:1543, 1985.
41. Federman, JL, Wilson, RP, Ando, F, Peyman, GA: Contact laser: thermal sclerostomy ab interna. Ophthal Surg 18:726, 1987.
42. Higginbotham, EJ, Kao, G, Peyman, G: Internal sclerostomy with the Nd:YAG contact laser versus thermal sclerostomy in rabbits. Ophthalmology 95:385, 1988.
43. Javitt, JC, O'Connor, SS, Wilson, RP, Federman, JL: Laser sclerostomy ab interno using a continuous wave Nd:YAG laser. Ophthal Surg 20:552, 1989.
44. Wilson, RP, Javitt, JC: Ab interno laser sclerostomy in aphakic patients with glaucoma and chronic inflammation. Am J Ophthal 110:178, 1990.
45. Jaffe, GJ, Williams, GA, Mieler, WF, Radius, RL: Ab interno sclerostomy with a high-powered argon endolaser. Am J Ophthal 106:391, 1988.
46. Jaffe, GJ, Mieler, WF, Radius, RL, et al: Ab interno sclerostomy with a high-powered argon endolaser. Clinicopathologic correlation. Arch Ophthal 107:1183, 1989.
47. Berlin, MS, Rajacich, G, Duffy, M, et al: Excimer laser photoablation in glaucoma filtering surgery. Am J Ophthal 103:713, 1987.
48. Brown, RH, Denham, DB, Bruner, WE, et al: Internal sclerectomy for glaucoma filtering surgery with an automated trephine. Arch Ophthal 105:133, 1987.
49. Brown, RH, Lynch, MG, Denham, DB, et al: Internal sclerectomy with an automated trephine for advanced glaucoma. Ophthalmology 95:728, 1988.
50. Sugar, HS: Experimental trabeculectomy in glaucoma. Am J Ophthal 51:623, 1961.
51. Cairns, JE: Trabeculectomy. Preliminary report of a new method. Am J Ophthal 5:673, 1968.
52. Rich, AM, McPherson, SD: Trabeculectomy in the owl monkey. Ann Ophthal 5:1082, 1973.
53. Spencer, WH: Histologic evaluation of microsurgical glaucoma techniques. Trans Am Acad Ophthal Otol 76:389, 1972.

54. Schmitt, H: Histological examination on disks obtained by goniotrephining with scleral flap. Klin Monatsbl Augenheilkd 167:372, 1975.
55. Taylor, HR: A histologic survey of trabeculectomy. Am J Ophthal 82:733, 1976.
56. Lalive d'Epinay, S, Reme, C, Witmer, R: Influence of different topographical locations of trabeculectomy specimens on regulation of intraocular pressure and the quality of the filtering bleb. Klin Monatsbl Augenheilkd 182:387, 1983.
57. Cairns, JE: Trabeculectomy. Trans Am Acad Ophthal Otol 75:1395, 1971.
58. Shields, MB, Shelburne, JD, Bell, SW: The ultrastructure of human limbal collagen. Invest Ophthal Vis Sci 16:864, 1977.
59. Shields, MB, Bradbury, MJ, Shelburne, JD, Bell, SW: The permeability of the outer layers of limbus and anterior sclera. Invest Ophthal Vis Sci 16:866, 1977.
60. Shields, MB: Trabeculectomy vs full-thickness filtering operation for control of glaucoma. Ophthal Surg 11:498, 1980.
61. Benedikt, O: The mode of action of trabeculectomy. Klin Monatsbl Augenheilkd 167:679, 1975.
62. Benedikt, O: Demonstration of aqueous outflow patterns of normal and glaucomatous human eyes through the injection of fluorescein solution in the anterior chamber. Graefe's Arch Ophthal 199:45, 1976.
63. Krasnov, MM: A modified trabeculectomy. Ann Ophthal 6:178, 1974.
64. Clemente, P: Goniotrepanation with triangular scleral flap. Klin Monatsbl Augenheilkd 177:455, 1980.
65. Dellaporta, A: Experiences with trepano-trabeculectomy. Trans Am Acad Ophthal Otol 79:362, 1975.
66. David, R, Sachs, U: Quantitative trabeculectomy. Br J Ophthal 65:457, 1981.
67. Welsh, NH: Trabeculectomy with fistula formation in the African. Br J Ophthal 56:32, 1972.
68. Hoskins, HD Jr, Migliazzo, C: Management of failing filtering blebs with the argon laser. Ophthal Surg 15:731, 1984.
69. Watson, PG: Surgery of the glaucomas. Br J Ophthal 56:299, 1972.
70. Watson, PG, Barnett, F: Effectiveness of trabeculectomy in glaucoma. Am J Ophthal 79:831, 1975.
71. Hollwich, F, Fronimopoulos, J, Junemann, G, et al: Indication, technique and results of goniotrephining with scleral flap in primary chronic glaucoma. Klin Monatsbl Augenheilkd 163:513, 1973.
72. Papst, W, Brunke, R: Goniotrepanation as a second fistulizing procedure. Klin Monatsbl Augenheilkd 176:915, 1980.
73. Smith, BF, Schuster, H, Seidenberg, B: Subscleral sclerectomy: a double-flap operation for glaucoma. Am J Ophthal 71:884, 1971.
74. Vasco-Posada, J: Glaucoma: esclerectomia subescleral. Arch Soc Am Oftal Optom 6:235, 1967.
75. Tomey, KF, Shamas, IV: Single snip trabeculectomy using a specially designed punch. Ophthal Surg 17:816, 1986.
76. Soll, DB: Intrascleral filtering procedure for glaucoma. Am J Ophthal 75:390, 1973.
77. Schimek, RA, Williamson, WR: Trabeculectomy with cautery. Ophthal Surg 8:35, 1977.
78. McGuigan, LJB, Luntz, MH, Freedman, J, Harrison, R: The role of subscleral Scheie procedure in glaucoma surgery. Ophthal Surg 17:802, 1986.
79. Beckman, H, Fuller, TA: Carbon dioxide laser scleral dissection and filtering procedure for glaucoma. Am J Ophthal 88:73, 1979.
80. Krasnov, MM: Sinusotomy. Foundation, results, prospects. Trans Am Acad Ophthal Otol 76:368, 1972.
81. Nesterov, AP: Role of the blockade of Schlemm's canal in pathogenesis of primary open-angle glaucoma. Am J Ophthal 70:691, 1970.
82. Ellingson, BA, Grant, WM: Trabeculotomy and sinusotomy in enucleated human eyes. Invest Ophthal 11:21, 1972.
83. Zimmerman, TJ, Kooner, KS, Ford, VJ, et al: Effectiveness of nonpenetrating trabeculectomy in aphakic patients with glaucoma. Ophthal Surg 15:44, 1984.
84. Zimmerman, TJ, Kooner, KS, Ford, VJ, et al: Trabeculectomy vs. nonpenetrating trabeculectomy: a retrospective study of two procedures in phakic patients with glaucoma. Ophthal Surg 15:734, 1984.
85. Weber, PA, Keates, RH, Opremcek, EM, et al: Two-stage neodymium-YAG laser trabeculotomy. Ophthal Surg 14:591, 1983.
86. Hara, T, Hara, T: Deep sclerectomy with Nd:YAG laser trabeculotomy ab interno: two-stage procedure. Ophthal Surg 19:101, 1988.
87. Lee, P-F, Shihab, ZM, Fu, Y-A: Modified trabeculectomy: a new procedure for neovascular glaucoma. Ophthal Surg 11:181, 1980.
88. Herschler, J, Agness, D: A modified filtering operation for neovascular glaucoma. Arch Ophthal 97:2339, 1979.
89. L'Esperance, FA Jr, Mittl, RN, James, WA Jr: Carbon dioxide laser trabeculostomy for the treatment of neovascular glaucoma. Ophthalmology 90:821, 1983.
90. Sinclair, SH, Aaberg, TM, Meredith, TA: A pars plana filtering procedure combined with lensectomy and vitrectomy for neovascular glaucoma. Am J Ophthal 93:185, 1982.
91. Egerer, I, Freyler, H: Aqueous outflow following seton operations. Klin Monatsbl Augenheilkd 174:93, 1979.

92. Krejci, L: Hydrogel capillary drain for glaucoma: nine years' clinical experience. Glaucoma 2:259, 1980.
93. Honrubia, FM, Gómez, ML, Hernádez, A, Grijalbo, MP: Long-term results of silicone tube in filtering surgery for eyes with neovascular glaucoma. Am J Ophthal 97:501, 1984.
94. Kuljaca, Z, Ljubojević, V, Momirov, D: Draining implant for neovascular glaucoma. Am J Ophthal 96:372, 1983.
95. Molteno, ACB: New implant for drainage in glaucoma. Clinical trial. Br J Ophthal 53:606, 1969.
96. Schocket, SS, Lakhanpal, V, Richards, RD: Anterior chamber tube shunt to an encircling band in the treatment of neovascular glaucoma. Ophthalmology 89:1188, 1982.
97. Schocket, SS, Nirankari, VS, Lakhanpal, V, et al: Anterior chamber tube shunt to an encircling band in the treatment of neovascular glaucoma and other refractory glaucomas. A long-term study. Ophthalmology 92:553, 1985.
98. Freedman, J: The use of the single stage Molteno long tube seton in treating resistant cases of glaucoma. Ophthal Surg 16:480, 1985.
99. Minckler, DS, Heuer, DK, Hasty, B, et al: Clinical experience with the single-plate Molteno implant in complicated glaucomas. Ophthalmology 95:1181, 1988.
100. Ancker, E, Molteno, ACB: Molteno drainage implant for neovascular glaucoma. Trans Ophthal Soc UK 102:122, 1982.
101. Ancker, E, Molteno, ACB: Surgical treatment of chronic aphakic glaucoma with the Molteno plastic implant. Klin Monatsbl Augenheilkd 177:365, 1980.
102. Fish, LA, Heuer, DK, Baerveldt, G, et al: Molteno implantation for secondary glaucomas associated with advanced epithelial ingrowth. Ophthalmology 97:557, 1990.
103. McDonnell, PJ, Robin, JB, Schanzlin, DJ, et al: Molteno implant for control of glaucoma in eyes after penetrating keratoplasty. Ophthalmology 95:364, 1988.
104. Billson, F, Thomas, R, Aylward, W: The use of two-stage Molteno implants in developmental glaucoma. J Ped Ophthal Strab 26:3, 1989.
105. Lee, P-F, Ward, RH: Aqueous-venous shunt for glaucoma. A further report. Arch Ophthal 99:2007, 1981.
106. Krupin, T, Podos, SM, Becker, B, Newkirk, JB: Valve implants in filtering surgery. Am J Ophthal 81:232, 1976.
107. Krupin, T, Kaufman, P, Mandell, A, et al: Filtering valve implant surgery for eyes with neovascular glaucoma. Am J Ophthal 89:338, 1980.
108. Krupin, T, Kaufman, P, Mandell, AI, et al: Long-term results of valve implants in filtering surgery for eyes with neovascular glaucoma. Am J Ophthal 95:775, 1983.
109. Folberg, R, Hargett, NA, Weaver, JE, McLean, IW: Filtering valve implant for neovascular glaucoma in proliferative diabetic retinopathy. Ophthalmology 89:286, 1982.
110. Krupin, T, Ritch, R, Camras, CB, et al: A long Krupin-Denver valve implant attached to a 180° scleral explant for glaucoma surgery. Ophthalmology 95:1174, 1988.
111. Haas, JS, Peyman, GA, Lim, J: Experimental evaluation of a posterior drainage system. Ophthal Surg 14:494, 1983.
112. Hitchings, RA, Joseph, NH, Sherwood, MB, et al: Use of one-piece valved tube and variable surface area explant for glaucoma drainage surgery. Ophthalmology 94:1079, 1987.
113. Blasini, M, Shields, MB, Hickingbotham, D: A temporary glaucoma valve for transient intraocular pressure elevation. Ophthal Surg 21:199, 1990.
114. Petursson, GJ, Fraunfelder, FT: Repair of an inadvertent buttonhole or leaking filtering bleb. Arch Ophthal 97:926, 1979.
115. Awan, KJ, Spaeth, PG: Use of isobutyl-2-cyanoacrylate tissue adhesive in the repair of conjunctival fistula in filtering procedures for glaucoma. Ann Ophthal 6:851, 1974.
116. Ferry, AP: Hemorrhage into the lens as a complication of glaucoma surgery. Am J Ophthal 81:351, 1976.
117. Bellows, AR, Chylack, LT Jr, Epstein, DL, Hutchinson, BT: Choroidal effusion during glaucoma surgery in patients with prominent episcleral vessels. Arch Ophthal 97:493, 1979.
118. Bellows, AR, Chylack, LT Jr, Hutchinson, BT: Choroidal detachment. Clinical manifestation, therapy and mechanism of formation. Ophthalmology 88:1107, 1981.
119. Swan, KC, Lindgren, TW: Unintentional lens injury in glaucoma surgery. Trans Am Ophthal Soc 78:55, 1980.
120. Kozart, DM, Eagle, RC Jr: Stripping of Descemet's membrane after glaucoma surgery. Ophthal Surg 12:420, 1981.
121. Kao, SF, Lichter, PR, Musch, DC: Anterior chamber depth following filtration surgery. Ophthal Surg 20:332, 1989.
122. Stewart, WC, Shields, MB: Management of anterior chamber depth after trabeculectomy. Am J Ophthal 106:41, 1988.
123. Fiore, PM, Richter, CU, Arzeno, G, et al: The effect of anterior chamber depth on endothelial cell count after filtration surgery. Arch Ophthal 107:1609, 1989.
124. Phillips, CI, Clark, CV, Levy, AM: Posterior synechiae after glaucoma operations: aggravation by shallow anterior chamber and pilocarpine. Br J Ophthal 71:428, 1987.
125. Hung, SO: Role of sodium hyaluronate (Healonid) in triangular flap trabeculectomy. Br J Ophthal 69:46, 1985.

126. Teekhasaenee, C, Ritch, R: The use of PhEA 34c in trabeculectomy. Ophthalmology 93:487, 1986.
127. Wand, M: Viscoelastic agent and the prevention of post-filtration flat anterior chamber. Ophthal Surg 19:523, 1988.
128. Simmons, RJ, Kimbrough, RL: Shell tamponade in filtering surgery for glaucoma. Ophthal Surg 10:17, 1979.
129. Weber, PA, Baker, ND: The use of cyanoacrylate adhesive with a collagen shield in leaking filtering blebs. Ophthal Surg 20:284, 1989.
130. Sugar, HS: Treatment of hypotony following filtering surgery for glaucoma. Am J Ophthal 71:1023, 1971.
131. Savage, JA, Condon, GP, Lytle, RA, Simmons, RJ: Laser suture lysis after trabeculectomy. Ophthalmology 95:1631, 1988.
132. Cohen, JS, Osher, RH: Releasable suture in filtering and combined procedures. In: Perspectives in Glaucoma, Shields, MB, Pollack, IP, Kolker, AE, eds. Slack, Inc., Thorofare, NJ, p. 157, 1988.
133. Stewart, RH, Kimbrough, RL: A method of managing flat anterior chamber following trabeculectomy. Ophthal Surg 11:382, 1980.
134. Fisher, YL, Turtz, AI, Gold, M, et al: Use of sodium hyaluronate in reformation and reconstruction of the persistent flat anterior chamber in the presence of severe hypotony. Ophthal Surg 13:819, 1982.
135. Fourman, S: Management of cornea-lens touch after filtering surgery for glaucoma. Ophthalmology 97:424, 1990.
136. Brubaker, RF, Pederson, JE: Ciliochoroidal detachment. Surv Ophthal 27:281, 1983.
137. Chylack, LT Jr, Bellows, AR: Molecular sieving in suprachoroidal fluid formation in man. Invest Ophthal Vis Sci 17:420, 1978.
138. Gressel, MG, Parrish, RK, Heuer, DK: Delayed nonexpulsive suprachoroidal hemorrhage. Arch Ophthal 102:1757, 1984.
139. Ruderman, JM, Harbin, TS, Jr, Campbell, DG: Postoperative suprachoroidal hemorrhage following filtration procedures. Arch Ophthal 104:201, 1986.
140. Givens, K, Shields, MB: Suprachoroidal hemorrhage after glaucoma filtering surgery. Am J Ophthal 103:689, 1987.
141. Canning, CR, Lavin, M, McCartney, ACE, et al: Delayed suprachoroidal haemorrhage after glaucoma operations. Eye 3:327, 1989.
142. Ariano, ML, Ball, SF: Delayed nonexpulsive suprachoroidal hemorrhage after trabeculectomy. Ophthal Surg 18:661, 1987.
143. Frenkel, REP, Shin, DH: Prevention and management of delayed suprachoroidal hemorrhage after filtration surgery. Arch Ophthal 104:1459, 1986.
144. Lakhanpal, V, Schocket, SS, Elman, MJ, Nirankari, VS: A new modified vitreoretinal surgical approach in the management of massive suprachoroidal hemorrhage. Ophthalmology 96:793, 1989.
145. Abrams, GW, Thomas, MA, Williams, GA, Burton, TC: Management of postoperative suprachoroidal hemorrhage with continuous-infusion air pump. Arch Ophthal 104:1455, 1986.
146. Maumenee, AE: External filtering operations for glaucoma: the mechanism of function and failure. Trans Am Ophthal Soc 58:319, 1960.
147. Kornblueth, W, Tenebaum, E: The inhibitory effect of aqueous humor on the growth of cells in tissue cultures. Am J Ophthal 42:70, 1956.
148. Herschler, J, Claflin, AJ, Fiorentino, G: The effect of aqueous humor on the growth of subconjunctival fibroblasts in tissue culture and its implications for glaucoma surgery. Am J Ophthal 89:245, 1980.
149. Radius, RL, Herschler, J, Claflin, A, Fiorentino, G: Aqueous humor changes after experimental filtering surgery. Am J Ophthal 89:250, 1980.
150. Jampel, HD: Ascorbic acid is cytotoxic to dividing human Tenon's capsule fibroblasts. A possible contributing factor in glaucoma filtration surgery success. Arch Ophthal 108:1323, 1990.
151. Albrink, WS, Wallace, AC: Aqueous humor as a tissue culture nutrient. Proc Soc Exp Biol Med 77:754, 1951.
152. Ledbetter, SR, Hatchell, DL (Van Horn), O'Brien, WJ: Secondary aqueous humor stimulates the proliferation of cultured bovine corneal endothelial cells. Invest Ophthal Vis Sci 24:557, 1983.
153. Litin, BS, Jones, MA, Herschler, J: Heat and protease treatment of aqueous humor: effect on cell DNA synthesis and growth. Graefe's Arch Ophthal 222:154, 1985.
154. Joseph, JP, Grierson, I, Hitchings, RA: Chemotactic activity of aqueous humor. A cause of failure of trabeculectomies? Arch Ophthal 107:69, 1989.
155. McGuigan, LJB, Cook, DJ, Yablonski, ME: Dexamethasone, d-penicillamine, and glaucoma filter surgery in rabbits. Invest Ophthal Vis Sci 27:1755, 1986.
156. Starita, RJ, Fellman, RL, Spaeth, GL, et al: Short- and long-term effects of postoperative corticosteroids on trabeculectomy. Ophthalmology 92:938, 1985.
157. Giangiacomo, J, Dueker, DK, Adelstein, E: The effect of preoperative subconjunctival triamcinolone administration on glaucoma filtration. I. Trabeculectomy following subconjunctival triamcinolone. Arch Ophthal 104:838, 1986.
158. Blumenkranz, MS, Claflin, A, Hajek, AS: Selection of therapeutic agents for intraocular proliferative disease. Cell culture evaluation. Arch Ophthal 102:598, 1984.
159. Gressel, MG, Parrish, RK II, Folberg, R: 5-Fluo-

rouracil and glaucoma filtering surgery: I. An animal model. Ophthalmology 91:378, 1984.
160. Heuer, DK, Parrish, RK II, Gressel, MG, et al: 5-Fluorouracil and glaucoma filtering surgery. II. A Pilot study. Ophthalmology 91:384, 1984.
161. Heuer, DK, Parrish, RK II, Gressel, MG, et al: 5-Fluorouracil and glaucoma filtering surgery. III. Intermediate follow-up of a pilot study. Ophthalmology 93:1537, 1986.
162. The Fluorouracil Filtering Surgery Study Group: Fluorouracil filtering surgery study one-year follow-up. Am J Ophthal 108:625, 1989.
163. Weinreb, RN: Adjusting the dose of 5-fluorouracil after filtration surgery to minimize side effects. Ophthalmology 94:564, 1987.
164. Ruderman, JM, Welch, DB, Smith, MF, Shoch, DE: A randomized study of 5-fluorouracil and filtration surgery. Am J Ophthal 104:218, 1987.
165. Krug, JH Jr, Melamed, S: Adjunctive use of delayed and adjustable low-dose 5-fluorouracil in refractory glaucoma. Am J Ophthal 109:412, 1990.
166. Heuer, DK, Gressel, MG, Parrish, RK II, et al: Topical fluorouracil. II. Postoperative administration in an animal model of glaucoma filtering surgery. Arch Ophthal 104:132, 1986.
167. Kando, M, Araie, M: Iontophoresis of 5-fluorouracil into the conjunctiva and sclera. Invest Ophthal Vis Sci 30:583, 1989.
168. Hasty, B, Heuer, DK, Minckler, DS: Primate trabeculectomies with 5-fluorouracil collagen implants. Am J Ophthal 109:721, 1990.
169. Lee, DA, Flores, RA, Anderson, PJ, et al: Glaucoma filtration surgery in rabbits using bioerodible polymers and 5-fluorouracil. Ophthalmology 94:1523, 1987.
170. Skuta, GL, Assil, K, Parrish, RK II, et al: Filtering surgery in owl monkeys treated with the antimetabolite 5-fluorouridine 5′-monophosphate entrapped in multivesicular liposomes. Am J Ophthal 103:714, 1987.
171. Alvarado, JA: The use of a liposome-encapsulated 5-fluoroorotate for glaucoma surgery: I. Animal studies. Trans Am Ophthal Soc 87:489, 1989.
172. Litin, BS, Jones, MA, Kwong, EM, Herschler, J: Effect of antineoplastic drugs on cell proliferation—individually and in combination. Ophthal Surg 16:34, 1985.
173. Chen, C-W, Huang, H-T, Sheu, M-M: Enhancement of IOP control. Effect of trabeculectomy by local application of anticancer drug. Act XXV Con Ophthal, pp. 1487, 1986.
174. del Vecchio, PJ, Bizios, R, Holleran, LA, et al: Inhibition of human scleral fibroblast proliferation with heparin. Invest Ophthal Vis Sci 29:1272, 1988.
175. Joseph, JP, Grierson, I, Hitchings, RA: Taxol, cytochalasin B and colchicine effects on fibroblast migration and contraction: a role in glaucoma filtration surgery? Curr Eye Res 8:203, 1989.
176. Fulcher, S, Lui, G, Houston, LL, et al: Use of immunotoxin to inhibit proliferating human corneal endothelium. Invest Ophthal Vis Sci 29:755, 1988.
177. Nevárez, JA, Parrish, RK II, Heuer, DK, et al: The effect of beta irradiation on monkey Tenon's capsule fibroblasts in tissue culture. Curr Eye Res 6:719, 1987.
178. Miller, MH, Grierson, I, Unger, WG, Hitchings, RA: The effect of topical dexamethasone and preoperative beta irradiation on a model of glaucoma fistulizing surgery in the rabbit. Ophthal Surg 21:44, 1990.
179. Miller, MH, Joseph, NH, Wishart, PK, Hitchings, RA: Lack of beneficial effect of intensive topical steroids and beta irradiation of eyes undergoing repeat trabeculectomy. Ophthal Surg 18:508, 1987.
180. Fourman, S, Vaid, K: Effects of tissue plasminogen activator on glaucoma filter blebs in rabbits. Ophthal Surg 20:663, 1989.
181. McGuigan, LJB, Mason, RP, Sanchez, R, Quigley, HA: D-penicillamine and beta-aminopropionitrile effects on experimental filtering surgery. Invest Ophthal Vis Sci 28:1625, 1987.
182. Fourman, S: Effects of aminoproprionitrile on glaucoma filter blebs in rabbits. Ophthal Surg 19:649, 1988.
183. Traverso, CE, Greenidge, KC, Spaeth, GL, Wilson, RP: Focal pressure: a new method to encourage filtration after trabeculectomy. Ophthal Surg 15:62, 1984.
184. Yablonski, M, Masonson, HN, El-Sayyad, F, et al: Use of therapeutic ultrasound to restore failed trabeculectomies. Am J Ophthal 103:492, 1987.
185. Ortiz, JR, Walker, SD, McManus, PE, et al: Filtering bleb thrombolysis with tissue plasminogen activator. Am J Ophthal 106:624, 1988.
186. Sherwood, MB, Spaeth, GL, Simmons, ST, et al: Cysts of Tenon's capsule following filtration surgery. Medical management. Arch Ophthal 105:1517, 1987.
187. Scott, DR, Quigley, HA: Medical management of a high bleb phase after trabeculectomies. Ophthalmology 95:1169, 1988.
188. Richter, CU, Shingleton, BJ, Bellows, AR, et al: The development of encapsulated filtering blebs. Ophthalmology 95:1163, 1988.
189. Sherwood, MB, Grierson, I, Millar, L, Hitchings, RA: Long-term morphologic effects of antiglaucoma drugs on the conjunctiva and Tenon's capsule in glaucomatous patients. Ophthalmology 96:327, 1989.
190. Schoenleber, DB, Bellows, AR, Hutchingson, BT: Failed laser trabeculoplasty requiring surgery in open-angle glaucoma. Ophthal Surg 18:796, 1987.

191. Feldman, RM, Gross, RL, Spaeth, GL, et al: Risk factors for the development of Tenon's capsule cysts after trabeculectomy. Ophthalmology 96:336, 1989.
192. Shingleton, BJ, Richter, CU, Bellows, AR, Hutchinson, BT: Management of encapsulated filtration blebs. Ophthalmology 97:63, 1990.
193. Loftfield, K, Ball, SF: Filtering bleb encapsulation increased by steroid injection. Ophthal Surg 21:282, 1990.
194. Pederson, JE, Smith, SG: Surgical management of encapsulated filtering blebs. Ophthalmology 92:955, 1985.
195. Ewing, RH, Stamper, RL: Needle revision with and without 5-fluorouracil for the treatment of failed filtering blebs. Am J Ophthal 110:254, 1990.
196. Van Buskirk, EM: Cysts of Tenon's capsule following filtration surgery. Am J Ophthal 94:522, 1982.
197. Soong, HK, Quigley, HA: Dellen associated with filtering blebs. Arch Ophthal 101:385, 1983.
198. O'Connell, EJ, Karseras, AG: Intraocular surgery in advanced glaucoma. Br J Ophthal 60:124, 1976.
199. Lawrence, GA: Surgical treatment of patients with advanced glaucomatous field defects. Arch Ophthal 81:804, 1969.
200. Lichter, PR, Ravin, JG: Risks of sudden visual loss after glaucoma surgery. Am J Ophthal 78:1009, 1974.
201. Aggarwal, SP, Hendeles, S: Risk of sudden visual loss following trabeculectomy in advanced primary open-angle glaucoma. Br J Ophthal 70:97, 1986.
202. Hitchings, RA, Grierson, I: Clinico pathological correlation in eyes with failed fistulizing surgery. Trans Ophthal Soc UK 103:84, 1983.
203. Swan, KC: Reopening of nonfunctioning filters—simplified surgical techniques. Trans Am Acad Ophthal Otol 79:342, 1975.
204. Cohen, JS, Shaffer, RN, Hetherington, J Jr, Hoskins, D: Revision of filtration surgery. Arch Ophthal 95:1612, 1977.
205. Kurata, F, Krupin, T, Kolker, AE: Reopening filtration fistulas with transconjunctival argon laser photocoagulation. Am J Ophthal 98:340, 1984.
206. Rankin, GA, Latina, MA: Transconjunctival Nd:YAG laser revision of failing trabeculectomy. Ophthal Surg 21:365, 1990.
207. Ticho, U, Ivry, M: Reopening of occluded filtering blebs by argon laser photocoagulation. Am J Ophthal 84:413, 1977.
208. Van Buskirk, EM: Reopening filtration fistulas with the argon laser. Am J Ophthal 94:1, 1982.
209. Praeger, DL: The reopening of closed filtering blebs using the neodymium:YAG laser. Ophthalmology 91:373, 1984.
210. Dailey, RA, Samples, JR, Van Buskirk, EM: Reopening filtration fistulas with the neodymium-YAG laser. Am J Ophthal 102:491, 1986.
211. Cohn, HC, Whalen, WR, Aron-Rosa, D: YAG laser treatment in a series of failed trabeculectomies. Am J Ophthal 108:395, 1989.
212. Ruderman, JM, Allen, RC: Simmons' tamponade shell for leaking filtration blebs. Arch Ophthal 103:1708, 1985.
213. Melamed, S, Hersh, P, Kersten, D, et al: The use of glaucoma shell tamponade in leaking filtration blebs. Ophthalmology 93:839, 1986.
214. Fourman, S, Wiley, L: Use of a collagen shield to treat a glaucoma filter bleb leak. Am J Ophthal 107:673, 1989.
215. Sinnreich, Z, Barishak, R, Stein, R: Leaking filtering blebs. Am J Ophthal 86:345, 1978.
216. Hattenhauer, JM, Lipsich, MP: Late endophthalmitis after filtering surgery. Am J Ophthal 72:1097, 1971.
217. Lobue, TD, Deutsch, TA, Stein, RM: *Moraxella nonliquefaciens* endophthalmitis after trabeculectomy. Am J Ophthal 99:343, 1985.
218. Freedman, J, Gupta, M, Bunke, A: Endophthalmitis after trabeculectomy. Arch Ophthal 96:1017, 1978.
219. Mandelbaum, S, Forster, RK, Gelender, H, Culbertson, W: Late onset endophthalmitis associated with filtering blebs. Ophthalmology 92:964, 1985.
220. Kanski, JJ: Treatment of late endophthalmitis associated with filtering blebs. Arch Ophthal 91:339, 1974.
221. Stern, GA, Engel, HM, Driebe, WT, Jr: The treatment of postoperative endophthalmitis. Results of differing approaches to treatment. Ophthalmology 96:62, 1989.
222. Olk, RJ, Bohigian, GM: The management of endophthalmitis: diagnostic and therapeutic guidelines including the use of vitrectomy. Ophthal Surg 18:262, 1987.
223. Sugar, HS: Cataract and filtering surgery. Am J Ophthal 69:740, 1970.
224. Marion, JR, Shields, MB: Thermal sclerostomy and posterior lip sclerectomy: a comparative study. Ophthal Surg 9:67, 1978.
225. Chauvaud, D, Clay-Fressinet, C, Pouliquen, Y, Offret, G: Opacification of the lens after trabeculectomy. Arch Ophthal (Paris) 36:379, 1976.
226. Fink, AJ, Boys-Smith, JW, Brear, R: Management of large filtering blebs with the argon laser. Am J Ophthal 101:695, 1986.
227. Scheie, HG, Guehl, JJ III: Surgical management of overhanging blebs after filtering procedures. Arch Ophthal 97:325, 1979.
228. Harris, LS, Galin, MA: Delayed spontaneous hyphema following successful sclerotomy with cautery in three patients. Am J Ophthal 72:458, 1971.
229. Namba, H: Blood reflux into anterior chamber after trabeculectomy. Jap J Ophthal 27:616, 1983.

230. Wilensky, JT: Late hyphema after filtering surgery for glaucoma. Ophthal Surg 14:227, 1983.
231. Michels, RG, Rice, TA: Bimanual bipolar diathermy for treatment of bleeding from the anterior chamber angle. Am J Ophthal 84:873, 1977.
232. Vela, MA, Campbell, DG: Hypotony and ciliochoroidal detachment following pharmacologic aqueous suppressant therapy in previously filtered patients. Ophthalmology 92:50, 1985.
233. Berke, SJ, Bellows, R, Shingleton, BJ, et al: Chronic and recurrent choroidal detachment after glaucoma filtering surgery. Ophthalmology 94:154, 1987.
234. Burney, EN, Quigley, HA, Robin, AL: Hypotony and choroidal detachment as late complications of trabeculectomy. Am J Ophthal 103:685, 1987.
235. Laatikainen, L, Syrdalen, P: Tearing of retinal pigment epithelium after glaucoma surgery. Graefe's Arch Ophthal 225:308, 1987.
236. Spaeth, GL, Rodrigues, MM: Staphyloma as a late complication of trabeculectomy. Ophthal Surg 8:81, 1977.
237. Putterman, AM, Urist, MJ: Upper eyelid retraction after glaucoma filtering procedures. Ann Ophthal 7:263, 1975.
238. Alpar, JJ: Acquired ptosis following cataract and glaucoma surgery. Glaucoma 4:66, 1982.
239. Deady, JP, Price, NJ, Sutton, GA: Ptosis following cataract and trabeculectomy surgery. Br J Ophthal 73:283, 1989.
240. Shammas, HF, Zubyk, NA, Stanfield, TF: Sympathetic uveitis following glaucoma surgery. Arch Ophthal 95:638, 1977.
241. Riss, B, Binder, S: Review of 402 goniotrephinations. Klin Monatsbl Augenheilkd 176:286, 1980.
242. Rehak, S, Hrochova, J, Rozsival, P: Long-term follow-up of scleral cauterization in glaucoma surgery. Klin Monatsbl Augenheilkd 181:283, 1982.
243. Jerndal, T, Lundstrom, M: 330 trabeculectomies—a follow-up study through ½–3 years. Acta Ophthal 55:52, 1977.
244. Wilson, P: Trabeculectomy: long-term follow-up. Br J Ophthal 61:535, 1977.
245. Schwartz, AL, Anderson, DR: Trabecular surgery. Arch Ophthal 92:134, 1974.
246. D'Ermo, F, Bonomi, L, Doro, D: A critical analysis of the long-term results of trabeculectomy. Am J Ophthal 88:829, 1979.
247. Zaidi, AA: Trabeculectomy: a review and 4-year follow-up. Br J Ophthal 64:436, 1980.
248. Jay, JL, Murray, SB: Characteristics of reduction of intraocular pressure after trabeculectomy. Br J Ophthal 64:423, 1980.
249. Watson, PG, Grierson, I: The place of trabeculectomy in the treatment of glaucoma. Ophthalmology 88:175, 1981.
250. Jerndal, T, Lundstrom, M: 330 trabeculectomies. A long time study (3–5½ years). Acta Ophthal 58:947, 1980.
251. Mills, KB: Trabeculectomy: a retrospective long-term follow-up of 444 cases. Br J Ophthal 65:790, 1981.
252. Inaba, Z: Longterm results of trabeculectomy in the Japanese: an analysis of life table method. Jap J Ophthal 26:361, 1982.
253. Shirato, S, Kitazawa, Y, Mishima, S: A critical analysis of the trabeculectomy results by a prospective follow-up design. Jap J Ophthal 26:468, 1982.
254. Drance, SM, Vargas, E: Trabeculectomy and thermosclerectomy: a comparison of two procedures. Can J Ophthal 8:413, 1973.
255. Lewis, RA, Phelps, CD: Trabeculectomy v thermosclerostomy. A five-year follow-up. Arch Ophthal 102:533, 1984.
256. Spaeth, GL, Joseph, NH, Fernandes, E: Trabeculectomy: a re-evaluation after three years and a comparison with Scheie's procedure. Trans Am Acad Ophthal Otol 79:349, 1975.
257. Spaeth, GL, Poryzees, E: A comparison between peripheral iridectomy with thermal sclerostomy and trabeculectomy: a controlled study. Br J Ophthal 65:783, 1981.
258. Watkins, PH Jr, Brubaker, RF: Comparison of partial-thickness and full-thickness filtration procedures in open-angle glaucoma. Am J Ophthal 86:756, 1978.
259. Blondeau, P, Phelps, CD: Trabeculectomy vs thermosclerostomy. A randomized prospective clinical trial. Arch Ophthal 99:810, 1981.
260. Wilson, MR: Posterior lip sclerectomy vs trabeculectomy in West Indian blacks. Arch Ophthal 107:1604, 1989.
261. Freedman, J, Shen, E, Ahrens, M: Trabeculectomy in a Black American glaucoma population. Br J Ophthal 60:573, 1976.
262. Ferguson, JG Jr, MacDonald, R Jr: Trabeculectomy in blacks: a two-year follow-up. Ophthal Surg 8:41, 1977.
263. David, R, Freedman, J, Luntz, MH: Comparative study of Watson's and Cairn's trabeculectomies in a Black population with open angle glaucoma. Br J Ophthal 61:117, 1977.
264. BenEzra, D, Chirambo, MC: Trabeculectomy. Ann Ophthal 10:1101, 1978.
265. Miller, RD, Barber, JC: Trabeculectomy in black patients. Ophthal Surg 12:46, 1981.
266. Thommy, CP, Bhar, IS: Trabeculectomy in Nigerian patients with open-angle glaucoma. Br J Ophthal 63:636, 1979.
267. Sandford-Smith, JH: The surgical treatment of open-angle glaucoma in Nigerians. Br J Ophthal 62:283, 1978.
268. Bakker, NJA, Manku, SI: Trabeculectomy versus Scheie's operation: a comparative retrospec-

tive study in open-angle glaucoma in Kenyans. Br J Ophthal 63:643, 1979.

269. Kietzman, B: Glaucoma surgery in Nigerian eyes: a five year study. Ophthal Surg 7:52, 1976.
270. Cadera, W, Pachtman, MA, Cantor, LB, et al: Filtering surgery in childhood glaucoma. Ophthal Surg 15:319, 1984.
271. Stewart, RH, Kimbrough, RL, Bachh, H, Allbright, M: Trabeculectomy and modifications of trabeculectomy. Ophthal Surg 10:76, 1979.
272. Kolozsvari, L: Trabeculectomy in cases of buphthalmos. Klin Monatsbl Augenheilkd 183:503, 1983.
273. Gressel, MG, Heuer, DK, Parrish, RK II: Trabeculectomy in young patients. Ophthalmology 91:1242, 1984.
274. Beauchamp, GR, Parks, MM: Filtering surgery in children: barriers to success. Ophthalmology 86:170, 1979.
275. Levene, RZ: Glaucoma filtering surgery factors that determine pressure control. Trans Am Ophthal Soc LXXXII:282, 1984.
276. Heuer, DK, Gressel, MG, Parrish, RK II, et al: Trabeculectomy in aphakic eyes. Ophthalmology 91:1045, 1984.

Chapter 37

CYCLODESTRUCTIVE SURGERY

All of the operations discussed in the preceding chapters lower the intraocular pressure (IOP) by improving the rate of aqueous outflow. An alternative approach is to reduce the rate of aqueous production by partly eliminating the function of the ciliary processes. These techniques are rarely the first operation of choice, because the results are hard to predict and damage to ocular structures or inflammation often lead to complications. However, the cyclodestructive procedures constitute a valuable adjunct in our surgical armamentarium for cases in which other operations have repeatedly failed or are thought to be contraindicated.

Overview of Cyclodestructive Procedures

Cyclodestructive operations differ according to (1) the destructive energy source and (2) the route by which the energy reaches the ciliary processes. In the 1930s and '40s, several energy sources were evaluated, including diathermy, beta-irradiation, and electrolysis, although only cyclodiathermy achieved clinical acceptance. Cryotherapy was introduced in the 1950s and is at present the most commonly used cyclodestructive procedure. However, more recent experience with laser cyclophotocoagulation suggests that this may soon become the preferred cyclodestructive operation. Other more recently evaluated cyclodestructive elements include ultrasound and microwaves.

Each of the energy sources noted above may be delivered via the transscleral route, in which the destructive element passes through conjunctiva, sclera, and ciliary muscle before reaching the ciliary processes. Transscleral cyclodestructive operations have the advantages of being noninvasive and relatively quick and easy, although significant disadvantages include the inability to visualize the processes being treated and damage to adjacent tissue, leading to unpredictable results and frequent complications. With the advent of laser energy as the cyclodestructive element, alternative delivery routes are possible, including transpupillary and intraocular.

Early Cyclodestructive Procedures

Penetrating Cyclodiathermy

Weve[1] introduced the concept of cyclodestructive surgery in 1933, using nonpenetrating diathermy to produce selective destruction of ciliary processes. Vogt[2,3] modified the technique by using a diathermy probe that penetrated the sclera, and this became the standard cyclodestructive procedure. The technique involves penetration of the sclera 2.5–5 mm from the corneolimbal junction with a 1.0–1.5 mm electrode, and the application of a diathermy current of 40–45 mA for 10–20 seconds.[3] This may be done with or without preparation of a conjunctival flap. One or two rows of diathermy lesions are generally placed several millimeters apart for approximately 180°. The mechanism of permanent IOP reduction is probably cell death within the ciliary body.[4] In addition, it may be that the more posteriorly placed lesions create a draining fistula in the region of the pars plana.

Early reports of experience with cyclodiathermy were encouraging.[5,6] However, subsequent study revealed a low success rate and a significant incidence of hypotony. In a review of 100 cases, 5% had lasting, useful reduction in IOP, while about the same number developed phthisis.[7] Results undoubtedly vary with the technique, and experience with a newer one-pole diathermy unit has been said to be encouraging.[8]

Other Early Cyclodestructive Procedures

Beta-Irradiation Therapy. In 1948, Haik and co-workers[9] reported the experimental application of radium over the ciliary body in rabbit eyes and in one clinical case. Although this was shown to produce a reduction in the vascular supply of the ciliary body, it also caused damage to the lens, and the technique was never adopted for clinical use.

Cycloelectrolysis. Berens and co-workers,[10] in 1949, described a technique that employs the use of low-frequency galvanic current to create a chemical reaction within the ciliary body. This leads to the formation of sodium hydroxide, which is caustic to the tissue of the ciliary body. Although this was shown in rabbit studies to produce destruction of ciliary processes,[11] the procedure did not seem to have significant advantages over penetrating cyclodiathermy and never achieved widespread clinical popularity.

CYCLOCRYOTHERAPY

The use of a freezing source as the cyclodestructive element was suggested by Bietti[12] in 1950. Cyclocryotherapy is generally considered to be somewhat more predictable and less destructive than penetrating cyclodiathermy and has gradually replaced the latter technique as the most commonly used cyclodestructive operation.

Mechanism of Action

Physical Principles of Cryosurgery.[13] The ability of a freezing source, or cryogen, to freeze tissue depends on the degree to which it removes heat, which is a function of the boiling point of the source. For example, liquid nitrogen boils at −195.6°C and is an excellent cryogen. When the freezing source is applied to a tissue, a hemispherical iceball will develop, composed of different thermogradients, or temperature zones. The temperature at any point within the iceball depends upon: (1) the distance from the cryogen, with gradually increasing temperatures at progressively greater distances resulting from a resupplying of heat by blood vessels; and (2) the rate of freezing, with a rapid freeze producing colder temperatures near the edge of the growing iceball.

Biologic Principles of Cryosurgery.[13] There are two phases of cryoinjury-induced in vivo cell death. Initially, freezing of extracellular fluid concentrates the remaining solutes, which leads to cellular dehydration and is the probable mechanism of cell death associated with a slow freeze. When the rate of cooling is rapid, intracellular ice crystals develop. Although these crystals are not always lethal to the cell, a slow thaw leads to the formation of larger crystals, which are highly destructive to the cell via an uncertain mechanism. Maximum cell death is achieved with a rapid freeze and a slow thaw. A second and later mechanism of cryoinduced cell death is a superimposed hemorrhagic infarction, which results from obliteration of the microcirculation within the frozen tissue. Ischemic necrosis is the histologic hallmark of cryoinjured tissue.

Cyclocryotherapy. Cyclocryotherapy presumably destroys the ability of ciliary processes to produce aqueous humor via the biphasic mechanism of intracellular ice crystal formation and ischemic necrosis as outlined above. Animal studies have revealed significant differences between the temperature of the cryoprobe and the temperature within the treated tissues.[14,15] In living eyes, a temperature of −60 to −80°C over the sclerolimbal area was shown to produce a temperature of approximately −10°C at the tips of the ciliary processes after a lag of 20–30 seconds.[15] The latter temperature is near the minimum thermogradient at which cryoinjury normally occurs.[15] Ciliary body blood flow in rabbits is reduced 50–60% when treated with −80°C cryoapplications for 60 seconds.[16] Histologic studies of eyes treated with cyclocryotherapy show destruction of vascular, stromal, and epithelial elements of the ciliary processes with replacement by fibrous tissue.[4,15,17,18] Ciliary epithelium has been observed to regenerate in monkeys eyes but not in those of humans.[18]

In addition to lowering the IOP, cyclocryotherapy may provide relief of pain via the destruction of corneal nerves. Wallerian degeneration of corneal nerve fibers was observed in rabbits following cyclocryotherapy, although regeneration began within 9–16 days.[19]

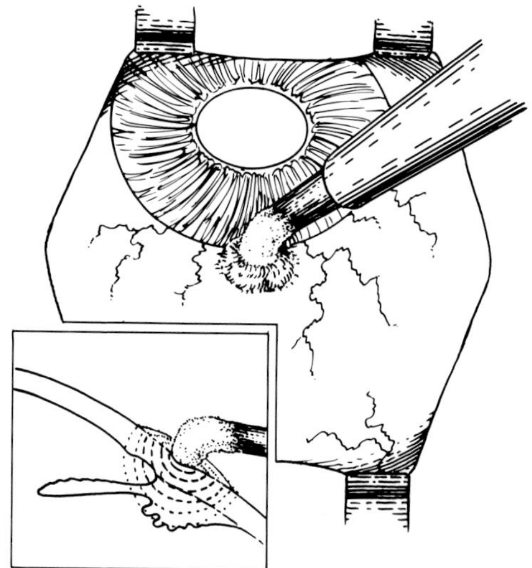

Figure 37.1. Cyclocryotherapy technique, showing placement of probe and shape of iceball (*inset*).

Techniques

Cryoinstruments. Either nitrous oxide or carbon dioxide gas cryosurgical units may be used. The diameters of the more commonly used cryoprobe tips range from 1.5 to 4 mm, and it has been suggested that 2.5 mm may be optimum for cyclocryotherapy.[20] A modified cryoprobe with a curved 3 × 6-mm tip has been developed to reduce the number of applications required.[21] An automatic timer to monitor the duration of each application has also been described.[22]

Cryoprobe Placement. With the 2.5-mm tip, placement of the anterior edge of the probe 1 mm from the corneolimbal junction temporally, inferiorly, and nasally, and 1.5 mm superiorly is believed to concentrate the maximum freezing effect over the ciliary processes (Figs. 37.1–37.3).[20] It has also been suggested that transillumination may be helpful by delineating the pars plicata,[23,24] although this is not usually necessary unless the anatomic landmarks are distorted, as with buphthalmos. The cryoprobe should be applied with firm pressure on the sclera, since this may reduce ciliary blood flow, thereby contributing to faster penetration of the iceball to the ciliary processes.[20] A device has been described that indicates the applicator contact pressure continuously during therapy, both optically and acoustically.[25]

Number of Cryoapplications. Most surgeons treat two to three quadrants, with three to four cryoapplications per quadrant. A study in cats showed that graded cyclocryotherapy of 90°, 180°, or 270° produced graded destruction of the ciliary epithelium and proportionally related changes in IOP and aqueous humor dynamics.[26] The number of cryolesions may be based to a degree on preoperative parameters, such as the type of glaucoma, the IOP level, and the number of previous cyclocryotherapy procedures. It has also been shown that younger patients generally require a larger number of cryoapplications than do older individuals to achieve satisfactory pressure reduction.[27] However, there are no precise guidelines by which an individual patient's response to therapy can be predicted, and it is best to err on the side of undertreatment rather than to run the risk of phthisis. One recommended approach is to limit each

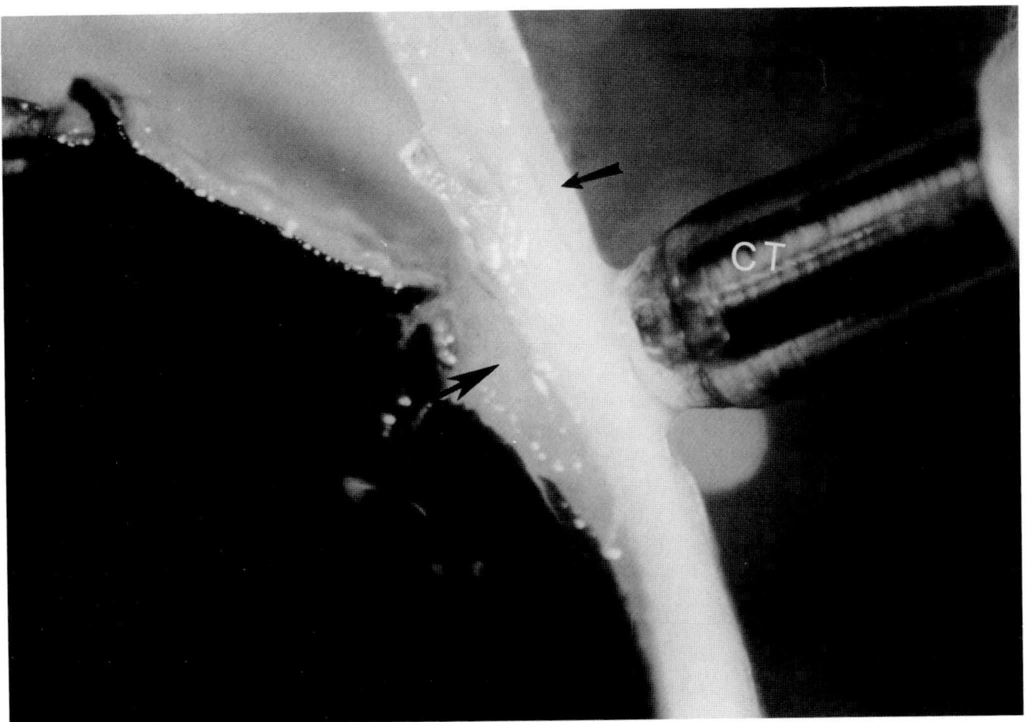

Figure 37.2. Section of human autopsy eye showing placement of cryoprobe tip (*CT*) in relation to ciliary body (*large arrow*) and anterior limbus (*small arrow*).

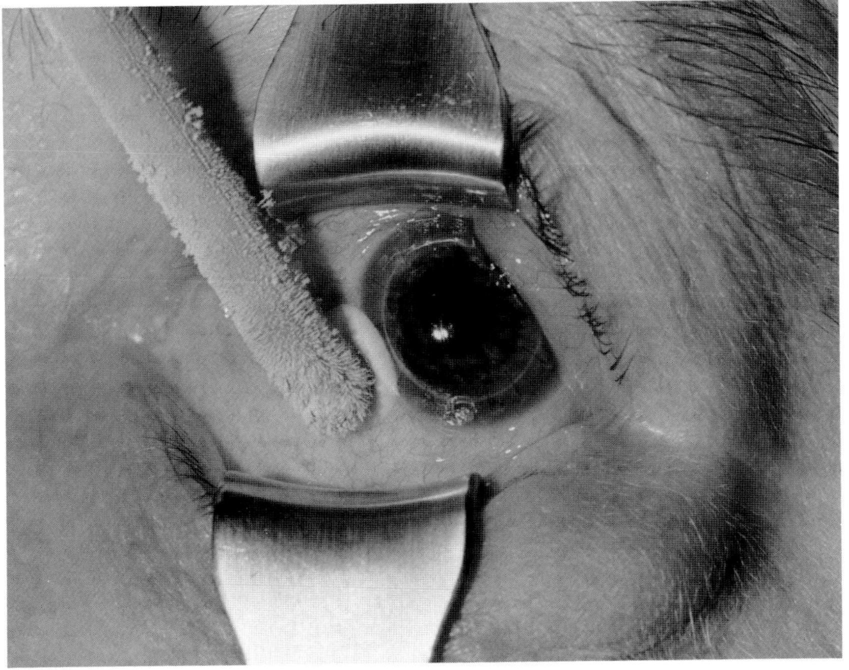

Figure 37.3. Typical appearance of iceball during cyclocryotherapy.

treatment session to six applications or fewer over 180° of the globe.[23]

Freezing Technique. Studies indicate that temperature levels warmer than −60 to −80°C or a duration of freeze less than 60 seconds does not provide adequate destruction of the ciliary process, while values much greater than these increase the risk of phthisis.[20] Therefore, most surgeons prefer −60 to −80°C applications for 60 seconds.[23,24,28] As previously noted, a rapid freeze and slow, unassisted thaw produce the maximum cell death.[13] Opinions differ as to the value of repeating the freeze in the same site. In the cryosurgical management of tumors, multiple freeze/thaw cycles have been shown to produce increasingly greater tissue destruction.[13] However, this does not necessarily imply optimum treatment, and no clear-cut advantage of the freeze-thaw-freeze technique has been shown for cyclocryotherapy. If the initial procedure does not adequately lower the IOP after approximately 1 month, cyclocryotherapy may be repeated one or more times as required. In one series of 61 eyes, 14 required two or more procedures.[28]

Postoperative Management. For approximately the first 24 hours, the patient may experience intense pain, and strong analgesics are often required. It has been noted that subconjunctival steroids at the end of the procedure also minimize the postoperative pain.[23] In addition, frequent topical corticosteroids, antibiotics, and a cycloplegic-mydriatic should be used routinely starting on the day of surgery. Since the IOP may remain elevated for a day or more after the treatment, it is advisable to keep the patient on the preoperative antiglaucoma medications, with the exception of miotics, until a pressure reduction is observed.

Complications

Transient IOP Rise. A marked rise in IOP may occur during cyclocryotherapy and in the early postoperative period. In one study, pressures of 60–80 mm Hg were recorded during the freezing phase, with return to baseline during the thawing phase.[29] The authors believed that this component of IOP elevation was due to volumetric changes, possibly related to scleral contraction, and they described a technique for controlling the complication with manometric regulation of the pressure during surgery. They also noted a second IOP rise that averaged 50 mm Hg and peaked 6 hours after the procedure. The mechanism for this component of the IOP elevation is unclear but is probably associated with the marked inflammatory response. Gonioscopic evaluation after cyclocryotherapy revealed frozen aqueous humor in the anterior chamber angle,[30] with the obvious consequences that this may have on the remaining conventional outflow system.

Uveitis. Uveitis occurs in all cases and is usually intense, with the frequent formation of a fibrin clot. One study suggests that the inflammation is prostaglandin-induced and might be minimized by pretreatment with aspirin.[31] However, a comparison of topical flurbiprofen, dexamethasone, and a placebo suggested that cyclocryotherapy-induced inflammation is hard to control with any topical medication.[32] A study in rabbits showed that an injection of heparin into the anterior chamber significantly reduced fibrin clots following cyclocryotherapy.[33] A chronic aqueous flare usually persists as a result of permanent disruption of the blood-aqueous barrier,[34] but this does not require treatment.

Pain. As previously noted, pain may be intense after cyclocryotherapy and may last for days. It is most likely a consequence of the IOP elevation and inflammation, both of which should be treated vigorously along with the use of strong analgesics.

Hyphema. This is a common complication, especially in eyes with neovascular glaucoma, and usually clears with conservative management.

Hypotony. A major disadvantage of all cyclodestructive procedures is that nothing can be done to reverse the hypotony or phthisis, if this should occur. Although this complication is less common with cyclocryotherapy than with cyclodiathermy,[28] it does occur and is best avoided by treating a limited area each time. It is far better to repeat the treatment several times than to produce phthisis by overtreatment.

Other Complications. Additional complications associated with cyclocryotherapy include choroidal detachment, which may lead to a flat anterior chamber.[35] Intravitreal neovascularization from the ciliary body, with vitreous hemorrhage, may follow cyclocryotherapy[36,37] and may regress after panretinal photocoagulation.[37] Anterior segment ischemia has been reported in eyes with neovascular glaucoma following 360° of cyclocryotherapy.[38] Proliferation of retinal glial cells and pigmented epithelial cells has been observed in rabbit eyes after cyclocryotherapy.[39] A subretinal fibrosis has been reported in one clinical case.[40] Other complications that have been reported include lens subluxation[41] and a possible case of sympathetic ophthalmia.[42] Ocular rigidity in rabbit studies was found to be low initially but then rose significantly after approximately 2 weeks, which is important to consider if indentation tonometry is being used.[43]

Indications

Cyclocryotherapy is usually reserved for situations in which other glaucoma operations have repeatedly failed or in which the surgeon wishes to avoid intraocular surgery. Two conditions in which this procedure is reported to have particular value are glaucoma after a penetrating keratoplasty[44,45] and chronic open-angle glaucoma in aphakia.[27,46] Good results were also reported in three eyes with marked buphthalmos and congenitally opaque corneas, in which limited cyclocryotherapy led to a reduction in the size of the eyes, allowing subsequent successful penetrating keratoplasty.[47] Cyclocryotherapy is believed by some surgeons to be useful in the management of neovascular glaucoma,[48,49] although others believe that the main benefit in this disease is relief of pain, since visual results are generally poor.[50–53]

TRANSSCLERAL CYCLOPHOTOCOAGULATION

Weekers and associates,[54] in 1961, employed light as the cyclodestructive element, using the transscleral application of xenon arc photocoagulation over the ciliary body. However, as with other operations that use light energy, it was the introduction of the laser that eventually led to the clinical application of cyclophotocoagulation. In 1969, Vucicevic and associates[55] reported transscleral cyclophotocoagulation in rabbits, using a *ruby laser* and a cytochemical to enhance laser absorption by the ciliary body. Other reports of transscleral laser cyclophotocoagulation followed,[56–59] and in 1984, Beckman and Waeltermann[60] reported a 10-year experience with 241 eyes treated by transscleral ruby laser cyclophotocoagulation. Their overall rate of IOP control was 62%, with 86% in eyes with glaucoma in aphakia and 53% in eyes with neovascular glaucoma. Chronic hypotony occurred in 41 eyes, with phthisis in 17 cases, although most eyes retained their preoperative level of vision. However, it was not until the availability of specially designed *neodymium:YAG* (Nd:YAG) lasers that widespread interest developed in transscleral cyclophotocoagulation.

Instruments

The Nd:YAG lasers used for transscleral cyclophotocoagulation may be operated in either a pulsed free-running, thermal mode or a continuous-wave mode and may be delivered by either a noncontact, slit-lamp system or a contact probe, fiberoptic system. The instrument that has been evaluated most extensively is the Lasag Microruptor 2, which provides slit-lamp delivery in a free-running mode of 20-millisecond (msec) pulses. It has two additional features that are needed to perform transscleral cyclophotocoagulation: (1) an adjustable offset between the focal points of the helium-neon (HeNe) aiming beam and the therapeutic beam, so the latter can be at a predetermined distance inside the eye when aiming on the conjunctiva (Fig. 37.4); and (2) high energy levels of up to 8–9 joules (J).

The other laser unit that has also been evaluated extensively is the Surgical Laser Technologies (SLT) CL60, which provides contact probe delivery in a continuous-wave mode of 0.1–10 seconds. A 2.2-mm sapphire-tipped, hand-held probe, which is focused at 1.5–2 mm in air, is coupled to a fiberoptic delivery system. The unit can provide powers in excess of 10 watts (W). (Note that energy in joules equals power in watts multiplied by duration in seconds.)

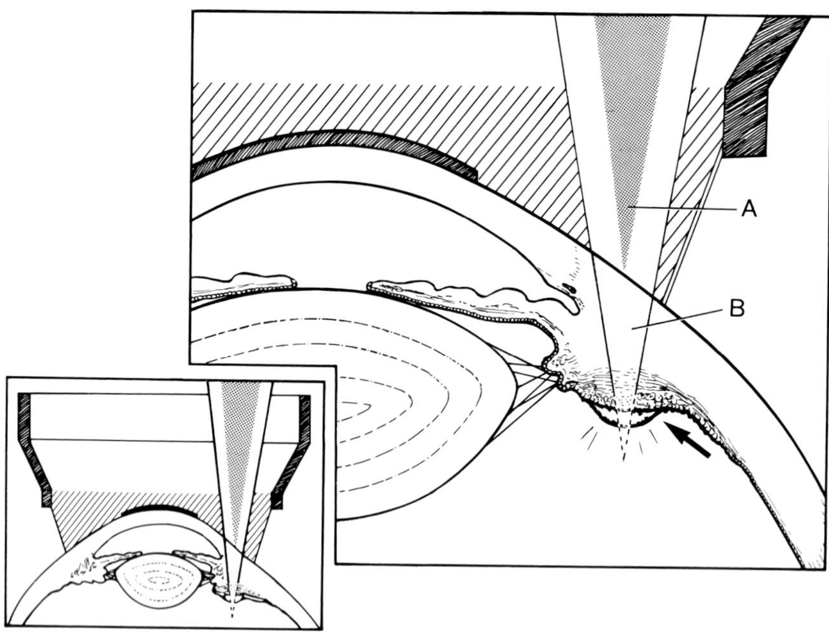

Figure 37.4. Noncontact transscleral Nd:YAG cyclophotocoagulation through a contact lens, showing HeNe aiming beam (*A*) focused on conjunctiva with therapeutic Nd:YAG beam (*B*) offset deep into ocular tissues and producing disruption of the ciliary epithelium (*arrow*).

Other lasers that have also been evaluated for transscleral cyclophotocoagulation include argon and krypton lasers[61] and a semiconductor diode laser.[62]

Theories of Mechanism

Initial rabbit studies showed that the transscleral application of Nd:YAG laser energy in the noncontact, free-running mode could damage the ciliary body and lower the IOP.[63,64] Histologic examination showed selective destruction of the ciliary epithelium.[64,65] In one study, the disrupted epithelium was elevated in a blister-like effect with sparing of ciliary muscle, sclera, and conjunctiva,[64] while another study showed damage to associated ciliary vessels in the immediate postoperative phase, followed by marked atrophy of the ciliary processes over the subsequent 4–8 weeks.[65] An incomplete regeneration of the epithelial layers and capillary network correlated with the level of sustained IOP reduction.[66] This histologic response was seen in pigmented, but not albino, rabbits,[67] and it is presumed that the laser energy is absorbed by melanin granules and converted to heat, which creates the observed response. Similar histologic changes have been described in rabbits treated with the contact, continuous-wave Nd:YAG laser, although there appears to be more of a coagulative necrosis of the epithelial layers[68] than is seen with the free-running mode. More posteriorly placed lesions over the pars plana or peripheral retina were also found to lower the IOP, which was believed to be related to the inflammatory response[69,70] or possibly to enhanced pars plana transscleral aqueous outflow.[71]

Studies of human autopsy eyes revealed structural changes of the ciliary body similar to those seen in rabbits. The gross appearance of lesions created by the noncontact, free-running Nd:YAG laser was a white elevation of the ciliary epithelium.[72] The histologic correlate was a blister-like elevation of the epithelial layers from the adjacent stroma with marked disruption primarily of the pigmented epithelium, but minimal change in the ciliary muscle and sclera in the path of the laser beam (Fig. 37.5).[73,74] In contrast, the histologic appearance of lesions created by the contact, continuous-wave Nd:YAG laser was a smaller,

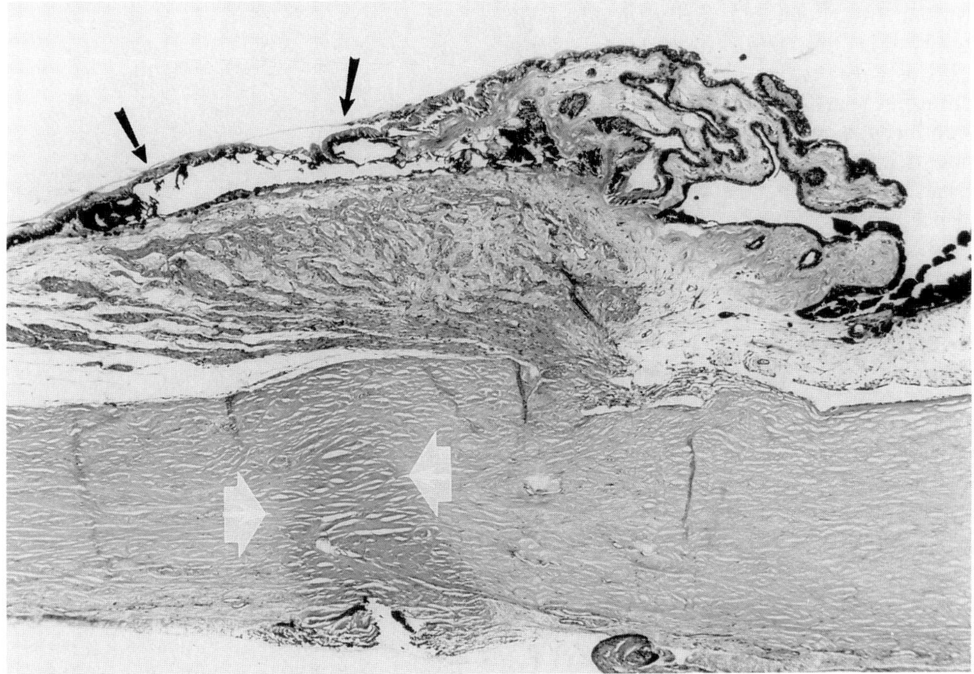

Figure 37.5. Light microscopic view of human autopsy eye treated with noncontact, free-running transscleral Nd:YAG cyclophotocoagulation showing blister-like elevation of disrupted ciliary epithelium (*black arrows*) with minimal ciliary muscle and scleral damage (*white arrows*). Defect on scleral surface was created by needle with India ink to mark center of laser track after laser application. (Reprinted from Hampton C, Shields, MB: Arch Ophthal 106:1121, 1988, with permission.)

more coagulative effect on the epithelium with less of the blister-like elevation.[74,75] One study showed a more full-thickness thermal effect, including sclera,[74] while another showed no scleral alteration.[75]

Histologic studies have also been performed on human eyes that were enucleated at some point after transscleral Nd:YAG cyclophotocoagulation. In one series of eyes treated with the noncontact, free-running Nd:YAG laser a few days before scheduled enucleation, the structural changes were the same as those seen in human autopsy eyes with the addition of fibrin and scant inflammatory cells between the disrupted epithelial layers and stroma.[76] No changes in ciliary body vasculature were observed. Histologic evaluation of another eye, which had received the same laser treatment 70 days before enucleation for hypotony and pain, revealed pigment disruption and granulomatous inflammation of the ciliary body.[77] Two eyes treated with contact, continuous-wave Nd:YAG transscleral cyclophotocoagulation 1 day before enucleation for melanomas revealed epithelial necrosis and partial capillary thrombosis of the ciliary body with slight scleral damage.[78]

These observations in animal and human eyes suggest that the most likely mechanism of IOP lowering by transscleral Nd:YAG cyclophotocoagulation is reduced aqueous production through destruction of ciliary epithelium. Alternative possibilities include ciliary vascular disruption with reduced inflow or chronic inflammation, which could influence either inflow or uveoscleral outflow.

Techniques

Pre- and Postoperative Management. Unlike most other laser procedures, the intraoperative pain associated with transscleral cyclophotocoagulation is such that retrobulbar anesthesia is usually required, although this has been omitted by some surgeons with the contact, continuous-wave technique.[78] Also unlike most other laser procedures, as well as other transscleral cyclodestructive procedures, postoperative IOP rise is not a frequent problem, and special pre- and postoperative measures, such as the use of topical apraclonidine, are usually unnecessary.

Postoperative inflammation can be a significant problem, requiring special prophylactic measures. One approach is to give a subconjunctival injection of a short-acting steroid at the end of the procedure and to prescribe topical atropine and steroid for approximately 10 days.[79] Preoperative glaucoma medications are continued, except for miotics, until IOP reduction allows discontinuation. Postoperative pain is typically mild, and a weak analgesic is usually sufficient. Intraocular pressure is usually checked a few hours after the procedure, the following day, and thereafter as required.

Laser Settings and Protocols. The histologic studies of human eyes, as previously described, have been used to establish protocols for clinical trials. However, preferred settings differ among surgeons, and the optimum protocol awaits long-term clinical experience.

Noncontact, pulsed, free-running techniques all use a pulse of 20 msec and a maximum offset between the aiming and therapeutic beams, which is 3.6 mm in air. Opinions differ regarding placement of laser lesions, but most agree that focusing on conjunctiva 1.0–1.5 mm behind the limbus is optimum for damaging the pars plicata.[72,73,76] Preferred energy levels also vary, with those reported ranging from 2 to 8 J.[79–83] With the patient at the slit lamp, and the eye fixed in the primary position, the laser beam will be slightly tangential to the scleral surface. The laser beam can be applied directly to the conjunctiva, although contact lenses have been designed for this operation. One provides the advantages of maintaining lid separation, compressing and blanching the conjunctiva, and providing measurements from the limbus (Fig. 37.6).[84] Compared with identical protocols without a contact lens, the use of the lens did not alter the histologic findings in human autopsy eyes[85] or the results in a clinical trial except for a higher incidence of phthisis.[86] Another contact lens for transscleral Nd:YAG cyclophotocoagulation with slit-lamp delivery is a glass cylinder with a truncated cone that is pressed against the conjunctiva.[87] It is likely that these lenses allow more laser energy to reach the ciliary body in the living eye by thinning and blanching the conjunctiva, as well as by reducing backscatter at the air-tissue interface, and lower laser settings may be advisable when using either lens. The total number of laser applications also varies among surgeons, with those reported ranging from 30 to 40 evenly-spaced lesions for 360°.[79–83]

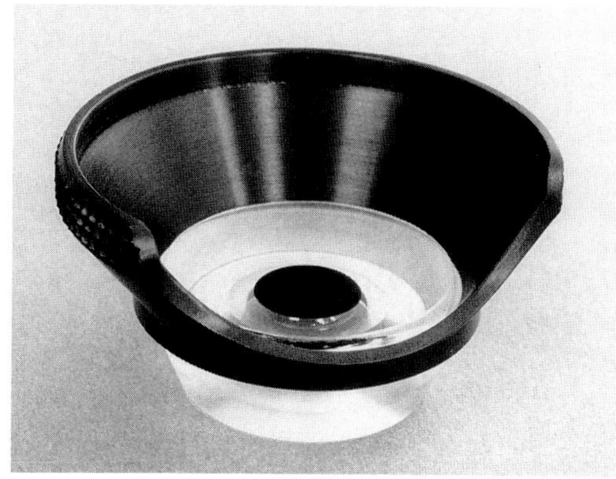

Figure 37.6. Contact lens for noncontact, free-running transscleral Nd:YAG cyclophotocoagulation. (Courtesy of Ocular Instruments, Inc., Bellevue, Wash.)

Contact, continuous-wave techniques generally use exposure times of 0.5–0.7 second. The laser focus is fixed by the design of the probe tip, which is held perpendicular to the surface of the conjunctiva with the anterior edge of the probe 0.5–1.5 mm behind the limbus. Power settings vary considerably among surgeons with a range of approximately 4–9 W (4 W at 0.5 sec provides an energy of 2 J, while 9 W at 0.7 sec delivers 6.3 J).[88,89] The reported number of applications also varies considerably from 16 for 360°[88] to 32–40 for 360° with sparing of the 3 and 9 o'clock positions.[89]

Clinical Experience

The patients in all reported clinical series, as with studies of other cyclodestructive

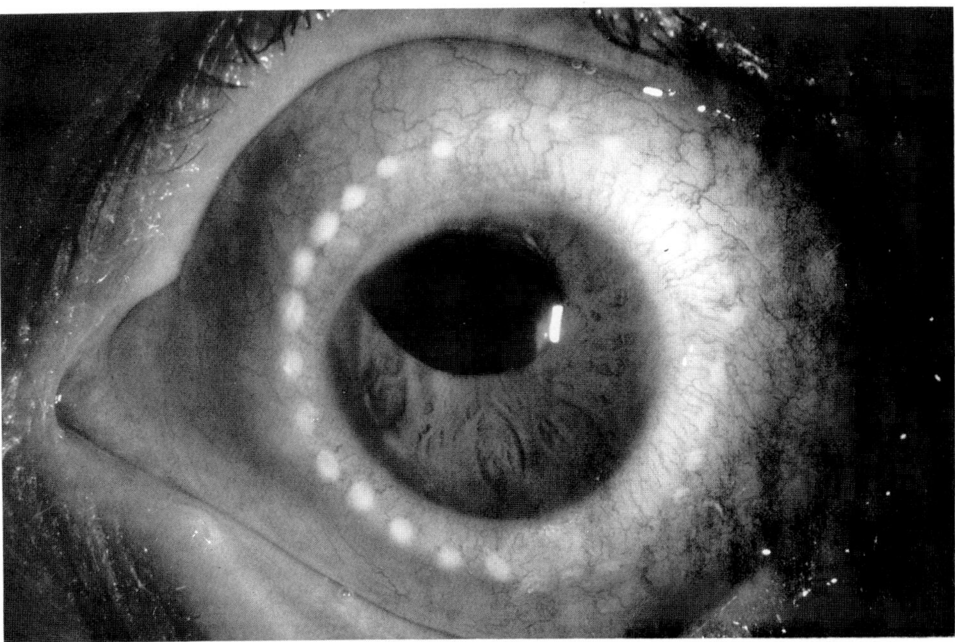

Figure 37.7. Slit-lamp view of conjunctival burns immediately after noncontact, free-running transscleral Nd:YAG cyclophotocoagulation. Note the larger lesions on the left half, in which the procedure was performed without a contact lens, as compared with the right side, in which the lens was used.

procedures, have refractory forms of glaucoma, such as glaucomas in aphakia or pseudophakia, neovascular glaucoma, glaucomas associated with inflammation, and glaucoma in eyes with multiple failed filtering procedures or following penetrating keratoplasty. With both the noncontact, free-running and the contact, continuous-wave techniques, transscleral cyclophotocoagulation provides satisfactory IOP reduction in approximately two-thirds or more of the cases following the initial treatment session, with most of the remainder coming under control with one or more retreatments.[79–83,88,89] Maximum pressure reduction is typically achieved in 1 month, and it is usually desirable to wait at least this long before retreating. The contact technique requires less total energy and appears to have a slightly better IOP success rate.[89] It also has the advantage of allowing treatment in a supine position, so that it can be performed under general anesthesia, if necessary.

In the immediate postoperative period, laser application sites are seen as white conjunctival burns, which can be minimized in the noncontact technique by use of the lens (Fig. 37.7).[86] These burns and the associated mild conjunctival hyperemia resolve in a few days. Significant advantages of transscleral cyclophotocoagulation over cyclocryotherapy include less transient IOP rise, less inflammation, and less pain, postoperatively.[79,89] However, reduced visual acuity remains a significant problem with the noncontact technique,[79] which may be another advantage of the contact, continuous-wave transscleral cyclophotocoagulation.[89] The reduced vision may be associated with postoperative inflammation, which is still marked in some eyes, with hypopyon and fibrin clots. Other reported complications have included hypotony with choroidal detachments and a flat anterior chamber,[90] hyphema, vitreous hemorrhages, cataracts, and possible sympathetic ophthalmia.[91,92]

Other Routes of Cyclophotocoagulation

Transpupillary Cyclophotocoagulation

Lee and Pomerantzeff,[93] in 1971, introduced the concept of argon laser cyclopho-

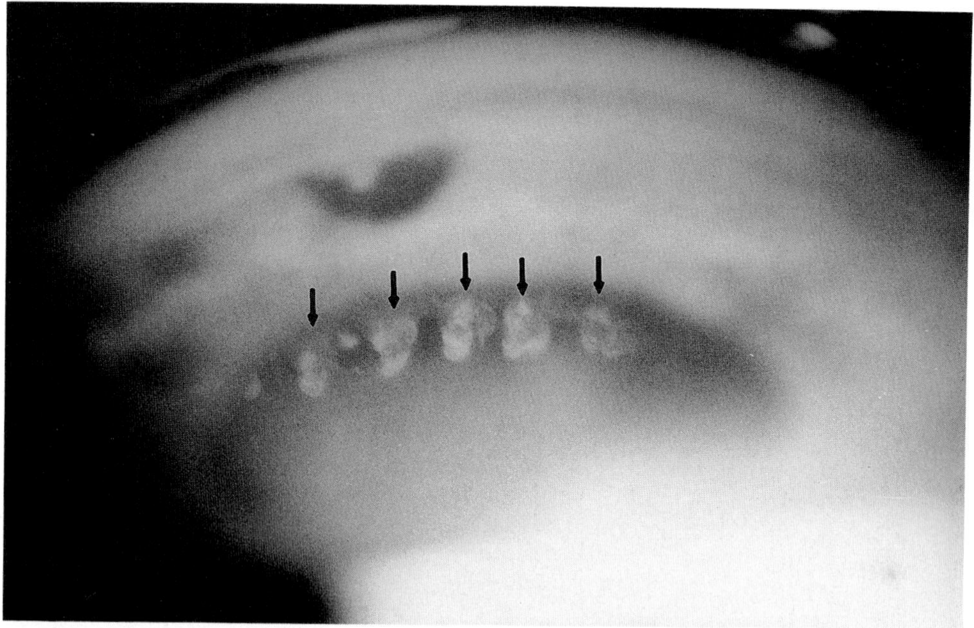

Figure 37.8. Gonioscopic view of ciliary processes (*arrows*) during transpupillary cyclophotocoagulation. Exposure of processes in this eye is due to retraction of iris by fibrovascular membrane of neovascular glaucoma.

tocoagulation via a transpupillary approach. Histopathologic studies in rabbit[93] and human[94] eyes confirmed the ability of direct laser application to selectively destroy ciliary processes.

Transpupillary cyclophotocoagulation is limited to those eyes in which a sufficient number of ciliary processes can be visualized gonioscopically. This is not possible in most eyes, especially those in which long-term miotic therapy prevents wide dilation. However, situations such as a large iridectomy or retraction of the iris, as in advanced neovascular glaucoma, may provide adequate visualization of ciliary processes (Fig. 37.8). Special contact lenses with scleral depressors have been developed to rotate the processes into better view. Typical argon laser settings are 0.1–0.2 seconds, 100–200 microns, and an energy level that is sufficient to produce white discoloration as well as a brown concave burn, often with pigment dispersion and/or gas bubbles (usually 700–1000 milliwatts). All visible portions of the ciliary process should be treated, which typically requires 3–5 applications per process. All visible processes should be treated up to a total of 180°. Additional processes can be treated at subsequent sessions if required.

The reported results with transpupillary cyclophotocoagulation have been variable.[95–100] Those cases in which the procedure fails may be due, in part, to the number of ciliary processes that can be visualized and treated[97] and to the intensity of the laser burns to each process,[95] although the number of treated processes and the intensity of treatment do not always correlate with the extent of the IOP reduction.[100] Another factor that may contribute to failure of transpupillary cyclophotocoagulation is the angle at which the processes are visualized gonioscopically. Even with scleral indentation, only the anterior tips of the ciliary ridges are usually exposed, preventing destruction of the entire ciliary process (Fig. 37.9).[100]

Intraocular Cyclophotocoagulation

An alternative to transscleral and transpupillary cyclophotocoagulation in eyes with glaucoma in aphakia is intraocular cyclophotocoagulation, using an endopho-

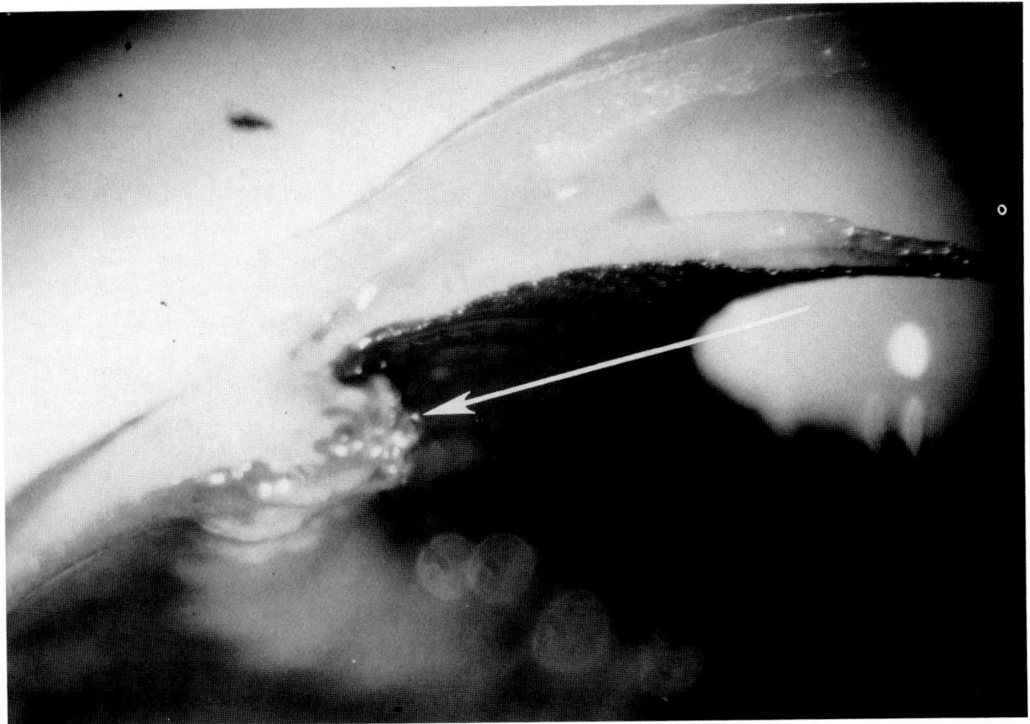

Figure 37.9. Section of human autopsy eye showing angle of ciliary process visualization during transpupillary cyclophotocoagulation (*arrow*), which provides view of only the anterior tip of the process. (Reprinted from Shields MB: Trans Am Ophthal Soc 83:285, 1985, with permission.)

tocoagulator through a pars plana incision. Visualization with this technique can usually be accomplished via the transpupillary route, although endoscopic visualization has also been evaluated.

Intraocular Cyclophotocoagulation with Transpupillary Visualization. Vitreoretinal surgeons have reported the use of argon laser endophotocoagulators via a pars plana incision for the treatment of retinal disorders under transpupillary visualization.[101–103] During the course of a vitrectomy in an aphakic eye, it is possible to lower the IOP and use scleral indentation to bring the ciliary processes into transpupillary view for the purpose of cyclophotocoagulation with the intraocular laser probe.[104–106]

After performing the vitrectomy, the vitreous instrument is removed and the endophotocoagulator is inserted through the same cannula. Scleral indentation in the opposite quadrants is then used to bring several ciliary processes into view, and the tip of the laser probe is positioned 2–3 mm from the processes (Fig. 37.10). With an exposure time of 0.1–0.2 seconds, laser therapy is applied to individual ciliary processes, using an energy level that is sufficient to produce a white reaction and a shallow tissue disruption (usually 1000 milliwatts). Three to five laser exposures are then applied to each process in the two quadrants opposite the entry site.

In one large series, three-fourths of the eyes had an IOP of 21 mm Hg or less with or without medications after one or two treatments, with an average follow-up of 13 months.[106] The primary value of this procedure is as an adjunct to pars plana vitrectomy in eyes with refractory glaucoma.

Intraocular Cyclophotocoagulation with Endoscopic Visualization. An ocular endoscope was modified for intraocular cyclophotocoagulation by attaching a laser fiberoptic, connected to a continuous-wave

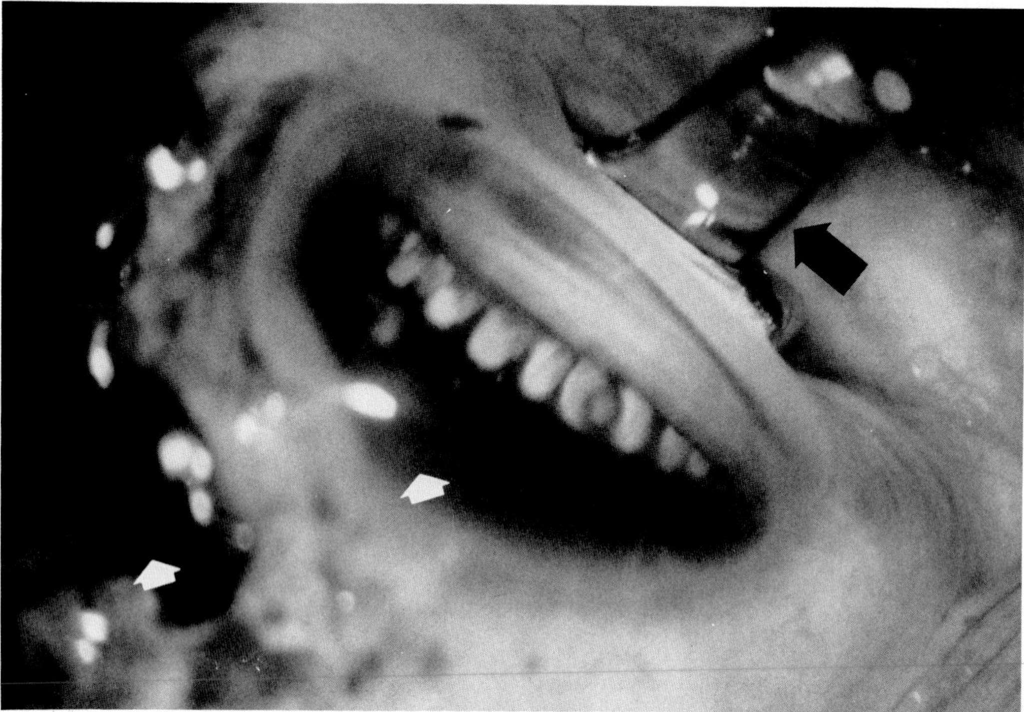

Figure 37.10. Intraocular cyclophotocoagulation with transpupillary visualization. Ciliary processes are brought into view with scleral depressor (*black arrow*) and treated with laser endophotocoagulator (*white arrows*) via a pars plana incision. (Reprinted from Shields MB: Trans Am Ophthal Soc 83:285, 1985, with permission.)

argon laser, to the tip of the instrument.[104,107,108] This allows direct visualization of ciliary processes via the pars plana incision with simultaneous application of the laser energy.

In a study with monkeys treated with a lensectomy, anterior vitrectomy, and endoscopic cyclophotocoagulation, histopathologic evaluation of the treated ciliary processes revealed variable degrees of epithelial layer destruction and late fibrosis of the ciliary processes.[107] A preliminary clinical trial demonstrated the ability of this technique to reduce IOP via selective photodestruction of ciliary processes.[108] However, the invasive nature and relative risks of the procedure make it less promising than transscleral cyclophotocoagulation.

Therapeutic Ultrasound

In 1964, Purnell and associates[109] introduced the concept of using focused transscleral ultrasonic radiation to produce localized destruction of the ciliary body in rabbit eyes. Coleman and co-workers, in 1985, reported the results of rabbit studies[110] and preliminary clinical trials[111] with high-intensity focused ultrasound.

The basic technique involves delivering an average of 6–7 exposures of ultrasound at an intensity level of 10 kW/cm^2 for 5 seconds each to scleral sites near the limbus.[111,112] The authors postulated that, in addition to reducing aqueous inflow via destruction of ciliary epithelium, this procedure may improve aqueous outflow via selective thinning of scleral collagen and via separation of the ciliary body from the sclera. The histologic evaluation of a human eye enucleated 8 months after therapeutic ultrasound revealed localized destruction of the ciliary epithelial layers, profound atrophy of the ciliary muscle, and loss of scleral collagen.[113] Several large clinical trials of therapeutic ultrasound in patients with refractory glaucomas, similar to those described in studies of other cyclodestructive procedures, revealed IOP reduction to the low 20s or less in one-half to two-thirds of the cases 6–12 months after a single treatment.[112,114,115] Reported complications of hypotony, phthisis, and reduced vision were low.

Other Cyclodestructive Procedures

Transscleral Microwave Cyclodestruction

The direct application of high-frequency electromagnetic radiation over the conjunctiva in rabbits produced heat-induced damage to the ciliary body with relative sparing of the conjunctiva and sclera.[116]

Excision of the Ciliary Body

In addition to the use of many cyclodestructive elements, as described above, other surgeons have sought to reduce aqueous production by removing a portion of the ciliary body. Several studies have revealed reasonable success and complication rates with this basic approach in eyes with unusually refractory glaucomas.[117–119]

SUMMARY

Cyclodestructive operations lower the IOP by partly eliminating the function of the ciliary processes, thereby reducing aqueous production. Destructive sources for the more commonly used procedures have included diathermy, cryogens, laser, and ultrasound. Each of these elements is delivered via the transscleral route, which provides a simple, quick, noninvasive technique but is associated with unpredictable results and a high rate of complications. With laser energy as the cyclodestructive source, alternative delivery routes include transpupillary and intraocular.

References

1. Weve, H: Die Zyklodiatermie das Corpus ciliare bei Glaukom. Zentralbl Ophthalmol 29:562, 1933.
2. Vogt, A: Versuche zur intraokularen Druckherabsetzung mittels Diatermieschadigung des Corpus ciliare (Zyklodiatermiestichelung). Klin Monatsbl Augenheilkd 97:672, 1936.
3. Vogt, A: Cyclodiathermypuncture in cases of glaucoma. Br J Ophthal 24:288, 1940.
4. Edmonds, C, de Roetth, A Jr, Howard, GM: Histopathologic changes following cryosurgery and diathermy of the rabbit ciliary body. Am J Ophthal 69:65, 1970.
5. Albaugh, CH, Dunphy, EB: Cyclodiathermy. Arch Ophthal 27:543, 1942.
6. Stocker, FW: Response of chronic simple glaucoma to treatment with cyclodiathermy puncture. Arch Ophthal 34:181, 1945.
7. Walton, DS, Grant, WM: Penetrating cyclodiathermy for filtration. Arch Ophthal 83:47, 1970.
8. Nesterov, AP, Egorov, EA: Transconjunctival penetrating cyclodiathermy in glaucoma. J Ocul Ther Surg July-Aug:216, 1983.
9. Haik, GM, Breffeilh, LA, Barber, A: Beta irradiation as a possible therapeutic agent in glaucoma. Am J Ophthal 31:945, 1948.
10. Berens, C, Sheppard, LB, Duel, AB Jr: Cycloelectrolysis for glaucoma. Trans Am Ophthal Soc 47:364, 1949.
11. Sheppard, LB: Retrociliary cyclodiathermy versus retrociliary cycloelectrolysis. Effects on the normal rabbit eye. Am J Ophthal 46:27, 1958.
12. Bietti, G: Surgical intervention on the ciliary body. New trends for the relief of glaucoma. JAMA 142:889, 1950.
13. Wilkes, TDI, Fraunfelder, FT: Principles of cryosurgery. Ophthal Surg 10:21, 1979.
14. de Roetth, A Jr: Ciliary body temperatures in cryosurgery. Arch Ophthal 85:204, 1971.
15. Quigley, HA: Histological and physiological studies of cyclocryotherapy in primate and human eyes. Am J Ophthal 82:722, 1976.
16. Green, K, Hull, DS, Bowman, K: Cyclocryotherapy and ocular blood flow. Glaucoma 1:141, 1979.
17. Ferry, AP: Histopathologic observations on human eyes following cyclocryotherapy for glaucoma. Trans Am Acad Ophthal Otol 83:90, 1977.
18. Smith, RS, Boyle, E, Rudt, LA: Cyclocryotherapy. A light and electron microscopic study. Arch Ophthal 95:284, 1977.
19. Wener, RG, Pinkerton, RMH, Robertson, DM: Cryosurgical induced changes in corneal nerves. Can J Ophthal 8:548, 1973.
20. Prost, M: Cyclocryotherapy for glaucoma. Evaluation of techniques. Surv Ophthal 28:93, 1983.
21. Machemer, R: Modified cryoprobe for retinal detachment surgery and cyclocryotherapy. Am J Ophthal 83:123, 1977.
22. Machemer, R, Lashley, R: Automatic timer for cryotherapy. Am J Ophthal 83:125, 1977.
23. Bellows, AR: Cyclocryotherapy: its role in the treatment of glaucoma. Pers Ophthal 4:139, 1980.
24. Wesley, RE, Kielar, RA: Cyclocryotherapy in treatment of glaucoma. Glaucoma 3:533, 1980.
25. Matthes, R, Koza, K-D, Heber, G, Matthaus, W:

A new device for glaucoma cryotherapy. Klin Monatsbl Augenheilkd 195:100, 1989.
26. Higginbotham, EJ, Lee, DA, Bartels, SP, et al: Effects of cyclocryotherapy on aqueous humor dynamics in cats. Arch Ophthal 106:396, 1988.
27. Brindley, G, Shields, MB: Value and limitations of cyclocryotherapy. Graefe's Arch Ophthal 224:545, 1986.
28. Bellows, AR, Grant, WM: Cyclocryotherapy in advanced inadequately controlled glaucoma. Am J Ophthal 75:679, 1973.
29. Caprioli, J, Sears, M: Regulation of intraocular pressure during cyclocryotherapy for advanced glaucoma. Am J Ophthal 101:542, 1986.
30. Strasser, G, Haddad, R: Gonioscopic changes after cyclocryocoagulation. Klin Monatsbl Augenheilkd 187:343, 1985.
31. Chavis, RM, Vygantas, CM, Vygantas, A: Experimental inhibition of prostaglandin-like inflammatory response after cryotherapy. Am J Ophthal 82:310, 1976.
32. Hurvitz, LM, Spaeth, GL, Zakhour, I, et al: A comparison of the effect of flurbiprofen, dexamethasone, and placebo on cyclocryotherapy-induced inflammation. Ophthal Surg 15:394, 1984.
33. Johnson, RN, Balyeat, E, Stern, WH: Heparin prophylaxis for intraocular fibrin. Ophthalmology 94:597, 1987.
34. Haddad, R: Cyclocryotherapy: experimental studies of the breakdown of the blood-aqueous barrier and analysis of a long term follow-up study. Wien Klin Wochenschr (suppl 126) 93:3, 1981.
35. Kaiden, JS, Serniuk, RA, Bader, BF: Choroidal detachment with flat anterior chamber after cyclocryotherapy. Ann Ophthal 11:1111, 1979.
36. Goldberg, MF, Ericson, ES: Intravitreal ciliary body neovascularization. Ophthal Surg 8:62, 1977.
37. Gieser, RG, Gieser, DK: Treatment of intravitreal ciliary body neovascularization. Ophthal Surg 15:508, 1984.
38. Krupin, T, Johnson, MF, Becker, B: Anterior segment ischemia after cyclocryotherapy. Am J Ophthal 84:426, 1977.
39. Yamishita, H, Sears, ML: Complications of cyclocryosurgery. Glaucoma 2:273, 1980.
40. Kao, SF, Morgan, CM, Bergstrom, TJ: Subretinal fibrosis following cyclocryotherapy. Arch Ophthal 105:1175, 1987.
41. Pearson, PA, Baldwin, LB, Smith, TJ: Lens subluxation as a complication of cyclocryotherapy. Ophthal Surg 20:445, 1989.
42. Sabates, R: Choroiditis compatible with the histopathologic diagnosis of sympathetic ophthalmia following cyclocryotherapy of neovascular glaucoma. Ophthal Surg 19:176, 1988.
43. Paterson, CA, Paterson, EF, Briggs, SA: Experimental cryosurgery. Effect upon ocular rigidity and intraocular pressure. Arch Ophthal 86:425, 1971.
44. West, CE, Wood, TO, Kaufman, HE: Cyclocryotherapy for glaucoma pre- or postpenetrating keratoplasty. Am J Ophthal 76:485, 1973.
45. Binder, PS, Abel, R Jr, Kaufman, HE: Cyclocryotherapy for glaucoma after penetrating keratoplasty. Am J Ophthal 79:489, 1975.
46. Bellows, AR, Grant, WM: Cyclocryotherapy of chronic open-angle glaucoma in aphakic eyes. Am J Ophthal 85:615, 1978.
47. Frucht-Pery, J, Feldman, ST, Brown, SI: Transplantation of congenitally opaque corneas from eyes with exaggerated buphthalmos. Am J Ophthal 107:655, 1989.
48. Feibel, RM, Bigger, JF: Rubeosis iridis and neovascular glaucoma. Evaluation of cyclocryotherapy. Am J Ophthal 74:862, 1972.
49. Klein, J, Kuechle, HJ: Cryotherapy of the ciliary body in cases of secondary glaucoma with poor prognosis. Klin Monatsbl Augenheilkd 179:470, 1981.
50. Faulborn, J, Birnbaum, F: Cyclocryotherapy of haemorrhagic glaucoma: clinical long time and histopathologic results. Klin Monatsbl Augenheilkd 170:651, 1977.
51. Krupin, T, Mitchell, KB, Becker, B: Cyclocryotherapy in neovascular glaucoma. Am J Ophthal 86:24, 1978.
52. Caprioli, J, Strang, SL, Spaeth, GL, Poryzees, EH: Cyclocryotherapy in the treatment of advanced glaucoma. Ophthalmology 92:947, 1985.
53. Benson, MT, Nelson, ME: Cyclocryotherapy: a review of cases over a 10-year period. Br J Ophthal 74:103, 1990.
54. Weekers, R, Lavergne, G, Watillon, M, et al: Effects of photocoagulation of ciliary body upon ocular tension. Am J Ophthal 52:156, 1961.
55. Vucicevic, ZM, Tsou, KC, Nazarian, IH, et al: A cytochemical approach to the laser coagulation of the ciliary body. Mod Probl Ophthal 8:467, 1969.
56. Smith, RS, Stein, MN: Ocular hazards of transscleral laser radiation: II. Intraocular injury produced by ruby and neodymium lasers. Am J Ophthal 67:100, 1969.
57. Vucicevic, ZM, Tsou, KC, Nazarian, IH, et al: A cytochemical approach to the laser coagulation of the ciliary body. Bibl Ophthal 79:467, 1969.
58. Beckman, H, Kinoshita, A, Rota, AN, Sugar, HS: Transscleral ruby laser irradiation of the ciliary body in the treatment of intractable glaucoma. Trans Am Acad Ophthal Otol 76:423, 1972.
59. Beckman, H, Sugar, HS: Neodymium laser cyclocoagulation. Arch Ophthal 90:27, 1973.
60. Beckman, H, Waeltermann, J: Transscleral ruby laser cyclocoagulation. Am J Ophthal 98:788, 1984.
61. Peyman, GA, Conway, MD, Raichand, M, Lin,

J: Histopathologic studies on transscleral argon-krypton photocoagulation with an exolaser probe. Ophthal Surg 15:496, 1984.
62. Schuman, JS, Jacobson, JJ, Puliafito, CA, et al: Experimental use of semiconductor diode laser in contact transscleral cyclophotocoagulation in rabbits. Arch Ophthal 108:1152, 1990.
63. Wilensky, JT, Welch, D, Mirolovich, M: Transscleral cyclocoagulation using a neodymium:YAG laser. Ophthal Surg 16:95, 1985.
64. Devenyi, RG, Trope, GE, Hunter, WH: Neodymium-YAG transscleral cyclocoagulation in rabbit eyes. Br J Ophthal 71:441, 1987.
65. England, C, van der Zypen, E, Fankhauser, F, Kwasniewska, S: Ultrastructure of the rabbit ciliary body following transscleral cyclophotocoagulation with the free-running Nd:YAG laser: preliminary findings. Lasers Ophthal 1:61, 1986.
66. van der Zypen, E, England, C, Fankhauser, F, Kwasniewska, S: The effect of transscleral laser cyclophotocoagulation on rabbit ciliary body vascularization. Graefe's Arch Ophthal 227:172, 1989.
67. Cantor, LB, Nichols, DA, Katz, LJ, et al: Neodymium-YAG transscleral cyclophotocoagulation. The role of pigmentation. Invest Ophthal Vis Sci 30:1834, 1989.
68. Brancator, R, Leoni, G, Trabucchi, G, Trabucchi, E: Transscleral contact cyclophotocoagulation with Nd:YAG laser CW: experimental study on rabbit eyes. Int J Tiss Reac 9:493, 1987.
69. Schubert, HD, Federman, JL: The role of inflammation on CW Nd:YAG contact transscleral photocoagulation and cryopexy. Invest Ophthal Vis Sci 30:543, 1989.
70. Schubert, HD, Federman, JL: A comparison of CW Nd:YAG contact transscleral cyclophotocoagulation with cyclocryopexy. Invest Ophthal Vis Sci 30:536, 1989.
71. Schubert, HD, Agarwala, A, Arbizo, V: Changes in aqueous outflow after in vitro neodymium:yttrium aluminum garnet laser cyclophotocoagulation. Invest Ophthal Vis Sci 31:1834, 1990.
72. Fankhauser, F, van der Zypen, E, Kwasniewska, S, et al: Transscleral cyclophotocoagulation using a neodymium YAG laser. Ophthal Surg 17:94, 1986.
73. Hampton, C, Shields, MB: Transscleral neodymium-YAG cyclophotocoagulation. A histologic study of human autopsy eyes. Arch Ophthal 106:1121, 1988.
74. Schubert, HD: Noncontact and contact pars plana transscleral neodymium:YAG laser cyclophotocoagulation in postmortem eyes. Ophthalmology 96:1471, 1989.
75. Allingham, RR, de Kater, AW, Bellows, AR, Hsu, J: Probe placement and power levels in contact transscleral neodymium:YAG cyclophotocoagulation. Arch Ophthal 108:738, 1990.
76. Blasini, M, Simmons, R, Shields, MB: Early tissue response to transscleral neodymium:YAG cyclophotocoagulation. Invest Ophthal Vis Sci 31:1114, 1990.
77. Shields, SM, Stevens, JL, Kass, MA, Smith, ME: Histopathologic findings after Nd:YAG transscleral cyclophotocoagulation. Am J Ophthal 106:100, 1988.
78. Brancato, R, Leoni, G, Trabucchi, G, Cappellini, A: Probe placement and energy levels in continuous wave neodymium-YAG contact transscleral cyclophotocoagulation. Arch Ophthal 108:679, 1990.
79. Hampton, C, Shields, MB, Miller, KN, Blasini, M: Evaluation of a protocol for transscleral neodymium:YAG cyclophotocoagulation in one hundred patients. Ophthalmology 97:910, 1990.
80. Devenyi, RG, Trope, GE, Hunter, WH, Badeeb, O: Neodymium:YAG transscleral cyclocoagulation in human eyes. Ophthalmology 94:1519, 1987.
81. Badeeb, O, Trope, GE, Mortimer, C: Short-term effects of neodymium-YAG transscleral cyclocoagulation in patients with uncontrolled glaucoma. Br J Ophthal 72:615, 1988.
82. Klapper, RM, Wandel, T, Donnenfeld, E, Perry, HD: Transscleral neodymium:YAG thermal cyclophotocoagulation in refractory glaucoma. A preliminary report. Ophthalmology 95:719, 1988.
83. Trope, GE, Ma, S: Mid-term effects of neodymium:YAG transscleral cyclocoagulation in glaucoma. Ophthalmology 97:73, 1990.
84. Shields, MB, Blasini, M, Simmons, R, Erickson, PJ: A contact lens for transscleral Nd:YAG cyclophotocoagulation. Am J Ophthal 108:457, 1989.
85. Simmons, RB, Blasini, M, Shields, MB, Erickson, PJ: Comparison of transscleral neodymium:YAG cyclophotocoagulation with and without a contact lens in human autopsy eyes. Am J Ophthal 109:174, 1990.
86. Simmons, RB, Shields, MB, Blasini, M, Wilkerson, M: Transscleral neodymium:YAG cyclophotocoagulation with a contact lens. A clinical trial. Am J Ophthal (submitted).
87. Dürr, U, Henchoz, P-D, Fankhauser, F, et al: Results and methods of transscleral laser cyclodestruction: a new contact lens for use with noncontact systems. Lasers Light Ophthal 3:123, 1990.
88. Brancato, R, Giovanni, L, Trabucchi, G, Pietroni, C: Contact transscleral cyclophotocoagulation with Nd:YAG laser in uncontrolled glaucoma. Ophthal Surg 20:547, 1989.
89. Schuman, JS, Puliafito, CA, Allingham, RR, et al: Contact transscleral continuous wave neodymium:YAG laser cyclophotocoagulation. Ophthalmology 97:571, 1990.
90. Maus, M, Katz, LJ: Choroidal detachment, flat

anterior chamber, and hypotony as complications of neodymium:YAG laser cyclophotocoagulation. Ophthalmology 97:69, 1990.
91. Edward, DP, Brown, SVL, Higginbotham, E, et al: Sympathetic ophthalmia following neodymium:YAG cyclotherapy. Ophthal Surg 20:544, 1989.
92. Brown, SVL, Higginbotham, E, Tessler, H: Sympathetic ophthalmia following Nd:YAG cyclotherapy. Ophthal Surg 21:736, 1990.
93. Lee, P-F, Pomerantzeff, O: Transpupillary cyclophotocoagulation of rabbit eyes. An experimental approach to glaucoma surgery. Am J Ophthal 71:911, 1971.
94. Bartl, G, Haller, BM, Wocheslander, E, Hofmann, H: Light and electron microscopic observations after argon laser photocoagulation of ciliary processes. Klin Monatsbl Augenheilkd 181:414, 1982.
95. Lee, P-F: Argon laser photocoagulation of the ciliary processes in cases of aphakic glaucoma. Arch Ophthal 97:2135, 1979.
96. Bernard, JA, Haut, J, Demailly, PH, et al: Coagulation of the ciliary processes with the argon laser. Its use in certain types of hypertonia. Arch Ophthal (Paris) 34:577, 1974.
97. Merritt, JC: Transpupillary photocoagulation of the ciliary processes. Ann Ophthal 8:325, 1976.
98. Lee, P-F, Shihab, Z, Eberle, M: Partial ciliary process laser photocoagulation in the management of glaucoma. Lasers Surg Med 1:85, 1980.
99. Klapper, RM, Dodick, JM: Transpupillary argon laser cyclophotocoagulation. Doc Ophthal Proc 36:197, 1984.
100. Shields, S, Stewart, WC, Shields, MB: Transpupillary argon laser cyclophotocoagulation in the treatment of glaucoma. Ophthal Surg 19:171, 1988.
101. Fleishman, JA, Schwartz, M, Dixon, JA: Argon laser endophotocoagulation. An intraoperative trans-pars plana technique. Arch Ophthal 99:1610, 1981.
102. Peyman, GA, Salzano, TC, Green, JL: Argon endolaser. Arch Ophthal 99:2037, 1981.
103. Landers, MB, Trese, MT, Stefánsson, E, Bessler, M: Argon laser intraocular photocoagulation. Ophthalmology 89:785, 1982.
104. Shields, MB: Cyclodestructive surgery for glaucoma: past, present and future. Trans Am Ophthal Soc 83:285, 1985.
105. Patel, A, Thompson, JT, Michels, RG, Quigley, HA: Endolaser treatment of the ciliary body for uncontrolled glaucoma. Ophthalmology 93:825, 1986.
106. Zarbin, MA, Michels, RG, de Bustros, S, et al: Endolaser treatment of the ciliary body for severe glaucoma. Ophthalmology 95:1639, 1988.
107. Shields, MB, Chandler, DB, Hickingbotham, D, Klintworth, GK: Intraocular cyclophotocoagulation. Histopathologic evaluation in primates. Arch Ophthal 103:1731, 1985.
108. Shields, MB: Intraocular cyclophotocoagulation. Trans Ophthal Soc UK 105:237, 1986.
109. Purnell, EW, Sokollu, A, Torchia, R, Taner, N: Focal chorioretinitis produced by ultrasound. Invest Ophthal 3:657, 1964.
110. Coleman, DJ, Lizzi, FL, Driller, J, et al: Therapeutic ultrasound in the treatment of glaucoma. I. Experimental model. Ophthalmology 92:339, 1985.
111. Coleman, DJ, Lizzi, FL, Driller, J, et al: Therapeutic ultrasound in the treatment of glaucoma. II. Clinical applications. Ophthalmology 92:347, 1985.
112. Burgess, SEP, Silverman, RH, Coleman, DJ, et al: Treatment of glaucoma with high-intensity focused ultrasound. Ophthalmology 93:831, 1986.
113. Margo, CE: Therapeutic ultrasound. Light and electron microscopic findings in an eye treated for glaucoma. Arch Ophthal 104:735, 1986.
114. Maskin, SL, Mandell, AI, Smith, JA, et al: Therapeutic ultrasound for refractory glaucoma: a three-center study. Ophthal Surg 20:186, 1989.
115. Valtot, F, Kopel, J, Haut, J: Treatment of glaucoma with high intensity focused ultrasound. Internat Ophthal 13:167, 1989.
116. Finger, PT, Smith, PD, Paglione, RW, Perry, HD: Transscleral microwave cyclodestruction. Invest Ophthal Vis Sci 31:2151, 1990.
117. Freyler, H, Scheimbauer, I: Excision of the ciliary body (Sautter procedure) as a last resort in secondary glaucoma. Klin Monatsbl Augenheilkd 179:473, 1981.
118. Demeler, U: Ciliary surgery for glaucoma. Trans Ophthal Soc UK 105:242, 1986.
119. Welge-Lussen, L, Stadler, G: Results with a modified ciliary body excision to reduce intraocular pressure. Klin Monatsbl Augenheilkd 189:199, 1986.

Chapter 38

SURGICAL APPROACHES FOR COEXISTING GLAUCOMA AND CATARACT

In the management of a patient with a cataract for which extraction is indicated, and coexisting glaucoma, there are three basic surgical approaches: (1) cataract extraction alone; (2) glaucoma filtering surgery alone, followed by cataract removal at a later date; and (3) combined cataract and glaucoma surgery as a single procedure. Combined procedures have a slightly greater risk of complications than does cataract surgery alone, as well as a lower chance of long-term glaucoma control than with a filtering operation alone. For these reasons, the surgeon should consider each of the basic surgical options and select the approach that seems to be most appropriate for each individual patient. We will first consider relative indications for the three basic approaches and then some of the surgical techniques.

INDICATIONS

Predicting Visual Potential

In each case, it is assumed that a cataract is present for which extraction is indicated, independent of the glaucoma. This is often difficult to determine in an eye with both a cataract and glaucoma, in which it is hard to know how much the glaucoma is contributing to the reduced vision. Several instruments have been developed to help predict the anticipated postoperative visual acuity. One focuses a miniaturized Snellen visual acuity chart on the retina (Potential Acuity Meter, or PAM) while others project stripe patterns from either a laser or white light (Visometer) source. In one study, the Visometer gave more accurate predictions than did the PAM in cataract patients with open-angle glaucoma, even with glaucomatous field loss.[1] In another study, the PAM was accurate if the glaucomatous damage was mild to moderate and the predicted visual acuity was better than 20/60, whereas the results with advanced visual field loss or a predicted reading worse than 20/60 were not reliable.[2]

When it is decided that cataract surgery is needed, the selection of the specific surgical approach is based primarily on the status of the glaucoma.

Cataract Extraction Alone

When the intraocular pressure (IOP) is under good control on a well-tolerated medical regimen, most surgeons prefer a cataract extraction alone. However, an extracapsular cataract extraction with a posterior chamber intraocular lens implantation can be associated with a significant IOP rise during the early postoperative course, especially in patients with preexisting glaucoma.[3–7] In one study, more than half of the patients had pressures greater than 25 mm Hg 2–3 hours postoperatively.[5] Although the pressure can usually be brought under control within the first few postoperative days, patients with advanced glaucomatous damage before surgery may suffer additional, irreversible loss of vision during this time. Therefore, moderate to advanced glaucomatous optic atrophy and visual field loss may argue against cataract surgery alone, despite the preoperative level of IOP.

Several studies have also looked at the IOP course in the intermediate and late postoperative periods among patients with preexisting glaucoma. In general, the extracapsular techniques with posterior chamber implants are tolerated better than intracapsular procedures,[4,8] although postoperative glaucoma control can be a significant problem with either technique. During the first 2–4 months after extracapsular surgery, many glaucoma patients will have pressures above the preoperative baseline, while others may be unchanged or even improved.[8–11] The cataract surgery does not appear to have a significant effect on the magnitude of IOP reduction obtained by means of preoperative argon laser trabeculoplasty,[9] although these patients are more likely to have pressure elevations during the first two postoperative months.[10] One to two years after extracapsular cataract surgery, patients with preexisting open-angle glaucoma actually have a small reduction in mean IOP and require fewer medications.[12–14] However, this trend may reverse with time,[15] and cataract surgery alone should not be relied upon as a means of treating uncontrolled glaucoma. On the other hand, when the IOP is well controlled on a low dose of well-tolerated medication with mild glaucomatous damage, extracapsular cataract surgery with posterior chamber intraocular lens implantation alone appears to be a reasonable choice. One specific situation in which this operation is reported to improve glaucoma control is primary angle-closure glaucoma after an iridectomy.[16]

Filtering Surgery Alone

When the glaucoma is uncontrolled despite maximum tolerable medical therapy and laser trabeculoplasty, the surgical procedure of choice is the one that has the greatest chance of controlling the IOP. In most cases, this is a filtering operation performed alone. If miotic therapy before the glaucoma surgery was aggravating the cataract-induced visual loss, it may be that eliminating the miosis postoperatively will improve the vision enough to delay the need for cataract surgery. In other cases, the cataract can be removed 4–6 months later, once the filtering bleb is well established, as the second part of a *two-stage approach*. In one study, patients who underwent the two-stage procedure had a greater percentage of long-term IOP reduction than did those who had cataract surgery alone or a combined cataract-glaucoma operation.[7] However, such results may vary among surgeons.

Combined Cataract Extraction and Glaucoma Surgery

Between the two extremes noted above (i.e., (1) those patients with good glaucoma control and (2) those with uncontrolled glaucoma that poses an immediate threat to vision), there is a third group of patients with borderline glaucoma status for whom a combined procedure may be indicated. There is often a fine line of judgement involved in selecting these cases, although the following situations are some in which such an approach might be preferred: (1) glaucoma under borderline control, despite maximum tolerable medical therapy and laser trabeculoplasty, especially when epinephrine is required or when the patient has significant drug-induced side effects; (2) advanced glaucomatous optic atrophy, despite adequate IOP control; or (3) uncontrolled glaucoma but an urgent need to restore vision or when two operations are not feasible.

The rationale for a combined procedure, as opposed to cataract surgery alone, in eyes with good IOP control but advanced damage is the risk of a transient pressure rise in the early postoperative period, as previously discussed. Even if laser trabeculoplasty has achieved good IOP control, it may still be necessary to add glaucoma surgery to the cataract extraction, since a good response to laser therapy before cataract surgery does not guarantee postoperative pressure control.[17] Studies have shown that the early postoperative pressure rise is significantly less after a combined procedure than after cataract surgery alone,[6,7] and this may actually be the primary benefit of the combined approach. However, reported long-term results following combined surgery are more variable, with some showing pressure control similar to that achieved with filtering surgery alone,[18–20] while others are less favorable.[7,21] As a result, some surgeons use the combined procedure in cases of uncontrolled glaucoma, while others reserve it for those indications noted above.

TECHNIQUES

Cataract Surgery in Eyes with Glaucoma

In some cases, the cataract operation can be performed in the surgeon's usual manner, with no special measures for the coexisting glaucoma. However, a common problem with cataract surgery in the glaucomatous eye is the irreversible *miosis* from chronic miotic therapy. This has become especially significant with the advent of extracapsular surgery, in which adequate pupillary dilation is needed for the anterior capsulotomy. One approach to the problem is to make a sector iridectomy above, often with two inferior sphincterotomies (Fig. 38.1),[22] or multiple sphincterotomies and a

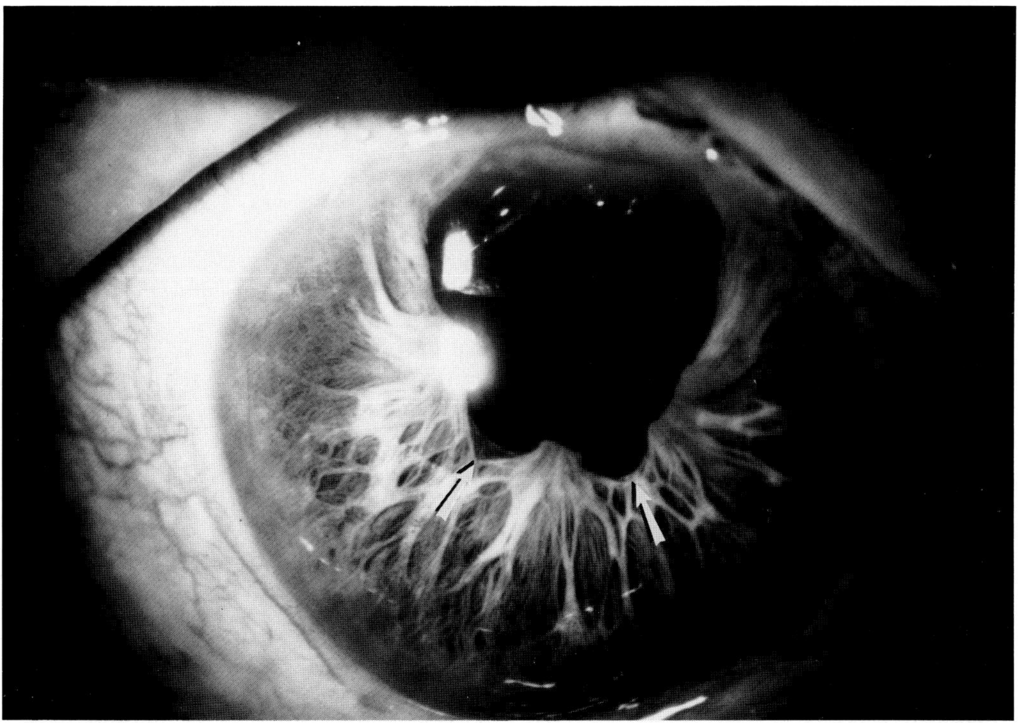

Figure 38.1. Slit-lamp view of glaucomatous eye following extracapsular cataract extraction in which superior sector iridectomy and inferior sphincterotomies (*arrows*) were created to facilitate anterior capsulotomy.

peripheral iridectomy.[23] If a sector iridotomy is made, some surgeons elect to close it with sutures after implanting the lens,[24] although it can be left open if the lens haptics are rotated away from the iridotomy. Other reported techniques for mechanically enlarging a miotic pupil include a micro-iris retractor, similar to the retinal tack,[25] and iris fixation sutures on a special needle.[26]

Viscoelastic substances, such as hyaluronic acid, should be used with caution in eyes with glaucoma. They are especially useful during the anterior capsulotomy, not only for maintaining a deep anterior chamber, but also for providing some additional pupillary dilation. However, they increase the risk of an early postoperative IOP rise and should be thoroughly aspirated and irrigated from the eye by the end of the procedure. If pupillary constriction is needed after lens implantation, intracameral *carabachol* may be preferable to acetylcholine, since the former is reported to be associated with better early postoperative pressure control.[27]

Selection of the proper *intraocular lens* is also important in eyes with glaucoma. Posterior chamber lenses appear to be very well tolerated, whereas anterior chamber lenses should probably be avoided in glaucomatous eyes. When loss of capsular support precludes the standard implantation of a posterior chamber lens, one option is to suture the lens in place. Several techniques have been described for this,[28–30] most of which use the basic principle of passing two 10-0 prolene sutures, attached to the lens haptics, through the ciliary sulcus and sclera and securing them beneath conjunctival and partial-thickness scleral flaps (Fig. 38.2).

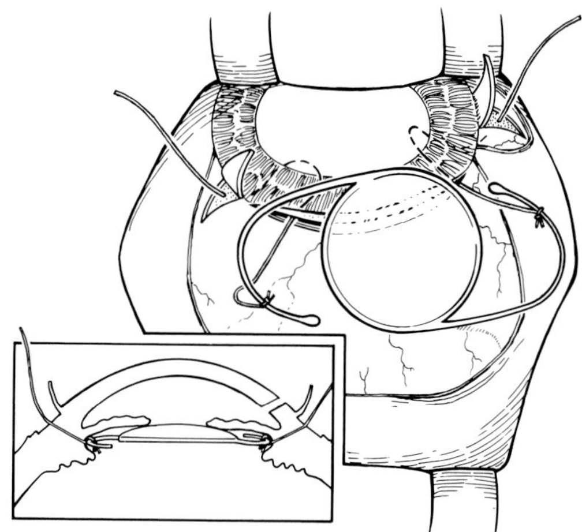

Figure 38.2. Technique for suturing posterior chamber intraocular lens in absence of capsular support. Two 10-0 prolene sutures on long, curved needles have been passed through the corneoscleral incision and pupil and brought out through the ciliary sulcus and sclera beneath small partial-thickness scleral flaps. After attaching the sutures to the lens haptics, the lens is inserted into the posterior chamber (*inset*) and the sutures are secured to the sclera beneath the protective flaps.

Cataract Extraction After Filtering Surgery

When extraction of the cataract becomes necessary in an eye with a functioning filtering bleb, surgeons generally prefer to make the cataract incision away from the bleb, either inferiorly[31–33] or through clear cornea superiorly (Fig. 38.3).[33–37] These two basic methods are comparable with regard to preserving function of the filtering bleb, although the clear cornea approach is technically easier for most surgeons. Other surgeons prefer a temporal limbal incision,[38] which is especially useful if the filtering surgery was performed in the superior nasal quadrant. Another reported technique is to make the incision through the filtering bleb and to create a new bleb adjacent to the original one.[39] In most reported series, the filtering bleb is preserved and the long-term IOP remains controlled, although it is common for the pressure to be slightly higher after the cataract surgery and for an increase in medications to be required.

Combined Cataract and Glaucoma Surgery

Early combined operations used full-thickness filtering procedures. However, the main problem with combining full-thickness glaucoma filtering techniques with a cataract extraction is the risk of a transient shallow or flat anterior chamber, which leads to significantly more complications in

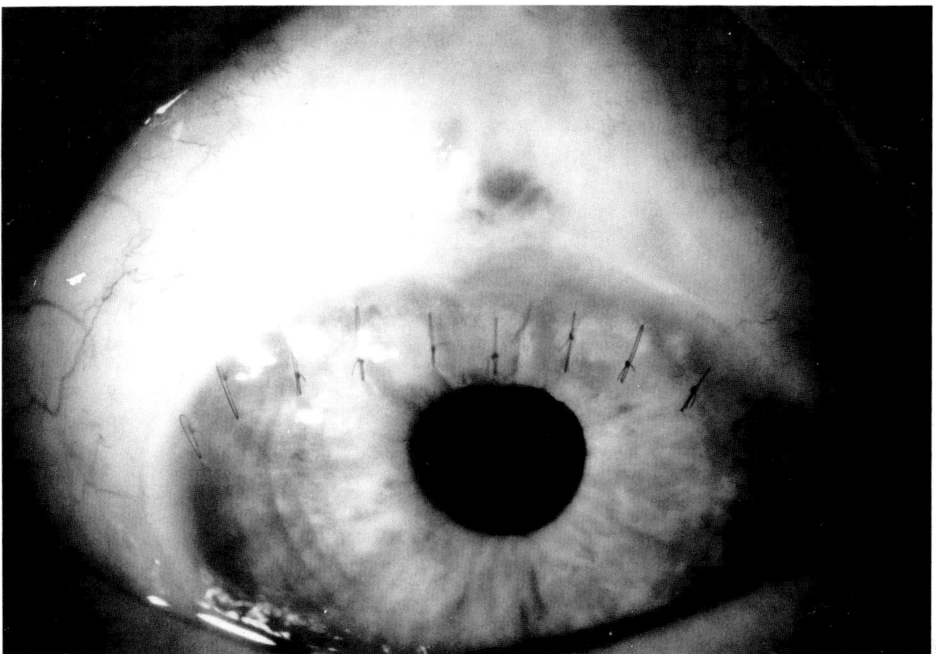

Figure 38.3. Slit-lamp view of eye with functioning glaucoma filtering bleb in which extracapsular cataract extraction and posterior chamber lens implantation were performed through a clear corneal incision to preserve the preexisting bleb. (Reprinted from *The Glaucomas,* ed. Ritch, Shields, Krupin, pg 701, C. V. Mosby, St. Louis, 1989, by permission.)

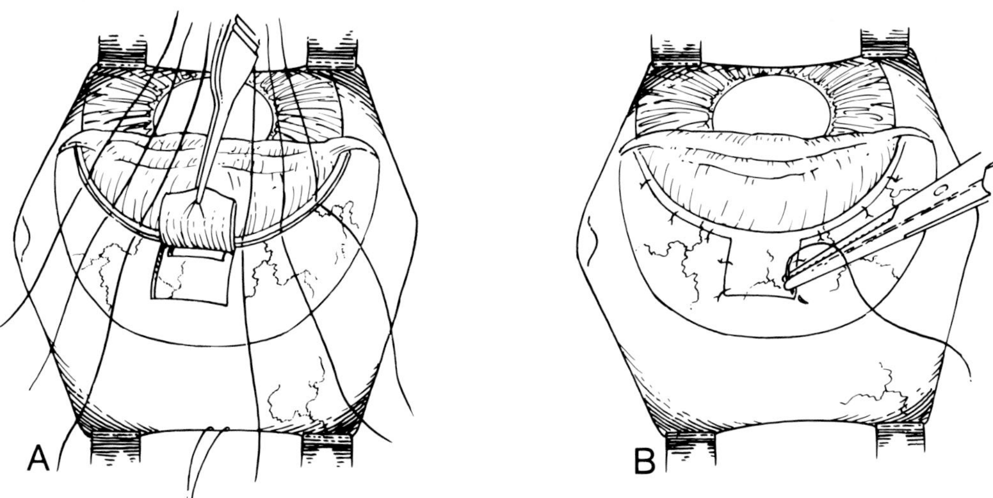

Figure 38.4. Trabeculectomy and cataract extraction: **A,** Partial-thickness scleral flap and deep limbal fistula are prepared and the cataract incision is extended from either side. **B,** Following lens extraction, the cataract incision and scleral flap are approximated with multiple sutures.

the inflamed, aphakic or pseudophakic eye. For this reason, the preferred combined operations employ a glaucoma procedure that is less likely to cause loss of the anterior chamber. In the vast majority of cases, this is some form of a guarded filtering procedure.

Trabeculectomy and Cataract Extraction. The protective scleral flap over a limbal fistula, which reduces the chances of an early postoperative flat anterior chamber, makes the guarded filtering operation particularly desirable for combined procedures. Several techniques have been described for combining a trabeculectomy with intracapsular cataract surgery[40–47] and subsequently with an extracapsular cataract extraction and posterior chamber intraocular lens implantation.[18–21,48–51] Implantation of a posterior chamber lens does not appear

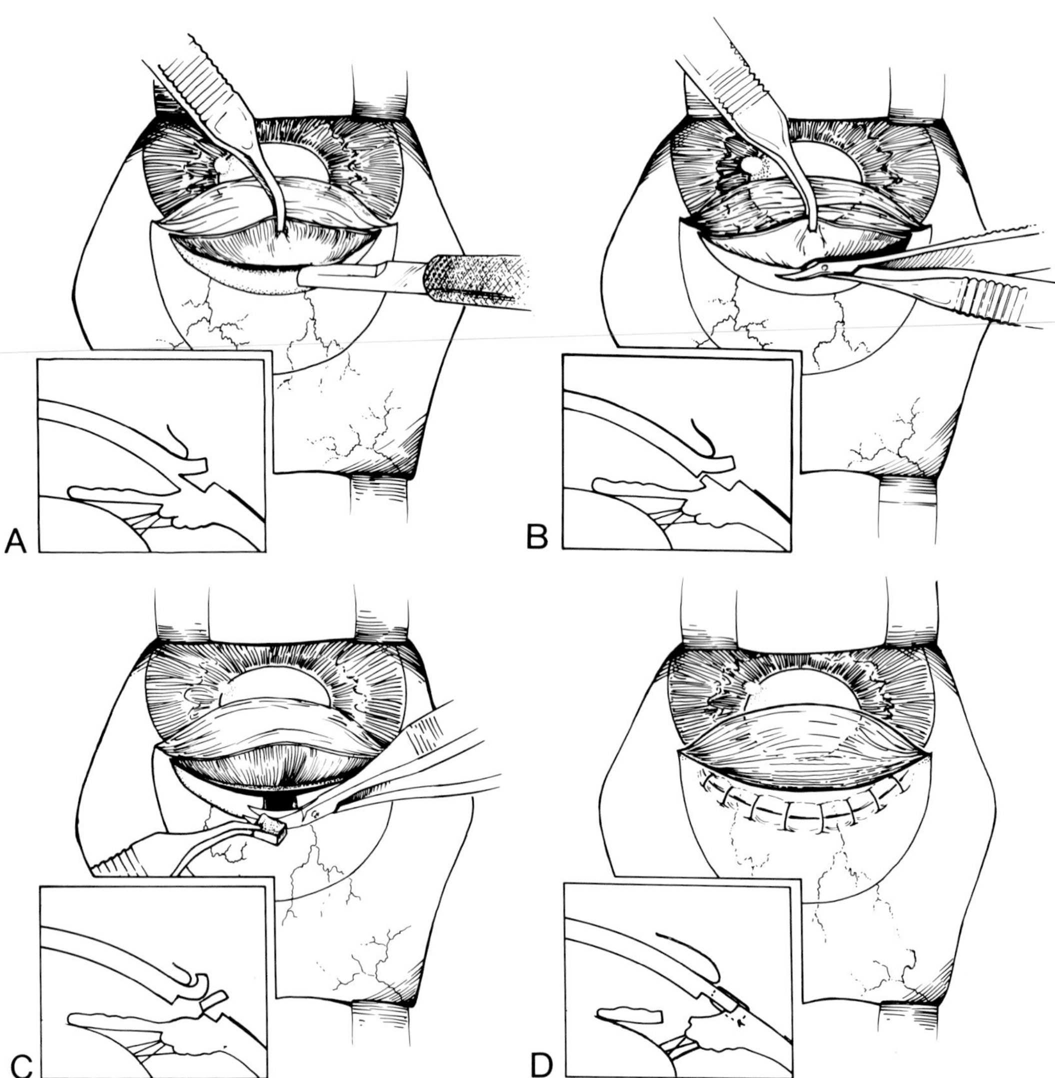

Figure 38.5. Guarded sclerectomy and cataract extraction: **A,** A beveled corneoscleral incision is created. **B,** The incision is extended full thickness with corneoscleral scissors. **C,** After cataract extraction and posterior chamber intraocular lens implantation, the glaucoma drainage fistula is created in the posterior lip of the corneoscleral incision. **D,** Approximation of the incision brings the anterior lip as a guard over the fistula.

to adversely affect the results of the combined procedure.[51]

The basic approach involves preparation of the partial-thickness scleral flap and limbal fistula in the usual manner, followed by extension of the corneoscleral incision from either side of the fistula (Fig. 38.4). After a standard extracapsular lens extraction and implantation of the posterior chamber lens, both scleral flap and corneoscleral incision are closed with multiple sutures. The conjunctival flap is closed in the manner described for glaucoma filtering procedures (Chapter 36). A limbal-based vs fornix-based conjunctival flap has not been found to influence the outcome of combined trabeculectomy and extracapsular cataract surgery.[21,50] Phacoemulsification has also been successfully used with trabeculectomy as a combined procedure.[52] The postoperative use of subconjunctival 5-fluorouracil has been shown to improve the postoperative IOP control following combined extracapsular cataract extraction and filtering surgery.[53]

Guarded Sclerectomy and Cataract Extraction. A simplified technique for creating a guarded fistula in conjunction with cataract surgery is to prepare a very beveled corneoscleral incision and create the fistula in the posterior lip of the incision with a scleral punch or scissors (Fig. 38.5). When the corneoscleral incision is approximated, the anterior lip of the incision covers the fistula, in the same manner as a trabeculectomy (Fig. 38.6). The procedure was originally described in conjunction with intracapsular cataract surgery[54,55] and was later modified for extracapsular techniques.[7,22,56] A comparison of limbal-based vs fornix-based conjunctival flaps revealed similar long-term IOP control and visual acuity, but better early postoperative pressure control with the limbal-based flaps.[56] The long-term results of the procedure are comparable to those with combined trabeculectomy and cataract extraction, although the guarded sclerectomy may require less surgical manipulation.

Cyclodialysis and Cataract Extraction. This has been used as a combined procedure for many years, with reports of good results.[57–60] However, in one large series, an analysis of the postoperative course suggested that the IOP reduction in many cases was due to the effect of the cataract surgery, rather than the cyclodialysis.[59] Since this effect may be lost with the newer techniques

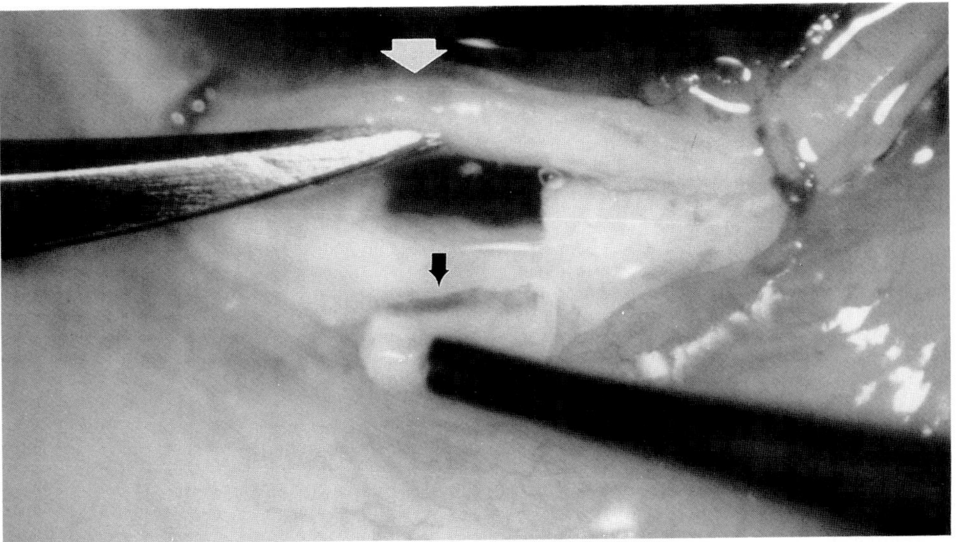

Figure 38.6. Intraoperative view during guarded sclerectomy and cataract extraction showing excision of fistula (*arrow*) from posterior lip of corneoscleral incision. (Reprinted from *The Glaucomas,* ed. Ritch, Shields, Krupin, pg 705, C. V. Mosby, St. Louis, 1989, by permission.)

of wound closure, and considering the unpredictable nature of cyclodialysis, most surgeons now prefer a guarded fistula for combined procedures.

Trabeculotomy and Cataract Extraction. McPherson[61] reported a technique in which a trabeculotomy is performed through a radial incision at 12 o'clock adjacent to a partial-thickness corneoscleral incision. The cataract wound is then extended full-thickness, and a cataract extraction is completed in a standard manner. Good results were obtained with the preliminary experience.

SUMMARY

In an eye with a cataract for which extraction is thought to be indicated, and coexisting glaucoma, the surgical approach is based primarily on the status of the glaucoma. In some cases, cataract extraction alone may be sufficient, whereas other eyes may require filtering surgery alone with cataract surgery at a later date. In other patients, a combined glaucoma and cataract operation may be the procedure of choice. The preferred technique for the glaucoma portion of a combined procedure is usually some form of guarded filtering surgery.

References

1. Spurny, RC, Zaldivar, R, Belcher, CD III, Simmons, RJ: Instruments for predicting visual acuity. A clinical comparison. Arch Ophthal 104:196, 1986.
2. Asbell, PA, Chiang, B, Amin, A, Podos, SM: Retinal acuity evaluation with the potential acuity meter in glaucoma patients. Ophthalmology 92:764, 1985.
3. McGuigan, LJB, Gottsch, J, Stark, WJ, et al: Extracapsular cataract e:traction and posterior chamber lens implantation in eyes with preexisting glaucoma. Arch Ophthal 104:1301, 1986.
4. Vu, MT, Shields, MB: The early postoperative pressure course in glaucoma patients following cataract surgery. Ophthal Surg 19:467, 1988.
5. Gross, JG, Meyer, DR, Robin, AL, et al: Increased intraocular pressure in the immediate postoperative period after extracapsular cataract extraction. Am J Ophthal 105:466, 1988.
6. Krupin, T, Feitl, ME, Bishop, KI: Postoperative intraocular pressure rise in open-angle glaucoma patients after cataract or combined cataract-filtration surgery. Ophthalmology 96:579, 1989.
7. Murchison, JF Jr, Shields, MB: An evaluation of three surgical approaches for coexisting cataract and glaucoma. Ophthal Surg 20:393, 1989.
8. Hansen, TE, Naeser, K, Rask, KL: A prospective study of intraocular pressure four months after extracapsular extraction with implantation of posterior chamber lenses. J Cat Ref Surg 13:35, 1987.
9. Brown, SVL, Thomas, JV, Budenz, DL, et al: Effect of cataract surgery on intraocular pressure reduction obtained with laser trabeculoplasty. Am J Ophthal 100:373, 1985.
10. Savage, JA, Thomas, JV, Belcher, CD III, Simmons, RJ: Extracapsular cataract extraction and posterior chamber intraocular lens implantation in glaucomatous eyes. Ophthalmology 92:1506, 1985.
11. McMahan, LB, Monica, ML, Zimmerman, TJ: Posterior chamber pseudophakes in glaucoma patients. Ophthal Surg 17:146, 1986.
12. Radius, RL, Schultz, K, Sobocinski, K, et al: Pseudophakia and intraocular pressure. Am J Ophthal 97:738, 1984.
13. Handa, J, Henry, JC, Krupin, T, Keates, E: Extracapsular cataract extraction with posterior chamber lens implantation in patients with glaucoma. Arch Ophthal 105:765, 1987.
14. Cinotti, DJ, Fiore, PM, Maltzman, BA, et al: Control of intraocular pressure in glaucomatous eyes after extracapsular cataract extraction with intraocular lens implantation. J Cat Ref Surg 14:650, 1988.
15. Sponagel, LD, Gloor, B: Does implantation of posterior chamber lenses lower intraocular pressure? Klin Monatsbl Augenheilkd 188:495, 1986.
16. Greve, EL: Primary angle closure glaucoma: extracapsular cataract extraction or filtering procedure? Int Ophthal 12:157, 1988.
17. Galin, MA, Obstbaum, SA, Asano, Y, et al: Laser trabeculoplasty and cataract surgery. Trans Ophthal Soc UK 104:72, 1984.
18. Percival, SPB: Glaucoma triple procedure of extracapsular cataract extraction, posterior chamber lens implantation, and trabeculectomy. Br J Ophthal 69:99, 1985.
19. Skorpik, C, Paroussis, P, Gnad, HD, Menapace, R: Trabeculectomy and intraocular lens implantation: a combined procedure. J Cat Ref Surg 13:39, 1987.
20. Raitta, C, Tarkkanen, A: Combined procedure for the management of glaucoma and cataract. Acta Ophthal 66:667, 1988.
21. Simmons, ST, Litoff, D, Nichols, DA, et al: Extracapsular cataract extraction and posterior chamber intraocular lens implantation combined with trabeculectomy in patients with glaucoma. Am J Ophthal 104:465, 1987.
22. Shields, MB: Combined cataract extraction and

guarded sclerectomy. Reevaluation in the extracapsular era. Ophthalmology 93:366, 1986.

23. Kolker, AE, Stewart, RH, LeBlanc, RP: Cataract extraction in glaucomatous patients. Arch Ophthal 84:63, 1970.
24. Saito, Y, Kiboshi, H: A new intra-anterior chamber iris suturing method. Am J Ophthal 105:701, 1988.
25. McCuen, BW II, Hickingbotham, D, Tsai, M, de Juan, E Jr: Temporary iris fixation with a microiris retractor. Arch Ophthal 107:925, 1989.
26. Murray, TG, Abrams, GW: A new self-sealing needle for iris suture fixation. Arch Ophthal 108:746, 1990.
27. Ruiz, RS, Rhem, MN, Prager, TC: Effects of carbachol and acetylcholine on intraocular pressure after cataract extraction. Am J Ophthal 107:7, 1989.
28. Hu, BV, Shin, DH, Gibbs, KA, Hong, YJ: Implantation of posterior chamber lens in the absence of capsular and zonular support. Arch Ophthal 106:416, 1988.
29. Stark, WJ, Gottsch, JD, Goodman, DF, et al: Posterior chamber intraocular lens implantation in the absence of capsular support. Arch Ophthal 107:1078, 1989.
30. Lindquist, TD, Agapitos, PJ, Lindstrom, RL, et al: Transscleral fixation of posterior chamber intraocular lenses in the absence of capsular support. Ophthal Surg 20:769, 1989.
31. Baloglou, P, Matta, C, Asdourian, K: Cataract extraction after filtering operations. Arch Ophthal 88:12, 1972.
32. Simmons, RJ, Thomas, JV, Singh, OS, Taheri, N: Surgical indications and options in the management of coexisting glaucoma and cataract. Glaucoma 4:92, 1982.
33. Kass, MA: Cataract extraction in an eye with a filtering bleb. Ophthalmology 89:871, 1982.
34. Riise, P: Influence of cataract operation on the pressure in glaucoma eyes operated with iridencleisis. Acta Ophthal 50:436, 1972.
35. Oyakawa, RT, Maumenee, AE: Clear-cornea cataract extraction in eyes with functioning filtering blebs. Am J Ophthal 93:294, 1982.
36. Wocheslander, E, Bartl, G: Follow-up examinations after trabeculectomy and cataract surgery. Klin Monatsbl Augenheilkd 183:323, 1983.
37. Binkhorst, CD, Huber, C: Cataract extraction and intraocular lens implantation after fistulizing glaucoma surgery. Am Intra-ocular Implant Soc J 7:133, 1981.
38. Antonios, SR, Traverso, CE, Tomey, KF: Extracapsular cataract extraction using a temporal limbal approach after filtering operations. Arch Ophthal 106:608, 1988.
39. Levene, R: Triple procedure of extracapsular cataract surgery, posterior chamber lens implantation, and glaucoma filter. J Cat Ref Surg 12:385, 1986.
40. Dellaporta, A: Combined trepano-trabeculectomy and cataract extraction. Trans Am Ophthal Soc 69:113, 1971.
41. Rich, W: Cataract extraction with trabeculectomy. Trans Ophthal Soc UK 94:458, 1974.
42. Bregeat, P: Cataract surgery and trabeculectomy at the same time. Klin Monatsbl Augenheilkd 167:505, 1975.
43. Jerndal, T, Lundstrom, M: Trabeculectomy combined with cataract extraction. Am J Ophthal 81:227, 1976.
44. Stewart, RH, Loftis, MD: Combined cataract extraction and thermal sclerostomy versus combined cataract extraction and trabeculectomy. Ophthal Surg 7:93, 1976.
45. Johns, GE, Layden, WE: Combined trabeculectomy and cataract extraction. Am J Ophthal 88:973, 1979.
46. Edwards, RS: Trabeculectomy combined with cataract extraction: a follow-up study. Br J Ophthal 64:720, 1980.
47. Praeger, DL: Combined procedure: sub-scleral trabeculectomy with cataract extraction. Ophthal Surg 14:130, 1983.
48. Ohanesian, RV, Kim, EW: A prospective study of combined extracapsular cataract extraction, posterior chamber lens implantation, and trabeculectomy. Am Intra-ocular Implant Soc J 11:142, 1985.
49. Jay, JL: Extracapsular lens extraction and posterior chamber intraocular lens insertion combined with trabeculectomy. Br J Ophthal 69:487, 1985.
50. McCartney, KL, Memmen, JE, Stark, W, et al: The efficacy and safety of combined trabeculectomy, cataract extraction, and intraocular lens implantation. Ophthalmology 95:754, 1988.
51. Neumann, R, Zalish, M, Oliver, M: Effect of intraocular lens implantation on combined extracapsular cataract extraction with trabeculectomy: a comparative study. Br J Ophthal 72:741, 1988.
52. Hansen, LL, Hoffmann, F: Combination of phacoemulsification and trabeculectomy—results of a retrospective study. Klin Monatsbl Augenheilkd 190:478, 1987.
53. Cohen, JS: Combined cataract implant and filtering surgery with 5-fluorouracil. Ophthal Surg 21:181, 1990.
54. Spaeth, GL, Sivalingam, E: The partial-punch: a new combined cataract-glaucoma operation. Ophthal Surg 7:53, 1976.
55. Shields, MB: Combined cataract extraction and glaucoma surgery. Ophthalmology 89:231, 1982.
56. Murchison, JF Jr, Shields, MB: Limbal-based vs fornix-based conjunctival flaps in combined extracapsular cataract surgery and glaucoma filtering procedure. Am J Ophthal 109:709, 1990.
57. Galin, MA, Baras, I, Sambursky, J: Glaucoma and cataract. A study of cyclodialysis-lens extraction. Am J Ophthal 67:522, 1969.

58. Shemleva, VV, Mukhina, EA: Combined cataract extraction and cyclodialysis. Vestn Oftalmol 85:30, 1972.
59. Shields, MB, Simmons, RJ: Combined cyclodialysis and cataract extraction. Trans Am Acad Ophthal Otol 81:286, 1976.
60. McAllister, JA, Spaeth, GL: Intracapsular cataract extraction with cyclodialysis. A useful procedure. Klin Monatsbl Augenheilkd 184:283, 1984.
61. McPherson, SD Jr: Combined trabeculotomy and cataract extraction as a single operation. Trans Am Ophthal Soc 74:251, 1976.

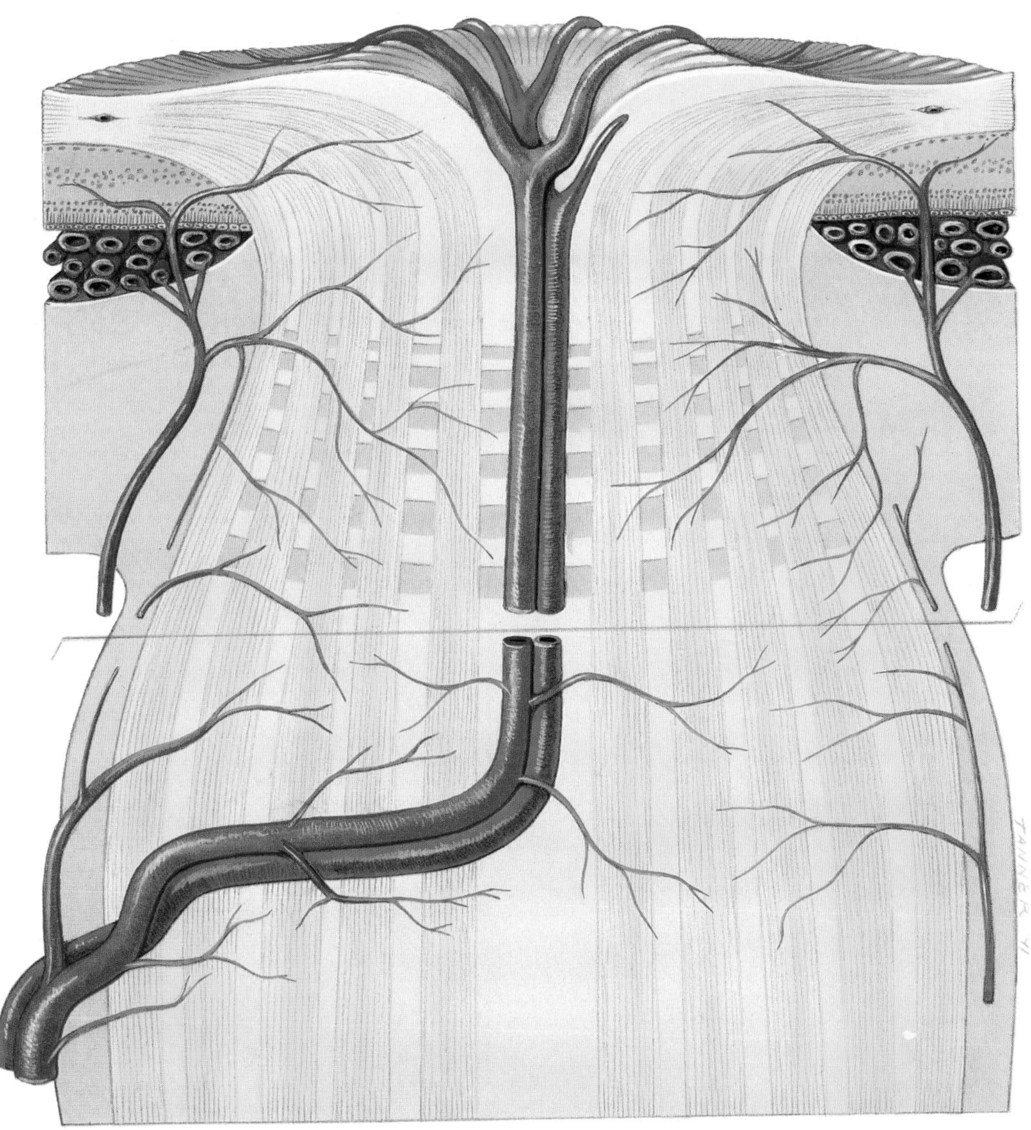

Cross-sectional schematic of optic nerve head
(See explanation in text, p. 86.)

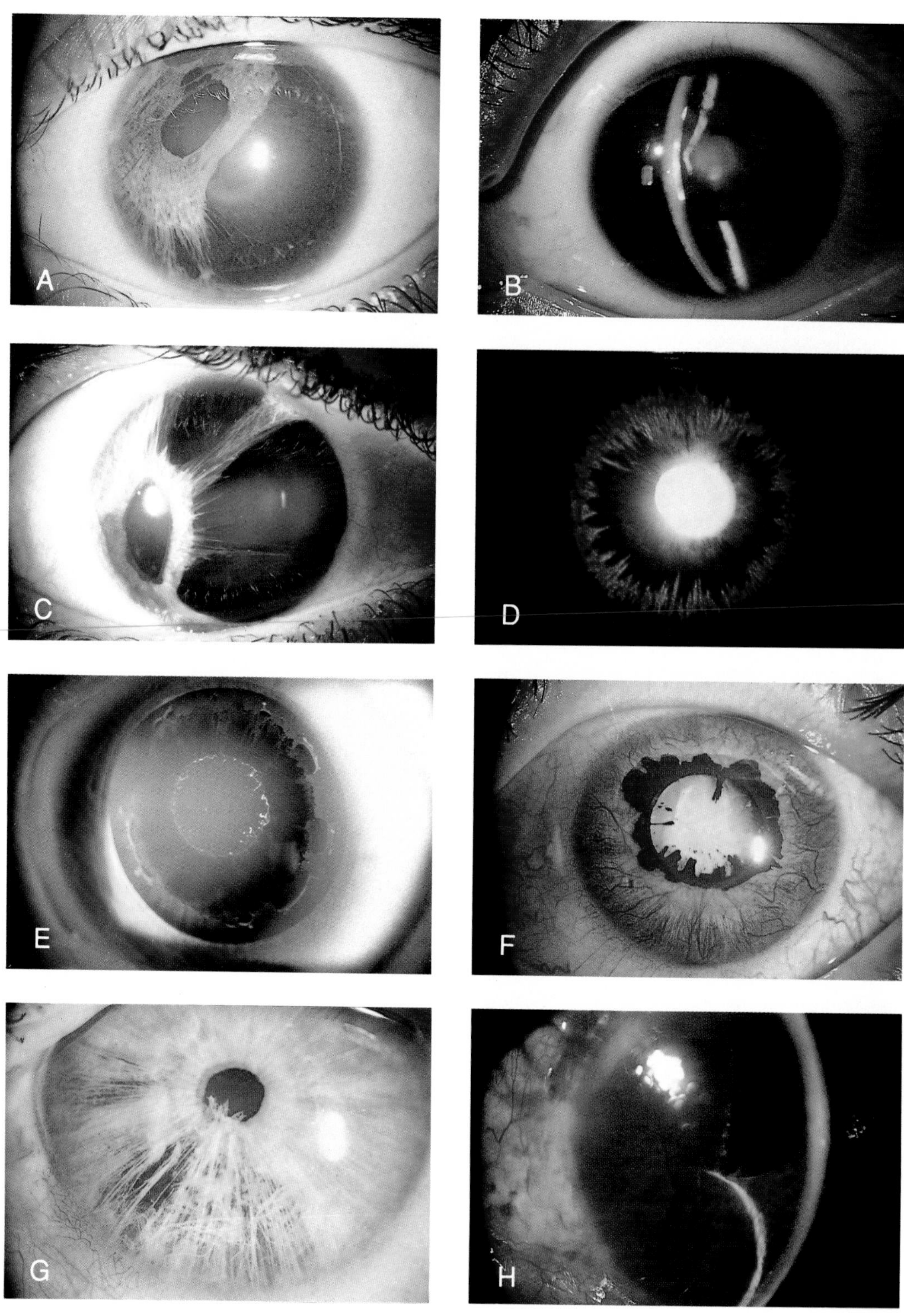

Optic disc photos: a) normal; b) large physiologic cups; c) oblique insertion and temporal crescents in myopic eyes with glaucomatous cupping (left photo); d) saucerization (left); e) focal cupping to inferior disc margin (right); f) baring of circumlinear vessel superiorly (left); g) cupping to superior and inferior disc margins (left) and to inferior margin (right) with inferotemporal nerve fiber layer defects in both eyes; h) disc hemorrhage inferiorly (right);

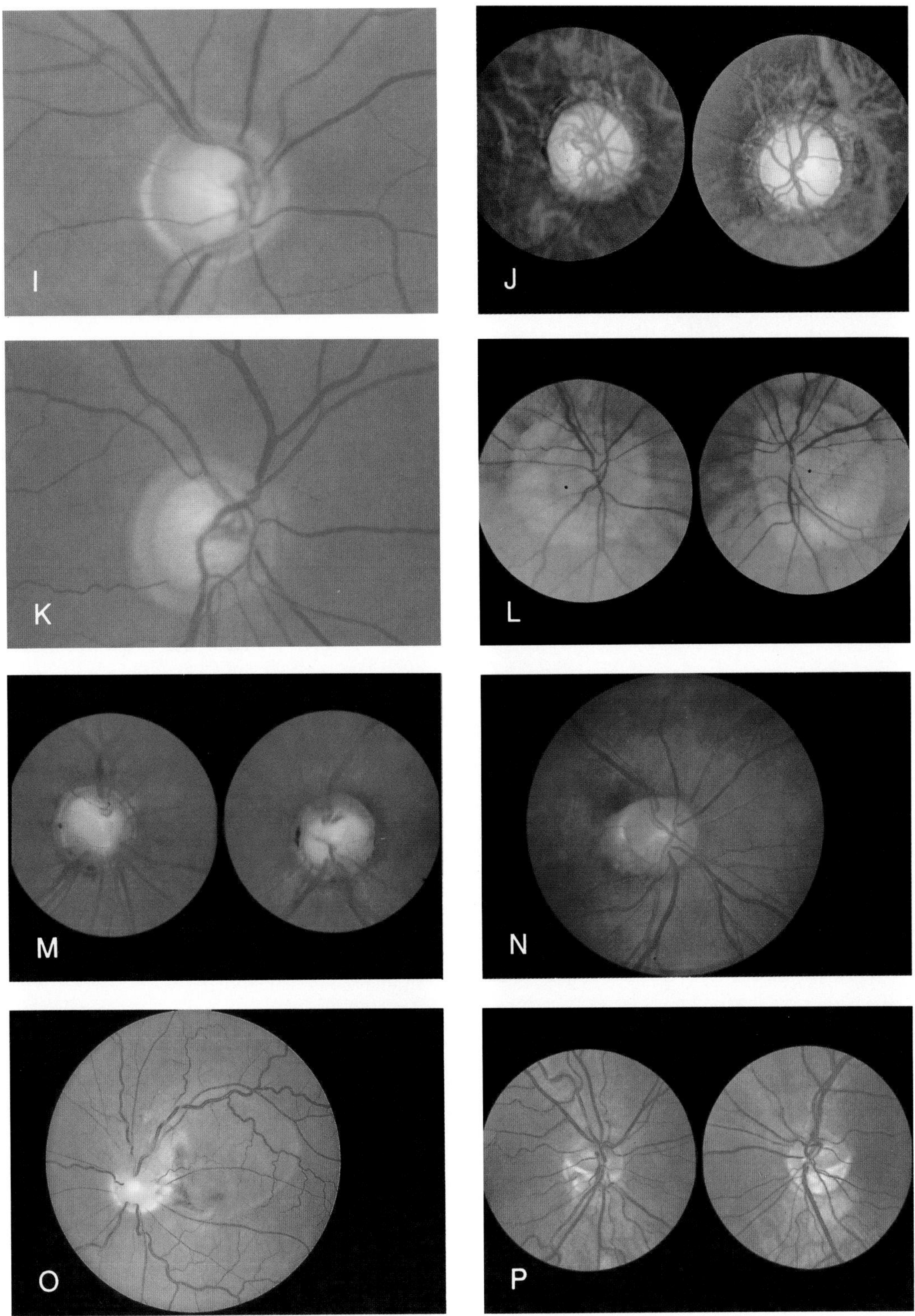

i) cupping to temporal disc margin with color in periphery of cup; j) total cup of both eyes with numerous shunt vessels (left); k) total deep cup and pallor with even peripapillary halo; l) wide, irregular peripapillary atrophy; m) colobomas of optic nerve heads; n) congenital optic pit; o) morning glory syndrome; p) tilted disc syndrome

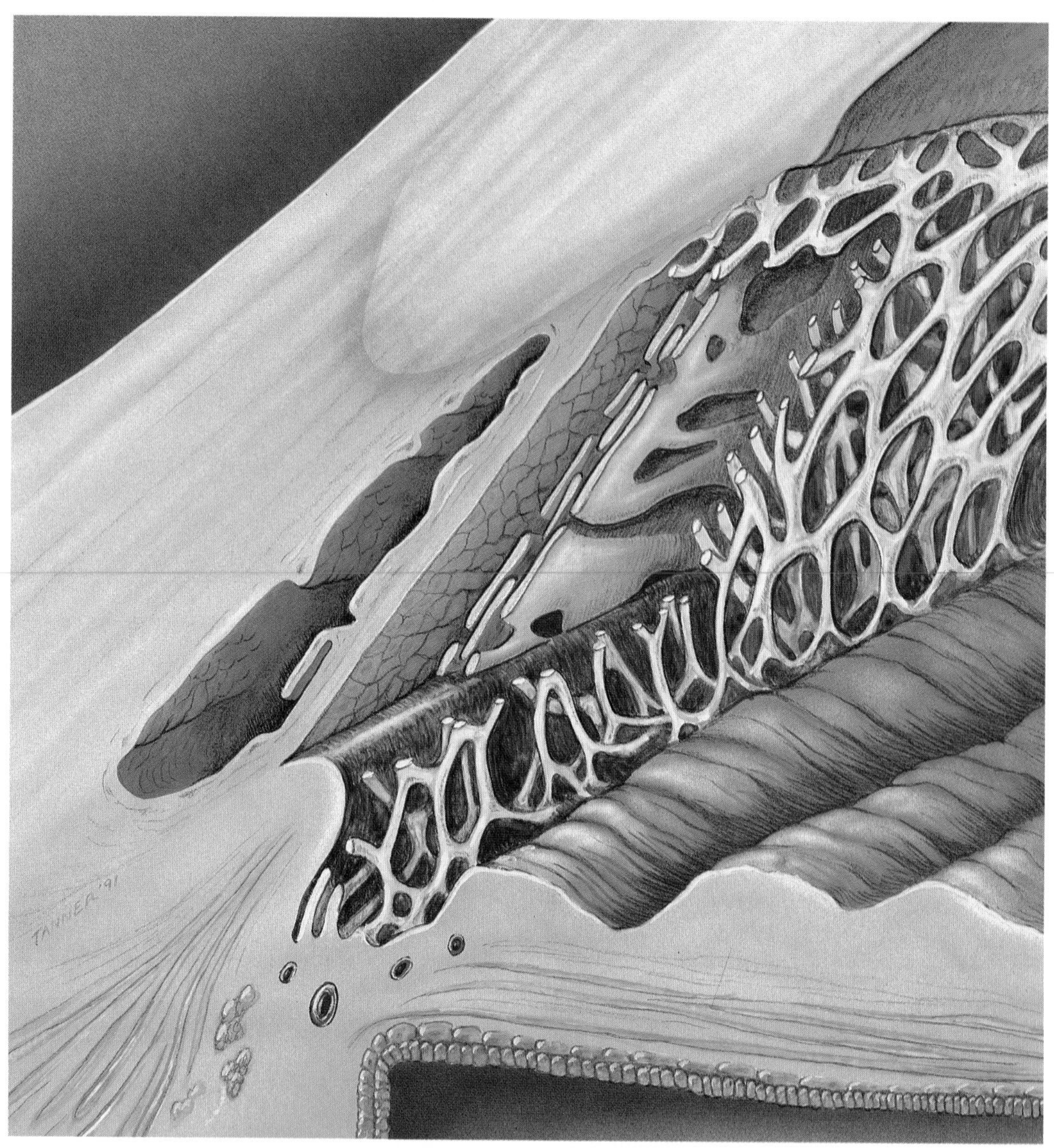

Schematic of internal anatomy of anterior ocular segment
(See explanation in text, p. 18.)

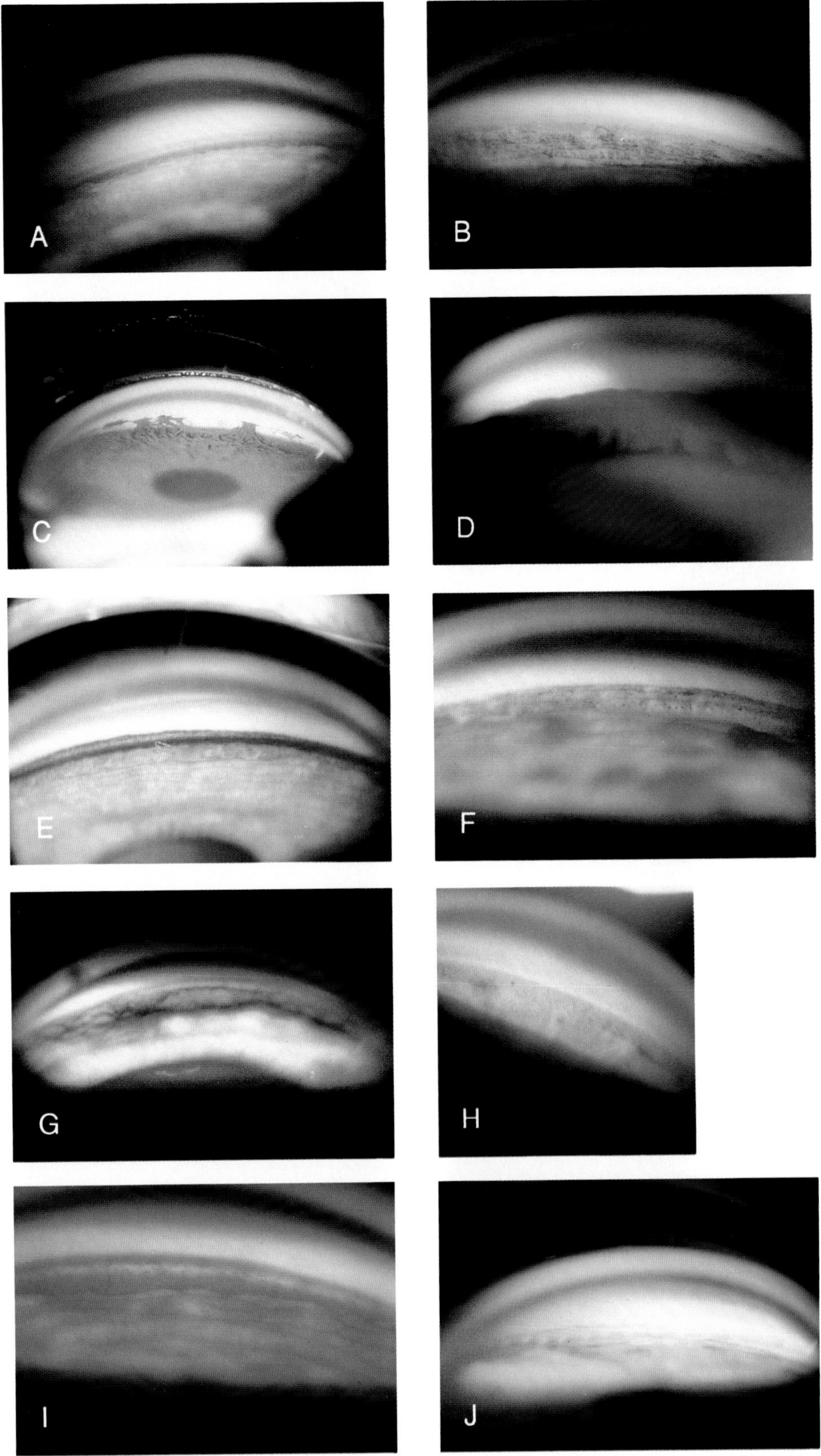

Gonioscopic photos: a) normal angle; b) congenital glaucoma; c) Axenfeld-Rieger syndrome; d) aniridia (note thin rudimentary iris and exposed ciliary processes); e) pigmentary glaucoma; f) exfoliation syndrome; g) ciliary body melanoma extending into anterior chamber angle; h) Fuchs' iridocyclitis with new vessels in angle; i) angle recession; j) argon laser trabeculoplasty (note blanched treatment sites on anterior trabecular meshwork)

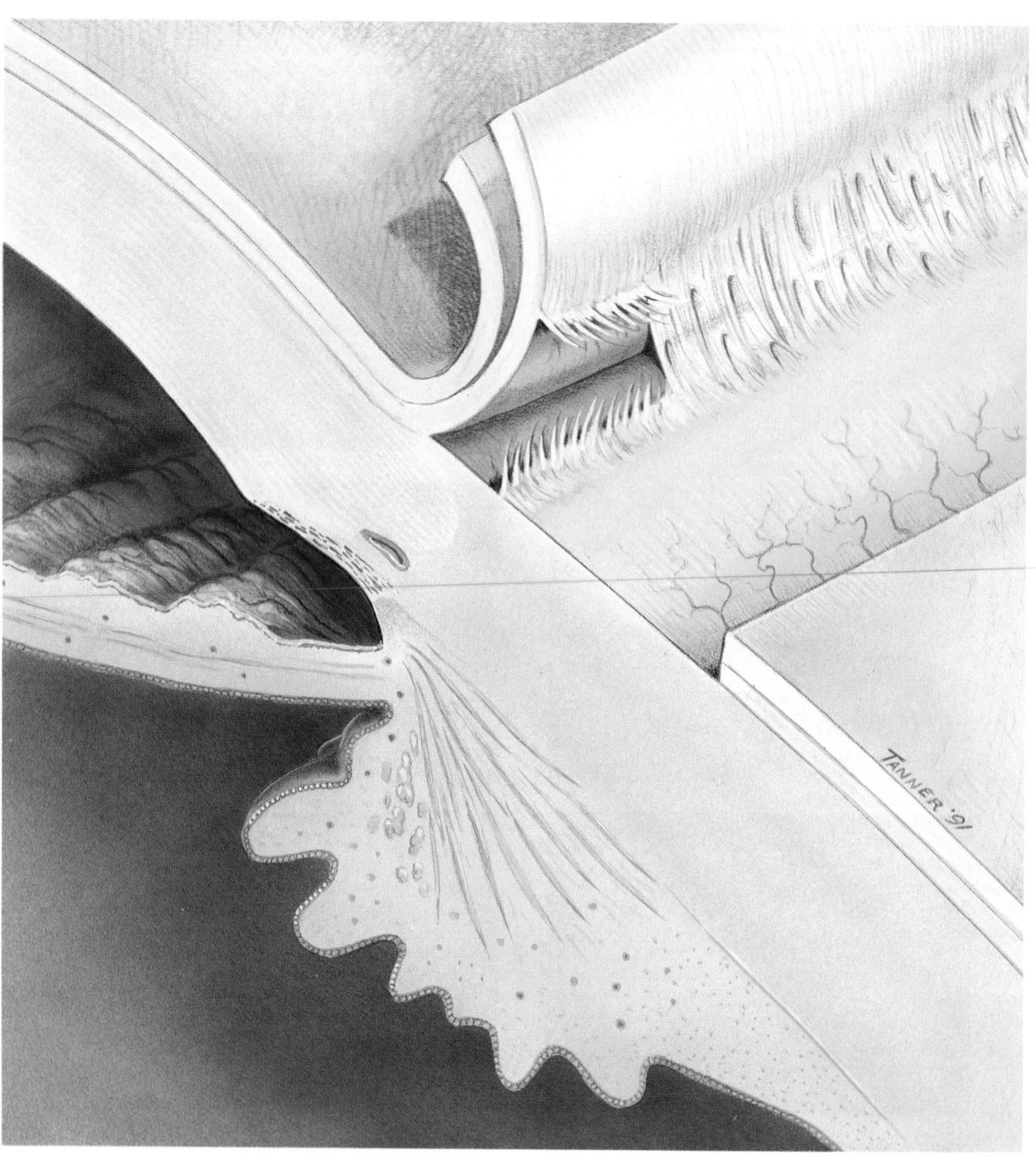

Schematic of external anatomy of anterior ocular segment
(See explanation in text, p. 525.)

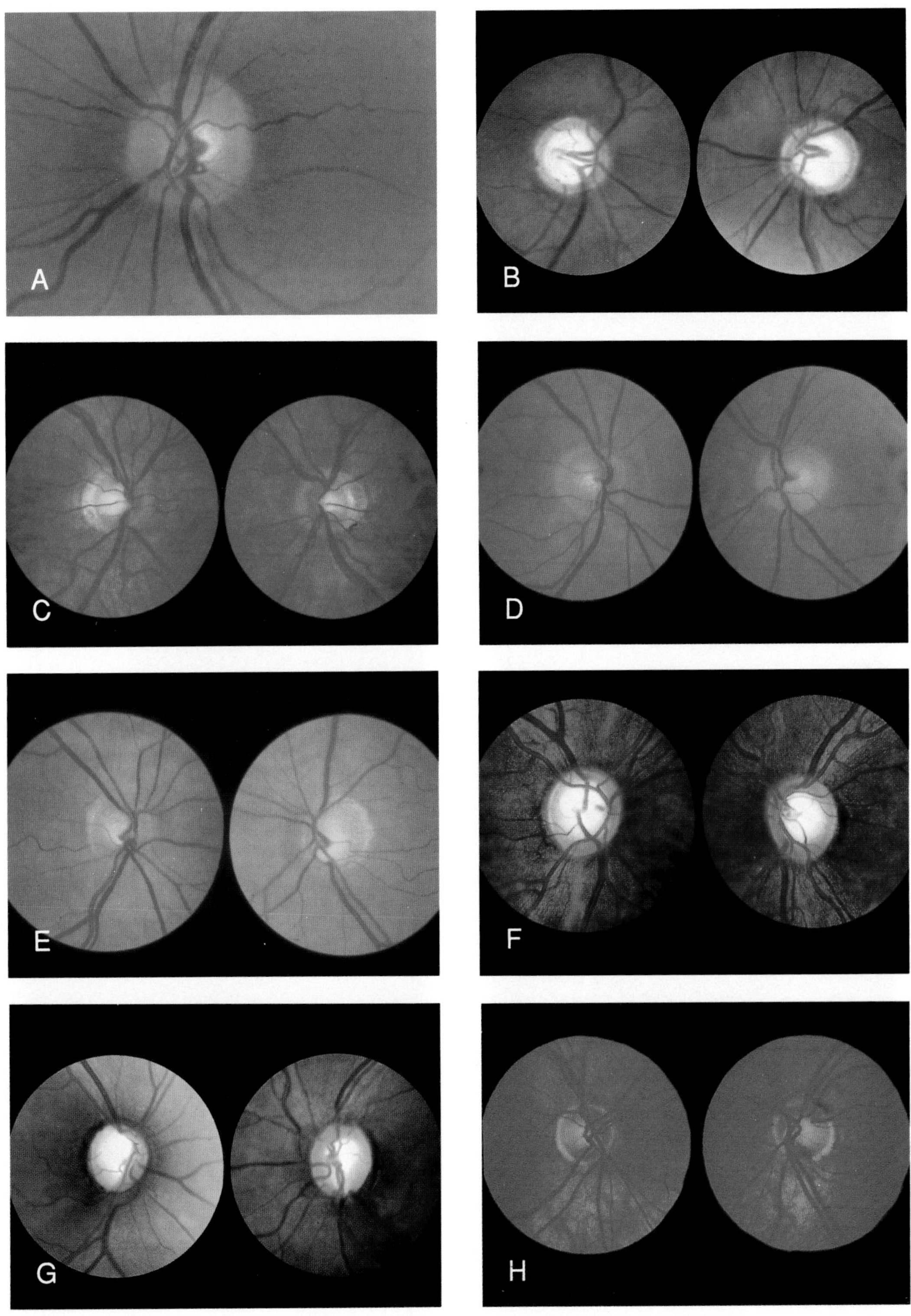

Slit lamp photos: a) Axenfeld-Rieger syndrome with prominent, anterior Schwalbe's line; b) Peters' anomaly with iris adhesion to opaque, central cornea; c) progressive iris atrophy variation of iridocorneal endothelial syndrome; d) midperipheral iris transillumination defects in pigmentary glaucoma; e) exfoliative material on anterior lens capsule in the exfoliation syndrome; f) neovascular glaucoma with ectropion uvea; g) iridoschisis of inferior iris quadrant; h) pupillary block in aphakia with iris bombé

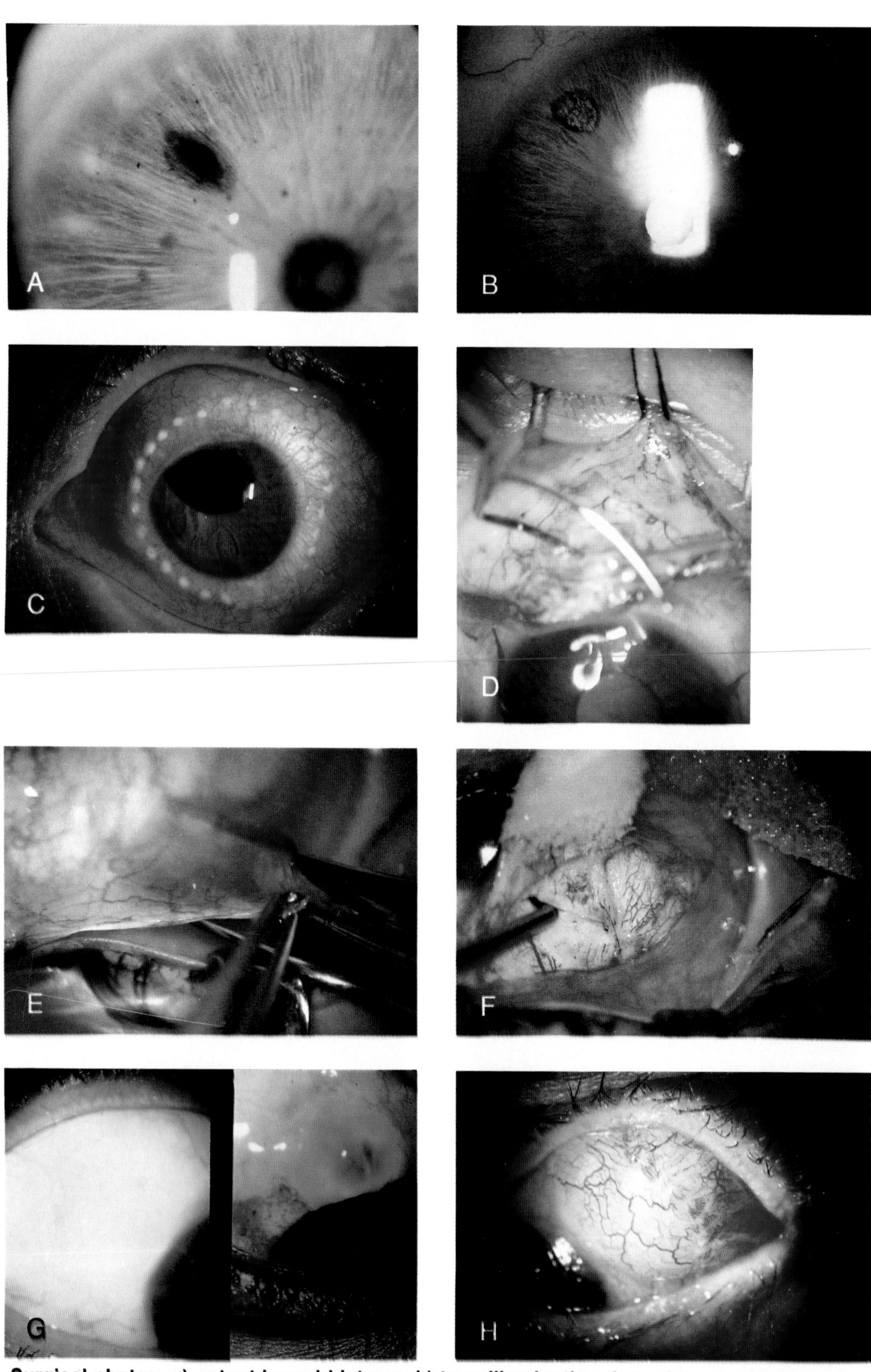

Surgical photos: a) patent laser iridotomy; b) transillumination through laser iridotomy despite intact iris stroma; c) conjunctival burns following transscleral Nd:YAG cyclophotocoagulation (performed with contact lens on right half and without on left); d) trabeculotomy with trabeculotome being rotated into the anterior chamber; e) preparation of conjunctival flap for filtering procedure with tips of scissors visualized through conjunctiva; f) triangular-shaped, partial-thickness scleral flap in trabeculectomy; g) functioning filtering blebs (elevated and localized on right and low and diffuse on left); h) encapsulated filtering bleb

INDEX

Page numbers in *italics* indicate figures; *t*, following a page number indicates a table.